SECOND EDITION

DRENNAN'S THE CHILD'S FOOT AND ANKLE

EDITORS

James J. McCarthy, MD

Associate Professor
Department of Orthopaedics and Rehabilitation
University of Wisconsin
Madison, WI

James C. Drennan, MD

Professor Emeritus of Orthopaedics and Pediatrics
University of New Mexico School of Medicine
Albuquerque, NM

Wolters Kluwer Health | Lippincott Williams & Wilkins

Philadelphia • Baltimore • New York • London
Buenos Aires • Hong Kong • Sydney • Tokyo

Acquisitions Editor: Robert Hurley
Product Manager: Dave Murphy
Senior Manufacturing Manager: Benjamin Rivera
Marketing Manager: Lisa Parry
Design Manager: Doug Smock
Production Service: KnowledgeWorks Global Ltd.

530 Walnut Street
Philadelphia, PA 19106 USA
LWW.com

Printed in China

Library of Congress Cataloging-in-Publication Data
Drennan's the child's foot and ankle / editors, James J. McCarthy, James C. Drennan. — 2nd ed.
p. ; cm.
Rev. ed. of: The Child's foot and ankle / editor, James C. Drennan. 1992.
Includes bibliographical references and index.
ISBN 978-0-7817-7847-3
1. Foot—Diseases. 2. Foot—Abnormalities. 3. Ankle—Diseases. 4. Ankle—Abnormalities. 5. Pediatric orthopedics. I. McCarthy, James J., 1962- II. Drennan, James C. (James Cyril), 1935- III. Title: Child's foot and ankle.
[DNLM: 1. Foot Deformities. 2. Adolescent. 3. Ankle Injuries. 4. Child. 5. Foot Injuries. 6. Infant. WE 883 D772 2009]
RD781.C45 2009
618.92′097585—dc22 2009033035

Care has been taken to confirm the accuracy of the information presented and to describe generally accepted practices. However, the authors, editors, and publisher are not responsible for errors or omissions or for any consequences from application of the information in this book and make no warranty, expressed or implied, with respect to the currency, completeness, or accuracy of the contents of the publication. Application of the information in a particular situation remains the professional responsibility of the practitioner.

The authors, editors, and publisher have exerted every effort to ensure that drug selection and dosage set forth in this text are in accordance with current recommendations and practice at the time of publication. However, in view of ongoing research, changes in government regulations, and the constant flow of information relating to drug therapy and drug reactions, the reader is urged to check the package insert for each drug for any change in indications and dosage and for added warnings and precautions. This is particularly important when the recommended agent is a new or infrequently employed drug.

Some drugs and medical devices presented in the publication have Food and Drug Administration (FDA) clearance for limited use in restricted research settings. It is the responsibility of the health care provider to ascertain the FDA status of each drug or device planned for use in their clinical practice.

To purchase additional copies of this book, call our customer service department at (800) 638-3030 or fax orders to (301) 223-2320. International customers should call (301) 223-2300.

Visit Lippincott Williams & Wilkins on the Internet: at LWW.com. Lippincott Williams & Wilkins customer service representatives are available from 8:30 am to 6 pm, EST.

10 9 8 7 6 5 4 3 2 1

CCS1009

To our families for their unwavering support and understanding.

To our mentors for giving us the gifts of clinical knowledge, skills and inquisitiveness. These men were pioneers in the field of pediatric orthopedics.

Charles H Herndon MD
G Dean MacEwen MD
WJW Sharrard FRCS

To the future generations of pediatric orthopedists may they build on this foundation and find the clinical joy of caring for children.

Jim Drennan and Jim McCarthy

CONTENTS

FOREWORD

It gives me great pleasure to introduce the second edition of *The Child's Foot and Ankle*. When the first edition was published in 1992, it was one of the first truly comprehensive textbooks where everything we knew about pediatric foot and ankle was assembled in one place. Drs. McCarthy and Drennan have continued this trend for the second edition. National and international experts have updated and rewritten every chapter to reflect what we now know about this most interesting anatomical area.

The child's foot is very complex and intricate and can be affected by disorders that are not found in adults. A fundamental understanding of these disorders is critical to all physicians who treat musculoskeletal disorders in children, from family practitioner to subspecialist. This comprehensive text builds on the first edition and includes information that is difficult to obtain from other sources, such as the chapters on reconstructive amputations, osteochondrodysplasias, and genetic conditions. New chapters have been added that focus on such topics as Ponseti casting, limb deficiencies and reconstruction, and adult consequences of pediatric foot disorders.

As with the first edition, this book emphasizes fundamental treatment principles as they are applied to a wide range foot and ankle disorders in children. It is a completed one source reference which combines decades of information into one location. My congratulation and thanks to Drs. McCarthy and Drennan for providing us with this most excellent book.

G. DEAN MACEWEN, MD

CONTRIBUTORS

Hadeel Abaza, MD Fellow in Pediatric Orthopaedic Surgery, Departments of Orthopaedic Surgery and Pediatrics, Rainbow Babies and Children's Hospital, Case Western Reserve University, Cleveland, OH

Alexandre Arkader, MD Assistant Professor of Clinical Orthopaedic Surgery, Keck School of Medicine, University of Southern California, Los Angeles, CA

John G. Birch, MD Assistant Chief of Staff, Texas Scottish Rite Hospital for Children, Dallas, TX

Danielle B. Cameron, BA Clinical Research Coordinator, Orthopaedic Surgery, Children's Hospital of Philadelphia, Philadelphia, PA

In Ho Choi, MD Professor, Department of Orthopaedic Surgery, Seoul National University College of Medicine, Seoul, Korea

Aaron Cook, BHB ChB FRACS (Ortho) Consultant Surgeon, Orthopadic Research, Tauranga Orthopaedic Research Society Inc., New Zealand

Julie A. Coplan, PT, DSc Clubfoot Clinic Coordinator, Sinai Hospital of Baltimore, Baltimore, MD

Marco Túlio Costa, MD Santa Casa Medical School and Hospitals, Santa Casa de Misericórdia de São Paulo, Departamento de Ortopedia e Traumatologia, São Paulo, Brasil

Jon R. Davids, MD Chief of Staff, Medical Director Motion Analysis Laboratory, Shriners Hospital for Children, Greenville, SC

John Delahay, MD FACS Peter and Rose Rizzo Professor of Orthopaedic Surgery, Vice Chairman, Department of Orthopaedic Surgery, Georgetown University School of Medical, Washington, DC

John P. Dormans, MD Chief, Division of Orthopaedic Surgery, The Children's Hospital of Philadelphia, Professor of Orthopaedic Surgery, University of Pennsylvania School of Medicine, Philadelphia, PA

James C. Drennan, MD Professor Emeritus of Orthopaedics and Pediatrics, University of New Mexico School of Medicine, Albuquerque, NM

Craig P. Eberson, MD Assistant Professor and Division Chief, Pediatric Orthopaedics and Scoliosis, Warren Alpert School of Medicine of Brown University, Providence, RI

Ricardo Cardenuto Ferreira, MD Departamento de Ortopedia e Traumatologia, São Paulo, Brasil

Gabriela J. Ferski, RN, MPH, MS Clinical Research Coordinator for Performance Improvement, Shriners Hospitals for Children - Twin Cities, Minneapolis, MN

Patricia M. de Moraes Barros Fucs, MD, PhD Associate Professor, Departamento de Ortopedia e Traumatologia, São Paulo, Brasil

Theodore J. Ganley, MD Director of Sports Medicine, The Children's Hospital of Philadelphia, Philadelphia, PA, Assistant Professor of Orthopaedic Surgery, The University of Pennsylvania School of Medicine, Philadelphia, PA

Gaia Georgopoulos, MD Department of Orthopaedic Surgery, University of Colorado Health Sciences Center, Denver, CO

H. Kerr Graham, MD, FRCS (Ed), FRACS Professor of Orthopaedic Surgery, Orthopaedic Department, The Royal Children's Hospital, The University of Melbourne and Murdoch Children's Research Institute, Melbourne, Australia

Walter B. Greene, MD Professor Emeritus University of Missouri, Columbia, MD

Leslie Grissom, MD Department Chair, Department of Medical Imaging, Alfred I. duPont Hospital for Children, Wilmington, DE

Dennis P. Grogan, MD Clinical Professor, Department of Orthopaedic Surgery, University of South Florida, Chief of Staff, Shriners Hospitals for Children, Tampa, FL

Kenneth J. Guidera, MD Chief of Staff, Pediatric Orthopedic Surgeon, Shriner's Hospital for Children, Twin Cities, Minneapolis, MN

Sigvard T. Hansen, Jr., MD Professor, Orthopedic Surgery and Sports Medicine, University of Washington, Seattle, WA.

Martin J. Herman, MD Associate Professor of Orthopedic Surgery, Drexel University College of Medicine, Philadelphia, PA

John E. Herzenberg, MD Head of Pediatric Orthopaedics, Sinai Hospital of Baltimore, Baltimore, MD

Mark A. Holowka, MSPO, CPO O&P Supervisor, Shriners Hospitals for Children—Philadelphia, Philadelphia, PA

Durga N. Kowtharapu, MD Research Fellow, Department of Orthopaedics, Alfred I. Dupont Hospital for Children, Wilmington, DE

S. Jay Kumar, MD Orthopaedic Surgeon, Department of Orthopaedics, Alfred I. Dupont Hospital for Children, Wilmington, DE

Mervyn Letts, MD Former Chief, Department of Surgery, Division of Pediotric Orthopaedics, Children's Hospital of Eastern Ontario, University of Ottowa; Consultant Pediatric Orthopaedic Surgeon, Sheikh Khalifa Medical City UAE.

James J. McCarthy Associate Professor, Department of Orthopaedics and Rehabilitation, University of Wisconsin, Madison, WI

Richard Miller, MD Professor for Department of Orthopaedic Surgery, University of New Mexico, Albuquerque, NM

Payam Moazzaz, MD Chief Resident for Department of Orthopaedic Surgery, UCLA Medical Center, Los Angeles, CA

Vincent S. Mosca, MD Associate Professor, Department of Orthopedics and Sports Medicine, University of Washington

Karen Myung, MD, PhD Assistant Professor of Orthopedic Surgery, Children's Orthopedic Center, Children's Hospital of Los Angeles, Los Angeles, CA

Professor Marek Napiontek, MD, PhD Department of Pediatric Orthopaedics and Traumatology, Karol Marcinkowski University of Medical Sciences, Poznan, Poland

Bradford Olney, MD Section Chief, Orthopaedic Surgery, Children's Mercy Hospital and Clinics, Kansas City, MO

Norman Y. Otsuka, MD Assistant Chief of Staff, Department of Pediatric Orthopaedic Surgery, Shriners Hospitals for Children Los Angeles, Los Angeles, CA

Ashish Ranade, MD Pediatric Orthopedic Surgery Fellow, St. Christopher's Hospital/Shriner's Hospital for Children Philadelphia, PA

Kenneth J. Rogers, PHD, ATC Senior Clinical Research Coordinator, Department of Orthopaedics, Alfred I. Dupont Hospital for Children, Wilmington, DE

Jonathan R. Schiller, MD Clinical Instructor, Orthopaedic Surgery, Warren Alpert School of Medicine of Brown University, Providence, RI

William F. Schrantz, MD Staff Orthopaedic Surgeon, Shriners Hospitals for Children, Philadelphia, PA

Hua Ming Siow, MBChB, MMed, FRCSEd Fellow, Department of Orthopaedic Surgery, The Children's Hospital of Philadelphia, Philadelphia, PA, Associate Consultant, Department of Orthopaedic Surgery, KK Women's and Children's Hospital, Singapore

Peter M. Stevens, MD Professor, Pediatric Orthopaedics, University of Utah School of Medicine, Salt Lake City, UT

Alan K. Stotts, MD Assistant Professor, Pediatric Orthopaedics, University of Utah School of Medicine, Salt Lake City, UT

Dinesh Thawrani, MD Research Fellow, Department of Orthopaedics, Alfred I. Dupont Hospital for Children, Wilmington, DE

G. H. Thompson, MD Professor, Orthopaedic Surgery and Pediatrics, Director Pediatric Orthopaedics, Departments of Orthopaedic Surgery and Pediatrics, Rainbow Babies and Children's Hospital, Case Western Reserve University, Cleveland, OH

John G. Tometz, MD Professor, Pediatric Orthopeadics, Medical College of Wisconsin, Millwaukee, WI

Frederick J. White[1] Department of Orthotics, Carrie Tingley Hospital, Albuquerque, NM

[1] *Deceased.*

Won Joon Yoo, MD Assistant Professor, Department of Orthopaedic Surgery, Seoul National University College of Medicine, Seoul National University Hospital, Seoul, Korea

PREFACE TO THE FIRST EDITION

Problems relating to the child's foot and ankle form a major portion of pediatric orthopaedics. They include a clinical spectrum ranging from abnormalities that spontaneously resolve to others that progress; and from isolated esoteric deformities to major functional disabilities associated with genetic syndromes or which develop secondary to a neuromuscular disease. Satisfactory pedal function is confirmed with each step and it is difficult to compensate for an unresolved foot deformity. The alignment of the lower extremities and gait abnormalities are frequently described in terms of the feet, which are the most visible portion.

Effective management is important, whether the goal is improved ambulation, satisfactory pedal positioning on a wheelchair footrest, or simply obtaining appropriate shoes. Recent changes in rehabilitation philosophy can be illustrated by the move from expensive "corrective" shoes to inexpensive flexible shoe gear as part of orthotic management. The physicians' objectives remain a painless plantigrade foot which can wear commercially available shoes, is cosmetically acceptable, and retains motion and sensation when possible.

This book is a culmination of my long interest in the pathophysiology of foot deformities combined with continual clinical exposure to the outcomes of unsatisfactory management. I did not initially envision a twenty-six chapter text, but recent advances in a variety of areas including gait analysis, orthotics, and our understanding of neuromuscular disorders has necessitated a book of this length. The reader is fortunate that a distinguished group of pediatric orthopaedists and associated medical colleagues have contributed their expertise on specific topics. These authors should be given the major credit for the content of the book as they share their clinical knowledge and insight regarding etiology and management of the myriad of problems.

The book provides the interested resident and practitioner with a clear understanding of the etiology and treatment of specific pedal deformities. The initial chapters provide basic information that can be applied to later clinical sections.

JAMES C. DRENNAN

PREFACE TO THE SECOND EDITION

The second edition of *Drennan's The Child's Foot and Ankle* is completely revised. It builds on the strengths of the first edition and remains comprehensive, serving as a single resource for pediatric foot and ankle disorders. All the chapters are rewritten, most by new authors, all of whom are experts in their fields. The contents have been expanded to reflect new techniques and knowledge. Several new chapters have been added, including Limb Deficiencies and Reconstruction, the Non-Operative Treatment of Congenital Clubfoot (including the Ponseti technique), Normal Function of the Ankle and Foot: Biomechanics and Quantitative Analysis, and Adult Consequences of Pediatric Foot Disorders. There is also an expanded trauma section. Unique chapters containing difficult-to-find information have been retained, such as the treatment of Poliomyelitis, Reconstructive Amputation of the Foot and Ankle, Macrodactyly, and Genetic Conditions.

Despite the additional chapters and updated information, the core principles of pediatric foot and ankle care remain. The goal is a painless platigrade foot, which can wear commercially available shoes, is cosmetically acceptable, and retains motion and sensation when possible. Pediatric foot and ankle disorders in the population with neuromuscular pathologies are frequently unique and deserve specific attention. The highest standard of treatment in childhood is critical for quality of life throughout the patient's lifetime.

This book provides the basic framework for interested resident and practitioners, offering a clear description of the etiology and treatment of specific pediatric foot and ankle deformities. These are details essential for the most specialized surgeons. We hope that this information will assist in the care of children today and for years to come.

ACKNOWLEDGMENTS

We would like to recognize the considerable contributions of several people in the development of the book. Dr Drennan's long time administrative assistant, Shirley Hagan, demonstrated great patience and professional skill in the revision of several complex chapters. Her ability to discern arrows and asterisks is uncanny. Dr McCarthy benefited from Barbara Wulf's incredible organizational skills and endless hard work to bring this project to completion.

We would both like to express our appreciation to our editor, David Murphy. He always maintained his sense of humor and grasp of the entire project in bringing the book to its conclusion.

CHAPTER 1

Anatomy

James C. Drennan

INTRODUCTION

The development of vertebrate limbs results from complex interactions between limb mesoderm and ectoderm. Multiple levels of control and regulation are needed between normal mesoderm and ectoderm to bring about the necessary interactions for normal proximodistal limb development.

The embryonic period comprises the first eight postovulatory weeks and has been divided into 23 stages (21). There is an important somite–somatopleure relationship that precedes the visible emergence of the limb bud. The somatopleural mesoderm is stimulated by the adjacent unsegmented somite mesoderm and becomes morphogenically active. Limb buds then emerge at four weeks of age (stages 12 and 13) as lateral thickenings of the somatopleure. The lower limb buds (stage 13) are initially located opposite somites 25 to 28. During the fifth week (stages 15 to 18), mammalian limb buds develop a thickened epithelium at their distal tips, the apical ectodermal ridge, which is the principal inducer of axial limb elongation. Experiments have demonstrated that further limb development stops when the ridge is removed and only established limb parts will continue to develop (22). The apical ridge is necessary both for the progressive specification of mesodermal limb parts as well as the promotion of axial growth through influencing cell division (measured by a relative proximodistal increase in the mitotic index of the dividing cells) (22). The ridge is the source of "morphogen" which is needed both for normal limb development and to effect a mitogenic influence on subjacent mesenchyme while suppressing differentiation of these cells (17). The apical ridge also acts to protect subridge mesodermal cells from necrosis during the active period of limb development (10).

The apical ridge is essential for the maintenance of the marginal vasculature in the developing limb. The primitive mesenchymal capillary network develops a peripheral component that results in the formation of an anterior and posterior marginal vein in the limb bud. The axial artery of the lower limb bud is visible by four weeks (stage 13), and practically, all the vessels of the adult limb are present by seven weeks (stage 20) (14). Proximodistal development of the appendicular skeleton is rapid when the mesenchyme becomes vascularized. During the fifth week, variations of vascular flow in the differentiating mesoderm result in the enlarging periphery of the limb bud retaining a rich vascularization, whereas the core mesoderm (presumptive zone of chondrogenesis) becomes a poorly vascularized region; this change in vascular flow may influence chondrogenesis. Nutrient availability from the vascular system causes the establishment of localized populations of cells that results in cytodifferentiation of the cartilaginous aspects of the limb. The precise spatial patterning of limb buds is brought about by a process of induction which transmits a unique morphogenic message to the rapidly dividing cells as they undergo specific differentiation.

Mesenchymal cells derived from the somite mesoderm limb bud give rise to the entire appendicular skeleton. The primordial cartilage of the larger lower limb bones can histologically be identified in the six-week-old embryo and begin as mesenchymal condensations. The initial phase of chondrification is termed precartilage and the mesenchymal cells at the periphery form a perichondrium outlining the skeletal anlage. The majority of the smaller bones of the foot can be identified during the seventh week and cartilage primority of all future bones of the appendicular skeleton are present by the eighth week.

The dual origin of the limb bud mesoderm is significant because muscle tissue develops from the cells of somite origin while tendons and cartilage form from somatopleural mesodermal cells. These precursor cells remain distinctive, and the cell types do not mix in the mesoderm of the developing limb. Cells with chondrogenic potential in the early limb bud are confined to the central core of the limb mesoderm while prospective myogenic cells form compartments surrounding the chondrogenic limb center (15). All skeletal muscles of the lower limb are present by the beginning of the eighth week. The lumbar and sacral plexuses are formed by five weeks (stage 15), and by stage 17, the tibial nerve enters the plantar region of the foot anlage, where it divides into a medial and lateral plantar nerve.

Spinal nerves grow into the developing limb and innervate the skeletal muscles. The adult pattern of dermatomes suggests that lumbar nerves supply the preaxial border of the limb bud, while the postaxial border is innervated by the first and second sacral nerves.

Collagen forms the major component of extracellular matrix and is produced by mesenchymal cells. Another group of macromolecules, proteoglycans, complex with collagen to play important roles in cell migration and chondrogenesis during limb development. These mesodermal condensations chondrify in a definite sequence and are eventually converted to bone. Each transitional step is characterized by the deposition of new histologically distinct collagen within the extracellularmatrix (12). In the early limb bud, hyaluronic acid is the major glycosaminoglycan chain of the proteoglycans and has its highest levels in the mesenchymal cells directly subjacent to the apical ectodermal ridge (9). There is a progressive decline in hyaluronate as cells become distanced from the ridge, and this may represent the first critical step in chondrogenesis (11). Chondrification of the skeletal elements of the foot follows, a definite pattern beginning at about six weeks and the number of chondrific centers increases for an additional two weeks. The tarsal bones develop by endochondral ossification and most of the tarsals ossify in postnatal life. The cartilage of the calcaneus calcifies and periosteal bone forms, and then vascular invasion and endochondral ossification begin. Endochondral ossification of the tubular bones, e.g., the metatarsi, grow by apposition from the perichondrium and by multiplication of cartilage cells already found in intracellular matrix. Ossification commences at the middle of the cartilaginous model with a thin layer of osteoid being laid down between the perichondrium and the hypertrophied cartilage cells of the shaft. The osteoid is rapidly calcified, and the innermost cells of the neoperiosteum differentiate into osteoblasts. Trabeculae begin to form and the primary bone collar gradually becomes multilayered. The primary bone collar is penetrated by blood vessels at several points to permit the formation of an ossific center. Osteoblasts and blood-forming cells develop and bone begins to be deposited about the residua of calcified cartilage matrix and endochondral ossification occurs. By the middle of prenatal life, endochondral ossification reaches the epiphyseal regions and the development of the growth plate becomes a reality. Changes in the mesenchyme located between centers of chondrification signal the beginning of the interzones which has two parallel chondrogenic layers separated by a less-dense layer. The primitive joint capsule also is formed. The peripheral portion of interzone mesenchyme forms Ihe synovium which becomes vascularized. Tiny spaces are needed in the intermediate zones which join together to form the joint cavity. The small joints of the feet may demonstrate a delay between interzone formation and cavitation.

Cell death is an essential part of normal development. Zones of necrosis are necessary to eliminate most or all interdigital mesodermal cells and to completely free human digits (6). There is a delicate balance between the digits growing by cell division and their separation by concomitant cell death occurring in the web tissue between the digits. The fact that cell deaths occur at precise time and placement may represent an end point for differentiation of the cells that die.

LOWER LIMB ROTATION

At five weeks of age, both the upper and lower limbs point laterally and caudally, and the future foot is paddle shaped. By six weeks, the knee joint is visible and points laterally while the leg and foot rotate so that the plantar surface of the foot faces the trunk. At eight weeks, an additional 90 degrees of proximal lower extremity torsion results in the knee pointing cranially, and at eight weeks, torsion of the lower limbs results in the twisting or "barber pole arrangement" which explains the "barber pole" cutaneous innervation (4).

Bohm (3) focused on the physiologic developmental phases of the embryonic foot. At five weeks, the embryonal foot is separated from the lower leg by a slight constriction and the paddle-shaped structure demonstrates 90 degrees of plantar flexion, is laterally rotated to lie in the sagittal plane, and functions as a direct extension of the lower leg in its long axis. Histologically the limb bud contains a talus lying between the distal ends of the fibula and tibia and the foot is adducted by the medial inclination of the calcaneus and talus. The navicular lies near the internal malleolus, and the metatarsi are progressively increasingly deviated toward the tibia in a position of forefoot adduction. The foot is flat and in the same plane as the transverse axis of the knee. Bardeen (1) also noted the marked equinus and that the cuboid appeared to be a direct extension of the calcaneus, while the navicular was a continuation of the talus. Bardeen noted at stage 20 that the talus was enlarging and extending beyond the calcaneus, thereby separating the navicular from the tibia and the foot began its deflections toward the position of abduction.

The second stage of Bohm's classification is reached when the length of the embryo exceeds 20 mm or has entered the third fetal month. The digits are well developed, initial heel protuberance is noted, and the foot continues to lie in the long axis of the leg, but there has been a rotation of the entire foot through 90 degrees to place it in a position of supination. The plane of the foot is perpendicular to the frontal plane of the lower leg, this change is caused by the position of the tarsal bones. A rudimentary plantar transverse arch is noted and adduction of the metatarsi persists. The calcaneus is also shifted plantarward and apposes the fibula. The third stage begins when the embryo length exceeds 35 mm and occurs in the middle of the third month. The most significant pedal change is the development of dorsiflexion of the ankle joint which changes the foot position from the previous extreme equinus. The foot persists in supination and forefoot adduction and mild hind foot equinus. The formation of the subtalar joints is completed and the calcaneus lies with its dorsal surface tilted laterally, and the plantar surface medially beneath the talus whose neck and head turn medially and plantarwards. The feet assume the "prayer position" during the fourth stage at the end of the third month. The soles are approximated and the feet placed in the midplane of the body and retain mild supination and slight persistent metatarsus adductus which is a position similar to the human adult. These changes occur gradually by continual transformation, and the fourth stage position is retained throughout fetal and neonatal life. The growth of the normal foot has been studied by Blais et al (2) (Figure 1-1).

SKELETON

The skeletal components of the ankle and foot include: the tibia and fibula, the tarsal and metatarsal bones, and the phalanges (Figure 1-2). The tibia contributes its inferior articular surface and medial malleolus whose lateral surface articulates with the trochlea tali. The malleolar sulcus, located posterior to the malleolus, is a groove through which tendons pass from the posterior aspect of the leg to the plantar surface of the foot. The lateral surface of the distal tibia has a fibular notch. The enlarged lower end of the fibula forms the lateral malleolus which has a medial facet for articulation with the talus.

There are seven tarsal bones which form the heel and the posterior portion of the foot (Figure 1-3). The calcaneus is the heel bone and is located beneath the talus. The calcaneus is the largest tarsal bone and its superior surface articulates with the talus by posterior and middle talocalcaneal joints which are separated by the sulcus calcanei containing the interosseous ligament. The sustentaculum tali bears the middle articular joint. The posterior aspect of the calcaneus is the downward-projecting tuber calcanei which has a specially roughened area on its superior surface for the attachment of the tendo Achillis. The groove for the tendon of the flexor hallucis longus passes posterior and beneath the sustentaculum tali. The flexor retinaculum and plantar aponeurosis are attached to the plantar medial tubercle and parts of the abductor hallucis and flexor digitorum breveis arise from this bony prominence. The short plantar ligament is attached to the anterior tubercle, while the long plantar ligament arises from a wide area on the inferior surface behind the anterior tubercle. The deltoid ligament and plantar calcaneonavicular ligament are attached to the medial margin of the sustentaculum tali.

The talus or ankle bone is composed of a body, head, and neck (Figure 1-4). The superior and lateral articular surfaces of the body form the trochlea tali which articulates with the medial and lateral malleolus and has a large articular convex superior surface for articulation with the inferior surface of the tibia. There are projections beneath the medial and lateral articular surfaces for the attachment of the medial and lateral ligaments of the ankle. The posterior talar process has an invagination for the tendon of the flexor hallucis longus muscle. The rough neck connects the expanded anterior head to the body, and the head has an anterior articular surface that articulates with the navicular

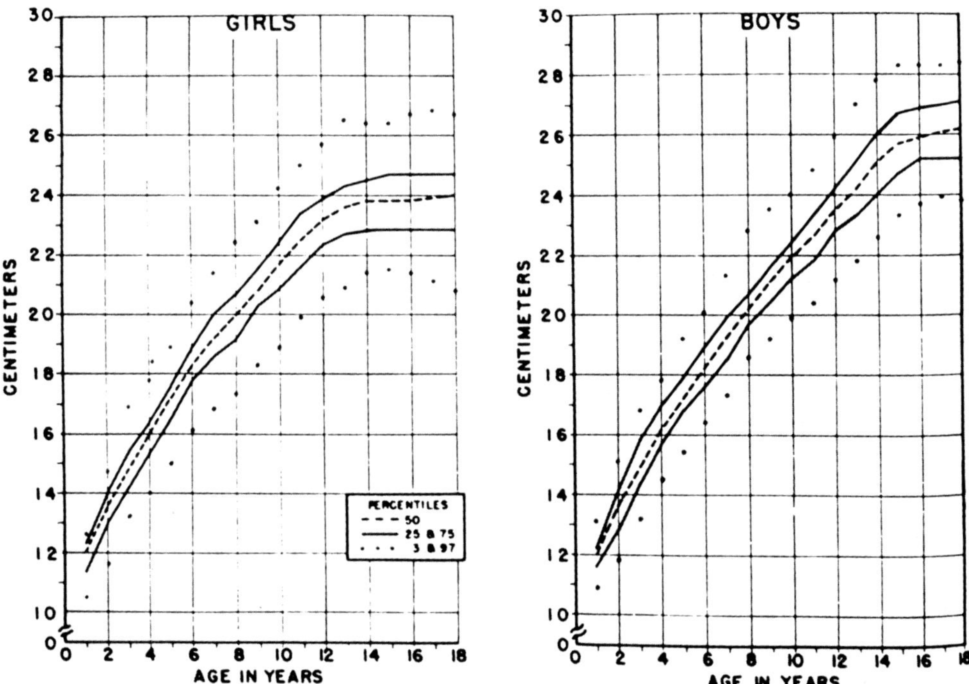

FIGURE 1-1 The length of normal foot determined by serial measurements of 512 children aged 1 to 18 years. Measurement was from the back of the heel to the tip of the hallux with the subject in a standing position. (From Blais MM, Green WT, Anderson M. Lengths of the growing foot. *Bone Joint Surg* 1956;38A: 998–1000, with permission.)

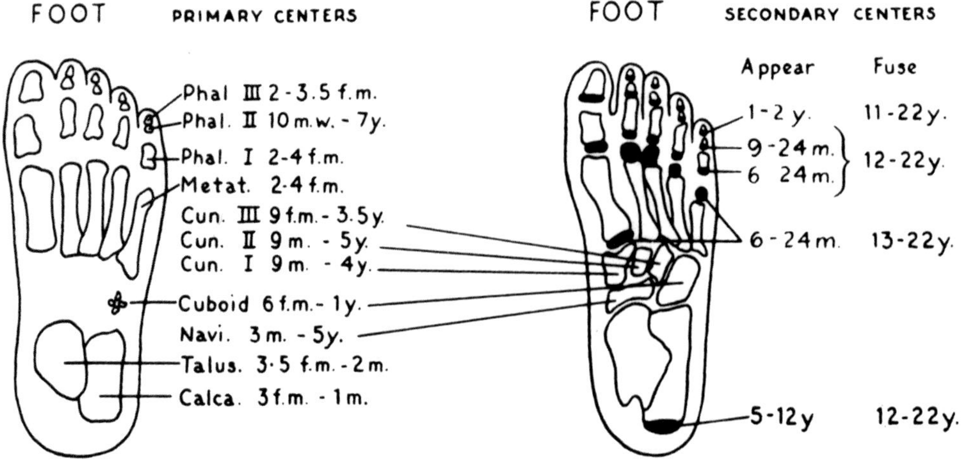

FIGURE 1-2 Schedule for appearance of primary and secondary ossification centers and fusion of secondary centers with the shafts in the heel. (From Caffey J. The extremities: anatomic variations. In: *Pediatric x-ray diagnosis,* 4th ed. Chicago: Year Book Medical, 1961;784 with permission.)

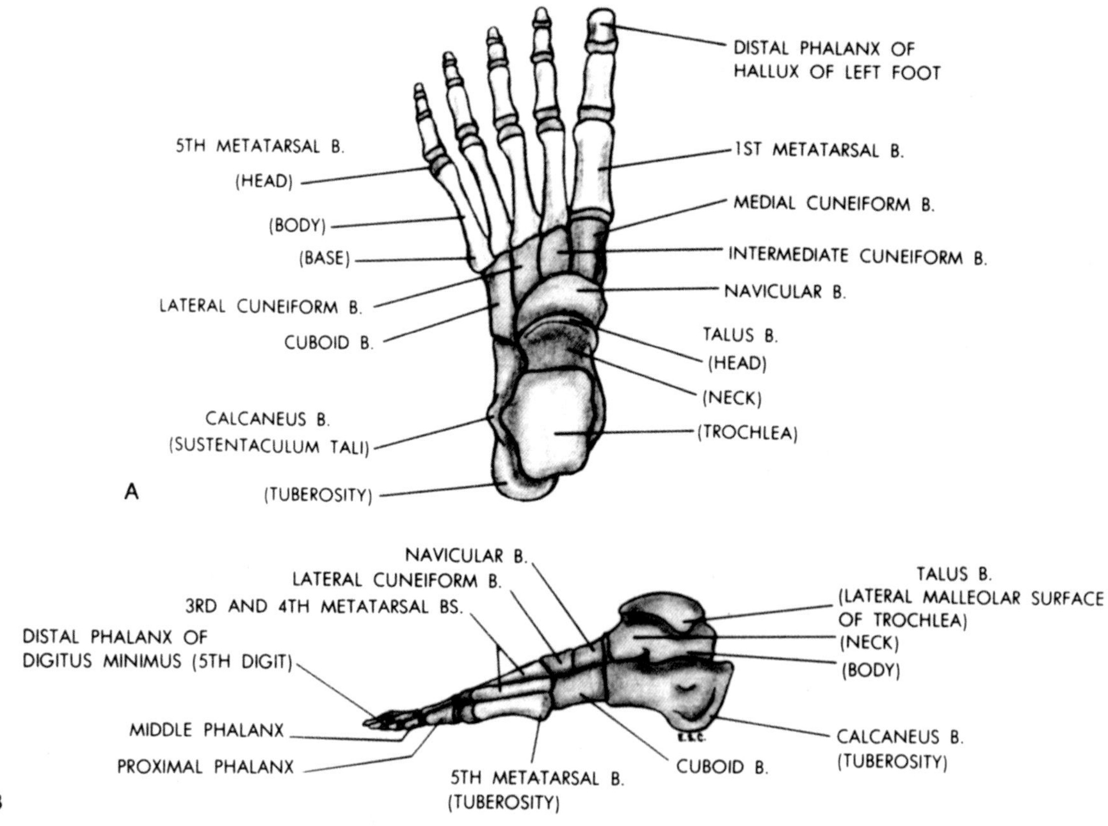

FIGURE 1-3 Dorsal (**A**) and lateral (**B**) drawings of the newborn pedal skeletal. Darker areas represent cartilage. (From Crelin ES. *Anatomy of the newborn: An atlas.* Philadelphia: Lea & Febiger, 1969;251:252; with permission.)

bone. Inferiorly, the oblique sulcus tali separates the larger posterior and smaller middle articular facets. The sinus tarsi forms a lateral depression between the two bones and extends posteriorly and medially beneath the neck of the talus to connect with the canal formed by the opposed sulcus calcanei and sulcus tali. The anterior capsule of the ankle joint attaches to the dorsal surface of the ankle.

The navicular extends in front of the talus, the cuboid in front of the calcaneus and the three cuneiform bones lie distal to the navicular and medial to the cuboid. The

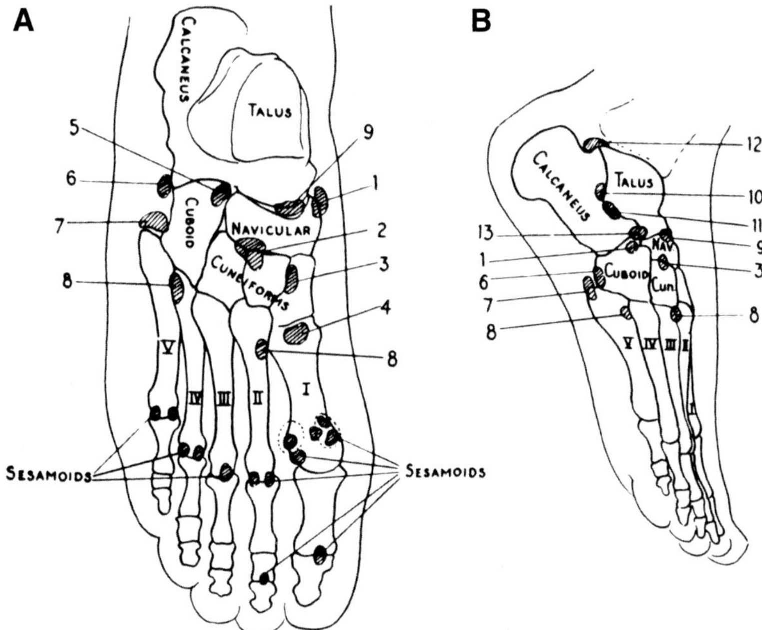

FIGURE 1-4 Common accessory bones in the foot. 1, os tibiale extremum; 2, processus uncinatus; 3, os intercuneiforme; 4, pars peronea metatarsalia I; 5, cuboides secundarium; 6, os peroneum; 7, os vesalianum; 8, os intermetatarseum; 9, accessory navicular; 10, talus accessories; 11, os sustentaculum; 12, os trigonum; 13, calcaneus secundarium. (From Caffey J. The extremities: anatomic variations. In: *Pediatric x-ray diagnosis,* 4th ed. Chicago: Year Book Medical, 1961;817, with permission.)

navicular has a concave proximal articular surface that accommodates the convex surface of the talar head and a slightly convex distal surface toward the three cuneiform bones. The medial surface has a tuberosity which serves as the insertion for the major portion of the tibialis posterior tendon. The plantar calcaneonavicular ligament stretches from the plantar surface of the navicular to the sustentaculum tali and additional anterior fibers of the deltoid ligament attach to the tuberosity. The cuboid bone lies between the calcaneus and the fourth and fifth metatarsi. Both its proximal and distal surfaces are wholly articular, and there is also a facet for the lateral cuneiform. Laterally and inferiorly, the cuboid tuberosity creates a sulcus for the tendon of the peroneus longus muscle.

The three cuneiform bones are wedge shaped and lie distal to the navicular and proximal to the three metatarsal bones. The medial cuneiform is the largest of these osseous structures and has a broader plantar surface than dorsal area and articulates with the navicular, intermediate cuneiform, first metatarsus, and the medial side of the base of the second metatarsus. The tibialis anterior attaches at its anterodistal aspect. The cuneiforms are stabilized by heavy interosseous ligaments. The intermediate cuneiform is the smallest and has a broader dorsal surface than plantar aspect. This bone articulates with the navicular, the second metatarsus, and the medial and lateral cuneiforms. Articulations of the lateral cuneiform includes the navicular, the inter-mediate cuneiform, the cuboid, and the third metatarsus, as well as small aspects of the second and fourth metatarsi. The only muscles attaching to the bones of the midfoot are the tibialis posterior to the navicular and medial cuneiform and the tibialis anterior to the medial cuneiform.

The metatarsi are the skeleton of the anterior part of the foot and consist of a base, a shaft, and a distally lying bead. The bases are firmly bound to the tarsi by ligaments at the tarsometatarsal joints. There is a gap between the medial and lateral cuneiforms and in front of the intermediate cuneiform in which the base of the second metatarsal bone fits and gains additional stability by this recession. The base of the first metatarsus is usually free, but all the remaining metatarsi have articular joints between them. The peroneus longus tendon attaches to the first metatarsus by a plantar tuberosity. Its shaft is heavy and articulates with the medial cuneiform. The first metatarsal head has two well-marked plantar grooves for articulation with the sesamoid bones. The remaining metatarsi have slender shafts and tend to be convex plantarward (7). Articular cartilage is limited to the distal and plantar aspect of the metatarsal heads for approximation with the phalanges at the metatarsophalangeal joints. The sides of the heads have grooves for attachment of the collateral ligaments of these joints. The phalanges contribute little to the length of the foot and represent a miniature long bone possessing both a shaft and two ends. The proximal phalanges have concave bases that articulate with the heads of the metatarsi and have slender bodies. Their heads have a central depression for articulation with the saddle-shaped base of the shorter middle phalanges. The distal phalanx of the great toe is large, while the others are miniature.

FASCIA, SUPERFICIAL NERVES, AND VESSELS

The superficial fascia of the dorsal of the foot is thin and permits mobility of the skin. However, on the plantar surface, it is thick and serves as padding between the skin and anchors the skin firmly to the underlying deep fascia.

Cutaneous Nerves

The saphenous nerve is the terminal branch of the femoral nerve and travels on the anteromedial portion of the leg with the great saphenous vein. The saphenous nerve supplies a series of medial crural cutaneous branches before coursing along the medial side of the foot and terminating at the hallucal metatarsophalangeal joint. Its terminal branches are distributed to the skin and fascia of the front and middle leg and posterior half of the dorsum and medial sides of the foot. The cutaneous component of the superficial peroneal nerve enters the anterolateral aspect of the foot and divides into two dorsal cutaneous nerves (Figure 1-5). The medial dorsal cutaneous supplies sensation to the medial side of the big toe and the adjacent second and third toes. The intermediate dorsal cutaneous nerve divides into two dorsal digital branches that supply the adjacent sides of the third, fourth, and fourth and fifth toes. The lateral and medial sural cutaneous nerves commonly join in the distal one-third of the leg and pass posterior and superficial to the peroneal retinaculum in close approximation to the peroneal tendons at the posterolateral aspect of the ankle, and then are directed onto the dorsal aspect of the lateral side of the foot and terminate in the lateral dorsal cutaneous nerve. The terminal sensory branch of the deep peroneal nerve supplies the dorsal digital nerves that service the adjacent sides of the first and second toes. The posterior tibial nerve passes behind to the medial malleolus and terminates under cover of the flexor retinaculum by dividing into the medial and lateral plantar nerves which supply the entire plantar surface of the foot. The plantar digital nerves are the terminal branch of the medial plantar nerve which supplies sensation to the medial three toes. The lateral plantar nerve innervates the remaining distal plantar surface through its superficial branch. The medial calcaneal branch of the posterior tibial nerve pierces the flexor retinaculum and supplies sensation to the skin and fascia of the heel and the posterior part of the sole of the foot.

The plantar venous arch receives the plantar superficial veins and communicating vessels pass between the metatarsi into the dorsal plexus of the foot. The dorsal metatarsal veins unite to form a dorsal venous arch. The long saphenous vein originates from the medial side of this arch, while the smaller saphenous vein originates from the lateral side. The long saphenous vein is accompanied by the saphenous nerve as it passes upward in front of the medial malleolus and then along the medial side of the leg. The short saphenous vein passes posterior to the lateral malleolus and proceeds proximally along the middle of the posterior calf.

Deep Fascia

The addition of transverse fibers to the deep fascia immediately proximal to the ankle creates the retinacula which are critical for the maintenance of the alignment of the tendons crossing the ankle joint. Anteriorly, the superior and inferior extensor retinacula are clearly separated. The superior extensor retinaculum is thin and stretches between the tibia and fibula just above the ankle. The more complex inferior extensor retinaculum arises from the lateral and upper surfaces of the calcaneus and extends over the talar neck and head (see Figure 1-3). This Y-shaped ligament divides into an upper limb which attaches to the medial malleolus and a lower limb which blends with the fascia on the medial side of the sole of the foot. The inferior extensor retinaculum contains three separate compartments for the entrance of the extrinsic tendons to the dorsum of the foot; these compartments contain tendon sheaths to permit gliding movement of the tendons. The peroneus tertius and extensor digitorum longus occupy the lateral compartment and the retinaculum then run superficial to the anterior tibial vessels and nerve before splitting again to enclose the tendon of the extensor hallucis longus and finally to enclose the tibialis anterior. The lower limb passes superficial to the tendons of the extensor hallucis longus and tibialis anterior and the dorsalis pedal artery. A band of fibers from the deep surface of the lower limb loops about the extensor digitorum longus and becomes attached to adjacent calcaneus and neck of the talus which binds the extensors in this area to the tarsal bones.

The flexor retinaculum spans the medial malleolus and the calcaneus. The bridged space contains four compartments created by three fibrous septa. The most anterior forms a tunnel for the tendon of the tibialis posterior. The other three contain the tendon of the flexor digitorum longus, posterior tibial nerve and vessels, and the most posterior is occupied by the tendon of the flexor hallucis longus. The tendons are provided with a synovial sheath that begins proximal to the retinaculum and extends slightly beyond the plantar surface of the inferior retinaculum. The superior peroneal retinaculum courses from the lateral malleolus to the calcaneus and binds the tendons of the peroneus longus and brevis and their common tendon sheath behind the malleolus. The inferior peroneal retinaculum is attached at both ends to the calcaneus, and dorsally, it blends with the lateral aspect of the inferior extensor retinaculum. It contains a septum which separates the two peroneal tendons.

DORSUM OF THE FOOT

The superficial nerves and vessels have already been described. Both the intrinsic and extrinsic muscles as well as the continuation of the deep peroneal nerve will be discussed. The intrinsic musculature includes the extensor hallucis brevis and extensor digitorum brevis (Figure 1-5). They share a common origin from the anterolateral aspect of the upper surface of the calcaneus and the deep surface of the inferior extensor retinaculum. The extensor hallucis

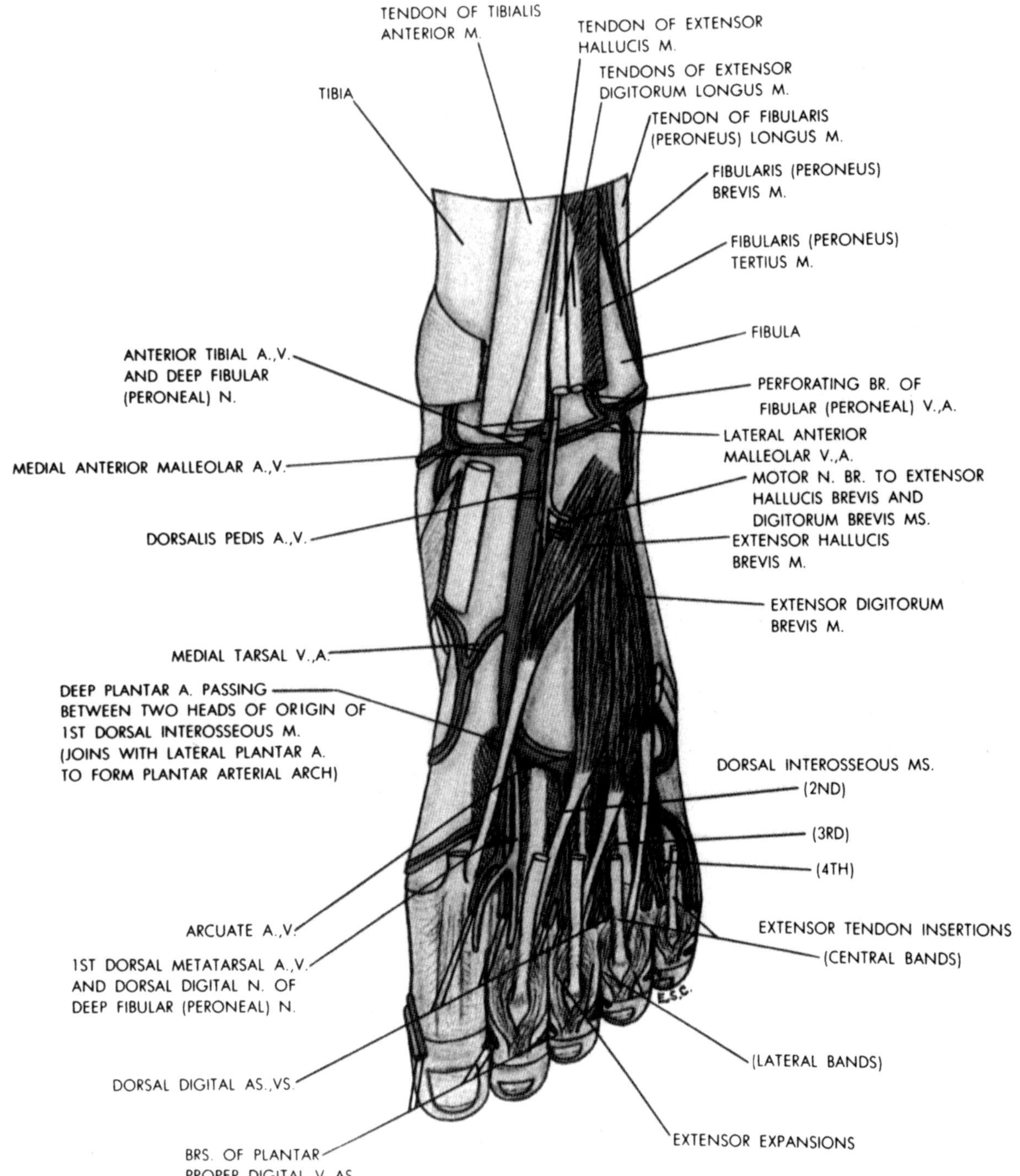

FIGURE 1-5 Arteries, muscles, and nerves of the dorsum of the foot and front of the ankle. (From Crelin ES. *Anatomy of the newborn: An atlas.* Philadelphia: Lea & Febiger, 1969;283. with permission.)

brevis is the more medial and larger muscle belly and crosses the dorsalis pedis artery before inserting on the proximal phalanx of the big toe. The extensor digitorum brevis separates into four divisions with tendons going to the second, third, and fourth toes and also joins the long toe extensors at the level of the metatarsal heads to insert with them into the middle and distal phalanges. Both of these muscles are supplied by the deep peroneal nerve which enters the foot between the tendons of the extensor hallucis longus and extensor digitorum longus. This nerve supplies a lateral branch to the short extensor muscles and gives sensation to the dorsal foot and intermetatarsal joints. The dorsalis pedis artery is a continuation of the anterior tibial artery and is located immediately medial to the deep peroneal nerve on the dorsum of the foot. It runs distally toward the innerspace between the first and second toes. It ends by dividing into a small transverse arcuate artery and a larger deep plantar artery that passes between the heads of the first dorsal interosseous muscle. These two branches supply the dorsal metatarsal arteries which in turn further divide into the minute dorsal digital arteries. The dorsalis pedis artery also gives off medial and lateral tarsal arteries which develop a collateral circulation with the arcuate artery and other hindfoot vessels. A perforating branch of the peroneal artery is a common anomaly when the anterior tibial artery fails to reach the foot (7) and courses beneath the interosseous membrane under the cover of the extensor digitorum longus and peroneus tertius muscles before anastomosing with the anterolateral malleolar branch of the tibialis anterior artery.

PLANTAR ASPECT OF THE FOOT

Fascia, Superficial Nerve, and Vessels

The weight-bearing skin of the foot is attached to tough subcutaneous tissue that continues around the sides of the foot to blend with the thin subcutaneous dorsal fascia at the borders of the foot. The tough subcutaneous tissue extends onto the plantar surface of the toes and surrounds the digital nerves, vessels, and flexor tendon sheaths. The plantar digital nerves and vessels present between slips of the plantar aponeurosis and become subcutaneous close to the bases of the proximal phalanges. The medial plantar nerve supplies the medial three toes, while the lateral plantar nerve supplies the remaining digits. The digital arteries arise from the plantar metatarsal arteries.

The deep fascia includes a dense central plantar aponeurosis that originates from the tubercle of the calcaneus and divides into slips which are directed toward the bases of the toes (Figure 1-6). The transverse fasciculi control the individual digitations in the midfoot and the plantar

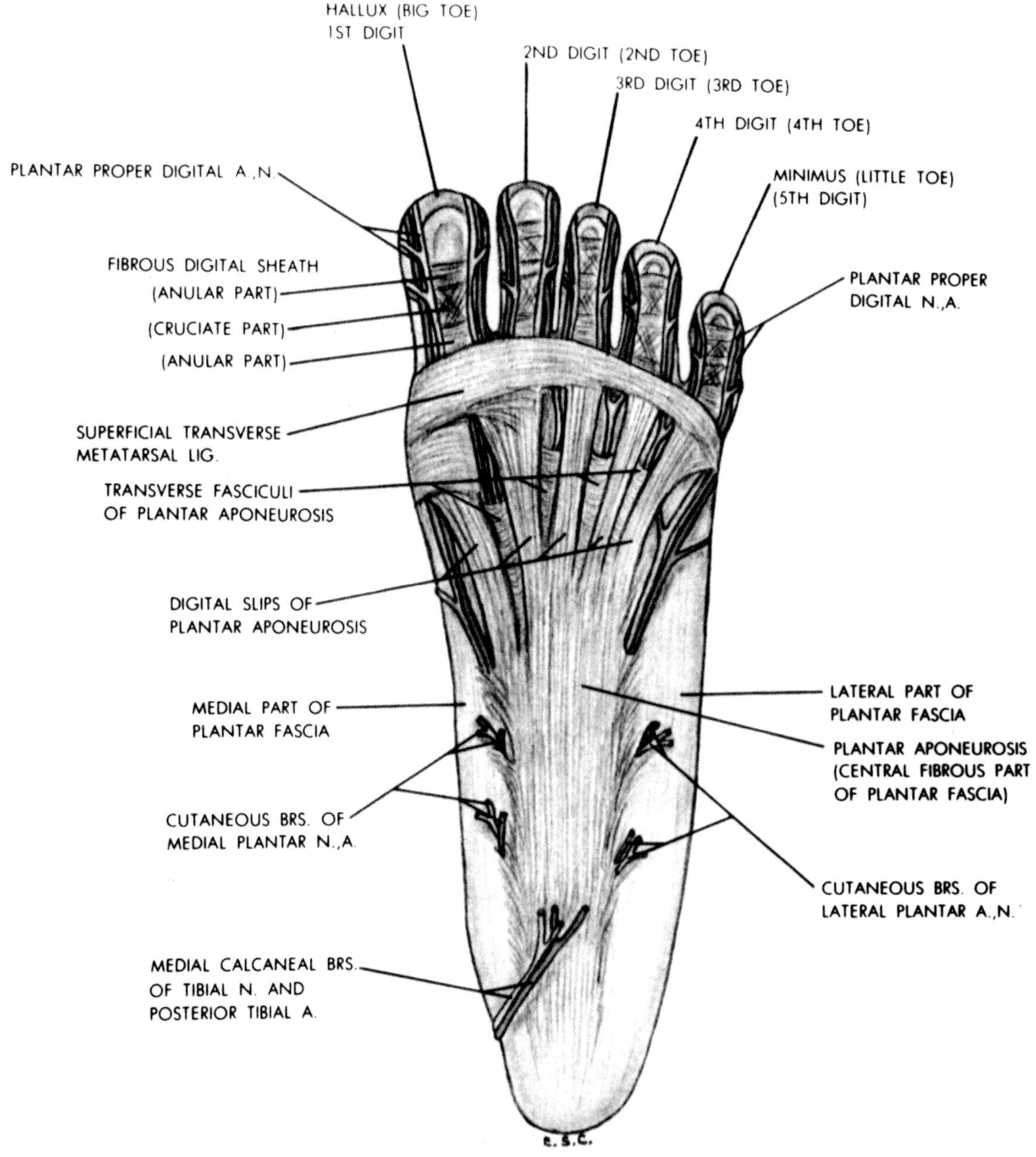

FIGURE 1-6 *(continued)*

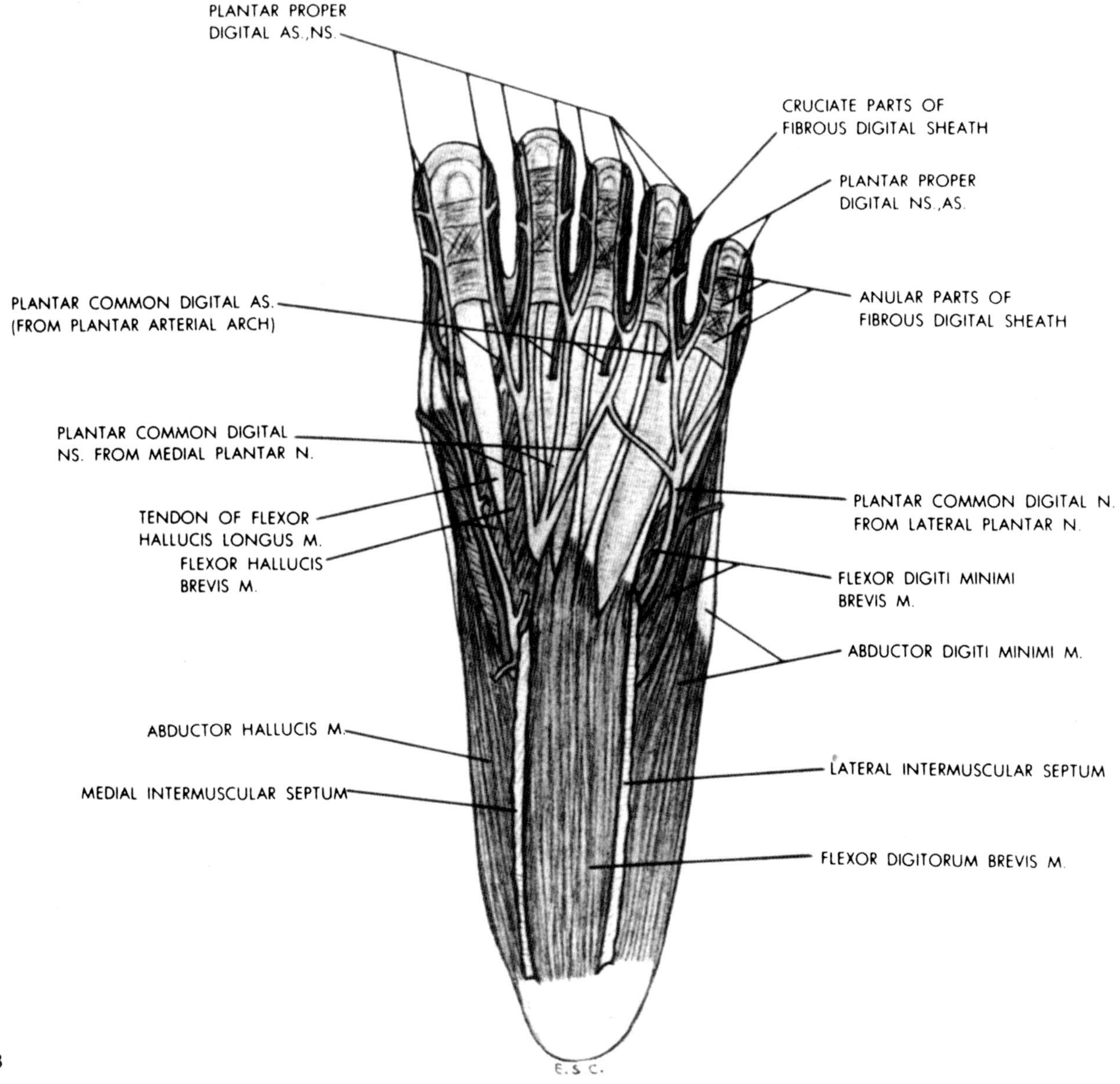

FIGURE 1-6 **A, B**: Plantar fascia and superficial layer of the plantar intrinsic muscles. (From Crelin ES. *Anatomy of the newborn: An atlas.* Philadelphia: Lea & Febiger, 1969;288;289, with permission.)

aponeurosis eventually splits to pass around the long toe flexor tendon sheaths before attaching on each side to the deep transverse ligaments and the base of the proximal phalanx. The superficial transverse metatarsal ligament connects the deep fascia of the first and fifth toes at the level of the heads of the metatarsi.

The medial and lateral edges of the plantar aponeurosis provide intermuscular septa which pass dorsally and divide the plantar foot into three compartments: lateral, intermediate, and medial. The lateral septum attaches over the tarsals proximally and extends to the fifth metatarsal distally and forms a special compartment for the muscles of the little toe. The medial intermuscular septum passes deep to the abductor hallucis to attach to the first metatarsal, while the intermediate contains the tendons of the long flexors.

MUSCLES AND RELATED STRUCTURES IN THE SOLE OF THE FOOT

Removal of the plantar aponeurosis exposes the digital nerves and common digital arteries as well as the superficial layers of the muscles of the sole (see Figure 1-6). The flexor digitorum brevis is the central presenting muscle and the medial plantar nerve and small artery pass on its medial side while the lateral plantar nerve and artery emerge on its lateral side. The medial plantar nerve and artery supply branches to the medial side of the big toe and the nerve divides into common digital sensory branches to the adjacent sides of the first, second, third, and fourth toes. This nerve also innervates the first lumbrical muscle. The lateral plantar nerve ends in a common digital branch that divides to form digital sensory nerves to the fourth and fifth toes. The lateral plantar artery joins the fourth plantar metatarsal artery before passing medially to end by anastomosing with the dorsalis pedis artery, forming the plantar arch.

Superficial Layer

The medial abductor hallucis, the central flexor digitorum brevis, and the lateral abductor digiti minimi comprise the superficial layer of muscles of the sole (Figure 1-7). All three arise from the calcaneus. The abductor hallucis originates from the medial tubercle and from the lower edge of the flexor retinaculum and inserts into the medial side of the base of the proximal phalanx of the hallux. The abductor also blends with the medial tendon of the flexor hallucis brevis into a combined tendon which inserts into the medial sesamoid. The medial and lateral plantar nerves and vessels enter the sole deep to the origin of this muscle. The lateral plantar nerve and artery turn laterally beneath the flexor digitorum brevis while the medial plantar nerve and vessel run forward deep to the abductor hallucis.

The flexor digitorum brevis arises from the medial process of the tuber calcanei and supplies four tendons that proceed toward the middle phalanges of the lateral four toes. These tendons are superficial to the tendons of the flexor digitorum longus and both flexors enter digital tendon sheaths on the toes. Within the sheaths, the tendons of the flexor brevis divide to allow the long flexor tendons to pass through to the distal phalanges. The slips then are reapproximated dorsal to the long tendons and insert into the middle phalanges. The abductor digiti minimi arises from both tubercles, the calcaneus, and adjacent fascia and inserts on the lateral side of the base of the proximal phalanx, it is the only superficial muscle that is innervated by the lateral plantar nerve.

Second Layer

The second layer consists of the tendons of the flexor hallucis longus and flexor digitorum longus and their associated muscles which include the quadratus planti and the four lumbrical muscles (Figure 1-8). The flexor digitorum longus passes anterior to the flexor hallucis longus at the ankle and crosses superficial to the tendon of the flexor hallucis longus which separates it from the spring ligament. The knot-of-Henry is formed at this point as the flexor hallucis gives a tendinous slip to the flexor digitorum. The four tendons of the flexor digitorum longus course distally to enter the fibrous flexor sheath of the toe where the tendon of the flexor digitorum brevis is perforated and the flexor digitorum longus inserts into the base of the distal phalanx. The flexor digitorum longus receives the insertion of the quadratus planti muscle before it divides into the four tendons which give origin to the lumbricales.

The quadratus planti originates from the medial and lateral sides of the plantar surface of the calcaneus and inserts into the lateral edge of the flexor digitorum longus tendon. This muscle is innervated by the lateral plantar nerve. The lumbrical muscles arise from the tendons of the flexor digitorum longus. The first lumbrical originates from the medial side of the tendon to the second toe, while the other three bipennate lumbricals arise from the adjacent sides of two tendons. They pass distally toward the tibial side of the lateral four toes and pass deep to the transverse metatarsal ligaments and then extend dorsally to the dorsal hood to join the extensor tendons on the proximal phalanx. The lateral three lumbricales are supplied by the lateral plantar nerve. The flexor hallucis longus enters the sole by passing deep to the flexor retinaculum and is enclosed in a synovial sheath. It passes deep to the flexor digitorum brevis and the flexor hallucis brevis and inserts at the base of the distal phalanx of the big toe.

Third Layer

The flexor hallucis brevis, the adductor hallucis, and the flexor digiti minimi brevis form the third layer. The flexor hallucis brevis originates from the cuboid and lateral

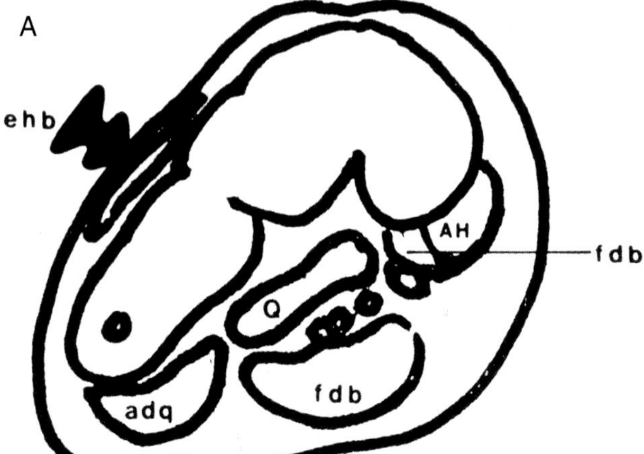

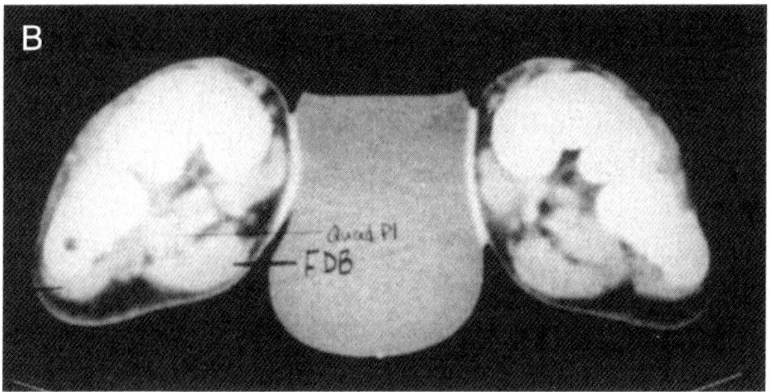

FIGURE 1-7 **A, B**: Computerized axial tomogram of midfoot demonstrating the coronal relationship of pedal intrinsic musculature. AH, abductor hallucis; fhb, flexor hallucis brevis; Q, quadratus planti; fdb, flexor digitorum brevis; adq, abductor digiti quinti; edb, extensor digitorum brevis.

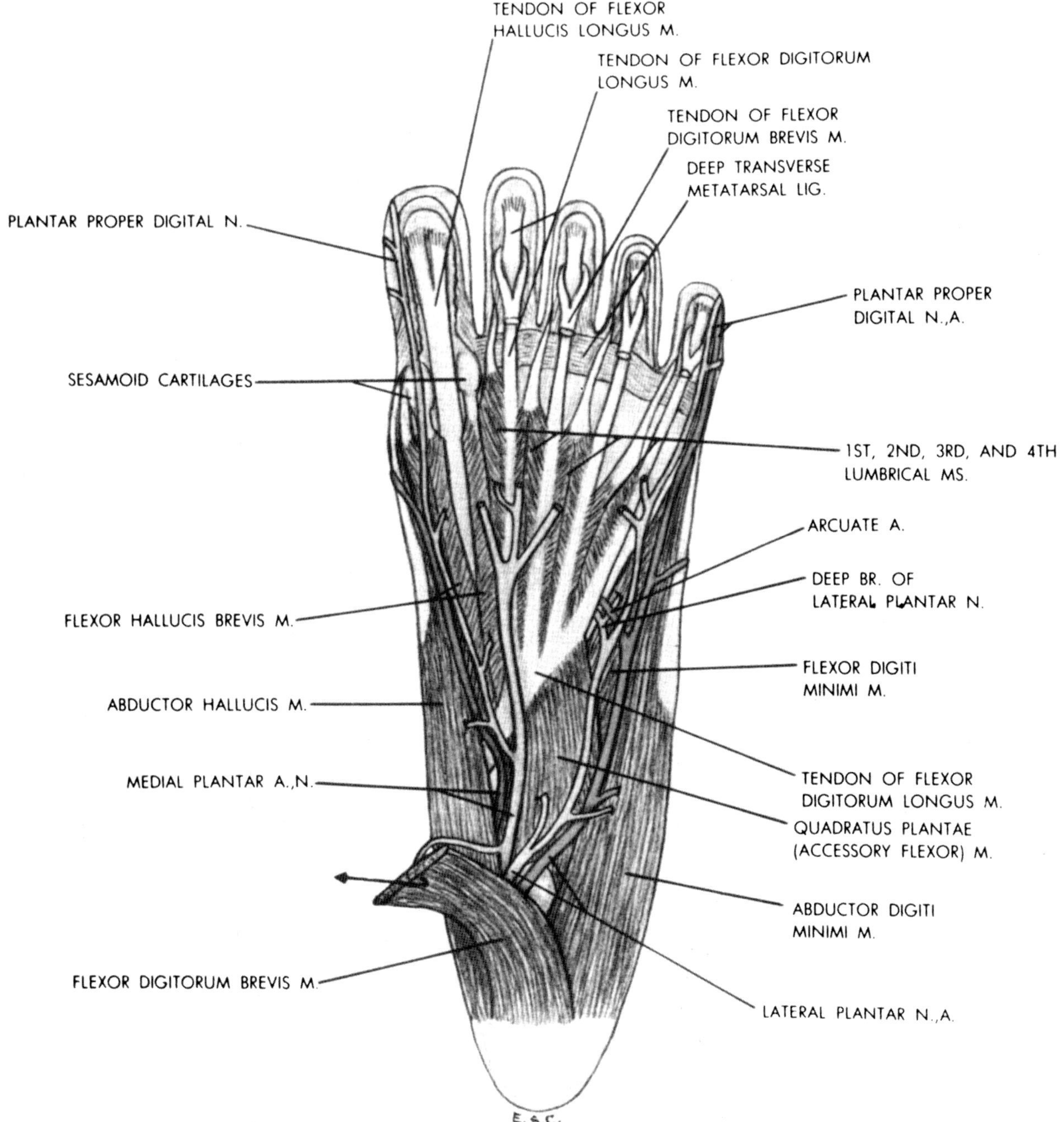

FIGURE 1-8 Second layer of plantar intrinsic muscles. (From Crelin ES. *Anatomy of the newborn: An atlas.* Philadelphia: Lea & Febiger, 1969;291, with permission.)

cuneiform bones and its muscle belly parallels the plantar surface of the first metatarsus before dividing at the level of the metatarsophalangeal joint to escort the tendon of the flexor hallucis longus. Its medial tendon blends with the insertion of the abductor hallucis and inserts into the medial sesamoid and medial aspect of the base of the proximal phalanx. The lateral tendon unites with the adductor hallucis and inserts into the lateral sesamoid as well as the lateral side of the base of the proximal phalanx. The medial plantar nerve innervates this muscle (Figure 1-9).

The adductor hallucis consists of both an oblique and transverse head. The larger oblique head arises from the bases of the second, third, and fourth metatarsals and the plantar sheath of the peroneus longus and runs obliquely to be inserted on the fibular side of the base of the proximal phalanx of the big toe. The smaller transverse head originates from the lateral metatarsophalangeal joint capsules and the deep transverse ligaments of the sole and runs transversely–medially beneath the flexor tendons to join the oblique head, inserting into the fibular side of the base of the proximal phalanx of the big toe.

The two heads also unite with the lateral tendon of the flexor hallucis brevis to insert into the lateral sesamoid. The flexor digit! minimi brevis originates from the sheath of the peroneus longus and the base of the fifth

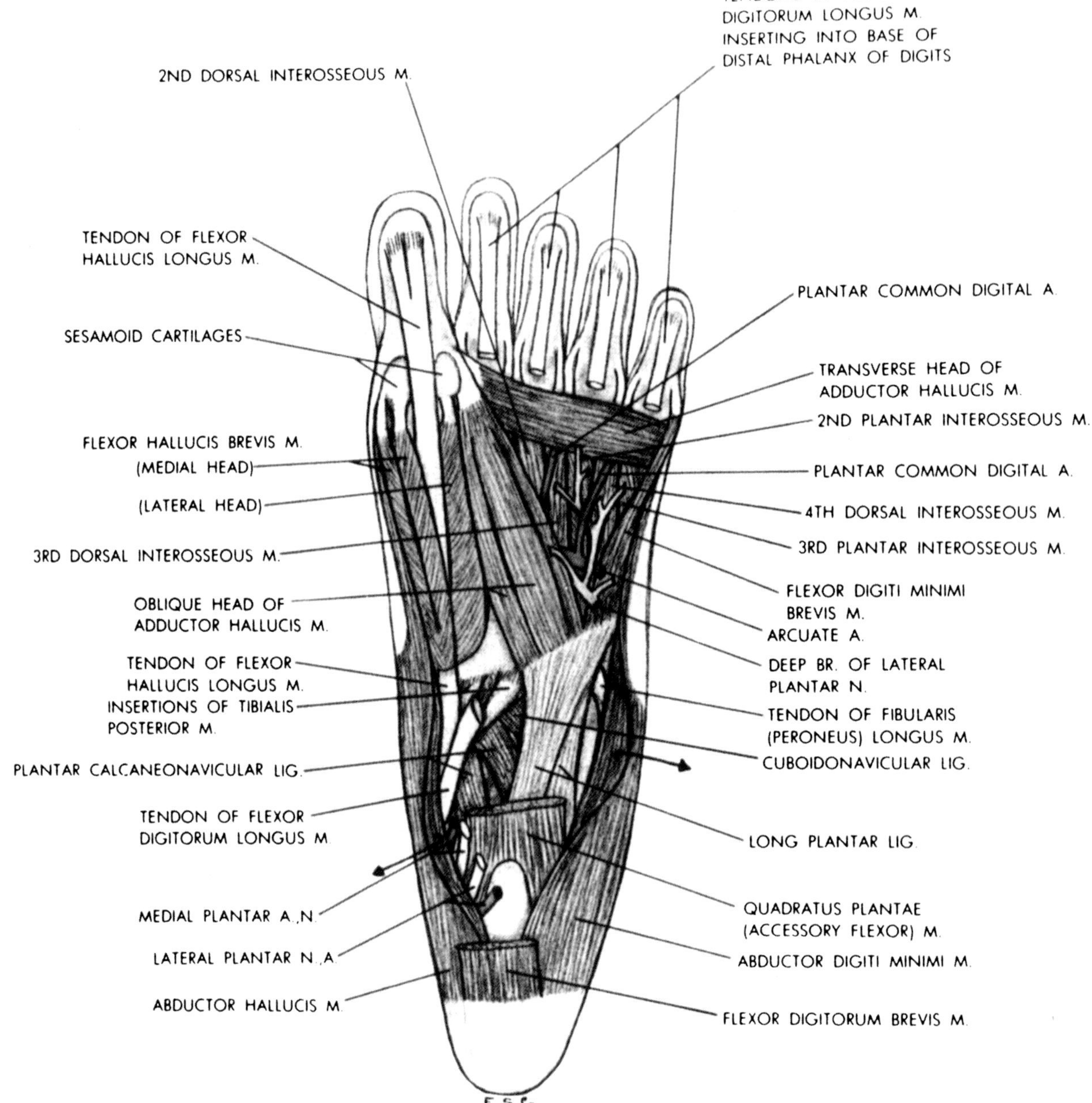

FIGURE 1-9 Third layer of plantar intrinsic muscles. (From Crelin ES. *Anatomy of the newborn: An atlas.* Philadelphia: Lea & Febiger, 1969;293, with permission.)

metatarsus and inserts into the fibular side of the base of proximal phalanx of the little toe. The latter two muscles are innervated by the lateral plantar nerve.

Fourth Layer

The fourth layer includes seven interossei divided into three plantar and four dorsal muscles and these occupy the interosseous spaces. They function to draw the digits toward the midline of the foot which is the midline of the second digit. The three plantar muscles lie in the lateral three interosseous spaces and arise from the medial side of the lateral three metatarsal bones. The dorsal interossei are bipennate and originate from the adjacent surfaces of the five metatarsi. The plantar interossei arise from a single bone which is a metatarsal with which it is associated. Each dorsal interossei arises from two metatarsals between which it lies. The interossei are arranged around the second digit as the midline. The plantar interossei therefore adduct the lateral three toes. They arise from the medial surface of the metatarsal and insert on the medial side of the base of the proximal phalanx of the same digit. The first two dorsal interossei attach on either side of the second toe while the third and fourth attach to the lateral side of their individual toes. All interossei are innervated by the lateral plantar nerve. Interossei are separated from the lumbrical muscles at the level of the metatarsal phalangeal joints by the deep transverse metatarsal ligament as they pass dorsal to these ligaments (Figure 1-10).

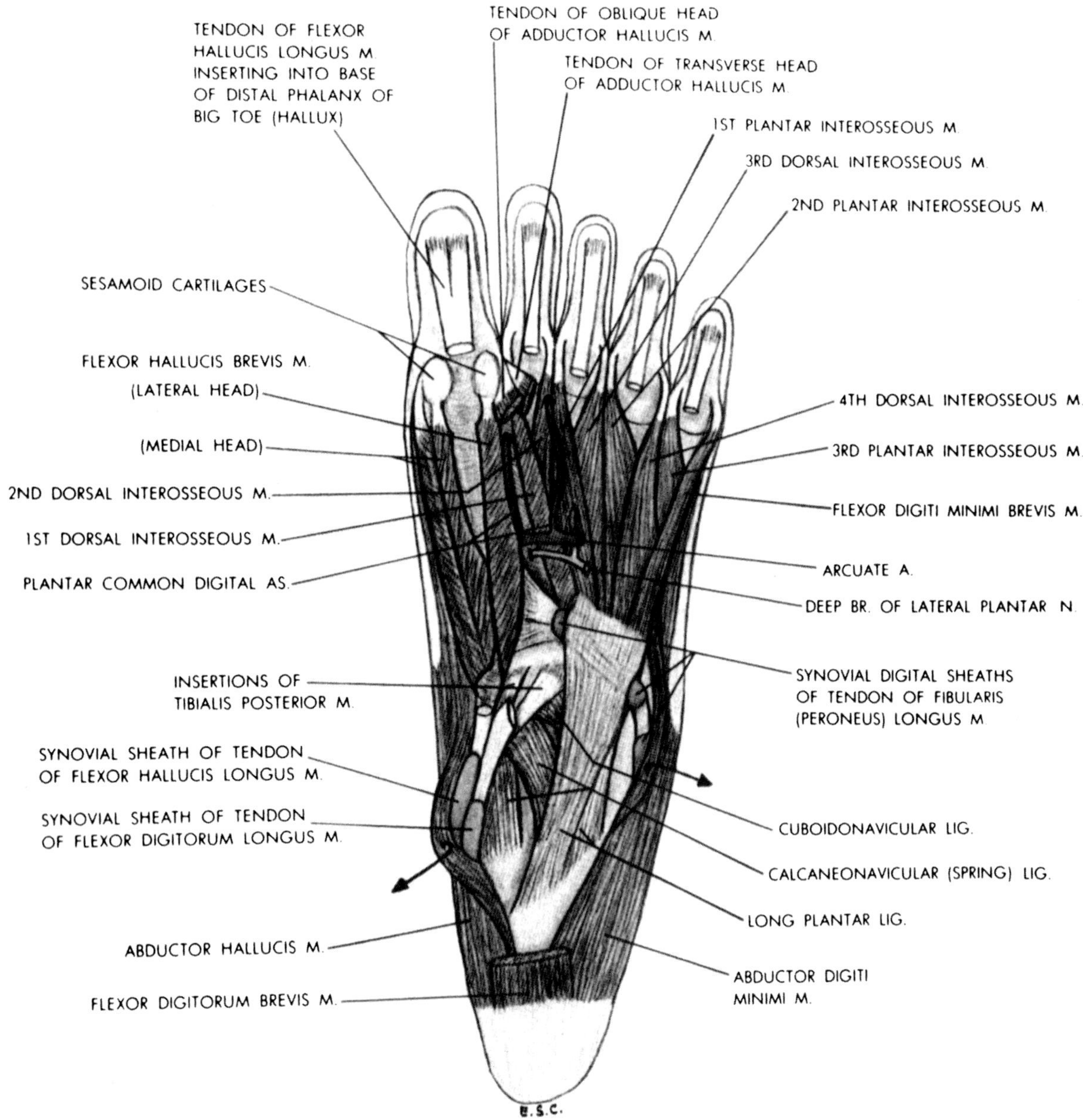

FIGURE 1-10 Fourth layer of plantar intrinsic muscles. (From Crelin ES. *Anatomy of the newborn: An atlas.* Philadelphia: Lea & Febiger, 1969;294, with permission.)

Vessels and Nerves

The posterior tibial artery and its accompanying venae comitantes divide into medial and lateral plantar vessels at the distal border of the flexor retkiaculum. The vessels enter the sole of the foot beneath the origin of the abductor hallucis and are accompanied by the medial and lateral plantar nerves. The medial plantar vessels and nerves course distally in the interval between the abductor hallucis and flexor digitorum brevis while the lateral structures diverge to pass deep to the flexor digitorum brevis. The smaller medial plantar artery supplies the muscles that surround it while its superficial branches supply the skin on the medial surface of the foot and give rise to the digital arteries. The lateral plantar artery is larger and crosses between the flexor digitorum brevis and the quadratus planti and then in the interval between the flexor digitorum brevis and abductor digiti minimi. At the base of the fifth metatarsal bone the lateral plantar artery abruptly turns medially toward the lateral side of the first metatarsus where it anastomoses with the dorsalis pedis artery to form the plantar arch. The plantar arch gives off four plantar metatarsal arteries that run forward on the interossei and develop collateral circulation with superficial branches of the medial and lateral plantar vessels. Bifurcation of the metatarsal arteries creates the common digital plantar arteries that then divide to form proper digital arteries. The plantar arch also gives off perforating branches that pass between the second, third, and fourth dorsal interossei to unite with the dorsal metatarsal arteries. The deep plantar branch of the dorsalis pedis passes between the heads of the first dorsal interosseous muscle and completes the medial plantar arch. This vessel may be very small in size.

The plantar digital veins drain into the metatarsal veins which form the plantar venous arch that supplies venous blood to the medial and lateral plantar veins that form the posterior tibial venae comitantes.

Slightly proximal to the flexor retinaculum, the posterior tibial nerve gives off a medial calcaneal branch to the medial and plantar surface of the heel. The tibial nerve then divides into the medial and lateral plantar nerves which enter the sole together beneath the tendon of origin of the abductor hallucis and in concert with the correspondingly named arteries (see Figure 1-9). The medial plantar nerve runs forward deep to the abductor hallucis in the company of the medial plantar artery. This nerve innervates the abductor hallucis and flexor digitorum brevis, and supplies the skin on the sole of the medial foot. It divides into four terminal plantar digital nerves which supply sensation to the medial three plantar surface toes and the first lumbrical. The lateral plantar nerves along with the lateral plantar artery pass between the flexor digitorum brevis and quadratus planti toward the base of the fifth metatarsal bone. This nerve innervates the quadratus planti and abductor digiti minimi, and ends by dividing at the base of the fifth metatarsal into a deep and superficial branch. The superficial branch innervates flexor digiti minimi and the third plantar and fourth dorsal interosseous before dividing into two digital branches applying sensation to the adjacent sides of the fourth and little toes. The deep branch runs medially with the lateral plantar artery and gives off muscular branches to both heads of the adductor hallucis as well as all the interossei not innervated by the superficial lateral plantar nerve.

JOINTS OF THE ANKLE AND FOOT

Talocrural Joint

The ankle joint has a hinge pattern and is formed by the trochlea tali and the lower ends of the tibia and fibula. Weight is transmitted from the distal surface of the tibia to the talus. The malleoli serve to secure the trochlea so that little lateral movement is possible. The narrower posterior part of the trochlea permits greater plantar flexion when it lies in the wider anterior part of the ankle joint. The tibia and fibula are approximated by the interosseous membrane and the anterior and posterior transverse tibiofibular ligaments as well as by the strong ligaments passing between the malleoli and the bones of the hindfoot. The medial (deltoid) ligament originates from the medial malleolus and fans out into several bands which are differentiated by their distal attachments (3). The tibionavicular, the tibiocalcaneal, and anterior and posterior tibiotalar bands unite the lower border of the medial malleolus to the specified bone. The anterior tibiotalar component is deep to the tibionavicular ligament. The tibiotalar bands are in a deeper plane than the other three and are commonly referred to as the deep deltoid ligament. The three bands of the lateral ligament of the ankle joint are distinct from each other and include the anterior and posterior talofibular and calcaneofibular ligaments. These bands fan out from their origin on the lateral malleolus. The anterior and posterior capsular ligaments are weak in order to permit a full range of dorsi- and plantarfiexion.

Joints of the Foot

The arches permit the foot to adapt itself to the ground in different positions and are capable of absorbing weight bearing. The arches are formed by the tarsal and metatarsal bones and are directed both longitudinally and transversely. The medial part of the longitudinal arch is higher than the lateral column. The posterior part of the calcaneus forms a common posterior cornerstone for both arches. This posterior pillar stabilizes the medial arch which is continued through the sustentaculum tali, the talar head, and the anterior component which is formed by the navicular, the three cuneiform bones, and medial three metatarsal bones. The lateral arch also begins with the tuber calcanei and passes forward through the body of the calcaneus, the cuboid, and the two lateral metatarsi. The body weight is transferred from the talus through the talocalcaneal joint to the lateral column and to the medial arch by the talocalcaneonavicular joint. The transverse arch can be located along the line of the tarsometatarsal joints and includes the anterior part of the tarsi and the posterior part of the metatarsi. Ligaments on the plantar concave side of these arches are strengthened to resist collapse of the arches. Preservation of the integrity of the arches ensures that the distribution of stress throughout the arch is strictly proportional to the relative heights of the various parts of the arch.

The tarsal joints include the talocalcaneal, the talocalcaneonavicular, the transverse tarsal, the calcaneocuboid, and the cuneonavicular joints. The talocalcaneal joint has a cylindrical shape with the talar facet being concave and the calcaneal convex. The capsular ligament is attached close to the articular surface circumferentially and is strengthened by the thicker portion termed the lateral and medial talocalcaneal ligaments. This joint is separated from the other portion of the subtalar joint by the tarsal canal which gives attachment to the posterior part of the capsule of the talocalcaneonavicular joint and the interosseous talocalcaneal ligament as well as the ligamentum cervicis, which is the strongest ligamentous attachment between the two bones (3). The functional subtalar joint allows inversion and eversion of the posterior part of the foot. The talocalcaneonavicular joint includes the convex talar head, the plantar surface of the talar neck that approximates the concave articular surface of the navicular, and the sustentaculum tali. This single synovial cavity includes the middle and anterior articular facets of the talus and calcaneus. There is an appreciable interval between the medial aspects of the navicular and calcaneus which is supported by the plantar calcaneonavicular ligament and to a lesser degree by the calcaneonavicular fibers of the bifurcated ligament. The plantar calcaneonavicular ligament supports the medial and inferior surfaces of the talar head and is attached behind to the sustentaculum tali and spreads out onto the plantar, medial, and superior surfaces of the navicular where it is joined by fibers from the deltoid ligament. The tendon of the tibialis posterior muscle passes into the sole beneath the ligament and acts as an additional sling. The calcaneonavicular part of the bifurcated ligament supports this complex joint on the lateral side. Its fibers arise from the anterior end of the calcaneus to the adjacent lateral surface of the navicular. The extensive ligamentous support to the talocalcaneonavicular socket limits its true capsule to weak posterior and dorsal components.

The calcaneocuboid joint is the highest point in the lateral longitudinal arch. The joint has additional plantar support from the plantar calcaneocuboid and the long and short plantar ligaments. The tendon of the peroneus longus also lends support to the joint as it passes beneath the cuboid. The calcaneocuboid ligament is a part of the bifurcated ligament. The short plantar ligament is attached to the calcaneocuboid joint and originates from the anterior-inferior surface of the calcaneus and attaches to the cuboid behind the ridge for the peroneal groove. The long plantar ligament is more superficial and arises from the entire plantar surface of the calcaneus and attaches by deep fibers to the cuboid while its more superficial fibers pass to the bases of the lateral three metatarsi.

Transverse Tarsal Joint

The irregular articular transverse plane formed by the talocalcaneonavicular and calcaneocuboid joints constitute the transverse talar joint. The cuneonavicular joint approximates the convex anterior surface of the navicular and the concave articular surfaces of the posterior aspects of the three cuneiform bones. The joint is surrounded by a capsular ligament and by weak dorsal cuneonavicular ligaments and more resolute plantar cuneonavicular ligaments. The transverse tarsal joint separates the forepart of the foot from the hindpart. This permits the forepart to move on the hindpart, in plantar and dorsiflexion, inversion and adduction, and eversion and abduction.

Tarsometatarsal Joints

The cuboid and three cuneiform bones articulate with the bases of the metatarsi. The first metatarsal bone articulates only with the anterior surface of the medial cuneiform bone, while the second metatarsi articulates in a socket with all three cuneiform bones. The fourth and fifth metatarsi articulate with the cuboid. The tarsometatarsal joint cavities are separated from each other by interosseous cuneometatarsal ligaments and short dorsal and plantar tarsometatarsal ligaments. The intermetatarsal joints are small synovial joints on the contiguous sides of the bases of the lateral four metatarsi. The bases are joined by the metatarsal interosseous ligaments. Usually, there is no joint cavity between the first and second metatarsi. The metatarsophalangeal joints include the convex metatarsal head and the cupped posterior end of the proximal phalanx. The capsule contains the thickened plantar ligament while its sides are reenforced by collateral ligaments. The plantar ligaments of the metatarsophalangeal joint of the big toe contain the two sesamoids of that joint. Plantar ligaments of all the metatarsophalangeal joints are connected by the deep transverse ligaments of the sole. The interphalangeal joints also have collateral and thickened plantar ligaments to strengthen their capsular attachments.

Movements of the Foot

Most of dorsifiexion and plantarflexion takes place at the talocrural joint while the subtalar and transverse tarsal joints allow eversion and inversion. Additionally, the forefoot can be flexed and extended on the hindfoot at the transverse tarsal joint.

The triceps surae is the dominant plantar flexor of the talocrural joint. Additional plantar flexors include long toe flexors, peroneus longus, peroneus brevis, and tibialis posterior. The principal dorsiflexors of the foot are the tibialis anterior and the extensor digitorum longus. The extensor hallucis longus is of secondary importance. The strongest inverters and adductors are the tibialis posterior and anterior; the triceps surae also inverts the hindfoot during plantar flexion. The extensor hallucis longus is a weak dorsiflexor during forefoot inversion. The peroneus longus and brevis function as everters and abductors. Dorsifiexion of the toes is accomplished by the long and short extensors of the toes. The long toe extensor is dependent on the lumbricals to stabilize the metatarsophalangeal joints or its action will be isolated to the hyperextension of the metatarsophalangeal joint and extension of the inteiphalangeal joints will not be accomplished (Figure 1-11). Flexion of the interphalangeal joints is the responsibility of the flexor digitorum longus and brevis and flexor hallucis longus with the extrinsic muscles acting strongly on the distal phalanges. The flexor digitorum brevis flexes the middle phalanges while flexion of the metatarsophalangeal joint is brought about by the intrinsic lumbricals and interossei.

STEM CELLS

Our understanding of skeletal biology has been greatly expanded by the increase of research in stem cells. These cells play a critical role in the development, tissue homeostasis, and regeneration of the musculoskeletal system. Stem cells are linked to growth via multiplication of cells rather than the enlargement of individual cells. They retain the capacity to self-renew as well as produce progeny that are more restricted in both mitotic potential and in the range of distinct types of differentiated cells to which they can give rise. The progeny have more than one differentiated phenotype and may be greatly expanded in an undifferentiated form (13).

The rate of production of new cells is at its highest during the periods of embryonic and fetal development (15). Once tissue differentiation begins, the proportion of cells engaged in proliferation declines. Neural progenerators replicate only in the embryo. The central nervous system lacks the progenitors to replace neurons lost to disease and trauma, and consequently, neural loss is irreversible.

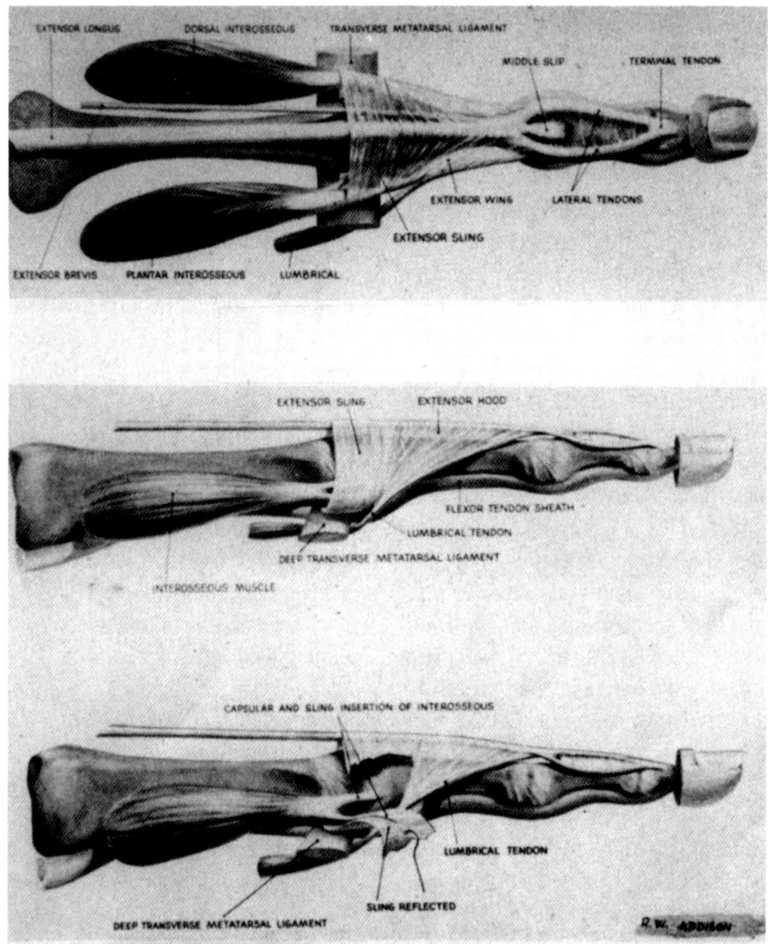

FIGURE 1-11 The lumbricals stabilize the metatarsophalangeal joint by their location on the plantar aspect of the metatarsophalangeal joint. They then join the extensor hood to act as accessory dorsiflexors of the interphalangeal joints. (From Pittinger MF, Marshak DR. *Mesenchymal stem cells of human adult bone marrow.* Cold Spring Harbor, NY: Cold Spring Harbor Laboratory Press, 2001; 40:349, with permission.)

Persistence of stems cells in the adult plays a major role in wound healing and is derived from the kinetics of normal tissue turnover. Stem cells are essential to the bone remodeling which occurs throughout life. The entire human skeleton is replaced every eight to ten years.

A promising research method uses human mesenchymal cells isolated from bone marrow and expanded *ex vivo.* These cells differentiate readily to multiple connective tissue lineages including osteoblasts, chondrocytes, myoblasts, tenoblasts, and adipocytes (16).

REFERENCES

1. Bardeen CR, Lewis WH. Development of the limbs, body-wall and back in man. *Anal 1901;1:1.*
2. Blais MM, Green WT, Anderson M. Lengths of the growing foot. *Bone Joint Surg* 1956;38A:998–1000.
3. Bohm M. Zur pathologie und rontgenologic des angeborenen klumpfusses. *Munchener Med Wehnschr 1928;75:1492.*
4. Crelin ES. The development of the human foot as a resume of its evolution. *Foot Ankle 1983;3:307–321.*
5. Hamilton W.
6. Hinchcliffe JR. Cell death in embryogenesis. In: Bowen ED, Locksin RA, eds. *Cell death in biology and pathology.* London: Chapman & Hall, 1981;35–78.
7. Hollingshead WH, Rosse C. *Textbook of anatomy, 4th ed.* Philadelphia: Harper & Row, 1985;438–456.
8. Hootnick DR, Levinson EM, Randall PS, Packard DS. Jr. Vascular dysgenesis associated with skeletal dysgenesis of the lower limb. *J Bone Joint Surg (Am) 1980;62:1123–1129.*
9. Kelly RW, Palmer GC. Regulation of mesenchymal cell growth during human limb morphogenesis through glycosaminoglycan adenylate cyclase interaction at the cell surface. *Ciba Found Symp* 1976;40:275–290.
10. Kelly RO, Fallon JF, Kelly RE. Jr. Vertebrate limb morphogenesis. In: Kalter H, ed. *Issues and reviews in teratology, vol* 2. New York: Plenum, 1984.
11. Kosher RA, Savage MP, Walker KH. A gradation of hyaluronate accumulation along the proximodistal axis of the embryonic chick limb bud. *J Embryol Exp Morphol 1981;63:85–98.*
12. Linsenmayer TF, Toole BP, Trelstad RL. Temporal and spatial transitions in collagen types during embryonic chick limb development. *Dev Biol* 1973;35:232–239.
13. Marshak DR, Gardner RL, Gottlieb D. *Stem cell biology.* Cold Springs Harbor Laboratory Press, Cold Spring Harbor, NY: 2001;40:1.

14. O'Rahilly R, Gardner E. The embryology of bone and joints. In: *Bone and joints*. International Academy of Pathology. Baltimore: Williams & Wilkins, 1976;1–16.
15. Park KS, Lee YS, Kang KS. In vitro neuronal and osteogene differentiation of mesenchymal stem cells from human umbilical cord blood. *J Vet Surg* 2006;7:343.
16. Pittinger MF Marshak DR. *Mesenchymal stem cells of human adult bone marrow*. Cold Spring Harbor Laboratory Press, Cold Spring Harbor, NY: 2001;40:349.
17. Rowe DA, Fallon KF. The proximodistal determination of skeletal parts in the developing chick leg. *JEmbryol Exp Morphol* 1982;68:1–7.
18. Rutz R, Haney C, Hauscbka S. Spatial analysis of limb bud myogenesis: a proximodistal gradient of muscle colony-forming cells in chick embryo leg buds. *Dev Biol* 1982;90: 399–411.
19. Sarafian SK, Toupouzin LIC. Anatomy and physiology of the extensor apparatus of the toes. *J Bone Joint Surg* 1969;51 A:669–679.
20. Sayeed SA, Khan FA, Turner NS, Kitakoa HB. Midfoot arthritis. *Am J Ortho* 2008;37:251.
21. Streeter GL. Development horizons in human embryos. A review of the histogenesis of cartilage and bone. *Contrib Embryol* 1949;33:149–167.
22. Summerbell D, Wolpert D. Cell density and cell division in the early morphogenesis of the chick wing. *Nature New Biology* 1972;239:24–26.

CHAPTER 2

Imaging of the Normal Foot

Leslie Grissom

INTRODUCTION

Imaging of the foot and ankle typically begins with anteroposterior (AP) and lateral radiographs. Other views including oblique, axial, Harris, sesamoid, Broder, and plantar flexion/dorsiflexion lateral views are added for specific indications. Ultrasound (US), computed tomography (CT), magnetic resonance imaging (MRI), and nuclear imaging are usually complementary but are increasingly used as the primary modality, particularly US and MRI for evaluation of masses, soft-tissue injury, and infection. To correctly diagnose imaging abnormalities, it is important to recognize the normal radiographic appearance and variants because normal developmental variants, accessory ossicles, and sesamoid bones around the foot and ankle can simulate pathology. It is also necessary to be familiar with the normal appearance of the foot and ankle in other modalities. In this chapter, the normal imaging findings, including normal development and normal variants, will be reviewed.

RADIOGRAPHY

Technique

Foot

Non–weight-bearing views are obtained for most indications; weight-bearing views are utilized for evaluation of alignment. Non–weight-bearing internal oblique views are added for improved visualization of the ankle mortise and the individual bones of the foot. The technical aspects are described in standard texts (1) and are summarized below.

Weight-bearing AP views of the feet are performed with 15 degrees angulation of the beam toward the heel to better visualize the hindfoot. The foot should be perpendicular to the tibia and not be pronated/supinated. The lateral view should be obtained with the ankle (not the foot) in the lateral position flexed 90 degrees. When weight bearing is not possible due to the age or medical condition of the patient, simulated weight-bearing views can be obtained by placing a paddle on the sole of the foot and flexing the foot 90 degrees with respect to the tibia, or by having the patient sit with the foot pressed on the table surface. It is important when using the paddle that the paddle be parallel to the beam and perpendicular to the x-ray cassette. Non–weight-bearing views should be performed with the ankle at least partially flexed for best visualization of the anatomy.

Oblique views of the foot are obtained with 45 degrees internal or external rotation; the metatarsals, calcaneonavicular joint, and tarsometatarsal joints are splayed out in the internal rotation view. This view is helpful for evaluation of fracture, calcaneonavicular coalition, and postoperative changes.

Axial views of the heel can be performed if calcaneal abnormality such as fracture or infection is suspected. Similar to the Harris view, this is obtained by angling anteriorly toward the plantar aspect of the foot with the foot in dorsiflexion. The angulation of the beam depends on whether or not the foot is dorsiflexed (25 degrees if dorsiflexed, 40 degrees if not). The Harris view is obtained with the patient standing and the beam angled downward anteriorly 35 and 45 degrees to visualize the talocalcaneal joint for possible talocalcaneal coalition. The normal medial and lateral facets are parallel; the medial facet is more superior than the lateral, and the joints are the same width. When there is foot deformity, the talocalcaneal joint may be excessively tilted or more horizontal than normal and not clearly demonstrated. CT or MRI can then be used for further evaluation. Another view used for visualization of the talocalcaneal joint (Broden view) is obtained without weight bearing, with the foot dorsiflexed and internally rotated 45 degrees and the beam angled 10–40 degrees.

Sesamoid views are performed on the tabletop by obtaining a view tangential to the metatarsophalangeal joints with the foot mildly plantar flexed and the toes dorsiflexed. The normal ossicles are smoothly corticated.

Plantar flexion and dorsiflexion lateral views are obtained for evaluation of movement and alignment between the hindfoot and the forefoot. These are most commonly used in pediatric patients to differentiate vertical talus from planovalgus deformity. In younger patients, these views are obtained by pressing on the dorsal or plantar aspect of the foot with a paddle, taking care to keep the foot in a lateral projection. In older patients, they can be performed with weight bearing. The talocalcaneal angle increases with dorsiflexion and decreases with plantar flexion. The talus is normally parallel to the metatarsals in plantar flexion (10).

A standard exam of the toes includes AP, lateral, and oblique views. The lateral view should be obtained with the digit in question separated from the others by pulling the remaining digits forward or back.

Ankle

The normal ankle views are AP, lateral, and oblique views. On the AP view, the tibia and fibula overlap, and the internal oblique view, obtained with 45 degrees internal rotation, separates the osseous structures. An additional mortise view is obtained with 15–20 degrees internal rotation. The talar dome should be square and congruous with the articular surfaces of the distal tibia and fibula. On the lateral view, the fibula projects over the posterior aspect of the tibia, and the rounded talar dome is seen.

Valgus and varus stress views of the ankles are obtained after inversion/eversion injury to demonstrate the integrity of the joint and its ligaments. Typically, both ankles are examined to compare the normal to the symptomatic side, and both rest and stress views are obtained. The views are performed in the AP position with a strap around the forefoot, everting and inverting the forefoot to determine if the ankle mortise is normally maintained. Normally, the ankle mortise does not widen more than 5 degrees, and it should be symmetric from side to side. A lateral stress view can also be done to assess tibio-talar instability (5).

NORMAL DEVELOPMENT

Development of the ossification centers and epiphyses of the foot and ankle usually follow an orderly sequence (Table 2-1). The ossification centers and epiphyses generally appear earlier and fuse earlier in girls than boys, and there are established ranges within each sex for each bone and its epiphysis. The metatarsals and phalanges ossify during early fetal development, and the talus and calcaneus ossify between 24 and 28 weeks' gestation. At 40 weeks' gestation, the talus, the calcaneus, the metatarsals, and usually the cuboid bone are seen. Sometimes the cuboid is not ossified at birth, but it should be present several months after birth, usually two months in girls and four months in boys. Most of the time all phalanges are present at birth, but some may be unossified. The bones of the mid-foot ossify later, the navicular last, between two and three years on average. None of the epiphyses of the foot or ankle are seen at birth (17).

At birth, the talus is normally plantar flexed and the calcaneus dorsiflexed. The talocalcaneal angle, measured by drawing lines through the mid-talus and the mid-calcaneus, is typically 25–50 degrees: higher in younger patients and lower in older children (7). Sometimes the osseous structures are small and the axis of the talus and calcaneus are difficult to determine, but as the child grows, the angle will become apparent. Normally, the talus will be parallel to the first metatarsal on the AP view and plantar flexed on the lateral view, parallel to the metatarsals, with the navicular bone (if ossified) seen between the two. On the AP view, the calcaneus should be parallel to the fourth metatarsal and dorsiflexed on the lateral view, forming the plantar arch. The plantar arch is measured on the lateral view by drawing lines along the longitudinal axis of the calcaneus or the inferior surface of the calcaneus and through the second or third metatarsal (3). Normally, this angle ranges from 150–175

TABLE 2-1

Age at Appearance of Selected Ossification Centers (Years–Months)

	Boys			*Girls*		
Centers	*5th*	*50th*	*95th*	*5th*	*50th*	*95th*
Cuboid	—	0 – 1	0 – 4	—	0 – 1	0 – 2
Lateral Cuneiform	0 – 1	0 – 6	1 – 7	—	0 – 3	1 – 3
Medial Cuneiform	0 – 11	2 – 2	3 – 9	0 – 6	1 – 5	2 – 10
1st Metatarsal	1 – 5	2 – 2	3 – 1	1 – 0	1 – 7	2 – 3
Middle Cuneiform	1 – 2	2 – 8	4 – 3	0 – 10	1 – 10	3 – 0
2nd Metatarsal	1 – 11	2 – 10	4 – 4	1 – 3	2 – 2	3 – 5
Navicular	1 – 1	3 – 0	5 – 5	0 – 9	1 – 11	3 – 7
3rd Metatarsal	2 – 4	3 – 6	5 – 0	1 – 5	2 – 6	3 – 8
4th Metatarsal	2 – 11	4 – 0	5 – 9	1 – 9	2 – 10	4 – 1
5th Metatarsal	3 – 1	4 – 4	6 – 4	2 – 1	3 – 3	4 – 11
Calcaneal apophysis	5 – 2	7 – 7	9 – 7	3 – 6	5 – 4	7 – 4

Adapted from Keats TE, Sistrom C, eds. *Atlas of Radiologic Mesasurement*, 7th ed. Elsevier: St. Louis, 2001;320–321, and Garn SM et al. *Med Radiogr Photog* 1967;43:45–66.

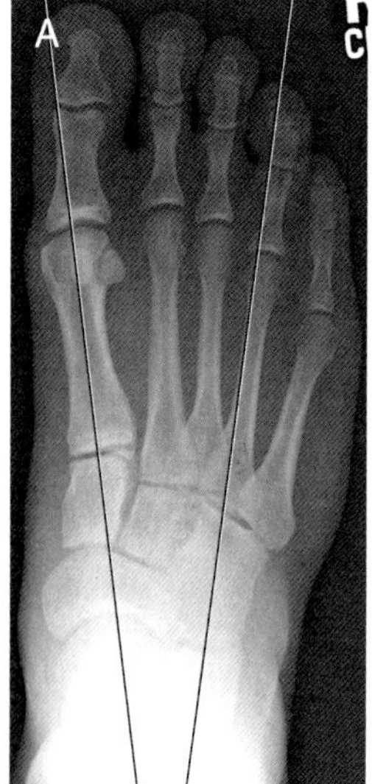

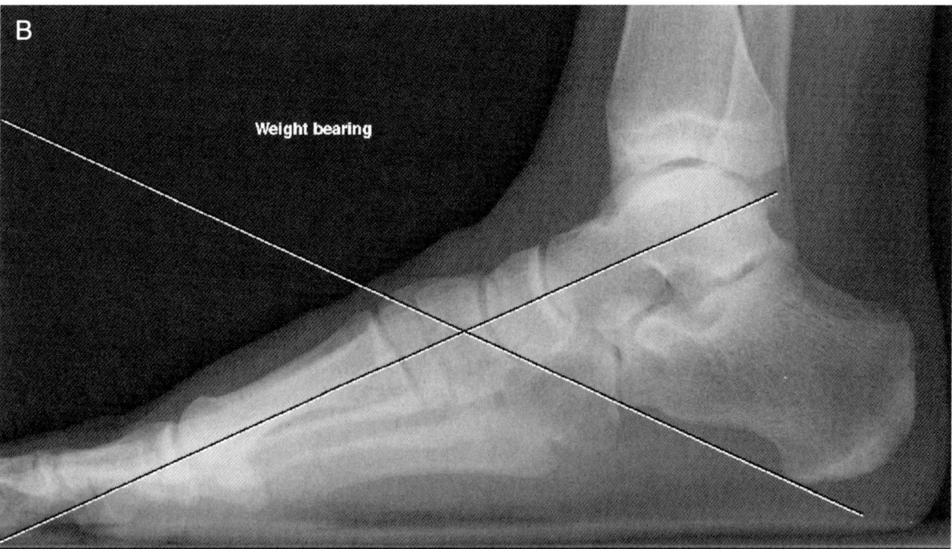

FIGURE 2-1 Normal weight-bearing views of the foot. **A.** Mid-talar line intersects the first metatarsal and calcaneal line passes through the base of the fourth metatarsal on the AP view. **B.** Mid-talar line is parallel to the metatarsals on the lateral view and with the calcaneal line forms the angle of the plantar arch on the lateral view.

degrees (Figure 2-1 A,B). At birth, there is often increased flexibility of the foot, and there may appear to be pes planus, which resolves as the child matures. On the AP view, the metatarsals are mildly splayed with overlapping of the bases, but there should be no more than 25 degrees angulation between the first and second metatarsals. On the lateral view, the metatarsals overlap distally. The digits are normally parallel to the corresponding metatarsals. The soft tissues of the foot and ankle consist of low-density subcutaneous tissue and higher-density deep soft tissue (muscles, fascia, and tendons). At the ankle, there is normally fat-density soft tissue anterior to the ankle joint and anterior to the Achilles tendon. Fluid in the ankle joint or in the retrocalcaneal bursa increases the density in these areas. Soft-tissue density along the posterior aspect of the distal tibia can be an accessory soleus muscle.

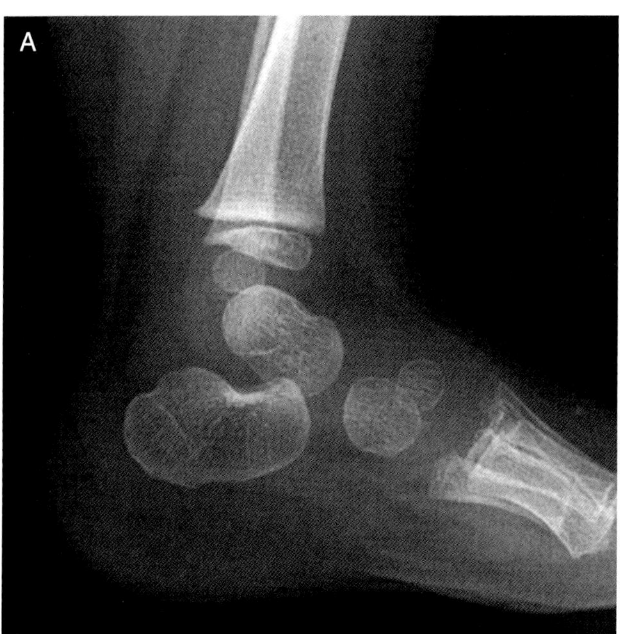

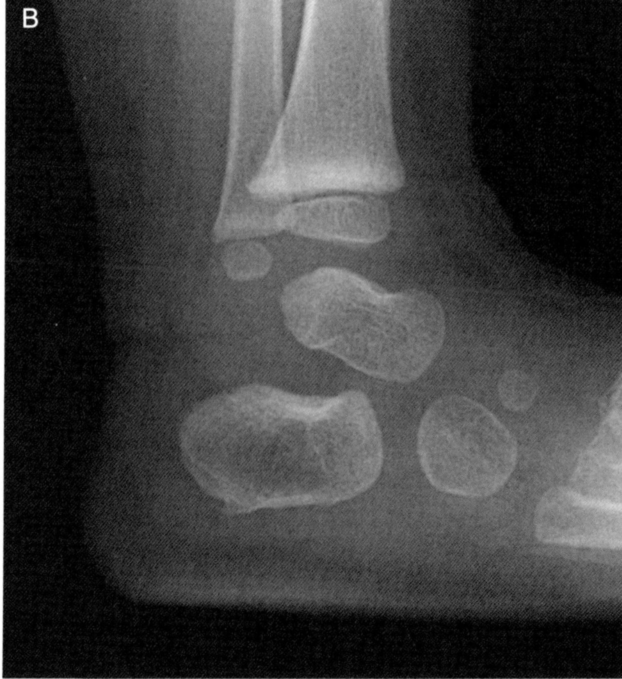

FIGURE 2-2 Lateral view of the foot. **A.** Line through the posterior calcaneus and mild contour deformity consistent with fusing calcaneal ossification centers. **B.** Small developmental spur on the plantar aspect of the calcaneus.

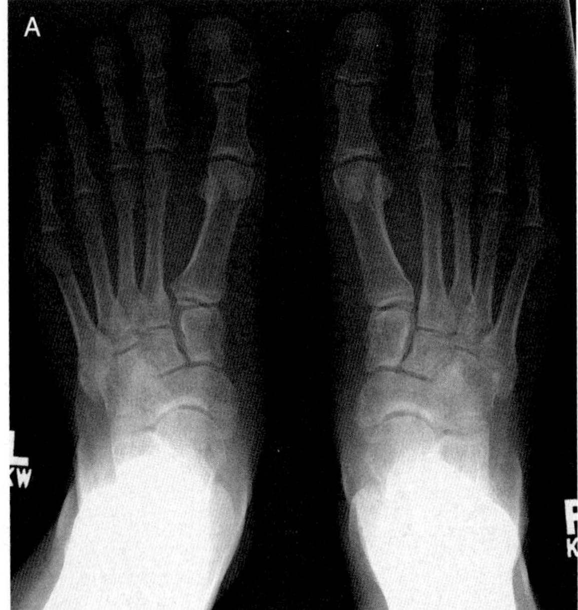

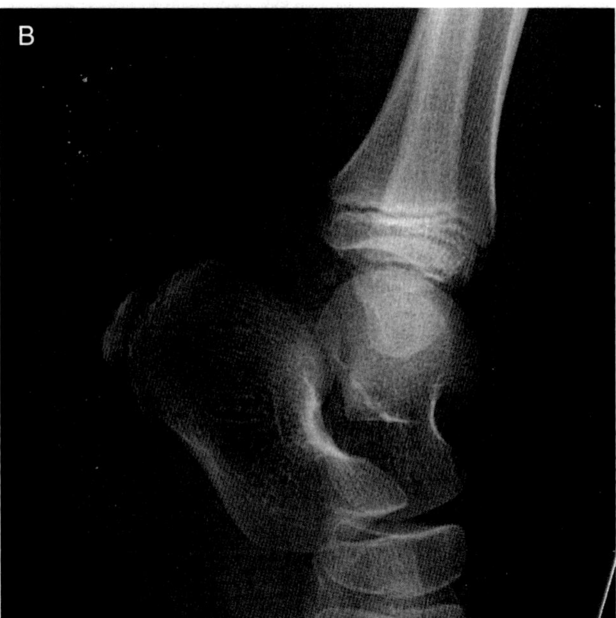

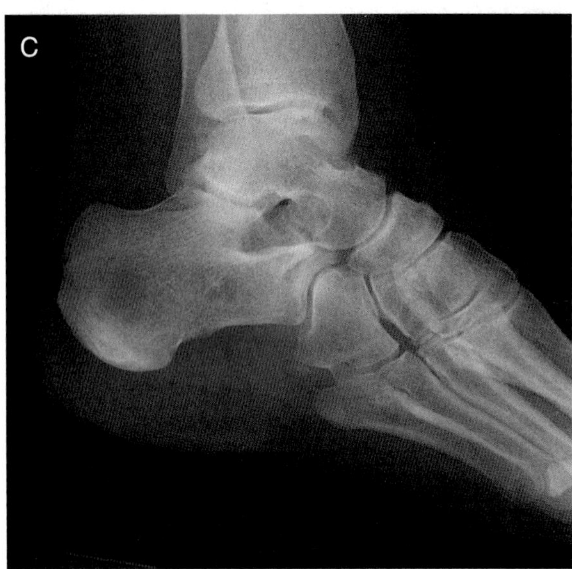

FIGURE 2-9 **A.** Bilateral os tibiale externum **B.** Os trigonum. Normal increased density of the calcaneal apophysis. **C.** Os perineum.

evaluated at some centers, focusing on the distance between the medial aspect of the navicular and the head of the talus, which is decreased in clubfoot when compared with normal (4).

Computed Axial Tomography (CT)

Computed axial tomography is often used for evaluation of fracture fragment alignment, post-traumatic physeal bar, coalition, infection, anomaly, and tumor (8,12). Axial cuts are obtained with dorsiflexion or plantar flexion, depending on the indication. Two-dimensional and three-dimensional reconstructed images can be produced and are valuable for assessing alignment and fragment displacement in alternate planes. CT scans can be performed on casted limbs; however, metallic hardware will cause streaking and limit the examination, particularly the reconstructions. Although the images may be degraded by metallic streak artifact, CT may be used to assess position of surgical hardware relative to joint spaces and fracture lines. The bony cortex is normally bright with fatty low-attenuation marrow. Increased density in the marrow is abnormal. Subcutaneous fat is also low in attenuation; muscles and tendons are brighter or higher in attenuation (Figure 2-12). The ability to differentiate between muscle, fluid, and tendons is limited with CT. Plantar tomography was used at one time, but CT has made it obsolete, and the equipment is no longer available.

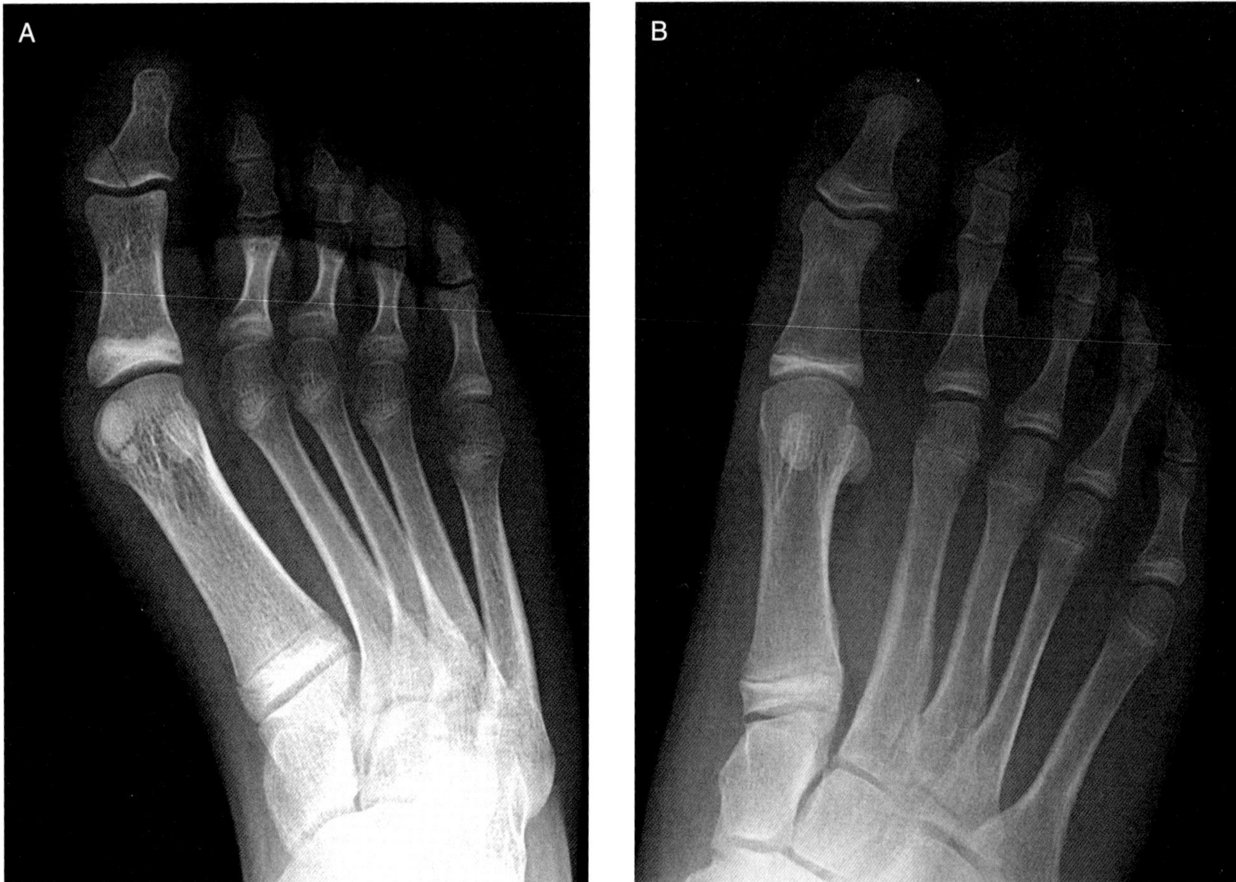

FIGURE 2-10 Two examples of variants of the sesamoids at the first metatarso-phalangeal joints.

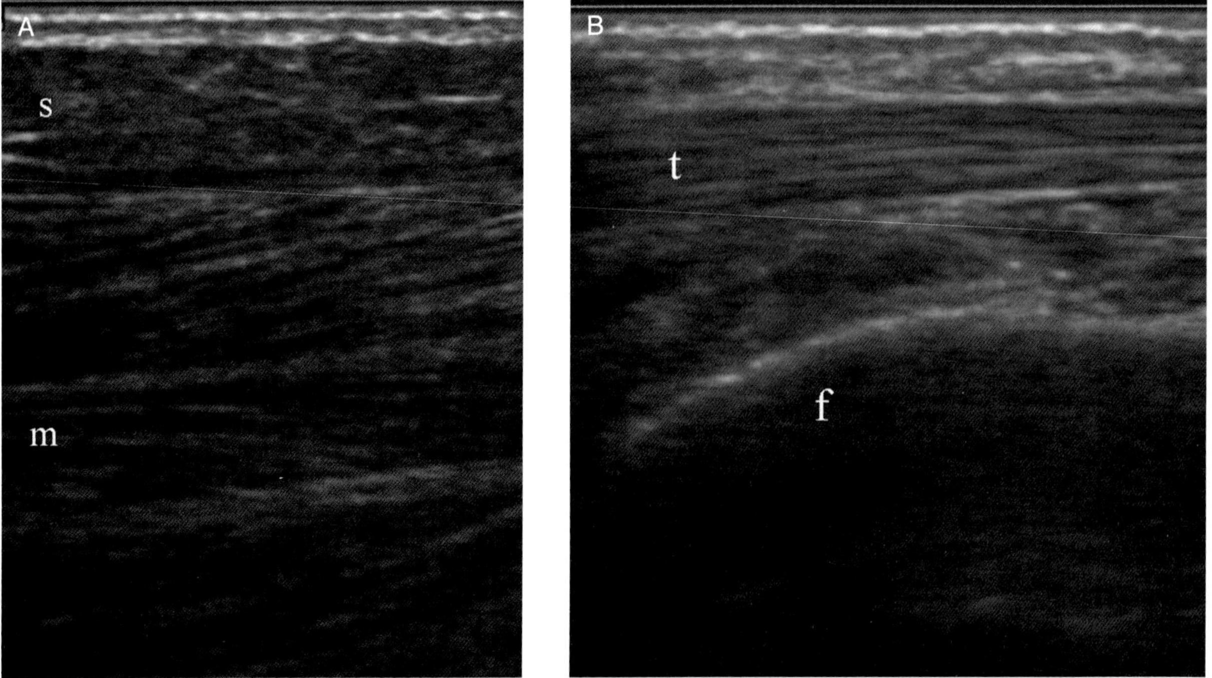

FIGURE 2-11 Ultrasound of the soft tissues. **A.** Normal muscle (*m*) and subcutaneous soft tissue (*s*). **B.** Peroneus longus tendon (*t*) overlying the fibula (*f*).

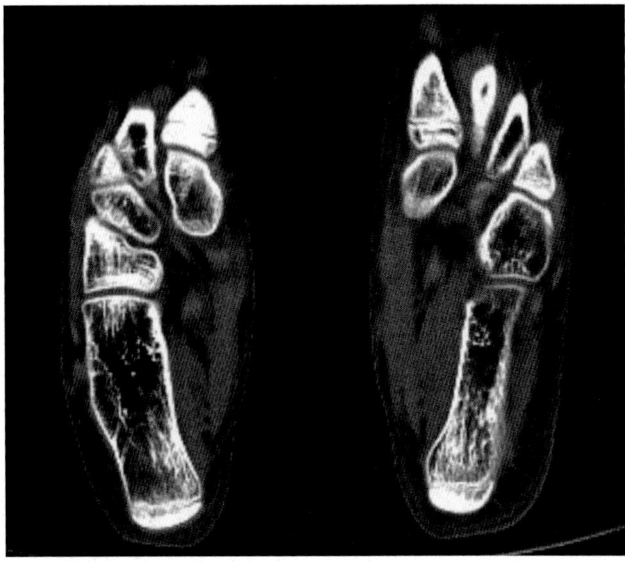

FIGURE 2-12 CT of the foot. Low-density fat in the subcutaneous tissues and the marrow, higher density muscles and tendons.

Magnetic Resonance Imaging (MRI)

Magnetic resonance imaging is increasingly used for evaluation of trauma, coalition, infection, masses, and internal derangement of the foot and ankle, and it is important to know the normal appearance. Because x-ray is relatively insensitive to early osteomyelitis and due to the exquisite sensitivity of MRI to edema in the marrow and soft tissues, MRI has increasingly become the primary modality in the diagnosis of infection and neoplasm. MRI also has the advantages of lack of ionizing radiation and direct multiplanar imaging. MRI is typically obtained in multiple planes and with multiple pulse sequences (13).

The technical aspects, including sequence parameters, coil selection, and field of view are complex and need to be optimized for the study to be useful. The most common sequences are T1 (fat bright), T2 (fat and fluid bright), and gradient echo (cartilage bright). STIR is a T2-weighted fat-suppressed image that is frequently used in musculoskeletal imaging because of the superior fat suppression although the resolution is not as good as on the T2-weighted images (Figure 2-13). Fat suppression is used on T2-weighted sequences to accentuate the fluid which is associated with most pathologic processes. Contrast (gadolinium chelate) will enhance many pathologic processes. When contrast is used, corresponding pre- and post- contrast T1-weighted images with fat suppression should be obtained in at least one plane to accurately assess enhancement.

The normal bone cortex is low in signal intensity on all sequences. The normal appearance of the marrow is variable in children due to the transition from hematopoetic marrow to fatty marrow (2). Frequently, the marrow signal in children is somewhat patchy and heterogeneous (15). The fatty soft tissues are hyperintense on the non–fat-suppressed images, and the tendons and muscles are relatively hypointense. It is essential to know the normal cross-sectional anatomy and its variations when interpreting MRI, and several texts are available for reference (11,18).

NUCLEAR MEDICINE

Bone scintigraphy has been used for many years for evaluation of infection, tumor, and trauma (16). A major advantage of the bone scan is that multiple areas of the body can be imaged during one test, so if the process is multifocal, all the abnormalities can be detected. Also, if there are no localizing signs, the bone scan can help define the pathology. Technetium-labeled phosphate agent is usually used. The tagged phosphate compound is adsorbed by hydroxyappatite crystals in bones. Typically, the entire body is scanned unless the symptoms are very focal. When scanning the feet, it is important to image both feet at the same time on each view obtained. This allows comparison of symptomatic and asymptomatic sides. Four-view imaging (anterior, posterior, medial-lateral and lateral-lateral) yields the most reliable results. Pathologic processes typically show increased uptake of tracer; they less often show decreased uptake. Areas in which there is increased bone turnover (e.g., the growth plates) will normally show more activity. This can be a limitation of bone scintigraphy in children as it may be difficult to distinguish normal activity from adjacent pathology. A bone scan of the feet where small bones and growth centers overlap often shows increased activity that is not pathological, making it difficult to distinguish normal from abnormal (Figure 2-14).

By performing a three-phase bone scan, soft tissue abnormalities can be separated from bone pathology. Three-phase imaging involves obtaining images of the

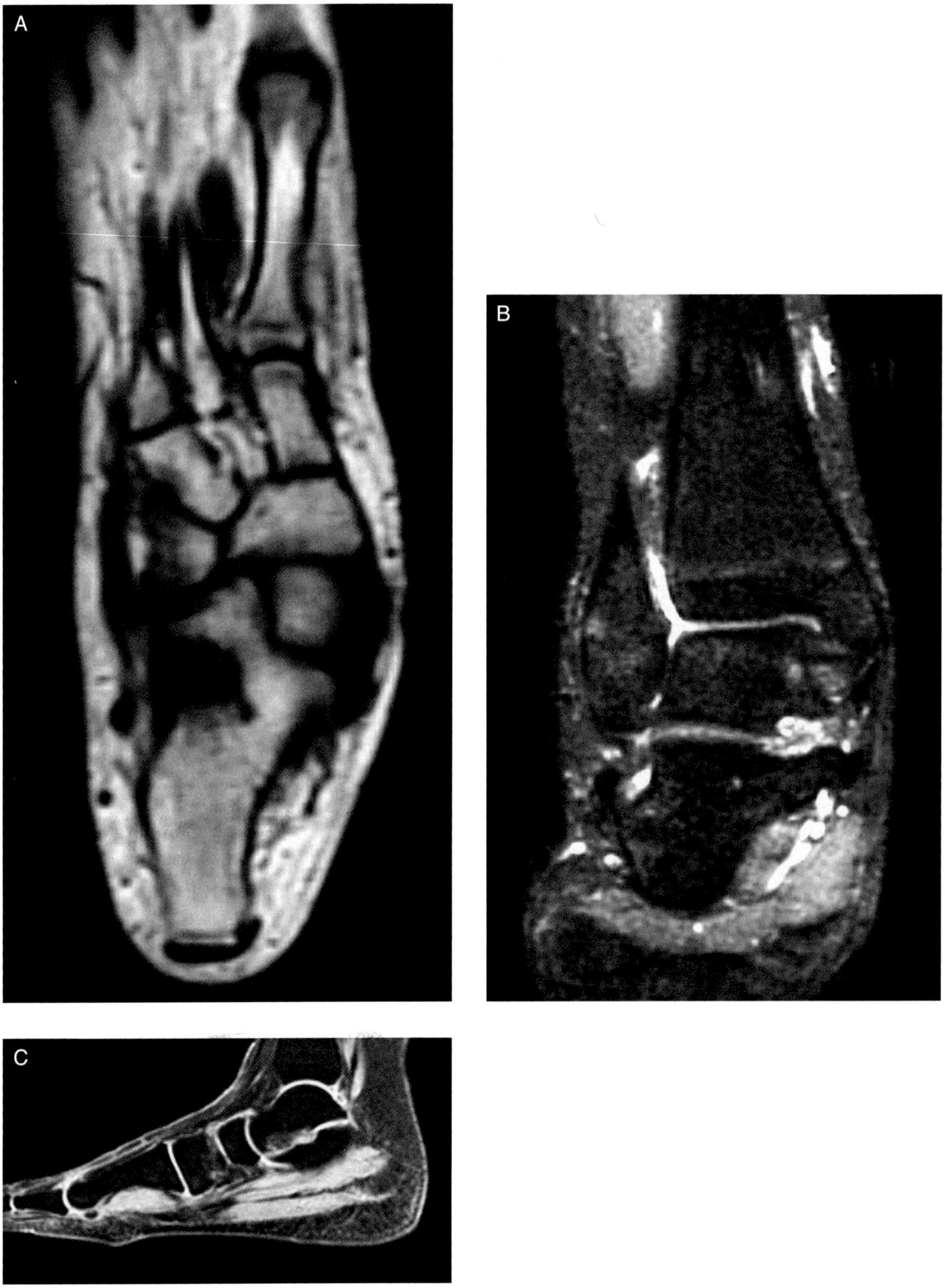

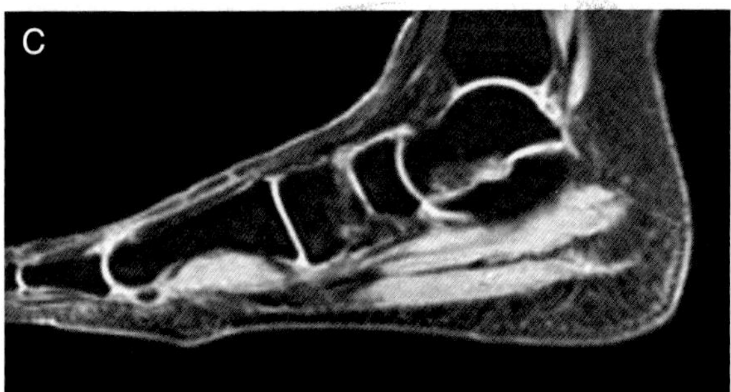

FIGURE 2-13 Normal MRI of the foot in an older child. **A**. T1: fat bright, marrow bright, muscles intermediate in signal. **B**. STIR: fat dark, vessels bright, muscles intermediate. **C**. Gradient echo fat suppressed: cartilage bright, fat dark, muscles bright.

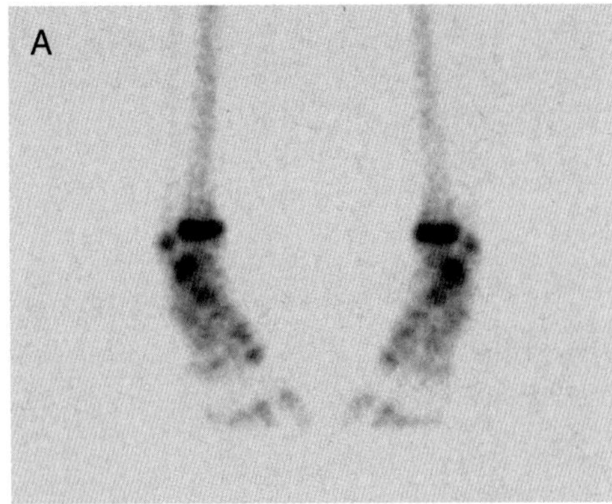

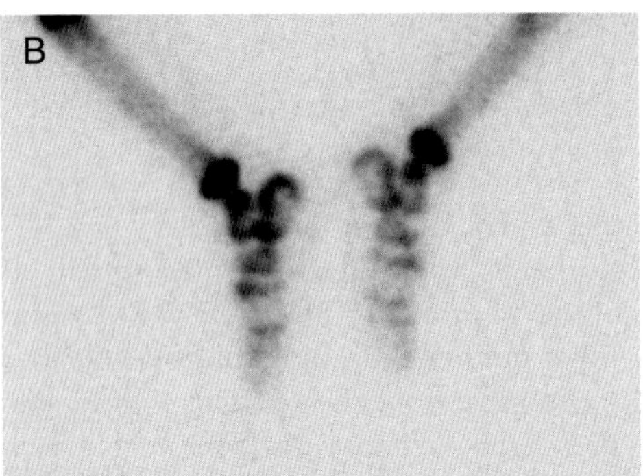

FIGURE 2-14 Bone scan. Delayed anteroposterior (**A**) and lateral (**B**) views show increased activity in the growth plates and multiple growth centers of the feet.

area of concern at the time of tracer injection, a few minutes after injection, and 1–2 hours post injection. Normally, the three-phase bone scan shows symmetric activity in all three phases: blood flow in the first phase, soft tissue and early bone activity in the second phase, and bone activity in the third phase. Other nuclear imaging, such as thallium, gallium, or positron emission tomography scans are not typically used for primary evaluation of the foot and ankle, but lower extremity images may be included on those scans if there is a need for information.

ARTHROGRAPHY

Arthrography is used in the foot and ankle for problem solving (e.g., to look for a loose body in osteochondritis dissecans or to look for post-traumatic incongruity of the joint space, epiphyseal exostoses, or coalition). The ankle and the joints of the hindfoot and mid-foot can be injected. In young children, the anterior subtalar joint may not communicate with the talonavicular joint, but in older patients, there is typically communication between the talocalcaneonavicular and the other tarsal joints. The posterior talocalcaneal joint is separate, divided by the tarsal sinus. Fluoroscopy is used to localize the tarsal or ankle joints for injection (10,13).

CONCLUSION

The normal imaging of the foot, including plain films, US, CT, MRI, nuclear medicine, and arthrography, has been reviewed. Again, it is important to recognize the normal appearance and normal variants to accurately diagnose abnormalities.

REFERENCES

1. Ballinger PW, Frank ED, eds. *Merrill's Atlas of Radiographic Positions and Radiologic Procedures.* St. Louis: Mosby, 2003.
2. Cohen MD, Edwards MK. *Magnetic Resonance Imaging of Children.* Philadelphia: B.C. Decker, 1990.
3. Davis LA, Hatt WS. Congenital abnormalities of the feet. *Radiology* 64:818, 1955.
4. Gigante C, Talente E, Turra S. Sonographic assesment of clubfoot. *J Clin Ultrasound* 32(5) 235–242, 2004.
5. Glasgow M, Jackson A, Jamieson A. Instability of the ankle after injury to the lateral ligament. *J Bone Joint Surg* 62B:196–200, 1980.
6. Keats TE, Anderson MW. *Atlas of Normal Roentgen Variants That May Simulate Disease, 7th ed.* St. Louis: Mosby, 2001.
7. Keats TE, Sistrom C. *Atlas of Radiologic Measurement, 7th ed.* St. Louis: Mosby 2001.
8. Lee JKT, Sagel SS, Stanley RJ, Heiken JP. *Computed Body Tomography with MRI Correlation, 4th ed.* Philadelphia: Lippincott-Raven, 2003.
9. Mandell GA. Nuclear medicine in pediatric orthopedics. *Semin Nucl Med* 28:95–115, 1998.
10. Ozonoff MB, ed. *Pediatric Orthopedic Radiology, 2nd ed.* Philadelphia: W.B. Saunders, 1992.
11. Pomeranz SJ. *MRI Total Body Atlas, Vol. III-Body.* Cincinnati: MRI-EFI Publications, 1996.
12. Resnick D. *Diagnosis of Bone and Joint Disorders, 4th ed.* Philadelphia: W.B. Saunders, 2002.
13. Resnick D, Kang HS, Pretterklieber ML: *Internal Derangements of Joints, Emphasis on MRI Imaging.* Philadelphia: W.B. Saunders, 2006.
14. Schmidt H, Freyschmidt J, Winter P, Kohler A, Zimmer EA. *Borderlands of the Normal and Early Pathologic Findings in Skeletal Radiography, 5th ed.* New York: Thieme, 1993.
15. Shabshin N. High-signal T2 changes of the bone marrow of the foot and ankle in children: red marrow or traumatic changes? *Pediatr Radiol* 36(7) 670–676, 2006.
16. Sirry A. The pseudo-cystic triangle in the normal os calcis. *Acta Radiol* 36(6): 516–520, 1951.
17. Standing S, ed. *Gray's Anatomy. The Anatomical Basis of Clinical Practice, 39th ed.* London: Elsevier, 2005.
18. Stoller DW. Magnetic Resonance Imaging in the Orthopaedics and Sports Medicine. Philadelphia: Lippincott-Raven, 1997.
19. van Holsbeeck MT, Introcaso JH, eds. *Musculoskeletal Ultrasound, 2nd ed.* St. Louis: Mosby, 2001.

CHAPTER 3

Bracing and Orthotics

Mark A. Holowka and Frederick J. White[1]

INTRODUCTION

An orthosis is defined as an external device that provides assistance, protection, support, substitution, and/or prevention of deformity to the musculoskeletal system via the application of biomechanical forces. The goals of management must be clearly defined and outlined in easily understandable terms when contemplating the provision of an orthosis for a particular patient. This should be accomplished by consensus when a multidisciplinary approach is practiced because the orthotic system will profoundly affect the rehabilitation efforts of all health care professionals working with the patient. The primary care team generally consists of the orthopedic surgeon or physiatrist, physical/occupational therapist, and orthotist.

The prescription is formulated to outline the parameters of the orthotic goals while giving the orthotist a document from which to work. The goals of orthotic management are:

1. To protect a joint or limb segment
2. To correct alignment in a flexible deformity
3. To substitute for functional loss
4. To enhance or promote function
5. To immobilize a segment of the body

It is imperative that the prescription be comprehensive, yet concise enough to provide the information critical to the design and implementation stages of orthotic construction (Figure 3-1).

The underlying diagnosis is the first critical piece of information necessary on the prescription form. While the diagnosis may not be all-inclusive, it does allow the orthotist to begin to categorize the patient in broad terms based on an understanding of natural history of the disease, prognosis, developmental implications, and empirical technical knowledge about the individual patient group.

The biomechanical considerations or goals should specifically address angular or biomechanical deformities, as well as other kinetic or kinematic deficits which will impact on orthotic design. The design of an orthosis will utilize one or more of the following functions: allow free motion, assist motion, resist motion, stop motion, hold motion, or lock motion. An example would be a patient with spastic diplegic cerebral palsy who demonstrates persistent dynamic knee flexion or crouch gait. Goals for the patient with spastic diplegia could include increased plantar flexion/knee extension coupling while resisting sagittal plane motion at ankle–foot complex and also controlling planovalgus deformity.

The prescription should describe the orthotic in as detailed a manner as possible, e.g., "bilateral polypropylene anterior floor reaction ankle foot orthotics (AFO) set at 90 degrees with full toe plates and carbon composite reinforcements at ankle mortise." It is obvious that such a comprehensive prescription can only be generated after a collaborative assessment by team members who have an established network of communication and an intimate knowledge of the patient in question.

Finally, it is extremely important for the health care team to look at the patient globally, assessing the entire musculoskeletal system and the surrounding support network. It is easy for the allied health professional to zero in and focus on the deformity or impairment and lose sight of how other parts of the body are affected by this impairment and vice versa. When the body is in contact with the ground there is a closed kinetic chain, meaning the application of an ankle-foot-orthosis (AFO) for example may have profound effects on the knee, hips, and back. In the pediatric world, it is also imperative that the health care team work with the social support network (family, social worker, school, etc.) to assess how orthotic intervention will affect the child. If the pediatric patient is unable to properly don or doff the device, the patient will require the assistance of the social support system. Another consideration is the changing needs and desires of the child. Just as the goals of the health care team for the child may change over time, the child's personal goals and desires will also change over time. For example, while cosmesis may not be very important to a three year old, it may be a very important aspect for a teenager.

[1] Deceased.

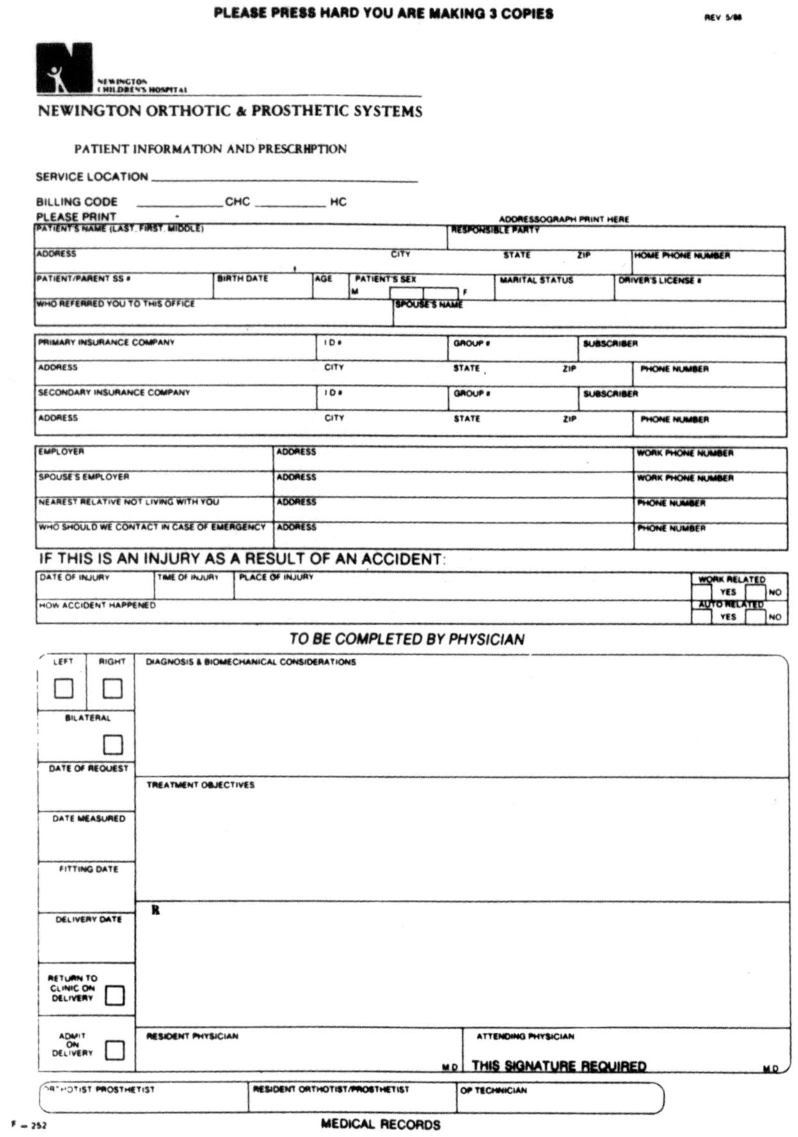

PLEASE PRESS HARD YOU ARE MAKING 3 COPIES

REV 5/96

NEWINGTON CHILDREN'S HOSPITAL

NEWINGTON ORTHOTIC & PROSTHETIC SYSTEMS

PATIENT INFORMATION AND PRESCRIPTION

SERVICE LOCATION ______

BILLING CODE ______ CHC ______ HC

PLEASE PRINT

ADDRESSOGRAPH PRINT HERE

PATIENT'S NAME (LAST, FIRST, MIDDLE) | RESPONSIBLE PARTY

ADDRESS | CITY | STATE | ZIP | HOME PHONE NUMBER

PATIENT/PARENT SS # | BIRTH DATE | AGE | PATIENT'S SEX M F | MARITAL STATUS | DRIVER'S LICENSE #

WHO REFERRED YOU TO THIS OFFICE | SPOUSE'S NAME

PRIMARY INSURANCE COMPANY | I D # | GROUP # | SUBSCRIBER

ADDRESS | CITY | STATE | ZIP | PHONE NUMBER

SECONDARY INSURANCE COMPANY | I D # | GROUP # | SUBSCRIBER

ADDRESS | CITY | STATE | ZIP | PHONE NUMBER

EMPLOYER | ADDRESS | WORK PHONE NUMBER

SPOUSE'S EMPLOYER | ADDRESS | WORK PHONE NUMBER

NEAREST RELATIVE NOT LIVING WITH YOU | ADDRESS | PHONE NUMBER

WHO SHOULD WE CONTACT IN CASE OF EMERGENCY | ADDRESS | PHONE NUMBER

IF THIS IS AN INJURY AS A RESULT OF AN ACCIDENT:

DATE OF INJURY | TIME OF INJURY | PLACE OF INJURY | WORK RELATED YES NO

HOW ACCIDENT HAPPENED | AUTO RELATED YES NO

TO BE COMPLETED BY PHYSICIAN

LEFT | RIGHT | DIAGNOSIS & BIOMECHANICAL CONSIDERATIONS

BILATERAL

DATE OF REQUEST | TREATMENT OBJECTIVES

DATE MEASURED

FITTING DATE

DELIVERY DATE | R

RETURN TO CLINIC ON DELIVERY

ADMIT ON DELIVERY | RESIDENT PHYSICIAN M.D. | ATTENDING PHYSICIAN THIS SIGNATURE REQUIRED M.D.

ORTHOTIST PROSTHETIST | RESIDENT ORTHOTIST/PROSTHETIST | OP TECHNICIAN

F – 252

MEDICAL RECORDS

FIGURE 3-1 Sample orthotic/prosthetic prescription outlining key areas of information.

The importance of an appropriate prescription is even more critical when patient care is fragmented between the various health care professionals. Very often a private orthotic facility is called on to service an outpatient clinic at a rehabilitation facility/hospital. This arrangement combined with outside physical and occupational therapists, and with orthopedic care provided by an in-house attending physician, can set the stage for poor communication, conflicting goals, and compromised patient care. Such eventualities can be precluded when distinct protocols are established and followed by the care team members regardless of their specific affiliations or base of operation.

MATERIALS

Throughout much of the 20th century, the orthotist relied heavily on the physical properties of metal and leather to solve most biomechanical problems. The widespread introduction of thermoplastics to the field of orthotics in the 1970s signaled the beginning of tremendous technological advances in brace design, versatility, and clinical application.

The most frequently used thermoplastics are crystalline polymers (polypropylene and polyethylene) which utilize a dense molecular packing. The tight molecular packing allows the crystalline polymer to remain stiffer and stronger until a given amount of heat is absorbed. The load-bearing capabilities of crystalline polymers can be increased by reinforcing them with fibers of glass or other materials. Another common type of thermoplastic used in the design of an orthosis is copolymer. Copolymer is formed from combining two different monomers in a polymerization reaction. The physical properties of the resultant copolymer will depend on the percentage and type of each monomer. The versatility and scope of thermoplastics bracing is now endless with the introduction of new polymer and copolymer plastics and the improvement of their application in the orthotic arena.

Thermoforming plastics enable the orthotist to achieve total contact, broad surface area control in a lightweight, aesthetically pleasing configuration. In

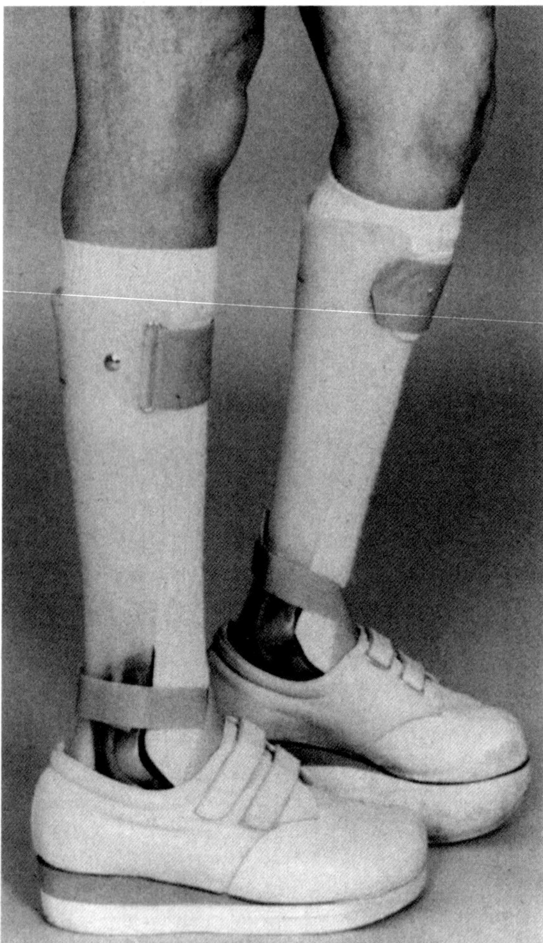

FIGURE 3-2 Polypropylene ankle foot orthosis with corrugations about the ankle mortise to increase the resistance against sagittal plane motion.

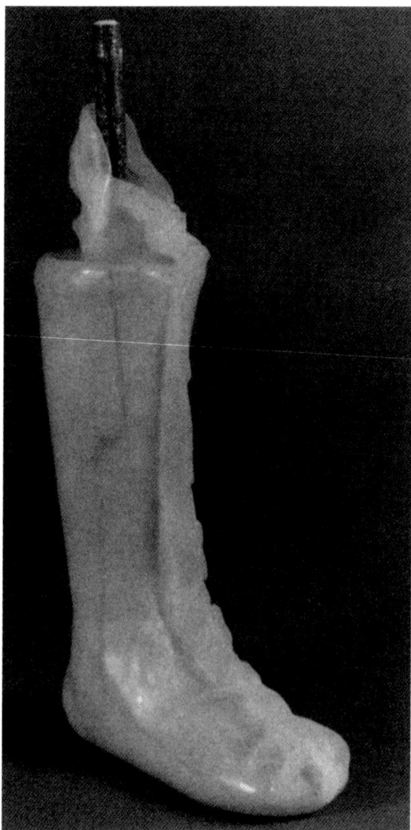

FIGURE 3-3 Modified plaster AFO model after vacuum forming. Plastic cut off and trimlines determined for final fitting on patient.

addition, the characteristics of strength, predictable deflection, and conformity under heat enable the provision of durable, infinitely adjustable, cost-effective devices whose strength or resistance to motion can be moderated by thickness, trimlines, reinforcements, articulating joints, or any combination of these (Figure 3-2).

Thermoplastic materials also have the advantage of being hypoallergenic, moisture- and bacteria-resistant, as well as sufficiently malleable to accommodate limited architectural changes of the extremity during the course of brace wear. This enables long-term utilization of a plastic orthosis with a very low incidence of fatigue, fracture, or material failure. In addition, the fact that the orthosis is fabricated from a negative model of the extremity and has been skillfully and accurately modified by the orthotist ensures a more accurate fit and accommodation for sensitive structures. The translucent nature of the vast majority of thermoplastics enables one to visualize key contact areas, observe inappropriate skin blanching, and ensure accurate donning and fitting techniques. These advantages are not inherent to a conventional metal orthosis attached to an orthopedic shoe. Strength and durability are unquestionably comparable to the conventional metal systems as long as thoughtful consideration is given to areas of stress, reinforcement, and fatigue. The broad application of biomechanical forces over a greater surface area physically and mathematically places the skin in less jeopardy following the equation:

$$\text{Pressure} = \frac{\text{Force}}{\text{Area}}$$

It has been our experience that the only true contraindications for the use of thermoplastics in orthotics are the presence of significant fluctuating edema in the limb or the inability of the skin to handle any pressure or shear. The presence of mild to moderate volume changes can be controlled by the adjunctive use of compressive vascular stockings, but in the presence of severe edema, the broad surface area coverage by the plastic orthosis makes consistent fitting precarious during a given day. Occasionally, a severe burn or scarring will make the skin extremely fragile and sensitive to pressure and shear and as a result can prevent the use of thermoplastics.

A consideration that is particularly relevant to the pediatric population is accommodating growth in the young child and elongating the effective lifespan of the brace. While the metal orthosis has a less intimate fit and can be constructed with overlapping uprights to facilitate incremental length changes (Figure 3-3), similar design considerations and adjustments can be incorporated into a plastic system.

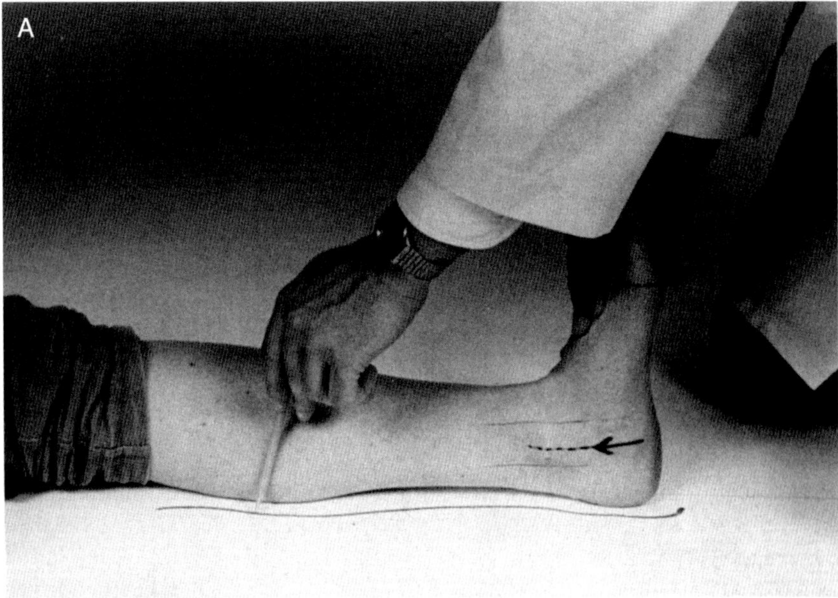

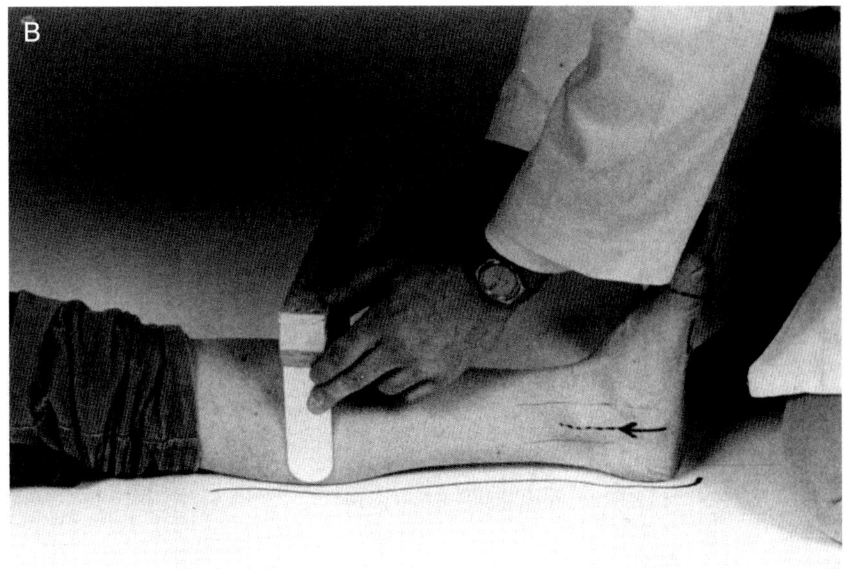

FIGURE 3-4 Typical delineation (*tracing*) of extremity to obtain outside shape (**A**) and dimension (**B**) prior to fabrication of conventional metal orthosis.

The inclusion of a foam liner which can be removed following growth, and the concomitant longitudinal shifting of joint attachment points can enable one to achieve the same accommodation for growth. It should be anticipated that a pediatric custom plastic orthosis will have a lifespan (in terms of fit) ranging between 10 and 18 months before necessitating replacement due to longitudinal or axial growth. This is not significantly different from the lifespan of a conventional metal orthosis, which in our experience will maintain fit between 12 and 20 months.

MEASUREMENT TECHNIQUES

Delineation

There are three fundamental methods for obtaining the necessary information to fabricate any orthosis. The traditional method used in the fabrication of a conventional metal orthosis is known as a tracing or delineation. This method involves generating a schematic outline along the periphery of the extremity in question as well as obtaining circumferential and medial-lateral dimensions at key points along the extremity (Figure 3-4A,B). The delineations are taken in a non–weight-bearing method with any desired alignment changes achieved in the frontal plane during the outlining process.

Following the initial tracing, the schematic is then modified to accommodate component sizes, padding, skin clearances, and joint clearances before fabrication is initiated in the laboratory. This process of delineation to obtain a blueprint for brace fabrication is two dimensional and achieves clinical success only after two or more fitting procedures at interim stages of fabrication. The conventional metal brace by virtue of its limited contact with the extremity lends itself well to this type of measurement technique (Figure 3-5).

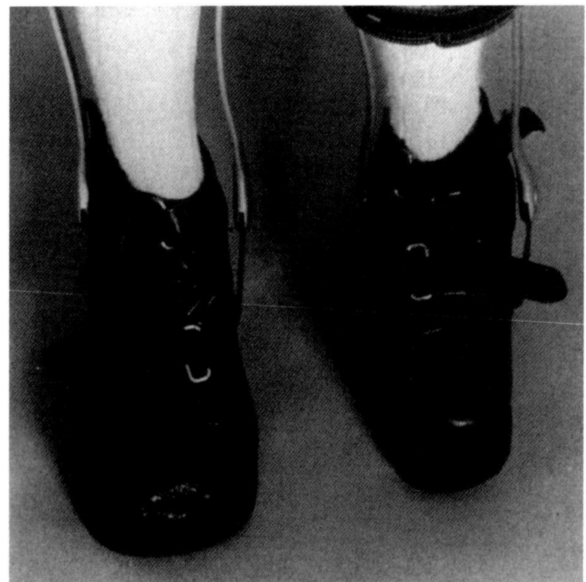

FIGURE 3-5 Relationship between metal uprights of conventional AFO and the extremity. Note the amount of clearance between the skin and the structural components.

Casting

Concurrent with the universal introduction of the thermoplastics to the field of orthotics was the introduction of plaster casting methodologies to obtain a positive model on which to fabricate the orthosis.

The process of obtaining an accurate negative plaster model of a body part is one of the most critical steps in ensuring successful application of a thermoplastic orthosis. The limb must be aligned in the desired position, avoiding undue distortion of the soft tissue or bony landmarks (Figure 3-6). It is generally desirable to take the mold in a partial or non–weight-bearing configuration, as full weight bearing during plaster curing lends itself to significant expression of the deformities that one is seeking to control (Figure 3-7). For example, when casting patients diagnosed with cerebral palsy or other neuromuscular diseases where high tone or muscle contractures may be present, non–weight-bearing positioning is essential to reduce the tone and place the extremity in a more suitable position.

After the negative plaster impression is removed from the patient, the negative model is filled to produce the positive plaster model. This model is then modified according to desired biomechanical goals. Plaster of Paris is strategically removed in areas where force is to be applied and conversely added where pressure-sensitive areas exist, such as bony prominences and superficial neural structures (Figure 3-8). This plaster modification process is critical to the eventual fit and function of any thermoplastic orthosis, as it determines all contact points, trimlines, and force application vectors on the extremity. The modified cast is then used as the positive model over which the heated plastic is vacuum formed in an effort to achieve intimate and accurate contouring around the subtle shapes and modifications inherent to the mold (see Figure 3-3).

Computer Aided Design

The third and most recent capture method patient information involves the use of computer aided design (CAD) and computer aided manufacturing (CAM). While CAD/CAM has been in use in a wide variety of industrial manufacturing, it wasn't until the late 1990s that it became a tool for the orthotist. CAD/CAM involves the use of a portable scanner which can capture a shape or image of the patient and send it to a computer. The orthotist then modifies the shape on the computer and then sends the image to a machine which will carve the shape out of a dense material. The shape will serve as the positive model which the orthotist will use to design the orthosis.

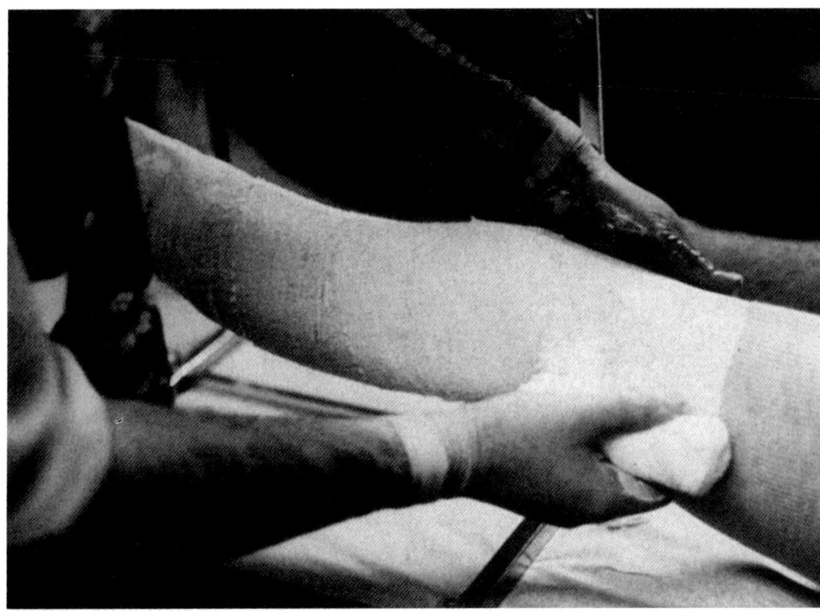

FIGURE 3-6 Typical application of plaster of Paris for negative impression of AFO.

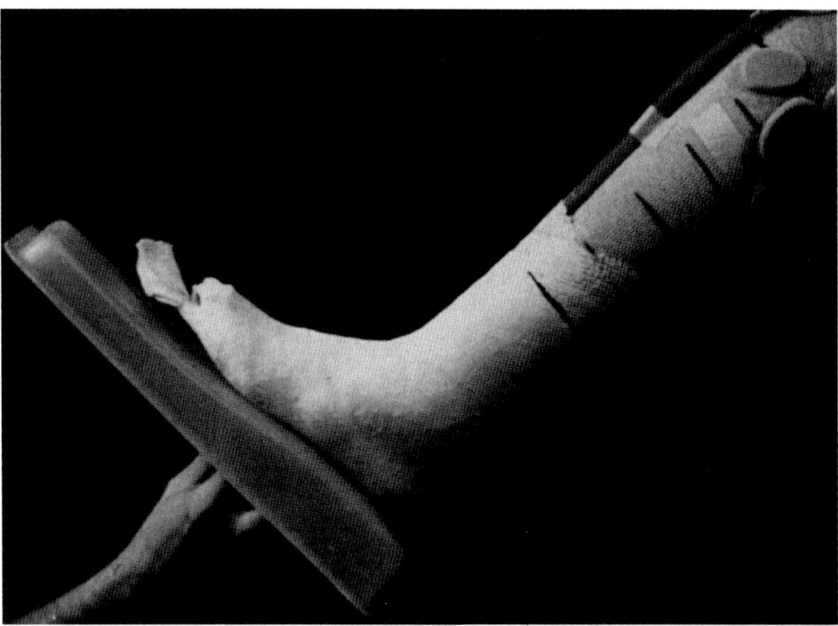

FIGURE 3-7 Non–weight-bearing mold with use of foot board for appropriate contouring of plantar surface.

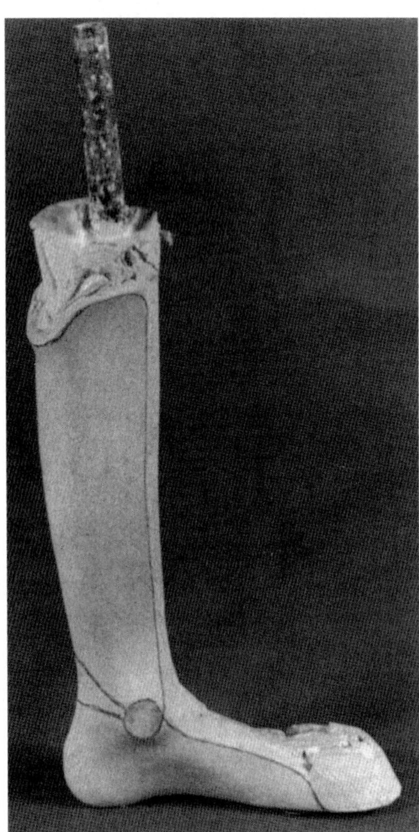

FIGURE 3-8 An example of a modified plaster model for fabrication of a plastic articulating AFO.

MANAGEMENT OF THE FOOT

The plantar surface of the foot as the primary weight-bearing structure represents a key area of consideration in all lower extremity orthotic management. Careful consideration must be given to supporting the medial longitudinal (ML) arch, the lateral longitudinal arch (LL), and the transverse metatarsal arch during the process of cast modification. It is important to reemphasize that the apex of support for the ML arch should fall directly under the sustentacular tali and not beneath the navicular or talar head which is often erroneously done. Support of the transverse metatarsal arch will ensure appropriate weight-bearing distribution between the metatarsal heads, thus reducing the incidence of callus formation and symptomatic weight bearing secondary to the development of metatarsalgia (Figure 3-9). The apex of the transverse metatarsal arch should be designed to fall behind the second metatarsal head with the deepest support point 15 mm posterior to a line connecting the apices of all the metatarsal heads.

In addition, any plantar surface abnormalities, such as prominent bony structures, callosities, or neuromas, must be addressed through the provision of proper relief, peripheral padding, or counterforce application. Regardless of the intricacy or scope of the brace design, a symptomatic or uncomfortable weight-bearing surface will preclude any possibility of successful orthotic application.

ARCH SUPPORTS

There are a myriad of arch support foot orthotic systems available on the market today ranging from generic, off-the-shelf forms to electrodynamically generated custom foot orthoses constructed from nylon-based plastic derivatives (Figure 3-10). Because of the constraints of this text, the general principles of foot management will be reviewed in lieu of discussing the relative merits of the various designs or materials.

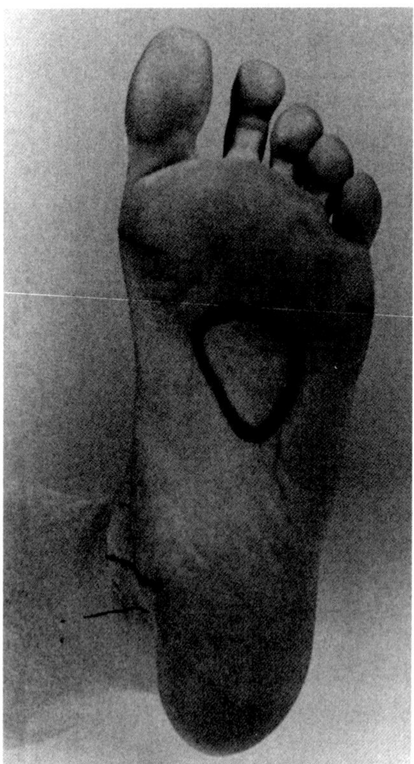

FIGURE 3-9 Placement of the transverse metatarsal arch support.

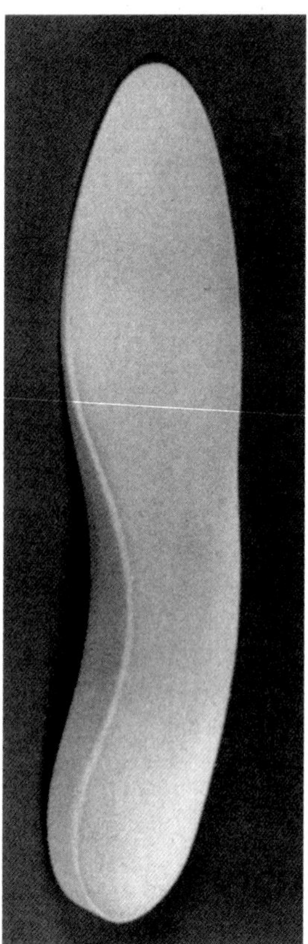

FIGURE 3-10 Sample arch support design to maintain the metatarsal longitudinal arch in weight bearing.

From an orthotic perspective, an arch support or foot orthosis is indicated when there is evidence of abnormal or poor foot biomechanics. The orthotist will select a corrective, semi-corrective, or accommodative foot orthosis according to the flexibility of the foot and condition of the skin. The direct application of forces to soft tissue is generally well tolerated, provided the foot mechanics relative to the bony structure are not significantly altered resulting in gross shifting of the center of gravity. This is particularly true in the case of the subtalar joint where a varus/valgus deformity can generate significant rotatory moments of deformity about the ankle mortise. In the event of such an occurrence, application of an arch support is inappropriate and will result only in the development of pressure areas where maximum control and support is attempted. Even the attempted use of wedging techniques in the arch support will prove inadequate in alleviating those symptoms that are secondary to profound subtalar malalignment.

In the pediatric population, dynamic subtalar instability can be managed very effectively through early intervention with a modified heel cup (Figure 3-11). This device is an inexpensive prefabricated plastic orthosis that grasps the calcaneus and through the use of strategic posting or wedging can provide biomechanical control of a varus or valgus deformity on weight bearing. It should be noted that the commercial heel cup is much more effective when used with the crepe wedge placed medially or laterally depending on deformity, as it extends the control lever arm, thus enhancing the ability to counter the deforming forces.

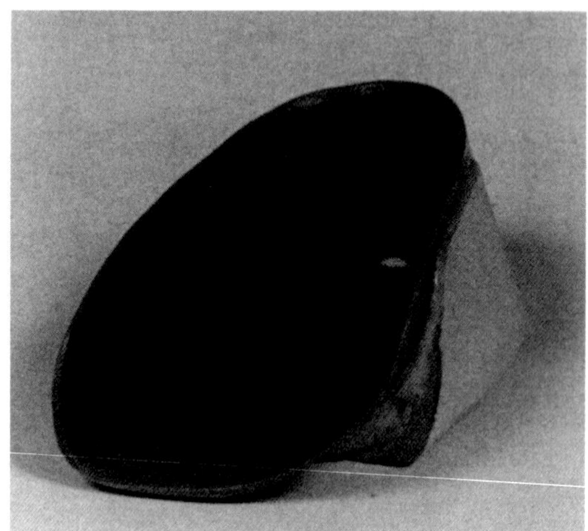

FIGURE 3-11 Commercial heel cup with five-eighths-inch crepe wedge adhered medially to extend biomechanical forces (varus producing) on weight bearing.

UCBL SHOE INSERT

The University of California Biomechanics Laboratory (UCBL) shoe insert was designed to correct flexible hindfoot deformities in patients who did not require sagittal motion control during stance (Figure 3-12). The orthosis was originally utilized in the treatment of pes planus in children. The UCBL insert applies correction to all three sections of the foot, rather than just to the calcaneus. Correction of the foot deformity with the use of the

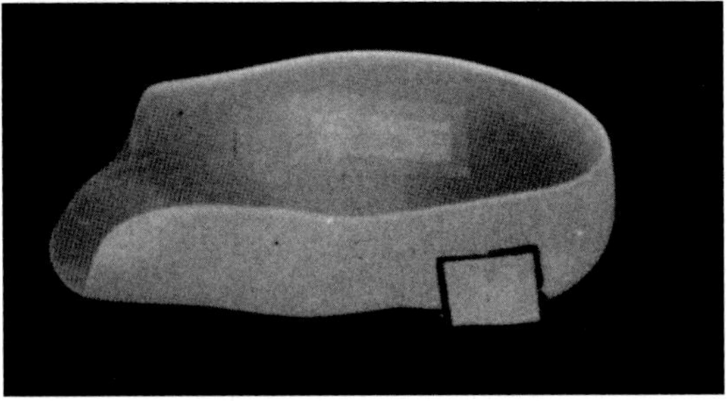

FIGURE 3-12 The University of California Biomechanical Laboratory (UCBL). UCBL with a Gillette modification used for medial weight-bearing stability.

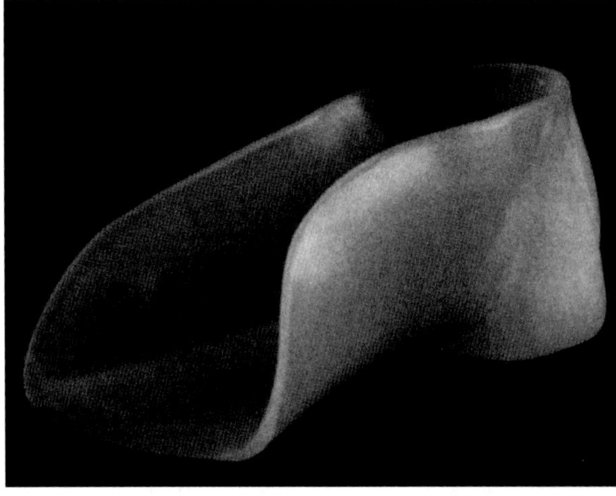

FIGURE 3-13 UCBL with Gillette modification for medial stability ground down to increase weight-bearing stability.

UCBL insert depends on one primary factor: the deformity must not be fixed and the foot must be sufficiently flexible to permit manipulation into the desired position of correction. An AFO should be recommended if increased three-point force is required to decrease the subtalar angulation. An AFO will increase the three-point force by providing a longer lever arm.

Casting for a UCBL is accomplished without a foot board. The forefoot is slightly adducted and the midfoot is maintained in subtalar neutral. Dorsiflexion of the metatarsophalangeal joints produces tension of the plantar fascia which elevates the longitudinal arch. The elevation is known as the windlass effect. This position helps create a close packed position of the tarsal bones and stability of the midfoot. As a result, this eliminates the need for muscle action of the foot intrinsics, mid-foot everters, and plantar flexors. The calcaneus is held in a perpendicular attitude and a varus or valgus corrective force may be fabricated into the orthosis. In most instances, a Gillette modification also is incorporated into the orthosis to increase the weight-bearing surface (Figure 3-13).

The trimlines of the UCBL are below the malleoli. The distal trimline for the footplate falls just proximal to the metatarsal heads unless the orthosis is correcting an additional flexible forefoot or metatarsus adductus. In this situation, the first metatarsal head is maintained within the trimline and lateral pressure is exerted to maintain the forefoot alignment. The UCBL is not indicated for fixed or rigid hindfoot deformities. The insert has proven less effective in patients with a tight or shortened tendo Achilles. Wedging the plantar aspect of the insert is not effective. The insert is contraindicated in the management of tarsal coalition.

ANKLE FOOT ORTHOSIS (AFO)

The ankle foot orthosis is the most widely prescribed lower extremity orthosis. Current design options include static or rigid ankle; semisolid ankle, motion assist, e.g., the posterior leaf spring (PLS) AFO; and the dynamic articulating or hinged form.

Taking the impression for the AFO is crucial. The foot and ankle must be positioned correctly during the casting process (see Figure 3-6). A foot board, equal in height to the plantar surface of the shoe the patient will wear, is used to duplicate the sole height and desired plantar flexion/dorsiflexion angle of the ankle. When the sole height is incorrectly measured, the patient will expend excessive, unnecessary kinetic energy because of abnormal flexion and extension moments produced at the knee. The correct degree of ankle dorsiflexion or plantar flexion provides adequate toe clearance during the swing phase of gait (Figure 3-14).

The AFO provides knee stability in the coronal and sagittal planes. Many patients requiring ankle stability also require sagittal plane stability at the knee. The correct ankle angle provides knee stability throughout the stance phase of gait and yet minimizes the knee flexion or extension moment at heel strike and throughout early stance phase. Knee stability during the latter part of the stance phase can be augmented by both the proper ankle angle and the trimline which modifies the length of the distal portion of the orthosis. The AFO functions as the biomechanical equivalent to an anterior and posterior pinstop, with a sole plate extending to the area of the metatarsal heads. The knee bending moment is modified during heel strike either by undercutting the heel of the shoe, or inserting a cushion wedge or a SACH (solid ankle cushion heel) to simulate controlled plantarflexion. The patient can change shoes when wearing the plastic AFO so long as the heel height and type of heel cushion material remain the same. When the heel height is changed, the biomechanical function of the orthosis is drastically altered (Figure 3-15).

The ankle trimlines are also crucial. The rigidity of the orthosis is affected by the malleolar location of trimlines. Alterations anterior to the malleoli increase brace rigidity, whereas cutting the trimlines posterior to the malleoli increase ankle flexibility (Figure 3-16). The location of the ankle trimline is dictated by the needs of the patient and includes the need for mediolateral stability and the desired sagittal plane motion during heel strike. Indications for the use of a solid ankle AFO with anterior trimlines include patients requiring a stabilizing mediolateral force or ankle joint immobilization. The solid ankle

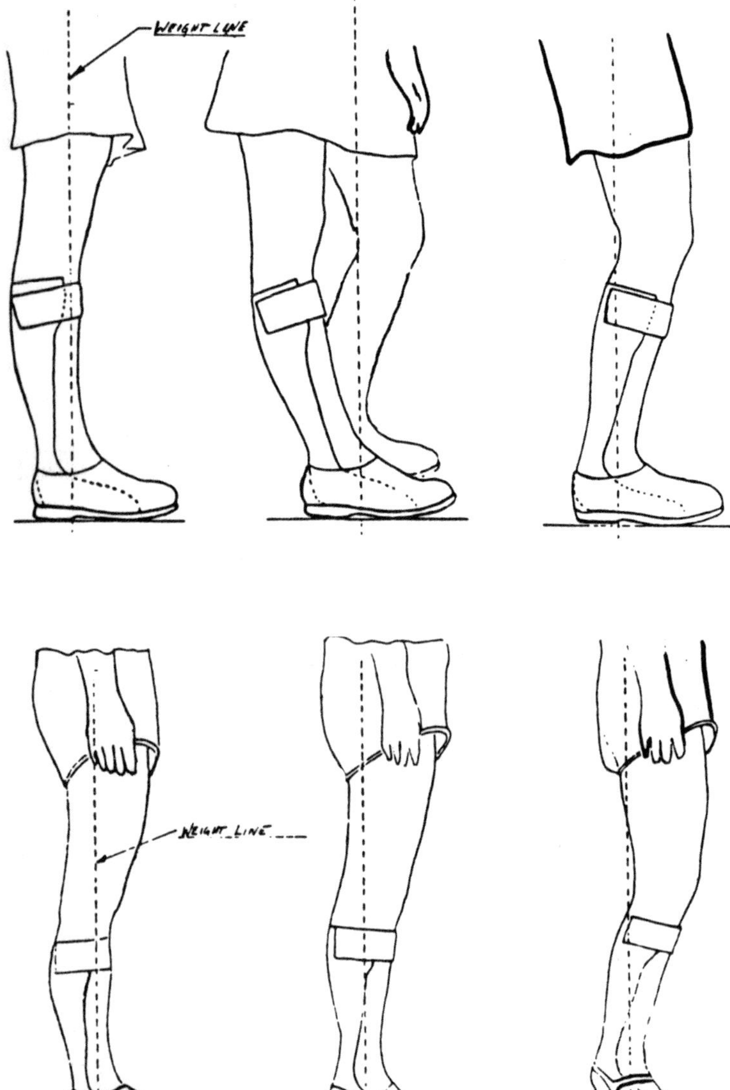

FIGURE 3-14 The effect of the forces exerted at the knee by the attitude of the ankle by an AFO.

FIGURE 3-15 The effect of a shoe heel height on the forces exerted at the knee by an AFO.

orthosis also may be indicated for patients who demonstrate mid-foot pronation and supination, flexible hindfoot calcaneovarus or valgus. Common clinical conditions requiring a solid ankle include patients with degenerative ankle arthritis, non-union of a hindfoot arthrodesis, distal tibial or fibular fractures, or when weight bearing on an unstable ankle is painful and restricted ankle motion is needed to permit comfortable ambulation.

The solid ankle AFO is frequently used as a nighttime orthosis. The AFO is utilized to maintain the ankle in a plantigrade position and is fabricated out of polyethylene or a non–weight-bearing material. Further modifications to the solid ankle AFO include the addition of aliplast or a foam interface and the trimlines are more anterior throughout the AFO (Figure 3-17).

The addition of carbon composite inserts and/or corrugations at the level of the ankle may be required as reinforcements to further restrict motion in the AFO. This type of modification must be vacuum formed into the AFO. An anterior calf shell may also be added to circumferentially restrict motion and assist in pain-free weight bearing (Figure 3-18).

Ankle trimlines may be cut back posteriorly to increase the ankle joint flexibility. The trimlines may bisect the malleoli when the patient requires less than rigid mediolateral stability. This trimline is most often indicated for a patient who does not evidence hindfoot varus or valgus or ankle mediolateral instability and who has controlled sagittal plane motion at the knee during stance. The semi-rigid ankle AFO may be indicated for patients with polio, closed head injury, cerebral palsy, or protection of mild ankle strains or sprains.

The orthosis will assist dorsiflexion at push off when the trimlines are posterior to the malleoli (posterior leaf spring orthosis trimline or PLS) (Figure 3-19A,B). The piano wire or single Klenzak brace serves as the metal counterpart for assistive dorsiflexion. This design reduces the extension moment at the knee at heel strike and requires

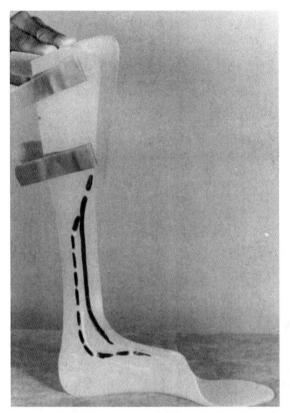

FIGURE 3-16 Variations in trimlines of an AFO. The solid line indicates semi-rigid ankle trimline and is bisecting the malleoli. The posterior leaf spring (PLS) is indicated by the dotted line. Note the trimline is posterior to the malleoli.

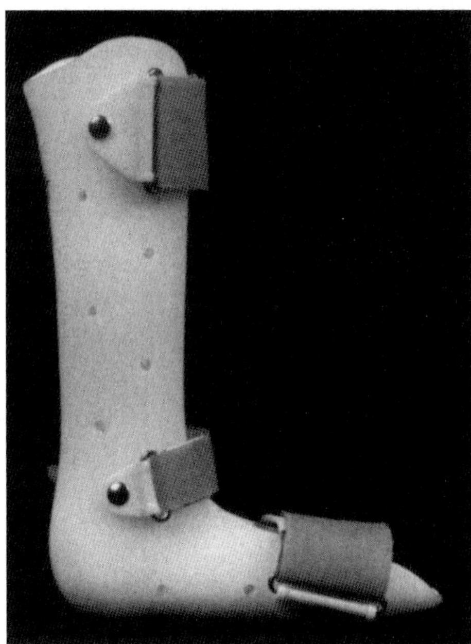

FIGURE 3-17 Solid ankle AFO nightsplint. Internal padding of soft foam and anterior trimlines for increased total contact.

corrugations posteriorly in the adult population to increase the durability of the plastic (Figure 3-20). Depending on the thickness of the plastic and the trimline, this orthosis allows the foot to move into limited plantar flexion and assists dorsiflexion in early swing phase.

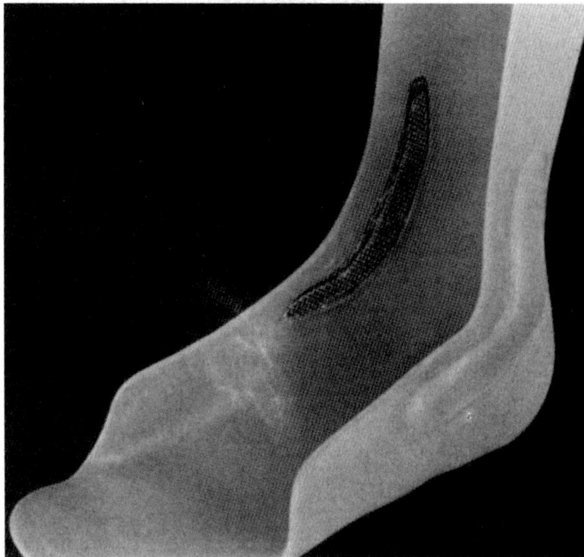

FIGURE 3-18 Solid ankle AFO with bilateral carbon fiber inserts for increased AFO rigidity and durability.

The mold can incorporate 5 to 7 degrees of ankle dorsiflexion to further increase the range of dorsiflexion and aid in knee flexion moment at heel off. However, this particular design has limited effectiveness in simulating push off and is not indicated for patients who lack knee sagittal plane stability in stance. A cerebral palsy patient with mild spasticity and minor knee recurvatum can benefit from this design of orthosis. Good quadriceps strength is required because of the limited knee extension moment. Patients with Charcot-Marie-Tooth and peroneal nerve palsy both benefit from this type of bracing.

SPECIAL MODIFICATIONS IN THE DESIGN OF AFOS

The previous discussion of trimlines emphasized ankle stability in the frontal and sagittal planes. The patient may also require additional support to control flexible hindfoot varus or valgus as well as displacement of the subtalar joint during weight bearing. A dynamic varus or valgus may necessitate either external posting of the AFO or utilization of a varus or valgus producing window at the level of the distal calf in order to prevent malleolar skin breakdown during weight bearing.

The Sabolich trimline can be used on either the lateral or medial aspect of the tibia midway between the knee center and the malleoli (Figure 3-21). This trimline incorporates a three-point pressure system to stabilize the tibia and prevents lateral or medial displacement of the subtalar joint. The length of the flange required to hold the tibia anteromedially or anterolaterally is determined by the size of the patient, the length of the tibia, and the amount of corrective force tolerated before skin embarrassment occurs. The longer flange or Sabolich trimline more evenly distributes the pressure required for correction. The orthotist may also need to modify the positive mold at the calcaneus and the

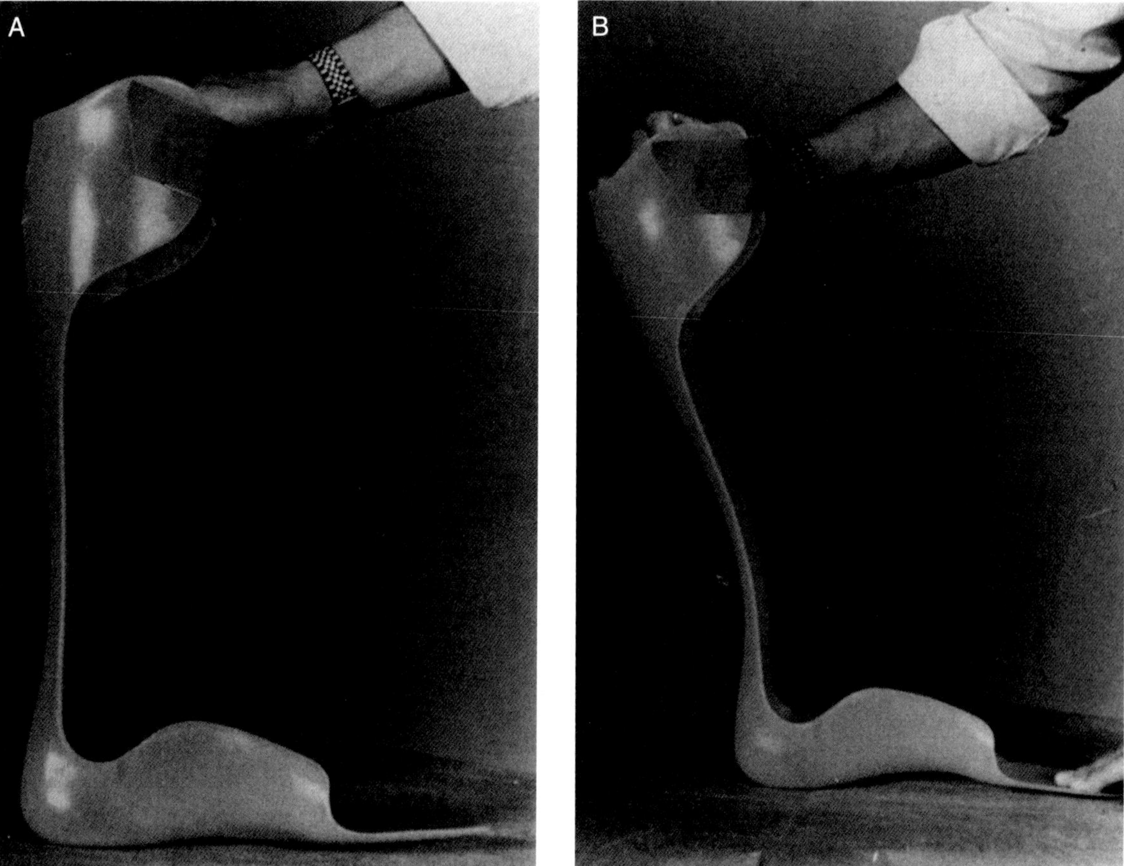

FIGURE 3-19 Posterior trimlines (**A**) and demonstration of flexibility (**B**) in a posterior leaf spring AFO.

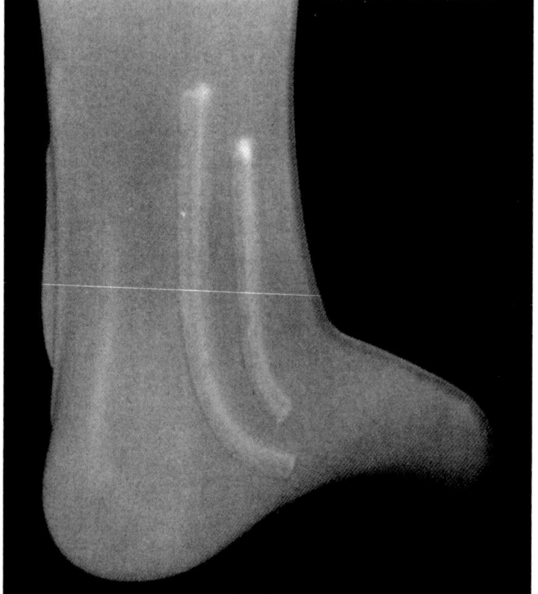

FIGURE 3-20 Ankle foot orthosis with bilateral corrugations for increased rigidity of the AFO. Increases the plastic durability to accommodate the posterior leaf spring (PLS) trimline.

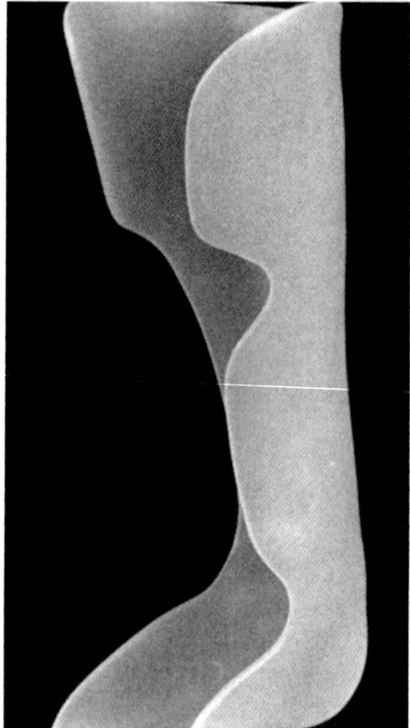

FIGURE 3-21 Solid ankle AFO with a lateral Sabolich trimline.

upper calf to create a three-point pressure system to maintain correction during stance. As an example, when a patient demonstrates a flexible hindfoot valgus deformity during midstance, the three-point pressure prescription would include: modification of the lateral aspect of the heel to push the calcaneus medially, the Sabolich trimline along the anteromedial aspect of the tibia, and the lateral aspect of the proximal calf. The trimline would incorporate a

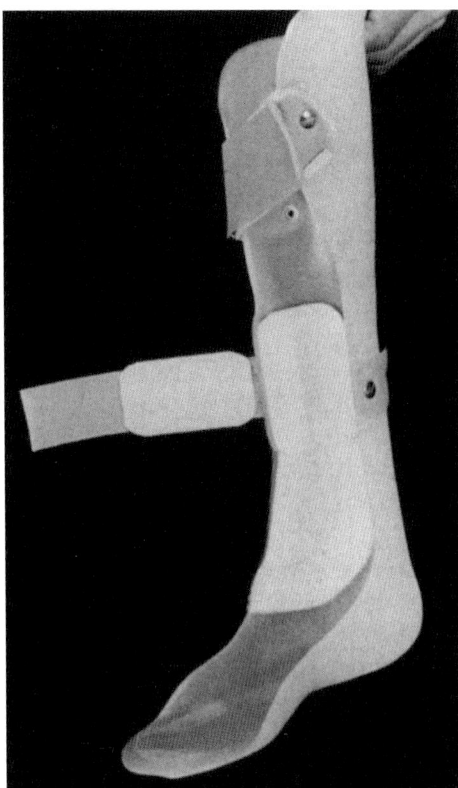

FIGURE 3-22 Solid ankle AFO with an internal varus door.

flange approximately six inches long that begins immediately proximal to the medial malleolus and extends midway between the medial malleolus and the proximal aspect of the orthosis. The trimline should wrap anteriorly but not impinge on the tibial crest.

The second modification that can be used to control the subtalar joint during ambulation incorporates a varus or valgus internal T-strap or control pad (5) (Figure 3-22). For example, the mold for correction of a varus deformity would include the removal of plaster from the positive model at the medial tibial flare, and the distal one-third of the shaft of the fibula. Plaster is also removed at the medial aspect of the os calcis distal to the medial malleolus. A small padded square is heated to conform to the cast in the area the pressure is to be distributed. The size and shape of the square determines the surface area over which the corrective force is applied. The principal corrective force is directed to the distal third of the fibular shaft and is adjustable with two Velcro™ straps. The incorporation of the internal varus or valgus strap has proven successful in eliminating pressure on the malleoli during active ambulation.

Posting is understood to be an external extension of the AFO or UCBL. External posting of the AFO or UCBL increases hindfoot stability and can be accomplished with the addition of a Gillette modification during the vacuum-forming process (see Figure 3-13). This additional flat wedge of plastic extends beyond the calcaneus either medially to control valgus or laterally to control varus and increases the weight-bearing surface of the AFO. When posting is added to an AFO, the orthotist strives to maintain the tibia in perpendicular alignment to the calcaneus and the ground throughout stance. The Gillette modification also incorporates a flat buttress. A buttress is considered an outflare to increase the medial and lateral stability of the AFO. The buttress may also be applied to the shoe externally to increase the medial lateral stability of the shoe.

The term "wedge" in orthotics indicates a material applied to the external aspect of the AFO or UCBL to maintain a fixed angle. For example, a wedge may be utilized when a patient demonstrates a tight tendo Achilles. The patient's ankle joint has a fixed plantar flexion angle and the AFO can be wedged to accommodate the fixed ankle angle and thus increase the weight- bearing surface of the AFO. Another example of this type of wedging would be the postoperative maintenance of a desired angle to protect tendo Achilles surgery. The wedge is eventually decreased or removed when healing of the tendon has occurred.

The presence of a severe internal or external rotary deformity may require the orthotist to control midfoot rotation within the AFO. The control of midfoot rotation can be aided by utilizing a wrap-around AFO design that has two essential components. The first component requires the fabrication of a more flexible supramalleolar (SMO) piece that intimately wraps around the both the plantar aspect and dorsum of the foot. It is essential that the SMO component be fabricated with the desired midfoot rotation built into the device. The second component is a standard AFO with standard trimlines that surrounds the SMO and holds it in place. The wrap-around design may or may not be articulated at the ankle joint.

Internal wedging of an AFO also may be indicated to maintain a specific angle of the ankle or foot. The involved extremity is maximally corrected during the casting process. When the plaster impression is modified for the relief of bony landmarks, a pelite or aliplast interface can be added to the plantar surface of the orthosis to maintain the tibia in the desired alignment. In this way, the wedged material is accommodating the foot deformity. Again, the wedge is ground down to maintain the foot alignment and the tibia perpendicular to the ground. After the correct amount of wedging is determined and incorporated onto the plaster impression, the plastic is vacuum formed over both the wedge material and the plaster impression. The finished product therefore accommodates the wedge inside the AFO to provide an even weight-bearing surface. Biomechanically, both internal and external wedges accomplish the same goals.

ARTICULATING HINGED ANKLE FOOT ORTHOSIS

Articulating AFOs are often prescribed for the patient who demonstrates passive range of motion of at least 5 degrees of dorsiflexion with the subtalar position maintained at neutral. Restriction of desired ankle motion can be avoided by the use of a hinged AFO which incorporates a posterior

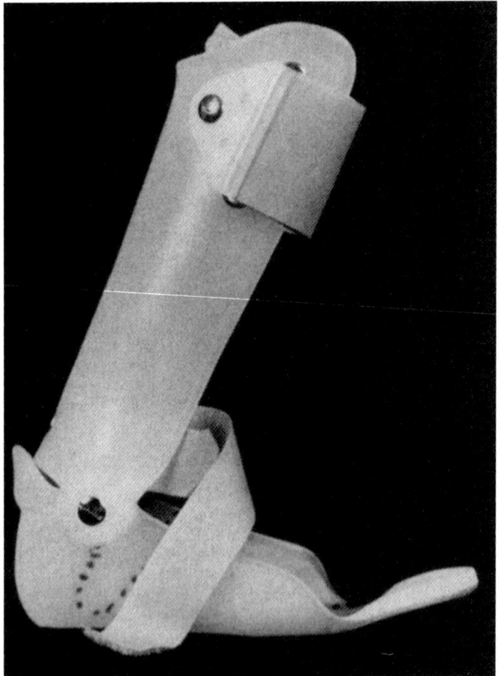

FIGURE 3-23 Articulating AFO.

overlap or stop which can be adjusted to allow for a limited or full range of plantar flexion. The articulated orthosis maintains subtalar frontal plane stability without prohibiting sagittal plane motion at the ankle. The design maintains the hindfoot and forefoot in appropriate alignment. The articulating AFO may be indicated for the patient who has independent voluntary control and will allow an effective range of motion at the ankle joint during the stance phase of gait. This permits the forward progression of the tibia and when indicated, push-off at the conclusion of stance phase. The stability of the midfoot with this type of brace is important because of the increased potential for skin breakdown when uncontrolled motion occurs during stance (Figure 3-23).

Articulating AFOs may incorporate a plantar flexion stop to control genu recurvatum or to break up the extension synergy patterns. As the patient gains voluntary control of push off in stance phase, the degree of ankle plantar flexion can be increased. Dorsiflexion may also be increased when the patient demonstrates voluntary knee extension as the lower extremity progresses over the foot during the stance phase. Hip and knee joint stability are therefore critical in assessing a child for an articulating AFO. Prerequisites include the child having satisfactory voluntary movement of the hip and knee independent of each other. Patients that have excessive ankle motion during early stance phase may develop compensatory gait patterns that may be difficult to overcome later in gait training.

There is a fine line in prescribing the permitted degree of dorsiflexion and plantar flexion in the hinged orthosis. Push-off becomes less effective in the latter part of the stance phase when dorsiflexion is decreased. When plantar flexion is increased, the paretic patient compensated by hip hiking and increased knee flexion during swing phase in order to clear the toes. Fortunately, new technology and design of the articulated brace allows the addition of discs to clinically titrate the desired range of motion. These discs are placed in the ankle section of the mold during fabrication and are known as dual action ankle joints.

Other indications for the articulating AFO include flexible pes planus, generalized hypotonia, ligamentous laxity, and calcaneal varus deviation that is correctable to neutral position in a weight-bearing position. When prescribing the hinged AFO for patients with upper motor neuron lesions, the orthosis must provide stabilizing forces for the pronated or supinated foot, and also prevent collapse of the medial longitudinal arch due to mid-foot instability. Chances of success with the articulating AFO are increased when the patient evidences a stable midfoot. Hinged AFOs are contraindicated when there is a fixed contracture of the plantar flexors, supinators, and or pronators allowing less then 5 degrees of dorsiflexion with the foot remaining in subtalar neutral. Contracted hamstrings, contracted hip flexors, or weak hip extensors which result in a crouch gait deformity also are contraindications for the use of articulating AFOs.

The posterior or rear-entry articulating AFO may also provide dorsiflexion control (Figure 3-24A,B). The stop is placed in the anterior section of the AFO. This limits dorsiflexion throughout stance and is thought to prevent crouch gait by assisting knee extension. This particular AFO is recommended for a very select population, including children with spastic diplegia who demonstrate a mild functional crouch gait with no associated fixed hip and knee flexion contractures. The AFO does provide good mediolateral stability without limiting ankle motion in the sagittal plane. The dorsiflexion can be increased by additional shaving of the anterior stop.

SUPRAMALLEOLAR ANKLE FOOT ORTHOSIS

The supramalleolar orthosis is designed to support the toes and the entire foot by extending the plastic trimlines proximal to the malleoli and distal to the toes (Figure 3-25). This design was originally used to accommodate the malleoli in neutral and included posting of the plantar aspect of the orthosis to stabilize the foot during stance. This type of orthosis will not control the knee in stance or in sagittal plane motion. The hindfoot and forefoot are secured. The height and width of the posterior trimlines allow plantar flexion by excluding the heel cord. Plantar flexion can be increased by modifying the posterior trimline to the mid-calcaneal or subtalar level. The orthosis is fabricated with even contact on the foot accomplished by a thin sheet of plastic. The supramalleolar design is accommodated by a slightly larger size tennis shoe.

Hylton advocated use of this orthosis for equinus-related pes valgus foot deformity (4). The intimate contact of this brace provides an exoskeletal effect and increases its ability to control frontal plane motion, while still allowing limited sagittal plane motion at the ankle.

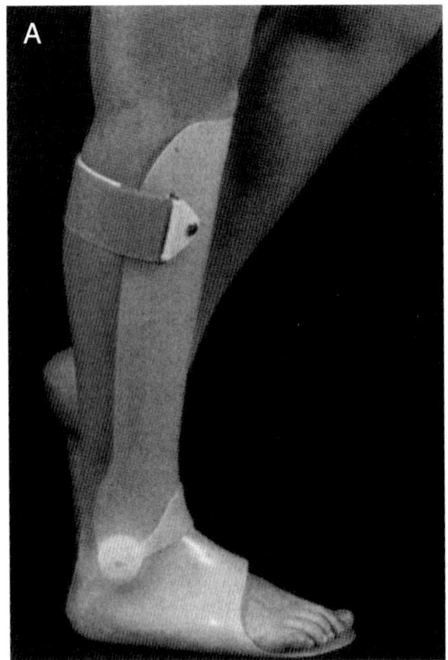

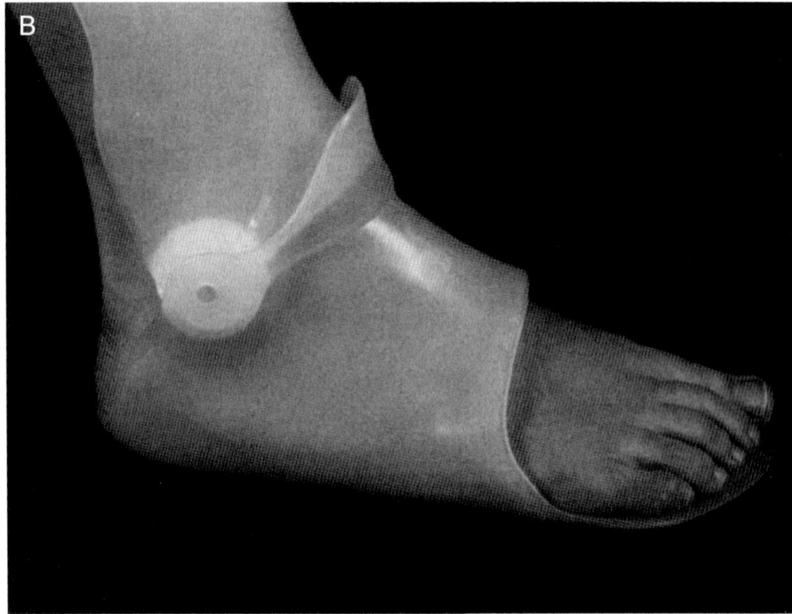

FIGURE 3-24 Posterior entry articulating AFO. **A.** Demonstrating the dorsiflexion stop. **B.** Demonstrating the plantar flexion range of motion.

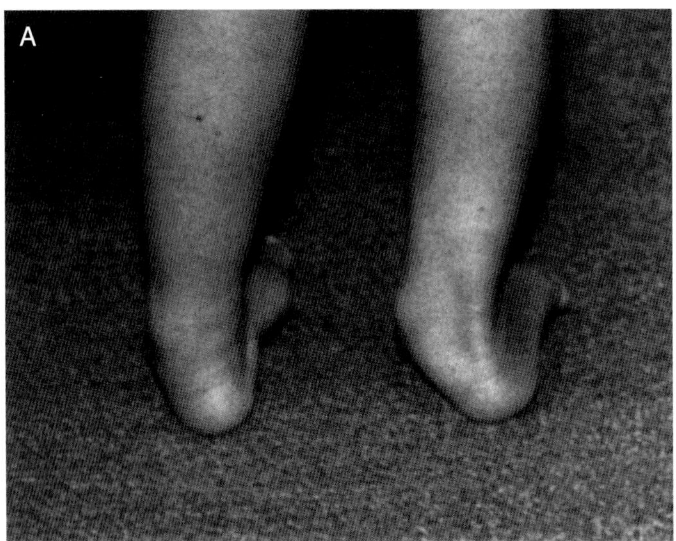

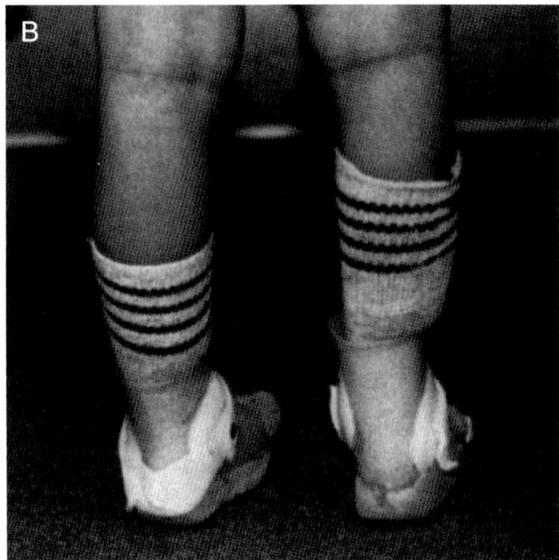

FIGURE 3-25 **A,B.** Supramalleolar AFO. Trimlines are more proximal than the UCBL. Posterior trimline modification for increased dorsiflexion. Both hindfoot valgus and varus can be controlled by the orthosis.

PATELLAR-TENDON BEARING ORTHOSIS (PTB)

McIlmurray and Greenbaum (6) introduced the concept of utilizing the patellar tendon and tibial condyles for weight bearing in the below-knee amputees to the discipline of orthotics, and this knowledge has led to the development of the patellar-tendon bearing orthosis (PTB). The orthotic foot and ankle section is molded to give total contact with the patient's foot and ankle (Figure 3-26). Special shoe modifications which include a SACH heel and rocker bottom help to simulate normal gait.

Indications for the PTB orthosis include conditions where weight bearing may produce pain or tissue damage such as delayed unions or non-unions, degenerative arthritis, ligamentous instability, and soft tissue insults including ulcers and the loss of heel pad.

Additional clinical reasons for utilizing this orthosis might include congenital or acquired loss of ankle or foot sensation, pedal infections, or avascular necrosis of the talar body. The PTB orthosis is contraindicated when fluctuating pitting edema is present; there is compromise of the peripheral vascular system; and the patient cannot tolerate circumferential pressure distal to the knee.

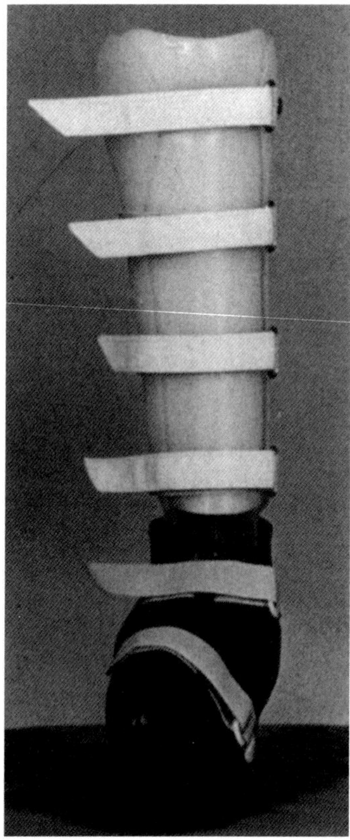

FIGURE 3-26 Patellar-tendon bearing (PTB) AFO with a modified shoe wedge. Note the tibia is perpendicular to the ground.

FLOOR REACTION ANKLE FOOT ORTHOSIS

The floor reaction orthosis was designed to stabilize the paralytic extremity without limiting knee motion (7). The orthosis extends to the midpatella and is constructed from rigid polypropylene with ankle carbon composite inserts. The principle behind the floor reaction AFO involves coupling of the plantarflexed forefoot floor reaction force to the anterior aspect of the proximal orthosis thereby assisting in stabilizing the knee joint into full extension (Figure 3-27). The AFO reacts as a first class lever and the plantar flexed attitude at the ankle takes advantage of the distal trimlines of the footplate at the metatarsal heads.

The floor reaction AFO is widely used for children with cerebral palsy who evidence a slight dynamic knee flexion due to overactive hamstrings or overlengthened Achilles tendon which results in a functional crouch gait. Children with myelomeningocele or cerebral palsy who demonstrate quadriceps weakness during midstance and have no fixed knee flexion contracture are ideal candidates. A minimum of grade 3 minus (good minus) quadriceps strength following overlengthening of the tendo Achilles represents another clinical indication for this form of bracing. Contraindications for floor reaction include fixed flexion contracture of the hip and knee, poor hip extensor strength, and adductor spasticity.

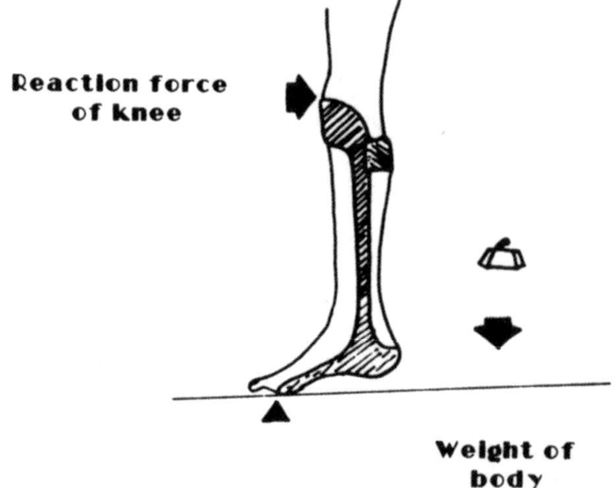

FIGURE 3-27 Extension forces of the floor reaction AFO. The weight line remains anterior to the knee to allow for an extension moment of the knee in stance.

MODERN TECHNOLOGY

The utilization of CAD/CAM to create a model of a patient has shown how the world of computers can impact the field of orthotics. Technological advancements will continue to revolutionize the orthosis in the future. As microprocessors become faster and continue to shrink in size, new orthotic designs are quickly embracing them. Wireless technology and laptop computers make it easy for both the patient and the orthotist to fine-tune and calibrate lower extremity devices relying on microprocessors. The incorporation of electrical stimulation, pressure sensors, and strain gauges in devices has provided the orthotist with an array of tools with which to work. Recent advances in material science have allowed the field of orthotics to embrace ultralight laminates, metallic alloys, and carbon fibers. Although these materials are extremely lightweight, they have limited pediatric applications due to their inability to be adjusted for growth. These technological tools allow the health care team to precisely tailor its care to each individual patient in the future.

SHOES

When treating pediatric foot and ankle disorders it is often necessary for the orthotist to make modifications to the patient's shoes in order to provide proper fit or to correct or accommodate a specific deformity. Successful treatment frequently depends on the selection of the appropriate type of footwear.

Function

Shoes can provide (11):

1. *Protection* for the foot from harm by the environment (cold, sharp objects, insects).
2. *Friction* between the foot and the ground.

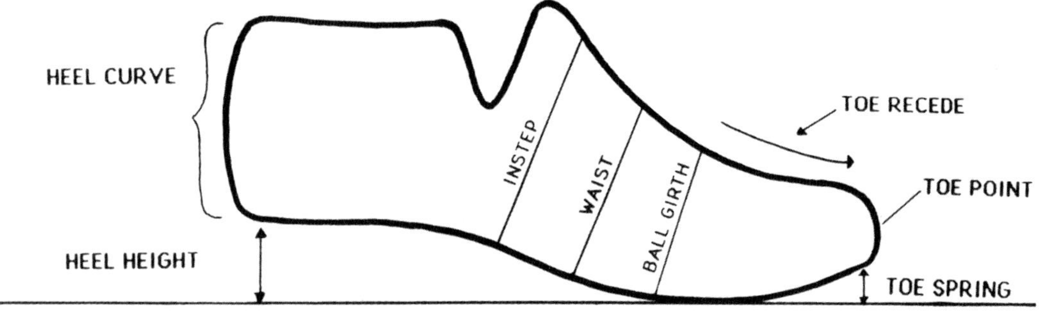

FIGURE 3-28 Some common terminology describing the shape of a shoe last.

3. *Support* for the foot during gait and assist in stabilizing the pedal joints.
4. *Relief of pain.* Shoe modifications can relieve pressure or stress from painful areas of the foot in many pedal disorders.
5. *Correction of foot deformities.* Appropriate shoes and modifications can maintain or accommodate various static foot deformities.
6. *Correction of leg length discrepancies* by the use of appropriate lifts or shoes.
7. *Cosmetic and/or functional improvements* for dissimilar feet, such as partial foot amputation.
8. *Function as a component of a lower extremity orthosis.*

Shoe Lasts

Shoes are formed over a last which acts as a positive mold of the foot. The final three-dimensional shape of the shoe is determined by the shape of the last; therefore, the last decides both the size and the style of the shoe. The form of the last is very critical to the eventual way that the shoe fits the foot.

Stock lasts are standardized for the dimensions of length, width, and girth at specific points. Styles also affect the shape of a last. Certain types of lasts remain fairly constant in design over the years, including those used for children and adult orthopedic shoes, work boots, and traditionally styled nurses' shoes (11). Some of the more basic last terminology and measurements are shown in Figure 3-28.

Shoe Construction and Components

There are three basic construction methods used to make shoes today.

Welt construction is a process in which the shoe upper, the insole, and the welt (a flat strip of leather) are first sewn together and then a lock-stitch outseam is used to attach the outsole to the welt. This type of construction often is used with orthopedic shoes because the outsole can be easily separated from the insole by cutting the outseam, thereby making it possible to insert wedges in any desired area. The outsole can then be re-stitched to the insole. Also, the entire outsole can be removed if necessary to make insole modifications or to replace the outsole as needed. The welt type of construction produces a durable shoe which resists splitting of the outsole from the upper.

Cement construction describes any footwear manufacturing process in which adhesives are used to permanently attach the outsole and the shoe upper (6). Typically, the edges of the upper are first cemented to the bottom of the insole and then the outsole is glued on. Many lightweight shoes and custom molded shoes are made by this process, as are many running shoes and athletic-type footwear.

Injection molded sole construction involves simultaneously molding and attaching the sole and heel component to the prefabricated upper. This method is popular for casual, inexpensive shoes. However, it is only available in limited widths and does not permit simple modification of the sole.

The principal components of the shoe include the upper, innersole, outersole, and the heel (Figure 3-29).

The upper section of the shoe covers the dorsum and sides of the foot and is attached to the sole of the shoe. Its major components are the vamp, quarter, lace stays, tongue, throat, heel counter, and toe box.

The *vamp* is the anterior portion of the upper covering the toes and forefoot. The *quarter* describes the posterior part of the upper. The *lace stays* are the parts of the upper on the dorsum of the foot used for shoe closure attachment purposes such as eyelets for laces. The *tongue* is a piece of material that attaches to or is continuous with the vamp and covers the dorsum of the foot underneath the lace stays. The *throat* is defined as the seam where the vamp and the quarter meet at the base of the tongue. The design and position of the throat will determine the maximum opening of the shoe.

The heel counter and the toe box act as reinforcements. The *heel counter* stiffens the back portion of the shoe and is used to provide mediolateral stability to the calcaneus and also helps preserve the shape of the back part of the shoe. The *toe box* is used to stiffen the toe of the shoe. It offers some protection to the toes and helps to maintain the shape of the upper of the toe area.

The *innersole* is a piece of material that is made to exactly fit the bottom of the last during manufacturing. Typically the innersole is first applied to the last, then the upper is fashioned over the last and the edges are attached to the innersole as previously described. The outersole is then attached to the innersole. Often there is a piece of leather or fabric attached to the dorsal surface

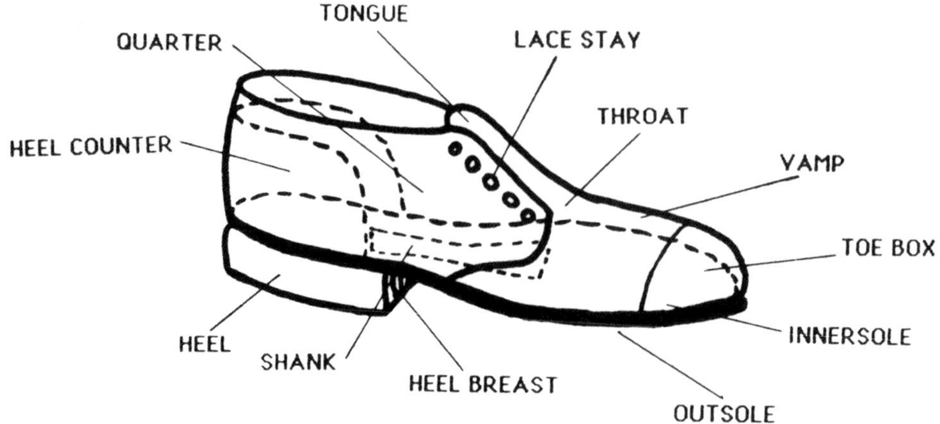

FIGURE 3-29 Components of a shoe.

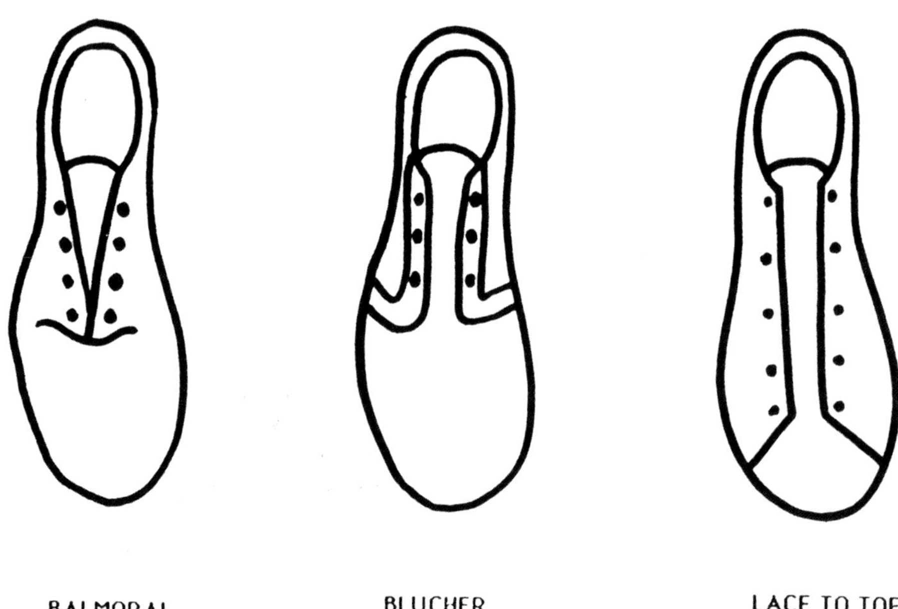

FIGURE 3-30 Shoe closure styles.

of the innersole after the removal of the shoe from the last. This sock lining covers any stitching or other attachments that would otherwise come in contact with the foot when worn. Many athletic shoes have a fabric covered foam insole covering the innersole, which provides cushioning for the foot. This insole frequently has a built-in foam medial longitudinal support.

The *outersole* is the layer which comes in direct contact with the ground. Outersoles provide traction for the shoe and are made of durable material. The flexibility of the shoe is determined by the material which is used to construct the outersole (11).

On shoes which have a heel, the *shank* is defined as the portion of the outersole that extends from the anterior edge of the heel to the ball of the shoe (11). The shank must be sufficiently rigid to prevent collapse of the shoe in this region and give support to the longitudinal arches of the foot. The shank is often reinforced with a shank piece, a long rectangular piece of spring steel or other reinforcement material which extends from mid-heel to within one-quarter to three-eighths inch of the ball or break of the foot. This shank is located between the innersole and outersole of the shoe.

The heel of an orthopedic shoe should be broad enough to provide a stable base of support to the subtalar joint in conjunction with a firm heel counter.

Shoe Styles

There are three main styles of shoe openings or lacing patterns to consider when selecting appropriate footwear (Figure 3-30). These are the Balmoral, the Blucher, and the lace-to-toe or surgical styles.

The Balmoral style has a more restrictive throat area caused by the two quarters coming together and being stitched to the vamp at the throat. This style can make shoe donning more difficult than the others, especially for someone with foot deformity. This difficulty can be increased by internal shoe modifications such as arch supports which decrease the depth of the shoe, the use of a plastic AFO, or in a patient who has a high instep or cavus type foot.

The Blucher style has a less confined throat area with open quarters which makes the task of putting the shoe on easier. This style of opening is recommended when inserts, supports, or plastic ankle foot orthoses are needed, or when significant foot deformity is present.

The lace-to-toe or surgical style opening is the easiest style to don. This is most often commercially available in a boot or high-top shoe configuration. It allows the forepart of the shoe to open fully for ease of donning and allows inspection of the toes to make sure they have not curled under. It is the recommended style for patients with insensitive feet or spastic toe musculature, such as children with myelomeningocele or cerebral palsy. This style also permits adjustment to accommodate feet that swell.

Style-conscious adolescents or their parents may have trouble accepting the style of the surgical boot, however. An athletic or running shoe often laces down more distally than a regular Blucher style and is a good compromise for ease of donning.

Shoe Selection Criteria

Infants and Young Children

Protection forms the major reason for shoe-wear for an infant with normal feet. The type of shoe worn is relatively unimportant before ambulation begins. General guidelines for selecting an infant's shoe include a soft, flexible sole and upper as well as a wide toe box area that does not restrict or put stress on the developing toes. A high-top shoe helps to prevent the child from kicking his or her shoes off. It is generally agreed that the pre-walker does not need shoes for foot support. An infant should spend a good deal of time without shoes to allow normal sensory stimulation of the feet and normal foot muscle development (1).

Shoes are necessary when the child begins to walk to protect the feet which are subjected to many environments. Opinions vary regarding the "correct" shoe for a toddler or young child with normal feet. It is generally agreed that the heel should be low or non-existent to assist in upright balance as well as to prevent heel cord contracture. The shoe should be straight lasted (Figure 3-31), which means that the last over which the shoe is made should be designed with a straight medial border and with the forepart of the shoe not deviating medially or laterally. Most shoes for pre-school age children are made on straight lasts.

The toe and ball area should again be broad to prevent any deforming forces from being applied by the shoe. The sole of the shoe should be flexible enough at the ball region to allow the metatarsophalangeal joint to dorsiflex during walking. The heel counter should be both narrow to grasp the calcaneus and firm to preserve the shape of the counter.

A high-top shoe should not be necessary for support of the normal ankle, but may help to keep the shoes on the flexible child's feet. Many sneakers or athletic-type footwear made today can fulfill these basic requirements.

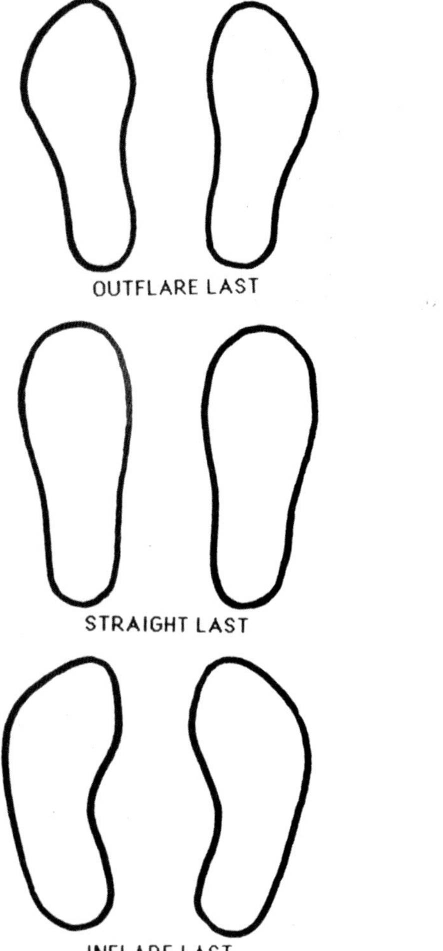

FIGURE 3-31 Common shoe last shapes for treating foot disorders of infants and children.

Older Children and Adolescents

Style plays an important role in the shoe selection for older children. Sneakers or running shoes are currently the most common styles for this age group. Special shoes may be required when severe foot deformity exists or when special modifications are necessary, for example, the attachment of conventional metal bracing to the shoes. The most important concern remains that the shoe fits the foot.

Fitting Criteria

It is important to measure and judge the fit of a shoe in a standing position as feet tend to lengthen and widen with weight bearing. A properly fitted shoe supports and conforms but does not compress the foot. The toe box should be broad and high enough to allow free movement of the toes and there should be approximately one-half inch space between the end of the toe box and the end of the longest toe to allow for the anticipated lengthening with weight bearing. The shoes for a growing child should be replaced when the toes touch the end of the toe box during weight bearing.

The vamp section should fit comfortably and not be excessively tight or loose on weight bearing and ambulation. The widest portion or ball of the vamp should coincide with the metatarsal heads of the foot to provide proper shoe break during ambulation.

The instep region should lace comfortably and have sufficient height and width. This can often be judged by observing the distance between the lace stays when tied. The Blucher pattern of lacing allows for better adjustability when fitting feet with significantly low or high instep (11).

The heel counter should be firm and properly fit the heel in order to prevent slipping during ambulation. Heel slipping can be caused by a shoe that lacks flexibility of the sole, improperly fitting heel counter (too low), or a shoe that is too large (10). One useful clinical technique is to check the shoe size to be certain that the heel counter snugly fits the heel before the shoe is laced.

Many children and adolescents with neuromuscular disorders require lower extremity bracing to provide support, promote ambulation, or prevent contractures. These plastic bracing systems may effectively increase the width of the foot and make the selection of appropriate shoes a major problem. Sneakers or running shoes are usually the wisest choices as the soft uppers help conform to the wider width and the longer lacing patterns allow easier donning. Some manufacturers do produce these types of shoes in wider than normal widths for children. Many have removable insoles that give extra room for the orthosis when removed. The lighter weight of these shoes is also beneficial, as is their contemporary style.

Whenever possible, it is wise to have shoes fitted after brace delivery to take into account the additional room needed to accommodate the orthosis.

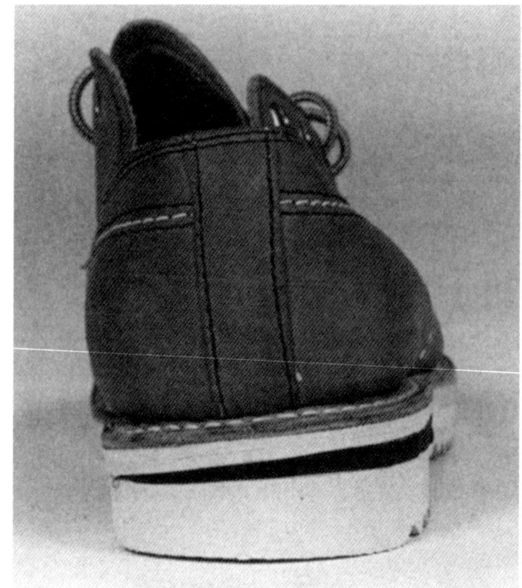

FIGURE 3-32 Heel wedge to create an inversion or eversion moment at the calcaneus.

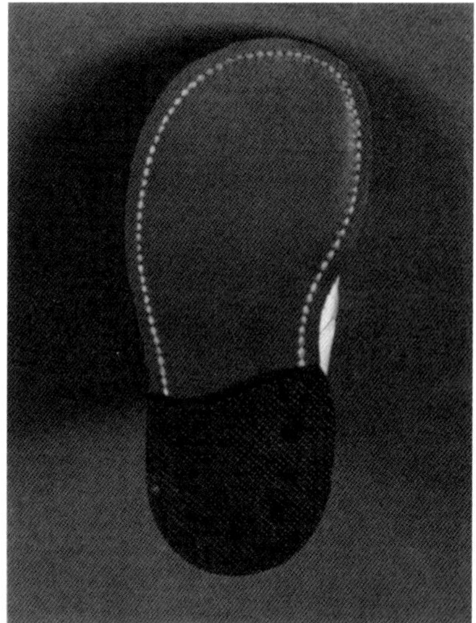

FIGURE 3-33 Thomas heel.

Special Shoes

Pronation is one of the more common pediatric problems. Mild pronation can be supported or corrected with the proper type of shoe previously described. Additional support can be gained in the young child by adding a longitudinal arch pad ("cookie") to support the medial side of the calcaneus and the medial longitudinal arch. Currently the use of a custom shoe insert is recommended. There is the occasional need for additional support that can be achieved with an external medial heel wedge coupled with a snug fitting heel counter (Figure 3-32). This combination tilts the hindfoot into slight varus during floor contact to control pronation.

The Thomas heel (Figure 3-33) can also be used on shoes made with separate heel construction. This style has an approximate one-half inch distal heel extension which helps to reinforce the shank on the medial side and supports the medial longitudinal arch of the foot. This modification is seldom used today.

Inflare Shoes

Shoes for treatment of pediatric pronation usually are inflare shoes, which are constructed on an inflare last (see Figure 3-31). This variety is designed to supinate the foot by inverting the heel, raising the longitudinal arch, and adducting the forefoot. In addition to being built on inflare lasts, these shoes usually incorporate medial heel wedges, rigid shanks, and Thomas heels. The heel counter is extended forward or distally on the medial side to further support the hindfoot. This style is rarely used today.

Outflare Shoes

Special children's shoes may be used to control a corrected metatarsus varus forefoot with an outflare shoe (see Figure 3-31). The forefoot of this shoe swings outward to hold the forefoot in the correct position. The patient often progresses to a straight last shoe after treatment with an outlast shoe.

Another unique treatment used for metatarsus varus is the Bebax orthosis from Camp International, Inc. (Figure 3-34). This orthosis has two locking swivel joints that allow the hindfoot and forefoot components to be adjusted in relation to one another and then locked in place with an Allen wrench. The orthosis is designed to

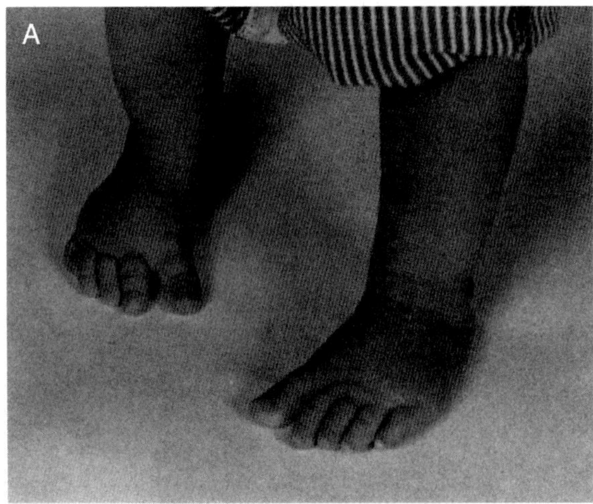

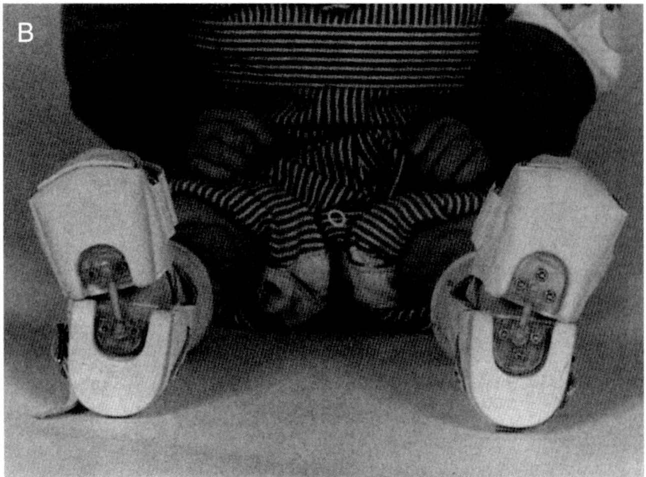

FIGURE 3-34 The Bebax orthosis for treatment of metatarsus varus. **A.** Metatarsus varus deformity. **B.** Treatment of same feet in a Bebax orthosis.

replace casting for metatarsus varus and allows removal for hygiene, examination, and stretching exercises.

When treatment for corrected clubfeet or metatarsus adductus involves the use of a Denis-Browne bar, special infant shoes are commercially available with steel screw receptacles in the sole of the shoe to allow attachment without clamps or rivets. The shoes should be attached to the bar to promote external rotation and slight dorsiflexion. The amount of external rotation and dorsiflexion should be specified by the physician. The Denis-Browne bar is typically worn 23 hours a day; therefore, it is imperative that the skin is checked regularly to prevent blistering or ulceration. A semi-rigid or rigid clubfoot may be difficult to maintain the inside the shoe and in those cases an internal heel counter may need to be added to tighten the anterior-posterior dimension proximal to the malleoli. As clubfoot treatment progresses successfully the wearing schedule of the Denis-Browne bar may be reduced to napping or nighttime wear only.

Shoe Modifications

Custom Molded Shoes

Severe foot deformity such as rigid talipes equinovarus can prevent the fitting of stock shoes. Custom molded shoes may be the best choice to accommodate the shape of the foot and to appropriately distribute the weight bearing. Other pediatric indications for molded shoes include significantly dissimilar size or shape of feet, insensitive feet, and feet with poor circulation. They are most commonly used for myelomeningocele foot deformities.

The plaster cast for custom molded shoes is taken with the foot in a partial weight-bearing configuration. The shoes often incorporate custom insoles, relatively thick lightweight outersoles, and soft leather uppers. Large opening and Velcro™ closures allow easy donning. These shoes offer good foot protection and support when properly constructed (Figure 3-35).

Custom molded shoes are occasionally used in conjunction with lower extremity bracing. It is possible to have them fabricated with the necessary attachment for conventional bracing. When plastic orthoses are used, the cast should be taken with the orthosis applied in order to allow proper room in the shoes for the brace.

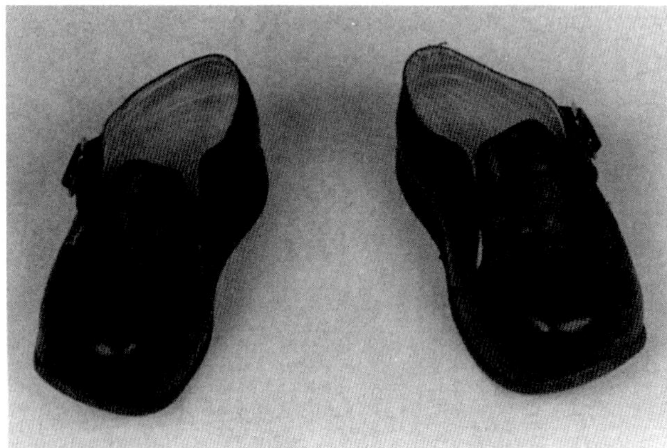

FIGURE 3-35 Custom molded shoes fabricated for a myelomeningocele patient with rigid equinovarus feet.

Toe or Foot Fillers for Shoes

Patients with marked deformity of one foot can often wear matched size shoes with the use of a toe filler or partial foot filler. This is a custom fabricated device typically incorporating a combination of plastic, foam materials, spring steel, and leather. Properly constructed, this can offer improved function and use of stock shoes for the individual patient (Figure 3-36 A,B,C).

Easier donning and extra shoe width for children using an orthosis can be accomplished by cutting the vamp to effectively locate the throat more distally, thus elongating the tongue. This modification also increases the width of the shoe in the throat and ball region enough to compensate for the additional width and depth needed when plastic AFOs or other foot orthoses are used (Figure 3-37A,B). This technique can also be useful when foot deformity or swelling makes the shoe too tight over the ball region.

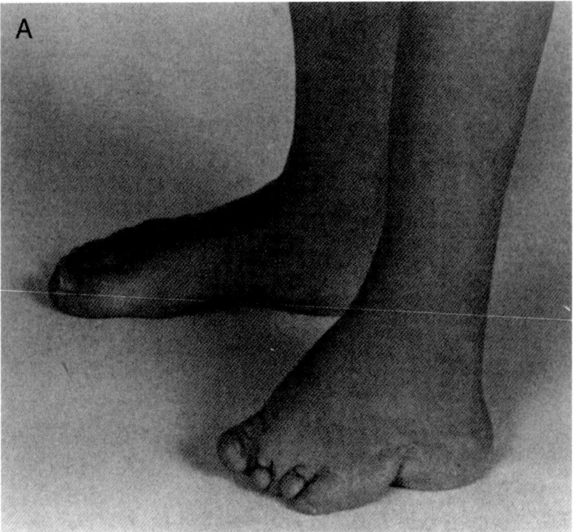

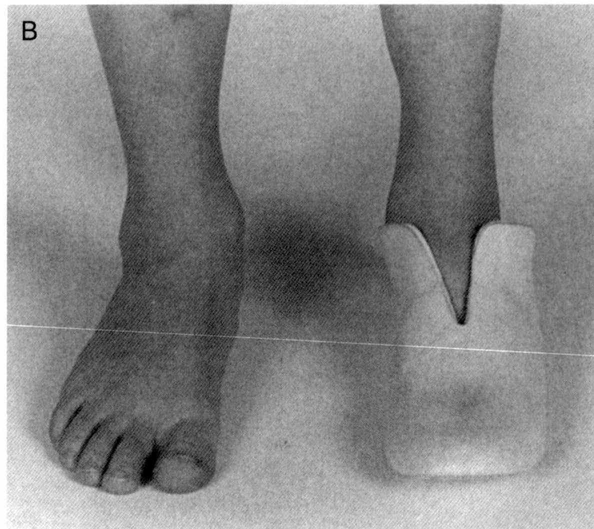

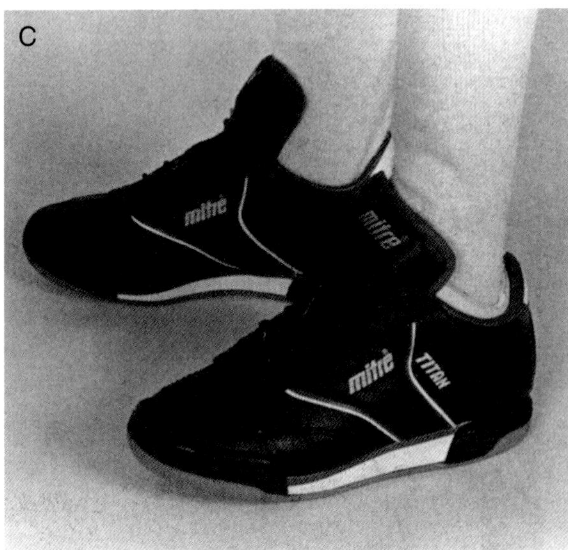

FIGURE 3-36 **A.** 10-year-old patient with congenital deformity of the left foot. **B.** Partial foot filler for the same patient. **C.** Patient wearing matched sneakers with partial foot filler from **B.**

Other modifications of the pediatric shoe upper include enlarging with a shoe stretcher to obtain a slightly greater width in the ball area or creating localized relief with a shoemakers' swan to relieve pressure from claw toes or other deformities. Only leather shoes can be relieved by stretching or spot relief.

Tongue pads can sometimes improve the fit of a shoe that is slightly too large or long. The self-adhesive pad is applied to the inside of the tongue to help push the foot back toward the heel. This is often used when one foot is slightly smaller than another and permits shoes of the same size to be used (Figure 3-38).

Innersole Modifications

There are many innersole modifications that can relieve pressure over a sensitive region of the foot or distribute weight bearing more effectively. These include custom shoe inserts or foot orthotics that have previously been described, and these inserts can be transferred to more than one pair of shoes. Modifications can be made to the individual shoe including the longitudinal arch pad "cookie," previously discussed, for mild pronation in younger children. A heel elevation pad can be glued inside the shoe to a maximum height of one-quarter inch. Any additional heel lift should be placed on the bottom of the shoe in order to preserve the fit of the heel counter.

One-eighth to one-quarter inch medial or lateral heel wedges can be added to the shoe to help control inversion or eversion. These modifications are more effective when applied to the outside of the heel of the shoe as the heel counter can then contribute to the control of inversion or eversion moment.

Metatarsal pads can be glued to the innersole to help relieve pressure on the metatarsal heads by transferring the weight-bearing force to the metatarsal shafts.

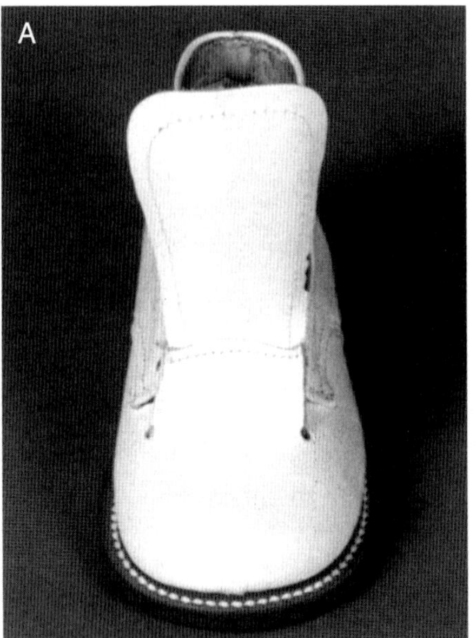

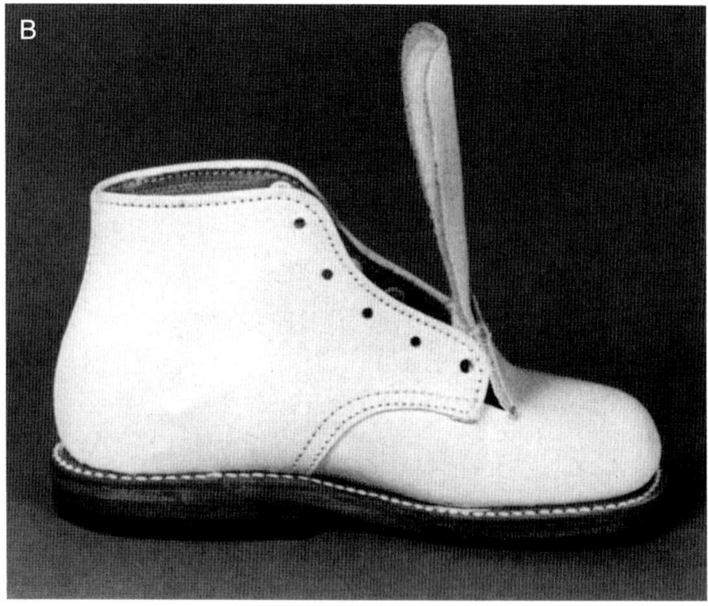

FIGURE 3-37 **A,B.** Modification to increase width in throat or ball region to accommodate plastic AFO use, provide more width in the ball region, or provide more ease in donning.

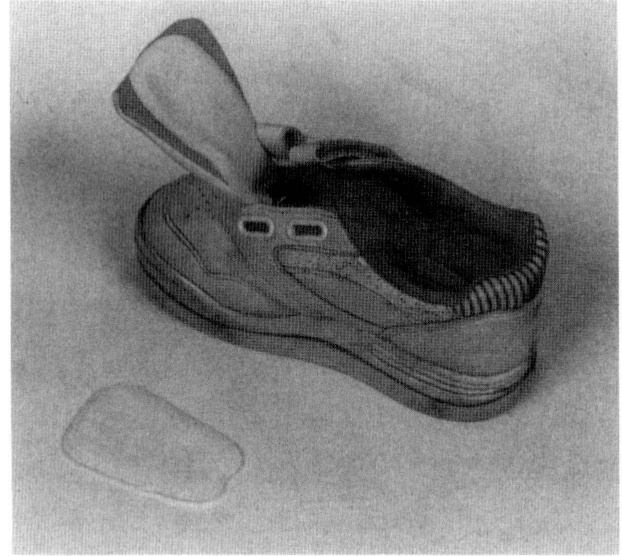

FIGURE 3-38 Tongue pad used to improve the fit of a slightly large shoe.

Toe crest (buttress) pads are often applied to the innersole to aid in the relief of forefoot pain and stress on hammer or claw toes. They can also help re-distribute weight across the metatarsals and reduce toe tip irritation within the shoe. Toe crest pads are commonly available off-the-shelf according to measurement or they may be custom molded in combination with an arch support.

Heel and Outersole Modifications

Outersole Modifications

Another common shoe modification for young children's shoes is a sole lift to accommodate for limb length discrepancy. For the growing child it is desirable to utilize a lift of the same thickness on the entire sole instead of limiting the lift to the heel. Lightweight crepe material is commonly used for the elevations on popular types of sneakers. Often the lift can simply be glued to the bottom surface of the sole (Figure 3-39A) using a neoprene-type adhesive or special vinyl shoe adhesive. However, these lightweight materials tend to wear faster than other soling materials and active children or those with gait deviations that create unusually hard sole wear will often distort or wear out the lift before the shoe is outgrown.

The soles of some lightweight sneakers or running shoes are constructed of lightweight foam covered with a thin, hard-wearing rubber treaded material cemented to the bottom. It is often possible to remove this bottom layer with solvent, cement on sufficient layers of the lightweight build-up material to provide the proper height lift, and then reglue the bottom treaded material thus preserving the wear characteristics of the sole. However, some sneakers have one-piece molded soles that cannot be removed from the upper. Here it is sometimes possible to slice off the bottom treaded surface of the sole carefully on a bandsaw (Figure 3-39B), cement on the appropriate lift, and then reglue on the removed tread, thereby preserving the original friction surface.

Rocker Sole Modifications

After a sole lift incorporates a rocker sole modification, the sole lift is tapered sharply distal to the ball of the shoe (Figure 3-40). This modification helps to facilitate walking when dorsiflexion is prevented such as when a solid ankle AFO that prevents dorsiflexion is worn. It is also used to reduce stress on the major joints of the foot during heel off to toe off, in particular the metatarsophalangeal joints.

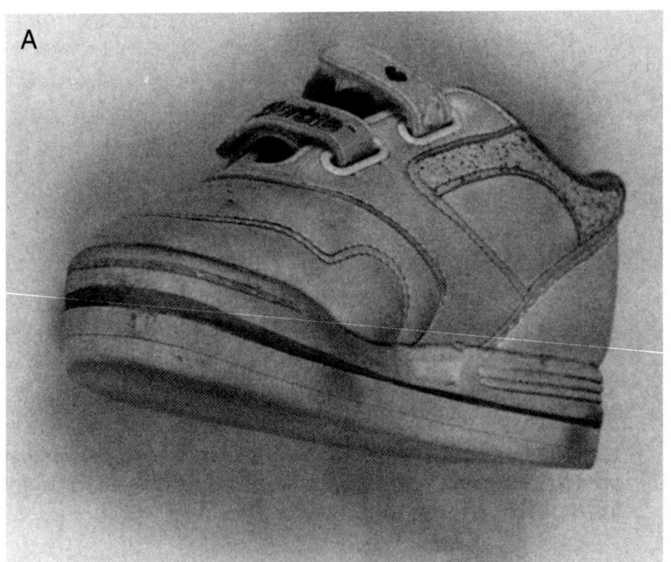

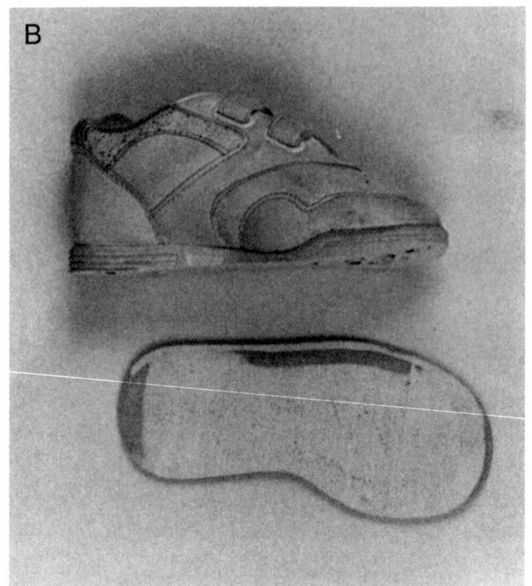

FIGURE 3-39 Shoe lifts for sneakers to accommodate limb length inequality. **A.** Lift applied to the bottom of the sole. **B.** Molded sole cut on a bandsaw to allow lightweight lift material to be added before replacing original soling material.

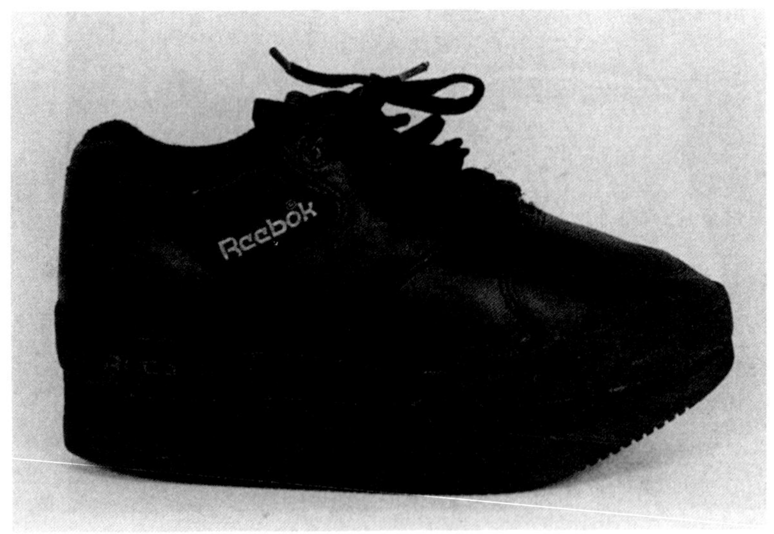

FIGURE 3-40 Rocker sole modification to facilitate rollover and reduce stress on metatarsophalangeal joints.

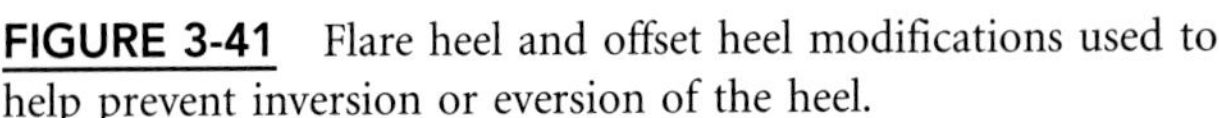

FIGURE 3-41 Flare heel and offset heel modifications used to help prevent inversion or eversion of the heel.

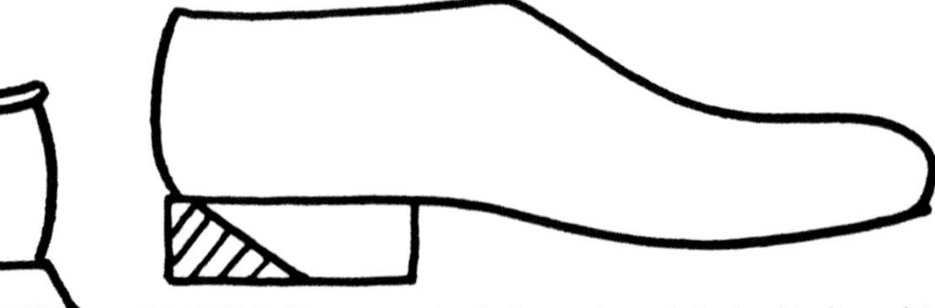

FIGURE 3-42 SACH heel: the section of the heel indicated is replaced with compressible foam rubber to simulate plantar flexion at heel strike.

Heel Modifications

Medial or lateral heel wedges (see Figure 3-32) are commonly used to impart inversion or eversion moments to the subtalar joint as previously described when small corrective forces are needed for better alignment for a flexible deformity. A flare heel modification (Figure 3-41) can be used by itself or in conjunction with a heel wedge to help prevent inversion or eversion by increasing the moment are of the heel. The offset heel modification (Figure 3-41) further prevents inversion or eversion by buttressing the heel counter as well. It should be noted that these heel modifications require a firm, well-fitting counter in the shoe.

A solid ankle custom heel (SACH) modification is used to simulate plantar flexion at heel strike to lessen the ground reaction force tending to flex the knee (Figure 3-42). This modification is commonly used with the rocker modification to smooth out the gait from heel strike to rollover. It is sometimes used when ankle motion is limited by an orthosis.

The roll heel is fabricated by leveling the heel and replacing the removed material with a compressible foam rubber. A thin layer of hard wearing material is usually added to the bottom of the heel for better wear characteristics.

ACKNOWLEDGMENTS

I wish to thank James M. Fezio, C.O., Robert S. Lin, C.P.O., and Kathleen T. Maginn, M.S.O.T.C.O., for their active support and technical assistance in preparing this chapter.

REFERENCES

1. Chong A. *Is your child walking right?* Wheaton, IL: Wheaton Resource Corporation, 1986.
2. Cusick BD. *Progressive casting and splinting for lower extremity deformities in children with neuromotor dysfunction.* Tucson, AZ: Therapy Skill Builders, 1990.
3. D'Amico JC. Developmental flatfoot. In: Ganley JV, ed. *Symposium on Podopediatrics—Clinics in Podiatry.* Philadelphia: WB Saunders, 1984;535–546.
4. Hylton N, Cusick B, Jordon RP. *Dynamic casting and orthotics.* Paper and instructional materials presented at the Neurodevelopmental Treatment Association annual meeting. Kansas City, MS, May 23, 1988.
5. Lin, RS. Application of varus T-strap principle to the poylpropylene ankle foot orthosis *Orthot Prost* 1982;36:67.
6. McIlmurray WJ, Greenbaum WA. A below-knee weight bearing brace. *Orthot Prosthet* 1974;28:14–20.
7. Saltiel, J. A one-piece laminated knee locking short leg brace *Orthot Prost* 23:69,1969.
8. Spencer AM, Person VA, Valmassay RL. Casting and orthotics for children. In: Ganley JV, ed. *Symposium on Podopediatrics—Clinics in Podiatry.* Philadelphia: WB Saunders, 1984;621–629.
9. Valmassay RL. Biomechanical evaluation of the child. In: Ganley JV, ed. *Symposium on Podopediatrics—Clinics in Podiatry.* Philadelphia: W.B. Saunders, 1984.
10. Weber D, ed. Foot wear. In: *Clinical aspects of lower extremity orthotics.* The Canadian Association of Prosthetists and Orthotists. Elgan Enterprises, Oakville, Ontario, Canada, 1990.
11. Wu KK. Principle and practice of pedorthotics. In: *Foot orthosis: Principles and clinical applications.* Baltimore: Williams & Wilkins, 1990;49–95.

CHAPTER 4

Normal Function of the Ankle and Foot: Biomechanics and Quantitative Analysis

Jon R. Davids

INTRODUCTION

The interaction between the ankle, foot, and the floor is a critical element of normal gait. Function of the ankle and foot is determined by a complex interaction of anatomy, physiology, and physics. Proper ankle and foot alignment is required for optimal function of the knee and hip during gait (10,19,20,27,29). Disruption of normal function of the ankle and foot may disrupt knee and hip function, compromising the energy efficiency of gait and, in extreme cases, precluding the ability to ambulate.

This review provides a focused biomechanical analysis of ankle and foot function during normal gait, utilizing standardized terminology and a four-segment model of the ankle and foot. Quantitative assessment of ankle and foot function is necessary to understand better and characterize the biomechanics of normal gait. Appreciation of normal gait facilitates the understanding of the pathomechanics of gait disruption associated with a variety of disease processes. Several quantitative techniques for the analysis of ankle and foot function (e.g., plain radiography, kinematics, and dynamic pedobarography) are considered.

ANKLE AND FOOT FUNCTION DURING NORMAL GAIT

The understanding of ankle and foot function during normal gait is facilitated by considering the lower leg as consisting of four segments: the tibial or shank segment; the hindfoot (talus and calcaneus) the midfoot (navicular, cuneiforms, and cuboid); and the forefoot (metatarsals and phalanges) (8,18,19,27). It is also helpful to consider the foot as consisting of two columns: the medial column (talus, navicular, cuneiforms, great toe metatarsal, and phalanges), and the lateral column (calcaneus, cuboid, lesser toe metatarsals, and phalanges). Standardized, consistent terminology is required to describe the alignment of the separate segments of the ankle and foot (28). Movement of the plantar aspect of the segment in question during the gait cycle is described as inversion (toward the midline) or eversion (away from the midline) (Figure 4-1). Movement of the distal aspect of the segment in question during the gait cycle is described as adduction (toward the midline) or abduction (away from the midline)(Figure 4-2). Supination is a combination of inversion and adduction. Pronation is a combination of eversion and abduction. Rotation of the segment about its longitudinal axis toward the midline is described as internal rotation. Rotation of the segment about its longitudinal axis away from the midline is described as external rotation.

The gait cycle is a period of time beginning with the initial contact of the reference foot with the ground, continuing through ipsilateral stance and swing phases until the subsequent ipsilateral initial contact. Stance phase occurs when the reference limb is in contact with the ground. Swing phase occurs when the reference limb is not in contact with the ground. The interaction of the ankle and foot with the ground during the stance phase of the gait cycle is described by the concept of three rockers (20,27,29). In normal gait, the heel is the first part of the foot to contact the ground at initial contact. The ground reaction force falls behind the ankle, creating an external plantar flexion moment. The ankle subsequently plantar flexes until the foot is flat on the floor. This motion is controlled by the eccentric activity of the ankle dorsiflexor muscle group, which generates an internal dorsiflexion moment. The first, or heel rocker, occurs from heel strike to foot flat during the loading response subphase of stance (Figure 4-3). As the body progresses forward over the foot, the ground reaction force moves progressively distally through the foot, creating an external dorsiflexion moment. The tibia advances forward over

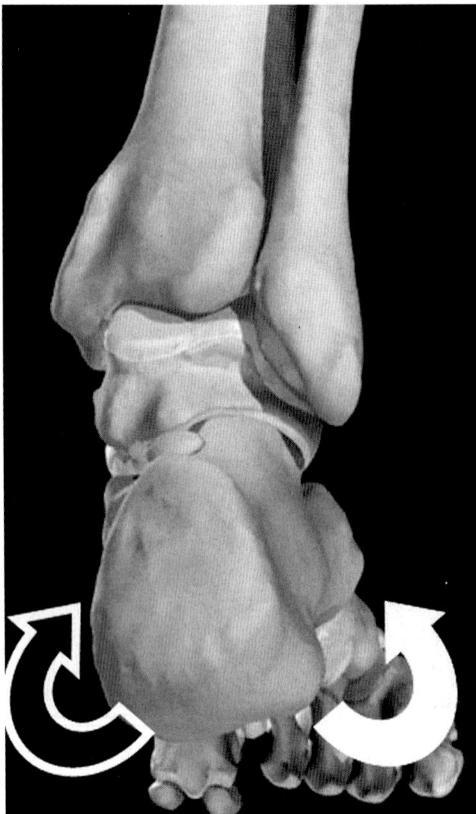

FIGURE 4-1 Terminology for describing foot segmental alignment. The hindfoot is seen from the posterior view. When the plantar aspect of the hindfoot is deviated toward the body's midline (open arrow), the segment is described as being inverted. When the plantar aspect is deviated away from the midline (solid arrow), the segment is described as being everted.

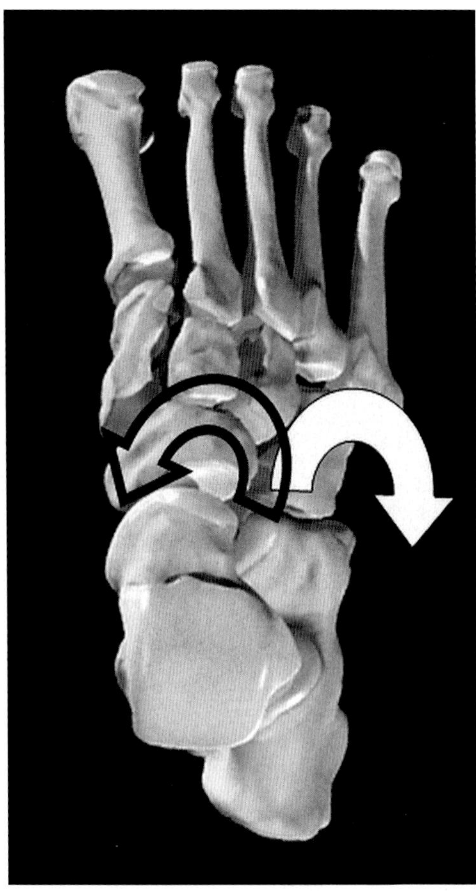

FIGURE 4-2 The hindfoot is seen from the cephalad view. When the distal aspect of the hindfoot is deviated toward the midline (open arrow), the segment is described as being adducted. When the distal aspect is deviated away from the midline (solid arrow), the segment is described as being abducted.

the foot, which is achieved by ankle dorsiflexion. This motion is controlled by eccentric activity of the ankle plantar flexor muscle group, which generates an internal plantar flexion moment. The second, or ankle rocker, occurs as the tibia advances over the foot during the midstance subphase of stance (Figure 4-4). With further forward progression, the ground reaction force remains distal to the ankle joint, creating an increasing external dorsiflexion moment. Immediately prior to the initial contact of the opposite foot, the heel of the reference foot rises off the ground and dorsiflexion occurs through the metatarsophalangeal joints of the forefoot. This motion is controlled by concentric activity of the ankle plantar flexor muscle group, which continues to generate an internal plantar flexion moment. The third, or forefoot rocker, occurs as the ankle begins to plantar flex during the terminal stance subphase of stance (Figure 4-5). This is an essential event during normal gait, as the largest moment generated by any single muscle group during the gait cycle is the internal plantar flexion moment generated by the ankle plantar flexor muscle group during third rocker in terminal stance (27,34).

In the stance phase of the normal gait cycle, the ankle and foot provide shock absorption during loading response (first or heel rocker), stability during midstance (second or ankle rocker), and a rigid lever during terminal stance (third or forefoot rocker)(18,20,27,29). During loading response, the tibial or shank segment rotates internally, and the ankle is plantarflexing. This results in eversion and abduction of the hindfoot, through the subtalar joint. Pronation of the hindfoot forces the talus to plantarflex, which "unlocks" the joints of the midfoot, which follows into pronation. This coupled movement of the hindfoot and midfoot results in maximum flexibility of the foot, which allows the joints to contribute to shock absorption. During midstance, the tibial or shank segment is rotating externally, and the ankle is dorsiflexing. This results in inversion and adduction of the hindfoot, through the subtalar joint. Supination of the hindfoot forces the talus to dorsiflex, which "locks" the joints of the midfoot, which follows into supination. This coupled movement of the hindfoot and the midfoot results in restoration of the longitudinal arch of the foot and maximum rigidity of the foot, which enhances stability. During terminal stance, the tibial or shank segment continues to rotate externally, and the ankle continues to dorsiflex. As the body progresses forward, the center of pressure beneath the foot advances distally into the

TABLE 4-1

Radiographic Measurements: Quantitative and Categorical Definitions

	Normal Mean ± 1 SD	*Abnormal High Value (> Mean + 1 SD)*	*Abnormal Low Value (< Mean − 1 SD)*
Hindfoot			
Tibio-Talar Angle (degrees)	1.1 ± 3.75	Eversion	Inversion
Calcaneal Pitch (degrees)	17 ± 6.0	Calcaneus	Equinus
Tibio-Calcaneal angle (degrees)	69 ± 8.4	Equinus	Calcaneus
Talo-Calcaneal Angle (degrees)	49 ± 6.9	Eversion	Inversion
Midfoot			
Naviculo-Cuboid Overlap (%)	47 ± 13.8	Pronation	Supination
Talo-Navicular Coverage Angle (degrees)	20 ± 9.8	Abduction	Adduction
Lateral Talo-First Metatarsal Angle (degrees)	13 ± 7.5	Pronation	Supination
Forefoot			
Anteroposterior Talo-First Metatarsal Angle (degrees)	10 ± 7.0	Abduction	Adduction
Metatarsal Stacking Angle (degrees)	8 2. ± 9	Supination	Pronation
Columns			
Medial-Lateral Column Ratio	0.9 ± 0.1	Abduction	Adduction

QUANTITATIVE ASSESSMENT OF ANKLE AND FOOT FUNCTION

Radiography (Quantitative Segmental Analysis)

Clinical decision making for the management of foot deformities in children is primarily based on the physical examination and the analysis of weight-bearing radiographs of the foot and ankle. Standing anteroposterior (AP) and lateral (LAT) views of the foot, and AP view of the ankle are utilized to assess the alignment of the segments of the ankle and foot. Multiple methods of analysis of weight-bearing radiographs of the foot for children have been described (1–3,22,31,32,35). Quantitative techniques are frequently incomplete, focusing primarily on assessment of hindfoot alignment. Qualitative techniques are more frequently utilized by experienced clinicians, but are subjective, have not been well described in the literature, and are difficult to apply when comparing management paradigms and intervention outcomes between or across centers.

Clinically useful classification systems should facilitate the prediction of the natural history of the disease process and guide in the selection of the most appropriate management strategy. Classification of ankle and foot alignment from the plain radiographs by segmental analysis is performed by determining the relative alignment of each segment, and the relative length of each column. The alignment of each segment may be determined relative to a global reference frame (e.g., the floor, calcaneal pitch); relative to the location of an adjacent segment (e.g., hindfoot relative to the tibia, tibio-calcaneal angle); or relative to the alignment between bones within the same segment (e.g., the talo-calcaneal angle). A comprehensive technique of quantitative segmental analysis of the ankle and foot has been developed, based on qualitative techniques derived from the foot model originally developed by Inman and colleagues (9). This technique of quantitative segmental analysis utilizes ten radiographic measurements to determine the alignment of the segments and the lengths of the columns of the ankle and foot. After establishing intra-and inter-observer reliability, normative values and ranges were determined from a cohort of 60 normal feet in children between the ages of 5 and 17 years (Table 4-1). Individual measures that fall beyond one standard deviation of the normal mean value are considered to be abnormal and can be utilized to describe segmental malalignment patterns.

Kinematics

Quantitative analysis of ankle and foot function during gait is performed in a motion analysis laboratory (12,14,27). The subject is instrumented and his or her movement is monitored by a measurement system as s/he walks along a smooth, level runway through the laboratory. Passive reflective markers are placed on the surface of the child's skin and aligned with respect to selected skeletal landmarks and joint axes. The locations of these markers are tracked by an array of cameras as the child walks through a designated, calibrated space. The camera data is processed by a central computer to determine the three-dimensional locations of the markers during the gait cycle. The marker position data is utilized to calculate the angular orientation of the various body segments, and the angles between adjacent body segments. This information, which describes the motions that occur, is represented in waveform plots, and is collectively referred to as "kinematics."

The calculation of the orientation of body segments and joint axes from the surface skin markers involves

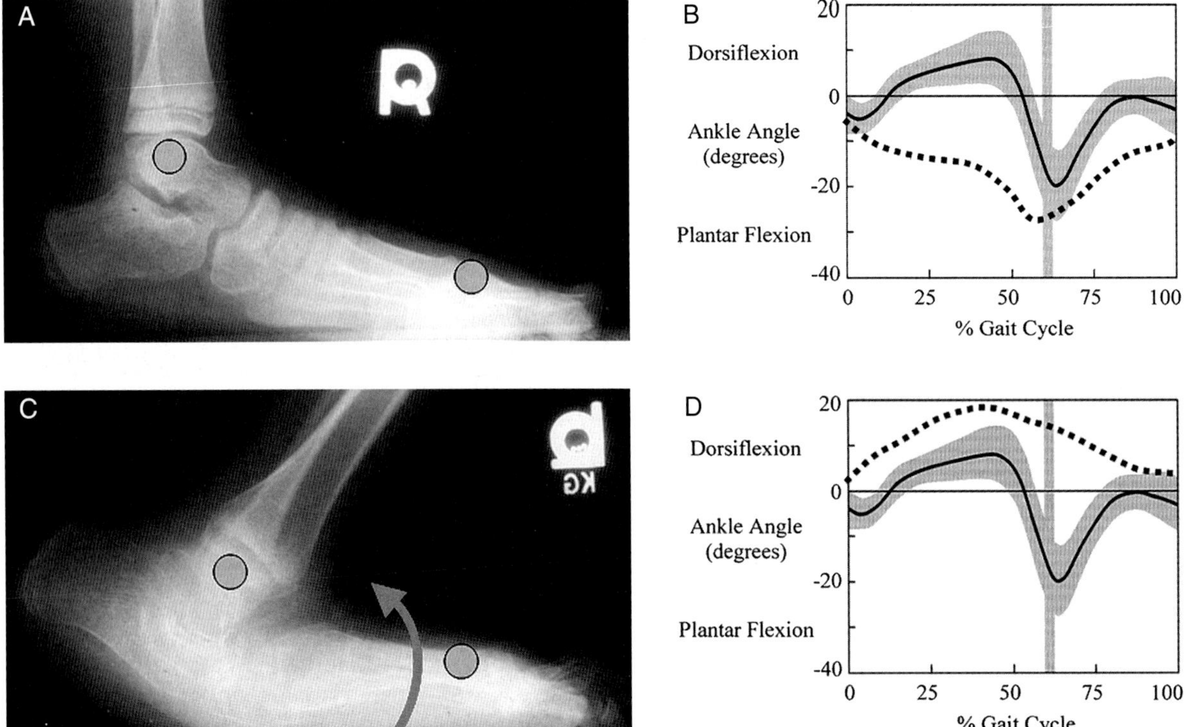

FIGURE 4-7 Effect of foot skeletal alignment on the measurement of ankle kinematics. Figure 4-7A shows a well aligned foot in equinus, with the standard marker placement (solid circles) associated with the single segment foot kinematic model. Figure 4-7B shows the sagittal plane ankle kinematic plot associated with the foot from Figure 4-7A (The normal curve is shown by the solid black line, and the subject's profile is shown by the dashed black line.) When the foot is well aligned, there will be agreement between observational gait analysis, which would show a toe–toe gait pattern; the clinical examination, which would show limited ankle dorsiflexion; and the kinematic profile at the ankle, which shows plantar flexion in both stance and swing phases. Figure 4-7C shows a foot with equinoplanovalgus segmental malalignment, with the standard marker placement (solid circles) associated with the single segment foot kinematic model. The hindfoot remains in equinus, but the forefoot is dorsiflexed (through the midfoot) relative to the hindfoot (solid curved arrow). Figure 4-7D shows the sagittal plane ankle kinematic plot associated with the foot from Figure 4-7C. (The normal curve is shown by the solid black line, and the subject's profile is shown by the dashed black line.) When the foot is malaligned, there will be apparent disagreement between observational gait analysis, which would show a toe–toe or flat foot gait pattern; the clinical examination, which would show limited ankle dorsiflexion; and the kinematic profile at the ankle, which shows dorsiflexion in both stance and swing phases. The deficiency in the kinematic data is a consequence of the simplistic, single-segment foot model.

modeling assumptions and approximations concerning the relationship between the markers and the underlying skeletal anatomy (12,14,27). The standard ankle and foot model most commonly used in clinical gait analysis was developed in the early 1980s (11,12). In this model, the orientation of the tibia is determined by the location of a vector between the calculated knee and ankle joint centers (as determined from distal femoral condylar markers and medial and lateral malleoli markers, respectively). The orientation of the foot is defined by a vector that passes from the calculated ankle joint center (medial and lateral malleoli markers) to the space between the second and third metatarsals (a single, dorsal forefoot marker). In this single-segment foot model, it is assumed that the foot segment is relatively rigid from the hindfoot to the forefoot. Ankle motion in the sagittal plane is calculated from the location of the foot axis relative to the tibial axis (Figure 4.7). Any motion between the forefoot marker and the malleolar markers in the sagittal plane is described by the computer as ankle dorsi- or plantar flexion. Any movement between the primary segments of the foot (e.g., hindfoot to midfoot, midfoot to forefoot) that occurs between these two marker groups will be captured by this simple foot model and described as ankle motion. Significant measurement artifact occurs when the integrity of the foot segmental alignment is compromised (e.g., equinoplanovalgus foot malalignment seen in children with cerebral palsy [CP]) (11). This creates apparent discrepancies between the data derived from the physical examination, observational gait analysis, and quantitative gait analysis, which may result in confusion for clinicians and compromise clinical decision making.

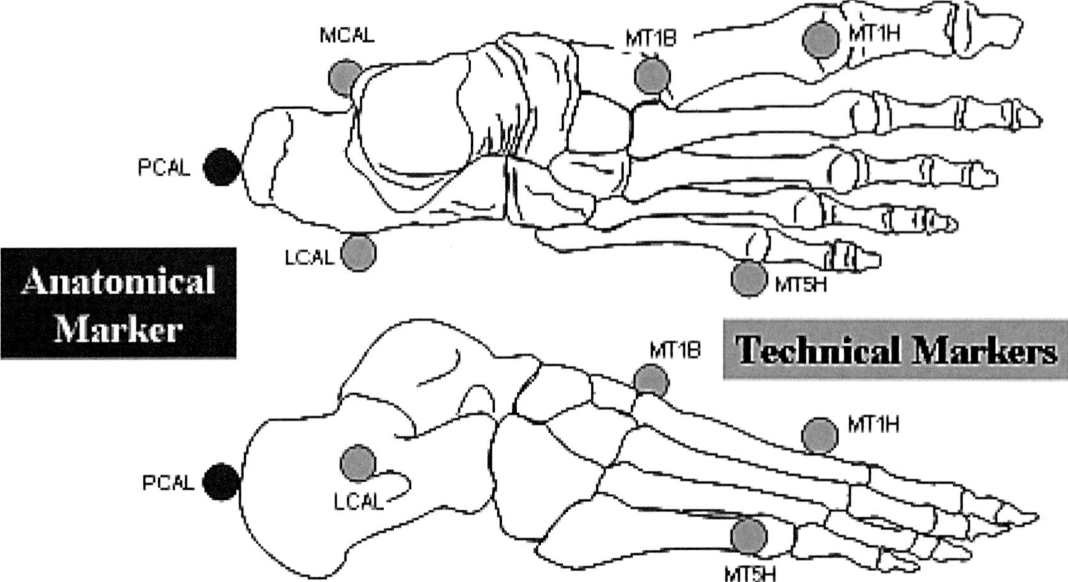

FIGURE 4-8 Diagram of the two-segment foot model. The single anatomical marker must be placed precisely over the posterior prominence of the calcaneus. The five technical markers require less precise positioning, and are utilized to determine virtual points that define the longitudinal axes of each segment (hindfoot and forefoot) of the model. (PCAL = posterior calcaneus, MCAL = medial calcaneus, LCAL = lateral calcaneus, MT1B = base of first metatarsal, MT1H = head of first metatarsal, MT5H = head of fifth metatarsal)

This simplistic, single-segment foot model was developed and adopted for clinical use in the 1980s because it was the best that movement measurement technology would allow at the time. Advances in marker, camera, and computer technologies now support improved spatial measurement resolution, potentially allowing more markers to be placed and tracked on a small limb segment such as the foot. This has created the opportunity to develop more sophisticated, multi-segment foot models that more accurately approximate the complex anatomy and biomechanics of the foot (6,11,24). The majority of these more advanced models have been developed for adult feet with easily identifiable skeletal landmarks that facilitate accurate marker placement. Unfortunately, children with conditions such as CP or clubfoot typically have very small feet (inter-marker distances are reduced beyond the ranges of resolution) that are deformed (segmental malalignment may obscure anatomical landmarks and compromise accurate marker placement). A foot model specifically for children, based on the Inman foot model discussed earlier, has been developed (11). This model consists of two segments (hindfoot and forefoot) that are tracked in three dimensions (Figure 4-8). The orientation of the two segments are calculated from a single anatomically precise marker, and five technical markers that require less precise positioning. These technical markers are clustered and utilized to determine virtual points that define the longitudinal axes of each segment (hindfoot and forefoot) of the model. This model should generate information that is clinically useful for clinical decision making for children regarding orthotic prescriptions, surgical planning, and post-intervention outcome assessment.

Dynamic Pedobarography

As noted above, clinical decision making for the treatment of ankle and foot deformities in children has been based primarily on the physical examination and static plain radiographs. The value of predicting dynamic function based on static alignment has been challenged by a study in adults which determined that only 35% of the variance in dynamic foot loading patterns, as determined by pedobarography, was explained by static foot alignment as determined by plain radiographs (7). Dynamic pedobarography is the measurement of the spatial and temporal distribution of force over the plantar aspect of the foot during the stance phase of the gait cycle. Pedobarography provides quantitative information regarding dynamic foot function, consisting of foot contact patterns, pressure distribution and magnitude, and progression of the center of pressure(25,30). In ambulatory individuals with peripheral neuropathies and diminished sensation, foot pressure distribution and magnitude have been utilized to predict regions of the foot that are at risk for overload and ulceration, and to assess the efficacy of various treatment interventions designed to offload such areas (4,16,17,23,30). In children, foot dysfunction during gait is primarily a consequence of skeletal segmental malalignment that compromises the shock absorption function during the first rocker, stability during the second rocker, and diminishes the moment arm available to the plantarflexor muscles during the third rocker in the stance phase of gait (13,15,26). This biomechanical disruption has been termed lever arm deficiency, and is best characterized by the center of pressure progression (COPP) relative to the foot.

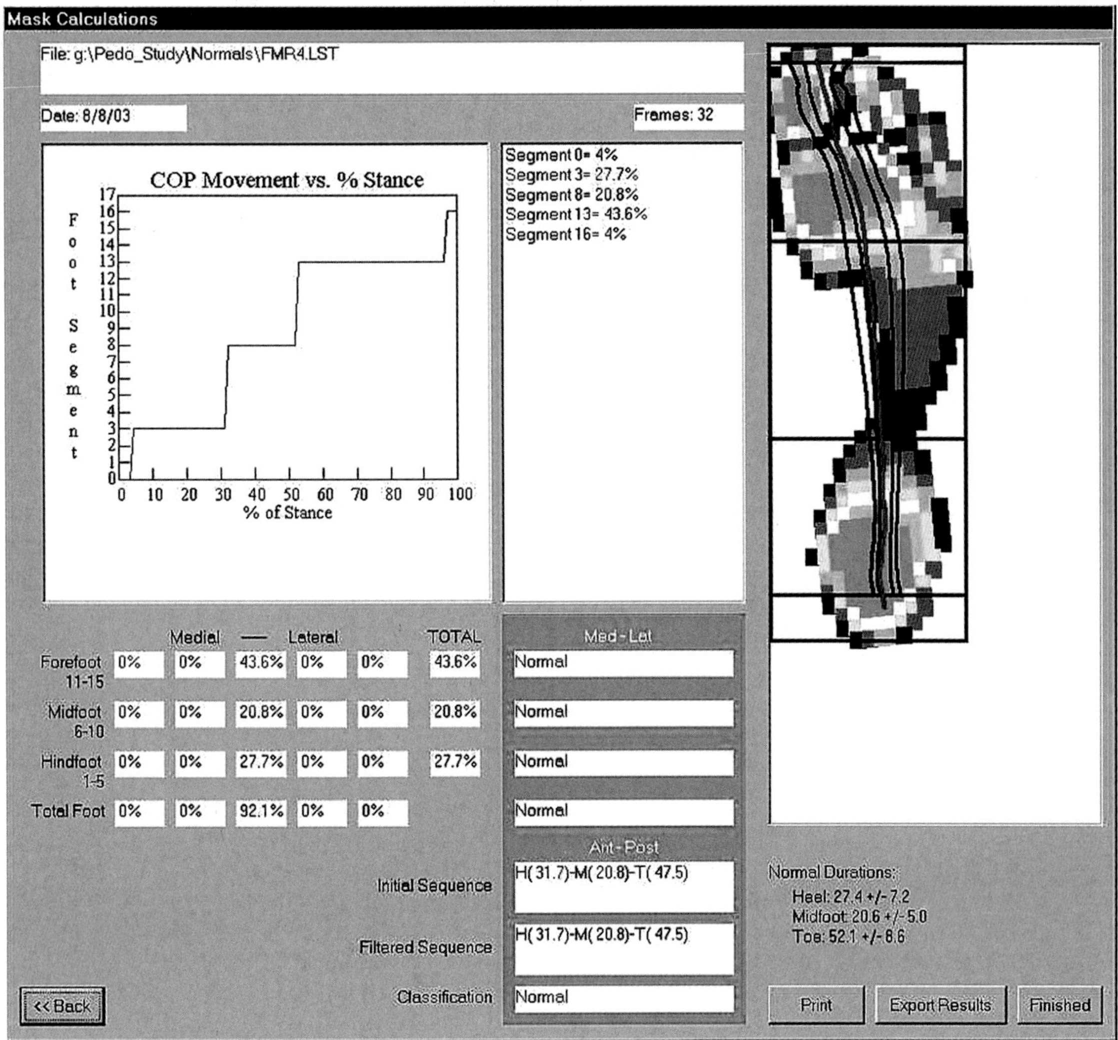

FIGURE 4-9 Representative pedobarograph display for a normal subject. The qualitative display of the data is seen in the upper right segment of the display. In this normal subject, the center of pressure progression (COPP, solid red line) passes through the middle segments of the hindfoot, midfoot, and forefoot. The quantitative display of the data is seen in the upper and lower left segments of the display. The graph in the upper left segment plots foot segment on the vertical axis and percent of stance phase on the horizontal axis. The normal center of pressure progression occurs in a stair step sequence from foot segment 3 to 8 to 13. The boxes in the lower left segment show the duration of the center of pressure, as percent of stance phase duration, in each of the foot segments. Automated pattern recognition analysis is shown in the middle lower segment. Foot loading patterns may be recognized in medial-lateral and anterior-posterior directions.

Although pedobarography has been utilized in quantitative clinical gait analysis for children, the collection, processing, analysis, and interpretation of the data varies widely (5,33). Pedobarographic assessment of dynamic foot function in children may be limited by the segmental malalignment of the foot and incomplete contact of the foot with the floor associated with pathologic gait. For use in patient care decision making, clinicians require a method of quantitative plantar pressure analysis that is practical, repeatable, and reliable for the routine clinical assessment in children with specific disease processes. A method for the application of dynamic pedobarography to children, focusing primarily on the COPP, has been developed (21). This technique utilizes the pedobarograph to document the location and duration of the COPP relative to the hindfoot, midfoot, and forefoot segments of the foot. The pedobarograph COPP data is presented both qualitatively and quantitatively, to facilitate utilization by clinicians for decision making (Figure 4-9). Location and duration of the COPP relative to the segments of the foot can be used to describe common abnormal loading patterns of the foot (Figure 4-10). Displacement of the COPP medially in a particular segment of the foot describes a valgus loading pattern, which might be the consequence of an everted, abducted, or pronated segmental malalignment of the foot segment. Displacement of the COPP laterally in a particular segment of the foot describes a varus loading pattern, which might be the consequence of an inverted, adducted, or supinated

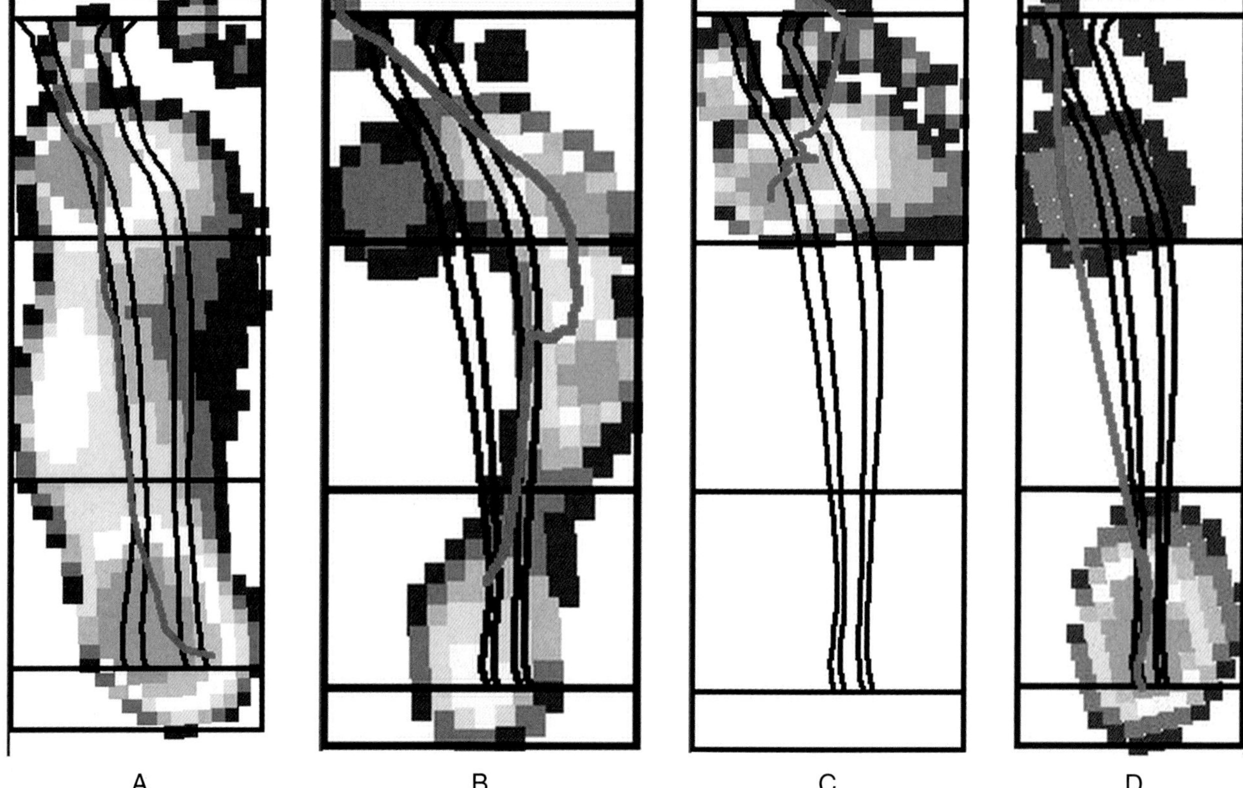

FIGURE 4-10 Abnormal foot loading patterns. (All examples are of the right foot.) Figure 4-10A shows displacement of the center of pressure progression (COPP, solid red line) medially, which describes a valgus loading pattern. Figure 4-10B shows displacement of the COPP laterally, which describes a varus loading pattern. Figure 4-10C shows displacement of the COPP distally, which describes an equinus loading pattern. Figure 4-10D shows displacement of the COPP proximally, which describes a calcaneus loading pattern.

segmental malalignment of the foot segment. Prolonged duration of the COPP in the forefoot segment describes an equinus foot loading pattern. Prolonged duration of the COPP in the hindfoot segment describes a calcaneus loading pattern. This standardized approach to the determination of foot loading patterns, based on normative data, should facilitate the characterization of abnormal foot loading patterns, clinical decision making, and the assessment of outcome following a variety of interventions.

SUMMARY

Proper alignment of the ankle and foot during the gait cycle is essential for optimal function and efficiency. The ankle and foot contribute to shock absorption in loading response, stability in mid stance, lever arm optimization in terminal stance, and clearance in swing phase. Ankle and foot alignment is tightly coupled to knee alignment, particularly in mid stance. Plain radiographs of the ankle and foot allow for a quantitative, static assessment of alignment, which may not be predictive of dynamic functional alignment during the gait cycle. Methods for the dynamic assessment of ankle and foot function include kinematics and pedobarography. Both techniques have significant limitations and require refinements for optimal application in children with disorders of the ankle and foot. Future work undoubtedly will focus on the correlations between static and dynamic methods for the assessment of ankle and foot alignment and function.

REFERENCES

1. Alman BA, Craig CL, Zimbler S. Subtalar arthrodesis for stabilization of valgus hindfoot in patients with cerebral palsy. *J Pediatr Orthop* 13:634–641, 1993.
2. Aronson J, Nunley J, Frankovitch K. Lateral talocalcaneal angle in assessment of subtalar valgus: follow-up of seventy Grice-Green arthrodeses. *Foot Ankle* 4:56–63, 1983.
3. Beatson TR, Pearson JR. A method of assessing correction in club feet. *J Bone Joint Surg Br* 48:40–50, 1966.
4. Betts RP, Franks CI, Duckworth T, et al. Static and dynamic foot-pressure measurements in clinical orthopaedics. *Medical & Biological Engineering & Computing* 18:674–684, 1980.
5. Bowen TR, Miller F, Castagno P, et al. A method of dynamic foot-pressure measurement for the evaluation of pediatric orthopaedic foot deformities. *J Pediatr Orthop* 18:789–793, 1998.
6. Carson MC, Harrington ME, Thompson N, et al. Kinematic analysis of a multi-segment foot model for research and clinical applications: a repeatability analysis. *J Biomech* 34:1299–1307, 2001.

7. Cavanagh PR, Rodgers MM, Iiboshi A. Pressure distribution under symptom-free feet during barefoot standing. *Foot & Ankle* 7:262–276, 1987.
8. Close JR, Inman VT, Poor PM, et al. The function of the subtalar joint. *Clin Orthop* 50:159–179, 1967.
9. Davids JR, Gibson TW, Pugh LI. Quantitative segmental analysis of weight-bearing radiographs of the foot and ankle for children: normal alignment. *J Pediatr Orthop* 25:769–776, 2005.
10. Davids JR, Rowan F, Davis RB. Indications for orthoses to improve gait in children with cerebral palsy. *J Am Acad Orthop Surg* 15:178–188, 2007.
11. Davis RB, Jameson EG, Davids J R, et al. The Design, Development, and Initial Evaluation of a Multisegment Foot Model for Routine Clinical Gait Analysis. In: Harris GF, Smith P and Marks R, eds. *Foot and Ankle Motion Analysis: Clinical Treatment and Technology.* Boca Raton: CRC Press, 425–444, 2007.
12. Davis RB, Tyburski D, Gage JR. A gait analysis data collection and reduction technique. *Human Movement Science* 10:575–587, 1991.
13. Gage JR. The clinical use of kinetics for evaluation of pathologic gait in cerebral palsy. *Instr Course Lect* 44:507–515, 1995.
14. Gage JR, DeLuca PA, Renshaw TS. Gait analysis: principle and applications with emphasis on its use in cerebral palsy. *Instr Course Lect* 45:491–507, 1996.
15. Gage JR, Novacheck TF. An update on the treatment of gait problems in cerebral palsy. *J Pediatr Orthop B* 10:265–274, 2001.
16. Holmes GB, Timmerman L, Willits NH. Practical considerations for the use of the pedobarograph. *Foot & Ankle* 12:105–108, 1991.
17. Hughes J. The clinical use of pedobarography. *Acto Orthopaedica Belgica* 59:10–16, 1993.
18. Inman VT. The human foot. *Manit Med Rev* 46:513–515, 1966.
19. Inman VT. The influence of the foot-ankle complex on the proximal skeletal structures. *Artif Limbs* 13:59–65, 1969.
20. Inman VT, Ralston HJ, Todd F. *Human Walking.* Baltimore: Williams & Wilkins, 1981.
21. Jameson EG, Davids JR, Anderson JP, et al. Dynamic pedobarography for children: use of the center of pressure progression. *J Pediatr Orthop* Accepted for publication 2007.
22. Keim HA, Ritchie GW. Weight-bearing roentgenograms in the evaluation of foot deformities. *Clin Orthop* 70:133–136, 1970.
23. Lundeen S, Lundquist K, Cornwall MW, et al. Plantar pressures during level walking compared with other ambulatory activities. *Foot & Ankle International* 15:324–328, 1994.
24. MacWilliams BA, Cowley M, Nicholson DE. Foot kinematics and kinetics during adolescent gait. *Gait Posture* 17:214–224, 2003.
25. Nicolopoulos CS, Giannoudis PV, Stergiopoulos KA. History and literature review of plantar pressure measurement studies and techniques. *Journal of Hellenic Association of Orthopaedics and Traumatology* 52;2001.
26. Ounpuu S, Bell KJ, Davis RB 3rd, et al. An evaluation of the posterior leaf spring orthosis using joint kinematics and kinetics. *J Pediatr Orthop* 16:378–384, 1996.
27. Perry J. *Gait Analysis: Normal and Pathological Function.* Thorofare, NJ: Slack Inc., 1992.
28. Ponseti IV, El-Khoury GY, Ippolito E, et al. A radiographic study of skeletal deformities in treated clubfeet. *Clin Orthop* 30–42, 1981.
29. Saunders JB, Inman VT, Eberhart HD. The major determinants in normal and pathological gait. *J Bone Joint Surg Am* 35–A:543–558, 1953.
30. Schaff PS. An overview of foot pressure measurement systems. *Clinics in Podiatric Medicine and Surgery* 10:403–415, 1993.
31. Simons GW. A standardized method for the radiographic evaluation of clubfeet. *Clin Orthop* 107–118, 1978.
32. Steel MW 3rd, Johnson KA, DeWitz MA, et al. Radiographic measurements of the normal adult foot. *Foot Ankle* 1:151–158, 1980.
33. Sutherland DH. Varus foot in cerebral palsy: an overview. *Instr Course Lect* 42:539–543, 1993.
34. Sutherland DH, Cooper L, Daniel D. The role of the ankle plantar flexors in normal walking. *J Bone Joint Surg Am* 62:354–363, 1980.
35. Vanderwilde R, Staheli LT, Chew DE, et al. Measurements on radiographs of the foot in normal infants and children. *J Bone Joint Surg Am* 70:407–415, 1988.

CHAPTER 5

Non-Operative Treatment of Congenital Clubfoot

Julie A. Coplan and John E. Herzenberg

INTRODUCTION

Idiopathic clubfoot is a common problem, affecting 1:1000 live birth (Figure 5-1) Today most orthopaedic surgeons agree that a system of clubfoot stretching, along with casting, bracing or strapping is the preferred initial method of clubfoot management in the newborn with congenital talipes equinovarus.

Historical Review

Hippocrates (460–377 BC) described the treatment of infant talipes equinovarus with manipulation and the use of a cloth bandage to secure the correction. Both Pare (1575) and Andry (1743) advocated manipulation and bandaging. Guerin (1836) was the first surgeon to use plaster casts. In 1921 Fiske (19) published the results of a questionnaire with 90% of respondents initiating care during the first month consisting of manipulation and casting.

Kite Method

Kite (1964)(28) became the first American whose non-operative technique of manipulation and casting received international acceptance. He utilized a dedicated clubfoot clinic and worked with trained nursing assistants who applied the plaster.

He employed gentle longitudinal traction with correction of the forefoot adduction occurring through the midtarsal joints. Kite grasped the forefoot with one hand and the heel with the other. He emphasized that the forefoot should be bent laterally without any twisting element. Next the heel was everted by putting pressure medially on the talar head with the thumb while attempting to reduce the navicular with the index finger of the opposite hand. This second step was discontinued when full forefoot abduction was accomplished. Dorsiflexion was attempted only after forefoot abduction and hindfoot inversion were fully corrected.

The cast was lightly padded. Kite initially created a plaster shoe which held the foot in as much abduction and dorsiflexion as the foot would be in when the cast was completed. The surgeon slipped his fingers out and set the foot on a plate glass. The foot was molded in abduction and under the arch and around the heel. The plaster extended beyond the toes and was carried by stages up to the mid thigh with the knee flexed 90 degrees.

Kite recommended weekly visits either with a cast change or a closing wedge taken out of the lateral cast and centered at the calcaneocuboid joint. He did not recommend day-time bracing following completion of casting. The patient used high-top laced brace shoes with a short leg brace and a valgus-producing T-strap at night. Parents stretched the foot in dorsiflexion twice daily. Recurrences were treated by the primary method.

Kite reported a 92% rates of success with 849 children with clubfeet using this non-operative method without the use of anesthesia or any form of surgery. An additional 73 patients initially treated by the Kite technique later underwent anesthesia. These included manipulation only (11), manipulation with tendo–Achillis lengthening (38) and tibialis anterior transfer (14). Other authors have not reported the same rate of success (2,50,53).

French Method

Bensahel (4) and Dimeglio introduced another non-surgical method of clubfoot management in 1972 which has been termed the French or functional method.

The French method describes progressive stretching and manipulation of the infant's foot (similar to the Ponseti manipulation), combined with stimulation of the peroneal muscles by a physical therapist. The manipulation/stimulation is done daily for 30 minutes per foot followed by non-elastic adhesive strapping to hold the position. The procedure is performed daily for 2 months then three times per week until the child ambulates. After the strapping has been completed a

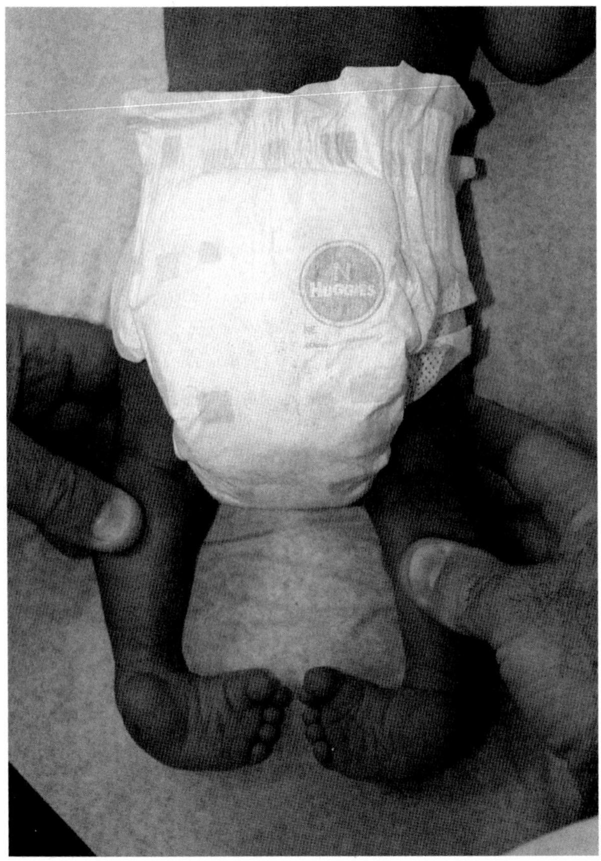

FIGURE 5-1 Idiopathic clubfeet in a newborn. Posterior view.

nighttime splint is used for an additional 2–3 years. The French method has also recently introduced the use of a CPM machine. In 1990 Bensahel et al (4) reported good success with this method (without CPM) in 48% of patients. With the use of the CPM, Richards (45) reported excellent or good results in 50%, fair in 29% and poor in 20% of patients. The French method is time consuming, costly due to the prolonged patient contact time required and dependent upon the quality of the manipulation perform by the physical therapist (46). For these reasons, it remains limited to specific geographic locations including France and Texas.

Ponseti (38) reviewed the outcomes of previous clubfoot care at the University of Iowa. Initial treatment consisted of some form of manipulation and casting, including the Kite method. Results were generally unsatisfactory and required extensive surgery which left the patient with "deep scarring, joint stiffness and weakness" (40). Although the rates of success in sort-term follow-ups of PMR surgery is described as good or excellent in 52% to 91% of cases, (9,10,33) long-term follow-ups of 10–15 years demonstrates less success with increasing foot pain and stiffness. (2,18,21,27). The unsatisfactory results from postero-medial releases (PMR) stimulated him to seek a better way to treat talipes equinovarus. The Ponseti method has recently gained international acceptance and is the most widely used technique today.

Ponseti Method

His method was based on his study of the pathoanatomy of talipes equinovarus. His protocol incorporates a program of anatomically-based foot manipulations, serial casting and bracing and is complimented by limited operative interventions.

From his study of the biomechanics, pathomechanics and structural physiology of talipes equinovarus, he deduced that the pronation mobilization Kite method actually served to lock the subtalar joint and prevented that joint from moving to a more anatomically normal position (44). He found that the forefoot needed to be lifted up to reduce the cavus, and align it with the hindfoot, and then the entire foot could be rotated (abducted) as a unit to correct the deformity through the normal range of movement of the subtalar joint. With the forefoot and rearfoot aligned, the midfoot and subtalar joint are unlocked, allowing abduction forces to move the foot through the subtalar joint, thus everting the calcaneus and allowing the calcaneus to rotate into eversion and abduction under the talus. The new idea of initiating clubfoot manipulation by lifting the first ray which bring the clubfoot into an even greater overall position of supination seemed counterintuitive to the practitioners of the Kite method.

His second major insight was into the problem of equinus. By the time the foot was thoroughly rotated externally through the subtalar joint, the equinus was only partly corrected. Ponseti realized that attempts to stretch the tight Achillis tendon were potentially dangerous, and could lead to crushing of the talus (the so-called 'nutcracker effect'). In order to deal with the residual equinus, Ponseti developed the concept of percutaneous Achillis tenotomy, which he applied in 90% of the cases. Immediately after the tenotomy the child was placed back in a long leg cast with the foot abducted for three weeks. The child used a Denis-Brown abduction orthosis for three months full-time and then for 10–14 hours per day. Ponseti estimated that in the United States in 2003, about 70% of clubfoot cases continue to be treated surgically, while about 30 percent are treated with the Ponseti Method (23).

Technique

The relaxed and quiet child can be positioned supine at the end of the plaster table or even in the mother's lap. The diaper needs to be undone from the limb to be casted in order to allow the cast to be extended high on the thigh. Raising the pelvis off the table by placing a small roll under it gives the practitioner better access to the limb. The mother should comfort the infant as needed, and feeding the infant during the casting often helps calm the baby.

Manipulation

The first cast manipulation is slightly different from all the following casts. In the first casting, the cavus is addressed by supinating and dorsiflexing the first metatarsal which brings the forefoot into alignment with the hindfoot. This places the metatarsals, navicular and cuneiforms in straight alignment which can be then be used as a lever arm for manipulating the foot out of inversion (Figure 5-2).

Once the forefoot has been aligned with the hindfoot, the foot is held in position with the first cast. Casts should be applied with an assistant holding the toes with only two fingers, and abducting the foot externally. One hand holds the baby at the level of the knee. The cast is applied with minimal padding, and wrapped snugly around the foot and less so around the calf and thigh. One week later (5–7 days) (36), the cast is removed either by soaking off the day of the clinic visit or carefully with a cast saw. The subsequent manipulations and castings are done by abducting the forefoot and applying counter-pressure to the neck of the talus to prevent a breach of the distal tibiofibular syndesmosis. It is important to apply the counter-pressure to the talus (sinus tarsi) and not to the calcaneus. This allows the entire foot to rotate laterally from underneath the talus. With counter-pressure on the talar head acting as a fulcrum the forefoot is abducted as a unit through force applied to the first metatarsal and cuneiform. As the navicular and cuneiform are displaced laterally, the anterior calcaneus is displaced anteriorly and upward correcting the varus deformity of the calcaneus without ever actually touching it. Manipulation continues in this manner until the foot is overcorrected into a position of 70 degrees of foot abduction (thigh foot angle) (Figure 5-3).

Casting

The cast should be snug, thinly padded and light weight. They are to be applied after performing the manipulations as described above. The practitioner should manipulate the foot gaining a good sense of how far the foot can be corrected on that day and to hold that idea in his mind as the cast is applied.

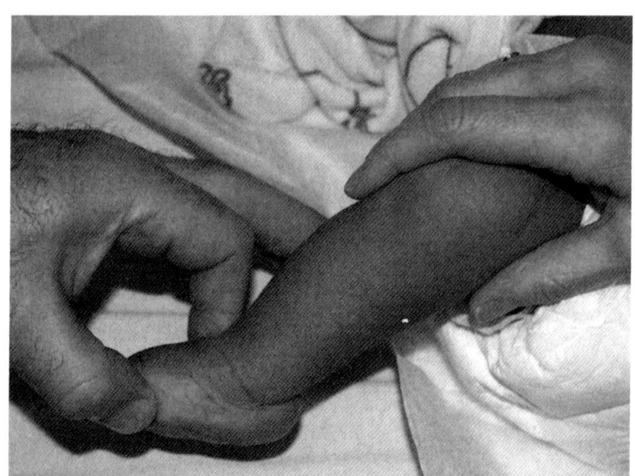

FIGURE 5-2 Elevation of first metatarsal.

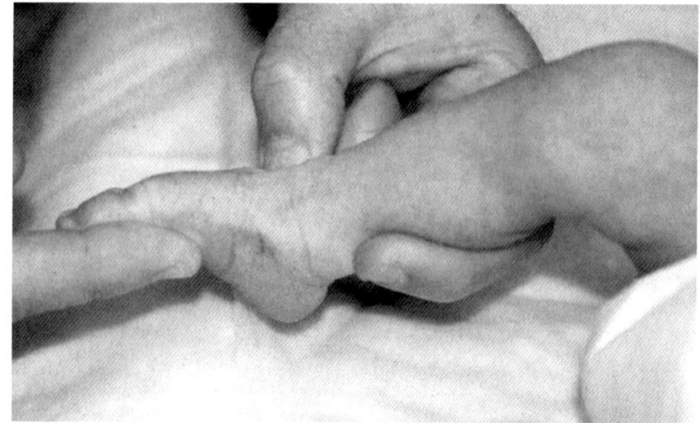

FIGURE 5-3 The basic Ponseti manipulation of abduction of the forefoot with counter pressure on the neck of the talus.

Two people are required to apply a cast. One holds the child's leg while the other applies the padding, plaster, and then molds the hardening cast. Throughout the cast application the child's leg should be held by the "holder" in the final casting position so that the padding and plaster do not bind when the child's knee is flexed 90 degrees. The foot is everted to the maximum position achieved comfortably and the tibia is slightly externally rotated. The "holder" sitting at the child's feet, holds the foot at the metatarsal heads/phalanges with only two fingers in alignment with the foot. This decreases interference of the fingers with the cast. The "holders" other hand is at the thigh keeping the knee flexed 90 degrees, and the tibia slightly externally rotated (Figure 5-4).

The "molder" may apply Tincture of Benzoin to sites on the leg to help keep the soft padding from slipping as the cast is applied. One of two layers of Soft Roll padding is applied. An extra layer or two can be added at the toes and the thigh to cushion the edges. Small longitudinal strips of cast padding can be judiciously used to cushion the malleoli, heel, and to create a strip along the medial and lateral sides of the cast to prevent cast saw burns. Cast saws are not used in Ponseti's clinic. Instead, the preferred method of removal is partial soaking in the clinic followed by removal with a cast knife (Figure 5-5).

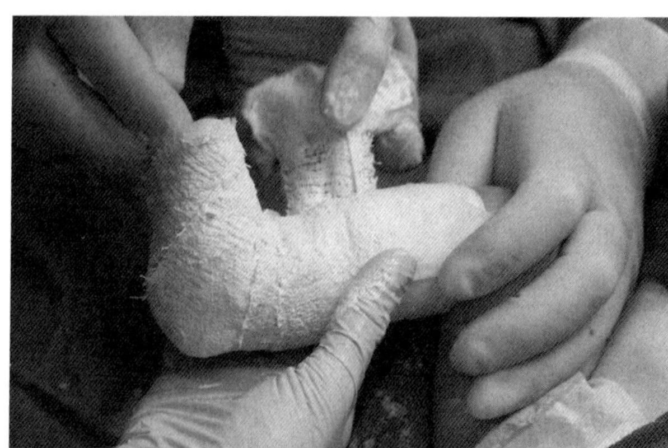

FIGURE 5-4 Holding the foot and rolling the plaster.

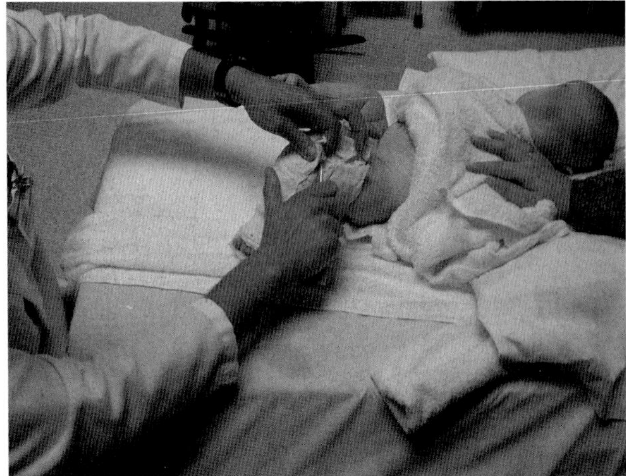

FIGURE 5-5 Removal of cast with cast knife after partial soaking.

Begin by applying a short leg cast. Too much padding or a loose cast will not hold the corrected position. While rolling the cast, tension must be snug at the foot and ankle and can be less at the tibia and femur. Once the short leg cast is applied, the molding begins. Pressure must be maintained consistently over the talar head. It is recommended to move the thumb gently around a small area of the talar head to reduce the risk of creating a pressure sore on the neck of the talus. Overhand and underhand techniques of holding are essentially equivalent. Once the short leg cast is fairly hard, it is then run up to a long leg cast, with the knee bent 90 degrees to prevent slippage, and with the knee slightly rotated externally (Figure 5-6). Trim the toe section to expose the fifth toe, but leave the plantar surfaces supported to help stretch out the toe flexors. A common beginner error is to leave the toes unsupported. Instruct the parents to check daily for signs of cast slippage. If the cast begins to slip, the parents should soak off the cast immediately. A slipped cast can cause swollen painful feet and pressure sores which will complicate the treatment, and even lead

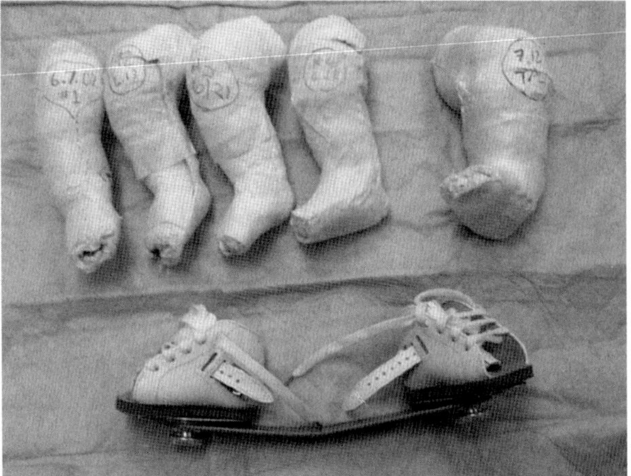

FIGURE 5-7 Series of casts, and boots and bars.

to the development of an iatrogenic atypical clubfoot (43). Five to six casts are required on average for a typical clubfoot. The observer can see the progression of improvement in foot alignment by comparing the series of casts (Figure 5-7).

Tenotomy

In most cases, after a series of 4–8 casts, depending on the severity of the foot, the position is markedly improved, the heel is in valgus, and up to 70 degrees of abduction is achieved. At this point, the foot is typically in neutral position, but not dorsiflexed. The residual equinus is now addressed with a percutaneous tenotomy. Only the mildest of feet can be managed without tenotomy. The practitioner must be careful that the foot does not cosmetically appear dorsiflexed due to breakdown of the structures in the mid foot causing a 'rocker bottom' foot. When dorsiflexion is in question an x-ray can quantitatively determine true dorsiflexion and the need for tenotomy. If the stress lateral dorsiflexion x-ray shows more "dorsiflexion" through the midfoot than the hindfoot, then a tenotomy should be done (14,44) (Figure 5-8).

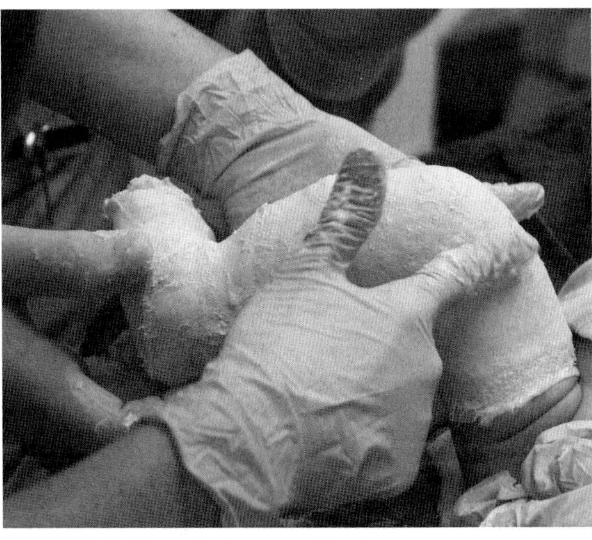

FIGURE 5-6 Long leg cast completed.

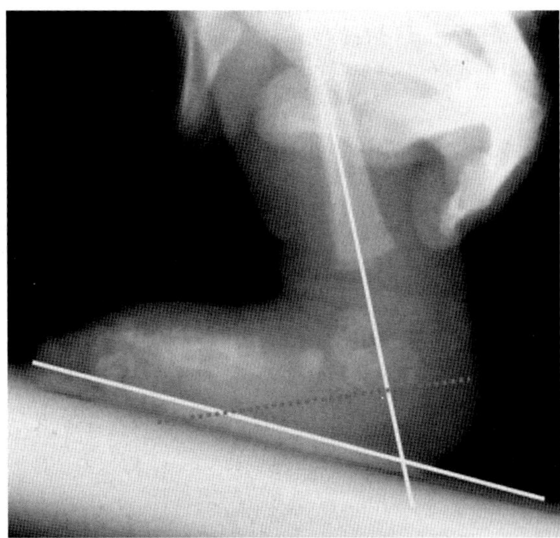

FIGURE 5-8 Pseudodorsiflexion in a mild clubfoot.

The tenotomy is typically done in the clinic with local anesthesia. The skin is cleansed, and Emla cream may be applied to the back of the Achillis tendon for 45 minutes for additional analgesia (6). The leg is prepped with Betadine and sterile towel drapes applied. The area just anterior and medial to the tendon about 10–15 mm above the calcaneus is infiltrated with a few tenths of a milliliter of 1 percent xylocaine. Do not use too much, or the anatomical landmarks will be obscured. It is a mistake to make the tenotomy too distal (at the calcaneal insertion) where the tendon is fanning out. The tenotomy itself is done with a 15 scalpel or a 64 Beaver blade. Insert the blade, palpate anterior and posterior to the tendon to define it, and then turn the blade 90 degrees to face posterior while dorsiflexing the foot. Be careful not to button hole through the posterior skin. When the tendon has been cut, there is a palpable "pop", and the foot can be dorsiflexed about 15 degrees more than preoperatively (Figure 5-9). If desired, stress lateral dorsiflexion radiographs can be made before and after the tenotomy to document the improvement in the dorsiflexion of the calcaneus (14,44) (Figure 5-10). Place either a band-aid or an absorbable stitch in the wound, and then apply a well padded, well molded Ponseti cast in maximum dorsiflexion. Inform the parents that bleeding on the cast should be minimal, no more than quarter sized and have them watch for or be aware of other bleeding complications, such as pseudoaneurysms, that can arise (8,17). The cast will be worn for three weeks.

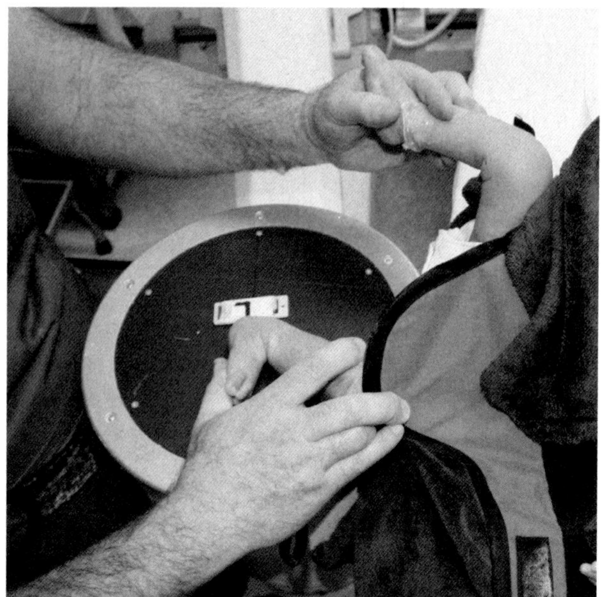

FIGURE 5-10 C-arm in the clinic for stress lateral dorsiflexion x-ray documentation.

Foot abduction brace program

On the day of the tenotomy, the child should be measured for shoes and a foot abduction brace (FAB). The family is instructed to bring the shoes and FAB with them when they return in three weeks to have the tenotomy cast removed.

There are two systems used with the FAB. The traditional shoe is either a Blucher or lace to the toes style and may have an open toe and open heel. The Mitchell and Ponseti shoe is often used and looks more like a sandal with three soft leathered buckle straps, and open toe and heel and is made of soft silicone (Figure 5-11). The shoes or sandals are securely attached to the rigid FAB. The shoes can be abducted on the bar with the distance between the heels of the shoes equal to the width of the child's shoulders. The bar is bent to have a slightly concave shape to place the feet in a dorsiflexed position. Recently, Dobbs has introduced a modified abduction bar that is articulated, and allows motion at the feet, thus increasing the comfort level and possibly the compliance with the bracing (11) (Figure 5-12).

The parents are taught how to apply the shoes and FAB. A break-in period may be used to acclimate the child to the FAB, but within 2–3 days, the baby should be wearing the shoes and bars for 23 hours per day, and continue for three full months. Then the child's wear time is reduced to nights and naps only. Recently, it has been advocated by the Iowa group that the transition from 23 hours per day to night time be gradual over a few months. When the Ponseti technique is initiated within the first few weeks of life then the child will be wearing

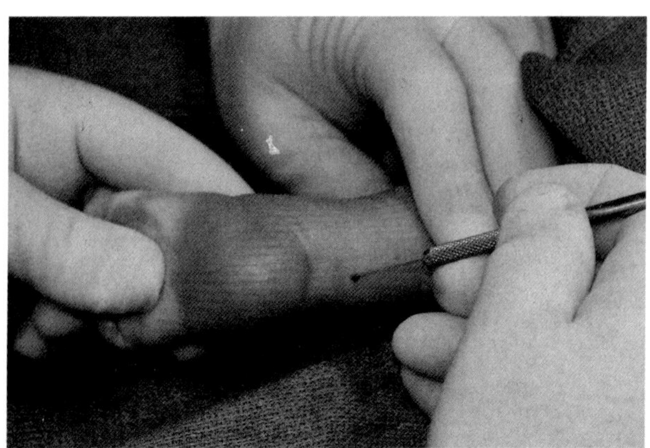

FIGURE 5-9 Percutaneous tenotomy with a 64 Beaver blade.

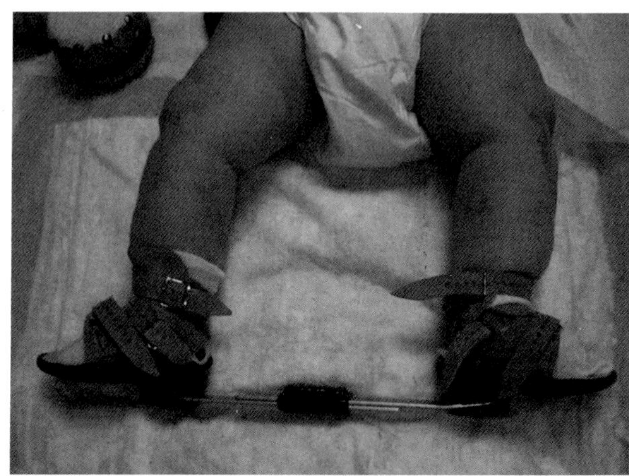

FIGURE 5-11 Mitchell Foot Abduction Brace.

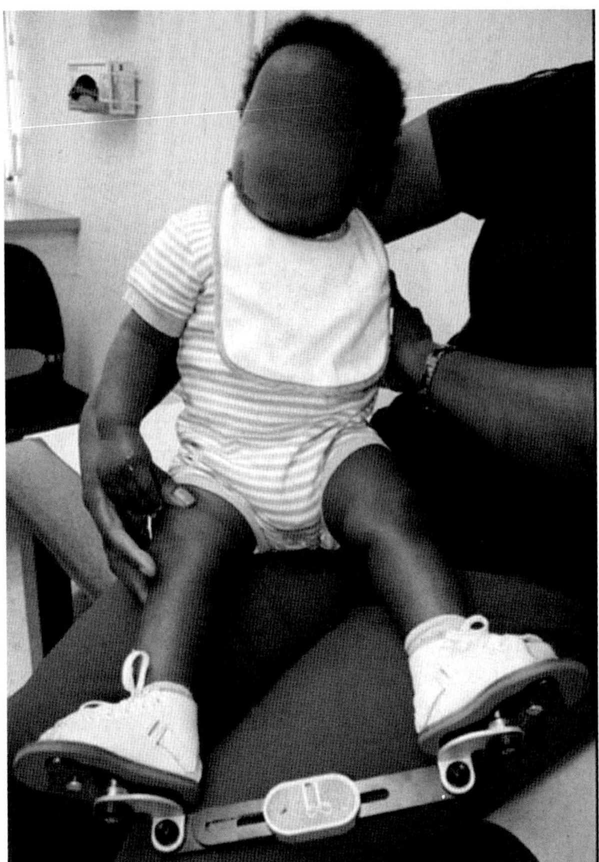

FIGURE 5-12 Dobbs articulated abduction bar with Markell shoes.

them for nights and naps only by four months of age. There seems to be no delay in motor or neurological development with this approach. Ponseti advises the shoes and FAB be worn for nights and naps until the child is four years of age, and in selected cases, longer.

Parent education

One of the most critical factors of success of the program is the family's ability to carefully follow the program. When the program is adhered to rigidly there is a 95% rate of success (25). Studies have shown that there is an 89% chance of relapse when the child stops wearing the shoes and bars prematurely (35). The Ponseti practitioner and family should work together to remove any barriers to adherence with the bracing program. The more the practitioner can do to enlist the parents full cooperation in the program the greater the chance of success. The earlier the parents begin to learn about clubfoot management, the sooner they feel empowered and better able to manage the child. It is possible to discuss these issues even during a prenatal consultation when clubfoot is discovered on routine prenatal ultrasound.

While not part of the formal Ponseti protocol, we recommend a series of simple home exercises to help maintain foot mobility during the bracing phase. These exercise include dorsiflexion with foot eversion, plantarflexion, and stimulation of the peroneal eversion reflex. The exercises should be performed twice daily, five repetitions each and the stretches should be held for 10 seconds. The exercises not only help to maintain foot mobility and flexibility but also bring the families' attention to the child's foot motion so that if there is an early relapse, it can be discovered earlier by the family. The family should be instructed to bring the child in for a check-up if the foot begins to lose mobility.

There is a great deal of information for the families of clubfoot babies to absorb. Educational hand-outs that the family can take home and review are helpful. Families should also be given practitioner contact information to assist them in managing problems that may occur. To this end, it is helpful in a busy clubfoot practice to have a nurse or physiotherapist to function as liaison and patient advocate. Indeed, it has been shown that a clubfoot clinic program administered by a dedicated physiotherapist can be more successful than one run by a harried orthopaedic surgeon (17). Many families find help and support from Ponseti parent support websites such as www.nosurgerv4 clubfoot.com.

RESULTS

Numerous studies have examined the efficacy of this technique and report rates of success from 90–95% (1,7,25,29,47). Ponseti's original publication in 1963 had 71% good results, 28% with slight residual deformity and 1 poor result (38). His protocol was modified to the more widespread use of tenotomies, and strict protocols for up to four years. His next publication had an 85-90% success rate (39).

Other Ponseti practitioners found similar success rates of the Ponseti method. Abdelgawad et al (1) reported a 93% success rate at 2 years with no need for extensive surgery. Herzenberg et al (25) reported a 96% success rate in avoiding PMR surgery with the Ponseti method (Figures 5-13 and 5-14). Cooper and Deitz (12) published a study of a 30 year follow-up of Ponsetis patients and

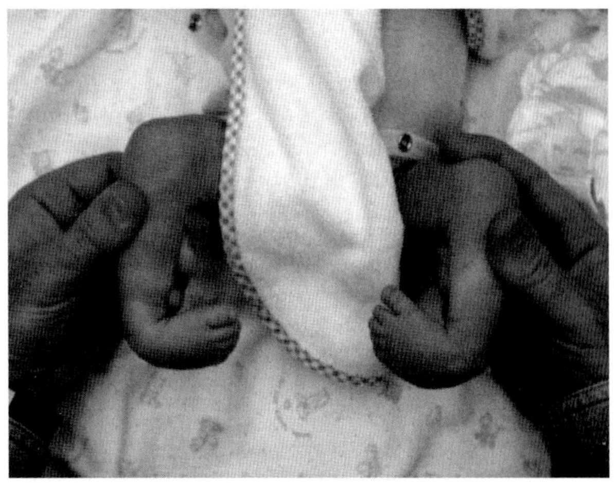

FIGURE 5-13 Idiopathic clubfeet before Ponseti casting.

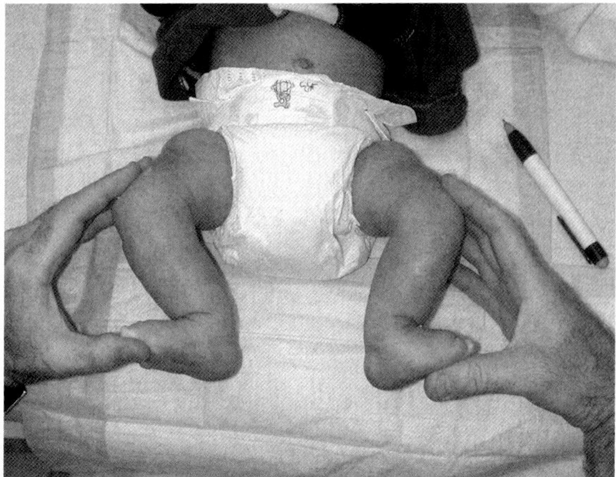

FIGURE 5-14 Idiopathic clubfeet after Ponseti casting and tenotomy.

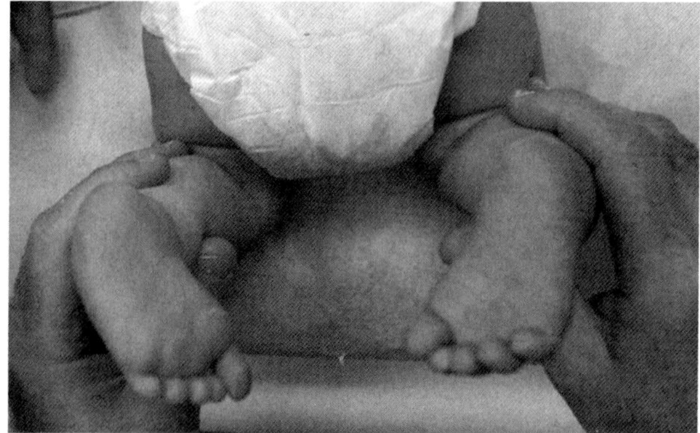

FIGURE 5-15 Relapsed clubfeet with internal rotation, adductus and varus.

found that 78% patients had an excellent or good functional and clinical outcomes compared to 85% of aged matched controls with no congenital foot deformity.

These results are in sharp contract to long-term surgical outcomes. Although the rates of success in short-term follow-up of PMR is described as good or excellent in 52% to 91% of cases (9,10,33). Long term follow-ups of 10–15 years demonstrate less success with an increasing incidence of foot pain and stiffness (2,18,21,27). Overcorrection and relapse may lead to the need to further surgery (3,30,50). Ponseti noted that the multiple chapters and articles on "complications of clubfoot surgery attest to the tragic failure of early surgery." (40).

RELAPSE MANAGEMENT

Recurrence of clubfoot is the return of one of the original primary clubfoot deformities which include equinus, varus, adduction and cavus. The most frequently recurring are equinus, calcaneo varus and over-active supination during gait (41). A study by Morcuende et al (35) in 2004 calculated the rate of relapse in 157 patients with 256 feet to be 11%. Only 1% of families compliant with the abduction brace experienced relapse where 89% of those families who were non-compliant experienced relapse. These statistics strongly supports the need for family compliance with the brace wearing schedule and the need for practitioners to frequently and firmly educate families about this need (15,16,24,35) (Figure 5-15). One of the prime pitfalls that Ponseti and others have observed in application of this technique is deviation from the originator's prescribed technique, which often leads to incomplete correction or relapse.

Relapse management in children younger than age two years is the same as the original treatment program. The child's foot is manipulated and recasted using the traditional method. One adjustment in the program is that the casts may be worn for two weeks instead of one week to give the older and stronger connective tissue more time to adapt. Typically relapse management requires only two to three casts before the desired 70 degrees of foot abduction is achieved. The child must then return to using the shoes and bars consistently for nights and naps or there is a high incidence of re-relapse.

Ponseti recognized the need for limited surgical management of clubfoot relapse and considers them part of the program. When a child experiences a relapse and after repeat casting does not achieve 15 degrees of dorsiflexion then a repeat percutaneous tenotomy or open Achilles tendon lengthening should be considered.

Tibialis anterior transfer

One of the common features of a clubfoot is the over-activity of the supinating muscles and under-activity of the everting muscles. Some children of walking age begin to demonstrate supination during swing and stance phase of gait due to this muscle imbalance. Such children may show excessive callus formation on the lateral border of the foot. Ponseti recommends an anterior tibial tendon transfer to the lateral cuneiform for these children over 2 1/2 years of age. The ossific nucleus of the lateral cuneiform must be visible on x-ray in order to effectively transfer the tendon. The tendon transfer may be done without preliminary casting when the foot is flexible but has a muscle imbalance. When the foot can be fully correctable passively, then it is imperative to initially cast the foot with classic long leg casts in order to obtain a well corrected foot prior to the tendon transfer. When necessary, an Achillis tendon lengthening and anterior tibialis tendon transfer can be performed at the same time.

Some families seem to have difficulty keeping their children in the shoes and FAB. After an anterior tibial tendon transfer, the shoes and FAB wear can be discontinued. A tendon transfer functions as a biologic brace, and may be a good solution for those families having difficulty with compliance wearing the orthotic.

Technique

The anterior tibial tendon is released from its insertion on the base of the first metatarsal and moved subcutaneously to an auxiliary anterolateral incision and reattached to the third cuneiform (Figure 5-16). By age 2 1/2 years

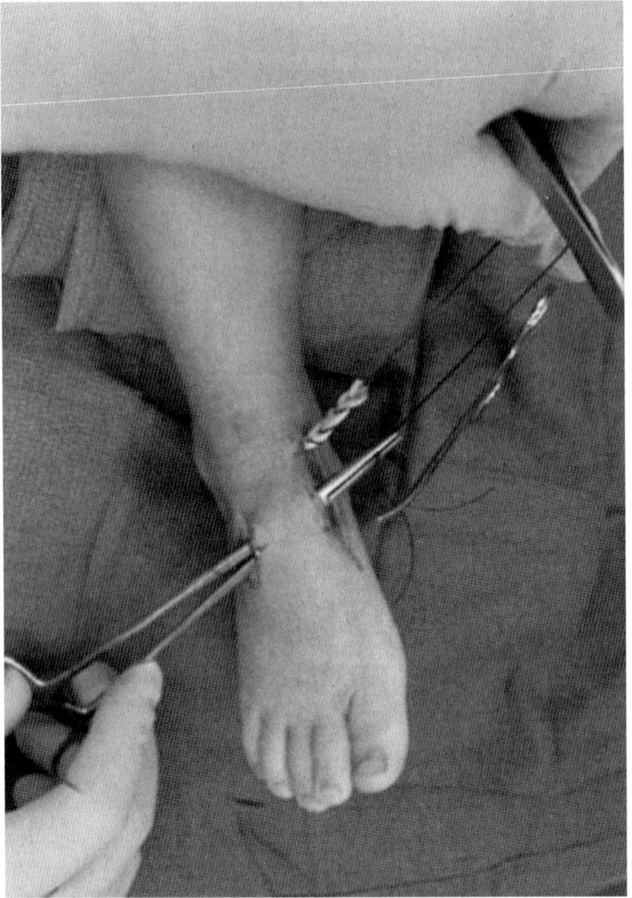

FIGURE 5-16 Anterior tibialis tendon about to be transferred subcutaneously to the lateral incision.

the ossific nucleus of the third cuneiform is sufficiently large to allow secure attachment of the anterior tibial tendon (15). The classical description by Garceau (20) called for pull out sutures tied over a sponge and button on the plantar surface of the foot. We have added an absorbable interference screw to help secure the tendon in addition to the pull out button. The screw makes it less necessary to tighten the pull out button very tightly on the skin, which can cause pressure sores.

Huang et al (26) questioned the need to wait to perform an anterior tibial tendon transfer until age 2 1/2 years of age. They demonstrated 91.8% good or excellent results in anterior tendon transfers in infants 6–12 months of age. Percutaneous tenotomies, Achilles tendon lengthening and anterior tibial tendon transfers are all joint sparing surgeries. Consequently they do not cause the joint stiffness and arthritis seen following PMRs and are considered part of the formal method. Success outcomes of 95 degrees are reported when the program is diligently followed (7).

THE ATYPICAL CLUBFOOT

Ponseti recently called attention to a small subset of clubfeet that are particularly stiff and resistant to manipulation (43). The feet do not respond well to casting and

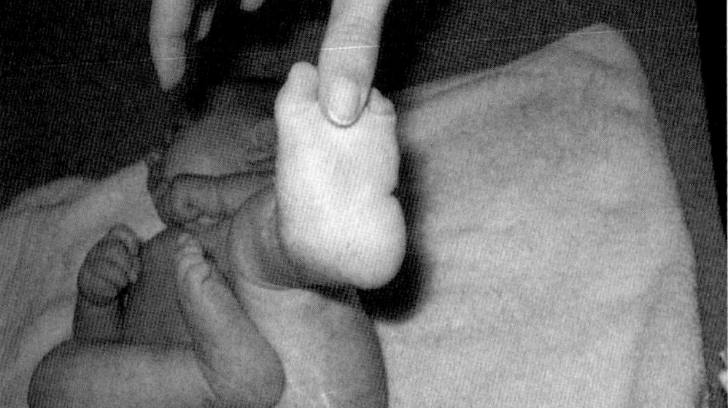

FIGURE 5-17 Atypical clubfoot demonstrating hyperabduction at Lisfranc joint.

usually appear short and fat with short metatarsals, rigid severe cavus and a hall mark deep transverse plantar crease. After two or three casts the metatarsals remain plantar flexed and the anterior tuberosity of the calcaneus remains caught under the head of the talus. Continued attempt to abduct the forefoot leads to hyperabduction of the forefoot alone and a lateral shift through the Lisfranc joint. The foot often becomes swollen and red. Ponseti called these feet atypical clubfeet (Figure 5-17).

He recognized the need to adjust the method of manipulations for these atypical clubfeet. If the foot is swollen and inflamed, he advised leaving the cast off for a week to allow the foot to settle down. He described an alternate manipulation ("Ponseti II") for the atypical clubfoot, consisting of pulling down on the dorsal talus with the fingers of both hands while pushing up on the metatarsal heads with both thumbs (Figure 5-18). The goal of foot abduction is reduced from 70 degrees to 40 degrees. An early tenotomy may be recommended. The post manipulation program remains similar to the typical clubfoot except for abducting the clubfoot to 40 degrees rather than 70 degrees in the foot ankle brace.

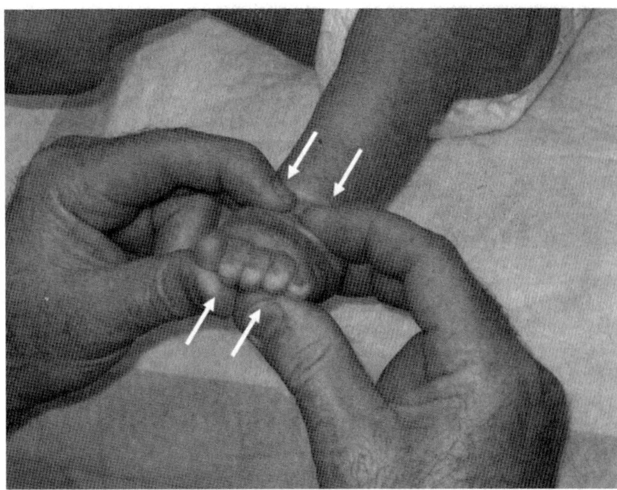

FIGURE 5-18 Ponseti II maneuver for atypical clubfoot.

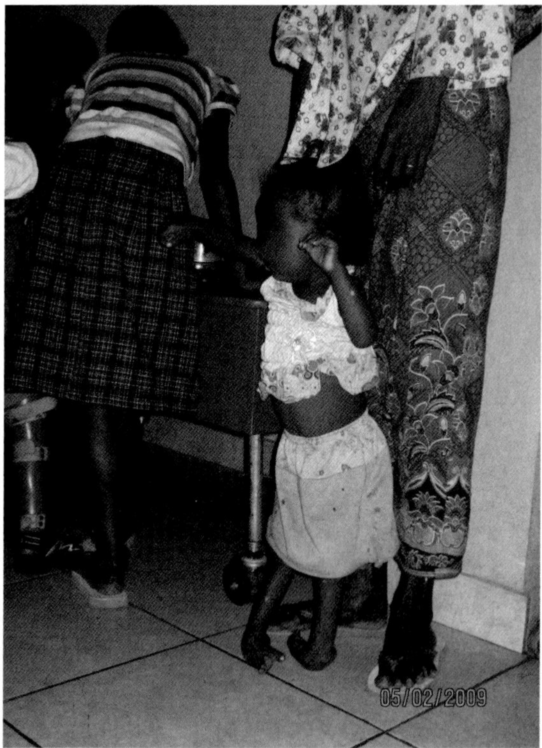

FIGURE 5-19 Neglected clubfeet in a child from East Timor.

TREATING THE OLDER CLUBFOOT

Neglected clubfeet are commonly seen in the developing world (Figure 5-19). Many of the 80,000 children with clubfeet have been under-treated or untreated because of the dearth of medical facilities and/or cost of treatment. As the Ponseti technique spreads to underdeveloped countries where surgical options are limited, some practitioners are using the method on older children with neglected clubfeet, often with very good outcomes (5,32,49). Additional studies are needed to determine a protocol for older children and find the optimal age where success is likely.

CLUBFOOT PROGRAM IN DEVELOPING COUNTRIES

In 1999 Pirani and Penny initiated the Uganda national clubfoot program. Their mission was to implement the Ponseti method of clubfoot treatment on a country-wide basis. They performed a pilot study (37) at Mulago Hospital, Makere University in Kampala. They treated 236 clubfeet in 155 consecutive patients who were 9 months of age or less using the method. One hundred eight infants with 182 clubfeet completed the corrective phase of the treatment. Of those 96.7% corrected well with the program. Three percent did not correct and underwent surgery. Twenty-three percent of infants with clubfeet did not complete the corrective phase of the treatment. Most of the infants in the study were treated by orthopaedic officers that were trained in the Ponseti method. An appropriate foot abduction brace was designed that could easily be made by local artisans for about $12 per brace (Figure 5-20).

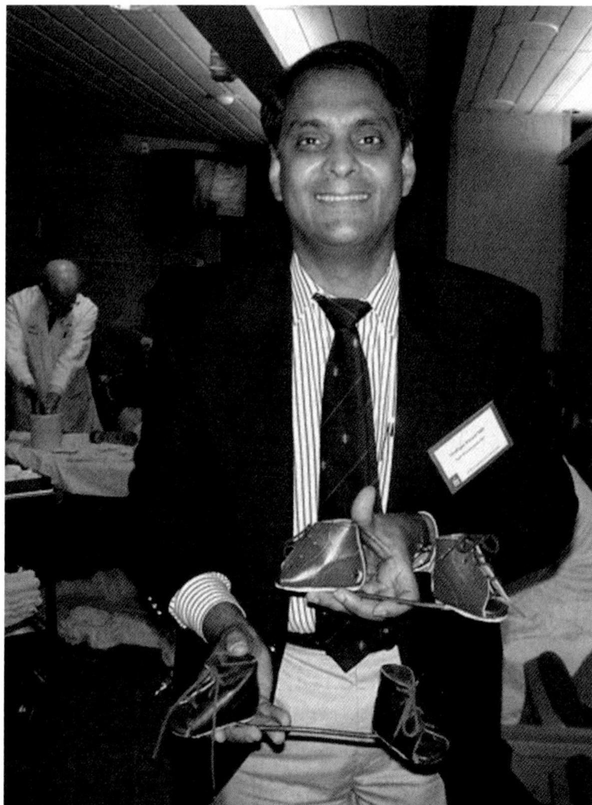

FIGURE 5-20 Dr. Shafique Pirani with the Steenbeek abduction orthosis made by local Ugandan artisans. Note Dr. Ponseti in the background, casting.

The developing world pilot data suggested a success rate of over 90% for infants who completed the Ponseti manipulation, casting and tenotomy treatment program (22,52). Resources and support are growing for a global initiative to eradicate the problem of the neglected clubfoot worldwide by introducing broad-based training of the Ponseti method, especially in the developing world (23,51).

REFERENCES

1. Abdelgawad AA, Lehman WB, van Bosse HJ, Scher DM, Sala DA. Treatment of idiopathic clubfoot using the Ponseti method: minimum 2-year follow-up. J Pediatr Orthop B. 2007 Mar; 16(2):98–105.
2. Aronson J, Puskarich CL. Deformity and disability from treated clubfoot. J Pediatr Orthop. 1990 Jan-Feb; 10(1):109–19.
3. Atar D, Lehman WB, Grant AD. Complications in clubfoot surgery. Orthop Rev. 1991 Mar; 20(3):233–9.Review.
4. Bensahel H, Guillaume A, Czukonyi Z, Desgrippes Y. Results of physical therapy for idiopathic clubfoot: a long-term follow-up study. J Pediatr Orthop. 1990 Mar-Apr; 10(2):189–92.

5. Bor N, Herzenberg JE, Frick SL. Ponseti management of clubfoot in older infants. Clin Orthop Relat Res. 2006 Mar; 444:224–8.
6. Bor N, Katz Y, Vofsi 0, Herzenberg JE, Zuckerberg AL. Sedation protocols for Ponseti clubfoot Achilles tenotomy. J Child Orthop. 2007 Dec; 1(6):333–5.
7. Bor N, Coplan JA, Herzenberg JE. Ponseti treatment for idiopathic clubfoot: minimum 5-year followup. Clin Orthop Relat Res. 2009 May; 467(5):1263–70.
8. Burghardt RD, Herzenberg JE, Ranade A. Pseudoaneurysm after Ponseti percutaneous Achilles tenotomy: a case report. J Pediatr Orthop. 2008 AprMay; 28(3):366–9.
9. Carroll NC, Gross RH. Operative management of clubfoot. Orthopedics. 1990 Nov; 13(11):1285–96.
10. Carroll NC. Clubfoot: what have we learned in the last quarter century? J Pediatr Orthop. 1997Jan-Feb; 17(1):l–2.
11. Chen RC, Gordon JE, Luhmann SJ, Schoenecker PL, Dobbs MB. A new dynamic foot abduction orthosis for clubfoot treatment. J Pediatr Orthop. 2007 Jul-Aug; 27(5):522–8.
12. Cooper DM, Dietz FR. Treatment of idiopathic clubfoot. A thirty-year follow-up note. J Bone Joint Surg Am. 1995 Oct; 77(10):1477–89.
13. Currier DP, Nelson RM. *Dynamics of Human Biologic Tissues.* Philadelphia, PA: F. A. Davis Company; 1992.
14. de Gheldere A, Docquier PL. Analytical radiography of clubfoot after tenotomy. J Pediatr Orthop. 2008 Sep; 28(6):691–4.
15. Dietz FR. Treatment of a recurrent clubfoot deformity after initial correction with the Ponseti technique. Instr Course Lect. 2006; 55:625–9. Review.
16. Dobbs MB, Rudzki JR, Purcell DB, Walton T, Porter KR, Gumett CA. Factors predictive of outcome after use of the Ponseti method for the treatment of idiopathic clubfeet. J Bone Joint Surg Am. 2004 Jan; 86-A(1):22–7
17. Dobbs MB, Gordon JE', Walton T, Schoenecker PL. Bleeding complications following percutaneous tendo Achilles tenotomy in the treatment of clubfoot deformity. J Pediatr Orthop. 2004 Jul-Aug; 24(4):353–7.
18. Dobbs MB, Nunley R, Schoenecker PL. Long term follow-up of patients with clubfeet treated with extensive soft-tissue release. J Bone Joint Surg Am. 2006 May; 88(5):986–96.
19. Fiske EW. Present tendencies in the treatment of clubfeet. J Orthop Surg. 1921 3:668–674.
20. Garceau Gl. Anterior tibial tendon transfer for recurrent clubfoot. Clin Orthop Relat Res.1972 May; 84:61–5.
21. Green AD, Lloyd-Roberts GC. The results of early posterior release in resistant club feet. A long-term review. J Bone Joint Surg Br. 1985 Aug; 67(4):588–93.
22. Gull A, Sambandam S. Results of manipulation of idiopathic clubfoot deformity in Malawi by orthopaedic clinical officers using the Ponseti method: a realistic alternative for the developing world? J Pediatr Orthop. 2007 Dec; 27(8):971.
23. Gupta A, Singh S, Patel P, Patel J, Varshney MK. Evaluation of the utility of the Ponseti method of correction of clubfoot deformity in a developing nation. Int Orthop. 2008 Feb; 32 (1): 75–9.
24. Haft GF, Walker CG, Crawford HA. Early clubfoot recurrence after use of the Ponsetimethod in a New Zealand population. J Bone Joint Surg Am. 2007 Mar; 89(3):487–93.
25. Herzenberg JE, Radler C, Bor N. Ponseti versus traditional methods of casting for idiopathic clubfoot. J Pediatr Orthop. 2002 Jul-Aug; 22(4):517–21.
26. Huang YT, Lei W, Zhao L, Wang 1. The treatment of congenital club foot by operation to correct deformity and achieve dynamic muscle balance. J Bone Joint Surg Br. 1999 Sep; 81(5):858–62.
27. Hutchins PM, Foster BK, Paterson DC, Cole EA. Long-term results of early surgical release in club feet. J Bone Joint Surg Br. 1985 Nov; 67(5):791–9.
28. Kite JH. The Clubfoot. 1964. New York: Grune & Sttatton.
29. Laaveg SJ, Ponseti IV. Long-term results of treatment of congenital club foot. J Bone Joint Surg Am. 1980 Jan; 62(1):23–31.
30. Lau JH, Meyer LC, Lau HC. Results of surgical treatment of talipes equinovarus congenita. Clin Orthop Relat Res. 1989 Nov; (248):219–26.
31. Lavy CB, Mannion S J, Mkandawire NC, Tindall A, Steinlechner C, Chimangeni S, Chipofya E. Club foot treatment in Malawi - a public health approach. Disabil Rehabil. 2007 Jun 15–30; 29(ll–12):857–62.
32. Lourenco AF, Morcuende JA. Correction of neglected idiopathic club foot by the Ponseti method. J Bone Joint Surg Br. 2007 Mar; 89(3):378–81.
33. McKay DW. New concept of and approach to clubfoot treatment: Section HJ-evaluation and results. J Pediatr Orthop. 1983 May; 3(2):141–8.
34. Morcuende JA, Egbert M, Ponseti IV. The effect of the internet in the treatment of congenital idiopathic clubfoot. Iowa Orthop J. 2003; 23:83–6.
35. Morcuende JA, Dolan LA, Dietz FR, Ponseti IV. Radical reduction in the rate of extensive corrective surgery for clubfoot using the Ponseti method. Pediatrics. 2004 Feb; l 13(2):376–80.
36. Morcuende JA, Abbasi D, Dolan LA, Ponseti IV. Results of an accelerated Ponseti protocol for clubfoot. J Pediatr Orthop. 2005 Sep-Oct; 25(5):623–6.
37. Penny IN, Pirani S, Morcuende JA, Schwentker E. The Ponseti Method of Clubfoot care: A vision for the developing world. Steps Charity, http://www.steps-charity.org.uk/downloads/A % 20Vision%20for%20the%20Developing%20World.pdf. Updated August 17, 2006. Accessed May 15, 2009.
38. Ponseti IV, Smoley EN. Congenital Club Foot: The Results of Treatment. J. Bone Joint Surg. Am., Mar 1963; 45:261–344.
39. Ponseti IV. Treatment of congenital club foot. J Bone Joint Surg Am. 1992 Mar; 74 (3): 448–54.
40. Ponseti IV. *Congenital Clubfoot: Fundamentals of Treatment.* New York, NY: Oxford University Press Inc.; 1996.
41. Ponseti IV. The Ponseti technique for correction of congenital clubfoot. J Bone Joint Surg Am. 2002 Oct; 84-A(l 0):1889–90; author reply 1890-1.
42. Ponseti IV, Morcuende JA. Current management of idiopathic clubfoot questionnaire: a multicenter study. J Pediatr Orthop. 2004 Jul-Aug; 24(4):448.
43. Ponseti IV, Zhivkov M, Davis N, Sinclair M, Dobbs MB, Morcuende JA. Treatment of the complex idiopathic clubfoot. Clin Orthop Relat Res. 2006 Oct; 451:171–6.
44. Radler C, Manner HM, Suda R, Burghardt R, Herzenberg JE, Ganger R, Grill F. Radiographic evaluation of idiopathic clubfeet undergoing Ponseti treatment. J Bone Joint Surg Am. 2007 Jun; 89(6):1177–83.
45. Richards BS, Johnston CE, Wilson H. Nonoperative clubfoot treatment using the French physical therapy method. J Pediatr Orthop. 2005 Jan-Feb; 25(1):98–102.
46. Richards BS, Faulks S, Rathjen KE, Karol LA, Johnston CE, Jones SA. A comparison of two nonoperative methods of idiopathic clubfoot correction: the Ponseti method and the French functional (physiotherapy) method. J Bone Joint Surg Am. 2008 Nov; 90(11):2313–21.
47. Segev E, Keret D, Lokiec F, Yavor A, Wientroub S, Ezra E, Hayek S. Early experience with the Ponseti method for the treatment of congenital idiopathic clubfoot. Isr Med Assoc J. 2005 May; 7(5):307–10.
48. Shack N, Eastwood DM. Early results of a physiotherapist-delivered Ponseti service for the management of idiopathic congenital talipes equinovarus foot deformity. J Bone Joint Surg Br. 2006 Aug; 88(8):1085–9.
49. Spiegel DA, Shrestha OP, Sitoula P, Rajbhandary T, Bijukachhe B, Banskota AK. Ponseti method for untreated idiopathic clubfeet in Nepalese patients from 1 to 6 years of age. Clin Orthop Relat Res. 2009 May; 467(5):1164–70.

50. Sud A, Tiwari A; Sharma D, Kapoor S. Ponseti's vs. Kite's method in the treatment of clubfoot—a prospective randomized study. Int Orthop. 2008 Jun; 32(3):409–13.
51. Tindall AJ, Steinlechner CW, Lavy CB, Mannion S, Mkandawire N. Results of manipulation of idiopathic clubfoot deformity in Malawi by orthopaedic clinical officers using the Ponseti method: a realistic alternative for the developing world? J Pediatr Orthop. 2005 Sep-Oct; 25(5):627–9.
52. Wilcox Carol. "A healing touch". *Iowa Alumni Magazine.* http://www.iowalum.com/magazine/feb03/exclusive/ponseti.html. Published February 2003. Accessed 30 Jun 2007.
53. Zimbler S. Practical considerations in the early treatment of congenital talipes equinovarus. Orthop Clin North Am. 1972 Mar; 3(1):251–9.

CHAPTER 6

Clubfoot: Operative Treatment

George H. Thompson and Hadeel Abaza

INTRODUCTION

Congenital talipes equinovarus (clubfoot) is one of the more common and complex pediatric foot deformities confronting the orthopaedic surgeon. Correction can be achieved through both nonoperative and operative methods. With the recent success of the Ponseti casting technique, however, there is agreement that the initial method of treatment should be nonoperative, regardless of the severity of the deformity. Recurrence of the deformity following the Ponseti technique is usually due to lack of compliance with appropriate bracing after correction has been achieved (17,23). Recurrence occurs most frequently during the first several years of life while the foot is rapidly growing. Repeat Ponseti casting may be beneficial in recurrent deformities. After failure of nonoperative treatment, extensive surgical releases have been shown to produce excellent or good results in a significant percentage of feet (12). The goal, regardless of method of treatment, is to achieve a functional, pain-free, plantigrade foot without the need for shoe-wear modifications. This section will deal with the initial operative treatment of resistant clubfeet. The treatment of recurrent deformities following surgery and their associated complications will be discussed in the next section.

PATHOANATOMY

Because the pathoanatomy of clubfoot deformities is complex, a thorough understanding is essential prior to undertaking surgical correction. Dissection studies and other analyses have helped to further our understanding (7,8,24,28,33,3447,48,50,56). These have identified the following major pathoanatomical abnormalities:

1. Lateral rotation of the body of the talus in the ankle mortise
2. Posterior deviation of the lateral malleolus
3. Talar and calcaneal equinus
4. Medial subluxation of the navicular on the head of the talus causing it to abut against the anterior aspect of the medial malleolus
5. Medial and plantar deviation of the talar neck
6. Medial rotation and supination (varus) of the calcaneus
7. Medial subluxation of the cuboid on the head of the calcaneus
8. Forefoot cavus
9. Soft-tissue contractures, especially the triceps surae, tibialis posterior, flexor hallucis longus, and flexor digitorum longus muscles and tendons which are short; the long and short plantar ligaments, spring ligament, posterior ankle capsule, the subtalar capsule, and the lateral ankle ligaments, and especially the posterior talofibular and calcaneofibular ligaments which are contracted.

Downey and Drennan (18) performed preoperative magnetic resonance imaging (MRI) studies on ten infants with congenital clubfeet and found essentially the same pathoanatomic abnormalities. They found MRI useful in defining cartilaginous anlage of the talus, calcaneus, and navicular. It was concluded that the primary problem in clubfeet is the deformity of the talar head and neck allowing the anterior aspect of the calcaneus to follow the deformed talus, causing a pivot about the interosseous ligament such that the posterior aspect of the calcaneus is forced laterally.

It was recently appreciated that significant calcaneocuboid subluxation is present in some clubfeet. Thometz and Springer (60) in 1990 demonstrated that the degree of subluxation can be radiographically estimated and that cases showing more than a minimal amount of subluxation require circumferential calcaneocuboid capsulotomy with reduction and pinning. In a review of 100 unoperated feet, they found 30% had no subluxation, 45% had mild subluxation, and 25% had moderate or severe subluxation. Only those with moderate or severe subluxation required treatment.

CLINICAL CHARACTERISTICS

The congenital clubfoot is characterized by: (i) the absence of other congenital anomalies; (ii) variable rigidity of the foot; (iii) mild calf atrophy; and (iv) mild

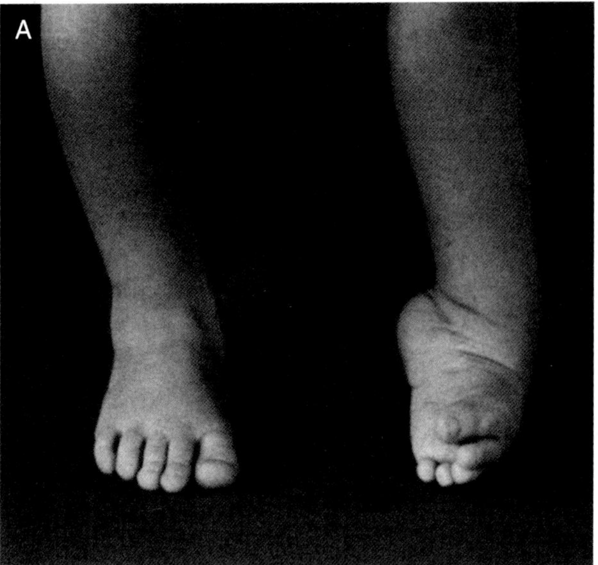

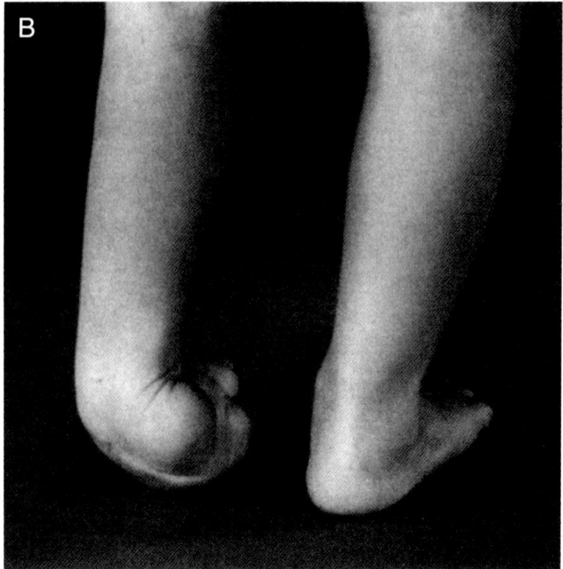

FIGURE 6-1 Preoperative anterior (**A**) and posterior (**B**) photographs of a two-year-old child with an untreated left congenital clubfoot.

hypoplasia of the tibia, fibula, and bones of the foot. The femur may be slightly short, but this is usually only demonstrable on scanographic evaluation.

Examination of the infant clubfoot demonstrates hindfoot equinus, hindfoot varus, forefoot adduction, and variable rigidity (Figure 6-1). All of these findings are presumably secondary to the medial subluxation of the navicular on the head of the talus. When the navicular is medially subluxed experimentally in fresh cadaver specimens, the clinical as well as the radiographic appearance of a congenital clubfoot is reproduced including functional rigidity (Figure 6-2A–D) (8,62).

In the older child, calf and foot atrophy are more obvious than in the infant regardless of how well corrected or functional the foot may be. These findings are due to the etiological aspects of clubfoot and not the methods of treatment, including surgery.

RADIOGRAPHIC EVALUATION

The preoperative radiographic evaluation of clubfeet is also controversial. The reasons include: (i) complexity of the deformities which occur in various planes; (ii) the immaturity of the ossification centers of the foot at the time of birth; the navicular does not ossify until the third year of life or later; the cuboid ossification center is not present until six or seven months of life, and the talar ossification center may be round at birth and may not be amenable to having its long axis accurately measured; (iii) Shapiro and Glimcher (48) demonstrated that the ossific nucleus of the talus is eccentrically located in the anterior talar neck, thus, a line bisecting the talar ossification nucleus may not represent the true longitudinal axis of the talus; (iv) surgeons may experience difficulty in taking, measuring, and interpreting the films; and (v) marking as many as half a dozen angles and axes on several radiographic views is laborious and time consuming.

There are situations in which plain radiographs are useful:

1. The documentation of reduction of talonavicular subluxation and the correction of forefoot adduction during nonoperative management
2. When a plateau has been reached in conservative treatment
3. Immediately before surgery
4. During surgery
5. Postoperatively at various intervals to assess maintenance of alignment and the effects of growth and development.

RADIOGRAPHIC TECHNIQUE

It is important to use a standard technique to obtain preoperative, intraoperative, and postoperative radiographs (51). These are weight-bearing or simulated weight-bearing anteroposterior (AP) and lateral radiographs of the involved foot. Non–weight-bearing radiographs are usually of minimal value. If the surgeon desires to evaluate the range of motion at the ankle joint, it is necessary to obtain lateral views with the ankle joint in full plantar and dorsiflexion (52,54,64). An intraoperative posteroanterior (PA) rather than the AP view may be taken when the patient is in the prone position. Measurement values are the same for both the PA and AP views. Clues that suggest improper technique or positioning are presented in Table 6-1.

Radiographic Measurements

Numerous radiographic measurements can be made on routine radiographs (Figures 6-3–6-8). The most common in the anteroposterior projection are illustrated in Figure 3A. On the lateral radiograph, the most common measurements are demonstrated in Figure 3B. The normal range for most of these measurements in children less than five years of age is presented in Table 6-2.

Measurements on the AP (or PA) View

The anteroposterior talocalcaneal angle is determined by measuring the angle between the long axes of the talus and calcaneus (6,13,14,25,32,44,58,59,66). Divergence between the anterior end of the talus and the calcaneus is also measured on this view (54,61). This describes the rotary motion of the talus over the calcaneus (see Figures 6-4 and 6-5). Overlap may also be utilized to evaluate the relationship between the posterior aspects of the talus and the calcaneus. If there is less than 50% overlap of the posterior one-half of the talus and calcaneus (as determined by visual estimate), translation of the talus beneath the calcaneus has occurred.

The navicular position is ascertained once it has ossified sufficiently to evaluate its location relative to the talar head (see Figure 6-6). In the normal relationship, the navicular ossification center lies centrally on the distal end of the talar head. When it lies medially, medial subluxation of the navicular is present; conversely, when it lies laterally, lateral subluxation of the talar head is present (54).

Before ossification of the navicular occurs, the relationship of the talar axis to the base of the first metatarsus indicates the position of the navicular. If the talar axis passes medial to the base of the first metatarsus, the navicular has been over-reduced into a lateral subluxated position. If the talar axis passes medial to the base of the first metatarsus, it indicates under-correction of the medial talonavicular subluxation (see Figure 6-6) (54).

The medial flare or extension on the medial side of the calcaneus indicates that ossification of the sustentaculum tali is taking place. When this is present, a line parallel with the long axis of the calcaneus, bisecting the medial border where the flare begins, serves as a useful marker for the assessment of calcaneocuboid subluxation. Before the flare appears, the medial line may be formed by drawing the tangent parallel with the long axis. The cuboid position can be evaluated by noting the relationship of the cuboid central point of the ossification center to the medial line (60). The central point of the cuboid ossification center normally lies on the long axis of the calcaneus. With mild subluxation, it lies between the long axis and the medial line. Once the central point of the ossification center moves medial to the medial calcaneal line, significant calcaneocuboid subluxation is present; this requires surgical correction (see Figure 6-7).

Finally, the first ray angle (see Figure 6-3A) described by Barriolhet (3) in 1990 indicates the amount of forefoot adduction present. This measurement is independent of supination as the forefoot is placed flat on the cassette when the radiographic view is exposed. This is measured by the angle formed between the first metatarsal axis and a line along the base of the metatarsi. The talar-first metatarsal angle can also be used to measure the amount of forefoot adduction.

Measurement on the Lateral View

The long axis of the talus is located by a similar technique used for the AP view. The calcaneal axis is most accurately obtained by drawing a line along its plantar surface, except during the first three to six weeks of life, when the posterior inferior surface may not be clearly ossified and the inferior surface may appear as an irregular V-shaped contour. In this case, the tracing technique can be used.

Both lateral talocalcaneal (6,25,32,44,58) and tibiocalcaneal angles (6,44,68) measure equinus of the hindfoot (see Figure 6-3B). The latter is probably a more accurate parameter for measuring equinus but the former is most commonly used at this time. The tibiotalar angle (6,32,44) must be evaluated by comparing maximum dorsiflexion and plantar flexion views to ascertain the true ankle range of motion. The navicular location is established by the same technique used to determine its position on the AP radiograph (see Figure 6-8) (54). Subluxation of more than one-third of the vertical height of the navicular above the dorsum of the talus is considered significant. The navicular ossification center is usually sufficiently ossified by the fourth or fifth year to permit direct evaluation of this measurement, whereas prior to ossification of the navicular, the talar axis relationship to the base of the first metatarsus is used (54). The talar-first metatarsal angle (see Figure 6-3B) described by Meary (37) in 1967 is a helpful measurement for rocker-bottom or cavus deformity. The angle is formed by the intersection of the talar and first metatarsal axes.

SURGICAL MANAGEMENT

Surgical treatment can be divided into three major categories: (i) soft-tissue releases; (ii) tendon transfers; and (iii) bone procedures, including arthrodeses. The latter two are rarely indicated in the initial operative treatment of resistant clubfeet

Soft-Tissue Releases

Posterior release and complete soft-tissue release are the two common methods of soft-tissue releases.

Posterior Release

Lengthening of the tendo-Achillis and release of the posterior aspect of the ankle and subtalar joint has been recommended for residual equinus when the mid-foot and forefoot deformities have been fully corrected by serial casting (2,22,27,38). The indications for a posterior release, other than Achilles tendon tenotomy during the Ponseti technique, rarely occur since the major deformity occurs at the talonavicular joint, which generally fails non-operative treatment.

Complete Soft-Tissue Releases

Currently, the recommended initial method of surgical management is a comprehensive or complete soft-tissue

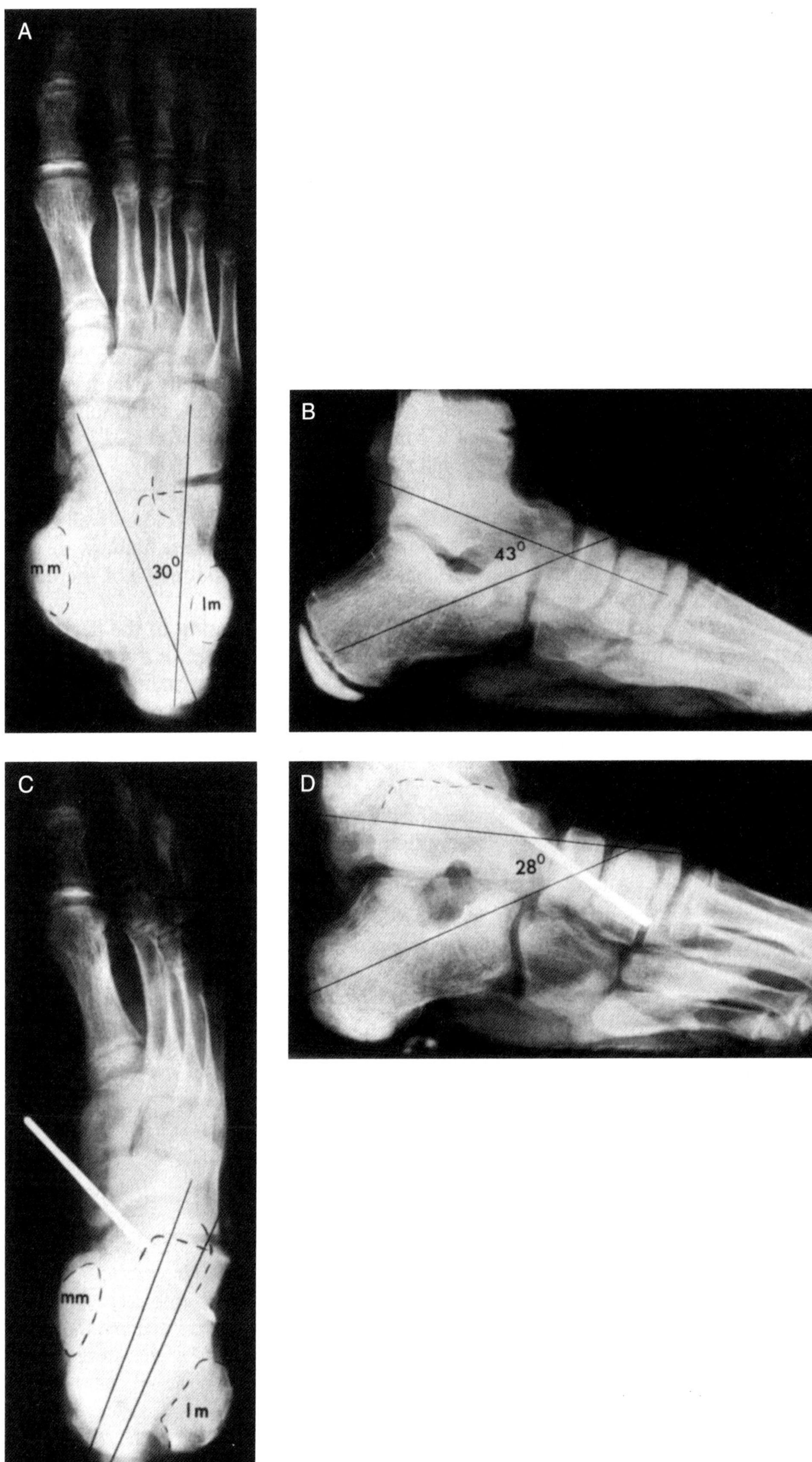
A
mm
30°
lm
B
43°
C
mm
lm
D
28°

TABLE 6-1

Radiographic Clues Which Suggest Improper Technique

Anteroposterior Radiographic
Talus and calcaneus heads at different levels
If the heads of these bones are more than 2–3 mm apart, the radiographic tibia was not positioned at 30 degrees, or the foot was malpositioned in plantar flexion.
Significant overlapping of the metatarsi
This suggests the foot was inverted. It will also decrease the talocalcaneal angle. This finding must be correlated with the clinical appearance of the foot.
Visualization of the tibial and fibular shafts
This suggests inadequate dorsiflexion of the foot or that significant equinus prevented dorsiflexion. This too will decrease the talocalcaneal angle. The film must be compared to the clinical appearance of the foot.
Lateral Radiographs
Extreme posterior positioning of the fibula with respect to the tibia
The hindfoot is positioned in external rotation. This will produce a false increase in the talocalcaneal angle. This may be due to improper positioning or significant medial deviation of the mid-foot and forefoot.
Loss of overlapped appearance of the metatarsi
The foot is inverted. The metatarsi are stacked and the talocalcaneal angle decreased. This film must be compared to the clinical appearance of the foot.
Lack of ankle dorsiflexion
Inadequate dorsiflexion due to positioning or equinus contracture. This is associated with a decreased talocalcaneal angle. Clinical correlation is necessary.

release including the posterior, medial, lateral, anterior, and possibly the plantar structures. Thompson et al. (62) in 1982 demonstrated the limited value of isolated procedures performed specifically to lengthen the tendo-Achillis or isolated releases of posterior or medial structures. There is an inverse relationship between the number of operative procedures performed and the final result with respect to function and appearance (9,29,62). Therefore, it is important that the initial procedure be definitive with a minimal risk for recurrence and need for additional surgery. Techniques for a complete release have been described by Turco (64,65); Thompson et al. (21); McKay (34,36); Simons (53,55); Carroll et al. (8,9); Bensahel et al. (4); Goldner (21); and Crawford et al (10).

The timing for initial surgery is controversial. Some surgeons prefer early intervention, between three and six months of age (9,15), while others prefer to delay until nine to twelve months of age (16,61,65). Neonatal surgery has been performed but is technically demanding and there is no evidence that these infants achieved better long-term results (42,45,57) Simons (53) felt the size of the foot is more important than age and recommends surgery when the foot is eight centimeters or longer in length. Those who advocate early surgery feel that the amount of pedal growth during the first year of life is considerable and that early correction permits this growth and remodeling of the talus, calcaneus, and navicular to occur in the corrected position, resulting in a more stable, congruous alignment. Those surgeons who prefer to wait list safer anesthesia, the larger size of the anatomical structures which are therefore easier to manage, and the benefits of early weight bearing on the corrected foot to help with maintenance of correction. Bilateral clubfeet can usually be corrected safely under the same anesthesia.

FIGURE 6-2 **A.** Anteroposterior radiograph of the amputated right foot of a ten-year-old male. Traumatic below knee amputation was sustained in a railyard accident. Radiograph demonstrates the normal relationships between the forefoot, midfoot, and hindfoot as well as the ankle. There is a 30-degree anteroposterior talocalcaneal angle and a 1+ talocalcaneal overlap. The relationship between the medial malleolus (*mm*) and lateral malleolus (*lm*) is easily visualized. **B.** Simulated lateral weight-bearing radiograph shows a 43-degree lateral talocalcaneal angle and a normal medial longitudinal arch. **C.** The anteroposterior radiograph following release of the talonavicular joint and medial subluxation of the navicular on the head of the talus. Stabilization with a Kirschner pin was necessary to maintain this relationship. Radiograph now demonstrates 3+ talocalcaneal overlap and parallelism between the long axis of the calcaneus and talus. There is posterior displacement of the lateral malleolus. There is also moderate forefoot adduction. **D.** Simulated lateral weight-bearing radiograph demonstrates a varus alignment of the hindfoot. The lateral talocalcaneal angle measured 28 degrees. There is the appearance of a flat-top talus and visualization directly through the sinus tarsi. There is mid-foot varus as demonstrated by the navicular overlying the cuboid and a varus forefoot with stacking of the metatarsi.

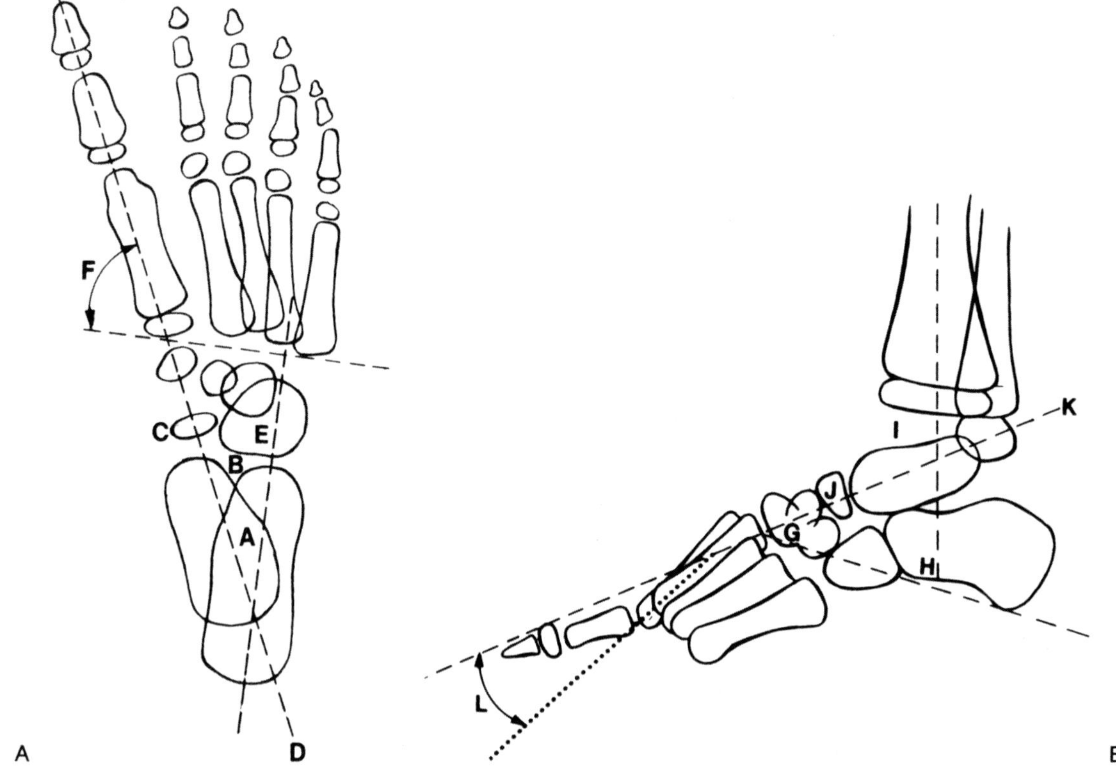

FIGURE 6-3 **A.** Radiographic measurements in the anteroposterior view of a child less than five years of age. These include: the talocalcaneal angle (*A*), the talocalcaneal divergence (*B*), the navicular position (*C*), the talar axis (*D*), the cuboid position (*D*), and the first-ray angle (*F*). **B.** Radiographic measurements for the lateral radiograph. These include: the lateral talocalcaneal angle (*G*), the tibiocalcaneal angle (*H*), the tibiotalar angle (*I*), the navicular position (*J*), the talar axis (*K*), and the talar-first metatarsal angle (*L*). (From Simons GW. Complete subtalar release in clubfeet. Part II. Comparison of less extensive procedures. *J Bone Joint Surg (Am)* 1985;67:1056–1065, with permission.)

Staged operative procedures separated by two to three weeks should be performed when the surgery on the first foot is difficult and the anesthetic is prolonged.

The type of skin incision is also controversial. Crawford et al. (10) described the transverse Cincinnati incision, which allows excellent visualization of the mid-foot,

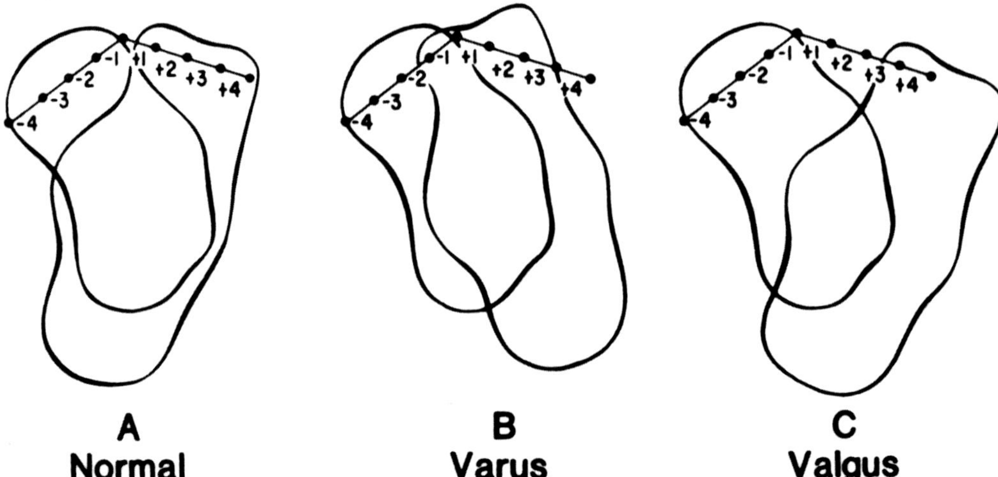

FIGURE 6-4 Talocalcaneal divergence is normal in children less than five years of age. Overlap of the distal ends of each bone is measured in negative one-quarter increments (−1 through −4); separation or divergence is measured in positive one-quarter increments (+1 to +4). (From Simons GW. Complete subtalar release in clubfeet. Part II. Comparison of less extensive procedures. *J Bone Joint Surg (Am)* 1985;67:1056–1065, with permission.)

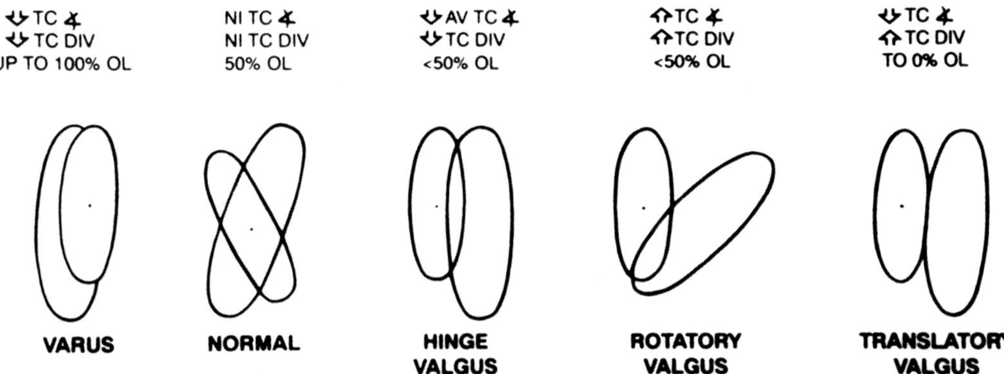

FIGURE 6-5 The characteristic TC angle (Δ), TC divergence (DIV), and overlap (OL) of the posterior half of the talus and calcaneus are given for varus of the uncorrected clubfoot; the normal relationship following complete correction; hinge valgus, where the subtalar joint hinges open like a book following release of the anterior, medial, and posterior subtalar capsules and interosseous ligament; rotary valgus following complete subtalar release with the calcaneus rotating into excessive valgus; and translatory valgus following complete subtalar release with the entire calcaneus translated into a valgus position.

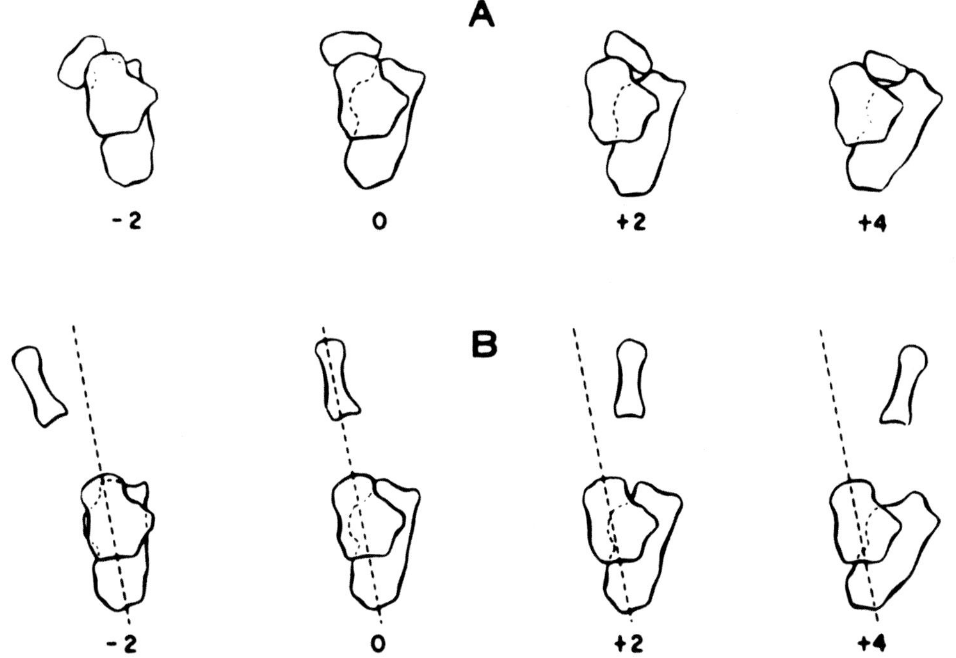

FIGURE 6-6 **A.** The ossified navicular is graded zero when centrally positioned on the talar head. Lateral (+1) or medial (−1) indicates displacement of the navicular by one-quarter of the talar head width. Additional displacement is measured in one-quarter increments of talar head width. Grade +1 or +2 is overcorrected but satisfactory, while grades +3 or +4 represent marked overcorrection and a complication. All minus (–) grades represent incomplete correction and a major complication. **B.** The unossified navicular is in normal alignment (grade 0) when the talar axis passes through the base of the first metatarsus. The talar axis deviates by $1/2$ of the width of the first metatarsal base in grade 1; medial is +1 while lateral is −1. The grade becomes +2 or −2 when the talar axis deviates from the width of the entire first metatarsal base. Grades of zero and +1 are considered normal, and +2 is considered satisfactory, while other ratings are considered to represent major complications. (From Simons GW. Complete subtalar release in clubfeet. Part II. Comparison of less extensive procedures. *J Bone Joint Surg (Am)* 1985;67:1056–1065, with permission.)

hindfoot, and ankle with minimal postoperative wound problems and is currently popular (5,33,34,55). Simons (55) has reported a slight increase in the incidence of wound edge necrosis when the Cincinnati incision is employed in children three years of age or older. Other common surgical approaches include a single curving, posteromedial incision (61) or the use of two or more incisions (9,53). The selection of incision is based primarily on the experience of the individual surgeon.

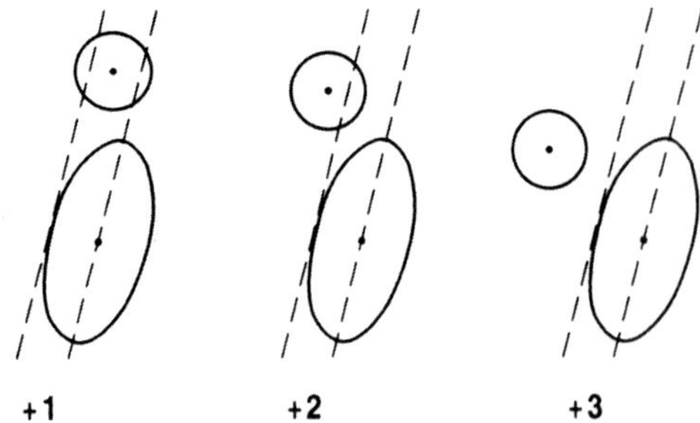

FIGURE 6-7 The calcaneal long axis is determined by a line parallel to its lateral border. A parallel medial line passes tangentially to the medial border of the calcaneus. Grade I (normal) demonstrates the midpoint of the cuboid ossification lying between the long axis and the medial line; grade 2 has the central point of the cuboid ossification lying medial to the medial line; grade 3 (severe) the central point of the cuboid ossification moving proximal to the distal end of the calcaneal ossification center.

The Cincinnati incision allows the procedure to be performed in the prone position, which allows better visualization of the pathologic anatomy, especially on the lateral aspect of the hindfoot (33,34,55). The other techniques usually require the child to be in the supine position. It must be remembered that these are only skin incisions, and their title does not reflect the surgical release that is employed once the wound is entered. Virtually any combination of soft-tissue releases can be employed through these incisions.

The critical aspects of the surgical anatomy include the recognition that: (i) the navicular is subluxated medially and articulates with the anterior aspect of the medial malleolus and (ii) the calcaneus is supinated and medially rotated about the axis of the talocalcaneal ligament and therefore its lateral portion is articulating with the posterior surface of the lateral malleolus (33,34,55). Thus, it must be appreciated that a clubfoot is a complex rotational abnormality of the subtalar complex (talonavicular, talocalcaneal, and calcaneocuboid joints).

The complete soft-tissue release involves extensive dissection of the posterior, medial, and lateral portions of the foot. The posterior release typically includes:

1. Achilles tendon lengthening
2. Release of the posterior ankle and subtalar joints, including the posterior talofibular ligament
3. Release of the thickened peroneal retinaculum and tendon sheaths posterior and inferior to the lateral malleolus
4. Lengthening, usually by recession, of the tendons of the flexor digitorum longus and flexor hallucis longus.

The medial release includes:

1. Z-plasty of the tibialis posterior tendon
2. Complete capsulotomy of the talonavicular join,
3. Recession of the abductor hallucis tendon
4. The possible release of the medial and plantar surface of the calcaneocuboid joint
5. Release of the medial aspect of the subtalar joint
6. Release of part or all of the interosseous ligament.

The lateral release involves:

1. Release of the lateral aspect of the subtalar joint
2. Release of the contracted calcaneofibular ligament
3. Perhaps complete release of the calcaneocuboid joint.

A plantar release is performed by incising the common origin of the plantar structures from the tuberosity of the calcaneus. This procedure is not performed routinely by

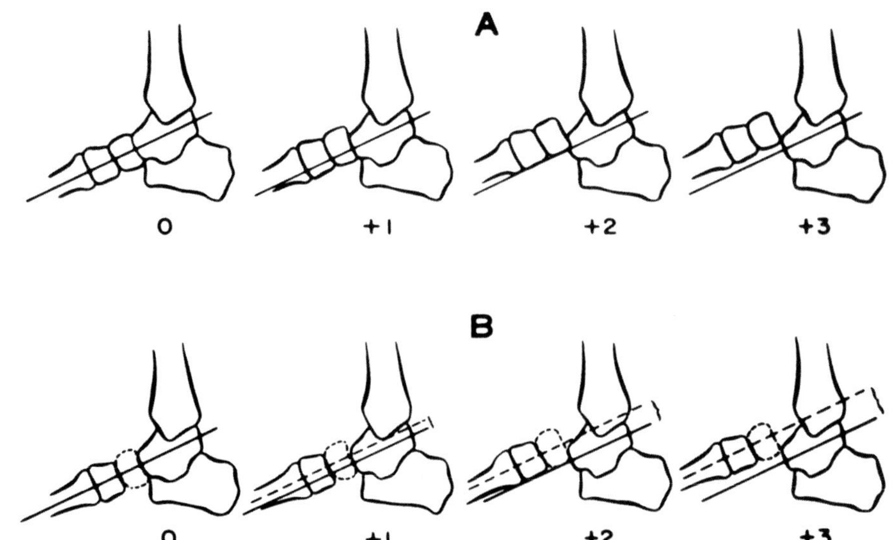

FIGURE 6-8 Talonavicular alignment in the ossified (**A**) and unossified (**B**) navicular. The normal position is graded as zero. Superior displacement of one-third or less of the ossified navicular is graded +1 with increments of additional 1/3 displacement graded as +2 or +3. Grade +1 is considered satisfactory whereas the latter two are unsatisfactory and a major complication. **B.** This grading system utilizes a line drawn through the talar and first metatarsal axis. The grading system is similar to (**A**) and is based on the distance between the two lines relative to the height of the talar head. More than +1 is considered unsatisfactory. (From Simons GW. Complete subtalar release in clubfeet. Part II. Comparison of less extensive procedures. *J Bone Joint Surg (Am)* 1985;67:1056–1065, with permission.)

TABLE 6-2

Radiographic Measurements of the Feet in Children Less Than Five Years of Age

	Anteroposterior radiograph	
Measurement	**Determines**	**Normal range**
A = Talocalcaneal angle	Rotatory or hinge varus/valgus	20–40°
B = Talocalcaneal divergence	Translatory or rotatory varus/valgus	0 to +1°
C = Navicular position	Talonavicular subluxation (medial/lateral)	Central
D = Talar axis	Talonavicular subluxation (medial/lateral)	Through base of first metatarsus
E = Cuboid position	Calcaneocuboid subluxation	0
F = 1st ray angle	Forefoot adduction/abduction	55–65°
	Lateral radiograph	
Measurement	**Determines**	**Normal range**
G = Talocalcaneal angle	Equinus/calcaneus	35–50°
H = Tibiocalcaneal angle	Equinus/calcaneus	DF 25–60°
I = Tibiotalar angle	Ankle range of motion	DF 70–100° PF 120–180° (total ROM > 30°)
J = Navicular position	Talonavicular subluxation (dorsal or volar)	Central
K = Talar axis	Talonavicular subluxation (dorsal or volar)	Through base of first metatarsus
L = Talar–first metatarsal angle	Cavus/rocker-bottom	0–20°

all authors but has been demonstrated to be effective in the correction of forefoot adduction and cavovarus components of the clubfoot deformity (61,9,39,49,67).

All of the techniques described for the complete release are similar. There are differences, especially regarding the partial (61,64,65) or circumferential (8,9,35,34,54,55) release of the subtalar joint, release of the deep portion of the deltoid ligament at the medial ankle joint (21), and the inclusion of a plantar release. Release of the talocalcaneal interosseus ligament also varies. Simons (54,55) recommends that this ligament always be released, it is usually released by McKay (34), rarely, if ever, released by Turco (65), and never released by Goldner (21). El-Deeb et al. (19) prospectively studied 66 idiopathic clubfeet treated by posteromedial release and found that releasing the talocalcaneal interosseous ligament was advisable to improve outcome in severe and very severe clubfeet. The ligament can be narrowed to enhance the medial rotation of the talus and eliminate the possible need for a talocalcaneal pin stabilization. In a comparative study of the techniques described by Turco, McKay, and Carroll, Magone and coworkers (31) found similar results from the various procedures both in clinical and radiographic evaluation. However, when these patients were placed into two groups of "excellent and good" and "fair and poor," the comparative evaluation demonstrated that McKay's procedure results in better outcomes. However, the authors were reluctant to recommend one procedure over another as the number of cases was small and the length of follow up short.

The use of postoperative internal fixation is common. Most surgeons employ a Kirschner wire, threaded or smooth, across the talonavicular joint, while others may also use a wire across the subtalar joint (35) and possibly the calcaneocuboid joint (53,55). In the study by Thompson et al. (62), no internal fixation was used and the feet were managed postoperatively with serial casting similar to that utilized preoperatively. They reported an 86% satisfactory long-term result in 93 feet without prior surgical treatment. The long-term results with and without pin fixation appear to be similar. The use of internal fixation is most beneficial in the early postoperative period when the foot is edematous and there could be difficulty in maintaining alignment.

Postoperative management consists of immobilization in either short leg (61) or long leg plaster casts (9,11,33,34,42,55) for six to twelve weeks. Turco (65), however, recommends four months of postoperative casting. The casts are changed at one- or two-week intervals. The type of plaster immobilization depends on the age of the child at surgery. Young children, three to six months of age, usually require long leg casts while older children can be satisfactorily immobilized in short leg casts. At the end of the casting period, supplemental bivalved casts, orthoses, or corrective shoes are commonly used for several months to a few years (9,53,54,61). Most authors now feel that long leg casts are necessary for all children following clubfoot surgery. The lower leg is placed in maximal external rotation and the leg is held in the cast with the knee flexed at 70 to 90 degrees. Simons allows no weight bearing. McKay (33,34) utilizes a long leg cast with the knee flexed at 90 degrees and a hinged foot section to encourage ankle motion, especially plantar flexion. McKay (36) also recommends passive stretching by the parents, exercises including toe-walking, and the use of regular shoes.

Common Soft-Tissue Operations

Posteromedial Plantar Release

The posteromedial plantar release, as initially described by Thompson, Richardson, and Westin (61) in 1982, has been modified from its original description and is generally performed at nine months of age. With the patient in

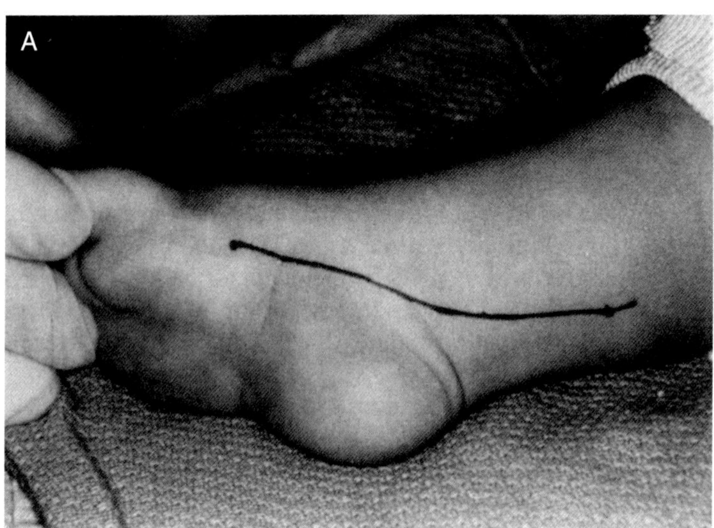

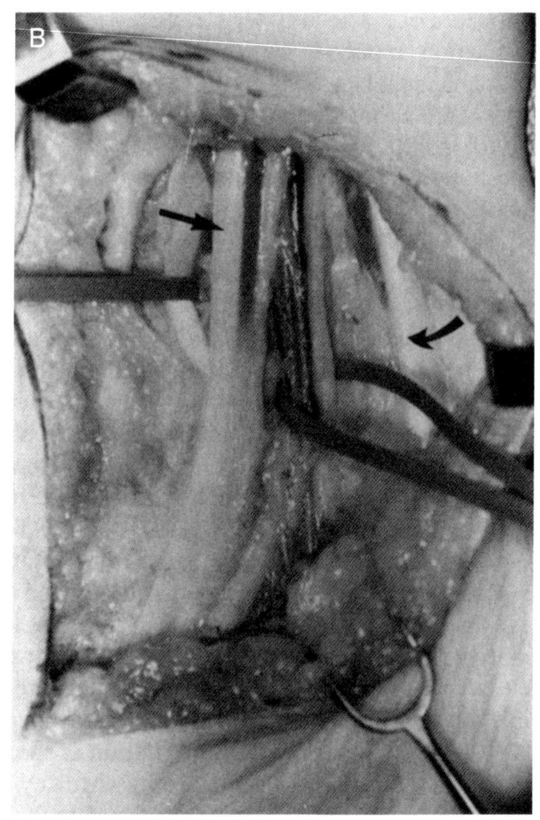

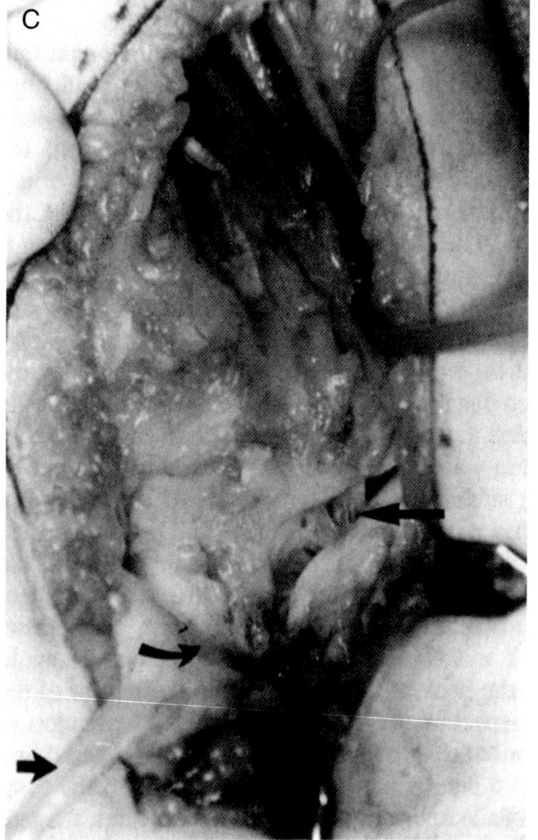

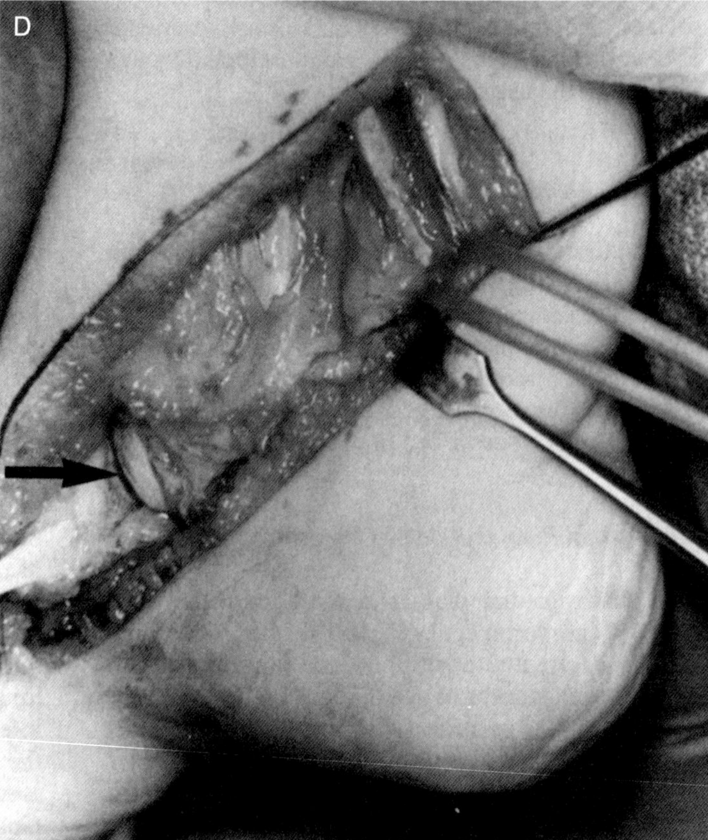

FIGURE 6-9 *(Continued)*

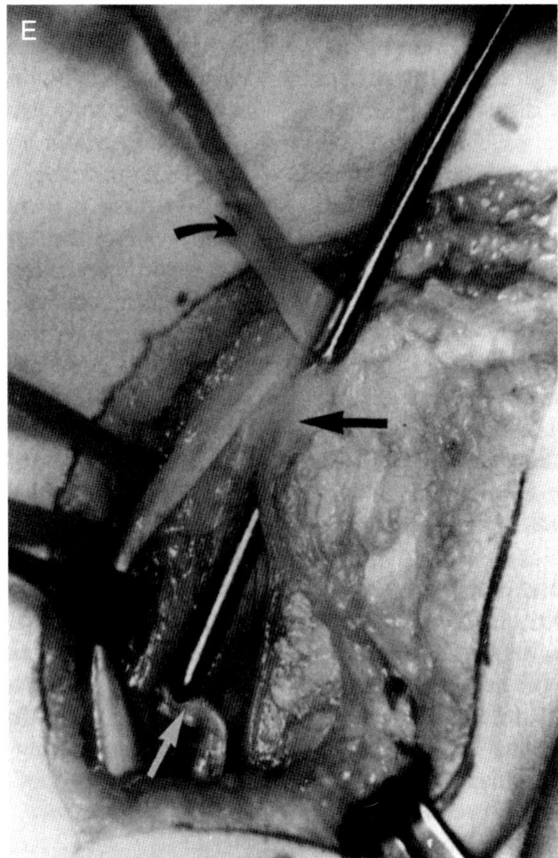

FIGURE 6-9 **A.** Skin incision for the posteromedial plantar release. A slightly curving incision is made over the posteromedial aspect of the foot and ankle. Care is taken to avoid extending the skin incision onto the plantar surface of the foot. **B.** Extensive dissection is carried out to identify all of the important structures that are proximal and posterior to the medial malleolus. The neurovascular bundle is isolated with a vessel loop. The tibialis posterior tendon is also identified by a second vessel loop. The flexor digitorum longus tendon (*straight arrow*) is anterior to the neurovascular bundle and the tendo-Achillis posterior (*curved arrow*). **C.** The subtalar joint is released circumferentially. The interosseous ligament (*long arrow*) is visible but is later partially released to enhance talocalcaneal rotation. The lateral aspect of the subtalar joint is released by working anteriorly and posteriorly to the interosseous ligament. The posterior aspect is easily visualized by gentle traction on the heel. This allows excellent visualization of the peroneal tendons and tendon sheath as well as the calcaneofibular ligament. The released talonavicular joint (*curved arrow*) and tibialis posterior tendon (*short arrow*) are also demonstrated. **D.** A 0.062 smooth Kirschner wire is inserted longitudinally through the body of the talus. Insertion begins posterolaterally and the pin exits through the talar head anteromedially. The navicular is centered onto the head of the talus (*arrow*). It is important that dorsal displacement does not occur. Once the navicular is in satisfactory position, the pin is advanced. The forefoot is held in the correct position, and the pin is advanced further. The pin will exit the foot percutaneously along the medial aspect of the head of the first metatarsus. The pin is withdrawn until the tip of the pin enters the body of the talus posteriorly. **E.** The distal end of the lengthened tibialis posterior tendon (*white arrow*) is then repassed through the slip of tendon sheaths at the tip of the medial malleolus (*black arrow*) and repaired to the proximal tendon (*curved arrow*) with the foot held in slight equinus. The tendo-Achillis is also repaired in a similar manner.

a supine position, a slightly curved posteromedial incision is made over the foot and ankle after the leg has been exsanguinated with an Esmarch bandage and a pneumatic tourniquet inflated, usually to 200 mm Hg. The incision begins anterior to the distal one-fourth of the Achilles tendon and passes approximately one centimeter posterior to the medial malleolus and then extends horizontally to terminate over the medial aspect of the first metatarsal-medial cuneiform joint. The subcutaneous tissues are bluntly divided and the investing fascia of the neurovascular bundle identified. The neurovascular structures are initially mobilized at the level of the medial malleolus and dissection proceeds proximally. A vessel loop is passed about these structures for retraction and protection.

The neurovascular bundle is then exposed distally and medially. The medial plantar nerve, which takes it origin from the posterior tibial nerve at approximately the level of the medial malleolus, is identified and followed distally until it passes deep to the abductor hallucis muscle origin. This muscle is mobilized from its calcaneal attachment and retracted plantarward. The nerve is followed into the plantar aspect of the foot where it is no longer held securely by the abductor hallucis muscle or soft tissues. The tendinous portion of the musculotendinous junction, of the abductor hallucis muscle is identified and released.

The Achilles tendon is exposed and Z-lengthened in the coronal plane. This is contrary to the traditional sagittal plane. This technique avoids the anterior muscle insertion of the musculotendinous junction, and an extensive lengthening of the Achilles tendon can be achieved without the interposition of muscle tissue at the time of repair.

The tibialis posterior and flexor digitorum longus tendons are identified proximal to the medial malleolus. The sheath of the flexor digitorum longus is completely incised from its musculotendinous junction into the plantar surface of the foot. Care is taken to avoid injury to the medial plantar nerve during this portion of the procedure. The sheath of the tibialis posterior tendon is opened proximal to the medial malleolus (Figure 6-9E). The tendon is Z-lengthened above the medial malleolus. A small portion, 5–7 mm, of the tendon sheath is preserved at the tip of the medial malleolus. The sheath is re-opened distally and the distal end of the tibialis posterior tendon extracted. A clamp is placed on this end of the tendon which is then used as a guide to identify the medially subluxated talonavicular joint. This is carried out by dissecting the medial, dorsal, and plantar capsule of this joint (see Figure 6-9C). Usually the tuberosity of the navicular abuts the anterior aspect of the medial malleolus. The plane of the talonavicular joint, as a consequence, is malaligned and care must be taken to avoid injuring the neck of the talus. During the release of the inferior aspect of the talonavicular joint, the tendon of the flexor hallucis longus is frequently encountered and is retracted plantarward to prevent injury. At the completion of the release of the talonavicular joint, the tendon of the flexor hallucis longus is mobilized proximally by incising its sheath as it passes inferior to the sustentaculum tali. The entire muscle-tendon unit is subsequently mobilized to allow it to be retracted medially.

The talocalcaneal or subtalar joint is released next. It is generally easier to open the joint posteriorly because its capsular structures are thin and easily entered. The dissection then progresses distally along its medial border (see Figure 6-9C). The talocalcaneal or interosseus ligament is preserved. This may be thinned circumferentially to enhance rotation during reduction. Once the medial aspect of the subtalar joint has been opened, the medial and plantar capsule of the calcaneocuboid joint is incised. This joint is easily reached through the posteromedial incision as it lies just plantar and lateral to the talonavicular joint. The subtalar joint is then released posteriorly to the level of the lateral malleolus. The tendon sheath of the peroneus longus and brevis are identified and released. With slight traction on the heel, it is possible to open the subtalar joint and visualize the lateral aspect of the subtalar joint, including the remaining peroneal muscle sheath. The proximal aspect of the lateral subtalar joint is opened by dissecting posterior to the interosseus ligament and the distal portion by dissecting anteriorly to this ligament.

Following the complete subtalar release, the ankle joint is released posteriorly. This extends from almost the tip of the medial malleolus to the lateral malleolus. The talus should now be free to rotate posteriorly into the ankle mortise when the foot is dorsiflexed.

A plantar release is performed working posterior to the neurovascular bundle. Small Metzenbaum scissors are passed bluntly between the tuberosity of the os calcis and the common origin of the plantar structures. Another plane is created between the subcutaneous tissue and the common plantar aponeurosis. The aponeurosis is then divided. This allows correction of any residual cavus deformity and forefoot adduction.

The foot should now be supple and easy to correct. A 0.062 mm smooth Kirschner wire is then inserted through the posterior aspect of the talus slightly lateral to its midline and is directed towards the head of the talus. When the pin is visible, the body of the talus is rotated medially and the talonavicular joint reduced (see Figure 6-9D). It is important that the navicular not be over-reduced. The navicular tuberosity is allowed to remain prominent basically in alignment with the medial malleolus to assure accurate reduction. It is also important to prevent dorsal subluxation of the navicular by adequately aligning the dorsal surface of the talar head and neck with that of the navicular. When the navicular is properly positioned, the pin is advanced to secure the talonavicular joint. The forefoot is then abducted to a neutral position and the pin is advanced. This will usually allow the base of the first metatarsus to be secured, thus correcting any residual forefoot adduction. The pin typically will exit the skin along the medial aspect of the first metatarsal head. The pin is then advanced sufficiently that its posterior tip is completely within the body of the talus.

The foot is carefully inspected at this time to assure alignment. Intraoperative anteroposterior and lateral simulated weight-bearing radiographs can be obtained to assess the alignment of the foot. Closure is begun when the foot is satisfactorily aligned both clinically and radiographically.

The tendon of the flexor hallucis longus is replaced in its groove inferior to the sustentaculum tali. The flexor digitorum longus is also replaced into its normal position. The distal end of the tibialis posterior tendon is passed back through its retinaculum at the tip of the medial malleolus (see Figure 6-9E). The Achilles and tibialis posterior tendons are repaired with absorbable sutures with the foot held in approximately 5 degrees of equinus. This ensures appropriate tension on the repair once the foot is brought to the neutral position. The tendinous portion of the musculotendinous junction of the flexor digitorum longus and flexor hallucis longus may be divided to correct any residual toe flexion deformity while maintaining continuity of the muscles.

The pneumatic tourniquet is deflated, hemostasis achieved, and the vascularity of the foot assessed. Usually there is prompt return of capillary filling and normal coloration. The subcutaneous tissues are closed in a single layer followed by a running subcuticular skin closure using absorbable suture material. The wound is supplemented with Steri-strips, sterile dressing, and a well-padded posterior long leg splint applied with the knee flexed 70 to 90 degrees, the foot externally rotated and in neutral position. Casting is not begun for one week to allow for the development and regression of soft-tissue swelling.

Postoperatively, immobilization is continued for 12 weeks. The talonavicular pin is removed at six weeks in the clinic. Casting is continued in a short leg weight-bearing cast for an additional six weeks. At the completion of the postoperative immobilization the child is usually ambulatory. Further support is continued following the Ponseti technique with straight or reversed last shoes and a Denis-Brown bar at nighttime until the child is two to four years of age. An ankle-foot-orthosis (AFO) is not utilized. Periodic anteroposterior and lateral weight-bearing radiographs are obtained to assess alignment of the foot with growth.

Complete Subtalar Release (CSTR) Using the Cincinnati Incision

This technique described by Simons (53,54,55) requires the surgeon to use operating lenses or loops because the operation is performed between the ages of three and six months and usually requires microvascular technique. The surgery is performed with the patient in the prone position and the foot and leg is prepped and draped so that the knee is free and the proximal tibial apophysis can be marked with an indelible pen (Figure 6-10). This helps in determining the proper alignment of the foot during the procedure and when it is repositioned on the lower leg (Figure 6-11A–E).

The tourniquet is inflated to approximately 150 mm Hg, but the veins are not fully exsanguinated to assist in identifying the neurovascular bundle. The Cincinnati incision extends from the mid-portion of the first metatarsus around the heel one centimeter proximal to the distal skin crease and terminates at the calcaneocuboid joint.

Medial dissection exposes the abductor hallucis which is reflected downward from the fascia overlying the first metatarsus. The muscle arcade may easily be released, allowing the neurovascular bundle to be fully exposed.

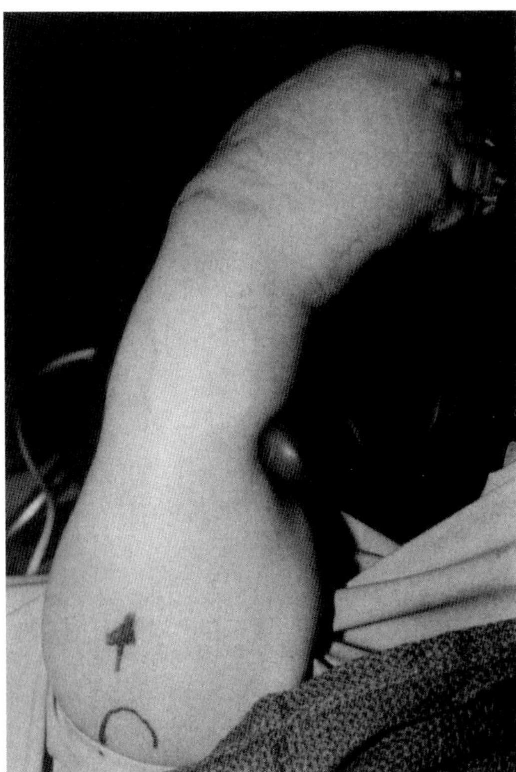

FIGURE 6-10 Lower limb of a child with a right clubfoot deformity who is in the prone position. The leg is draped above the knee. The proximal tibial apophysis and anterior border of the tibia have been marked with an indelible pen to serve as references for realigning the foot at the end of the procedure.

The neurovascular bundle is then dissected distally (see Figure 11A,B). The calcaneal branch of the posterior tibial nerve is carefully dissected from its surrounding fascia. Umbilical tape is then passed around the neurovascular bundle for protection and retraction.

The flexor digitorum longus tendon is dissected from its sheath up to the level of Henry's knot, which is incised. The tibialis posterior tendon sheath is opened from the proximal extent of the wound to the level of the posterior aspect of the medial malleolus distally and lengthened (see Figure 6-11C). Next the tendon of the flexor hallucis longus is exposed.

The Achilles tendon is Z-lengthened either in the sagittal or coronal plane. There is a tendency to insufficiently lengthen the heelcord which would require ankle plantar flexion to permit satisfactory tendon approximation. A minimum of four centimeters of lengthening is recommended.

The posterior capsule of the ankle joint is located and incised (see Figure 6-11D) from the peroneal tendons laterally to the tibialis posterior tendon sheath medially. The posterior talofibular ligament is divided. Once this ligament has been incised, the ankle joint will open significantly unless there is a flat-top talus present. The subtalar joint capsule is now divided laterally to the peroneal tendons but not through their sheath. Medially, this incision extends to the flexor hallucis longus (see Figure 6-11D).

Lateral dissection is now performed. The sural nerve is dissected free at the level of the subtalar joint. The peroneal tendons are identified and a circumferential incision is made in their sheath parallel to the subtalar joint. It is imperative that this incision not be made vertically, as the tendons then tend to subluxate anteriorly. Entrance to the lateral subtalar joint is easily achieved anterior to the tendons and the capsular incision then carried posteriorly. A hemostat may be inserted beneath the calcaneofibular ligament and exit through the lateral capsule posterior to the peroneal tendons and the ligament is divided by cutting down onto the hemostat. The release of this ligament is critical for the correction of the calcaneal rotation described by McKay (see Figure 6-11E) (37). The lateral subtalar joint incision is then carried distally. Dissection extends around the talar head with care taken to avoid injury to the blood supply coming from the lateral side of the neck and includes the entire lateral talonavicular joint. The capsular incision is extended across the dorsum of the foot by tunneling beneath the overlying tendons and neurovascular structures. If a calcaneocuboid joint release is required, it can be performed at this time.

The medial dissection includes passage of a probe down the tibialis posterior tendon sheath to the navicular insertion. A small vertical incision is made and the distal end of the tendon passed beneath this preserved portion of the sheath and extracted distally. Retraction of this tendon permits palpation of the subluxed navicular and its articulation with the medial malleolus. The actual talonavicular joint lies deep to the navicular. The dissection across the dorsum of the talonavicular joint is completed with scissors which also divide the spring ligament and the other structures on the inferior surface (see Figure 6-11E).

The tendon of flexor digitorum longus is retracted anteriorly providing direct access to the superficial deltoid ligament which is completely incised to release the medial subtalar joint. Locating the anterior subtalar joint line can be facilitated by viewing the subtalar joint through the posterior wound and recognizing a small medial talar column projecting downward which is actually part of the inferior surface of the talar head and neck that overlies the sustentaculum tali. The surgeon should release the interosseous ligament in its entirety, if visualization is difficult.

Medial dislocation of the foot from the talar head facilitates placement of the Kirschner wire, and avoids the need to sublux the neurovascular bundle and tendons to the lateral side of the foot.

The hindfoot can now be reduced and wires inserted unless supplemental procedures are necessary. These may include: (i) calcaneocuboid capsulotomy, (ii) calcaneal osteotomy, (iii) cuneiform and cuboidal osteotomy, and (iv) plantar release. The results of metatarsal osteotomies and tarsometatarsal capsulotomies as a part of the primary procedure have been disappointing and are no longer performed at the same time as the complete subtalar release.

Supplemental Procedures

Calcaneocuboid Capsulotomies

Calcaneocuboid capsulotomy is indicated for persistent calcaneocuboid subluxation intraoperatively following complete

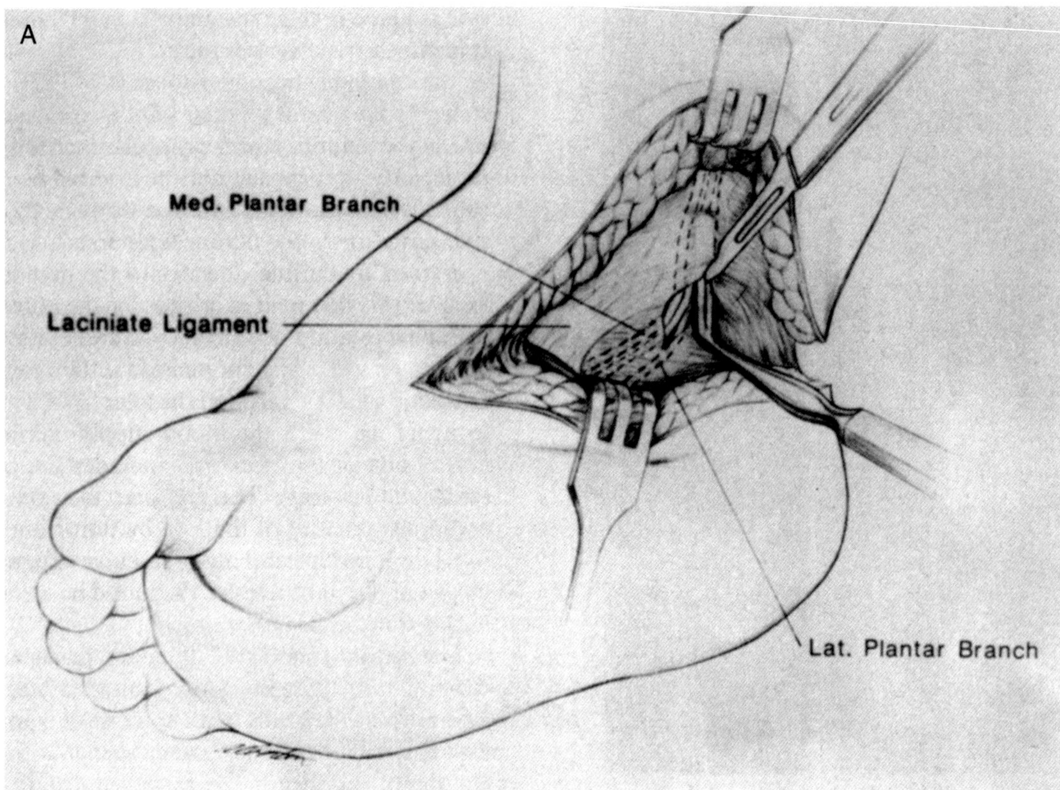

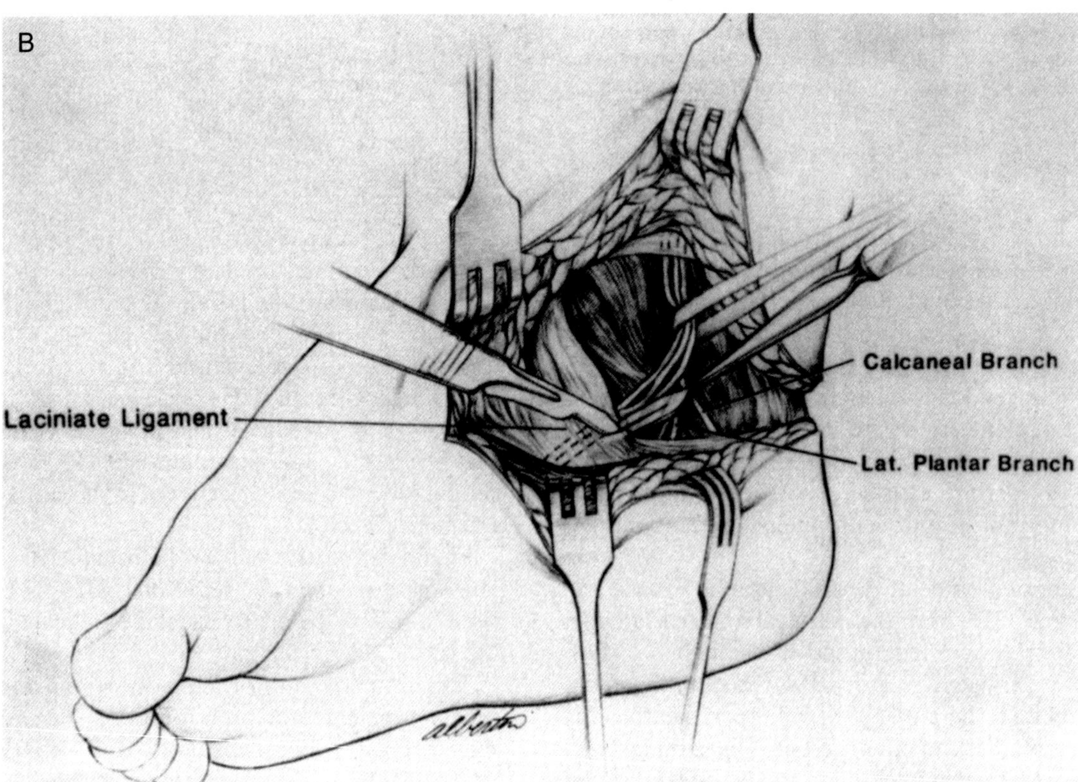

FIGURE 6-11 **A.** The laciniate ligament is incised from the medial malleolus proximally to the proximal end of the incision. **B.** The laciniate ligament is incised from the mid-malleolus distally to the area where it passes into the midfoot. **C.** Flexor digitorum communis or longus tendon lying within its sheath, which has been opened down to and including, Henry's knot. The posterior tibial tendon is lengthened by the Z-lengthening technique. **D.** The hindfoot following posterior capsulotomy of the ankle joint and a posterior subtalar capsulotomy. The posterior talofibular ligament has been incised. The ankle and subtalar joints can now open widely and are seen easily. **E.** The technique for releasing the calcaneofibular ligament. The hemostat is passed beneath this ligament from

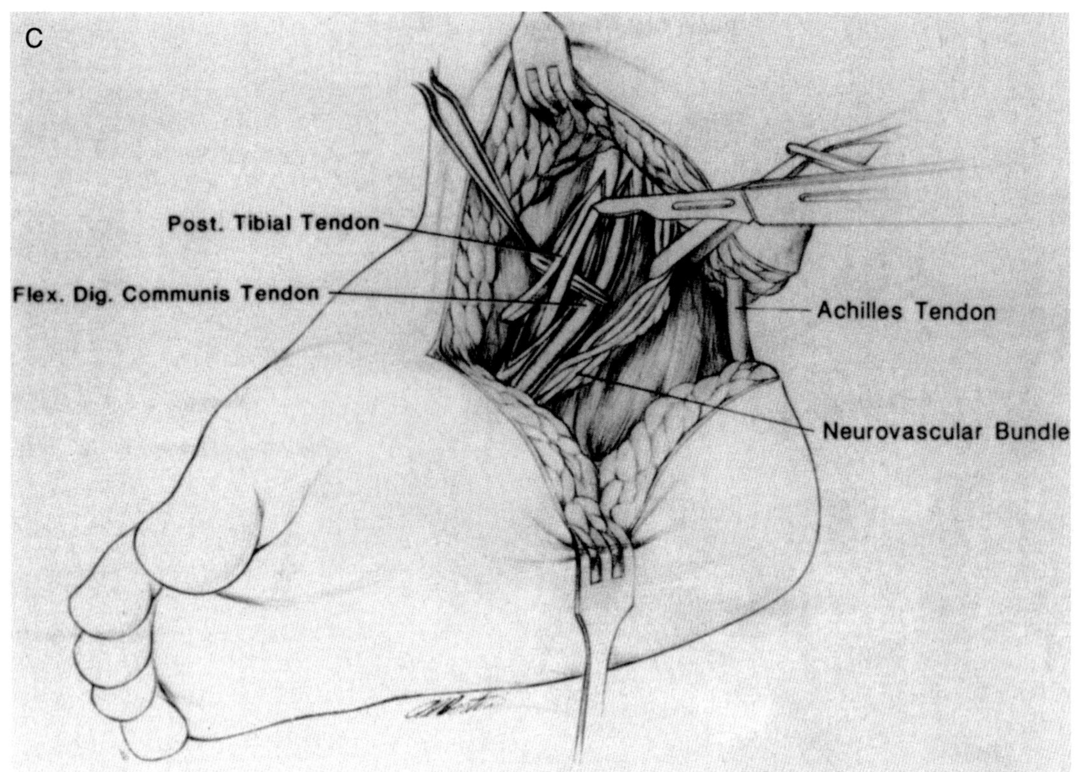

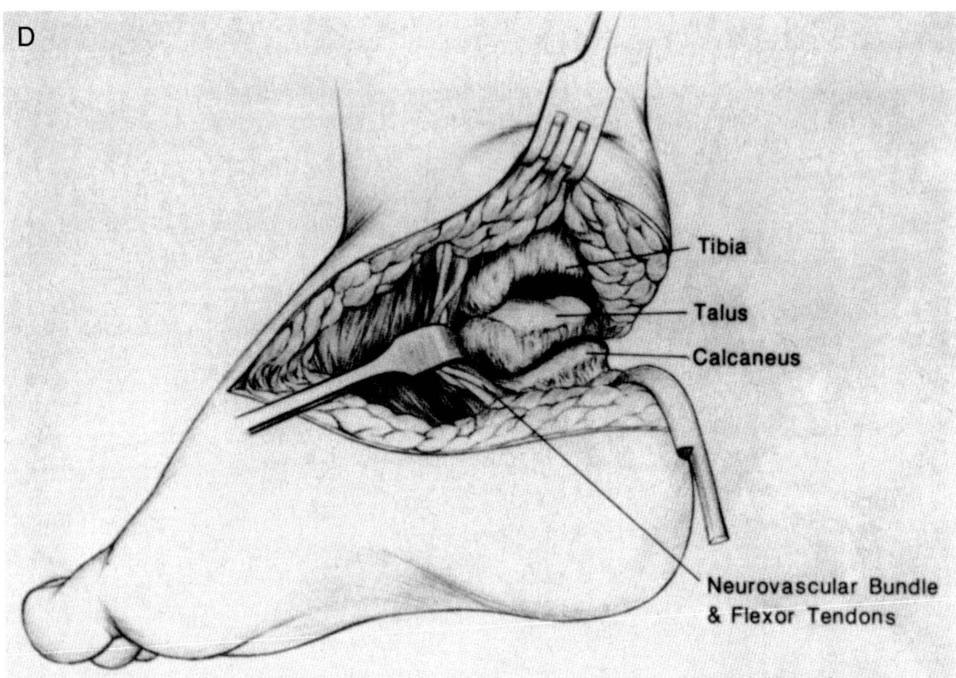

the posterior wound to the lateral wound. A scalpel is used to cut through the ligament into the underlying hemostat. **F.** Dissection across the talonavicular joint on the dorsum of the foot. The scissors are on the capsule at all times and are used to spread the tissues underneath the dorsal tendons and neurovascular bundle. The medial incision is extended to meet the lateral incision across the dorsum of the talonavicular joint. The plantar surface of the talonavicular joint is dissected in a similar manner, and the spring ligament and associated ligaments are incised.

subtalar release. Mild degrees do not require realignment. The extent of the calcaneocuboid subluxation can be assessed by PA intraoperative radiograph (see Figure 6-7). Surgical reduction is indicated when there is +2 or +3 calcaneocuboid subluxation. The distal portion of the lateral incision may need to be extended to perform this circumferential capsulotomy. A small Homan retractor is very helpful in retracting the peroneal tendons. A plantar release may also be performed if tightness of the medial plantar structures becomes more pronounced when the calcaneocuboid joint is reduced (60).

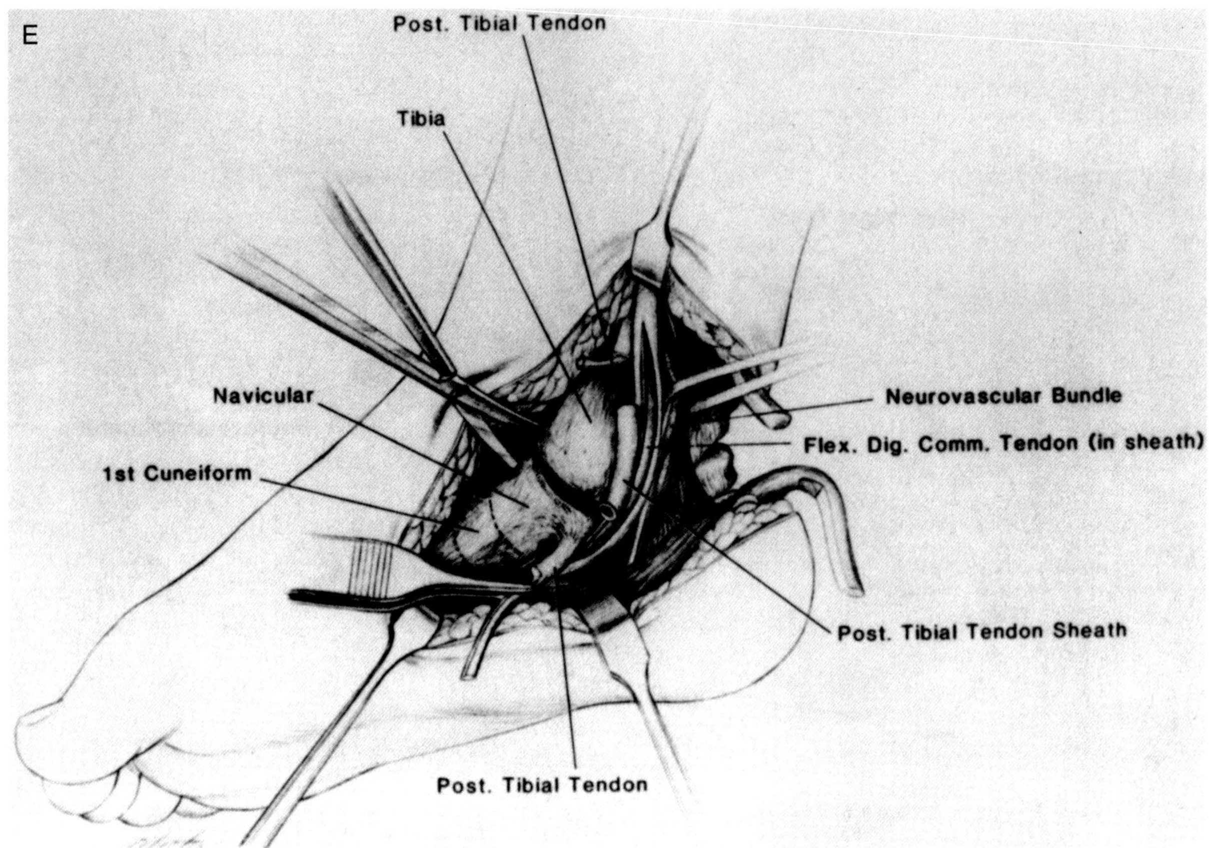

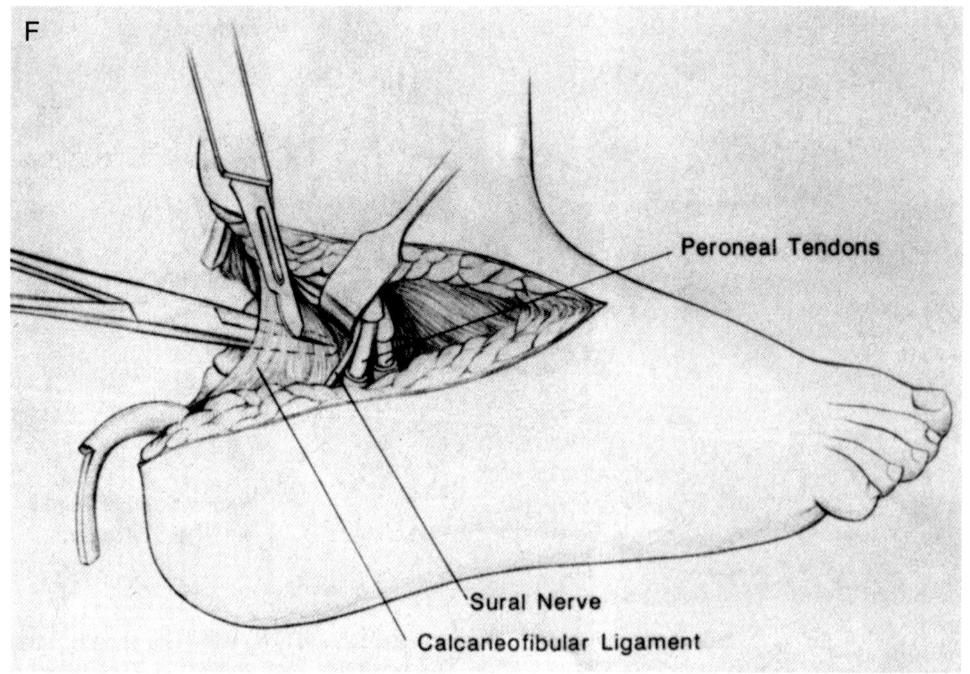

FIGURE 6-11 (*Continued*)

Cuneiform and Cuboid Osteotomies

Combined medial cuneiform and cuboid osteotomies are limited to children over five years of age at initial surgery or those who have significant residual forefoot adduction following CSTR (46). The cuneiform ossification center is too small before this age to permit satisfactory fusion of the inserted bone graft. A medial opening wedge osteotomy of the first cuneiform is combined with a lateral closing vertical wedge osteotomy of the cuboid. The removed cuboid wedge is inserted into the cuneiform osteotomy and a significant degree of correction of the forefoot adduction can be expected (1). Before five years of age, a plantar release is recommended to correct forefoot adduction.

Calcaneal Osteotomy

Lundburg (30) found that a calcaneal osteotomy, as described by Dwyer, was beneficial in preventing recurrent hindfoot varus when performed during a complete soft tissue release in infants one year of age or less. Toohey and Campbell (63) also found this osteotomy to be beneficial in younger patients with resistant clubfeet.

Plantar Release

A plantar release may be indicated for: (i) forefoot adduction, (ii) cavus deformity, or (iii) subluxation of the calcaneocuboid joint. Definite contraindications for plantar release include flatfoot or rocker-bottom deformity. A plantar release is accomplished medially in the axilla between the calcaneal branch and the neurovascular bundle. The scissors are directed toward the bony surface of the calcaneus as well as posteriorly to avoid injury to the lateral plantar vessels and nerve (Figure 6-12).

Internal Fixation

The foot can be realigned and pinned following the CSTR. Two or three smooth or threaded Kirschner wires are used depending upon the number of joints released (Figure 6-13A,B). Insertion of the talonavicular pin is facilitated by medially dislocating the foot. Accurate repositioning of the foot on the talus is critical to the success of the procedure. In the three- to six-month-old child this may be a matter of just two or three millimeters. The important clinical steps for repositioning include: (i) the navicular tuberosity must protrude a short distance medially; (ii) the dorsal surface of the navicular should correspond to the dorsal surface of the talar head and neck; (iii) the talus must be in longitudinal alignment with the navicular and midfoot; (iv) the talonavicular joint should not have a step-off laterally; and (v) the posterior aspect of the subtalar joint should be closed.

The calcaneocuboid joint is fully dislocated and the wire is driven in retrograde fashion through the calcaneus. The joint is reduced, and three-point pressure is applied to maintain reduction, while the wire is drilled into the cuboid.

A calcaneotalar pin crosses the subtalar joint into the talus, but does not extend into the ankle joint, while gentle lateral pressure is applied to the heel to push the calcaneus away from the fibula.

The position of the foot should be checked by flexing the knee and holding the foot at a right angle to the leg. The alignment of the foot is compared with the previously marked knee. The foot should appear to be absolutely plantigrade and with normal rotation so that it is in 0–20 degrees of external rotation with respect to the tibial apophyseal landmark (Figure 6-14).

Before radiographs are taken, the tension in the flexor tendons should be ascertained. The flexor hallucis longus frequently requires lengthening by recessing the musculotendinous junction whereas the flexor digitorum longus seldom requires lengthening. Before the radiographs are obtained the pneumatic tourniquet is deflated and hemostasis achieved. It is imperative that the position of the foot be checked radiographically during surgery after pin placement. The child should have intraoperative posteroanterior (PA) and lateral views. The cassette is placed on the

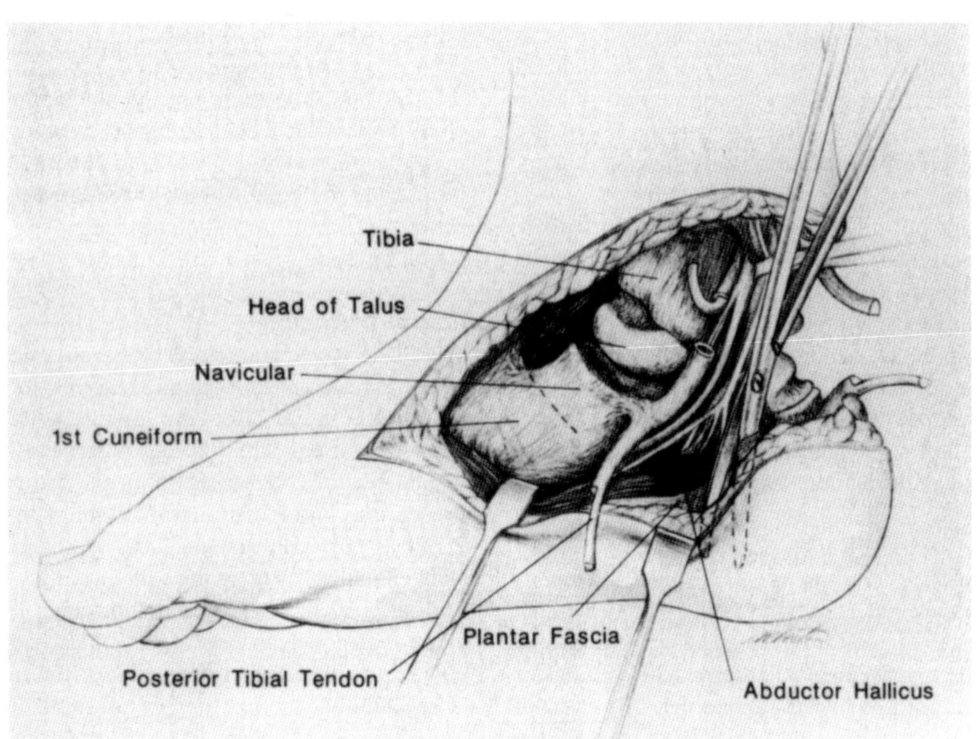

FIGURE 6-12 Technique of performing a plantar release.

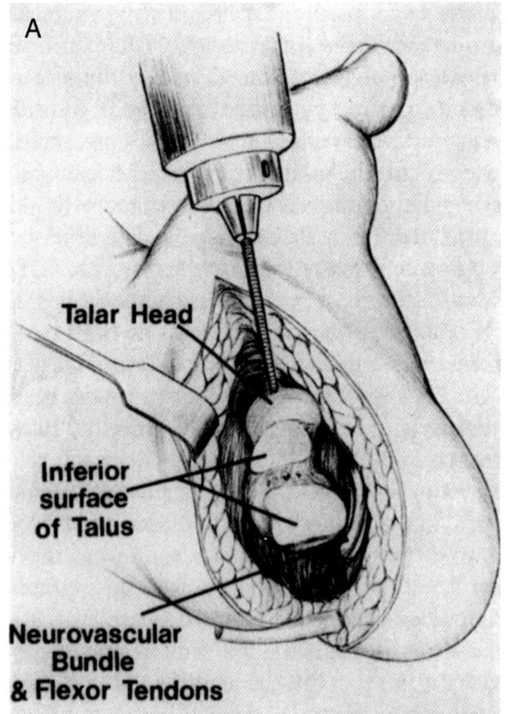

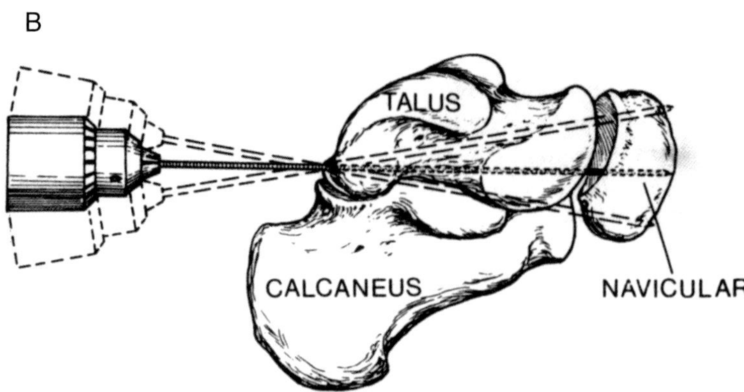

FIGURE 6-13 **A.** Technique of pin insertion into the central portion of the talar head which is preferred to inserting the pin from posteriorly to anteriorly. **B.** Improper pin insertion techniques. If the pin is inserted through the posterior end of the talus, it is unlikely that the pin will exit through the exact center of the talar head. Subsequent pinning of the navicular may be eccentric, and the pin may pull loose, causing loss of reduction of the talonavicular joint. (From Simons GW. Complete subtalar release in clubfeet. Part I. A preliminary report. *J Bone Joint Surg [Am]* 1985;67:1044–1055, with permission.)

table beneath the foot and the dorsum of the foot is laid on the cassette (Figure 6-15A,B). The head of the radiographic unit is perpendicular to the foot and the beam is angled between 27 and 30 degrees from the vertical position. A routine cross-table lateral projection is obtained with the foot held in the position of maximum dorsiflexion and parallel to the cassette (see Figure 6-15B). The radiographs should document satisfactory correction of all components of the deformity (see Table 6-1). As the PA view is essentially a midfoot-hindfoot projection, the forefoot should be over-exposed. This allows the entire circumference of the ossification centers of the talus and calcaneus to be visualized and measured in the young child.

The wires can be left percutaneous and bent or cut off just beneath the surface of the skin. The tibialis posterior tendon is replaced through its tunnel beneath the medial malleolus. The flexor hallucis longus is placed back into its canal and the other tendons are repaired with absorbable sutures.

Tendon Transfers

Tendon transfers are not commonly utilized in the initial surgical correction of resistant clubfeet. They are usually performed in the management of recurrent deformities or for salvage in the older child or adolescent. However, in very selected cases, they may be beneficial as part of the initial complete soft-tissue release.

McKay (33) has transferred the flexor hallucis longus tendon to the peroneus longus tendon when peroneal weakness could be documented preoperatively. This is difficult to evaluate in infants and young children. It is more commonly performed in older children or those with only one recurrence following surgery when there is no extensive scar formation.

The one indication for initial tendon transfer is the clubfoot associated with congenital absence of the tibialis posterior muscle and tendon. In these rare instances (4), transfer of the tibialis anterior tendon into the second or third cuneiform has maintained adequate muscle balance to the foot and prevented recurrence.

Ilizarov Technique

The Ilizarov technique has been an excellent means of treating relapsed or residual clubfeet following surgical correction. It has also been useful in treating neglected clubfeet in the older child that otherwise would have been candidates for osteotomies or triple arthrodesis. It is not used in the initial treatment of clubfeet in young patients. It allows correction at the focus of the deformity that is slow enough to protect the soft tissues, as well as allowing multilevel correction without shortening the foot. The Ilizarov technique can be used in children under the age of eight to distract soft tissues without the need for osteotomies, although above the age of eight, bony procedures are often needed as bones and joints are less capable of remodeling (40). Although several studies have found using an Ilizarov a useful tool with satisfactory outcomes (20,26,40,43).

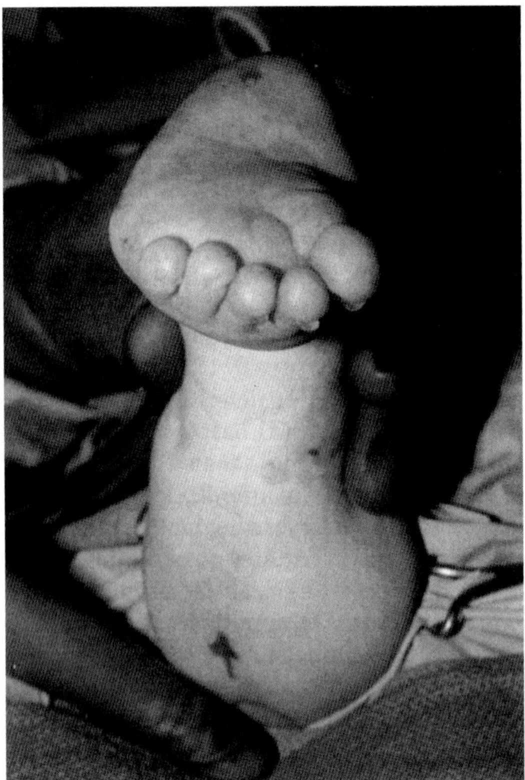

FIGURE 6-14 The position of the corrected foot with respect to the knee landmarks during surgery. The patient is prone position and the knee flexed at 90 degrees. The foot should be rotated around the talus until is aligned with the knee, and then it is properly aligned in other planes. (From Simons GW. Complete subtalar release in clubfeet. Part I. A preliminary report. *J Bone Joint Surg [Am]* 1985;67:1044–1055, with permission.)

RESULTS

Satisfactory long-term results have been reported in approximately 72% to 88% of cases following a complete soft-tissue release, including feet in young children with previous but less extensive surgery (10,19,34,41,54,61,65). A satisfactory result can be defined as a foot that is: (i) plantigrade and straight, (ii) has an adequate range of ankle motion including more than 10 degrees of dorsiflexion and 20 degrees of plantar flexion, (iii) no residual in-toeing, (iv) satisfactory radiographic measurements (see Table 6-2), and (v) requires no additional treatment (Figure 6-16A-F). Feet with unsatisfactory results or those that require additional treatment are usually secondary to extrinsic muscle imbalance rather than incomplete correction. Thompson et al. (61) demonstrated that radiographic findings that correlated the best with long-term results included the anterior talocalcaneal overlap or divergence, the lateral talocalcaneal angle, and the positions of the navicular and calcaneus.

ASSOCIATED DEFORMITIES

Other congenital anomalies can be associated with congenital clubfeet (Figure 6-17A-C). These can include: (i) polydactyly (see Figure 6-17A); (ii) overlapping fifth toe (see Figure 6-17B); (iii) accessory muscles (see Figure 6-17C); (iv) absence of the tibialis posterior muscle; and (v) anomalous insertions, such as the tibialis posterior tendon into the medial malleolus; and others. The treatment of these is individualized. Accessory muscles are usually excised while the tibialis anterior tendon is transferred to the dorsum at the foot when there is an absent or anomalous insertion of the tibialis posterior tendon.

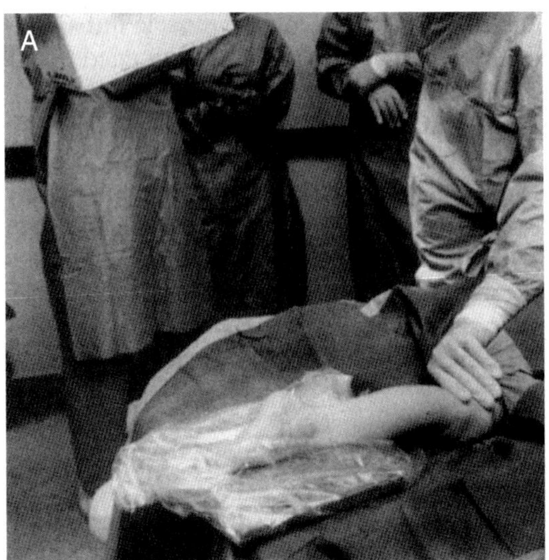

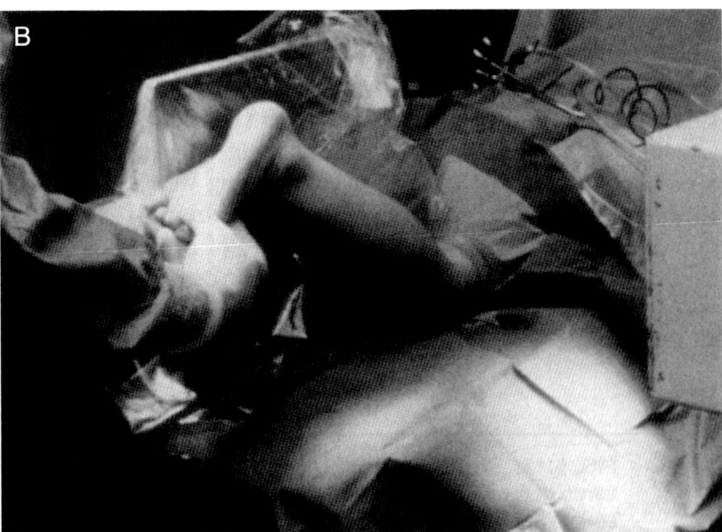

FIGURE 6-15 **A.** The technique of obtaining the intraoperative AP x-ray. The dorsum of the foot lies on the cassette in full dorsiflexion. The x-ray tube is angled at 27-30 degrees from the vertical position and the beam aimed at the talar head. **B.** The technique of taking the intraoperative lateral radiograph. The foot is held against the side of the cassette so that the hindfoot is parallel with the cassette. The x-ray tube is perpendicular to the foot and the cassette.

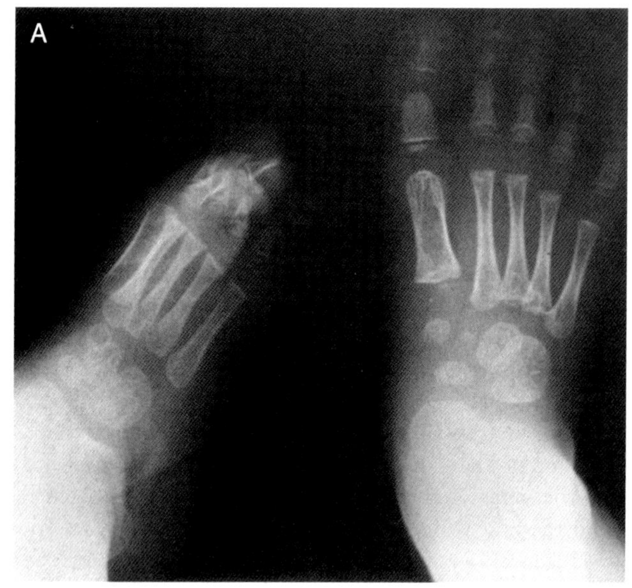
A

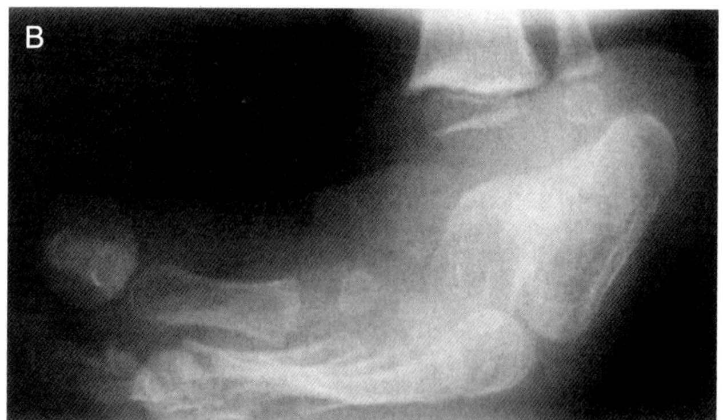
B

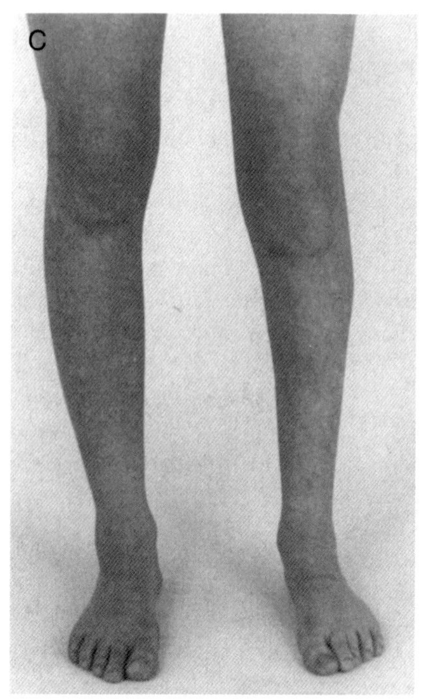
C

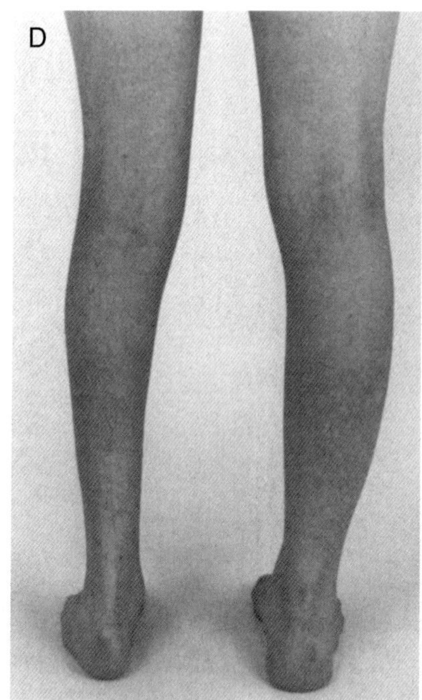
D

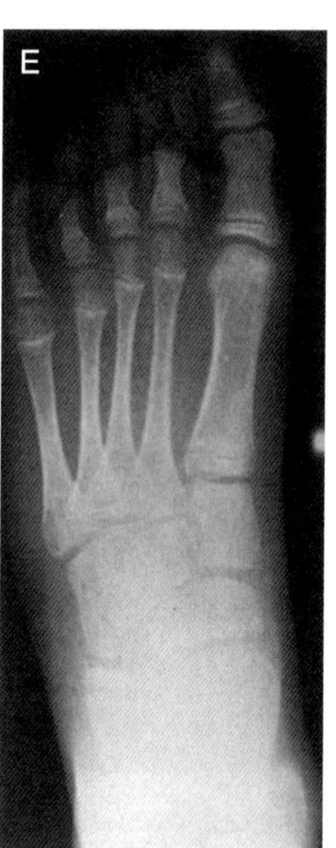
E

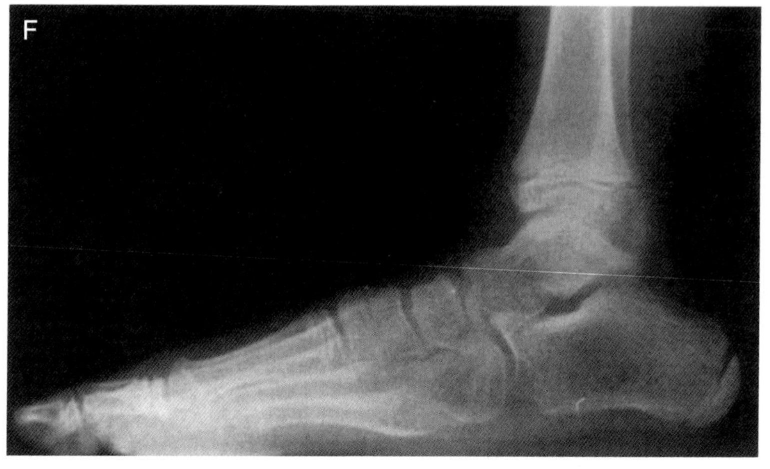
F

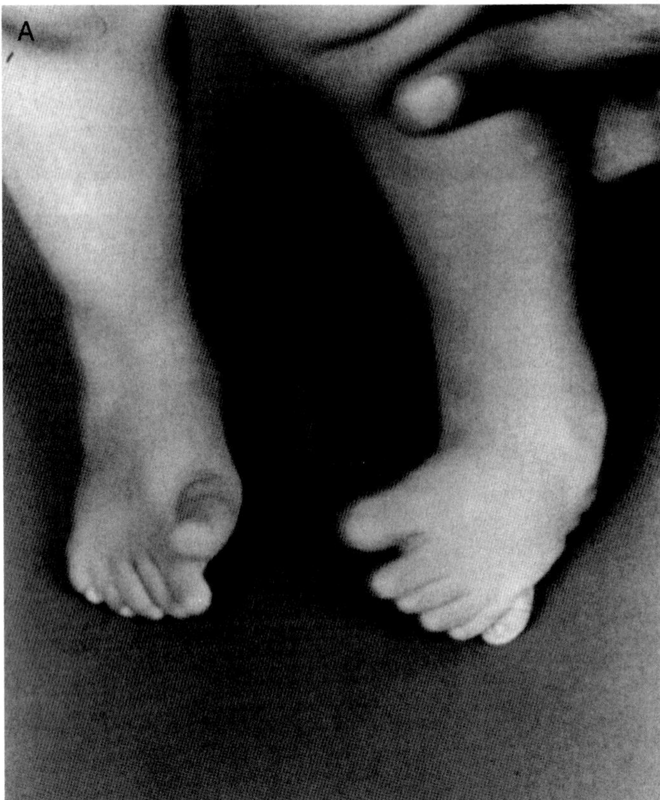

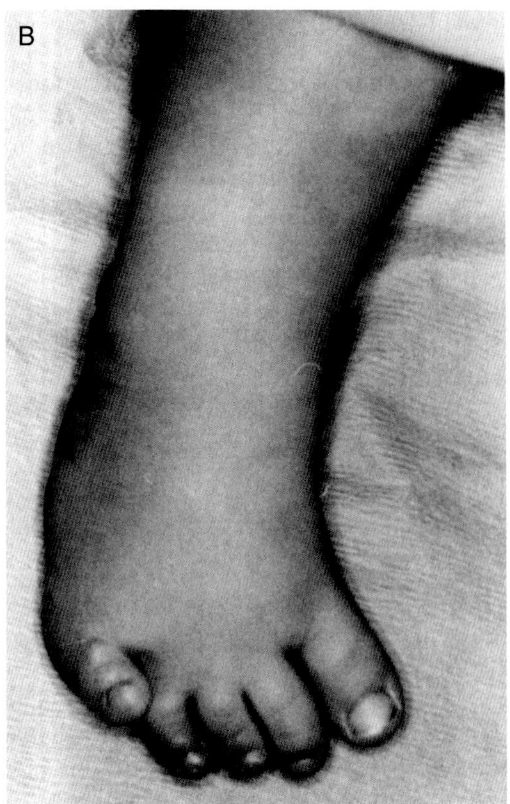

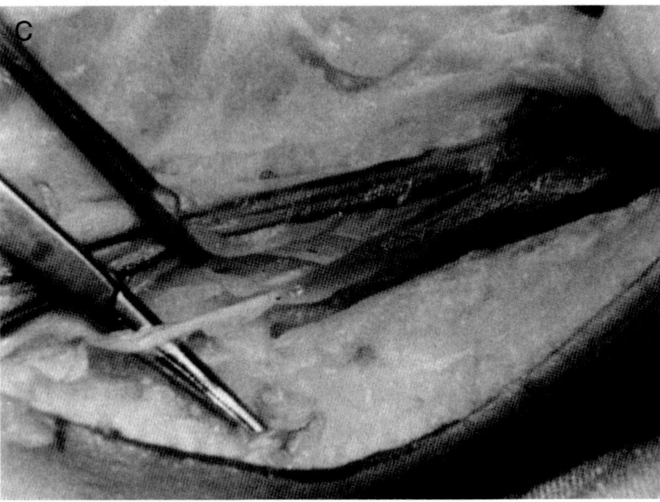

FIGURE 6-17 **A.** Clinical photograph of a nine-month-old male with a left congenital clubfoot associated with bilateral polydactyly. **B.** Clinical photograph of a nine-month-old female with a right congenital clubfoot and overlapping fifth toe. **C.** Intraoperative photograph of an accessory muscle. The muscle belly overlies the neurovascular bundle. Its small tendon inserts into the medial aspect of the calcaneus.

FIGURE 6-16 **A.** Preoperative AP (**A**) and lateral (**B**) weight-bearing radiographs showing the severe equinovarus deformity of the left foot and the normal appearing right foot. The lateral view also demonstrates severe forefoot supination. **C.** Clinical photograph obtained ten years following a left posteromedial plantar release. The foot is corrected with excellent mobility. There is moderate calf atrophy and an involved extremity. **D.** The posterior view demonstrates that the hindfoot is smaller and the calf atrophy and tibial shortening are more apparent in this view. **E.** Weight-bearing radiograph of the left foot ten years after surgical correction. The AP views demonstrates 1+ talocalcaneal overlap, a 20-degree talocalcaneal angle, and a centralized navicular indicating satisfactory correction. **F.** The lateral view demonstrates a neutral appearing calcaneus and a lateral talocalcaneal angle of 34 degrees.

COMPLICATIONS

Complications following clubfoot surgery occur in approximately 5% of cases. Overcorrection and under-correction are usually the result of extrinsic muscle imbalance, such as dynamic supination and dorsal subluxation at the navicular from a strong tibialis anterior muscle. True complications include marginal skin necrosis, wound dehiscence, pin tract infection, and avascular necrosis of the talus. These will be discussed in greater detail in subsequent chapters.

REFERENCES

1. Anderson D, Schoenecker P. *Combined lateral column shortening and medial column lengthening in the treatment of severe forefoot adductus.* Paper presented at the First International Congress on Clubfeet, Milwaukee, WI, Sept 5–6, 1990.
2. Attenborough CG. Early posterior soft-tissue release in severe talipes equinovarus. *Clin Orthop* 1972;84:71–78.
3. Barriolhet JL. *The first ray angle.* Paper presented at the First International Congress on Clubfeet, Milwaukee, WI, Sept 5–6, 1990.
4. Bensahel H, Csukonyi Z, Desgrippes Y, Chaumien JP. Surgery in residual clubfoot: one-stage medioposterior release "a la carte." *J Pediatr Orthop* 1987;7:145–148.
5. Brougham DI, Nicol RO. Use of the Cincinnati incision in congenital talipes equinovarus. *J Pediatr Orthop* 1988;8:6:696–698.
6. Cabanac J, Petit P, Maschas A. Le traitment de pied bot varus equin congenital. *Rev Chir Orthop* 1952;38:314.
7. Campos de Paz A Jr, De Souza V. Talipes equinovarus: Pathomechanical basis of treatment. *Orthop Clin North Am* 1978;9:171–185.
8. Carroll NC, McMurtry R, Leete SF. The pathoanatomy of congenital clubfoot. *Orthop Clin North Am* 1978;9:225–232.
9. Carroll NC. Pathoanatomy and surgical treatment of the resistant clubfoot. *Insrtuc Course Lect* 1988;37:93–106.
10. Crawford AH, Marken JL, Osterfeld DL. The Cincinnati incision: A comprehensive approach for surgical procedures of the foot and ankle in childhood. *J Bone Joint Surg (Am)* 1982;64:1335–1358.
11. Cummings RJ, Lovell WW. Current concepts review; operative treatment of congenital idiopathic club foot. *J Bone Joint Surg (Am)* 1988;70:1108–1112.
12. Davidson, RS. Clubfoot Salvage: A review of the past decade's contributions. *J Pediatr Orthop* 2003;23:410–418.
13. Davis LA, Hatt WS. Congenital abnormalities of the feet. *Radiology* 1955;64:318.
14. Debrunner H. Die Terapie des Angeborenem Klumpfusses. *Orthop* 1957;88:1–182.
15. DeDuy J, Drennan JC. Correction of idiopathic clubfoot: a comparison of results of early versus delayed posteromedial release. *J Pediatr Orthop* 1989;9:44–48.
16. DeRosa GP, Stepro D. Results of posteromedial release for the resistant clubfoot. *J Pediatr Orthop* 1986;6:590–595.
17. Dobbs MB, Rudzki JR, Purcell DB, Walton T, Porter KR, Gurnett CA. Factors predictive of outcome after use of the Ponseti method for treatment of idiopathic clubfeet. *J Bone Joint Surg (Am)* 2004;1:22–27.
18. Downey DJ, Drennan JC, Garcia JF. Magnetic resonance imaging findings in congenital talipes equinovarus. *J Pediatr Orthop* 1992; 12:224–228.
19. El-Deeb KH, Ghoneim AS, El-Adwar KL, Khalil AA. Is it hazardous or mandatory to release the talocalcaneal interosseous ligament in clubfoot surgery? A preliminary report. *J Pediatr Orthop* 2007;27:517–521.
20. Ferreira RC, Costa MT, Frizzo GG, Santin RA. Correction of severe recurrent clubfeet using a simplified setting of the Ilizarov device. *Foot Ankle Int* 2007;28(5):557–568.
21. Goldner JL. Congenital talipes equinovarus—Fifteen years of surgical treatment. *Current Practice of Orthopaedic Surgery* 1969;4:61–123.
22. Green ADL, Lloyd-Roberts GC. The results of early posterior release in resistant clubfeet. *J Bone Joint Surg (Br)* 1985;76:588–593.
23. Haft GF, Walker CG, Crawford HA. Early clubfoot recurrence after use of the Ponseti method in a New Zealand population. *J Bone Joint Surg (Am)* 2007;89:437–493.
24. Herzenberg JE, Carroll NC, Christofersen MR, Lee EH, White S, Munroe R. Clubfoot analysis with three-dimensional computer modeling. *J Pediatr Orthop* 1988;8:257–262.
25. Heywood SWB. The mechanics of the hindfoot in clubfoot as demonstrated radiographically. *J Bone Joint Surg (Br)* 1964;46:102–107.
26. Hoffman AA, Constine RM, McBride GG, Coleman SS. Osteotomy of the first cuneiform as treatment of residual adduction of the fore part of the foot in club foot. *J Bone Joint Surg (Am)* 1984;66:985–990.
27. Hutchins PM, Foster BK, Patterson DC, Cole EA. Long-term results of early surgical release in club feet. *J Bone Joint Surg (Br)* 1985;67:791–799.
28. Irani RN, Sherman MS. The pathological anatomy of idiopathic clubfoot. *Clin Orthop* 1972;84:14–20.
29. Laaveg SJ, Ponseti IV. Long-term results of treatment of congenital club feet. *J Bone Joint Surg (Am)* 1980;62:23–31.
30. Lundberg BJ. Early Dwyer operation in talipes equinovarus. *Clin Orthop* 1981;154:223–227.
31. Magone JB, Torch MA, Clark RN, Kean JR. Comparative review of surgical treatment of idiopathic clubfoot by three different procedures at Columbus Children's Hospital. *J Pediatr Orthop* 1989;9:49–58.
32. Marique P, Meuter DEW. Le controle radiographique au cours du traitment de pied bot par la methode de Denis Browne. *Rev Chir Orthop* 1951;37:250.
33. McKay DW. New concepts of an approach to clubfoot treatment. Section II. Principles and morbid anatomy. *J Pediatr Orthop* 1983;3:10–21.
34. McKay DW. New concepts of an approach to clubfoot treatment. Section III. Principles in morbid anatomy. *J Pediatr Orthop* 1983;3:141–148.
35. McKay DW. New concepts of and approach to clubfoot treatment. Section I. Principles in morbid anatomy. *J Pediatr Orthop* 1982;2:347–356.
36. McKay DW. Surgical correction of clubfoot. *Instr Course Lect* 1988;37:87–92.
37. Meary R. Le pied creux essential. Symposium. *Rev Chir Orthop* 1967;53:389.
38. Nather A, Bose K. Conservative and surgical treatment of clubfoot. *J Pediatr Orthop* 1987;7:42–48.
39. Ostremski I, Salam R, Khermosh O, Weintraub S. An analysis of the results of a modified one-stage posteromedial release (Turco operation) for the treatment of clubfoot. *J Pediatr Orthop* 1987;7:149–151.
40. Paley, D. The correction of complex foot deformities using Ilizarov's distraction osteotomies. *Clin Orthop Rel Res* 1993;293:97–111.
41. Porat S, Kaplan L. Critical analysis of results in club feet treated surgically along the Norris Carroll approach: Seven years of experience. *J Pediatr Orthop* 1989;9:137–143.
42. Pous JG, Dimeglio A. Neonatal surgery in clubfoot. *Orthop Clin North Am* 1978;9:233–240.
43. Premm H, Zenios M, Farrell R, Day JB. Soft tissue correction of congenital talipes equinovarus- 5 to 10 years postsurgery. *J Pediatr Orthop* 2007;27:220–224.
44. Reimann I. *Congenital idiopathic clubfoot.* Copenhagen: Munnksgaard, 1967.
45. Ryoppy S, Sairanen H. Neonatal operative treatment of clubfoot: a preliminary report. *J Bone Joint Surg (Br)* 1983;65:320–325.

46. Schaefer D, Hefti F. Combined cuboid/cuneiform osteotomy for correction of residual deformity in idiopathic and secondary club feet. *J Bone Joint Surg (Br)* 2000;82-B:881–884.
47. Settle GW. The anatomy of congenital talipes equinovarus. Sixteen dissected specimens. *J Bone Joint Surg (Am)* 1963;45:1341–1354.
48. Shapiro F, Glimcher MJ. Gross and histological abnormalities of the talus in congenital clubfoot. *J Bone Joint Surg (Am)* 1979;61:522–530.
49. Sherman FC, Westin GW. Plantar release in the correction of deformities of the foot in childhood. *J Bone Joint Surg (Am)* 1981;63:1382–1389.
50. Simons GW, Sarrafian S. The microsurgical dissection of a stillborn fetal clubfoot. *Clin Orthop* 1983;173:275–283.
51. Simons GW. A standardized method for the radiographic evaluation of clubfeet.
52. Simons GW. Analytical radiography of clubfoot. *J Bone Joint Surg (Br)* 1977;59:485–489.
53. Simons GW. Complete subtalar release in clubfeet. Part I. A preliminary report. *J Bone Joint Surg [Am]* 1985;67:1044–1055.
54. Simons GW. Complete subtalar release in clubfeet. Part II. Comparison of less extensive procedures. *J Bone Joint Surg (Am)* 1985;67:1056–1065.
55. Simons GW. The complete subtalar release in clubfeet. *Orthop Clin North Am* 1987;18:667–688.
56. Smith RB. Dysplasia and the effects of soft-tissue release in congenital talipes equinovarus. *Clin Orthop* 1983;174:303–309.
57. Somppi E, Sulumaa M. Early operative treatment of congenital club foot. *Acta Orthop Scand* 1971;42:513–520.
58. Templeton AW, McAlister WH, Zim ID. Standardization of terminology and evaluation of osseous relationships in congenitally abnormal clubfeet. *Am J Roentgenol* 1965;93:374–381.
59. Thomasen E. Der Angeborenem Klumpfuss. Uber die Machanik der Deformitat und ihre Primare Behandlung. *Acta Orthop Scand* 1941;12:33.
60. Thometz JG, Simons GW, Springer M. *Calcaneocuboid joint deformity in talipes equinovarus.* Paper presented at the annual meeting of the Pediatric Orthopaedic Society of North America. San Francisco, CA, May 6–9, 1990.
61. Thompson GH, Richardson AB, Westin GW. Surgical management of resistant congenital talipes equinovarus deformities. *J Bone Joint Surg (Am)* 1982;64:652–665.
62. Thompson GH. Comprehensive review of congenital clubfeet. *Adv Orthop Surg* 1991;14:245–260.
63. Toohey JS, Campbell P. Distal calcaneal osteotomy in resistant talipes equinovarus. *Clin Orthop* 1985;197:224–230.
64. Turco VJ. Resistant congenital clubfoot. *Instr Course Lect* 1975;24:104–121.
65. Turco VJ. Resistant congenital clubfoot-one-stage posteromedial release with internal fixation: A follow-up report of 15 years experience. *J Bone Joint Surg (Am)* 1979;61:805–814.
66. Wisbrun W. Neue Gesichtspunkle zum Redressement des Angeborenem Klumpfusses und Daraus such Ergebende Schlussfolgerungen Bezuglich der Atiologie. *Arch Orthop Unfallchir* 1932;31:451.
67. Yoneda B, Carroll NC. One-stage management of resistant clubfoot. *J Bone Joint Surg (Br)* 1984;66:302.
68. Zadek I, Barnett ELL. The importance of the ligaments of the ankle in correction of congenital clubfoot. *JAMA* 1917;69:1057.

CHAPTER 7

Complications in the Management of Talipes Equinovarus

Payam Moazzaz and Norman Y. Otsuka

INTRODUCTION

With an estimated occurrence of one to two clubfeet per 1,000 live births, talipes equinovarus represents the most common congenital orthopaedic anomaly. Historically management includes an initial trial of manipulations and serial casting (37,43). Thirty percent to fifty percent of feet did not respond to treatment with manipulations and required surgical correction (20,43,48,76,81). Given 3.75 million annual births in the United States this implies that over 2,000 patients annually would have surgery recommended due to failure of nonoperative treatment. Surgery historically involved a one-stage complete soft-tissue release between three and twelve months of age. Initial surgical treatment is successful in 50% to 87% of cases, however the average failure rate is considerable at 25% (13% to 50%).

Coleman stated that "despite meticulous care and attention to detail occasional untoward results are inevitable even with the most conscientious treatment of some congenital clubfeet" (8). These "untoward results" determine the failure rate (32). They consist of complications that may occur before, during and after surgery. Some of them are preventable.

More neently the Ponseti technique of casting and other manipulative methods have become the current standard of core. This technique and the complications are discussed in chapter 5

COMPLICATIONS OF NON–SURGICAL TREATMENT OF THE CLUBFOOT

Complications occurring from non–surgical management of the clubfoot must not be overlooked. Vigorous manipulations and casting are not innocuous and must be done meticulously to prevent pressure sores, stress fractures, infections from ingrown toenails, and deformities of the toes due to cast pressure. In addition, the challenging "rocker bottom" deformity may be seen as a result of an exceedingly vigorous attempt at before the prerequisite correction of the talus and calcaneus has occurred.

Kite employed a technique combining gentle manipulation and serial cast treatment, and this is still commonly used today. This technique is complicated by the development of pressure sores which preclude not only the continuation of this technique but also interrupt the corrective treatment to allow the wounds to heal. Surgical treatment may also be compromised by scarring and infected skin which may necessitate alteration of the surgical approach (37). He recommended the use of soft felt protective pads placed at locations under the cast, where the surgeon's fingers would exert pressure.

Great care is required in the application of any clubfoot cast in order to prevent loss of proper positioning and cast slippage. The foot is casted and molded into the appropriate position over the proper amount of cotton or Webril padding. Once this portion of the cast has hardened, the more proximal leg portion is added. The leg and foot are then externally rotated to force the forefoot out of adduction and the cast is continued up to the groin with the knee flexed 40–60 degrees. This type of cast effectively forces the foot into the corrected position while maintaining satisfactory alignment of the ankle. The above knee cast also prevents displacement or loss of the cast in the "wiggling baby" (43).

Keim described damage to the "soft" bones of the foot, especially the dome of the talus, which may occur when the un-giving foot is manipulated (36). The "nutcracker" treatment of the clubfoot should be avoided, and gentle manipulation should be performed in the proper sequence to avoid the creation of a stress fracture (Figure 7-1). Denham's words should be remembered: "In the infant hard tissues (bone and cartilage) should be regarded as soft and the soft tissues (tendon and ligaments) as hard" (12). Fractures of the leg and foot caused by excessive manipulation may not be recognized unless x-rays are taken following the manipulation (79). An iatrogenic hallux valgus deformity

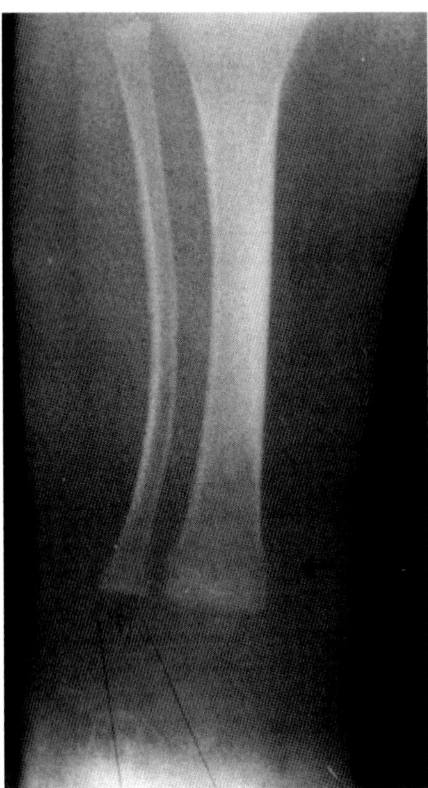

FIGURE 7-1 Stress fracture of the tibia following clubfoot manipulations.

may also be created by excessively vigorous casting (Figure 7-5). Severe deformity will respond only to surgical release.

Toenail Infections

Infections from ingrown toenails can be devastating in the infant and result in bacteremia. The "ingrown" toenail usually involves the hallux and is caused by the cast pressing the skin against the toenail. These infections are very resistant to treatment once they occur. Management includes the cessation of casting, warm soaks, packing the overlying eponychium away from the nail, or excising a portion of the nail. All casting, manipulations, and surgery must be delayed or modified once the complication of an ingrown toenail occurs.

Rocker-Bottom

The dreaded "rocker bottom" deformity has been found to occur in up to 3.2% of patients managed with conservative treatment of idiopathic congenital clubfoot (38). The "rocker bottom" foot can be avoided if correction of the equinus hindfoot is not attempted until the calcaneus has been de-rotated from the talus (Figure 7-2). When spurious clinical correction occurs at the calcaneo-cuboid and talonavicular joints (Chopart's joints), the result is a mid-foot weight-bearing pressure area which will continually break down (Figures 7-3 and 7-4). This complication is difficult to correct and requires manipulating the foot back to its original deformity before correcting the malrotation of the calcaneus on the talus. Often surgical correction is also required to correct this challenging deformity.

COMPLICATIONS OF SURGICAL MANAGEMENT OF CLUBFOOT SURGERY

Infections

Infection is the bane of the clubfoot surgeon. The most carefully performed surgical release will be doomed by the development of a subsequent infection (Figure 7-12). Preoperative casting should be stopped at least two weeks prior to surgery to allow the skin to be stretched and cleansed with soap and water twice daily. Perioperative antibiotics are recommended. Intravenous antibiotics are begun prior to surgery and maintained for 36 to 48 hours postoperatively. Currently cephalosporin is utilized at the

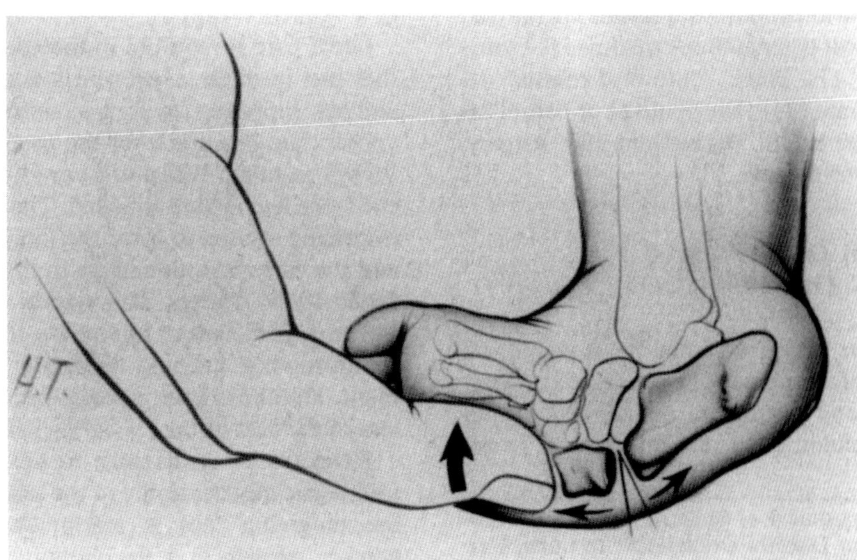

FIGURE 7-2 "Rocker bottom" foot. Manipulation of the foot has not brought the heel down out of equinus and because the calcaneus has not rotated around the talus the foot is being "broken" at Chopart's joint (calcaneocuboid and talonavicular joints).

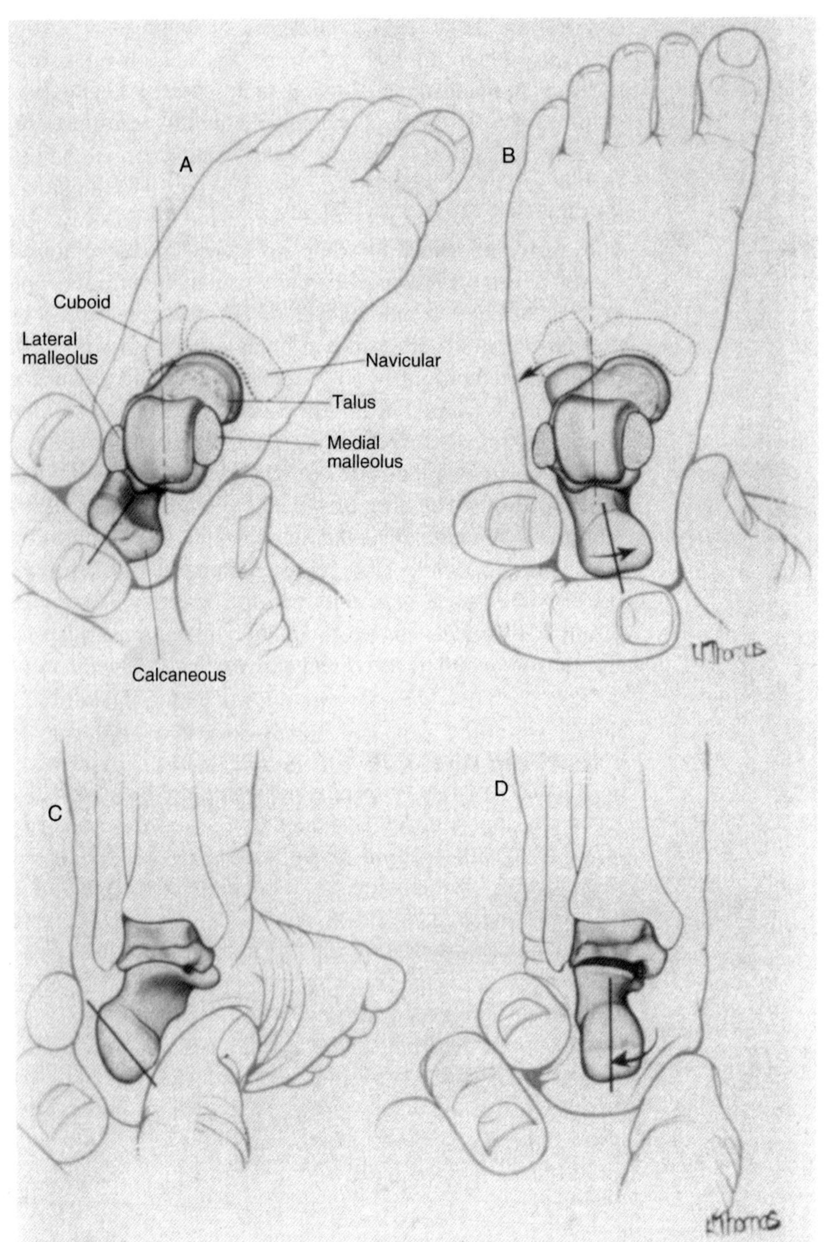

FIGURE 7-3 Derotating of the calcaneus. The deformed medial pointing talus with the navicular displayed medially and calcaneus fixed in an inverted medial rotated position at the subtalar joint (**A**). The calcaneus rotated laterally with the navicular and cuboid at the subtalar joint allowing dorsiflexion of the foot to bring the heel out of equinus (**B**) at the same time allowing eversion of the heel to occur at the subtalar joint (**C,D**).

Shriners Hospitals for Children Los Angeles, and we suggest that the antibiotic choice be made by the infectious disease consultant at your institution. Postoperative adhesive strips are placed over the incision without use of tincture of benzoin which may be contaminated. An iodine impregnated dressing is used to cover the wound prior to the addition of sterile padding and plaster casting. The use of this protocol has led to a minimal number of post-operative infections at our institution.

A temperature elevation of > 38.5 degrees Celsius on the third to fourth postoperative day usually indicates infection. The wound should be cleaned, cultured, and appropriate antibiotics should be given. The infection may be related to the pin sites (18) and necessitate their removal. Wound dehiscence, skin sloughs, and wound infection usually result in excessive scarring which may unfortunately lead to recurrence of the deformity.

Skin Incisions and Wound Healing

Many incisions have been devised for clubfeet surgery. Selecting an incision that provides satisfactory exposure and is associated with prompt wound healing may be difficult, especially in a foot that has experienced previous incisions. Consideration of the vascular territories supplied by the arteries of the ankle and foot (angiosomes) (46) (Figure 7-6) indicate that certain incisions are safer than others (Figure 7-7). The Cincinnati and circumferential incisions (9,53,67,77) extend across the vascular supply of the skin and involve adjacent angiosomes. Skin slough should be anticipated, especially over the age of two years (9,55) (Figure 7-8). The posterior longitudinal incision is safe; however, problems with wound healing and excessive scar formation are common, and exposure is limited to the medial and lateral sides of the foot (22,33,60). The posteromedial incision combined with a

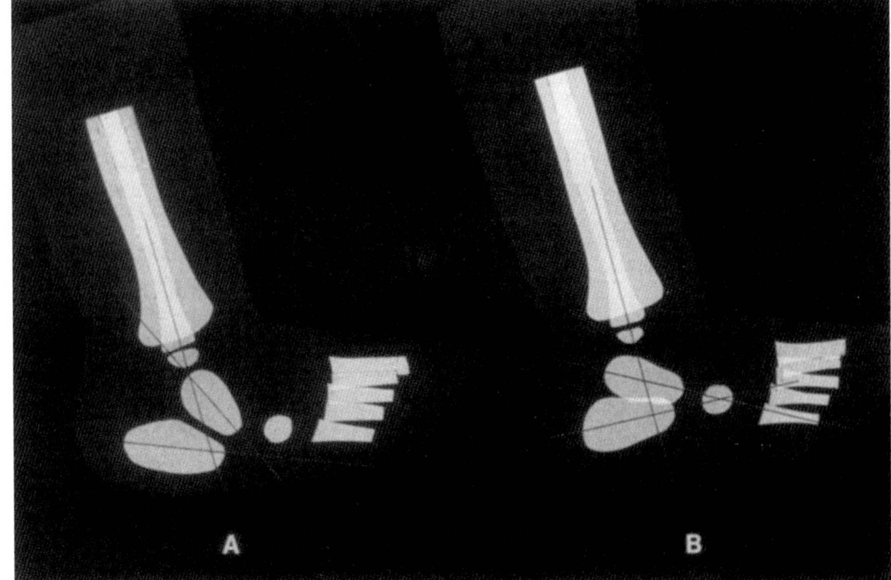

FIGURE 7-4 Diagrammatical representation of an x-ray (**A**) of a clubfoot being forced into dorsiflexion and the correction occurring at Chopart's joint (false correction) and (**B**) showing dorsiflexion correcting the equinus of the heel if the calcaneus as shown in Figure 7-3 is rotated laterally at the subtalar joint.

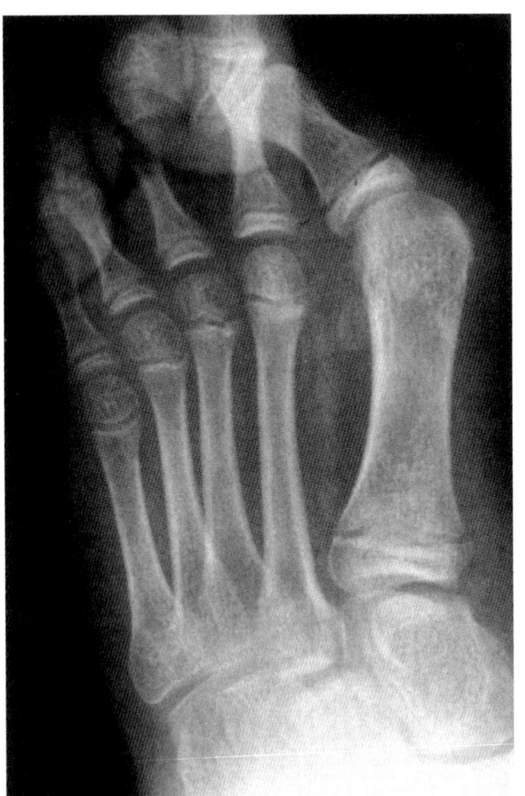

FIGURE 7-5 Hallux valgus deformity as a result of clubfoot casting.

vertical lateral or anterolateral incision, when necessary, is probably the safest approach which allows for extensile exposure (4,24,43,46).

Wound dehiscence can be prevented by preoperative stretching of the contracted soft tissues, gentle handling of the tissues during surgery, and careful hemostasis prior to skin closure (65).

The foot may be left in a partially corrected position when the skin incision cannot be approximated with the foot in the fully corrected position and Kirschner wires have not been used to stabilize the hindfoot correction. Weekly or biweekly cast changes are then performed, gradually changing the position of the foot while the soft tissue heals. When fixation is used to maintain proper alignment of the talonavicular and talocalcaneal joints, it may be necessary to remove one or both wires to allow skin approximation and follow this with staged manipulations and casting to allow the foot to reach the desired position. In some cases, a dorsolateral skin incision may allow the movement of redundant lateral skin medially which is commonly found after operative correction (5,6,24) (Figure 7-9). Alternatively, closure may be obtained by a Z-plasty skin closure (Figure 7-10).

Preoperative myocutaneous or fasciocutaneous flaps or a balloon tissue expander may be considered when skin problems are anticipated (2,24,62) (Figure 7-11). A local transpositional flap can also be utilized at the time of wound closure in older patients with severe clubfoot deformity (35). The application of human skin allograft may also be used for open wounds in severe cases in which the incision may not be closed primarily. The allograft skin affords protection to the underlying tissue while allowing granulation tissue formation and wound contraction (64).

There is consensus that scarring of tendon repairs and skin may cause a recurrence of the clubfoot deformity. The choice of material and technique to repair tendons and skin incisions is debated. The authors recommend repairing tendons with small caliber bioabsorbable sutures while using small needles (P-3). The flexor hallucis longus and flexor digitorum longus tendons should be lengthened at their musculocutaneous junction when necessary (3). Minimal subcutaneous sutures are recommended to avoid compromising the dermal blood supply. A subcuticular

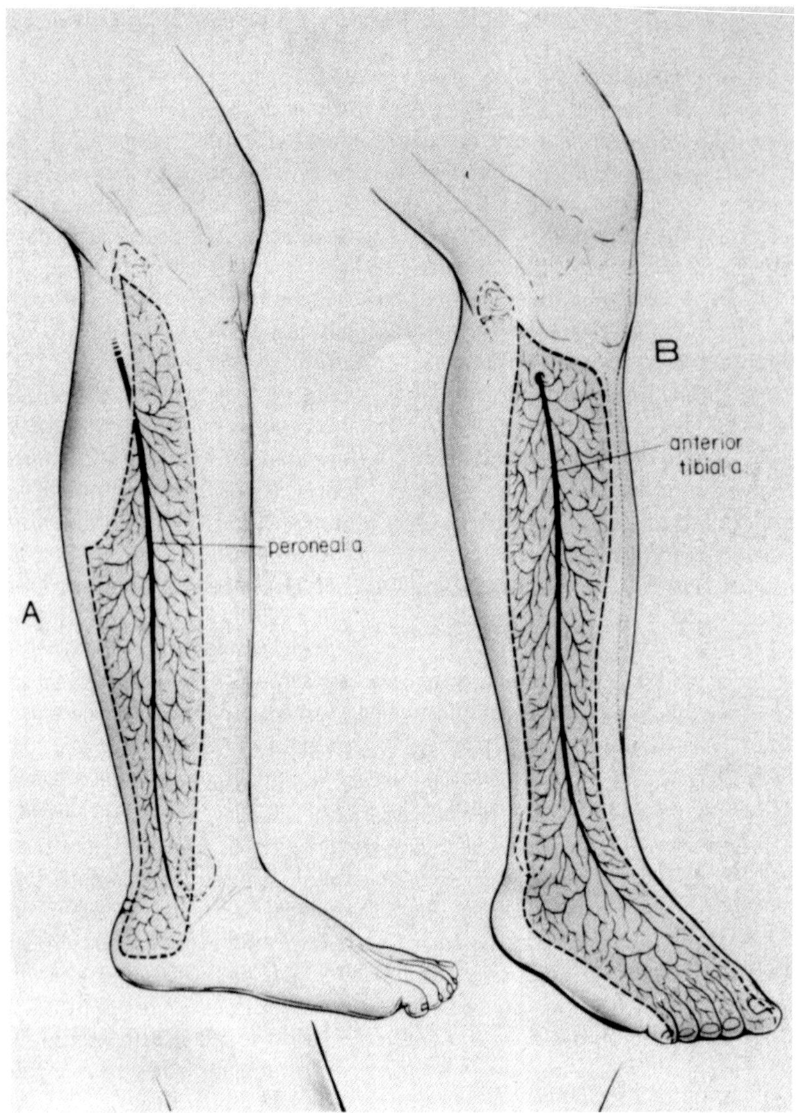

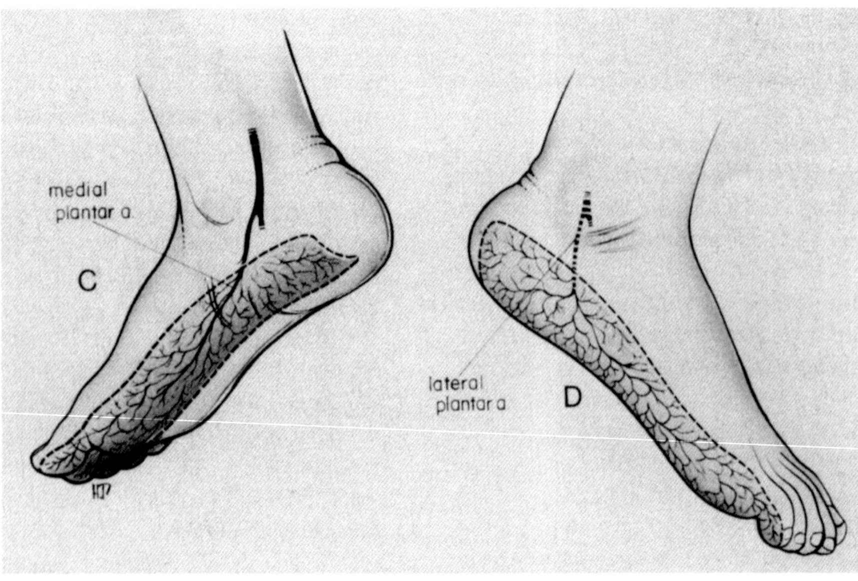

FIGURE 7-6 Angiosomes (vascular territory) of the foot. **A.** Peroneal artery, a branch of the popliteal artery supplying the lateral side of the leg just below the fibula malleolus. **B.** The anterior tibial artery, a branch of the popliteal supplying the anterolateral part of the leg and dorsum of the foot. **C.** Medial plantar artery supplying the medial part of the sole of the foot. **D.** Lateral plantar artery supplying the lateral part of the sole of the foot. **E,F.** Posterior tibial artery. A branch of the popliteal artery supplying the posteromedial part of the leg and a small strip of skin on the medial side of the foot and big toe and a large part of skin on the posterior part of the heel.

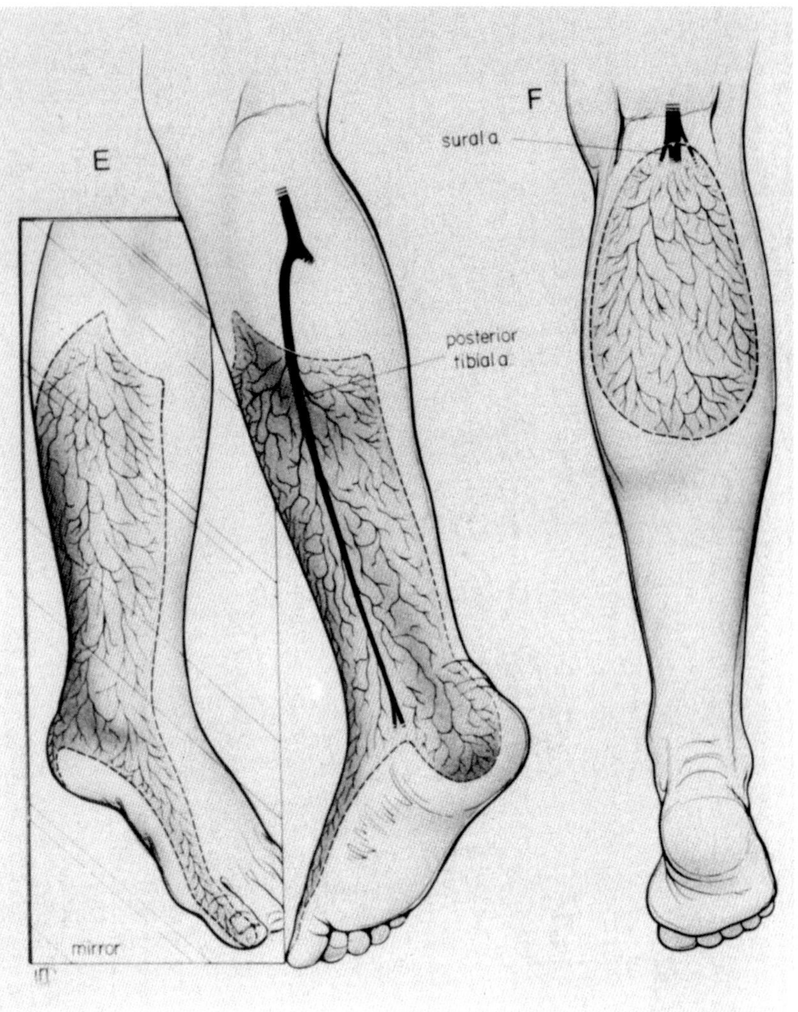

FIGURE 7-6 (*Continued*)

skin closure is appropriate even though this is time consuming. Alternatively, interrupted sutures of non–absorbable material may be required when postoperative manipulations will be necessary to help avoid wound dehiscence. Scar is the enemy of a good result—it must be avoided every step of the way.

Existing skin incisions will test the ingenuity of any surgeon involved in revision clubfoot surgery. As a general rule, crossing existing skin incisions should be avoided. The previous approaches should be utilized and reopened in order to avoid additional dermal compromise. Auxiliary vertical incisions may be added.

When pullout buttons are utilized over the sole of the foot with anterior or posterior tibial tendon transfer for persistent muscle imbalance, plantar skin necrosis may occur. This may be avoided by padding the undersurface of the button with soft rubber tubing instead of cotton, or using an absorbable suture that will dissolve by itself, allowing the button to eventually fall off.

Damage to the Neurovascular Bundle

The neurovascular bundle is carefully identified, dissected, and mobilized before the remainder of the clubfoot surgery is performed. The blood supply of the foot depends largely or entirely on the patency of the posterior tibial artery since the dorsalis pedis artery is absent or abnormal in many clubfeet. Vascular compromise should be anticipated in any clubfoot operation. Complete transaction of the posterior tibial artery and tibial nerve has been described (7). Injury to the peroneal artery and the lesser saphenous vein are also known complications of percutaneous tendo-Achilles tenotomy (15). Transfixing pins may also puncture the neurovascular bundle or its branches during surgery. These vessels should then be coagulated and change of the pin position may possibly be required. When skin blanching occurs because of excessive stretching of the neurovascular bundle the foot should be placed in an under-corrected position until skin color returns. The tourniquet should be released and all bleeding controlled before skin closure. Hemostasis should be maintained throughout the procedure. The position of the foot which allows for an uncompromised dermal vascular supply should be maintained in the cast or posterior plaster splint postoperatively. Excessive stretching of the posterior tibial artery by casting the foot in a forcibly corrected position may result in soft tissue necrosis when the dorsalis pedis artery is absent. There has been at least one report of a compartment syndrome

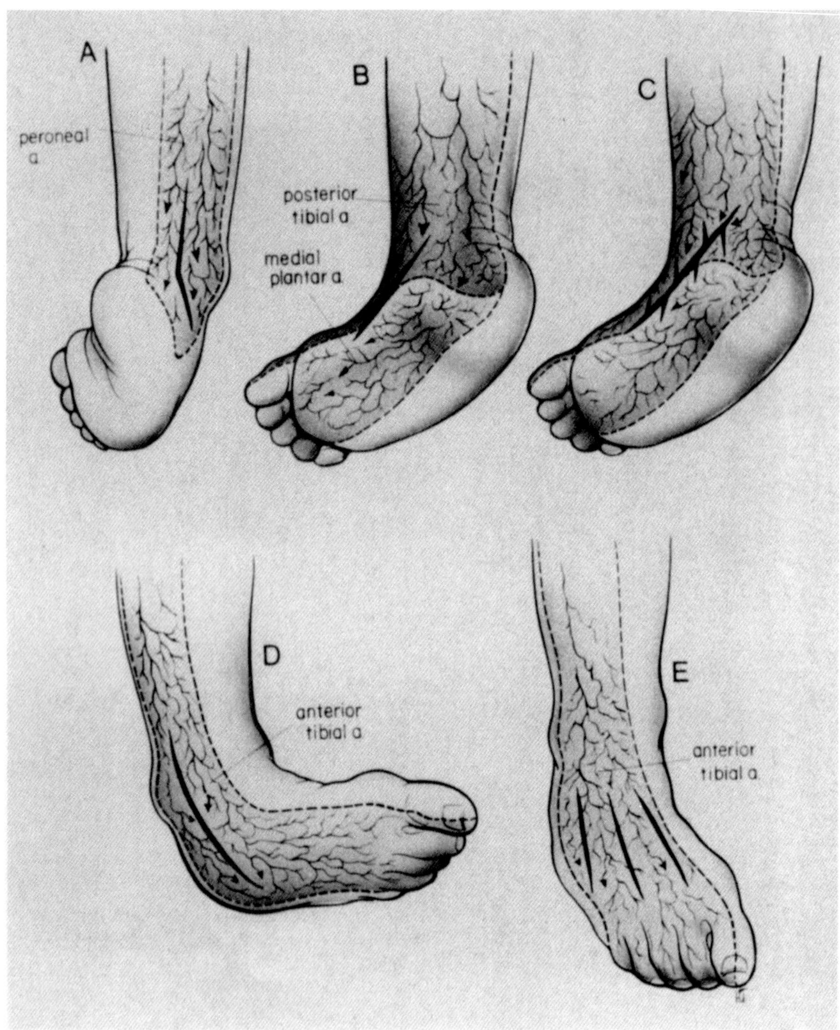

FIGURE 7-7 Vertical incisions of the foot are anatomically best and safest to avoid crossing angiosomes. **A.** Posterolateral incisions. **B.** Posteromedial incision. **C.** Z-plasty posteromedial incision. **D.** Vertical anterolateral incision (for approach to the lateral side of the foot including the calcaneo-cuboid joint and sinus tarsi). **E.** Dorsal vertical incisions of the foot.

in after clubfoot surgery (68). Pseudoaneurysm presenting as an enlarging, pulsatile mass two to three months after the index procedure has also been described and requires treatment with ligation and excision (41,57). Postoperative avascular changes may result in amputation (14,30,31) and underlines the importance of preventing vascular injury during or following surgery. It is suggested that eye loupes of 2–3 times magnification be used in young children to avoid vascular embarrassment.

Torniquet Use

The amount and duration of tourniquet pressure is important. The recommended pressure is 50–75 mmHg above the systolic pressure obtained by the anesthesiologist in the operating room. The use of the tourniquet makes the surgical procedure technically less demanding and minimizes blood loss. The use of an Esmarch or Martin bandage to exsanguinate the extremities is probably unnecessary and simple elevation of the leg for 3–4 minutes before tourniquet inflation is sufficient to decompress the vessels. Visualization of the partially emptied vessels by this technique will assist the surgeon during dissection. The tourniquet can be safely inflated for at least one hour and probably up to an hour and a half. It is recommended that the tourniquet be released after one hour to allow the leg to be perfused for 2–3 minutes and can then be reapplied. There have been several reports of skin blisters and dermal necrosis under the tourniquet when iodine compounds have been used to prepare the skin. These chemical burns can cause severe soft tissue necrosis and unsightly scarring. We would recommend the use of an alcohol-water-soap preparation for the skin. The application of a tourniquet may be difficult in infants because of the very short length of the thigh and prove inadequate for the duration of the surgical procedure and may necessitate a change or adjustment of the tourniquet. We have found a sterile tourniquet above the drape to be helpful since it is accessible for possible adjustment and change. Monitoring of the blood pressure should be done by the anesthesiologist and is easier when the tourniquet is in view and not obscured by drapes (19). The neurovascular bundle may be inadvertently transected, most commonly during the dissection of a badly scarred reoperated clubfoot. Any nerve laceration should be promptly repaired. The tourniquet is then released to evaluate the blood flow to the foot. Vascular integrity is

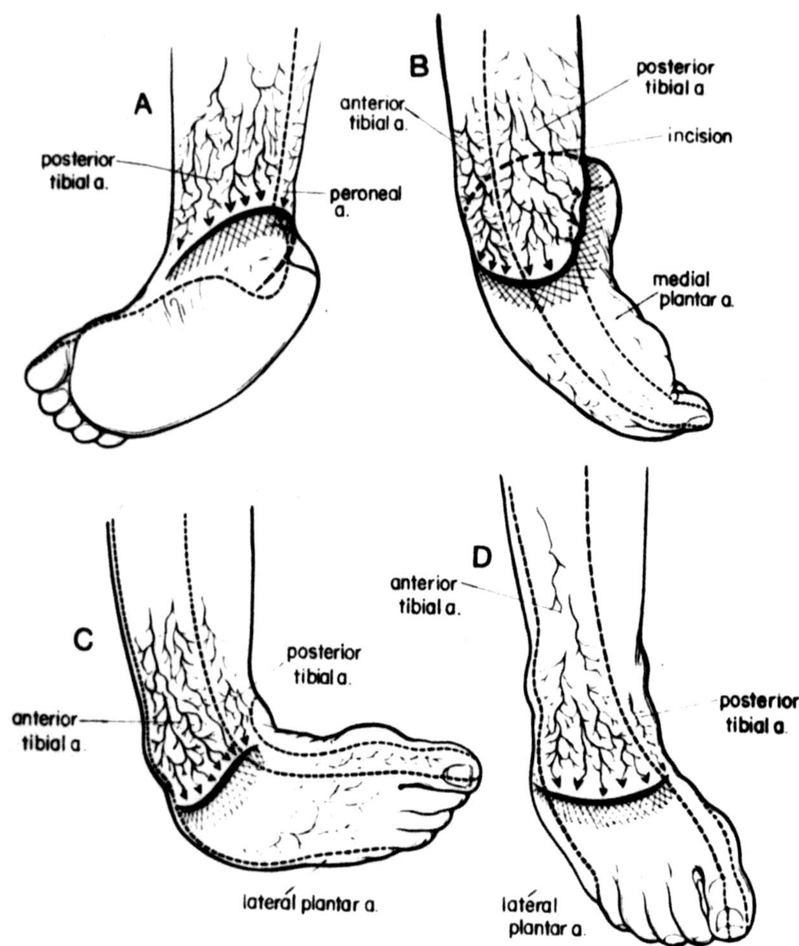

FIGURE 7-8 Horizontal incisions although extensile cross angiosomes and will compromise skin noted by the cross hatching. **A.** Horizontal or transverse incision. **B.** Circumferential incision. **C,D.** Typical lateral sinus tarsi incision.

generally adequate and therefore the vessel most likely will not require repair. Vessel repair should be attempted when blood flow appears inadequate. The tourniquet should be released and all bleeding controlled before skin closure.

Postoperative immobilization begins with sterile, soft cast padding which should be completely applied from the toes to the thigh, followed by application of the plaster cast which is also split or bivalved. In our institution, we have found it best to simply utilize a posterior plaster splint and delay the definitive cast until a few days later especially when there is considerable postoperative swelling on the dorsum of the foot (68).

Injury to Bones and Joints

Inadvertent transection of the sustentaculum tali and the talar head may occur during the surgical dissection. There are almost no sequelae to these complications when recognized and treated promptly. The sustentaculum tali can be transected during medial subtalar release, especially when a fibrous or cartilaginous talocalcaneal bar is present (25). The detached part should be repositioned and fixed with Kirschner wires or sutures. The talar head may be divided during an attempt to open the talonavicular joint and should be similarly repositioned and fixed with Kirschner wires or sutures.

Avascular Necrosis

Extensive surgical dissection may cause avascular necrosis of the talus and the navicular (1,8,42). The vascularity of the talus in children has been described as more vulnerable than that of adults (34). Osteonecrosis of the talus has been reported in 0.5% of cases, and more commonly occurs with the more severe types of clubfoot (18,42,66). This complication can be prevented by refraining from lateral dissection of the subtalar joint and sinus tarsi during the posteromedial release (1,42). Nine cases of flattening of the talar dome or hypolasia of the talar head or neck were recently reported in 96 patients following McKay soft tissue release. The absence of normal talar growth lines and bone-within-the-bone appearance of the talus at any time during follow up was always associated with an abnormality of the talus in this study (11). The

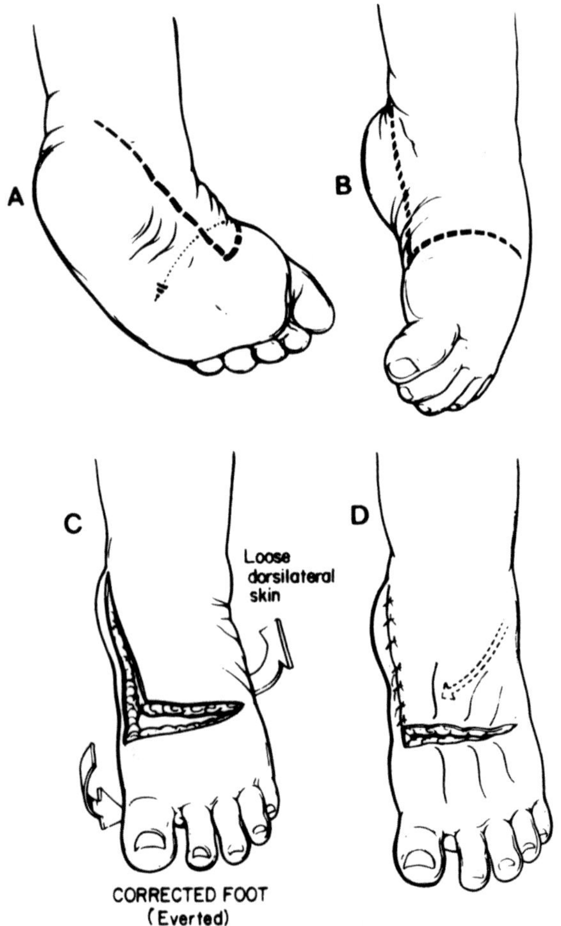

FIGURE 7-9 Lateral skin release. After foot is placed in corrected position, a dorsal incision is made releasing a dorsal flap of skin to be moved medially due to the extra skin folds laterally in the clubfoot.

treatment of talar aseptic necrosis is supportive; patellar tendon bearing brace until re-ossification of the talus is sufficient. Long-term results are poor, often requiring arthrodesis because of pain.

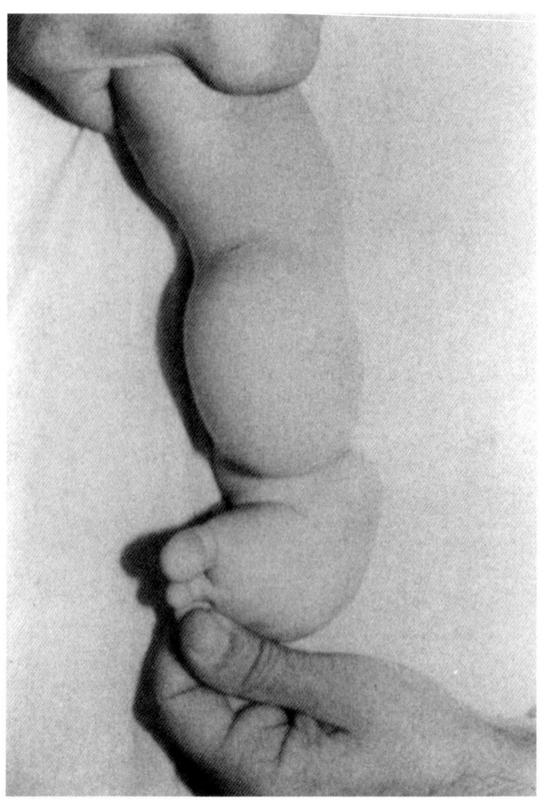

FIGURE 7-11 Balloon tissue expander. A sterile subcutaneous balloon with a water reservoir has been inserted in the foot to obtain more skin foreclosure.

The navicular in a normal child may be radiographically asymmetric in size, shape and density. Since the navicular usually does not ossify until two to four years of age, it is not unusual for a normal navicular to demonstrate a fragmented appearance as it ossifies. Wedging and flattening are not uncommon in the treated clubfoot. Two cases of navicular aseptic necrosis in 81 surgical cases were recently reported. This study also noted an additional seven feet demonstrated fragmentation of the navicular associated with either delayed ossification or multiple ossification

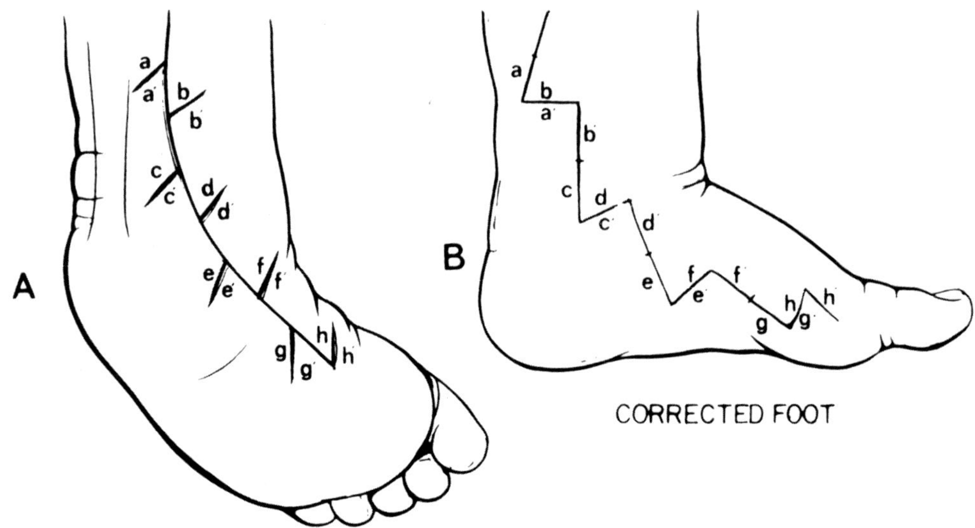

FIGURE 7-10 Z-plasty skin release.

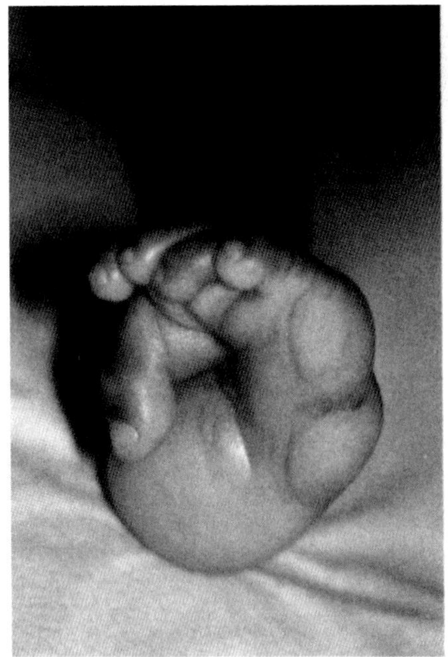
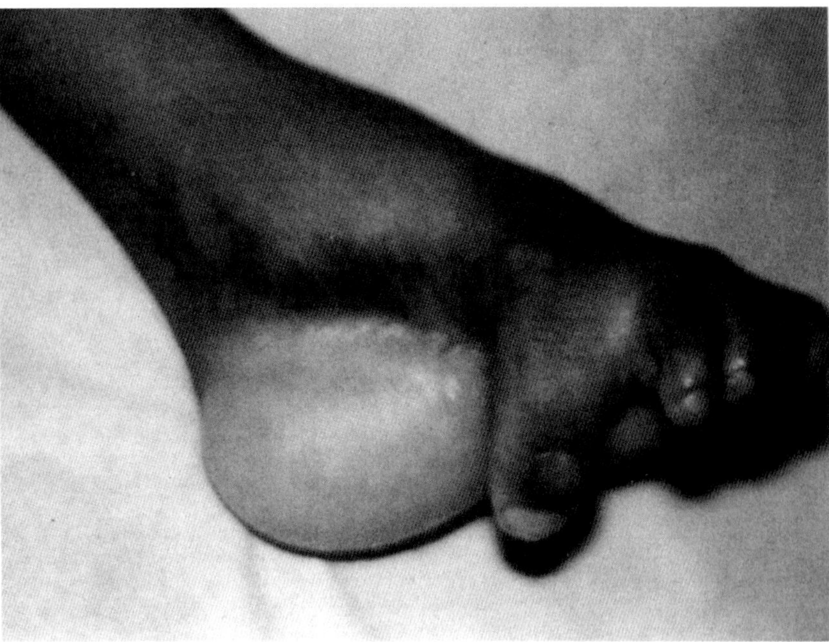

FIGURE 7-12 Postoperative complete soft tissue clubfoot release following skin infection. **A.** Sole of foot. **B.** Medial view of foot.

centers (66). Another report found that 20 out of 24 feet surgically corrected showed wedging and truncation of the navicular which may be caused by aseptic necrosis (58). Avascular necrosis of the navicular causes no functional impairment early. The bone will re-ossify. Long-term effects of the abnormal ossified navicular have not been reported.

Excessive surgical dissection with damage to the subtalar articular surfaces will result in stiffness. It may also cause the creation of an iatrogenic talocalcaneal bar which may cause gradual recurrent inversion of the heel requiring repeated clubfoot surgery (45). Meticulous release of the subtalar joint is recommended and consideration given to avoidance of the use of pin fixation so that the feet can be manipulated frequently to avoid stiffness. It is not certain whether stiffness of the subtalar joints is related to surgical dissection or the use or non–use of transfixing pins. Pin site infections, pin migration, and pins puncturing vessels or causing tendon impingement must be recognized and the pins adjusted (13).

Injury to Growth Plates

The posterior tibial physis may be damaged during posterior capsulotomy. An increasing equinus or varus or valgus deformity of the ankle may result. Treatment includes excision of the osseous bar with fat graft interposition or supramalleolar wedge osteotomy in the older child (Figure 7-13).

The distal fibular physis may also be violated during the posterior release (section of the calcaneofibular ligament), resulting in ankle valgus. Treatment includes bar excision with fat graft interposition, fibular lengthening or supramalleolar varus osteotomy of the tibia in the older child.

The first metatarsal physis may be injured during capsulotomy of the cuneiform-first metatarsal. A short first metatarsal may result, which mechanically places the stress of weight bearing on the second and third metatarsal heads. Varus or valgus deviation of the first metatarsal may occur when the physis is only partially damaged. Treatment includes physeal bar resection with fat interposition or first metatarsal lengthening or osteotomy.

Persistent Equinus

Persistent equinus may result from inadequate posterior release and can be prevented by obtaining intraoperative radiographs. The restoration of the normal lateral talocalcaneal angle documents adequate posteromedial release (43) (Figure 7-14). This deformity can also result from inadequate postoperative cast management or non–compliant parents. It usually necessitates repeat surgical intervention.

Calcaneus Deformity (Heel Walker)

Over-lengthening of the Achilles tendon is the most common cause of this deformity. This complication may occur even with experienced surgeons (55, 80) (Figure 7-15). Conservative treatment includes passive stretching of the ankle capsule and the dorsiflexor muscles as well as active exercise program for the plantar flexors. Surgical intervention may be necessary when conservative management fails and can include anterior ankle release (capsule, toe extensors, and peroneus tertius), posterior transfer of the anterior tibial or posterior tibial tendon or both to the calcaneus, shortening of the Achilles tendon, or calcaneal osteotomy (80). Results of surgical correction of this deformity were recently examined in thirteen patients with seventeen feet undergoing surgical intervention. The authors concluded that if any objective benefit from surgery is to be gained, reconstruction should be performed

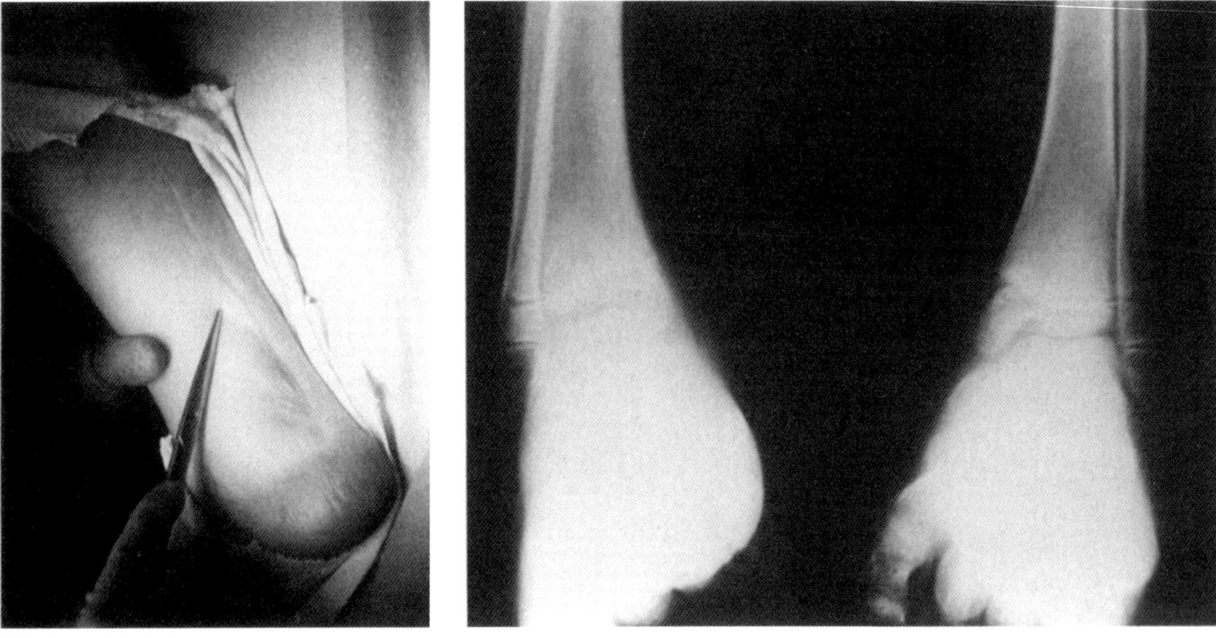

FIGURE 7-13 Posteromedial tibial physis injury from a posterior clubfoot release requiring osteotomy. **A.** Posterior incisions. **B.** Physeal closure.

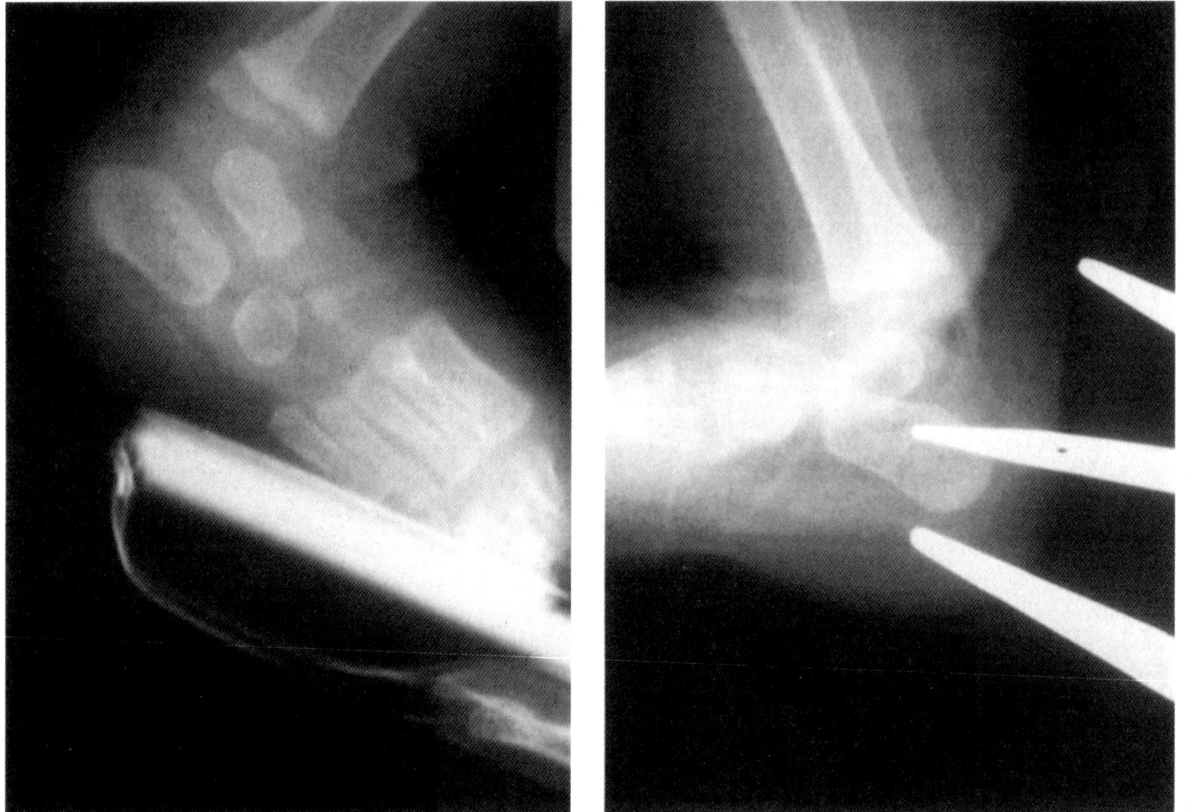

FIGURE 7-14 Intraoperative lateral radiographs demonstrating preoperative equinus of heel and parallel talus and calcaneus (**A**), and postoperative correction of subtalar joint (**B**)—the heel is out of equinus and the anteriosuperior portion of the calcaneus overlaps the inferior anterior portion of the talus indicating that the heel has been rotated around the talus.

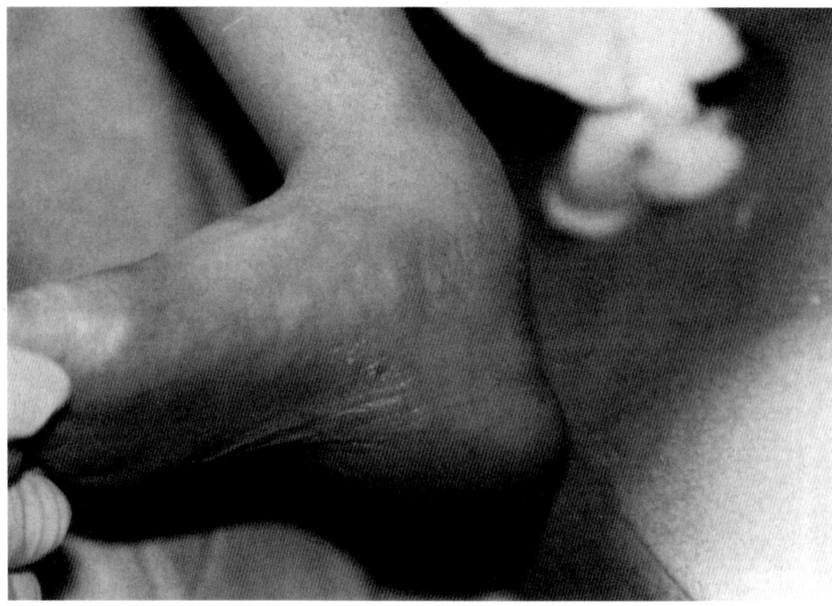

FIGURE 7-15 Calcaneus deformity postoperative extensive clubfoot release.

prior to the age of six years and that this complication of clubfoot surgery is far better avoided than salvaged by attempted reconstruction (61).

Pes Planus

Most clubfeet have varying degrees of pes planus immediately after soft tissue release. The following types are prone to flat feet: preoperative rocker bottom clubfoot, excessive plantar flexion, excessive ligamentous hyperlaxity, and underdevelopment of sustentaculum tali. The interosseous ligament is only partially divided to permit the unlocking of the calcaneus and to correct the subtalar deformity (75). Complete transection of the talocalcaneal interosseous ligaments may produce a severe pes planus with hindfoot valgus or translocation of the heel and this technique probably should be avoided unless talocalcaneal fixation is used for a minimum of six weeks holding the heel in a neutral position. Transection of the tibialis posterior during soft tissue release has been cited as a cause of residual flat foot. Transection of the posterior tibial tendon in the child less than two years of age will usually not result in pes planus. Lengthening of the posterior tibial tendon is preferable over the age of two years. Residual flexible pes planus is usually only a cosmetic problem and very infrequently a functional problem at maturity (75).

Pes Cavus

This is the result of inadequate plantar release. Re-intervention and thorough surgical plantar release is indicated in a young child. Dorsal wedge osteotomy (tarsal or tarsometatarsal) is the treatment of choice in the child older than 8 years of age (Figure 7-16).

Heel Varus

This deformity results from incomplete release of the subtalar joint which may include division of the interosseous ligament and calcaneal cuboid joint capsule in severe rigid clubfeet. Re-intervention permits the accomplishment of a complete release. Rigid heel varus in the older child can be treated by calcaneal wedge osteotomy or triple arthrodesis.

Forefoot Adduction

Forefoot adduction, or metatarsus varus, often results from failure to adequately release the talonavicular joint capsule, thus blocking the centralization of the navicular on the talus. This deformity can also result from an inadequate release of the abductor hallucis or of the navicular cuneiform first metatarsal capsule. Mild deformity can be treated by manipulations, casts, and splinting. Moderate deformity requires capsulotomies of the navicular-cuneiform-first metatarsal with abductor hallucis tenotomy at its insertion or, more commonly, repeat surgical release of the talonavicular joint and repositioning of the navicular into its appropriate position (51). Several authors have stated that forefoot adduction deformity gradually improves and at maturity there may be a mild residual deformity but that the patient has cosmetically acceptable "pigeon toe" gait (4,75,81). The severe deformity in the older child should be treated by metatarsal osteotomies or first cuneiform osteotomy (29). Shortening of the lateral column with lengthening of the medial column is an effective means of treating fixed forefoot adduction deformities (41,49). Tarsometatarsal capsulotomies are not recommended because of the persistent pain and the development of a dorsal bunion (4,71). Forefoot adduction and negative foot progression angle gait may also respond to supramalleolar osteotomy after age eight years.

Skew Foot (Serpentine Foot)

Improperly corrected forefoot adduction may be associated with overcorrection of the hindfoot resulting in a skew foot. Conservative treatment includes manipulation and casts to invert the heel and abduct the forefoot. Surgery is considered when conservative treatment fails. Correction

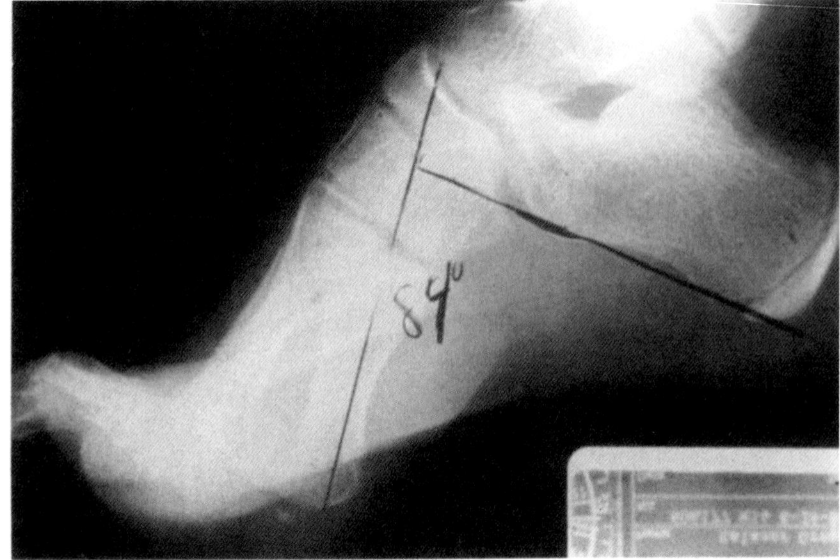

A

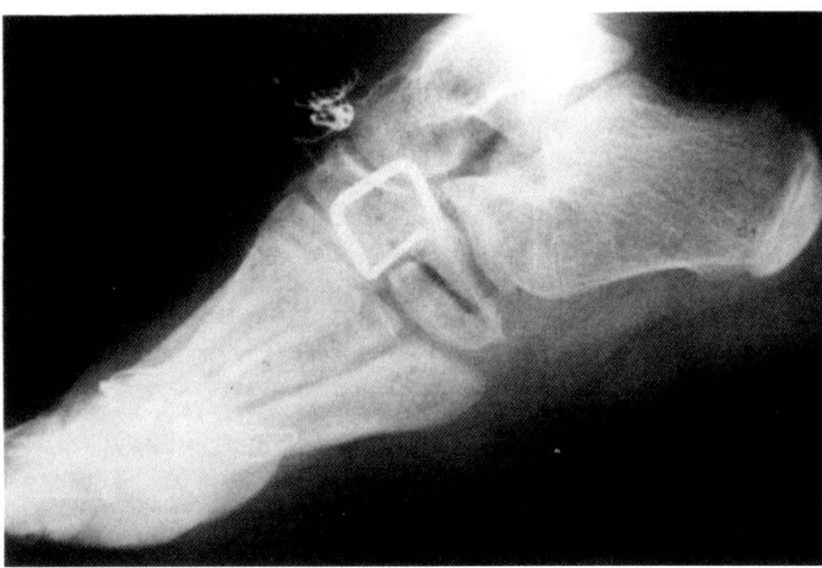

B

FIGURE 7-16 Residual cavus deformity post-clubfoot surgery. **A.** Cavus deformity. **B.** Post-midtarsal osteotomy.

of forefoot adduction combined with a plantar release is recommended when the hindfoot is flexible. With a fixed hindfoot valgus, a subtalar fusion (Grice or Dennyson) with plantar release or metatarsal osteotomies combined with a Dwyer calcaneal osteotomy or triple arthrodesis (over age eight years) should be considered (44).

Forefoot Supination

Residual supination of the forefoot may result from muscle imbalance between the strong tibialis anterior and the persistent weakness of the peronei. Orthotic management can be attempted. Split tibialis anterior tendon transfer is indicated when this treatment fails. Midtarsal or metatarsal osteotomies or triple arthrodesis is required for fixed deformity over the age of eight years.

Tarsal Navicular Subluxation (Dorsal, Plantar Medial, Lateral)

The treatment and the maintenance of the reduction of the talonavicular joint influences the final result. Turco stated that the surgeon can only "eyeball" the placement of the navicular (76). The dorsal surface of the navicular should be placed at the same level as the talus and the medial surface of the navicular should protrude medially 2–3 mm in the infant and 5–7 mm in the older child at the time of joint thinning.

Simons (67) has recently published radiographic measurements to distinguish insignificant minor complications from clinically relevant complications that may require further surgery. Anteroposterior radiographs should demonstrate alignment of the navicular with respect to the talar head. Lateral displacement of up to one-half of the talar head may occur in hypermobile flat feet and therefore, although considered overcorrection, represent only a minor clinical complication since an orthosis will control the midfoot subluxation. Medial navicular displacement up to one-quarter of the talar head is under-correction but considered a minor problem, whereas more pronounced medial displacement is considered a major complication. The central navicular position on the lateral radiograph is again considered normal. Up to one-third dorsal subluxation of the navicular on the talar head is considered overcorrection but only a minor complication consistent with a satisfactory result. Dorsal subluxation to a greater degree or any navicular plantar subluxation is thought to be a major complication.

The medially subluxed navicular generally produces an unsatisfactory residual forefoot adduction which may necessitate re-intervention. The majority of cases displaying lateral navicular subluxation were rated as satisfactory clinical results (66,74). An incidence of 15% to 54% of dorsal navicular subluxation has been reported (42,58,66). However, even the extreme subluxation that may give the foot a cavus like appearance need not necessarily preclude a satisfactory result and corrective surgery is not recommended for this problem (66). For patients with refractory midfoot pain and dorsal-lateral subluxation of the talonavicular (TN) joint with a secondary forefoot cavovarus deformity, talo-navicular arthrodesis has been described to result in satisfactory clinical improvement (78).

Sinus Tarsi Syndrome

Correction of the equinovarus attitude of the calcaneus during soft tissue clubfoot release may place the bone into a valgus position that often closes down the sinus tarsi during weight bearing. This compression may result in pain over the sinus tarsi (23,42). The lateral sural nerve may also be compressed or severed during surgery and release of surrounding scar tissue or excision of the neuroma may help decrease pain. Ingrowth of nearby cutaneous nerves will usually result in a return of sensation. Causalgia or reflex sympathetic dystrophy secondary to a nerve injury is rare and very difficult to treat.

Dorsal Bunion (Hallux Flexus)

Dorsal bunion deformity is usually attributed to muscle imbalance, originally being described as a sequela of anterior poliomyelitis. The imbalance between elevation (tibialis anterior) and depression (peroneus longus) of the first metatarsal, and between hallucal flexors and extensors, leads to the deformity. The first metatarsal head is prominent dorsally ("the bunion"), with the great toe sharply flexed at the metatarsophalangeal joint. The metatarsophalangeal joint may sublux with increasing flexion. The dorsal articular surface of the metatarsal head may develop chondromalacia and flexion contracture of the metatarsophalangeal joint capsule and short hallucal flexors, producing a rigid painful deformity. McKay reported the deformity in 11 children who underwent posteromedial release for clubfeet (52). He attributed the deformity to the deterioration of the triceps surae in patients after clubfeet release. The bunion develops as the patient tries to push off with the toe flexors to compensate for the triceps weakness.

While others advocate flexor hallucis longus (FHL) transfer to the base of the first metatarsal, McKay proposed transfer of the short flexors (flexor hallucis brevis, abductor and adductor hallucis) to the dorsal surface of the first metatarsal head to produce depression while leaving the flexor hallucis longus (FHL) undisturbed (82). Rigid deformity requires bony correction which may include osteotomy at the base or neck of the first metatarsal. An alternative procedure would include osteotomy of the proximal phalanx and possibly even partial resection of the base of the proximal phalanx or head of the metatarsal in patients over the age of eight years.

Hallux Valgus

Hallux valgus is uncommon in clubfoot. The deformity usually occurs after skeletal maturity but may be seen in early childhood secondary to excessively vigorous casting which forces the big toe laterally. Hallux valgus is more likely to occur in children with the most severe deformity who have undergone multiple manipulations and operations (Figure 7-17). Hallux valgus is often associated with a flexion contracture of the interphalangeal joint of the big toe and interphalangeal fusion may be necessary to eliminate the painful callosity and deformity of the interphalangeal joint. Hallux valgus has also been observed in the normal foot of a unilateral clubfoot deformity.

Hallux Varus

Hallux varus is often associated with contracture of the flexor hallucis brevis and abductor hallucis leading to a medial pointing toe. Treatment includes lengthening of the flexor hallucis brevis and abductor hallucis just proximal to their insertions as well as capsulotomy of the metatarsophalangeal joint. Internal fixation for six weeks is required.

Claw Toes

When the foot is placed into dorsiflexion after completion of soft tissue release, the flexor hallucis longus and the flexor digitorum may be placed under tension which causes clawing of the toes. Turco believes that the tendons will lengthen spontaneously (76). However, the deformity sometimes persists. Many surgeons advocate formal lengthening of the flexor tendons during soft tissue procedures. This can be accomplished by fractional lengthening of the flexor tendons proximal to the ankle joint in order to avoid scar formation (3). Cicatrix may cause adherence of the tendons on the medial side of the foot and necessitate a repeat soft tissue release.

Overcorrection

Overcorrection of clubfeet will lead to valgus inclination of the hindfoot and pronation of the forefoot (54). A recent report established the association between generalized joint laxity and the incidence of overcorrection in surgically treated clubfeet (28). Immediate overcorrection may result from an associated anterior tibial tendon transfer being placed lateral to the second metatarsal. This complication can be salvaged only by releasing the anterior tibial tendon or retransferring the muscle to the middle cuneiform. The overcorrected foot may also result from excessive lateral placement of the navicular on the talus; excessive subtalar

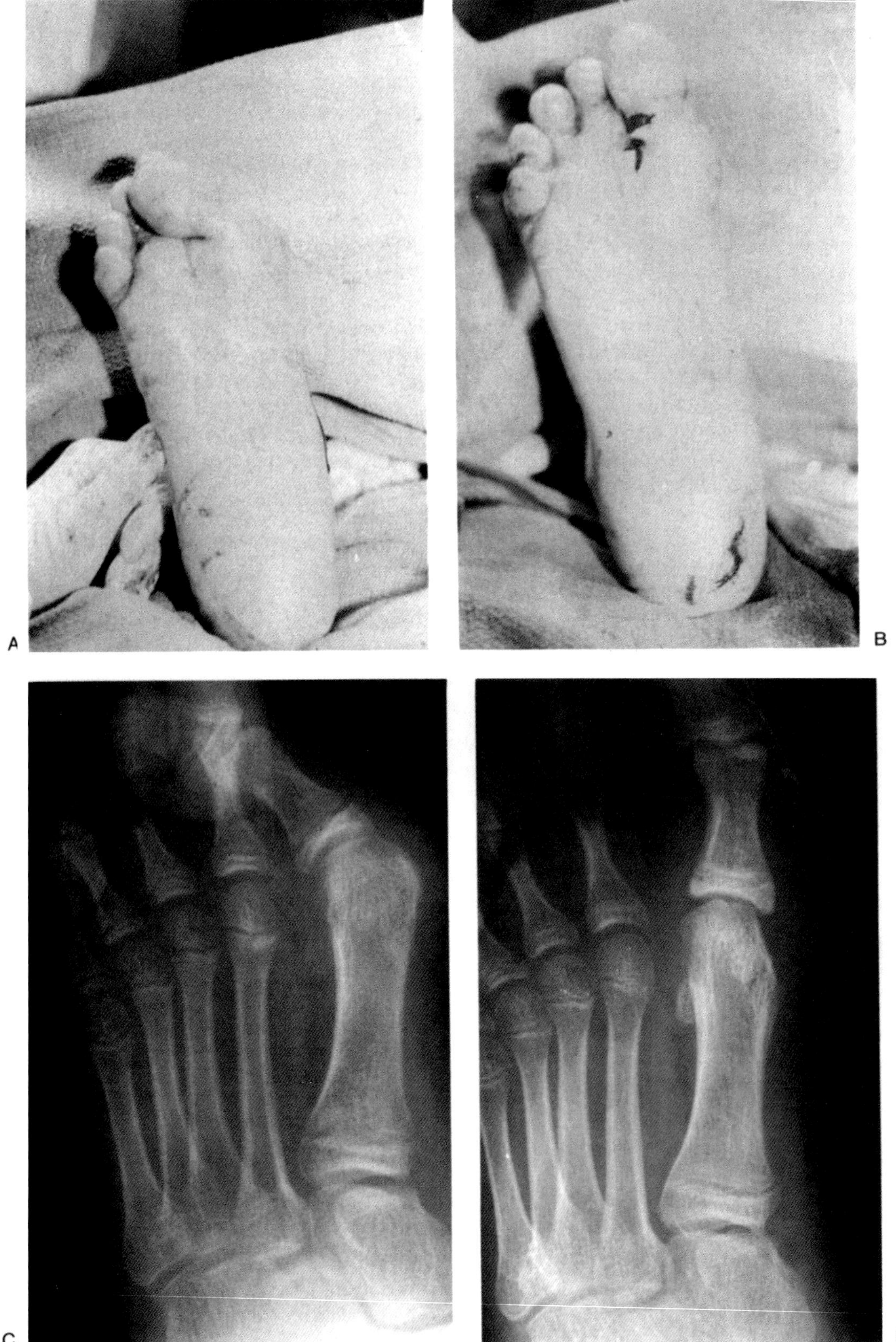

FIGURE 7-17 Hallux valgus is a result of too vigorous casting of a clubfoot. **A.** Preoperative. **B.** Postøperative following Z-plasty of the skin on the lateral side of the big toe and standard bunion soft-tissue repair and fixation with a pin. **C.** Preoperative x-ray. **D.** Postoperative x-ray.

release placing the foot in eversion; postoperative eversion casting for a prolonged period of time; compression of the lateral part of the distal tibial physis by inappropriate casting; or severance of the deep deltoid ligament without adequate repair (Figure 7-18).

Forefoot abduction is usually a delayed complication and may occur after metatarsal osteotomies, tarsometatarsal capsulotomies, or a Dillwyn-Evans procedures (posteromedial release combined with calcaneo-cuboid fusion) done before age six years. Conservative treatment includes stretching exercises and bracing. Metatarsal osteotomies or midfoot corrective osteotomy may be indicated.

Iatrogenic hindfoot valgus may be produced at either the ankle or subtalar joints. Division of the medial part of the deep deltoid (tibiotalar) ligament may cause the deformity at the ankle joint. Prompt repair should be performed when the problem is recognized at the time of surgery.

Overzealous release of the subtalar joint can lead to overcorrection of the hind foot especially when the talocalcaneal interosseous ligament is completely divided. Division of the interosseous ligament should be limited to the decrease necessary to unlock the calcaneus and correct the deformity (75). However, a recent report suggests that release of the talocalcaneal interosseous ligament can be performed in severe and very severe clubfeet while maintaining the lateral subtalar capsule without causing extreme overcorrection (17). Over-corrected feet are sometimes asymptomatic. Lau reported 66% of the overcorrected feet had unsatisfactory function (42).

Treatment for patients less than four years of age who have a flexible deformity include, a heel cup; from age four to ten years, subtalar arthrodesis (Grice or Dennyson); and patients over ten years may require triple

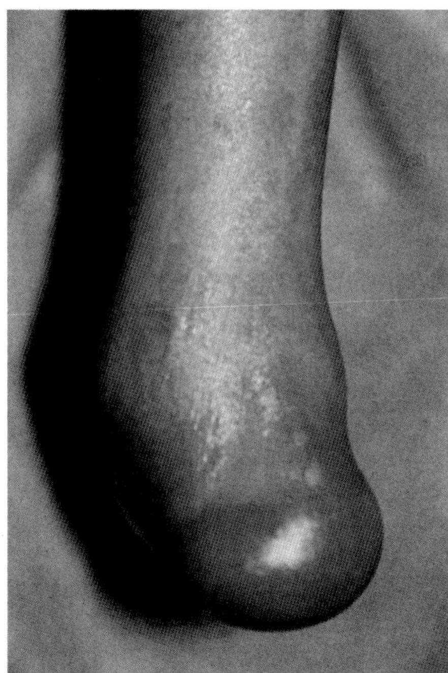

FIGURE 7-18 Overcorrected clubfoot due to severed deep deltoid ligament.

arthrodesis. A repeat soft-tissue release is recommended for patients less than four years of age with rigid deformity. This approach is combined with subtalar arthrodesis for the four to ten year age group, while triple arthrodesis is the procedure of choice for the older patients (4).

Ankle and Subtalar Pain

There is a very low incidence of pain in the young postoperative patient (3–6 months to 2–3 years). Pain may or may not be a frequent problem in the older child with the level of activity being a major factor. Overuse symptoms may be treated with limited activity and shoe modification including heel cups and molded supports. Callous formation on the heel and lateral side of the foot is related to a recurrent deformity. Late osteoarthritic pain from the subtalar joint and subsequently from the ankle joint will usually respond to cushioned shoeing, anti-inflammatory medication and modification of activity. Occasionally, there will be the need for limited fusion of the subtalar joint or a triple arthrodesis. Rarely, significant symptomatic arthritis will be treated by ankle arthrodesis.

Calf Atrophy

All patients with clubfeet have calf atrophy and weakness following soft tissue release. These findings are related to the Achilles lengthening as well as the underlying neuromuscular disorder that resulted in the clubfoot deformity. The weakness may improve over time as muscle power increases with the return of normal function. Asymmetric calf muscle development is noted in the unilateral deformity (39).

Small-Sized Foot

The unilateral clubfoot is generally smaller than the opposite foot and may demonstrate a one-half to two shoe size difference (39). Some of this discrepancy in shoe size may resolve during growth, but damage to the cartilage model of the foot during surgery will result in further shortening. Very little can be done unless severe shortening occurs and then foot lengthening could be considered. Lambs wool placed in the toe box serves as a soft bumper and may prevent the shorter foot from excessive movement in the shoe.

Leg Length Discrepancy

Leg length discrepancy is usually not severe. The unilateral clubfoot will frequently have 1 to 2 cm leg shortening, but this very rarely needs correction unless the distal tibial physis was damaged during management.

Recurrence of the Deformity

Recurrent clubfoot deformity often is due to incomplete initial surgical correction. However, late relapses in patients with idiopathic clubfoot may represent the onset of a previously undiagnosed neuromuscular disease, and should be thoroughly evaluated (49). Most studies report that infant clubfoot surgery has a 5% to 20% incidence of recurrent deformity even in the hands of an experienced

TABLE 7-1

Algorithm for re-surgical intervention in clubfeet

Age at revision	*Method of treatment*
Six months to two years	1. Re-soft tissue release 2. If prominent plantar crease, add plantar release. 3. If forefoot adduction not corrected—add capsulotomies: Navicular-cuneiform-first metatarsal as needed.
Two years to four years	Follow steps 1, 2, 3 4. If forefoot adduction not corrected, add excision of cartilage of calcaneo-cuboid joint or decancellectomy of cuboid.
Four years to eight years	Follow steps 1, 2, 3 5. If forefoot adduction not fully corrected, add A. Fusion calcaneal cuboid joint (Dilwyn-Evans) B. *or* excision of distal calcaneus (34) C. *or* cuboid decancellation D. *or* open wedge osteotomy first cuneiform E. *or* tarso metatarsal capsulotomies F. *OR* metatarsal osteotomies (over age five) 6. If overacting tibialis anterior vs. weak peroneal—add tibialis anterior transfer or split anterior tibialis transfer. 7. If heel varus still not corrected, add Dwyer osteotomy.
Over age eight	Up to age 10 possible to start with steps 1, 2 and then proceed according to deformity remaining Calcaneus: stage 7 Forefoot adduction: stage 5, A, B, C, F 8. Persistent cavus-midtarsal osteotomy 9. Distraction osteogenesis (Ilizarov) as the only procedure 10. Over age 10 years—triple arthrodesis as the only procedure 11. Supramalleolar tibial osteotomy

clubfoot surgeon (22,40,56,67,76). Treatment of the resistant or recurrent clubfoot deformity represents a significant challenge to the clubfoot surgeon. The use of the Ilizarov method of external fixation and gradual distraction is one of many corrective procedures that have been described. Work by the senior author demonstrated that this method often results in poor outcomes associated with residual or recurrent deformity, often requiring revision surgery (21).

Intraoperative anteroposterior and lateral radiographs demonstrating the accomplishment of normal talocalcaneal relationship may help to ensure the completeness of the soft tissue release. In some cases, after formal complete soft tissue release, lack of concentric reduction of the navicular may result in overcorrection or in residual mid and forefoot adduction or cavus. Awareness of the possibility of a deformed talus (head and neck may be in medial, lateral, or plantar tilt in relation to the talar body) may require talar osteotomy in rare cases and usually is recognized late (72).

Loss of surgical correction may occur during the immediate postoperative period due to inadequate internal fixation (pins or soft tissue repair), inadequate external fixation (cast), or after premature discontinuation of the cast. When pins are not used, we recommend that postoperative care include manipulation of the foot and cast change at three and six weeks following surgery. When pins are employed, the initial cast should remain for six weeks. A long leg cast is retained for an additional six week period and then replaced by outflare shoes with Denis-Browne bar or ankle-foot-orthosis (AFO) as needed accompanied by frequent manipulation by the parents for two years (16,58). As in clubfoot deformity treated nonoperatively, the final result of clubfoot surgery is extremely dependent on postoperative maintenance of the position of the foot and manipulative exercises for a long period of time (27).

A comprehensive approach for revision surgery in clubfeet in outlined in Table 7-1 (4,70).

REFERENCES

1. Aplington JP, Riggle CD. Avascular necrosis of the body of the talus after combined medial and lateral release of congenital clubfoot. *South Med J* 1976;69:1037.
2. Atar D, Grant AD, Silver L, Lehman WB. The use of tissue expander in clubfoot surgery. *J Bone Joint Surg [Br]* 1990;72:574–577.
3. Atar D, Lehman WB, Grant AD, Strongwater A. Fractional lengthening of the flexor tendons in clubfoot surgery. *Clin Orthop* 1991;264:267–269.
4. Atar D, Lehman WB, Grant AD, Strongwater A. Revision clubfoot surgery. *Bulletin of the Hospital for Joint Disease* 1990;60(2):149.

5. Bethem D, Weiner D. Radical one-stage posteromedial release for the resistant clubfoot. *Clin Orthop* 1978;131:214–223.
6. Breed A. Partial wound closure in clubfoot surgery. In: *Proceedings of the International Congress on Clubfeet.* Milwaukee, 1990.
7. Changulani M, Garg N, Bruce CE. Neurovascular complications following percutaneous tendoachillis tenotomy for congenital idiopathic clubfoot. *Arch Orthop Trauma Surg* 2007;127:429–430.
8. Coleman SS. *Complex foot deformities in children.* Philadelphia: Lea & Febiger, 1983.
9. Crawford AH, Marxsen JL, Osterfield DF. The Cincinnati incision: a comprehensive approach to surgical procedures for the foot and ankle in childhood. *J Bone Joint Surg (Am)* 1982;64:1355.
10. Cummings J, Lovell WW. Current concept review: operative treatment of congenital idiopathic clubfoot. *J Bone Joint Surg [Am]* 1988;70:1108–1112.
11. Cummings RJ, Bashore CJ, Bookout CB, Elliott MJ. Avascular necrosis of the talus after McKay clubfoot release for idiopathic congenital clubfoot. *J Pediatr Orthop* 2001;21:221–224.
12. Denham RA. Congenital talipes equinovarus. *J Bone Joint Surg (Br)* 1967;49:583.
13. Depuy T, Drennan JC. Correction of idiopathic clubfoot. A comparison of results of early versus delayed posteromedial release. *J Pediatr Orthop* 1989;9:44–48.
14. Devalano PG, Ruiz DG. Reporte preliminar al hallazode le avsenica vascular en efermus con pies equino cavo varo aducto cogneito. *Rev Orthop Latin Am* 1968;8:27–34.
15. Dobbs MB, Gordon JE, Walton T, Schoenecker PL. Bleeding complications following percutaneous tendoachilles tenotomy in the treatment of clubfoot deformity. *J Pediatr Orthop* 2004;24:353–357.
16. Edelson JG, Husseini N. The pulseless clubfoot. *J Bone Joint Surg (Br)* 1984;66:700–702.
17. El-Deeb KH, Ghoneim AS, El-Adwar KL, Khalil AA. Is it hazardous or mandatory to release the talocalcaneal interosseous ligament in clubfoot surgery?: A preliminary report. *J Pediatr Orthop* 2007;27:517–521.
18. Epps GH, Kahn A. Complications and salvage procedures in surgery of the foot. In: *Complications in orthopaedic surgery,* 2nd ed. Philadelphia: JB Lippincott, 1984;1259–1267.
19. Exner GU. Tourniquet lesions and their prevention in clubfoot surgery. In: *Proceedings of the International Congress on Clubfeet.* Medical College of Wisconsin, Milwaukee. CME Conference Inc. Cherry Hill, NJ, 1991.
20. Franke J, Hein G. Our experience with the early treatment of congenital clubfoot. *J Pediatr Orthop* 1988;8:26–30.
21. Freedman JA, Watts H, Otsuka NY. The Ilizarov method for the treatment of resistant clubfoot: Is it an effective solution? *J Pediatr Orthop* 2006;26:432–437.
22. Ghali NN, Smith RB, Clayder AD. The results of pantalar reduction in the management of congenital talipes equinovarus. *J Bone Joint Surg (Br)* 1983;65:1–7.
23. Giorgini R, Bernard R. Sinus tarsi syndrome in a patient with talipes equinovarus. *J Am Podiatr Med Assoc* 1990;80:218–222.
24. Goldner JL, Fitch RD. Idiopathic congenital talipes equinovarus (clubfoot). In: Jahss, ed. *Disorders of the foot and ankle: medical and surgical management,* 2nd ed. Philadelphia: WB Saunders. 1991;771–829.
25. Grant AD, Lehman WB. Talocalcaneal coalition in arthrogryposis multiplex congenita. *Bull Hosp Jt Dis Orthop Inst* 1982; 42(2):236.
26. Greider MD, Siff SJ, Gerson D. Arteriography in clubfoot. *J Bone Joint Surg (Am)* 1982;64:837–840.
27. Haft GF, Walker CG, Crawford HA. Early clubfoot recurrence after use of the Ponseti method in a New Zealand population. *J Bone Joint Surg Am* 2007;89:487–493.
28. Haslam PG, Goddard M, Flowers MJ, Fernandes JA. Overcorrection and generalized joint laxity in surgically treated congenital talipes equino-varus. *J Pediatr Orthop B* 2006;15:273–277.
29. Hoffman AA, Costine RM, McBride GC, Coleman SS. Osteotomy of the first cuneiform as treatment of residual adduction of the fore part of the foot in clubfoot. *J Bone Joint Surg (Am)* 1984;66:985–990.
30. Hootnick DR. Necrosis leading to amputations following clubfoot surgery. In: *Proceedings of the International Congress on Clubfeet.* Medical College of Wisconsin, Milwaukee. CME Conference Inc. Cherry Hill, NJ, 1991.
31. Hootnick DR, Packard DS, Levinsohn ME. Necrosis leading to amputation following clubfoot surgery. *Foot Ankle* 1990;10:312–316.
32. Hutchins RM, Foster BK, Paterson OD, Cole EA. Long-term results of early surgical release in clubfeet. *J Bone Joint Surg (Br)* 1985;67:791–799.
33. Hsu WK, Bhatia NN, Raskin A, Otsuka NY. Wound complications from idiopathic clubfoot surgery: a comparison of the modified Turco and the Cincinnati treatment methods. *J Pediatr Orthop* 2007;27:329–332.
34. Huber H, Galantay R, Dutoit M. Avascular necrosis after osteotomy of the talar neck to correct residual club-foot deformity in children. A long-term review. *J Bone Joint Surg (Br)* 2002;84-B:426–430.
35. Kamath BJ, Bhardwaj P. Local flap coverage following posteromedial release in clubfoot surgery in older children. *Int Orthop* 2005 Feb;29:39–41.
36. Keim HA, Ritchie GW. "Nut-cracker" treatment of clubfoot. *JAMA* 1964;189:613.
37. Kite JH. Non-operative treatment of congenital clubfoot. A review of 100 cases. *South Med J* 1930;23:345.
38. Koureas G, et al. The incidence and treatment of rocker bottom deformity as a complication of the conservative treatment of idiopathic congenital clubfoot. *J Bone Joint Surg Br* 2008;90:57–60.
39. Kránicz J, Than P, Kustos T. Long-term results of the operative treatment of clubfoot: A representative study. *Orthopedics* 1998;21:669–74.
40. Kumar J. The role of footprints in the management of clubfeet. *Clin Orthop* 1979;140:32–36.
41. Kuo KN, Smith PA. Correcting residual deformity following clubfoot releases. *Clin Orthop Relat Res*;2008 Dec 17. [Epub ahead of print].
42. Lau JHK, Meyer LC, Lau HC. The results of surgical treatment comparison of results of early versus delayed posteromedial release. *Clin Orthop* 1989;248:219.
43. Lehman WB. *The clubfoot.* Philadelphia: JB Lippincott, 1980.
44. Lehman WB. Skewfoot. In: Jahss, ed. *Disorders of the foot and ankle: medical and surgical management,* 2nd. ed. Philadelphia: WB Saunders, 1991;840–847.
45. Lehman WB, Atar D, Grant AD, Strongwater A. Re-do clubfoot: surgical approach and long-term results. *Bull NY Acad Med* 1990;66:601–617.
46. Lehman WB, Silver L, Grant AD, Strongwater A, Oskar W. The anatomical basis for incisions around the foot and ankle in clubfoot surgery. *Bull Hosp Jt Dis Ortho Inst* 1990;24:218–227.
47. Lichtblau S. A medial and lateral release operation for clubfoot; a preliminary report. *J Bone Joint Surg (Am)* 1973;55:1377–1384.
48. Lloyd-Roberts GC. *Orthopaedic surgery in infancy and childhood.* London: Butterworth's, 1971.
49. Lourenco AF, Dias LS, Zoellick DM, Sodre H. Treatment of residual adduction deformity in clubfoot: the double osteotomy. *J Pediatr Orthop* 2001;21:713–718.
50. Lovell ME, Morcuende JA. Neuromuscular disease as the cause of late clubfoot relapses: Report of 4 cases. *Iowa Orthop J* 2007;27:82–84.
51. Lowe LW, Hannon MA. Residual adduction of the forefoot in treated congenital clubfoot. *J Bone Joint Surg (Br)* 1973;55:809.
52. McKay DW. Dorsal bunions in children. *J Bone Joint Surg (Am)* 1983;65:975–980.
53. McKay DW. New concept of an approach to clubfoot treatment. Section II. Correction of clubfoot. *J Pediatr Orthop* 1983;3:10.
54. McKay DW. Correction of the overcorrected clubfoot. In: *Proceedings of the International Congress on Clubfeet.* Medical College of Wisconsin, Milwaukee. CME Conference Inc., Cherry Hill, NJ, 1991.

55. Magone J, Torch MA, Clark RN, Kean JR. Comparative review of surgical treatment of the idiopathic clubfoot by three different procedures at Columbus Children's Hospital. *J Pediatr Orthop* 1989;3:49–58.
56. Main BJ, Crider RJ, Polk M, Lloyd-Roberts GC. The results of early operation in talipes equinovarus: a preliminary report. *J Bone Joint Surg (Br)* 1988;59:337–341.
57. Mardjetko SM, Lubicky JP, Kuo KN, Smrcina C. Pseudoaneurysm after foot surgery. *J Pediatr Orthop* 1991;11:657–662.
58. Miller WE, Bernstein S. The roentgenographic appearance of the corrected clubfoot. *Foot Ankle* 1986;5:177.
59. National Center for Health Statistics. *Monthly Vital Statistics Report* 1989;36(13).
60. Nistor L, Foster BK, Paterson OD, Cole EA. Long-term results of early surgical release in clubfeet. *J Bone Joint Surg (Br)* 1985;67:791–799.
61. O'Brien SE, Karol LA, Johnston CE 2nd. Calcaneus gait following treatment for clubfoot: Preliminary results of surgical correction. *J Pediatr Orthop B* 2004;13:43–47.
62. Ponten B. The fasciocutaneous flap: Its use in soft tissue defects of the lower leg. *Br J Plast Surg* 1981;34:215.
63. Reinman I, Becker-Anderson H. Early surgical treatment of congenital clubfoot. *Clin Orthop* 1974;102:200–206.
64. Rockwell WB, Daane S, Zakhireh M, Carroll KL. Human skin allograft used to treat open wounds after club foot release. *Ann Plast Surg* 2003;51:593–597.
65. Rosselli P, Reyes R, Medina A, Céspedes LJ. Use of a soft tissue expander before surgical treatment of clubfoot in children and adolescents. *J Pediatr Orthop* 2005;25:353–356.
66. Schlafly B, Butler JE, Sherwin J. The appearance of the tarsal navicular after posteromedial release of clubfoot. *Foot Ankle* 1985;5:222–237.
67. Simons GW. Complete subtalar release in clubfeet. Part II. Comparison with less extensive procedures. *J Bone Joint Surg (Am)* 1985;67:1056–1065.
68. Simons GW. Compartment syndrome in clubfoot. In: *Proceedings of the International Congress on Clubfeet.* Medical College of Wisconsin, Milwaukee. CME Conference Inc. Cherry Hill, NJ, 1991.
69. Somppi E, Sulamaa M. Early operative treatment of congenital clubfoot. *Acta Orthop Scand* 1971;42:513.
70. Spire TD, Gross RH, Low W. Management of the resistant myelodysplastic or arthrogrypotic clubfoot with the Verebelyi-Ogston procedure. *J Pediatr Orthop* 1987;4:705–710.
71. Stark JG, Johnston JE, Winter R. The Heyman-Herndon tarsometatarsal capsulotomy for metatarsus adductus. Results in 48 feet. *J Pediatr Orthop* 1987;7:305–310.
72. Tachdjian MO. Congenital talipes equinovarus. In: *Pediatric orthopaedics.* Philadelphia: WB Saunders, 1990;2428–2541.
73. Tayton K, Thompson P. Relapsing clubfeet—later results of delayed operation. *J Bone Joint Surg (Am)* 1978;61: 474–480.
74. Thompson GH, Richardson AB, Westin GW. Surgical management of the resistant congenital talipes equinovarus deformities. *J Bone Joint Surg (Am)* 1982;64:652–664.
75. Turco VJ. Clubfoot. In: *Current problems in orthopaedics.* New York: Churchill Livingstone, 1981.
76. Turco VJ. Surgical correction of the resistant clubfoot. *J Bone Joint Surg (Am)* 1971;53:477–497.
77. Watts H. *Personal communication.*
78. Wei SY, Sullivan RJ, Davidson RS. Talo-navicular arthrodesis for residual midfoot deformities of a previously corrected clubfoot. *Foot Ankle Int* 2000;21:482–485.
79. Weseley M, Barenfeld P, Barret N. Complications of the treatment of clubfoot. *Clin Orthop* 1972;84:93.
80. Wijensinha S, Mennelaus M. Operation for calcaneus deformity after surgery for clubfoot. *J Bone Joint Surg (Br)* 1989;71:234–236.
81. Wynne-Davis R. Talipes equinovarus. A review of eighty-four cases after completion of treatment. *J Bone Joint Surg (Br)* 1964;46:464–476
82. Yong SM, Smith PA, Kuo KN. Dorsal bunion after clubfoot surgery: outcome of reverse Jones procedure. *J Pediatr Orthop* 2007;27:814–820.

CHAPTER 8

Metatarsus Adductus and Metatarsus Varus

George H. Thompson and Hadeel Abaza

INTRODUCTION

Metatarsus adductus or adduction of the forefoot is one of the most common foot deformities of childhood (29,31). Unfortunately, the diagnosis can be confusing as some authors use the terms metatarsus varus, hooked forefoot, skewfoot, z-foot, serpentine foot, or metatarsus adductovarus when discussing metatarsus adductus. A review of the literature indicates that metatarsus adductus and metatarsus varus are two distinct deformities that may appear to be clinically similar, especially during the first several years of life (3). Metatarsus varus is the more severe and complex deformity, while metatarsus adductus is relatively benign. In this chapter, we will distinguish between these two disorders as they have different prognoses. Kite (23) suggested that metatarsus adductus was one-third of a congenital clubfoot deformity. Peterson (37) felt that metatarsus varus, which he called skewfoot, was the opposite deformity of the congenital clubfoot. While these statements are not true etiologically or pathoanatomically, it is a major reason these disorders are frequently discussed together. In fact, Wynne-Davies (48) noted an increased incidence of clubfeet in siblings of children with metatarsus varus. Undoubtedly, most of these patients had metatarsus adductus.

METATARSUS ADDUCTUS

In true metatarsus adductus, there is only forefoot adduction. The metatarsals are adducted at the tarsometatarsal joints. There is relatively normal alignment of the midfoot and hindfoot.

Etiology

Because a significant percentage of metatarsus adductus will resolve spontaneously, it appears to be the result of *in utero* positioning (10,41) and is more common in first born than in subsequent births (3). This has been attributed to greater molding from the primigravida uterus and abdominal wall. Others have disagreed and favored muscle imbalance and soft-tissue contracture theories (10,14,21,22,23,27,32,). The confusion between metatarsus adductus and metatarsus varus undoubtedly has been a major factor. Wynne-Davies (48) found that this disorder occurs in approximately 1 per 1,000 live births. She found no correlation between maternal age and birth order suggesting no association with *in utero* factors. When a child has the deformity, there is approximately a 5% chance of subsequent siblings having the deformity (38,41,48). Metatarsus adductus occurs equally in males and females, and in approximately 50% of cases, there will be bilateral involvement (23). The incidence of metatarsus adductus appears to be increasing over the past decade. This most likely represents increased awareness (38).

A relationship between metatarsus adductus and acetabular dysplasia has been observed by some authors (3,18,26). Jacobs (18) reviewed 300 consecutive children with metatarsus adductus and found that 30 children (10%) had associated hip dysplasia. Kumar and MacEwen (26), however, reported only a 1.53 % incidence of hip dysplasia in 720 children with metatarsus adductus. The relationship between metatarsus adductus and hip dysplasia has been felt to be due to in utero positioning and molding. However, recently Bielski et al. (5) examined the relationship between 13 orthopedic conditions and intrauterine crowding in multiple gestation pregnancies and found only one condition, torticollis, to have a greater incidence compared to single gestation pregnancies. There was a 0% incidence of hip dysplasia in the 261 patients followed over a 10-year period. They concluded that routine ultrasound screening in children with foot deformities are not recommended unless there are positive physical findings. It is therefore important that any child with a metatarsus adductus deformity have a careful hip examination.

Pathoanatomy

In a study by Morcuende and Ponseti in 1996 (33), two fetuses (16 and 19 weeks' gestation) that had metatarsus adductus were studied by taking histologic sections through the feet. They found the shape of the medial cuneiform was altered, and the first cuneometatarsal joint was tilted medially and dorsally. Although the first metatarsal appeared normal, they found the other metatarsals were deformed in slight adduction at the metaphyseal level. They did not observe any subluxation at the other cuneometatarsal joints or the naviculocuneiform joint, as well as no tendon abnormalities. In addition, there was also no evidence of medial or lateral displacement of the navicular in relation to the talus. Based on these findings, they concluded that the pathogenic factor causing metatarsus adductus was the abnormal development of the medial cuneiform.

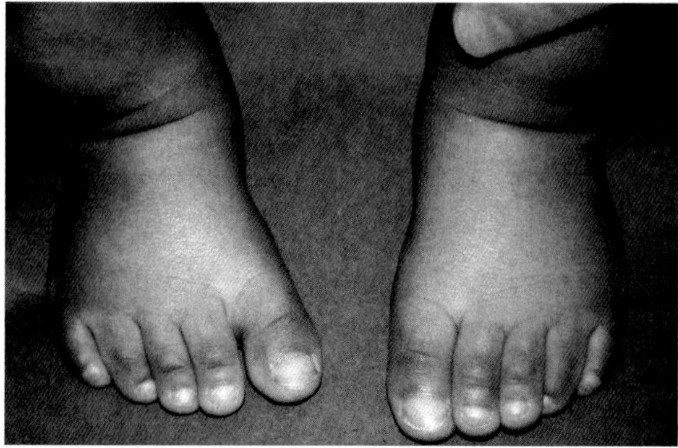

FIGURE 8-1 Metartarsus adductus of the right foot in a two-year-old male. It has improved considerably over the last year. No treatment was rendered.

Clinical Characteristics

The clinical features of metatarsus adductus are relatively consistent except for the degree of forefoot flexibility. The forefoot is typically adducted and slightly supinated (Figure 8-1). The lateral border of the foot is convex with increased prominence of the base of the fifth metatarsus. The medial aspect of the foot is concave. Usually, there are no associated transverse skin creases in the concavity. The hindfoot is in a neutral or slight valgus position. Ankle and subtalar joint mobility is typically normal and there is no equinus contracture. The medial longitudinal arch may be slightly elevated in height. Occasionally, a separation will occur between the first and second toes. The major feature which allows classification of metatarsus adductus is the flexibility of the forefoot. Internal or medial tibial torsion of varying degrees is commonly present.

Classification

Approximately 86% of children with metatarsus adductus resolve satisfactorily without treatment (41). Assessing the flexibility of the forefoot allows a clinical method of classification of the deformity, which is useful prognostically and in determining which feet will benefit from treatment. Several classifications based on flexibility have been used. Most recently, Crawford and Gabriel (10) reported a useful three-group clinical classification based on active and passive mobility. Stroking the lateral border of the foot will cause peroneal muscle contractions which will demonstrate the degree of active forefoot mobility. The type I metatarsus adductus is very flexible and the forefoot will correct past neutral into a slightly overcorrected position. A type II deformity has partial flexibility and does not correct to neutral actively but does passively. The type III deformity is rigid and does not correct to neutral even with passive stretching. The type I deformity usually does not require treatment, while the type II deformity may benefit by passive stretching or corrective shoes. The type III deformity requires more active treatment such as serial casting. Bleck (6), however, disagrees with flexibility grading systems. He found no correlation between poor results using a severity and flexibility grading system.

Radiographic Findings

Routine radiographs are not usually required in the assessment or management of metatarsus adductus (31). Radiographs are indicated only in difficult or severe cases or for a patient undergoing serial cast treatment who is not responding. Berg (3), however, has recommended anteroposterior and lateral standing or simulated weight-bearing radiographs in all infants and children with forefoot adduction. He recognized two radiographic types of both metatarsus adductus and metatarsus varus—simple and complex. The radiographic measurements and values for normal infants and children have recently been published by Vanderwilde et al. (46). In a normal foot, the long axis of the first metatarsus parallels or diverges laterally from the long axis of the talus (normal, 0 to +20 degrees). With forefoot adduction, the first metatarsal line is medial to the talar line (negative value). The first metatarsus is usually more deviated than the lateral metatarsi. There is a normal anteroposterior talocalcaneal angle as well as normal overlap of the heads of the talus and calcaneus. The lateral radiograph will demonstrate a normal lateral talocalcaneal angle. In simple metatarsus adductus, the first metatarsal line diverges medially to the talar line but the midfoot and hindfoot have normal alignment. In complex metatarsus adductus, the midfoot is laterally translated as demonstrated by lateral displacement of the cuboid from the calcaneal line.

The radiographic classification of Berg has not gained much popularity because of the variability of ossification of the talus and calcaneus. This makes the accuracy of measurements unreliable. Cook et al. (9) reported significant extraobservor and intraobserver measurement variability for the anteroposterior and lateral talocalcaneal angle using this classification.

Treatment

The treatment of metatarsus adductus can be both non-operative and operative. The type of treatment and its success is based on the patient's age when treatment is initiated.

Nonoperative Treatment

Infants less than six months of age with flexible metatarsus adductus type I and type II deformities may be observed (10,14,31,38). These will typically resolve over the next six to twelve months. The majority of the improvement begins after the child pulls to stand and walks independently. Rushforth (41) reported that 86% of 83 children (130 feet) who were observed were normal or had only mild residual forefoot adduction by three years of age. The deformity was graded by initial clinical photographs, but all feet corrected to neutral with passive stretching. Ponseti and Becker (38) observed that only 44 (11.6%) of 379 patients had rigid deformities and required active treatment. Of the 335 patients observed, there was a tendency to progress slightly until one or two years of age and then improve over the next two years. Dynamic hallux varus may be observed after satisfactory correction of the forefoot adduction but this also resolves over an additional one to two years.

Infants with type I or type II feet that present after the age of six months or who are not improving under observation may require: (i) passive stretching exercises, (ii) corrective shoes or othoses, or (iii) serial casting.

Passive Stretching Exercises

Crawford and Gabriel (10) recommended stretching exercises for type II deformities in children younger than walking age. Others have also recommended exercises under similar circumstances. The success of this method of treatment is controversial as there is no evidence that it alters the natural history of relatively flexible metatarsus adductus.

Stretching exercises are performed by stabilizing the hindfoot with one hand with firm pressure being applied over the cuboid. The forefoot is manipulated laterally by the opposite hand with pressure being applied over the first metatarsal head and neck. Pressure should not be applied to the great toe as this will not correct the forefoot. Usually, 20 repetitions are performed with each diaper change. The forefoot is held in the corrected or abducted position for approximately five seconds with each repetition. This stretches the medial soft tissues, especially the abductor hallucis muscle. Tachdjian (45) as well as Ponseti and Becker (38) do not recommend passive stretching exercises because they felt they were poorly performed by the parents.

Corrective Shoes or Orthoses

Shoes may be either straight or reversed-last (10,31). These are usually high top with the toes exposed. Reversing normal high top shoes should not be performed because of the improper alignment within the heel portion of the shoe which may result in skin irritation and ulceration. The shoes are worn 20 to 22 hours a day and may be removed for baths and for play activities. Serial casting may be considered when no significant improvement has been achieved after six to eight weeks of shoewear. However, the majority of type I and type II deformities will respond satisfactorily to this simple technique. Commercially available orthoses can also be utilized.

Serial Casting

Type III or rigid metatarsus adductus deformities require manipulation and serial casting (6,10,31,38). Corrective shoes should not be attempted because of the risk for skin irritation and pain. Bleck (6) found the results of serial cast treatment to be statistically better when treatment was initiated before eight months of age. Thus, it is important to treat these rigid deformities early rather than observing for spontaneous improvement with growth. The majority of children with type III feet will correct after six to eight weeks with serial casting. Kite (21–24) recognized three criteria for corrected metatarsus adductus. These include: (i) the base of the fifth metatarsus is no longer prominent, (ii) the forefoot is straight and active abduction is present, and (iii) the convex appearance of the lateral border of the foot has been corrected. Holding casts for an additional one to two months or corrective shoes are required.

Usually, a short leg or below-knee plaster cast is employed for serial casting and may be applied in either one or two sections. It is important that the techniques are followed precisely to prevent increased hindfoot valgus. Katz et al. (19) demonstrated that below-knee casts are as effective as above-knee or long leg casts (6,13,21,38) in the treatment of metatarsus adductus (19,21–24,31). Proper technique permits stabilization of the hindfoot in a neutral position with one hand while the opposite hand molds the plaster cast with pressure being applied over the metatarsal head and neck. The forefoot is gently manipulated into the corrected position while the plaster is allowed to set. This technique maintains the hindfoot in the neutral position while allowing correction of only the forefoot. The casts are changed at one- to two-week intervals depending on the size of the child and the associated rate of pedal growth. Satisfactory correction is usually obtained in six to eight weeks. Holding casts or perhaps corrective shoes can be used thereafter depending on the degree of correction and the flexibility.

Recurrent deformities can occur once nonoperative treatment has ceased (6,23,30). The incidence of reported recurrence is variable. Kite (23) found that approximately 20% of his 2,818 children with metatarsus varus (actually adductus) required additional casting. Bleck (6) reported that 29 of 265 feet treated (11%) had some recurrence of their deformities. McCauley et al. (30) reported that 23 of 63 feet (37%) had one or more recurrences following cast treatment. These recurrences usually develop within one to two months after cessation of initial casting. Recurrent deformities are managed with a second series of correcting casts.

The use of a Denis-Browne bar following serial casting is controversial. Berg (3) reported a significant incidence (63%) of a flatfoot deformity associated with the use of this splint. He attributed this deformity to increased hindfoot valgus produced by the splint and suggested that the bar be bent into an inverted-V shape to decrease the valgus force on the hindfoot. Ponseti and Becker (38) also did not recommend Denis-Browne bars for the same reason.

Operative Management

The upper limit for the use of serial casting is controversial. Serial casting should be the initial method of treatment for resistant or persistent deformities in children up to four years of age. Children less than one year of age have a high incidence of satisfactory results. However, there will be declining rate of success with conservative treatment in the older child. Patients between four and six years of age or younger children who have failed serial casting may benefit from soft-tissue releases such as: (i) recession of the abductor hallucis muscle, (ii) medial release, or (iii) a tarsometatarsal and intermetatarsal release. Older children require multiple metatarsal osteotomies or other osseous procedures to achieve correction.

Abductor Hallucis Recession

This procedure, can be performed by either percutaneous or open surgery and has been recommended by Mitchell (32) and others (10,27). This procedure may be helpful when the abductor hallucis tendon is tight when the first metatarsus is abducted or manipulated laterally (27). After the musculotendinous junction is released, serial casting is performed for eight to ten weeks to stretch the remaining medial soft tissues. This procedure is most successful in younger children. It is important that the contracted abductor hallucis muscle be the sole cause of the deformity since more complex abnormalities may not correct satisfactorily following its release.

Medial Release

This release is performed through a longitudinal incision over the medial aspect of the foot (2,45). The musculotendinous junction of the abductor hallucis muscle is recessed. The first metatarsal-medial cuneiform and medial cuneiform-navicular joint are released dorsally, medially, and on the plantar surface. This usually affords excellent flexibility of the foot. Short leg casts are applied and maintained for six to eight weeks. Corrective shoes are not usually required postoperatively, but occasionally, a child may benefit by the use of a straight last shoe for several additional months. The older the child, the more likely they are to require corrective shoes in order to hold the foot in the corrected position to permit subsequent growth and development in the corrected position to occur. Ghali et al. (14) reported 23 patients with 38 feet with metatarsus adductus treated by an anteromedial release. They did not release the musculotendinous junction at the abductor hallucis muscle but did section the portion of the tibialis anterior tendon that inserted into the medial and plantar aspects of the medial cuneiform, which they felt was abnormal and responsible for persistent adduction of the forefoot. They reported uniformly excellent results with respect to appearance, function, and radiographic assessment. Their mean age at surgery, however, was only one year eight months (range, nine months to five years six months). Postoperatively, these feet were immobilized for three months. The postoperative follow up averaged 4.4 months.

Asirvatham and Stevens (2) reported improved talo-first metatarsal angles in 12 feet with metatarsus adductus at a mean follow-up of 3.6 years following a medial release including recession of the abductor hallucis muscle. An internal fixation pin was used for four weeks postoperatively to maintain correction. A below-knee walking cast was used for an additional four weeks. Corrective or reverse last shoes were then used for several months.

Tarsometatarsal and Intermetatarsal Release

This procedure was described by Heyman et al. in 1958 (15) and consisted of a release of the tarsometatarsal and intermetatarsal joints through a transverse incision over the dorsum of the foot. The operation was recommended for resistant metatarsus adductus and for residual forefoot adduction in clubfeet in children three to seven years of age. Postoperatively, the child required three months of immobilization in short leg weight-bearing casts in order to allow for adequate remodeling. Heyman et al. reported excellent or good results in all nine feet (five patients) with persistent metatarsus adductus treated by this procedure. In 1970, Kendrick et al. (20) described further experience with this technique as well as additional follow-up of Heyman's initial patients who demonstrated no changes in their ratings with this further follow-up. They stressed the need to leave intact the lateral two-thirds of the metatarsal-cuneiform capsule to prevent a dorsal bunion and the lateral aspect of the fifth metatarsal-cuboid joint to prevent overcorrection. They recommended that each foot be immobilized for four months. Complications reported in this second study included skin slough, avascular necrosis of the second and third cuneiforms, dorsal prominence of the first metatarsal-cuneiform joint, and late degenerative changes in this joint. Pain was not mentioned. However, Stark et al. (42) have recently reported a high incidence of unsatisfactory results following this procedure. Only 8 of 15 feet (52%) with metatarsus adductus had satisfactory results. The mean age at surgery was 5.4 years with 11.4 years of follow up. There was no correlation whether the surgery was performed before four years of age or in older children. Crawford and Gabriel (10) now recommend this procedure for children less than five years of age. They pin the first and fifth metatarsi in a slightly overcorrected position to help prevent recurrence of the deformity. Most current authors favor multiple metatarsal osteotomies with internal fixation.

Metatarsal Osteotomies

In children six to eight years of age or older, metatarsal osteotomies with internal fixation is the procedure of choice (4,10,15,42,43). This consists of performing an osteotomy at the base of all five metatarsals either

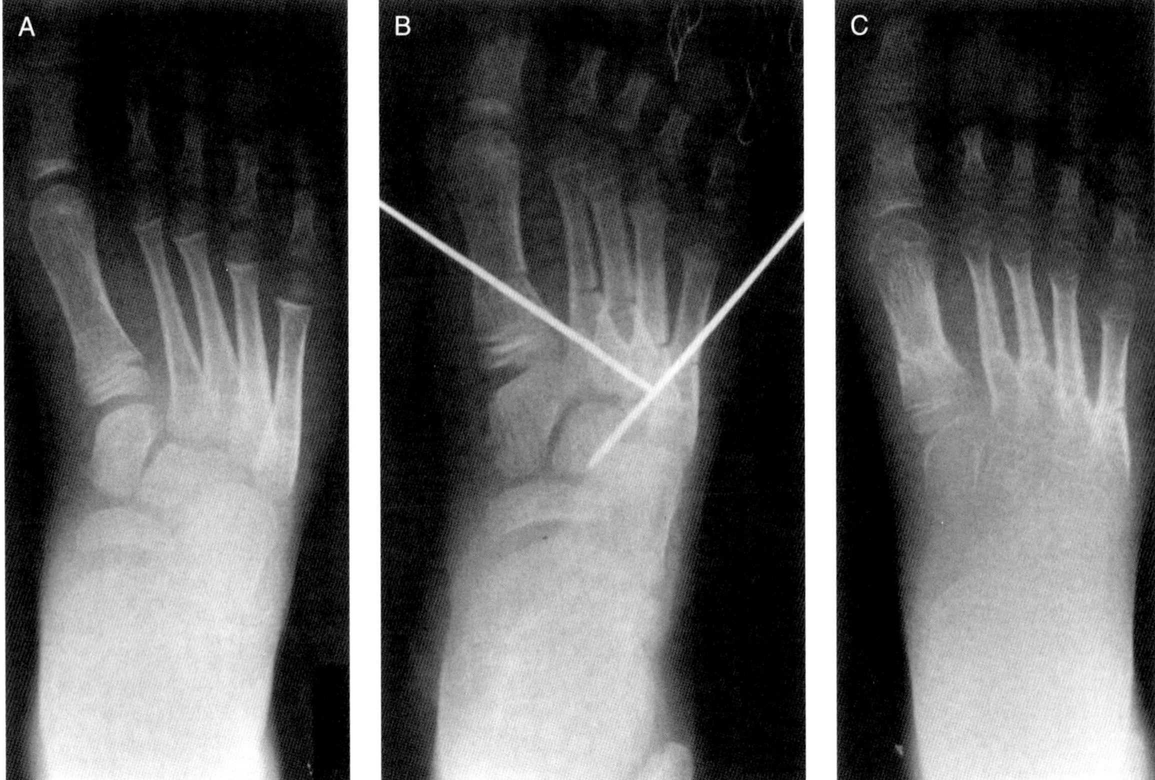

FIGURE 8-2 **A.** Weight-bearing anteroposterior radiograph of the right foot of a six-year-old male with persistent metatarsus adductus. There is a normal talocalcaneal angle of 25 degrees, the navicular is centered on the head of the talus, and there is adduction at the tarsometatarsal articulation. The talar-first metatarsal angle measures −22 degrees. The first metatarsus is more adducted than the other four. **B.** Correction of the metatarsus adductus by closing wedge osteotomies at the base of all five metatarsi. The first and fifth metatarsi were stabilized by internal fixation with Kirschner wires. The middle three metatarsi were stable. **C.** Six weeks postoperatively following pin removal. The osteotomies are well healed and there is complete correction. (Talar-first metatarsal angle is zero degrees.)

through a transverse dorsal incision or two longitudinal incisions. The former has a slight risk for distal skin necrosis but affords better exposure. The risk for skin necrosis can be minimized by preserving the veins over the dorsum of the foot. Care is taken to avoid injury to the proximal physeal plate of the first metatarsus. The osteotomies can either be dome-shaped or a closing wedge type. With the forefoot held in the corrected position, Kirschner wires or Steinmann pins are used to secure the first to the second metatarsus and then a second pin to stabilize the fourth to the fifth metatarsus (Figure 8-2A–C). This maintains alignment and allows preservation of the normal medial arch of the metatarsi. The third metatarsal is usually sufficiently stable that no fixation is required. Care must be taken to avoid creating a cavus or flatfoot deformity. Pin placement and alignment must be checked by intraoperative radiographs. Approximately, six to eight weeks of short leg cast immobilization is required before adequate union is achieved. Berman and Gartland (4) reported that 17 of 18 feet (94%) with metatarsus adductus treated by multiple metatarsal osteotomies and internal fixation had excellent or good results. Their mean age at surgery was 9.1 years and they had a mean follow-up of 4.1 years.

Other Osseous Procedures

Other operative procedures for the older child that have recently been described include an opening wedge osteotomy of the first or medial cuneiform (25,28). Occasionally, this may be combined with a closing wedge osteotomy of the cuboid (1). This corrects any malalignment between the medial cuneiform and first metatarsus as well as shortens the lateral column of the foot. Osteotomy limited to the first and second metatarsi may provide satisfactory correction in feet with milder deformities. The lateral three metatarsi frequently have sufficient mobility that they do not require surgical correction.

Complications

The complications of treated metatarsus adductus are usually minimal. With conservative treatment the major complication has been recurrent deformity or pronation.

The incidence of recurrence has varied between 11% to 37% (6,23), and these patients will usually benefit from a second series of corrective casts. Pronation or flatfoot represents overcorrection due to prolonged casting or the use of a Denis-Browne bar (3,38).

The complications following surgical treatment are predominantly failure to achieve complete intraoperative correction. There is always the risk for a postoperative wound infection, pin tract infection, or marginal skin necrosis. Non-unions following osteotomies are uncommon but can also occur (4). Shortening of the first metatarsus from a non-union or physeal injury has been reported and this may lead to abnormal weight bearing (16).

METATARSUS VARUS

Metatarsus varus deformities appear similar to metatarsus adductus but are more severe and fortunately uncommon (26,44). There is malalignment of the metatarsal and tarsal bones. The metatarsals are adducted at the tarsometatarsal joints; there is a medial subluxation of the metatarsals, lateral subluxation of the navicular on the head of the talus, and hindfoot valgus. There is also a rotational component to the forefoot deformity that occurs as a consequence to the hindfoot valgus (2,3,37). This has also been called a skewfoot or z-foot deformity. This combination of deformities produces a pronounced flatfoot appearance. Berg and others feel that there is a spectrum between metatarsus adductus and severe metatarsus varus (3,31). Kite (23) found only 12 of 2,818 feet with metatarsus adductus could actually be classified as metatarsus varus. Peterson (37) in his 1986 review of skewfoot documented only 50 cases in the world literature. However, he distinguished skewfoot from metatarsus varus. He felt the latter was associated with hindfoot varus and forefoot inversion. Meehan (31) has suggested that milder forms of metatarsus varus may be more frequent than appreciated and may be responsible for the cases of metatarsus adductus that are resistant to serial casting.

Etiology

Reimann and Werner (39) performed dissection studies on 14 normal feet in stillborns and concluded that congenital metatarsus varus is a primary medial subluxation of the tarsometatarsal joints occurring *in utero* when the foot is dorsiflexed. The soft-tissue contractures and adaptive bone changes are secondary deformities. In a later study (40), they demonstrated a contracture of the tibialis anterior muscle in an autopsy study performed on a newborn infant with a metatarsus varus deformity. This was associated with deformity of the medial cuneiform, subluxation between the middle and lateral cuneiforms and the second and third metatarsals, and additional soft-tissue contractures. Muscle histology was normal. They hypothesized that metatarsus varus develops in utero and results in secondary alterations of the developing bones and soft-tissue contractures. Peterson (37) stated that calf atrophy may be observed in children three years of age or older with a skewfoot. Browne and Paton (7) found anomalous insertions of the tibialis posterior tendon in 14 of 15 feet with resistant metatarsus varus. These studies suggest that perhaps there is a subtle underlying neuromuscular aspect to this disorder.

Clinical Characteristics

Clinical features in metatarsus varus are similar to metatarsus adductus. The deformity is usually more severe and there may be an associated deep transverse skin crease along the medial aspect of the foot over the tarsometatarsal joint (Figure 8-3A–C). Metatarsus varus deformities are typically less flexible than the metatarsus adductus deformities. Hindfoot valgus is present, but this can be difficult to assess in a non-ambulatory infant. The tendo-Achilles is not contracted.

Classification

Tachdjian (45) classified metatarsus varus based on flexibility, which is similar to the method used to classify metatarsus adductus. He felt that true metatarsus varus was a rigid deformity. He also described a functional metatarsus varus which was a dynamic deformity secondary to overactivity of the abductor hallucis muscle. He recognized a positional metatarsus adductus in which only the forefoot was deformed and the foot was correctable both actively and passively. These latter two deformities are essentially identical to metatarsus adductus.

Radiographic Findings

Anteroposterior and lateral standing or simulated weight-bearing radiographs are necessary to distinguish metatarsus varus from metatarsus adductus. In metatarsus varus, there is adduction of the forefoot and increased hindfoot valgus. The midfoot may be displaced laterally, but this is a variable finding. Typically the anteroposterior talocalcaneal angle exceeds 35 degrees, and there is no talocalcaneal overlap. On the lateral radiograph, there is also an increase in the lateral talocalcaneal angle. When the navicular becomes ossified, it usually is subluxated slightly laterally on the talar head.

Berg (3) distinguished a simple from complex skewfoot. In the simple form there is adduction of the forefoot, a valgus hindfoot but the midfoot is normal. In the complex skewfoot, the forefoot adduction is combined with lateral translation of the midfoot as well as the hindfoot valgus.

Hubbard et al. (17) from MRI studies of patients with skewfeet felt that if the base of the first metatarsal is lateral to the mid-talar axis, lateral subluxation of the navicular is to be expected and this distinguishes metarsus adductus from metatarsus varus or skewfoot.

Treatment

As with metatarsus adductus, the treatment can be either nonoperative or operative.

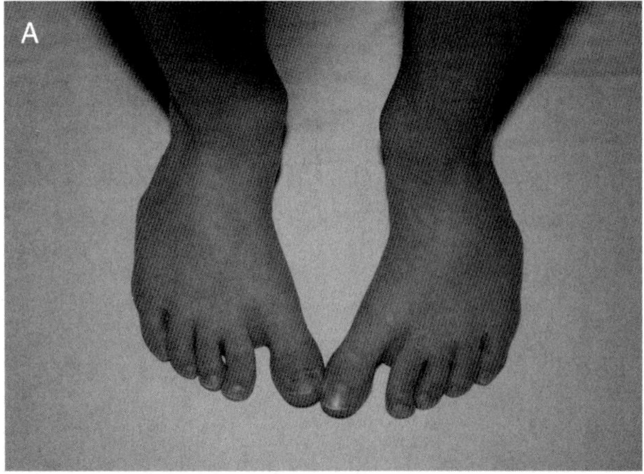

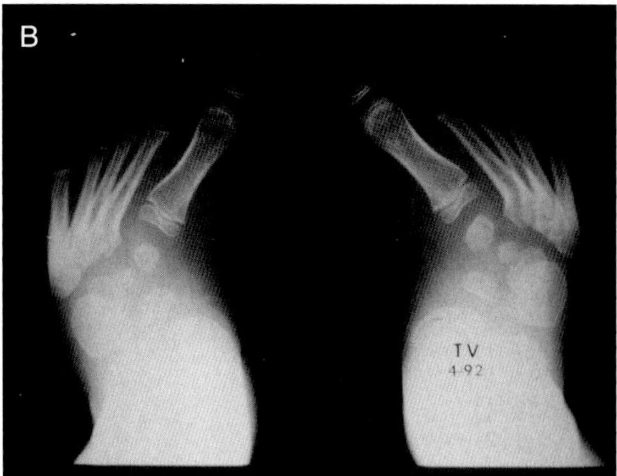

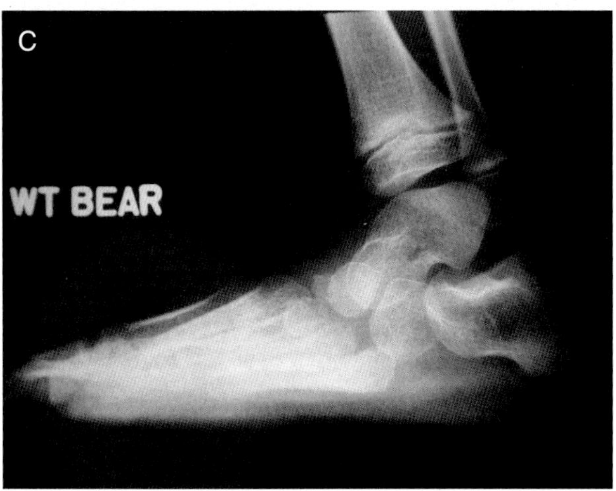

FIGURE 8-3 **A.** Bilateral metatarsus varus or skewfoot in a four-year-old male. His feet are asymptomatic but have not been improving with growth. **B.** The AP weight-bearing radiograph demonstrates the valgus hindfoot, neutral midfoot and forefoot adduction. **C.** The lateral weight-bearing radiograph demonstrates the hindfoot valgus confirming the diagnosis of metatarsus varus.

Nonoperative Treatment

Because there are few true cases of metatarsus varus as well as the confusion about the terms metatarsus adductus and metatarsus varus, it is difficult to determine whether nonoperative treatment plays a role in this deformity. Tachdjian (45) recommended serial casting using a long leg cast for children 12 months of age or less and felt the results were satisfactory using this approach. Similar outcomes were reported by Berg, but he found a significant increase in the duration of casting between metatarsus adductus and metatarsus varus, as well as between the simple and complex forms of the latter (3). The mean duration of treatment was 3.7, 6.0, 7.0, and 7.3 weeks for simple metatarsus adductus, complex metatarsus adductus, simple skewfoot, and complex skewfoot, respectively. Peterson (37) also felt that serial casting may be successful in infancy if the heel is held in varus, medial pressure applied to the navicular, and lateral pressure to the first metatarsal head. This position is difficult to achieve and maintain in small feet. As a consequence, nonoperative treatment is usually unsuccessful.

Serial casting is an appropriate initial procedure for children less than one year of age. The casting technique is similar to metatarsus adductus with the hindfoot maintained in neutral or slight varus and the forefoot abducted. Satisfactory correction usually takes longer because the deformity is more severe. This is usually eight to ten weeks followed by holding casts.

Operative Treatment

Operative treatment is typically used for children over one year of age who have radiographic documentation of a metatarsus varus deformity. Browne and Paton (7) performed transfer of the tibialis posterior tendon to the navicular tuberosity combined with a medial release. No ages were presented, but their patients had anomalous insertions of the tibialis posterior tendon to the plantar surface of the foot. Tachdjian recommended a similar approach to children with metatarsus adductus (35) and used a medial release for resistant deformities between one and two years of age; tarsometatarsal and intermetatarsal release for children three to seven years of age; and multiple metatarsal osteotomies for children eight years of age or older (Figure 8-4A–C).

Meehan recommended extensive soft-tissue releases in children between five and seven years of age (31). He

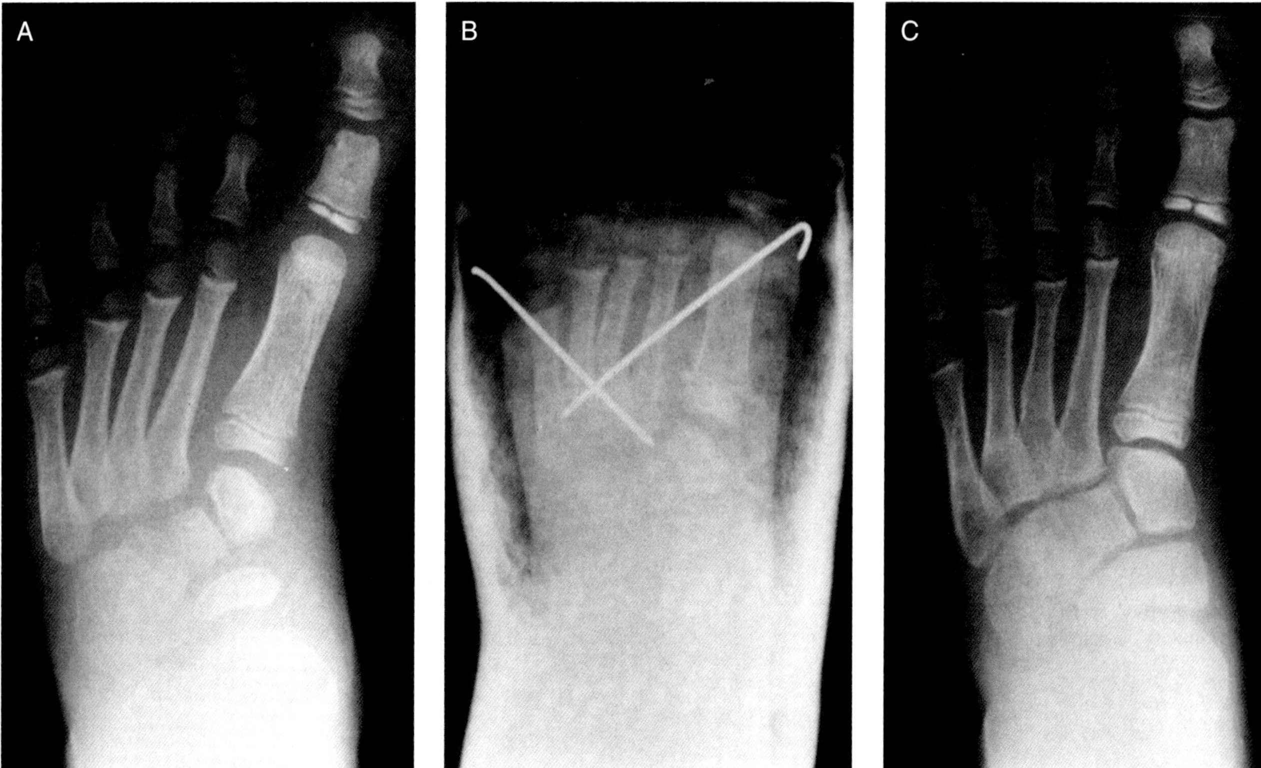

FIGURE 8-4 **A.** Weight-bearing anteroposterior radiograph of the left foot of an eight-year-old male with a metatarsus varus or skewfoot deformity. The talocalcaneal angle measures 33 degrees, the navicular is mildly subluxated laterally on the head of the talus, and the metatarsals are adducted. There is progressive adduction from medial to lateral. **B.** Multiple metatarsal osteotomies were performed. Kirschner wires stabilize the osteotomies. The medial pin transfixes the first and second metatarsi while the lateral pin stabilizes the fifth and fourth metatarsi. **C.** Two years later the foot remains improved. The lateral subluxation of the navicular persists, but hindfoot valgus has decreased to 25 degrees.

identified six anatomical abnormalities that must be addressed at the time of surgical treatment. These include: (i) severe forefoot adduction; (ii) deformity of the medial cuneiform; (iii) soft-tissue contractures especially of the tendo-Achilles, flexor digitorum longus, flexor hallucis longus, tibialis posterior, and occasionally of the tibialis anterior muscles and plantar fascia; (iv) lateral subluxation of the navicular; (v) lateral displacement of the calcaneus beneath the talus; and (vi) a long, lateral column of the foot. He felt that these children would benefit by an extensive soft-tissue release that would allow adequate realignment of the foot. While similar to the clubfoot release, the surgery also included a more extensive medial release as well as tarsometatarsal and intermetatarsal releases. This allowed the calcaneus to be reduced beneath the talus and the navicular to be reduced onto the talar head as well as correcting forefoot adduction. Internal fixation was necessary especially for the talonavicular and talocalcaneal joints.

Other procedures have also been described for correction of the skewfoot deformity in this age group. Coleman (8) recommended a plantar release and opening wedge medial cuneiform osteotomy. This has also been demonstrated to secondarily improve hindfoot alignment (47). Others have advocated hindfoot stabilization with a Grice extra-articular subtalar fusion followed by tarsometatarsal release or multiple metatarsal osteotomies (20,37). In the older child, Meehan has suggested a calcaneal osteotomy to correct the hindfoot valgus (31). In the adolescent, he recommended extensive soft-tissue releases followed by a triple arthrodesis and metatarsal osteotomies.

Currently, the combination of a calcaneal lengthening osteotomy, as described by Evans, combined with an opening wedge osteotomy of the medial cuneiform is the procedure of choice for symptomatic flatfoot and skewfoot (12,34,35). Mosca reported successful results in 9 of 10 children tracked after six years of age (34). Napiontek et al. (36) recently reported that a medial cuneiform osteotomy could be satisfactorily performed even in children less than four years of age and before ossification occurs. They had now growth disturbance in 37 feet in 25 children, although only four children had metatarsus adductus or skewfoot.

Results and Complications

It is difficult to discuss the results of treatment for the true metatarsus adductus or skewfoot as so few patients have been documented and treated by a standardized manner. The complications have been mainly undercorrection. It is therefore important that a distinction be made between metatarsus adductus and metatarsus varus when contemplating surgical intervention. The diagnosis can typically be made by physical examination, but occasionally, radiographs will also be necessary.

REFERENCES

1. Anderson D, Schoenecker P. *Combined lateral column shortening and medial column lengthening in the treatment of severe forefoot adductus.* Paper presented at the First International Congress on Clubfeet, Milwaukee, WI, Sept 5–6, 1990.
2. Asirvatham R, Stevens P. Idiopathic forefoot-adduction: medial capsulotomy and abductor hallucis lengthening for resistant and severe deformities. *J Pediatr Orthop* 1997;17:496–500.
3. Berg EE. A reappraisal of metatarsus adductus and skewfoot. *J Bone Joint Surg (Am)* 1986;68:1185–1196.
4. Berman A, Gartland JJ. Metatarsal osteotomy for the correction of adduction of the forepart of the foot in children. *J Bone Joint Surg (Am)* 1971;53:498.
5. Bielski RJ, Gesell MW, Teng AL, Cooper DH, Muraskas JK. Orthopaedic implications of multiple gestation pregnancy with triplets. *J Pediatr Orthop* 2006;26(1):129–131.
6. Bleck EE. Metatarsus adductus: classification and relationship to outcomes of treatment. *J Pediatr Orthop* 1983;3:2–9.
7. Browne RS, Paton DF. Anomalous insertion of the tibialis posterior tendon in congenital metatarsus varus. *J Bone Joint Surg (Br)* 1979;61:74.
8. Coleman SS. *Complex foot deformities in children.* Philadelphia: Lea and Febiger, 1983;267.
9. Cook DA, Breed AL, Cook T, DeSmet AD, Muehle CM. Observor variability in the radiographic measurement and classification of metatarsus adductus. *J Pediatr Orthop* 1992;12:86–89.
10. Crawford AH, Gabriel KR. Foot and ankle problems. *Orthop Clin North Am* 1987;18:649–666.
11. Duckworth T. The hindfoot and its relation to rotational deformities of the forefoot. *Clin Orthop* 1983;177:39.
12. Evans, D. Calcaneo-valgus deformity. *J Bone Joint Surg* 1975;57B:270.
13. Farsetti, P, Weinstein SL, Ponseti, IV. Long term functional and radiographic outcomes of untreated and non-operatively treated metatarsus adductus. *J Bone Joint Surg (Am)* 1994;76:257–265.
14. Ghali NN, Abberton MJ, Silk FF. The management of metatarsus adductus et supinatus. *J Bone Joint Surg (Br)* 1984;66:376.
15. Heyman CH, Herndon CH, Strong JM. Mobilization of the tarsometatarsal and intermetatarsal joints for the correction of resistant adduction of the forepart of the foot in congenital clubfoot or congenital metatarsus varus. *J Bone Joint Surg (Am)* 1958;40:299–310.
16. Holden D, Siff S, Butlers, Cain T. Shortening of the first metatarsal as a complication of metatarsal osteotomies. *J Bone Joint Surg (Br)* 1984;66:582.
17. Hubbard AM, Davidson RS, Meyers JS, Mahboubi S. Magnetic resonance imaging of skewfoot. *J Bone Joint Surg (Am)* 1996;78:389–397.
18. Jacobs JE. Metatarsus varus and hip dysplasia. *Clin Orthop* 1960;16:203–212.
19. Katz K, Rami D, Soudry M. Below-knee plaster cast for the treatment of metatarsus adductus. *J Pediatr Orthop* 1999;19:49–50.
20. Kendrick RE, Sharma NK, Hassler WL, Herndon CH. Tarsometatarsal mobilization for resistant adduction of the forepart of the foot. *J Bone Joint Surg (Am)* 1970;52:61.
21. Kite JH. Congenital metatarsus varus. *Instr Course Lect* 1950;7:126.
22. Kite JH. Congenital metatarsus varus. *J Bone Joint Surg (Am)* 1964;46:525.
23. Kite JH. Congenital metatarsus varus. *J Bone Joint Surg (Am)* 1967;49:388.
24. Kite JH. Congenital metatarsus varus. Report of 300 cases. *J Bone Joint Surg (Am)* 1950;32:500–506.
25. Kling TF Jr, Schmidt TL, Conklin Mi. Open *wedge osteotomy of the first cuneiform for metatarsus adductus.* Paper presented at the annual meeting of the Pediatric Orthopaedic Society of North America. San Francisco, CA, Aug 6–9, 1990.
26. Kumar SJ, MacEwen GD. The incidence of hip dysplasia with metatarsus adductus. *Clin Orthop* 1980;164:234–235.
27. Lichtblau S. Section of the abductor hallucis tendon for correction of metatarsus varus deformity. *Clin Orthop* 1975;110: 227–232.
28. Lincoln CR, Wood KE, Brigg EI. Metatarsus varus corrected by open wedge osteotomy of the first cuneiform bone. *Orthop Clin North Am* 1976;7:795–798.
29. Lincoln TL, Suen PW. Common rotational variations in children. *J Am Acad Orthop Surg* 2003;11:312–320.
30. McCauley J Jr, Lusskin R, Bromley J. Recurrence in congenital metatarsus varus. *J Bone Joint Surg (Am)* 1964;46:525–532.
31. Meehan P. Other conditions of the foot. In: Morrissy RT, ed. *Lovell and Winter's Pediatric Orthopaedics.* Philadelphia: JB Lippincott, 1990;991–1021.
32. Mitchell GP. Abductor hallucis release in congenital metatarsus varus. *Int Orthop* 1980;3:299–304.
33. Morcuende JA, Ponseti IV. Congenital metatarsus adductus in early human fetal development: a histologic study. *Clin Orthop Relat Res* 1996;333:261–266.
34. Mosca VS. Calcaneal lengthening for valgus deformity of the hindfoot. Results in children who had severe symptomatic flatfoot and skewfoot. *J Bone Joint Surg (Am)* 1995;77: 500–512.
35. Mosca VS. Flexible flatfoot and skewfoot. *Instr Course Lect* 1996;45:347–354.
36. Napiontek M, Kotwicki T, Tomaszewski M. Opening wedge osteotomy of the medial cuneiform before age 4 years in the treatment of forefoot adduction. *J Pediatr Orthop* 2003;23: 65–69.
37. Peterson HA. Skewfoot (forefoot adduction and heel valgus). *J Pediatr Orthop* 1986;6:24–30.
38. Ponseti IV, Becker JR. Congenital metatarsus adductus: the results of treatment. *J Bone Joint Surg (Am)* 1966;48:702–711.
39. Reimann I, Werner HH. Congenital metatarsus varus. A suggestion for possible mechanism and relation to other foot deformities. *Clin Orthop* 1975;110:223.
40. Reimann I, Werner HH. The pathology of congenital metatarsus varus. A post- mortem study of a newborn infant. *Acta Orthop Scand* 1983;54:847–849.
41. Rushforth GF. The natural history of hooked forefoot. *J Bone Joint Surg (Br)* 1978;60:530–532.
42. Stark JG, Johnson JE, Winter RB. The Heyman-Herndon tarsometatarsal capsulotomy for metatarsus adductus: results in 48 feet. *J Pediatr Orthop* 1987;7:305–310.
43. Steytler JCS, VanderWalt ID. Correction of resistant adduction of the forefoot in congenital clubfoot and congenital metatarsus varus by metatarsal osteotomy. *Br J Surg* 1966;53:558.
44. Sullivan JA. Pediatric flatfoot: evaluation and management. *J Am Acad Orthop Surg* 1999;7:44–53.
45. Tachdjian MO. In: *Pediatric orthopaedics. The foot and leg.* Philadelphia: WB Saunders, 1990;2612–2626.
46. Vanderwilde R, Staheli LT, Chew DE, Malagon V. Measurements on radiographs of the foot in normal infants and children. *J Bone Joint Surg (Am)* 1988;70:407–415.
47. Viehweger E, Jacquemier M, Launay F, Giusiano B, Bollini G. First cuneiform osteotomy alters hindfoot architecture. *Clin Orthop* 2005;441:356–365.
48. Wynne-Davies R. Family studies and the cause of congenital club foot. Talipes equinovarus, talipes calcaneovalgus and metatarsus varus. *J Bone Joint Surg (Br)* 1964;46:445–463.

CHAPTER 9

Congenital Vertical Talus/Oblique Talus

Marek Napiontek

INTRODUCTION

Congenital vertical talus (CVT) is rare disorder of the foot, often coexisting with neurological and genetic syndromes. The diagnosis has to be confirmed by X-ray. The treatment is difficult. The nonoperative treatment restricted exclusively to manipulations and casts almost always fails. The classic primary operative treatment option was one-stage open reduction with tendons lengthening and/or transposition in the first year of the life. Currently, a combined treatment consisted of manipulations and casting followed by limited surgery is a new option in management of the deformity.

Synonyms: congenital vertical talus, congenital flat foot, congenital convex pes valgus, rocker bottom foot, talipes convex pes valgus.

DEFINITION

The terms "vertical talus" or "oblique talus" are more widly used than congenital convex pes valgus which defines the anatomic or radiographic position of the talus in the ankle joint in the sagittal plane. The talus is visible on lateral radiographs in a fixed plantar flexed attitude. There is a dorsal and lateral dislocation of the midfoot in relation to the talus and calcaneus. This causes the clinical appearence of a convex plano-valgus foot with shortening of the Achilles tendon and the long extensors. The pedal disorder may be associated with a variety of conditions. It may be a primary congenital deformity known as congenital vertical talus, which can occur as an idiopathic form or associated with multiple malformation syndromes, an *in utero* deformity or a component of chromosome aneuploidy states. It may also be a secondary deformity to neuromuscular abnormalities such as a peripheral or central nervous system disease, after prolonged bed rest, as iatrogenic deformation especially after nonoperative treatment of congenital clubfoot, and with a deficient tibialis posterior tendon.

HISTORICAL REVIEW

Theodor Essau first described pathologic anatomy of congenital vertical talus in 1856 (27), while Henken in 1914 presented its radiological and clinical picture (16). Lamy and Weissman in 1939 described the malformation and its treatment in the English literature (19).

EPIDEMIOLOGY

Until today the frequency of occurrence of the deformity has not been clearly determined. Pick and Chicote-Campos (29), on the basis of the data found in the literature, state it comprises 0.24% to 0.4% of all foot deformities. Jacobsen and Crawford (17) reported that CVT accounts for less than 4% of all pedal deformities. A vertical talus constitutes 10% of foot deformities in myelomeningocele. Boys are affected slightly more often than girls. The deformity is unilateral in half the reported cases.

ETIOLOGY

The etiology is unknown but has been hypothesized to result from a neuromuscular imbalance *in utero*. In myelomeningocele, Drennan and Sharrard (11) thought it was due to an imbalance between a weak tibialis posterior and strong dorsiflexors, whereas Specht (33) found deficient intrinsic muscles. Approximately one-half of cases of CVT are associated with systemic neurologic, muscular or skeletal disorders, such as arthrogryposis, spina bifida, mental retardation, Down syndrome, and trisomy 13–15 and 17–18.

Isolated CVT can be transmitted as an autosomal dominant trait with variable expression and incomplete penetrance (34). Hereditary and familial occurrence has been rarely observed and is found mainly in idiopathic CVT

(14). Few familial cases have been reported, and no chromosomal location or candidate gene has previously been identified. There is a report of four generations family with radiographically demonstrated CVT in whom a HOXD10 gene mutation was identified (8). The reported familial cases are consistent with an autosomal dominant mode of inheritance with incomplete penetrance (20).

PATHOLOGIC ANATOMY

The hindfoot is locked in equinus and the talus generally assumes a vertical position relative to the ankle joint. Displacement through the transverse tarsal articulation includes medial column dislocation with the navicular moving dorsally and laterally relative to the talar head and neck. There is similar displacement of the cuboid relative to the anterior part of the calcaneus when the lateral column of the foot is involved. The forefoot is abducted and may also demonstrate pronation or supination (18). The navicular becomes triangular in shape with the plantar half hypoplastic. Eventually secondary osseous and articular surface changes develop, especially in the calcaneo-talo-navicular and calcaneo-cuboid joints. Shortening of the lateral column of the foot may also affect the outcome of surgical treatment.

The mid-tarsal displacement is associated with contractures of the posterior, dorsal, and lateral ligaments, tendons, and capsular structures, while the medial soft tissue structures are frequently overstretched. Shortening of the Achilles tendon and peroneal muscles may be found. Both the shortened peronei as well as the attenuated tibialis posterior may displace anterior to malleollei causing them to act as foot dorsiflexors (28). This may be an additional factor decreasing the push-off power in an untreated deformity. Shortening of the extensors of all toes, as well as tibialis anterior muscle is observed.

DIAGNOSIS

The defect is diagnosed as soon as the baby is born, especially if the deformity occurs as a part of genetic and chromosomal syndromes. Often the acquired type (group 3 according to Lichtblau [21]) or idiopathic type (group 5 according to Hamanishi [13]), are overlooked as in these cases an initial erroneous diagnosis of postural calcaneovalgus deformity had been made. It is essential to take a lateral radiograph in full plantar flexion, and only if the first metatarsal, lateral cuneiform, or navicular remain dorsally dislocated in relation to the talar head, a true CVT deformity can be considered CVT (Figures 9-1 and 9-2).

CLINICAL FEATURES

CVT is characteried by equinus position of the hindfoot, abduction of the forefoot, and a flattening or convexity of the expected medial longitudinal arch. The most prominent part of the sole is the talar head and anterior part of the calcaneus. The convexity on the medial border of the foot is done by protruding navicular bone. (This is the author's intraoperative observation.) Diminished calf girth and, in older children, a characteristic position of the toes with the second toe rising vertically and over-riding the third and great toe are also part of the clinical presentation. CVT can be considered as a complex of rotational disturbances, in which the subtalar complex consisting of the calcaneus, cuboid, and navicular together with the cuneiforms, metatarsals, and phalanges rotates outward in the horizontal and coronal planes. Additionally, a part of the subtalar complex anteriorly to the calcaneus rotates more in those both planes and dorsally in sagittal plane. Observations concerning forefoot supination in CVT were done by Król and Marciniak (18) and may have clinical importance, especially in attempted correction of the hindfoot equinus and eversion. The true congenital deformity is incorrectable without surgery.

IMAGING

The navicular does not ossify until age 2.5 years. In newborns and infants, ossification center of the medial (13) or lateral cuneiform (1) can be utilized on lateral radiograph to demonstrate the abnormal relationship of the midfoot to the long axis of the plantar flexed talus. However, on the same view, the ossific nucleus of the talus may have a rounded contour making measurements difficult. Careful observation of the soft tissue outline on the plantar surface of the foot will delineate the rocker-bottom deformity.

Radiographs

Standard weight-bearing AP and lateral x-rays should be obtained, in younger patients position should mimick weight bearing. Additionally, maximum dorsiflexion and plantar flexion lateral views are necessary to confirm the talonavicular dislocation. A lateral x-ray in maximum dorsiflexion confirms the fixed equinus position of the calcaneus and talus relative to the tibia caused by shortening of the Achilles tendon. This information aids the surgeon in decision making about its lengthening. A talar axis-first metatarsal base angle (TAMBA) and calcaneal axis-first metatarsal base angle (CAMBA) (14) are used to differentiate an oblique talus from navicular displacement and tendon Achilles shortening. An AP view demonstrates abduction of the forefoot at the midtarsal joint and also in Lisfranc joint. Interestingly the AP talocalcaneal angle generally is in an acceptable range (4) and measured a mean of 34 degrees (23). In toddlers, the talus acquires an hourglass shape brought about by the pressure that the navicular exerts on its neck. The anterior part of the calcaneus becomes slim and bent in a beak-like fashion,, and looks like a Dutch clog (18). Both the lateral and AP

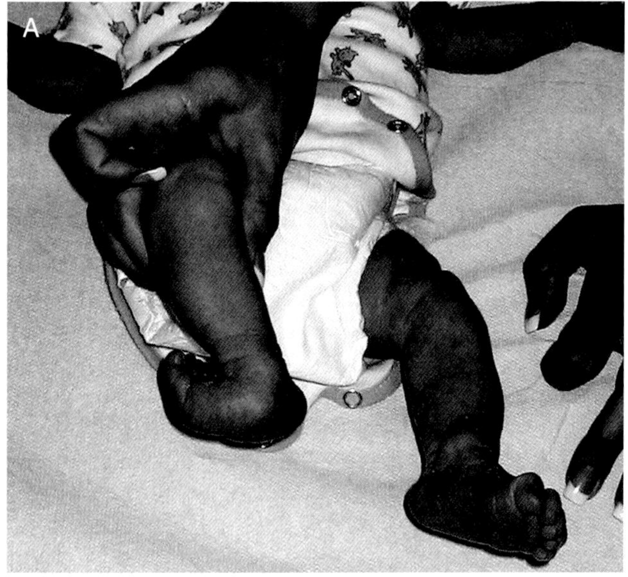

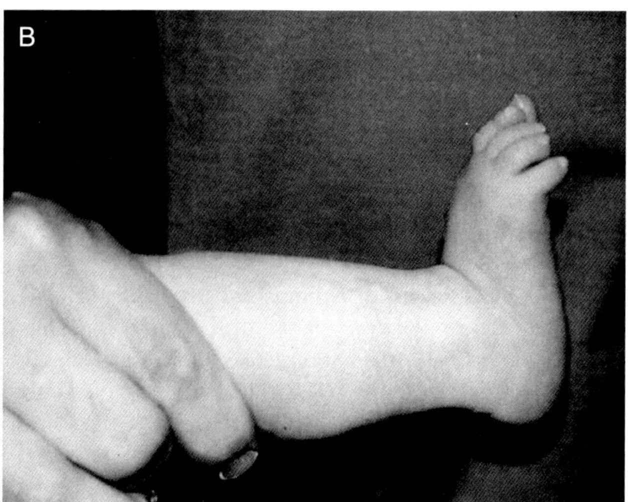

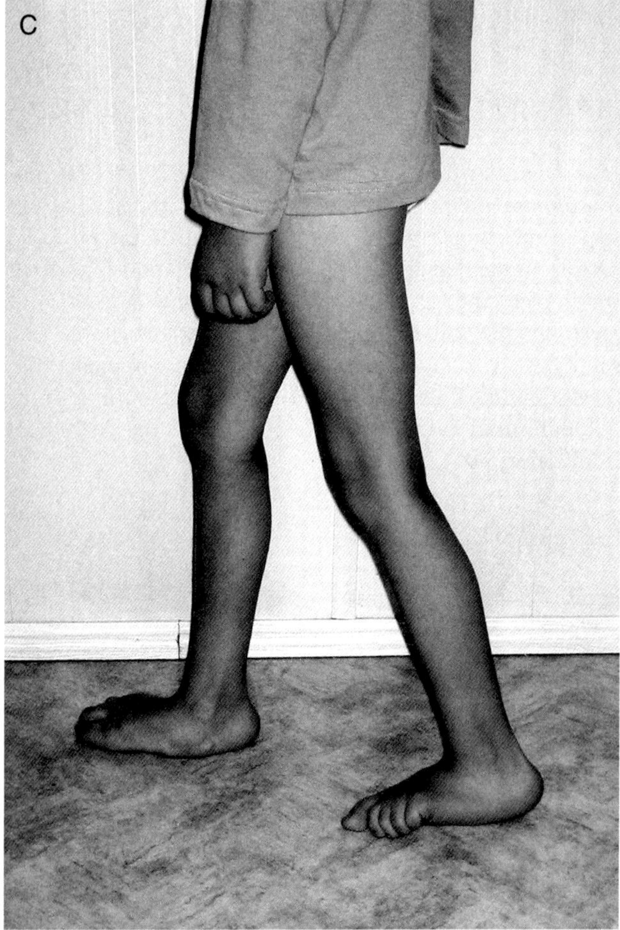

FIGURE 9-1 Idiopathic type of the CVT (group 3 according to Lichtblau and group 5 according to Hamanishi) in **A.** a newborn; **B.** a six-month-old child; **C.** a seven-year-old boy. Appearance of the foot may be mistaken for calcaneovalgus deformity (**A** and **B**) or flexible flatfoot (**C**).

radiographs reveal a dorsal and lateral dislocation, of the navicular in relation to the talar head and of the cuboid to the anterior part of the calcaneus respectively. The way of evaluating was presented by Napiontek (23) but its use for appraisal of the outcome of the treatment is applicable only in older children. In the deformities of neurogenic origin, the characteristic thin and elongated shapes of the talar and calcaneal bones are apparent.

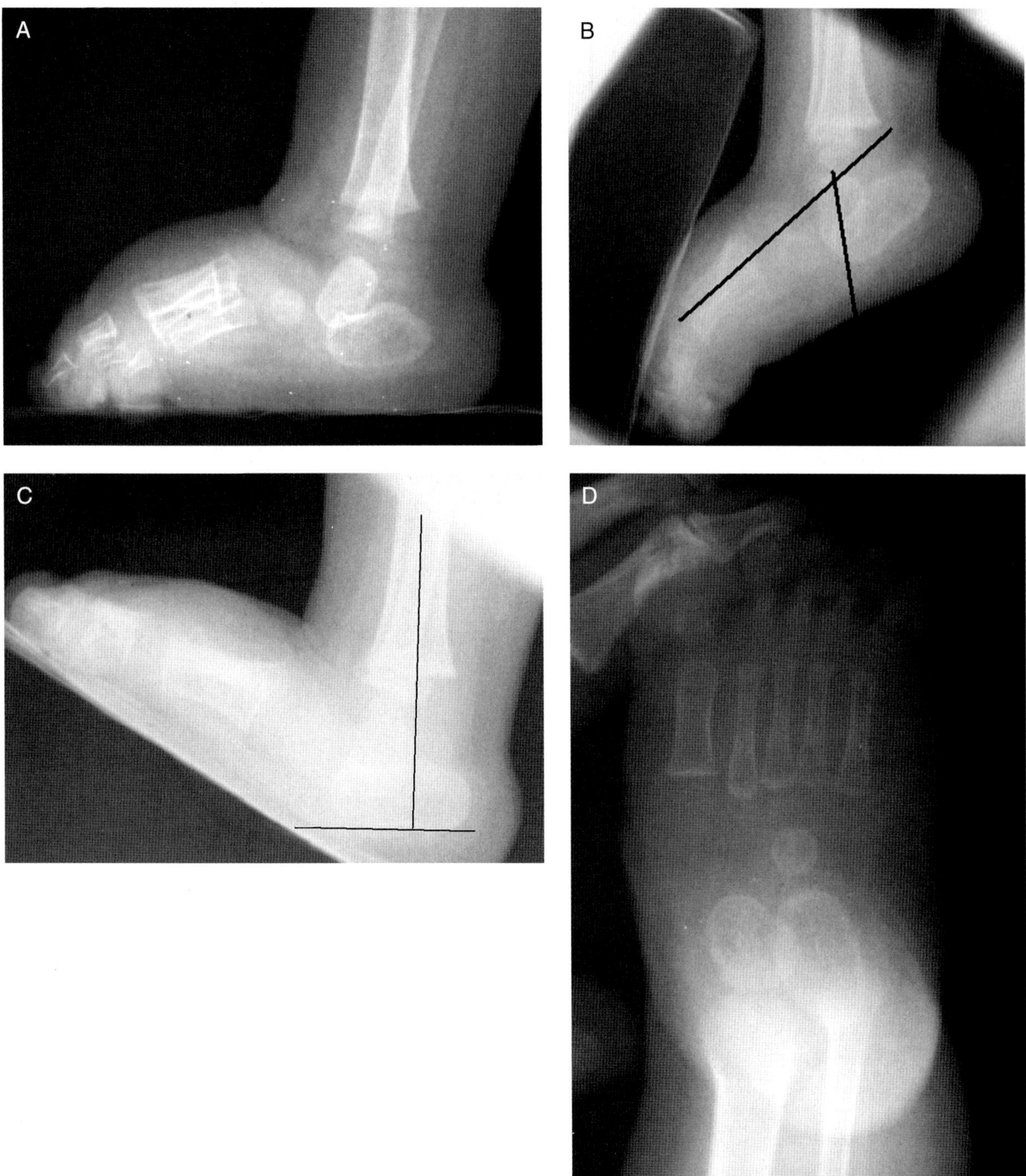

FIGURE 9-2 A. Lateral mimicking standing or standing radiograph of idiopathic CVT: In the normal foot, the center of cuboid lies on the calcaneus axis. The axis of the talus and first metatarsal is common. B. Lateral radiograph in maximum plantar flexion confirms persisted dorsal dislocation of the first metatarsal towards longitudinal axis of the talus as well cuboid towards anterior part of the calcaneus. C. Lateral radiograph in maximum dorsal flexion reveals equinus position of the hindfoot (diminished tibio-calcaneal angle). D. Dorsal-plantar view shows abduction of the forefoot (Navicular is unvisible on x-ray).

Ultrasound

This technique can be a useful supplement to radiological evaluation in infancy (31). Hamel and Becker (15) developed assessment of the talonavicular malalignment before ossification of the navicular.

CLASSIFICATION

Etiologic classifications given independently by Lichtblau (21) and Hamanishi (14) are the most useful. The first one is simple and practical, the second is more detailed.

Lichtblau's Classification

Group 1. Teratogenic type
genetic etiology, often familial history, bilateral, associated defects (developmental dislocation of the hip, mental retardation), recognized at birth as "Persian slipper deformity," the foot rigid and resisitant to passive manipulation, tight extensors and heel cord (Figure 9-3).

Group 2. Neurogenic type
muscle imbalance, myelomeningocele or neurofibromatosis, unilateral, it seems correctible in the infant, more rigid in the older child.

Group 3. Acquired type
from temporary malposition *in utero*, not familial, no other defects except an opposite equinovarus foot or developmental dislocation of the hip, unilateral, partially correctible and not severely rigid (may be mistaken for calcaneovalgus foot), hindfoot may not be fixed in equinus, the extensors permit manipulation of the forefoot into equinus.

Hamanishi's Classification

Group 1
CVT associated with neural tube defects and spinal anomalies. There are varying degrees of paralytic imbalances of the extrinsic and intrinsic muscles, which are considered to initiate the deformities, and an intrauterine postural effect may fix them secondarily.

Group 2
CVT associated with wide varieties of neuromuscular disorders without spinal anomalies (includes arthrogryposis multiplex congenita, neurofibromatosis, cerebral damage and cerebral palsy).

Group 3
CVT as a major part of the skeletal abnormalities of known malformation syndromes (includes Freeman-Sheldon syndrome).

Group 4
CVT with chromosomal aberrations.

Group 5
Idiopathic CVT subdivided into four groups in accordance with the patterns of other skeletal abnormalities and inheritance:

Group 5A - intrauterine molding or deformation
Group 5B - digitotalar dysmorphism
Group 5C - familial occurrence of CVT or oblique talus
Group 5D - sporadic and unassociated

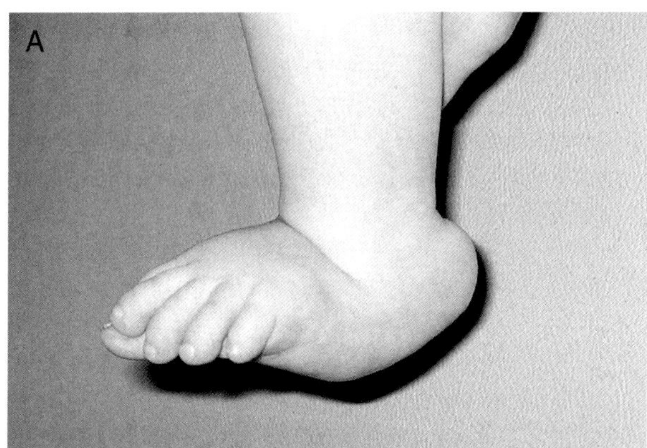

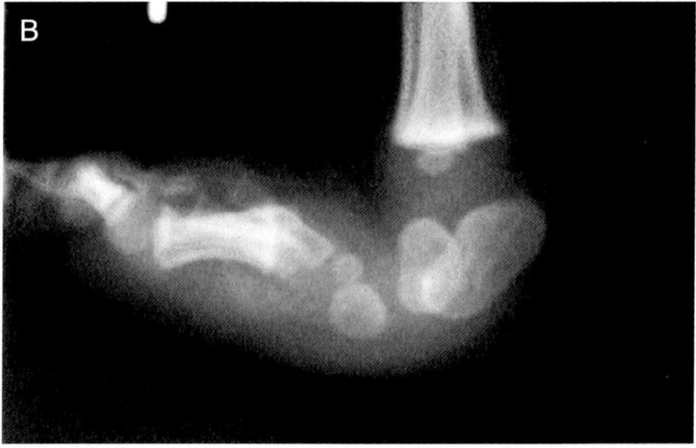

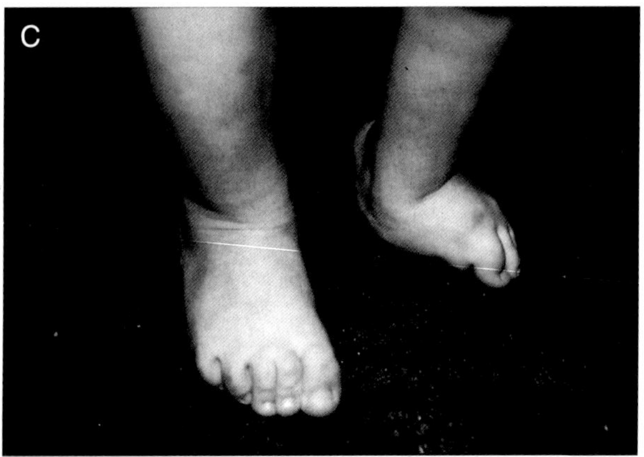

FIGURE 9-3 A teratogenic type of the CTV (group 1 according to Lichtblau or group 1 according to Hamanishi). **A.** In a six-month-old boy. **B.** Lateral radiograph of the same foot made immediately after birth. **C.** Extreme rocker bottom deformity in untreated 3-year-old girl.

Two other classification system offer additional insight into the problems.

Król and Marciniak classification (18) divides severe and mild type of CVT into two groups: with forefoot supination and forefoot pronation.

Coleman and Jarrett classification (2) divides the deformity into two groups as well: with and without a dislocation in the calcaneocuboid joint. In their opinion, the deformity is associated with a dislocation of the lateral column and is more difficult to treat.

DIFFERENTIAL DIAGNOSIS

In newborns, the calcaneovalgus foot especially with forefoot abduction can be misdiagnosed as CVT. A radiograph may not prove useful because in a lateral view the ossification centre of the talus maybe ideally spherical and the navicular is invisible. In older children, flexible or paralytic flatfoot (especially both with shortening of the Achilles tendon) with the oblique talus on the lateral standing radiograph can imitate CVT (Figure 9-4). Additionally oblique or vertical talus arising later in childhood

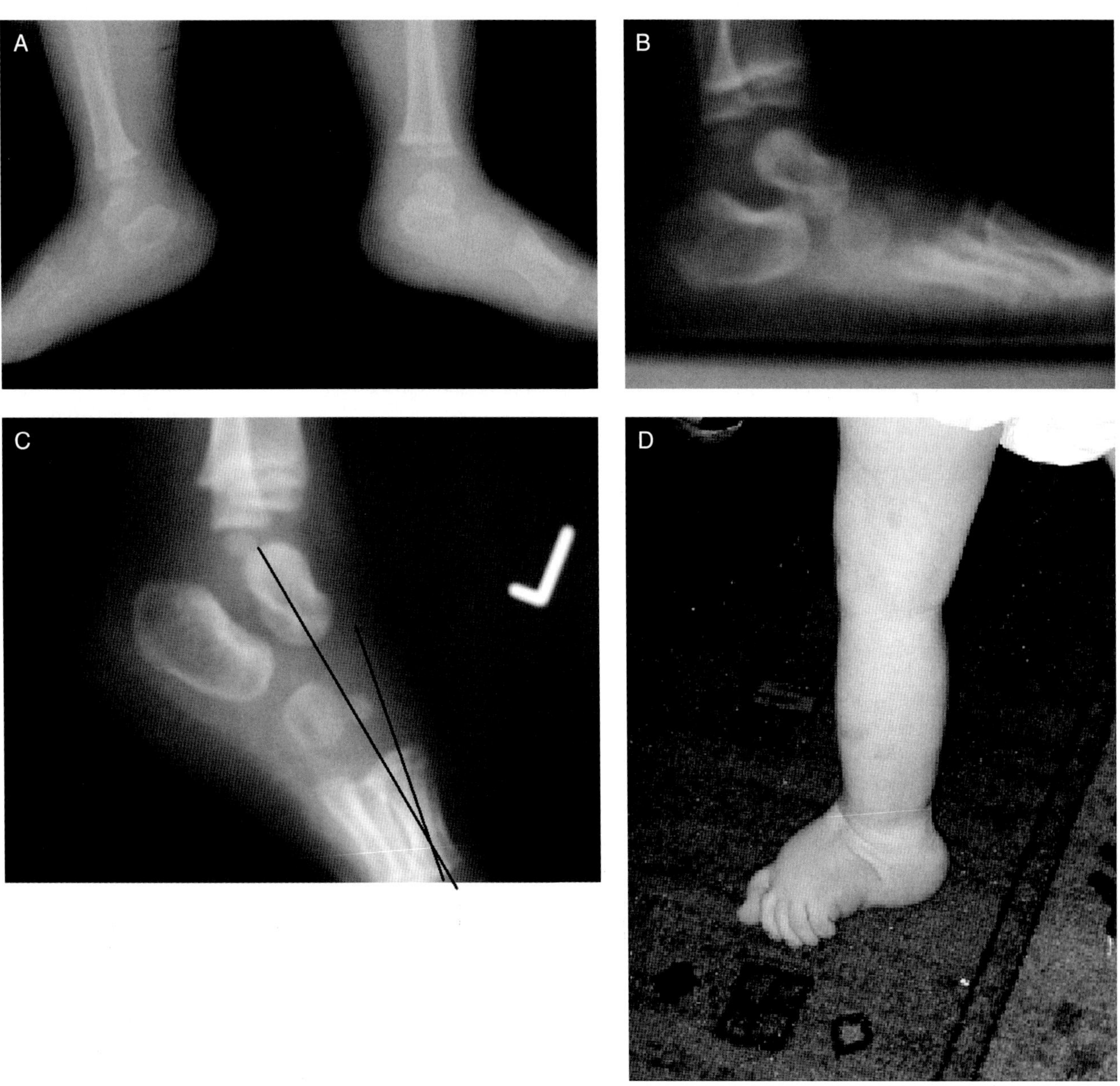

FIGURE 9-4 Oblique talus in the left foot misdiagnosed as CVT and treated by casting and manipulation. **A.** Lateral radiographs both feet before treatment. **B.** Lateral standing radiograph at improper qualification for surgery. **C.** Lateral radiograph in maximum plantar flexion – there is no talo-navicular and calcaneo-cuboid dislocation. **D.** Clinical appearance at age one year reveals forefoot abduction.

may besecondary to neuromuscular disorder such as poliomyelitis or cerebral palsy should be considered.

MANAGEMENT

The treatment of CVT should begin immediately after birth with serial manipulation and casting. The frequency and duration of it is similar to that used in congenital talipes equino-varus. The above-knee plaster cast is applied in maximum plantar flexion and supination of the foot. This nonoperative treatment is rarely sucessful.

Manipulation and Casts Combined with Limited Operative Treatment

Dobbs et al. (7, 9) proposed a new approach to management of idiopathic form of CVT. They reported success with serial manipulation and cast treatment combined with minor surgical intervention as the definitive treatment of idiopathic congenital vertical talus.

The principles of manipulation and treatment with plaster cast are similar to those used in Ponseti method of clubfoot correction, but the forces are applied in the opposite direction. All components of the deformity are corrected simultaneously, except for the equinus, which should be corrected last. The foot is stretched into plantar flexion and inversion while counterpressure is applied to the medial aspect of the talus. An average of five to six above-knee casts were required to reduce the forfoot onto the talar head in their study. By the time that last cast is applied, the foot presents equinovarus deformity. Once the forefoot is seen radiographically to be reduced on the head of the talus (a talar axis-first metatarsal base angle in maximum plantar flexion of $<30°$) the reduction is held by a Kirschner-wire passing percutaneously accross the talonavicular joint with the foot in maximum plantar flexion. The wire is placed retrograde from navicular into the talus while the foot is held in maximum plantarflexion. If the talo-navicular joint is not reduced radiographically, Kirschner wire in the navicular can be used to lever the bone into proper position and Kirschner wire is placed into the talus in retrograde manner while the forefoot is held in maximum plantar flexion. If the joint cannot be reduced closed then a small incision is made over the joint and dorsal capsulectomy of talo-navicular joint is performed. Once the forefoot is held in reduced positiom, the hindfoot equinus can be corrected by percutaneous Achilles tenotomy. Rarely the peroneus brevis tendon and/or tibialis anterior tendon must be fractionally lengthened.

Two above knee plaster casts are applied for two and three weeks. The first one with the foot in neutral position and the ankle in 5° of dorsiflexion. A second one with the ankle in 10°–15° of dorsiflexion. Following cast removal Dobbs recommends a solid ankle-foot orthosis with 15° of plantar flexion at the mid-tarsal joint be worn full time until the child starts walking and then for walking until the age of two years to maintain forefoot plantar flexion. That prevents recurence of the deformity. They state that patients with neuromuscular and genetic disorders tend to have more rigid deformities and are less amenable to this form of treatment.

OPERATIVE TREATMENT

The last 30 years have brought one-stage operative procedures (3,4,6,10,12,23,30,32,36,37,38) consisting basically of an open reduction of the dislocated joints, lengthening of the Achilles tendon, peroneals, and extensors. The K-wire stabilization is obligatory. The operation is best performed during the first year of age using the Cincinnati approach (3), as it ensures the best view of the anatomic structures of the hindfoot and midfoot.

One-stage Open Reduction Used by the Author (25)

The recommended child's age for this technique is nine months to 2 and a half years. With the child placed prone, the Cincinnati approach is used. However with children over 18–24 months, wound closing is difficult and it is highly advisable to use a double incision, either posteromedial and lateral, or posterolateral and medial (Figure 9-5).

The lateral release

The belly of the short toe extensors is released. The sheaths of the peroneous tendons are opened, distal to the lateral malleolus and the tendons are lengthened by Z technique. The capsulotomy of the calcaneocuboid joint is completed while the talonavicular joint is opened only from its lateral side. The talocalcaneal interosseus ligament as well as the calcaneofibular ligament are divided and the joints between the talus and the calcaneus are opened.

The posterior release

The Achilles tendon is lengthened by the Z technique. The procedure may be troublesome when the muscular belly of the triceps surae descends considerably low, causing shortness of the visualized tendon. Posterior capsulotomy of the ankle joint is optional and depends on the degree of fixed hindfoot equinus. During the posterior capsulotomy, both the posterior talofibular ligament and the posterior fibers of the deltoid ligament are divided.

The medial release

The foot the sheath of the tibialis posterior tendon is opened and the tendon is shortened by the Z technique. Both the tendon of the flexor digitorum longus and flexor hallucis longus are identified just below the talar head and navicular and are separated from the spring ligament. The spring ligament is then incised longitudinally parallel to the sheath of the posterior tibial muscle tendon. A transverse incision is added at the level of the talonavicular

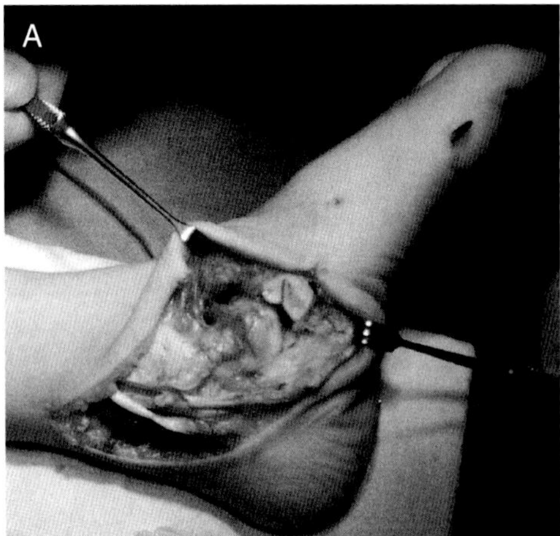

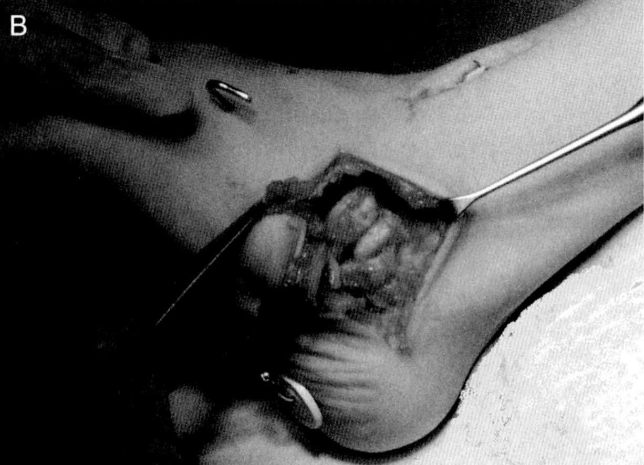

FIGURE 9-5 Author's method of operative treatment of CVT. **A.** Medial approach. **B.** Lateral approach with visible opening wedge osteotomy of the anterior part of calcaneus (bone graft from fibula). Anterior incision was done for extensors lengthening.

joint, proximal to the prominent navicular After exposing the head of the talus, all the tendinous and capsular components dorsal to the midtarsal joint should be divided completely. This is followed by lengthening of the tendon of the extensor digitorum longus and anterior tibial muscle, when these muscles are contracted. The last maneuver is best done from a separate incision above the ankle joint. In some incorrigible deformities, the capsule and ligaments between the talus and calcaneus must be cut thus the completing the subtalar release. This release makes possible a three-dimensional reduction of the subtalar complex in relation to the talus, and equalizes the medial and lateral columns of the foot. This occurs because during the talonavicular reduction the calcaneus moves a bit forward in relation to the talus.

Reduction

After such a release, the retrograde Kirschner wire is inserted into the true center of the talar head, and not into the center of its false articular surface, and exits at the posterior aspect of the talus. The drill is now attached to the posterior end of the wire which acts as a lever and the talus precisely onto the navicular (Figure 9-6). After the reduction, the wire exits on the dorsum of the foot. The reduction can be monitored radiologically, particularly when the surgeon is not experienced with the procedure. The appearance of the calcaneocuboid joint indirectly testifies to the correct talonavicular reduction, because of the plantar displacement of the cuboid, the anterior part of the calcaneus is entirely revealed. The displacement is so great that it seems incorrect. Particular attention should be paid to the talonavicular reduction in the horizontal plane. The difference in length between the medial and lateral columns of the foot is the reason why obtaining the correct shape of the foot in the horizontal plane (i.e., neutral position of the forefoot) is always connected with the medial displacement of the navicular bone in relation to the head of the talus (23). A correct reduction in this plane leaves the surgeon somewhat dissatisfied, because of some persistent abduction of the forefoot. It can be corrected by an opening wedge osteotomy of the anterior part of the calcaneus, but only when the talo-navicular joint has become stable, thus avoiding iatrogenic medial dislocation of the navicular. The calcaneocuboid joint may require stabilization with the Kirschner wire. Though the

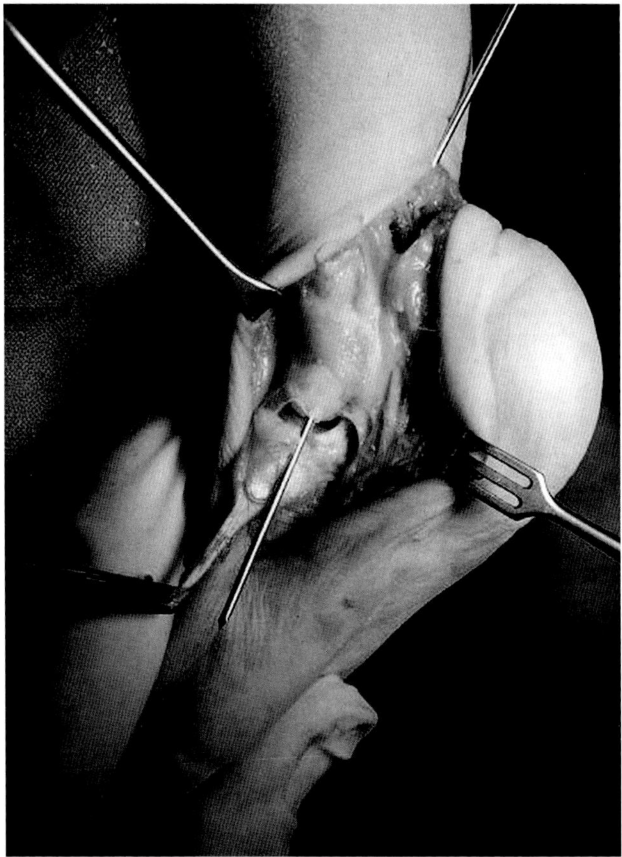

FIGURE 9-6 A way of proper reduction of the acquired/idiopathic CVT with one-stage surgical procedure from Cincinnati approach with K wire acting as a lever reducing the talus and navicular.

stabilization of the lateral column of the foot is occasional, the calcaneo-talar stabilization of the medial column is compulsory.

The procedure is completed with suturing of the tibialis posterior tendon and the lengthened tendons when they had been tense. An above-knee plaster cast is applied for six weeks. Then, after removing the K-wires (without anesthesia), a below-knee plaster cast is applied for another eight weeks (2 × 4 weeks). Normal shoes are worn immediately after removing the cast, with standard support of the longitudinal arch. In paralytic deformity, an ankle-foot-orthosis may be worn.

Techniques Complementary to Open Reduction

- Resection of the navicular bone (29) is especially useful in arthrogrypotic CVT in small children.
- Extra-articular talocalcaneal arthrodesis according to Grice (23), can be used from the age of 2.5 years on.
- Opening wedge of the anterior part of the calcaneus (25)
- Opening wedge with fibular graft inserted into the calcaneo-cuboid joint (22).
- Transposition of tendons, e.g.: the peroneus brevis onto the tibialis posterior tendon in paralytic deformity.

Salvage Procedures

- Resection of the talar head and cutting the tendons
- Dega's technique: resection of the talar head and closing-wedge osteotomy of the anterior part of the calcaneus (5)
- Triple arthrodesis

In some forms of CVT, such as Lichtblau's group 1 (teratologic) or Hamanishi's groups 2 (arthrogrypotic), 3 (malformation syndroms), and 4 (chromosomal aberrations), reconstruction of the normal anatomic relations is associated with tension of the soft tissues that can cause occlusion of the vessels on the dorsum of the foot. These may interfere with the blood supply and cause problems with the healing of the wound or with avascular necrosis, of the navicular and talar head. For that reason, in small children, it seems safer to consider naviculectomy which will relax the foot, equalize the rays, and enable an easy reduction. In older children, between four and six years of age, resection of the talar head with closing wedge osteotomy of the anterior part of the calcaneus coupled with tendo Achilles lengthening (5), will be a better solution. In rigid arthrogryposis or myelomeningocele, dividing the contracted tendons would not be a mistake.

COMPLICATIONS

Non-specific complications are associated with improper surgical technique and tight plaster cast application after the procedure. It may result in skin necrosis, avascular necrosis of the bones, or compartment syndrome. Specific complications are associated with the nature of the deformity. These include deficiency of the skin on the anterolateral aspect of the foot after the correction of the deformity: stretching and occlusion of the dorsalis pedis artery after the reduction of the stiff deformity causing skin necrosis and avascular necrosis of the talus and/or navicular. Avascular bone necrosis develops not only because of vascular compromise but may be due to the increased pressure in the talonavicular joint after its reduction. It is caused by elongation of the first ray of the foot. Weakening of push-off power can result of from overlegnthening of the tendo Achilles also from a calcaneal position of the hindfoot caused by lack of reduction and dorsal dislocation of the forefoot (in the sagittal plane the forefoot is shifted dorsally in relation to the hindfoot) (23). In some cases, Grice extra-articular arthrodesis can result in overcorrection, especially when there is primary supination of the forefoot (22).

LITERATURE REVIEW

Almost all authors report advantages of the one-stage procedure consisting of soft-tissue release, open reduction, tendon lengthening, and stabilization with the K-wires (4,6,10,12,23,26,30,32,36). Most of the authors emphasize good or satisfactory results associated with this method of treatment. Unfortunately, most studies include cerebral palsy and myelomeningocele patients. Additionally, only two of the mentioned papers contain radiographic criteria for evaluation of the talonavicular displacement. None present criteria for evaluation of the cuboid displacement at the calcaneo-cuboid joint. The criteria for clinical and radiographic evaluation are different in individual reports.

In this author's operative technique, restored normal appearanceto the foot and radiographic alignment, but a tendency for overcorrection has been observed. Pedobarographic analysis of operated feet differs from healthy feet with plantar pressure values higher on the lateral border of the foot and diminished on the heel (24).

Open reduction can be used in all types of deformities, irrespective of their etiologies. Varying the technique according to the etiology is possible in older children in whom the muscular imbalance may be estimated. It includes extending the release and as well as the transposition of the tendons. The last point concerns patients with paralytic deformity.

NO TREATMENT AS AN OPTION

Some authors state that different types of idiopathic form of CVT do not require surgical treatment because persistent talonavicular displacement seen on radiographs does not correlate with unacceptable foot shape, pain, or disability (1,22).

In the future, the natural history of untreated idiopathic CVT should be studied.

REFERENCES

1. Clark MW, D'Ambrosia RD, Ferguson AB. Congenital vertical talus. *J Bone Joint Surg [Am]* 59:816–824, 1977.
2. Coleman SS, Jarrett J. Congenital vertical talus: pathomechanics and treatment. *J Bone Joint Surg [Am]* 48:1026, 1966.
3. Crawford AH, Marxen JL, Osterfeld DL. The Cincinnati incision: a comprehensive approach for surgical procedures of the foot and ankle in childhood. *J Bone Joint Surg [Am]* 64:1355–1358, 1982.
4. Daumas L, Filipe G, Carlioz H. Le pied convexe congenital. Technique et resultats de la correction operatoire en un seul temps. *Rev Chir Orthop Appareil Moteur* 81:527–537, 1995.
5. Dega W. Pes planus taloflexus congenitus. Wrodzona płaskość stopy (Pes planus taloflexus congenitus. Congenital flattening of the foot). *Chir Narz Ruchu Ortop Pol* 20:281–283, 1955.
6. DeRosa P, Ahlfeld S. Congenital vertical talus: the Riley experience. *Foot & Ankle* 5:118–124, 1984.
7. Dobbs MB, Purcell DB, Nunley R, et al. Early results of a new method of treatment for idiopathic congenital vertical talus. *J Bone Joint Surg [Am]* 88:1192–2000, 2006.
8. Dobbs MB, Gurnett CA, Pierce B, et al. HOXD10 M319K mutation in a family with isolated congenital vertical talus. *J Orthop Res* 24(3):448–453, 2006.
9. Dobbs MB, Purcell DB, Nunley R, et al. Early results of a new method of treatment for idiopathic congenital vertical talus. Surgical technique. *J Bone Joint Surg [Am]* 89 Pt 1 Suppl 2:111–121, 2007.
10. Dodge LD, Ashley RK, Gilbert RJ. Treatment of the congenital vertical talus: a retrospective review of 36 feet with long-term follow-up. *Foot & Ankle* 7:326–332, 1987.
11. Drennan JC, Sharrard WJW. The pathological anatomy of convex pes valgus. *J Bone Joint Surg [Br]* 53:455–461, 1971.
12. Drennan JC. Congenital vertical talus. *Instruct Course Lect* 45:315–322, 1996.
13. Eyre-Brook AL. Congenital vertical talus. *J Bone Joint Surg [Br]* 49:618–627, 1967.
14. Hamanishi C. Congenital vertical talus: classification with 69 cases and new measurement system. *J Pediatr Orthop* 4:318–326, 1984.
15. Hamel J, Becker W. Sonographische Diagnostik bei Talus verticalis im Saugligs- und Kleinkindesalter. *Ultraschall Klin Prax* 9:185–189, 1995.
16. Henken R. *Contribution a l'etude des formes osseuses du piedplat valgus congenital.* Paris et Lyons. Lyons, 1914.
17. Jacobsen ST, Crawford AH. Congenital vertical talus. *J Pediatr Orthop* 3:306–310, 1983.
18. Król J, Marciniak W. Pes planus taloflexus congenitus - patologia i obraz kliniczny (Congenital flatfoot - its pathology and clinical picture). *Chir Narz Ruchu Ortop Pol* 31:587–592, 1966.
19. Lamy L, Weissman L. Congenital convex pes valgus. *J Bone Joint Surg* 21:79–91, 1931.
20. Levinsohn EM, Shrimpton AE, Cady RB, et al. Congenital vertical talus in four generations of the same family. *Skeletal Radiol* 33(11):649–654, 2004. Epub 2004 Sep 11.
21. Lichtblau S. Congenital vertical talus. *Bull Hosp Joint Diseases* 39:165–179, 1978.
22. Marciniak W. Die operative peritalare Reposition mit verlongerung des lateralen Fussstrahles bei angeborenen Plattfuss (Talus verticalis). *Beitr Orthop Traumatol* 34:426–432, 1987.
23. Napiontek M. Congenital vertical talus: a retrospective and critical review of 32 feet operated on by peritalar reduction. *J Pediatr Orthop Part B* 4:179–187, 1995.
24. Napiontek M., Walczak M. Idiopathic form of congenital vertical talus (CVT) treated by one stage open reduction. A clinical, radiographic and pedobarographic study. Abstract. 2nd Joint Meeting of International Federation of Foot and Ankle Societies, IFFAS. Naples, Italy September 15–18, 2005.
25. Napiontek M. Vertical talus. In: Fitzgerald, Kaufer, Malkani, eds. *Orthopaedics.* Philadelphia: W.B. Saunders Company, 1489–1495, 2002.
26. Oppenheim W, Smith C, Christie W. Congenital vertical talus. *Foot & Ankle* 5:198–204, 1985.
27. Osmond-Clarke H. Congenital vertical talus. *J Bone Joint Surg (Br)* 38:334–341, 1956.
28. Patterson WR, Fitz DA, Smith WS. The pathologic anatomy of congenital pes valgus. *J Bone Joint Surg (Am)* 50:458–466, 1968.
29. Pick CF, Chicote-Campos F. *Der angeborene Plattfuss mit Talus verticalis.* Ferdinand Enke Verlag, Stuttgart, 1979.
30. Raab P, Krauspe R. One-stage procedure for surgical correction of congenital vertical talus. In: Epeldegui T., ed. *Flatfoot and forefoot deformities.* A. Madrid Vicente, Ediciones, 253–258, 1995.
31. Schlesinger AE, Deeney VFX, Caskey PF. Sonography of the nonossified tarsal navicular cartilage in an infant with congenital vertical talus. *Pediatr Radiol* 20:134–135, 1989.
32. Seimon LP. Surgical correction of congenital vertical talus under the age of 2 years. *J Pediatr Orthop* 7:405–411, 1987.
33. Specht EE. Congenital paralytic vertical talus. An anatomical study. *J Bone Joint Surg [Am]* 57:842–847, 1975.
34. Stern HJ, Clark RD, Stroberg AJ, et al. Autosomal dominant transmission of isolated congenital vertical talus. *Clin Gen* 36:427–430, 1989.
35. Stone KH. Congenital vertical talus: a new operation. *Proc R Soc Med* 56:12–14, 1963.
36. Stricker S, Rosen E. Early one-stage reconstruction of congenital vertical talus. *Foot&Ankle International.* 18:535–543, 1997.
37. Tachdjian MO. *Pediatric orthopedics.* Philadelphia: WB Saunders, 1359–1372, 1972.
38. Zorer G, Bagatur AE, Dogan A. Single stage surgical correction of congenital vertical talus by complete subtalar release and peritalar reduction by using the Cincinnati incision. *J Pediatr Orthop B.* 11:60–67, 2002.

CHAPTER 10

Flexible Flatfoot and Skewfoot

Vincent S. Mosca

FLEXIBLE FLATFOOT

Flatfoot is the term used to describe a weight-bearing foot shape in which the hindfoot is in valgus alignment, the midfoot sags in a plantar direction with reversal of the longitudinal arch, and the forefoot is supinated in relation to the hindfoot. Flexibility refers to the mobility of the subtalar joint and the longitudinal arch, and the ability of both to reverse their alignments. The flexible, or hypermobile, flatfoot was determined to be the normal contour of a strong and stable foot by Harris and Beath (51) in their 1947 study of foot problems in 3,600 recruits in the Royal Canadian Army. No one before or since then has provided scientific evidence to refute their claim. Yet there are very few foot conditions that remain as controversial and poorly understood as the flexible flatfoot. This foot shape is common, often familial, rarely painful, and even more rarely disabling, yet the flexible flatfoot generates interest, investigation, and controversy.

Epidemiology

The true incidence of flatfoot is unknown, primarily because there is no agreement on strict clinical or radiographic criteria for defining a flatfoot. At the root of this dilemma is the lack of a universally accepted definition of a "normal," in contrast to an "average height," longitudinal arch. Traditionally, a flatfoot has been defined as a foot having an abnormally low or absent longitudinal arch in weight bearing. This description is based solely upon the static anatomic comparison of the height of the arch and is comparable to the description of stature, the height of an individual. Taking this analogy a step further, one would not automatically consider someone whose stature is below the fifth percentile as pathologic without more information. Yet the word flatfoot implies pathology to some health care providers and, in their clinical judgment, mandates the need for treatment. This anatomic definition fails to take into consideration the etiology of the flatfoot, the functional relationships between the bones, and the presence or evidence-based expectation of future pain or disability. It also ignores normal anatomic variations in arch height among adults (51), between children and adults (14,46,90,135,141,144), and between racial groups. It is well recognized that there is a higher incidence of flatfeet in blacks (15,77,131,139) than Caucasians and that these flatfeet, like those in Caucasians, rarely cause disability.

Despite the lack of a strict definition, it is believed that most children (14,46,90,135,141,144) and at least 20% of adults (51) have flatfeet, most of which are flexible. Harris and Beath (51) used their own definition when they identified flatfeet in approximately 23% of their adult study subjects. They subdivided flatfeet into three types: flexible flatfeet (FFF); flexible flatfeet with short tendo-Achilles (FFF-STA); and peroneal spastic or rigid flatfeet. They found that the flexible variety accounted for approximately two-thirds of all flatfeet and, in contrast to the latter two types, rarely caused disability. They emphasized that the flatness of the arch in weight bearing was of less importance than the mobility of the joints and tendons (51,52). They identified contracture of the Achilles tendon in association with flexible flatfeet in 25% of the total and noted that this type was often accompanied by pain and functional disability (51,52). The third and least common type, accounting for approximately 9% of all flatfeet, had restricted motion of the subtalar joint. These were most commonly caused by tarsal coalitions and were occasionally symptomatic.

Morley (90) evaluated the heel-to-arch width ratio on the footprints of children in the first decade of life and found that nearly 100% of 2 year olds were flatfooted while the same pattern was seen in only 4% of 10-year-old children. Though he and other authors (14,141) believed that many of these flatfeet actually had an arch that was obscured by a fat pad, Gould (46) and others (104,142) refuted the fat pad theory with radiographic evidence of actual flattening of the medial longitudinal arch. Staheli (135) used the footprint technique to evaluate the shape of the plantar surface in 882 asymptomatic feet in normal people aged 1 to 80 years. He

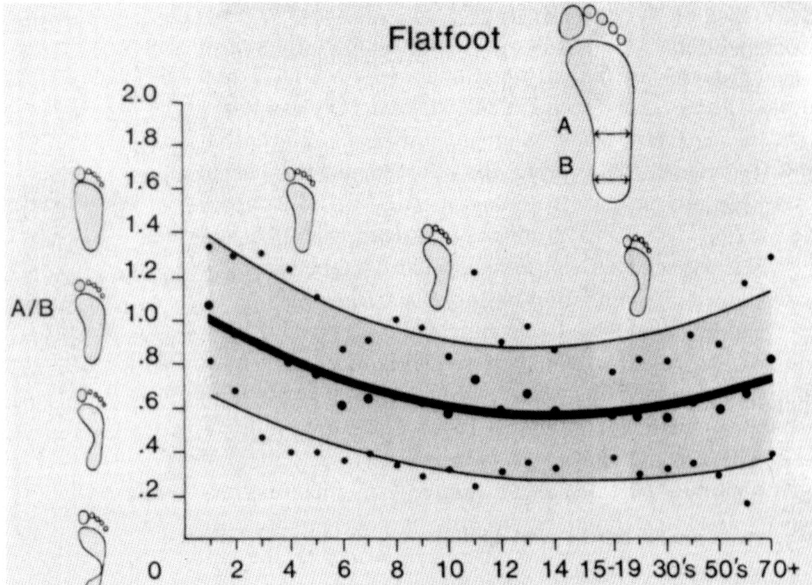

FIGURE 10-1 Normal development of the longitudinal arch. Average and two standard deviations for people of all ages determined by the ratio of arch-to-heel width on footprints. (From Staheli LT, Chew DE, Corbett M. The longitudinal arch. A survey of eight hundred and eighty-two feet in normal children and adults. *J Bone Joint Surg [Am]* 69:426–428, 1987, with permission.)

demonstrated that most infants are flatfooted, that the arch develops spontaneously during the first decade of life in most children, and that flatfeet are within the normal confidence limits for arch height in adults as well as children (Fig. 10.1). Vanderwilde, Staheli, and colleagues (144) confirmed these findings with the first comprehensive study on normative radiographic measurements of the foot in children. Average values and 2 standard deviation ranges for several AP and lateral measurements were determined from radiographs of normal feet in children aged 6 months to 10 years. It was found that there is a large spectrum of normal values for children of different ages, that these normal values are different from adult normal values, and that these normal values change spontaneously with age into the adult norms.

Comprehensive, normative radiographic values have recently become available for the adult foot (138). Wide variations were found in all measurements. Because all feet of these adult study subjects were painless and therefore "normal" despite their anatomic variations, the authors concluded that radiographs can quantify variations from average, but should not direct treatment even if the values are beyond the normal range. This opinion is shared by most authors of radiographic studies of the foot in children and adults. Radiographs can define the static relationships between bones, but they cannot provide clinical information on pain, flexibility, or function. Therefore, the information provided should not, in isolation, be used as the indication for treatment (138,144).

Pathogenesis

There are two main theories explaining the pathogenesis of FFF, that type of flatfoot that is present from birth and is accompanied by normal muscle function and good joint mobility. In 1959, Duchenne (31) utilized Faradic stimulation of the peroneus longus muscle to produce a longitudinal arch in a child's flatfoot. He felt that subclinical muscle weakness was responsible for the flexible flatfoot. Several authors since then have supported the theory that coordinated and normal function of the muscles of the foot and ankle is responsible for the maintenance of the longitudinal arch (50,58,62,63,101).

This theory, however, was refuted by Basmajian (6,47). His electromyographic assessment of the muscles of the foot and ankle showed little or no muscular activity when physiologic loads were applied to the static plantigrade foot. Muscular activity could be demonstrated only when very heavy loads were applied to the subjects. He concluded that the height of the longitudinal arch is determined by the bone-ligament complex, and that the muscles maintain balance, accommodate the foot to uneven terrain, protect the ligaments from unusual stresses, and propel the body forward. Proponents of this bone-ligament theory believe that the shape of the longitudinal arch under static loads is determined by the shapes and interrelationships of the bones, coupled with the strength and flexibility of the ligaments (6,17,51,52,56,57,61,78). Harris and Beath (52) strongly supported this position and presented anatomic specimens to substantiate their theory. They were unable to determine whether the abnormal shapes of individual bones and joints represented a primary or secondary reflection of a long-standing flatfoot.

Most current authors conclude that excessive ligamentous laxity is the primary abnormality in FFF and that bone deformities are secondary. Muscles are necessary for function and balance, but not for structural integrity. Mann and Inman (78) confirmed that muscle activity is not required to support the arch in static weight bearing. They also found that the intrinsic muscles are the principal stabilizers of the foot during propulsion, and that greater intrinsic muscle activity is required to stabilize the transverse tarsal and subtalar joints in a flatfooted individual than in one with an average height arch.

There are no long-term prospective studies on the natural history of untreated FFF regarding the development of pain, just the cross-sectional study of Harris and Beath (51,52). They found that, whereas FFF is rarely a cause for concern, FFF-STA often causes pain and disability. It is unknown whether the short tendo-Achilles in these feet is a primary pathologic feature or a secondary deformity. Harris and Beath (52) believed that FFF and FFF-STA are separate entities, although documentation of early clinical differentiation has not been reported.

While it is possible to document the number of individuals with painful FFF (with or without short tendo-Achilles) that seek medical attention, it is not possible to accurately document the much larger number of individuals with asymptomatic FFF who do not seek medical attention and, therefore, go uncounted. It is thus impossible to accurately estimate the risk of pain or disability from this very common foot shape. Nevertheless, the risk has been estimated to be small, even according to proponents of most surgical procedures for painful flatfeet. Therefore, treatment of people with asymptomatic FFF does not seem reasonable, though there are health care providers who ignore the evidence and treat these feet non-operatively and operatively. One must ask these providers what are the goals of their treatments. There are no controlled prospective studies documenting elevation of the longitudinal arch by non-operative methods or avoidance of long-term pain or disability by prophylactic non-operative or operative treatment of asymptomatic FFF.

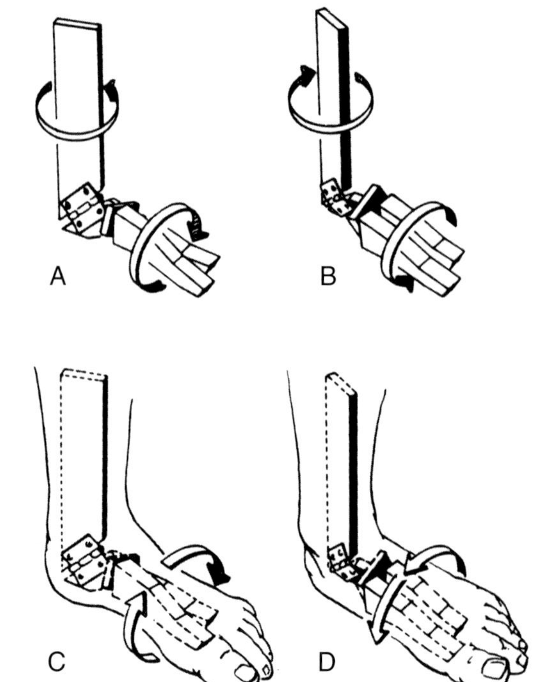

FIGURE 10-2 Mitered hinge representation of subtalar joint (with transtarsal joint added to model). The oblique axis of the subtalar joint couples rotation with angulation. **A, C.** "Locked" position as during late stance phase of gait. **B, D.** "Unlocked" position as during early stance phase. (From Close JR, Inman VT, Poor PM, et al. The function of the subtalar joint. *Clin Orthop* 50:159–179, 1967, with permission.)

Biomechanics/Pathomechanics

The functions of the foot include provision of a stable, but supple, platform that adapts to the ground during the early stance phase of gait, followed by conversion to a rigid lever during push-off (21,22,35,60,76). Several authors have represented the complex interrelationships between the bones of the mid- and hindfoot as a mitered hinge (21,22,60,76,79) (Figure 10-2), though that analogy is too simplistic. Using that as a first approximation or basic foundation, one must add a thorough understanding of the shape, structure, relationships, and motions of the subtalar joint complex to truly understand the biomechanics of the foot.

The subtalar joint complex is comprised of three bones (possibly four, if one includes the cuboid), several important ligaments, and multiple joint capsules that function together as a unit. Almost 200 years ago, Scarpa (126) saw similarities between the subtalar joint complex and the hip joint. He compared the femoral head to the talar head, and the pelvic acetabulum to his so-called acetabulum pedis. The latter is a cup-like structure made up of the navicular, the spring ligament, and the anterior end of the calcaneus and its facets. Although it is not a perfect comparison, I believe that the two anatomic areas share certain features that make the comparison both valid and worthwhile. The hip, a pure ball-and-socket joint with a central rotation point, is comprised of two bones, one intra-articular ligament, and a joint capsule. The subtalar joint is not an independent ball-and-socket joint, though the combined motions of the subtalar joint and the immediately adjacent ankle joint give the impression of a ball-and-socket. In fact, the subtalar joint has an axis of motion that is in an oblique plane that is neither frontal, sagittal, nor coronal, thus creating motions that are best described with the unique terms inversion and eversion. The stable structure in the hip joint is the acetabulum (the socket), while the stable structure in the subtalar joint complex is the talus (the ball). Inversion is comprised of plantar flexion, supination, and internal rotation of the acetabulum pedis around the head of the talus (32). Eversion is a combination of dorsiflexion, pronation, and external rotation of the acetabulum pedis around the talar head. The static position of inversion of the subtalar joint is called hindfoot varus and is found in cavovarus feet and clubfeet. Hindfoot valgus is the static position of the everted subtalar joint and is seen in flatfeet and skewfeet.

The tibia and talus internally rotate during the first half of the stance phase of the gait cycle while the subtalar joint complex everts. The talar head plantar flexes because of the lost support from the acetabulum pedis. The foot becomes quite supple, or unlocked, and flattens (see Figure 10-2B,D). During the latter part of the stance phase, the tibia and talus externally rotate while the subtalar joint complex inverts and the acetabulum pedis once again supports the head of the talus. The talus dorsiflexes and the entire foot becomes more rigid, or locked (see Figure 10-2A,C). This diminishes stress on the muscles and ligaments during push-off.

The flexible flatfoot begins stance in an unlocked, everted position, and does not completely invert to a rigid lever during the latter portion of stance. Theoretically, this should lead to muscle fatigue and pain, however, this seems to occur only in some flatfooted individuals (128).

Clinical Features

Flexible flatfeet rarely cause pain or disability in infancy and childhood. Children in this age group usually present for evaluation because of their parents' concern about the cosmetic appearance of the feet or because of a family history of special shoe wearing during childhood. The clinical assessment of an individual with a flatfoot should consist of a general examination of the musculoskeletal system, in addition to the specific foot and ankle examination. The general examination is aimed at assessing torsional and angular variations of the lower extremities and the walking pattern. The physician should examine the patient for evidence of generalized ligamentous laxity which can include touching the thumb to the volar forearm, hyperextension of the metacarpo-phalangeal joints of the fingers to 90 degrees, hyperextension of the elbows and/or knees into recurvatum, and touching the palms to the ground with knees extended. It is often rewarding to inquire about familial flatfeet and to examine the feet of other family members who have accompanied the child to the clinic visit. Flexible flatfeet may cause rapid and uneven shoe wear in older children and adolescents, so the child's shoes should be examined.

Assessment of the foot and ankle begins with the recognition, as first clearly stated by Mosca (96), that "*the foot is not a joint.*" Though simplistic and seemingly apparent, this fact does not appear to be universally recognized. Yet, it is the foundation for the understanding and appropriate management of foot deformities in children. There are at least two segmental deformities, often in opposite directions from each other, in all congenital and developmental deformities of the child's foot (96). For example, a flatfoot is not a single deformity. It is a combination of deformities that includes valgus deformity of the hindfoot and supination deformity of the forefoot. These are rotationally opposite direction deformities that, according to Mosca (96), give the impression that the foot has been "*wrung out like a towel.*" In a symptomatic flatfoot, there is also a contracture of the gastrocnemius or the Achilles tendon.

The clinical appearance of a flatfoot is more complicated than the simple depression or absence of a longitudinal arch. There is a straight or convex medial border of the foot. The midfoot sags and touches the ground in weight bearing (Figure 10-3A). The foot appears externally rotated in relation to the leg. The hindfoot is in valgus alignment (see Figure 10-3B) and the weight-bearing axis of the lower extremity is medial to the mid-axis of the foot. The patients or their parents are frequently most concerned about the hindfoot valgus, which they interpret as an apparent ankle deformity. These clinical features have been difficult to quantify and, therefore, a foot was deemed flat if it looked flattened. An attempt at a clinical classification of the longitudinal arch according to the footprint made in full weight bearing is shown in Figure 10-4, though it has not been universally acknowledged and utilized.

The flexibility of a flatfoot refers to the motion of the subtalar joint complex. It is a more important feature than the static shape of the foot and requires careful assessment. The subtalar joint will invert to neutral and a longitudinal arch can be observed in a flexible flatfoot that is dangling in the air while the individual is seated. A longitudinal arch can also be demonstrated by toe-standing (Figure 10-5) and by dorsiflexion of the great toe (Figure 10-6). This so-called toe-raising test, initially

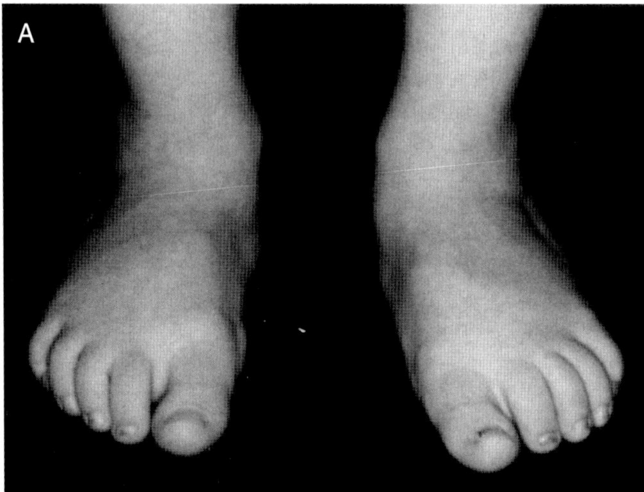

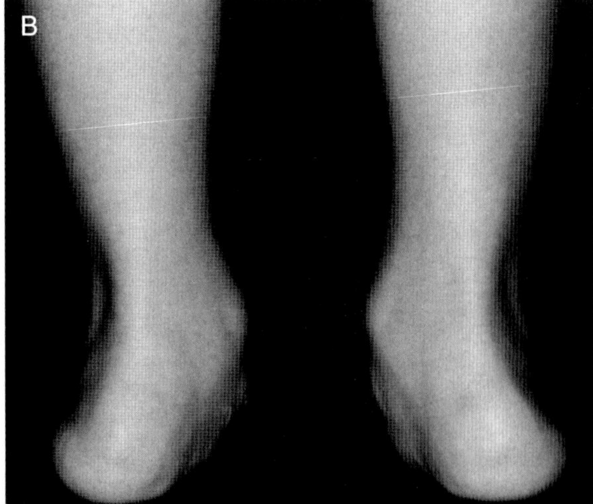

FIGURE 10-3 Flexible flatfeet. **A.** Convex medial border with midfoot sag. **B.** Valgus hindfoot. (From the private collection of Vincent Mosca, MD.)

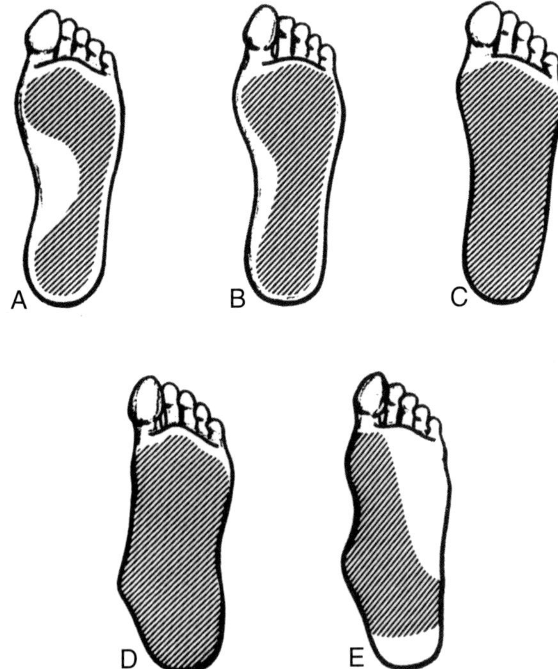

FIGURE 10-4 Classification of flatfeet based on increasing convexity of the medial border of the footprint. **A.** Normal arch with C-shaped footprint. **B.** Mild, or first degree, flatfoot. **C.** Moderate, or second degree, flatfoot. **D.** Severe, or third degree, flatfoot. **E.** Rocker-bottom deformity. (From Tachdjian MO. *The child's foot.* Philadelphia: WB Saunders, 556–597, 1985, with permission.)

described by Jack (61) and explained by Hicks (57), is due to the "windlass action" of the plantar fascia. The plantar fascia originates on the plantar aspect of the calcaneus and inserts into the plantar aspect of the toes through multiple interconnections. Great toe dorsiflexion pulls the plantar fascia distally under the pulley of the head of the first metatarsal. Because the plantar fascia is of fixed length, the great toe can only fully dorsiflex if the calcaneus is pulled distally toward the metatarsal heads, thereby shortening the foot, elevating the longitudinal arch, and inverting the subtalar joint. This windlass effect is also demonstrated during toe-standing by means of the same biomechanics.

Supination deformity of the forefoot on the hindfoot is revealed when the valgus hindfoot is passively inverted to neutral, though preoperative assessment does not directly correlate with the rigidity of the supination deformity or the need for operative reconstruction (Figure 10-7). It should be apparent that this separate, rotationally opposite, segmental deformity exists in a flatfoot. If not, a flatfooted individual would stand on the plantar-medial aspects of the hindfoot and forefoot with the lateral forefoot elevated off the ground. This does not happen. Instead, forefoot supination places all metatarsal heads on the ground for shared weight bearing when the hindfoot is in valgus alignment.

A flexible flatfoot with short tendo-Achilles (FFF-STA) has the same subtalar joint mobility as a FFF but is differentiated from that deformity by its limitation of ankle dorsiflexion. STA should be considered a proxy for

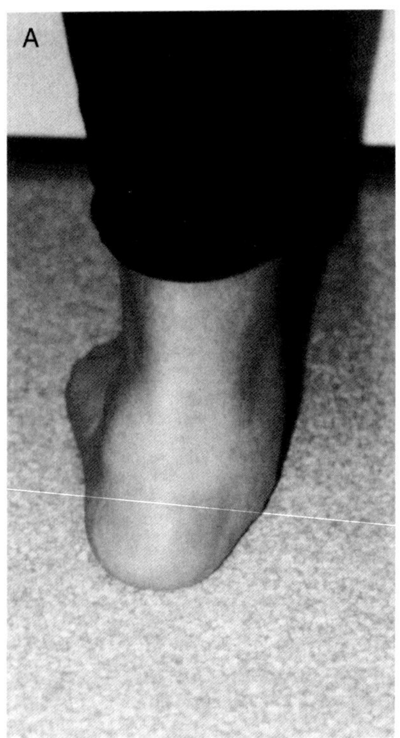

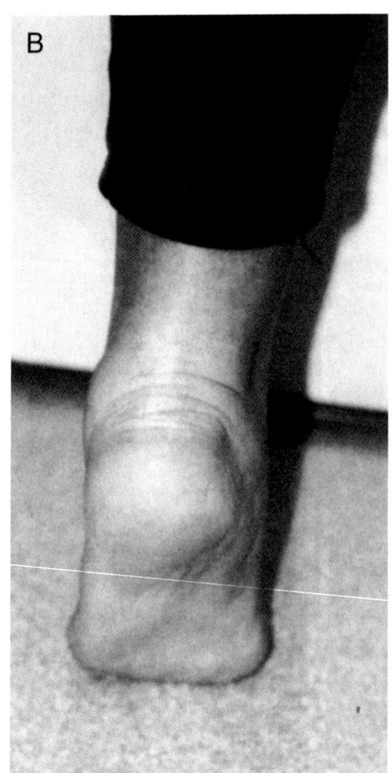

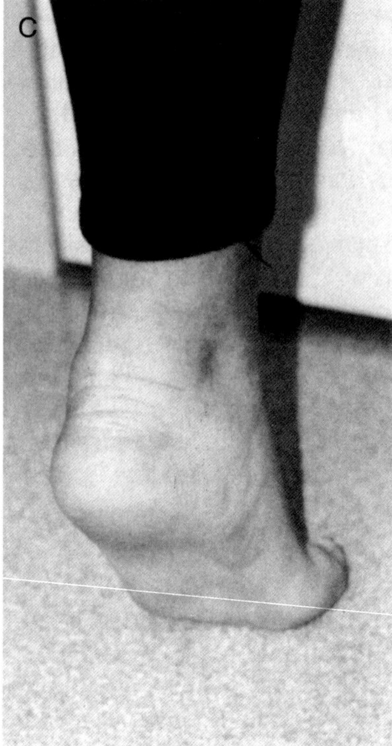

FIGURE 10-5 **A.** Weight-bearing left FFF. **B, C.** In toe-standing, heel valgus converts to varus and the longitudinal arch can be seen. (From the private collection of Vincent S. Mosca, MD.)

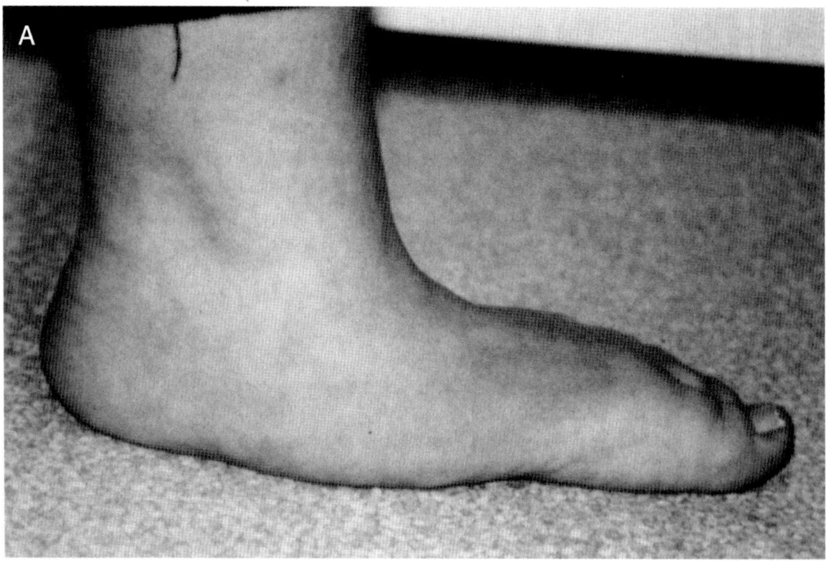

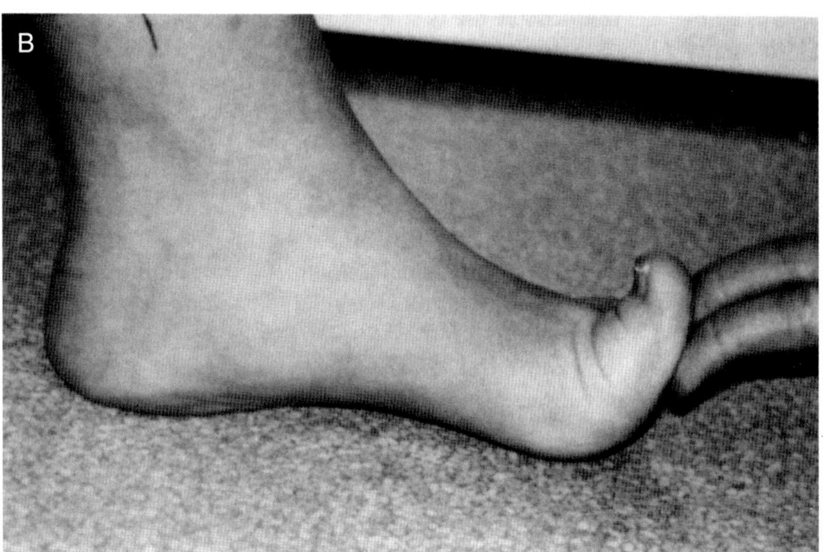

FIGURE 10-6 **A,B.** Jack's toe-raising test. An arch is created in a FFF by the windlass action of the great toe and plantar fascia. (From the private collection of Vincent S. Mosca, MD.)

contracture of either the gastrocnemius alone or the entire tendo-Achilles, as both prevent the talus from dorsiflexing in the ankle joint during the stance phase of gait. With a STA, the dorsiflexion force is shifted to the subtalar joint which, as a component of eversion, enables dorsiflexion of the calcaneus (acetabulum pedis) in relation to the talus. This *false* dorsiflexion often results in foot and ankle pain. Harris and Beath (51,52) observed that FFF-STA was much more likely to cause pain than the simple FFF. It is conceivable that the controversies regarding the understanding and management of the FFF are based on an historical failure to differentiate FFF from FFF-STA.

Assessment of true ankle dorsiflexion is important yet difficult to evaluate accurately. The subtalar joint complex must be locked in a neutral position by inversion, in order to isolate and assess the motion of the talus in the ankle joint. The knee is flexed and the ankle is dorsiflexed while maintaining neutral alignment (inverted from its valgus position) of the subtalar joint. Dorsiflexion is measured as the angle between the plantar-lateral border of the foot and the anterior tibial shaft. Less than 10 degrees of dorsiflexion indicates contracture of the soleus muscle, which equates to contracture of the entire tendo-Achilles. The knee is then extended while maintaining neutral alignment of the subtalar joint and trying to maintain dorsiflexion of the ankle joint. Dorsiflexion is remeasured. If more than 10 degrees of dorsiflexion was possible with the knee flexed, but less than 10 degrees of dorsiflexion is possible with the knee extended, the gastrocnemius alone is contracted (Figure 10-8). One should differentiate contracture of the gastrocnemius from contracture of the entire triceps surae (tendo-Achilles), because both can cause pain that justifies surgical management, but the surgical technique obviously varies between them.

A rigid flatfoot demonstrates restriction in subtalar motion. The arch remains flat when the foot is dangling in the air while the individual is seated as well as during toe-standing and the toe-raise test. This type of flatfoot

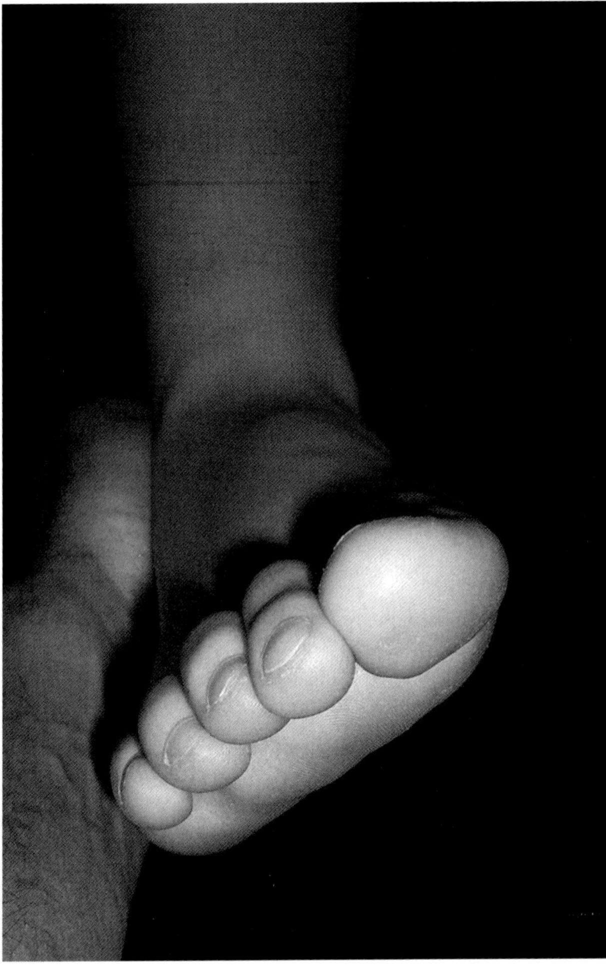

FIGURE 10-7 Forefoot supination can best be appreciated when the hindfoot is inverted to neutral, though preoperative assessment does not directly correlate with the rigidity of the deformity or the need for operative reconstruction. (From the private collection of Vincent S. Mosca, MD.)

can also cause pain and disability. The rigid flatfoot is discussed elsewhere in this text.

It is important to rule out other congenital and neuromuscular flatfoot etiologies when a patient with apparent FFF has pain as the presenting complaint. It is also imperative to exclude acquired and environmental causes of foot pain which may occur with any underlying foot shape, including FFF. Pain from FFF-STA is usually located on the plantar-medial aspect of the midfoot and occasionally in the sinus tarsi area. Pain from rigid flatfoot may be experienced at several sites, including the medial hindfoot, the sinus tarsi area, and occasionally the plantar-medial midfoot.

The orthopedist is urged to avoid the use of the term pronated as a substitute for the term flatfoot. While it is true that pronation is a component of the hindfoot deformity in this condition, the subtalar joint is dorsiflexed and externally rotated, the midfoot is abducted, and the forefoot is supinated in relation to the hindfoot. The term flatfoot encompasses all of these multi-site three-dimensional deformities and is, therefore, a better choice of terms.

Radiographic Evaluation

Radiographs of the flatfoot are not necessary for diagnosis, but they may be indicated to help with the assessment of pain or decreased flexibility, and for surgical planning. Weight-bearing anteroposterior (AP) and lateral views of the foot are generally sufficient to evaluate the flexible flatfoot, whereas the addition of the oblique and axial, or Harris, views is necessary to evaluate the rigid flatfoot. Without weight bearing, or at least simulated weight bearing, the radiographic relationships between the bones will not represent the true clinical deformities. An AP view of the ankle is also necessary, in most cases, to assess varus or valgus deformity at that adjacent joint. The lateral

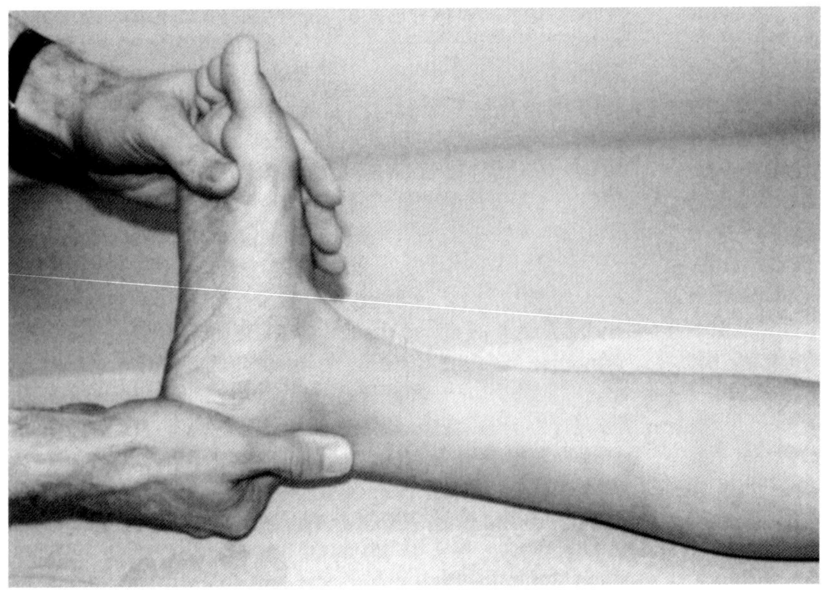

FIGURE 10-8 The subtalar joint must be held in neutral position and the knee extended in order to accurately assess ankle dorsiflexion. (From the private collection of Vincent S. Mosca, MD.)

appearance of the ankle can be appreciated on the lateral image of the foot.

The lateral radiograph of a flatfoot reveals plantar flexion of the calcaneus, measured by the calcaneal pitch (38), and an even greater degree of plantar flexion of the talus, measured by the talo-horizontal angle (13) (Figure 10-9). Meary (86) defined a normal longitudinal arch as having a continuous straight line formed by the lines drawn through the mid-axis of the talus and the mid-axis of the first metatarsal on a standing lateral radiograph. He defined a flatfoot as one with a plantar sag where those two lines intersect, but there is in fact a range of normal values that includes a few degrees of plantar sag.

The lateral view can also be used to identify the site of the midfoot sag, i.e., the site of the angular deformity. Although the foot is not a single bone, Paley's (105) concept of the center of rotation of angulation (CORA) can be applied to the foot in a modified version. The site of intersection of the axis of the talus and that of the first metatarsal in a flatfoot is most often located in the head of the talus or at the talo-navicular joint, which indicates the mid-foot sag is at the talo-navicular joint (Figure 10-10B). But the CORA can alternatively be located at the naviculo-cuneiform joint, or within the body of one of the mid-tarsal bones.

Interpretation of the AP radiograph is more challenging than the lateral. The navicular is laterally positioned on the head of the talus in a flatfoot. Because the navicular does not normally ossify until age three to four years and because its early ossification is asymmetric toward the lateral aspect of the cartilaginous anlage, assessment of talo-navicular joint alignment must be made indirectly. The AP talus-first metatarsal angle has been used as an alternative means of evaluating that relationship, but it may be unreliable as well. As discussed in the skewfoot section of this chapter, abduction or adduction at the tarso-metatarsal joints will falsely exaggerate or minimize the apparent deformity at the talo-navicular joint if assessed using the talus-first metatarsal angle (92,94). Using the CORA method, the true site or sites of deformity can be determined. In a simple flatfoot, the CORA should be in the head of the talus or at the talo-navicular joint, which indicates eversion of the subtalar joint that is manifest as abduction at the talo-navicular joint (see Figure 10-10 A). Knowledge of the CORA on the AP and lateral radiographs has implications for surgical treatment.

Treatment

One can currently conclude from published data that the typical FFF has a normal, but not average, longitudinal arch height. There is no reason to treat that which is normal. Some FFF have arches that are clinically and radiographically beyond two standard deviations from average. These are technically abnormal, in the same way that stature below the fifth percentile is abnormal, but there is no evidence that they will necessarily cause disability, so there is no absolute indication for treatment. There may, in fact, be some specific advantages to having flatfeet. Giladi et al. (42) found that military recruits with flatfeet had significantly less risk of stress fractures than those with average or high arches.

Yet despite the absence of scientific evidence for any derived benefit, treatment of asymptomatic FFF has been advocated for years. Several authors believed that muscle weakness was responsible for flatfootedness and recommended muscle strengthening exercises with the goal of developing an arch in a child's foot (11,58,74,150). Basmajian (6) showed that muscles are not responsible for the height of the arch and, therefore, these exercises are of no physiologic benefit.

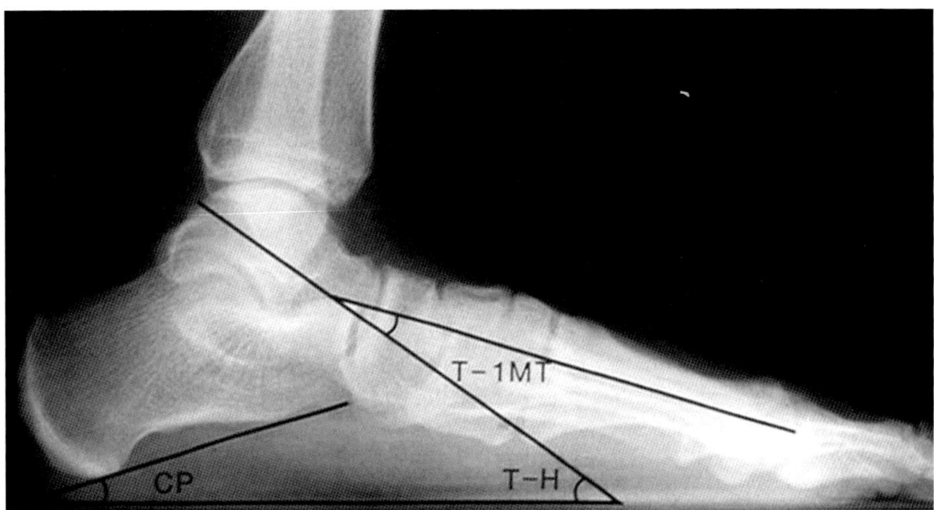

FIGURE 10-9 Standing lateral radiograph showing 3 fairly reliable angular measurements: the calcaneal pitch (*CP*), talo-horizontal angle (*T-H*), and Meary's talus-first metatarsal angle (*T-1MT*). (From Mosca VS. Calcaneal lengthening for valgus deformity of the hindfoot: Results in children who had severe, symptomatic flatfoot and skewfoot. *J Bone Joint Surg* [*Am*] 77: 500–512, 1995, with permission.)

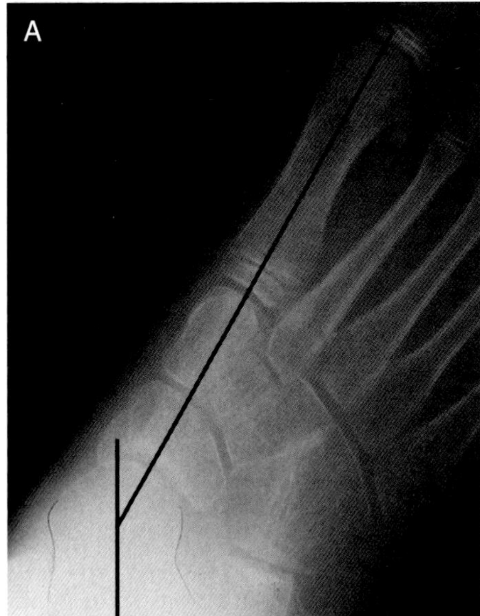

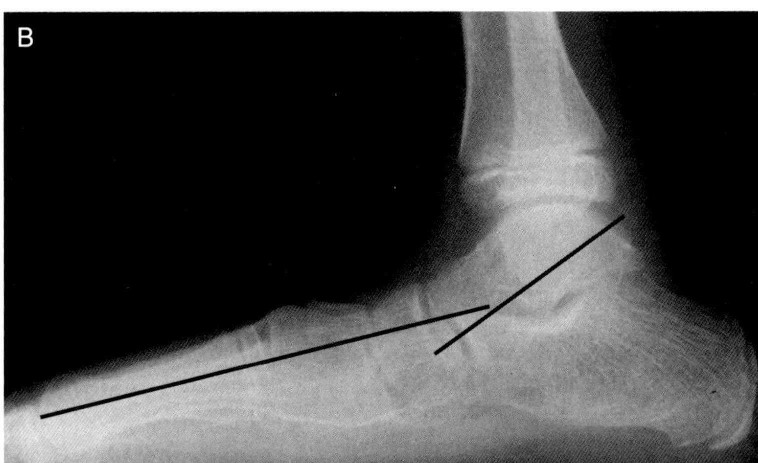

FIGURE 10-10 Standing radiographs of a flatfoot showing talus and first metatarsal axis lines crossing at the CORA in the center of the head of the talus, indicating a single deformity at the talo-navicular joint. **A.** Anteroposterior view. **B.** Lateral view. (From the private collection of Vincent S. Mosca, MD)

Controversy surrounds the management of asymptomatic FFF with "corrective shoes," over-the-counter and custom-molded arch supports, custom orthoses and heel wedges. The often reported goal of these interventions is to increase the height of the arch. Several uncontrolled studies in the United States have reported that definite permanent increases in arch height can be achieved both clinically and radiographically by the use of shoe modifications and inserts (13,16). However, the effect of any intervention cannot be determined without appropriate untreated matched controls. And several scientific clinical and radiographic studies (14,46,90,104,135,144) have shown that the height of the longitudinal arch increases spontaneously during the first decade of life.

A number of critical investigations of these treatment modalities have shown no positive treatment effect (7,12,46,53,87,108,118,119,131,136,147). Penneau et al. (108) found no significant radiographic differences between barefeet and those same feet when four types of special shoe modifications and inserts were donned. Rose (118,119) showed that shoe heel wedges did not change the shape of the foot. The foot maintained its original shape by shifting through the heel pad fat unless the forefoot was also supinated. He further noted that the foot remained flat despite years of using the devices. Helfet (53) stated that arch supports are actually dangerous since they lead to dependency, or what he called a life sentence. The foot remains flat and discontinuation of the device later in life increases the likelihood of symptoms. In the best prospective, randomized study on this topic ever reported, Wenger et al. (147) was unable to show a treatment effect for shoe modifications and inserts on the development of the longitudinal arch in normal children followed for three to five years when compared with untreated matched controls.

A potentially negative effect of extrinsic factors on the shape and development of the longitudinal arch is suggested, but not proven, by studies from developing countries. In 1958, Sim-Fook and Hodgson (131) reported that the flatfeet in their non–shoe-wearing Chinese study subjects were asymptomatic, mobile, and flexible. Somewhat surprisingly, they found a slightly higher incidence of flatfeet among the shoe-wearing population, some of which were painful and exhibited restricted mobility. Rao and Joseph (114), in 1992, similarly reported that flatfoot was more common in children in India who wore close-toed shoes than in those who did not wear shoes or who wore slippers or sandals.

Refuting the often heard comment that at least these devices do no harm is the study by Driano et al. (30) who reported long-term negative psychologic effects on adults who had worn shoe modifications as children compared with controls who did not. Nevertheless, the practice remains commonplace among some health care providers. Most pediatric orthopedic surgeons recommend soft, comfortable sneakers as standard shoe wear for children. This is based on the lack of evidence that one can create an arch using special shoes and orthotics, and the reported evidence that FFF is a normal variation of shape.

Occasionally, flexible flatfeet in a young child are associated with diffuse activity-related pain, cause early fatigue, create medial foot calluses, and lead to rapid shoe breakdown. Diffuse, non-localized, and nocturnal pain is also occasionally associated with FFF in these young children. These leg aches, or growing pains, are believed to represent an overuse, or fatigue, syndrome (110). This is consistent with the findings of Mann and Inman (78) that flatfooted individuals demonstrate greater intrinsic muscle activity than normal. Both soft over-the-counter and firm custom-molded shoe inserts have been shown to relieve or diminish symptoms, and to increase the useful life of shoes without a simultaneous permanent increase on the height of the arch (7,13,16,87,143). There is little information available to recommend one device over another, but there is probably little justification for the more expensive custom-molded orthotics except in more severe and symptomatic deformities.

The exact diagnosis must be established before prescribing orthotic devices. Their use with FFF-STA and rigid flatfeet could actually worsen the symptoms. The talus in an FFF-STA cannot dorsiflex normally because of the tendo-Achilles contracture. Therefore, an orthotic device that is designed to invert the subtalar joint by elevating the anterior end of the talus will meet resistance and increase pressure under the head of the talus, thereby creating more pressure and pain than originally existed. By definition, the shape of a rigid flatfoot will not change with an orthotic device or any other non-surgical intervention. As with the FFF-STA, an orthotic will merely increase pressure and pain under the head of the talus.

It seems reasonable to try to convert a symptomatic FFF-STA to an asymptomatic FFF by heelcord stretching exercises, which can be performed by parents when children are very young and can be easily monitored by parents when children are older. There have been no long-term studies on the effectiveness of this program, but it conforms with present knowledge, does no harm, and costs nothing. Therapists are not required. Heelcord stretching is accomplished with the knee in extension and the subtalar joint in neutral alignment to slight inversion. It is important, though difficult, to achieve this position of the subtalar joint during stretching. Doing so avoids *false* dorsiflexion through the everted subtalar joint and concentrates the stretch at the ankle joint.

Surgery is rarely, if ever, indicated for flexible flatfoot. If the goal of surgery is to change the shape of the foot, a shape that does not necessarily create problems, the documented risks and complications related to surgery must be weighed against the generally benign natural history of the foot shape itself. Nevertheless, numerous surgical procedures to correct flatfoot have been proposed during the last century. The indications for these procedures, whether for correction of deformity, relief of symptoms, or prophylaxis against anticipated pain and disability, are often difficult to ascertain from review of the literature. Therefore, the absolute and comparative success of these procedures is unclear because the reported series: used inconsistent surgical indications; likely included at least some patients with diagnoses other than idiopathic FFF; had patients of significantly different ages; lacked standardized evaluation criteria; and frequently had short follow up. The procedures can be categorized as soft tissue plications, tendon lengthenings and transfers, osseous excisions, osteotomies, arthrodesis of one or more joints, and interposition of bone or synthetic implants into the sinus tarsi. Combinations of these procedures have been reported.

Isolated soft-tissue procedures (44,62,70,111,117,122, 149) have had routinely unreliable results leading to their virtual abandonment. The failure of tendon transfer procedures underscores our understanding of the insignificant role of muscles in the maintenance of the arch. The lack of success with soft-tissue plications should be expected since the surgical scar tissue cannot be expected to develop the same strength as the original ligaments which themselves were not able to support the arch.

Isolated tendo-Achilles lengthening has been suggested to convert a painful FFF-STA to a painless FFF when performed before secondary adaptive or degenerative joint changes (potential sequelae of FFF-STA) have occurred (52). However, unsatisfactory results have led most surgeons to combine heelcord lengthening with a concurrent procedure that changes the shape of the foot.

Bone excision operations (26,45,140) have been abandoned because of their obvious destructive nature.

Arthrodesis of one or more of the joints in the subtalar complex has been abandoned as treatment for FFF, because of the detrimental effect of eliminating the shock-absorbing function of that important joint complex. Talonavicular (75), subtalar (48), and triple (1,3,123) arthrodeses shift stress to the ankle and mid-tarsal joints, leading to premature degenerative arthrosis at those sites (1,3,29,82,120,123,127,129,132,134).

Pseudoarthrodesis, or so-called arthroereisis, procedures were introduced by Chambers (20), Haraldsson (50), LeLievre (71), and Miller (88) between 1946 and 1977 as variations on a method to restrict excessive subtalar joint eversion by placing a bone block in the sinus tarsi. The bone grafts occasionally underwent resorption with recurrence of the deformity, or remained and resulted in restriction of subtalar motion (essentially a pseudoarthrodesis) with its associated problems. Arthroereisis by means of synthetic implants was started in the late 1970s because of the reported problems and complications associated with the bony arthroereisis procedures. No less than 10 types of synthetic implants and methods for insertion have been reported, most with follow-up of less than two years (40,41,49,59,80,81,99,100,103,125,151). Reported problems and complications have led to an ongoing search for a better implant and a better method for implanting it. The variety and succession of past implant materials and designs have prevented a validation study from being performed to determine the overall effectiveness of the procedure or even to validate the concept of the procedure (100). It should be clearly noted that the concept of arthroereisis has not been expanded to any other joint in the body.

There is no clear consensus among proponents on the indications for arthroereisis. Nevertheless, many are performed and the reported complication rate with the use of synthetic implants is 3.5% to 30%, with the most recent studies reporting rates of 3.5% to 11% (40,41,49,80,81,99,100,103,125,151). The complications include those associated with inappropriate implantation (obviously not counted, but certainly a major issue, especially if one considers the often-reported indication of performing the operation in an asymptomatic physiologic FFF in a young child); surgeon error (malpositioning, overcorrection, undercorrection, extrusion of implant, wrong size of implant); biomaterials problems (breakage, degradation); and biologic problems (foreign body reaction, synovitis, infection, persistent and recurrent pain, implant-induced sinus tarsi impingement pain, intraosseous ganglion cyst within the talus, osteonecrosis of the talus, peroneal spasm, calcaneus fracture) (40,41,49,80,81, 99,100,103,125,151).

The Maxwell Brancheau Arthroereisis (MBA) implant, a large cylinder-shaped titanium screw (80,81), and the Giannini Flatfoot Expanding Implant, a Teflon/stainless steel expansion drywall anchor design (40,41), are perhaps the most commonly used implants at the present time, based on the number of articles in the literature. According to published descriptions, both are inserted into the sinus tarsi anterior to the posterior facet along the trajectory of the tarsal canal (also known as the calcaneal sulcus and the sinus canalis) between the posterior and middle facets. The originators of these implants (40,41,80,81), as well as other authors (49,99,100,103,125,151) and even the product technique manuals, are evasive regarding the depth to which the implants enter the tarsal canal, though they certainly appear to enter it. Nevertheless, proponents consider them to be extraarticular, if inserted properly, because they do not technically touch articular cartilage, though they clearly encroach on it. The term extraarticular, when applied to other joints, means outside or adjacent to a joint. An example is a metaphyseal osteotomy that corrects angular deformity of a bone to correct malorientation of the adjacent joint. Another use of the term extraarticular is in lateral collateral ankle ligament reconstruction in which the procedures attempt to return normal stability and motion to a joint that has excessive motion and instability secondary to injury. The implication of these extraarticular procedures is that they do not restrict normal motion within the joint. They either re-orient the joint in space or return joint motion to normal. The arthroereisis implants mechanically block eversion but also decrease total subtalar joint motion (59,151), indicating that their effect is in fact intraarticular. Furthermore, an MRI study of the subtalar joint in adults with these implants found that the tarsal canal is smaller in height and length than the sizes of implants generally used (125), again suggesting encroachment.

In published studies on subtalar and triple arthrodeses, stress transfer to adjacent joints with the development of degenerative arthrosis was not seen for at least 10 years, which is longer than the follow-up in any of the reports on arthroereisis. Additionally, these implants, not surprisingly, lead to resorption of the adjacent cortical surfaces of the talus and calcaneus (Figure 10-11), the long-term effects of which are unknown. And no one has demonstrated or reported what happens to the implant during inversion and eversion of the subtalar joint. Does the implant stay with the calcaneus or with the talus as the beak of the calcaneus moves away from and then back towards the lateral process of the talus? Does it matter? Does it relate to long term success?

Both the MBA and Giannini arthroereisis implants are now offered as bioabsorbable implants made of poly-L lactic acid (PLLA), but the original metal designs seem to be used most often and the bioabsorbable implants have even shorter follow-up than the original designs. Based on MRI findings, Giannini (40) reported complete resorption of the implant by four years after implantation in 21 adolescents. Saxena et al. (125) found MRI evidence of residual bioabsorbable implant at greater than 4 years after implantation. These authors stated that there were no cystic changes noted in the bones, but acknowledged that granuloma formation from PLLA can appear in a delayed fashion. Additionally, their MRI study of the subtalar joint in adults with these implants found that the tarsal canal is smaller in height and length than the implant sizes generally used. They felt that this was a particular problem for the metal implants, and less so for the bioabsorbable ones, unless one considers that children and adolescents have an even smaller canal than the ones they studied. Finally, they questioned the benefit of the bioabsorbable implants because half of their patients required or were recommended to have explantation.

The bottom line seems to be that more information and, in particular, long-term studies are needed before arthroereisis can be recommended for children with painful flatfeet. And even more important is the need for the proponents of arthroereisis to clarify surgical indications based on the best scientific evidence available.

The most popular procedures used to correct FFF during the last century were the many modifications of Hoke's limited mid-tarsal arthrodeses (17,18,23,25,33,39, 58,61,89,129). Hoke (58) felt that the greatest abnormality in painful FFF was localized to the navicular and the two medial cuneiform bones. He reported favorable short-term results with the fusion of these three bones combined with tendo-Achilles lengthening. The Hoke procedure modifications combine arthrodesis of one or more mid-tarsal joints with soft tissue plication across the talonavicular joint. Tendo-Achilles lengthening was performed with all of the Hoke procedure modifications when 10–15 degrees of dorsiflexion could not be demonstrated after correction of the deformity. Favorable short-term results were consistently reported with these procedures, but unsatisfactory long-term results were reported in 49% of cases by Butte (17), 50% by Seymour (129), and 7 of 9 cases by Crego and Ford (25). The unsatisfactory feet in these series frequently showed persistence or recurrence of pain and deformity, and degenerative changes at the talonavicular and subtalar joints. The originators of these

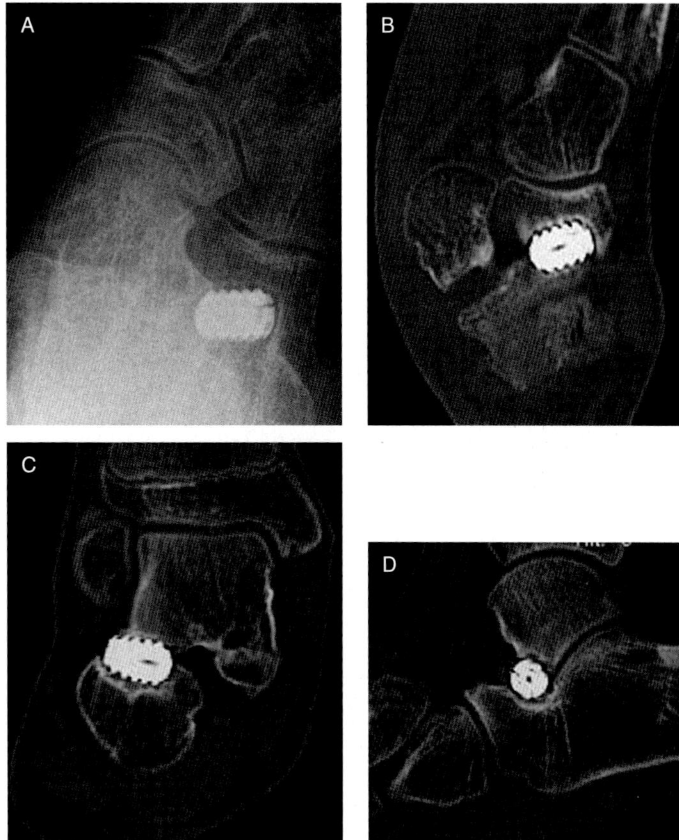

FIGURE 10-11 Radiographic and CT Scan images showing resorption of adjacent cortical surfaces of talus and calcaneus due to the presence of an MBA implant. (From the private collection of Vincent S. Mosca, MD.)

techniques acknowledged that the procedures were not capable of correcting severe hindfoot valgus deformity. This should not have been too surprising because these procedures do not directly correct the pathologically malaligned subtalar joint, but instead address the secondary forefoot supination deformity. The authors recommended triple arthrodesis for severe deformities and for persistent or recurrent postsurgical pain.

Osteotomy is the last category of procedures that has been used to treat flatfeet. This is a biologic approach that does not depend on soft tissues, that are known to stretch out, and it avoids arthrodeses/arthroereisis and the known complications of those procedures. There are two types of osteotomies of the calcaneus that address valgus deformity of the hindfoot. Gleich (43) and, later, Koutsogiannis (67) described an oblique osteotomy of the posterior calcaneus in which the posterior fragment is displaced medially to correct the apparent heel valgus. It does not actually correct the malalignment of the subtalar joint, but merely creates a compensating deformity to improve the valgus angulation of the heel. Recalling Scarpa's analogy to the hip (126), I believe the posterior calcaneal displacement osteotomy is the Chiari osteotomy of the acetabulum pedis. Koutsogiannis reported successful "correction" of valgus deformity in 30 of 34 feet, but arch restoration rarely occurred. Other authors confirmed these same results in FFF (74) as well as in paralytic flat feet (130). The posterior calcaneus osteotomy does not correct the multiple components of subtalar joint eversion, such as external rotation and dorsiflexion of the acetabulum pedis. Rathjen and Mubarak (115) reported good correction of flatfoot deformities by combining a modification of this osteotomy (medially based closing wedge with medial displacement) with a closing wedge osteotomy of the medial cuneiform, an opening wedge osteotomy of the cuboid, and medial reefing of the talonavicular joint (Figure 10-12).

The Dwyer (34) lateral opening wedge osteotomy of the posterior calcaneus represents another attempt to correct severe heel valgus. The Dwyer procedure is performed less frequently than the medial displacement osteotomy because it does not correct the deformity as completely. The reason is that the location of the osteotomy is not at the CORA (105). The CORA is located at the subtalar joint, so an adjacent angular osteotomy must be combined with translation of the posterior fragment. Alternatively, one can use translational displacement alone, as with the Koutsogiannis procedure, to center the plantar aspect of the posterior calcaneus under the mid-axis of the tibia.

The other osteotomy for correction of valgus deformity of the hindfoot is the calcaneal lengthening osteotomy, conceptualized by Evans (36) and elaborated by Mosca (94,98). Evans believed that the lateral column of the flatfoot was shorter than the medial column, a situation exactly opposite to that found in a cavo-varus foot.

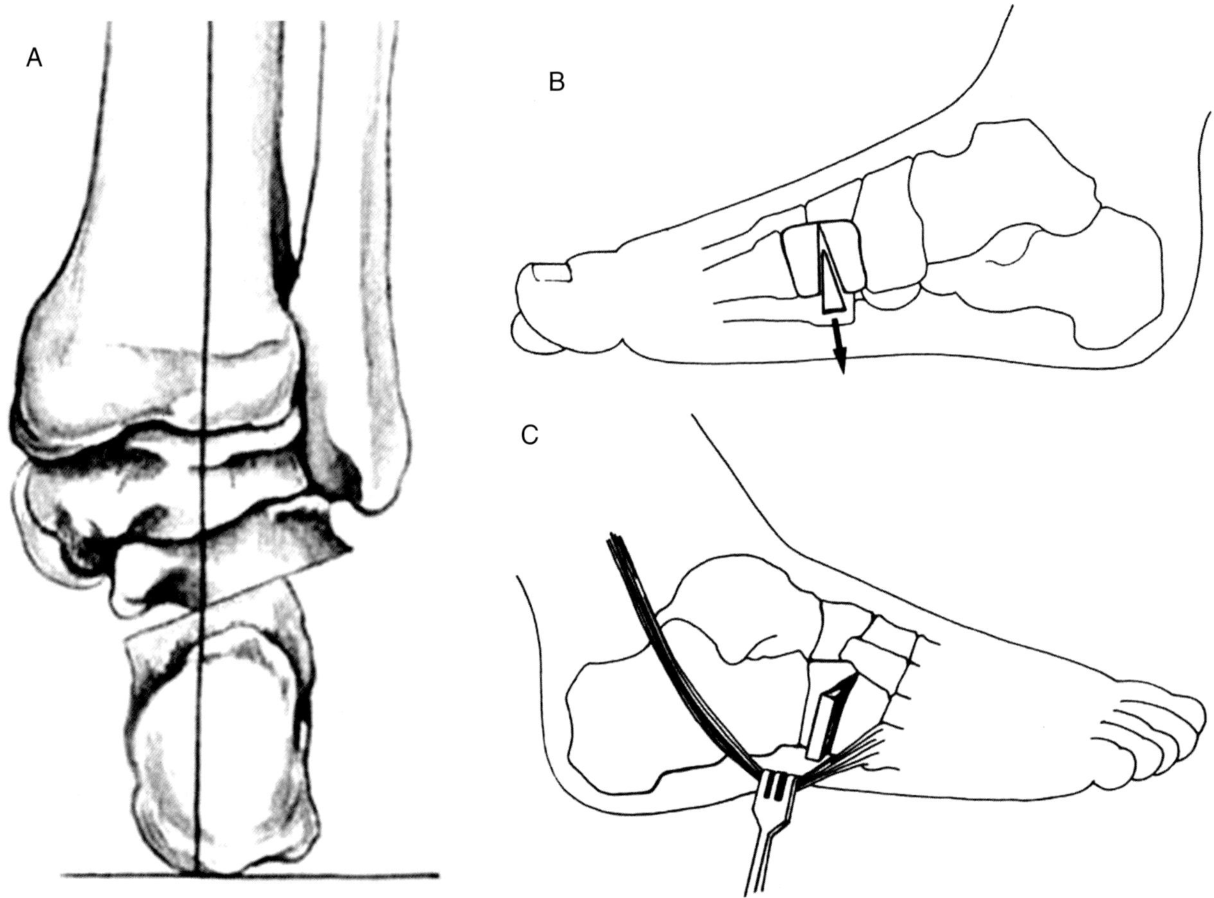

FIGURE 10-12 Calcaneo-cuboid-cuneiform osteotomies for correction of flatfoot. **A.** Medially-based closing wedge and medial displacement posterior calcaneus osteotomy (With permission from the private collection of Scott J. Mubarak, MD). **B.** Closing wedge osteotomy of the medial cuneiform. **C.** Opening wedge osteotomy of the cuboid. (B and C from Rathjen K, Mubarak S. Calcaneo-cuboid-cuneiform osteotomy for the correction of valgus foot deformities in children. *J Pediatr Orthop* 18:775–782, 1998, with permission.)

For painful flatfeet, he equalized the length of the columns by inserting a corticocancellous graft into an osteotomy of the anterior calcaneus that was made 1.5 cm proximal to, and parallel with, the calcaneocuboid joint. That was the entire extent of his description. By lengthening the calcaneus in this way, he showed that the heel valgus, talonavicular sag, and lateral subluxation of the navicular on the head of the talus could all be simultaneously corrected. Armstrong (5) recommended the technique and highlighted its advantages to be: correction of hindfoot valgus without need for arthrodesis, preservation of some subtalar motion, versatility for pronated and abducted feet of different etiologies, and simplicity of execution. Phillips (112) reported a 7- to 20-year (average 13 years) follow up of Evans' patients. Seventeen of the 23 feet had good to very good results when assessed by strict criteria. Anderson and Fowler (2) also reported very good results with this procedure in nine feet followed for an average of six and a half years. They reaffirmed the correction of all components of the hindfoot deformity by this simple technique and advised performing the procedure between ages six and ten years in appropriate individuals to allow remodeling of the tarsal joints, a consideration not mentioned by Evans.

In 1995, Mosca (94) reported the short-term results of calcaneal lengthening for valgus deformity of the hindfoot from various underlying etiologies in 31 feet in 20 children. He reported correction, at the site of deformity, of all components of even severe eversion of the subtalar joint complex, including dorsiflexion, pronation, and external rotation of the acetabulum pedis around the talar head. Function of the subtalar joint was restored, symptoms were relieved, and, at least theoretically, the ankle and mid-tarsal joints were protected from early degenerative arthrosis by avoiding arthrodesis. He stressed the need for strict indications for surgery, specifically a flexible or rigid flatfoot with Achilles or gastrocnemius contracture and intractable pain in the medial midfoot and/or sinus tarsi despite prolonged attempts at conservative management.

As noted above, Evans provided very little information on the technique, which made interpretation difficult and surgical success inconsistent by those who read his article. Mosca thoughtfully considered Evans' concept and applied an understanding of foot biomechanics and the principles of foot deformity-correction surgery to develop a reliable method for achieving consistently good surgical outcomes. His published contributions (32,94,97,98,124) include: the location of the skin incision (modified Ollier), the specific location and direction of the osteotomy (exiting medially between the anterior and middle facets), the shape of the bone graft (trapezoidal), management of the soft tissue constraints along the plantar-lateral border of the foot (lengthened) and the soft tissue redundancy along the plantar-medial border (plicated), stabilization of the calcaneo-cuboid joint to prevent subluxation (using a Steinmann pin), the need to recognize and concurrently manage rigid forefoot supination deformity if present (plantar-based closing wedge osteotomy of the medial cuneiform), and the importance of lengthening the Achilles or gastrocnemius tendon if contracted (which is usually the case in the symptomatic FFF) (Fig. 10-13).

Ragab et al. (113A) performed a descriptive anatomic study of cadaver bones and found that 33% of whites and 60% of blacks (46% of the total) had conjoined anterior and middle calcaneal facets. Although this was merely a description of the anatomic shapes of the bones, they used their findings to condemn the calcaneal lengthening osteotomy. Despite presenting no clinical data, they argued that the osteotomy is intra-articular and would likely cause degenerative changes in the subtalar joint. This result has not been born out by any published data.

Evans (36) may, in fact, have created a true intra-articular osteotomy in most cases. He wrote that the osteotomy should be performed 1.5 cm proximal to, and parallel with, the calcaneocuboid joint. In most adolescent feet, that location is within the middle facet. Nevertheless, in the average 13 year follow-up study of Evans' patients, Phillips (112) reported some cases with degenerative changes in the calcaneo-cuboid joint, but not the subtalar joint. And a possible explanation for the calcaneo-cuboid joint arthritis is that Evans did not protect that joint from subluxating with a longitudinal wire, as is recommended by Mosca (94,98).

Mosca (94) reasoned that it would be best to perform the osteotomy between the anterior and middle facets of the calcaneus to preserve the facets and to maintain the structural stability of the acetabulum pedis. The very fact that there are so many anatomic variations in the size, shape, and even existence of the anterior facet speaks to the possible insignificance of that structure (98A). Furthermore, the anterior facet does not support the head of the talus, even in the neutrally aligned subtalar joint. It is plantar-lateral and seems to act merely as an attachment point for the spring ligament (98A).

Additionally, the major displacement of the calcaneal fragments occurs laterally, away from the facets. The only potential problem in separating the conjoined or separate facets would be vertical translation of the calcaneal fragments (98A) which, I believe, can be avoided by attention to the details of the procedure as they have been described in the literature (94,98).

Other authors have subsequently confirmed the efficacy of the calcaneal lengthening osteotomy for relieving pain and correcting deformity in painful flatfeet (4,8,27,28,102,106,145,148,152).

In summary, if the requisite indication for the calcaneal lengthening osteotomy is intractable pain in a flatfoot with a short Achilles tendon, the relative risk of an intra-articular osteotomy compared with the reported excellent clinical results of the procedure is obviated.

I prefer this operative technique for the rare painful adolescent FFF with short tendo-Achilles who has failed prolonged conservative treatment, and has unacceptably rapid shoe wear. Tricortical iliac crest allograft bone is used for its strength, rapid incorporation, and low morbidity (146). Medial plication of the talonavicular joint capsule and tibialis posterior tendon is recommended to eliminate the redundant soft tissues and reset tension on the musculotendinous unit. Temporary stabilization of the calcaneo-cuboid joint with a retrograde longitudinally inserted Steinmann pin prevents subluxation and excessive intraarticular pressures in that joint. In the older adolescent, there is often a fixed supination deformity of the forefoot that is best managed by a plantar-based closing wedge osteotomy of the medial cuneiform. My experience with several hundred calcaneal lengthening osteotomies for idiopathic, neuromuscular, and other acquired flatfeet (including tarsal coalitions) has been favorable and I have consistently found very good to excellent clinical and radiographic correction of deformity, preservation of subtalar joint motion, elimination of pain and calluses, continued growth of the calcaneus, and elimination of shoe breakdown and brace intolerance.

Obviously, more long-term critical follow-up studies are needed for this procedure and all other conservative and surgical methods of treatment for symptomatic FFF. The Evans/Mosca procedure is unique, however, in that it corrects all components of even the most severe valgus deformities of the hindfoot while preserving subtalar joint motion. If degenerative changes occur later, arthrodesis of the anatomically corrected foot should be fairly straightforward.

SKEWFOOT

Skewfoot is the term used most commonly to designate a rare and poorly defined foot shape that combines adduction deformity of the forefoot with valgus deformity of the hindfoot, i.e., metatarsus adductus plus flatfoot. This is a consensual definition that has been recently accepted in the medical literature (19,92,93,94,95,109). Inconsistent terminology for this deformity was used in the three seminal articles in the English literature. In 1933, Peabody and Muro (107) reported an abnormality consisting of forefoot adduction coupled with valgus deformity of the hindfoot. They presented a series of 14 feet and reviewed the European literature extending over the preceding four decades in which they noted the presence of inconsistent

appearance of the foot in the frontal and sagittal planes, a feature that changes with age in some children.

Young children with persistent and rigid forefoot adductus deformity occasionally present with pain and callus formation at the base of the fifth metatarsal or the medial side of the hallux. They do not report, nor do they manifest, hindfoot symptoms. Parents report that the children do not like to stay in their shoes, though the reason is unclear.

Valgus deformity of the hindfoot, with adductus of the forefoot, can be better appreciated in the older child, adolescent (Figure 10-15.A,B), and adult. In these older individuals, the hindfoot has usually converted to the typical valgus deformity seen in a flatfoot, with full eversion of the subtalar joint and loss of the longitudinal arch with a midfoot sag. There is now concordance in the clinical appearance of the foot in the frontal and sagittal planes (Figure 10-15). Shortening of the tendo-Achilles is noted in the older child, adolescent, and adult with symptomatic skewfoot (92,93,94,95,96,97,98). Their symptoms are identical to those seen in individuals with flexible flatfoot with short tendo-Achilles, i.e., pain and callus formation under the head of the talus and, occasionally, impingement pain in the sinus tarsi region.

So it seems that symptomatic skewfoot in the younger child is related to the midfoot/forefoot deformity, whereas

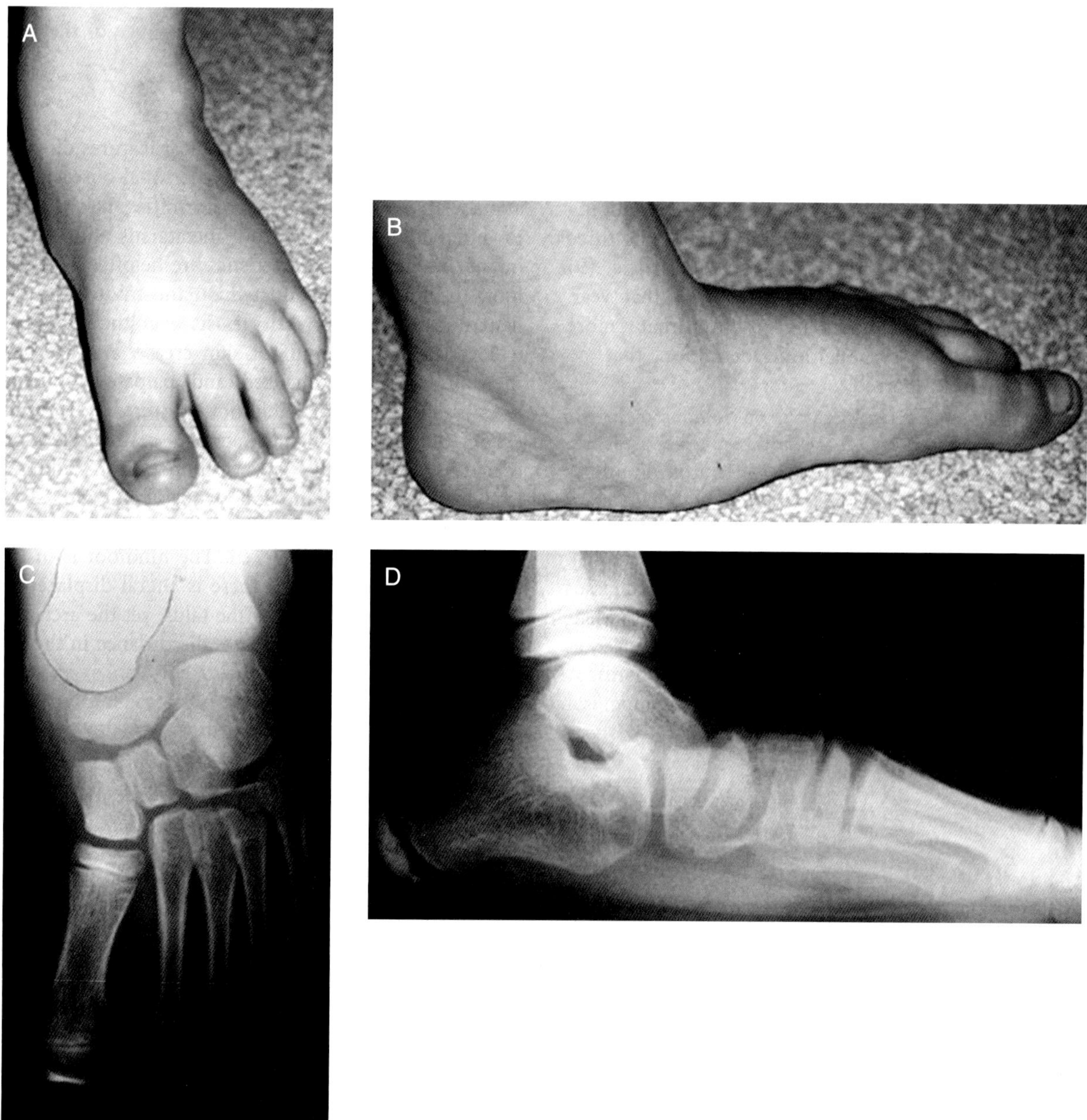

FIGURE 10-15 Adolescent skewfoot. Eversion of the subtalar joint with flat longitudinal arch. Adduction of the forefoot. Trapezoid-shaped medial cuneiform. **A,B.** Clinical photographs. **C,D.** Radiographs. (From Mosca VS. The Foot. In: Morrissy RT, Weinstein SL, eds.: *Lovell and Winter's Pediatric Orthopaedics.* 5th ed. Philadelphia: Lippincott Williams & Wilkins, 1151–1215, 2001, with permission.)

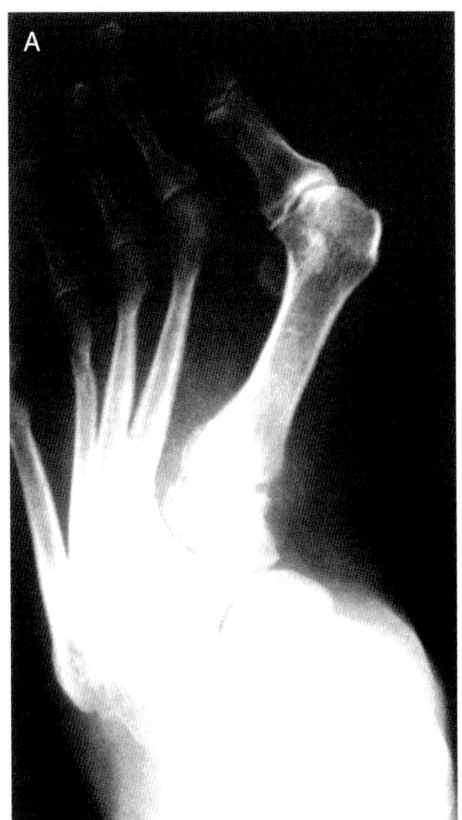

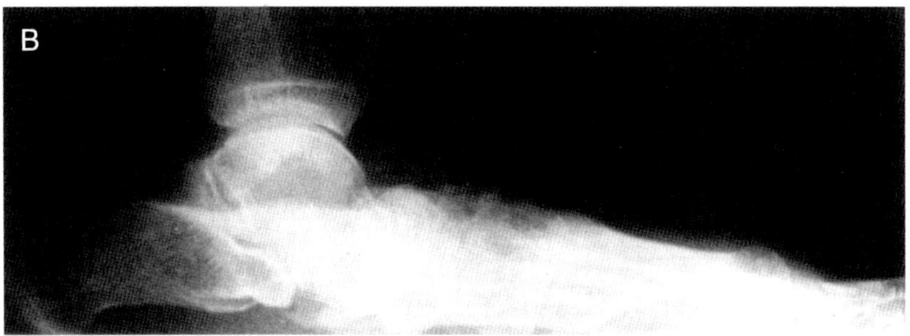

FIGURE 10-16 **A,B.** Painful skewfoot in a 45-year-old woman with severe deformity. Note degenerative changes at proximal and distal joints of first metatarsal. (From the private collection of Vincent S. Mosca, MD.)

symptomatic skewfoot in the older child, adolescent, and adult is usually related to the hindfoot deformity.

A careful clinical examination of the hips of a child with an apparent skewfoot should be performed, because of the reported 1.5% incidence of congenital hip dysplasia in children with metatarsus adductus (68). Because of the difficulty in differentiating these two foot deformities in infants, some of the so-called metatarsus adductus feet in these studies might have actually been skewfeet.

Radiographic Evaluation

The limitations of radiographic evaluation of the child's foot have been discussed earlier in this chapter. The navicular does not ossify until approximately age three years, and then begins ossifying eccentrically towards the lateral side of the cartilage anlage. This delayed and eccentric ossification makes identification of lateral talonavicular subluxation difficult, especially when the forefoot is adducted, as it is in a skewfoot. Berg (9) attempted to classify metatarsus adductus and skewfoot radiographically. Cook et al. (24) found the classification system to have poor interobserver and intraobserver reliability. The system was not valid, in part, because it was based on the radiographic assessment of the relationship of the navicular to the talus at age 5.5 months, an age at which the navicular is not yet ossified.

Standing anteroposterior and lateral radiographs of the foot in the older child, adolescent, and adult will confirm the deformities that are appreciated clinically, i.e., adductus of the forefoot on the midfoot and valgus deformity of the hindfoot (see Figure 10-15 C,D and Figure 10-16). The talus-first metatarsal angle has been used to assess the alignment between the forefoot and the hindfoot in older individuals, and has been considered a vital measurement in the young child before the navicular fully ossifies. Mosca (92,94) identified a flaw in using the talus-first metatarsal angle to assess skewfoot deformities: the skewfoot has two angular deformities between the talus and the first metatarsal that are in opposite directions from each other, resulting in two CORAs. He was also the first author to note that the skew, or zigzag, deformity is present in both the frontal and sagittal planes (92,94) (see Figure 10-15 C,D and Figure 10-17 A,D). Previous authors commented only on the frontal (anteroposterior) plane deformities in skewfeet. The two intervening angular deformities between the talus and first metatarsal create lateral and dorsal translation of the first metatarsal in relation to the talus (92,94). These intervening angular deformities tend to diminish the measured talus-first metatarsal angle despite large angular deformities at both intervening sites in both planes. For that reason, a skewfoot with severe valgus deformity of the hindfoot and

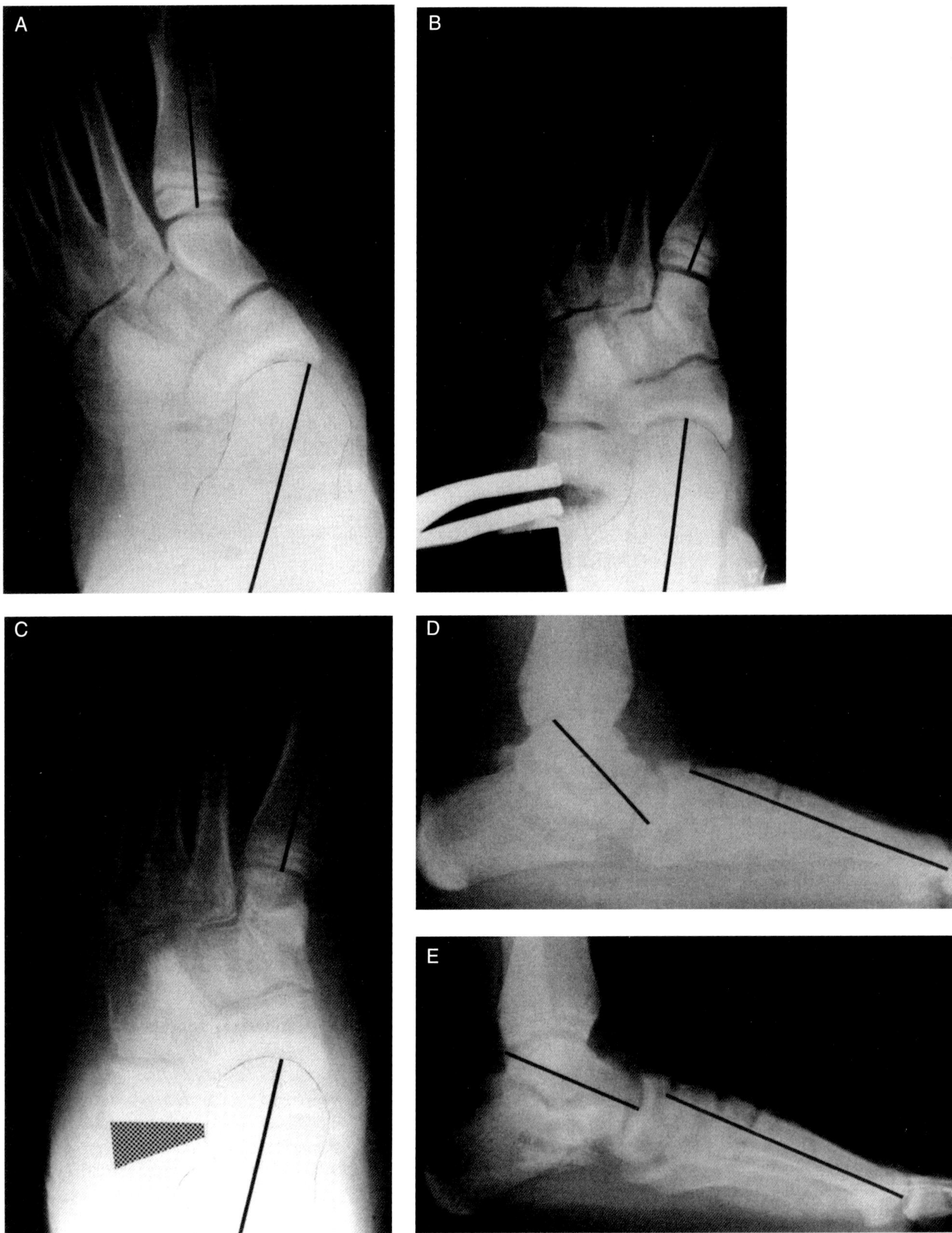

FIGURE 10-17 Painful skewfoot in a 13-year-old boy. **A.** Anteroposterior view showing skew, or zig-zag, deformity. **B.** Laminar spreader in anterior calcaneus osteotomy showing good correction of talonavicular joint subluxation. Note apparent exaggeration of forefoot adductus. Medial cuneiform is trapezoid-shaped with proximal and distal joints converging medially. A transverse osteotomy has been made at the waist of the medial cuneiform. **C.** Hatched area highlights calcaneal graft. Medial cuneiform graft is well seen. Talus and first metatarsal lines are now parallel. **D.** Lateral preoperative radiograph showing skew, or zig-zag, deformity in this plane as well. **E.** Postoperative correction of midfoot sag and low calcaneal pitch. Slight residual dorsal translation of metatarsal line is due to mild midtarsal cavus. (From the private collection of Vincent S. Mosca, MD.)

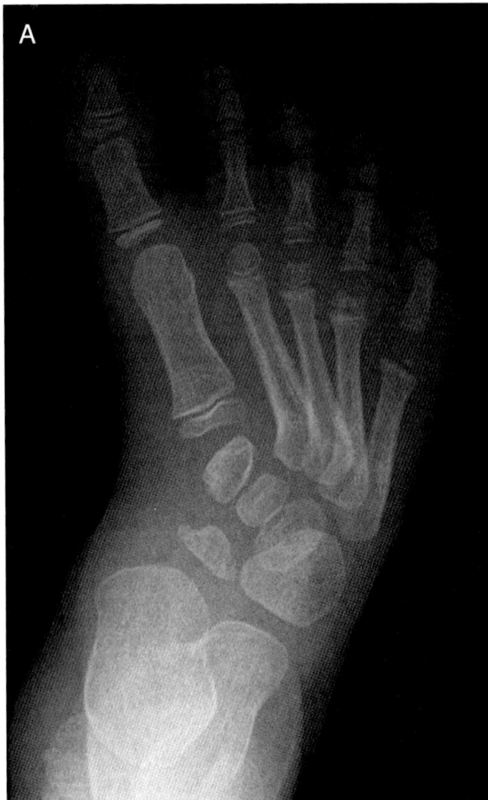

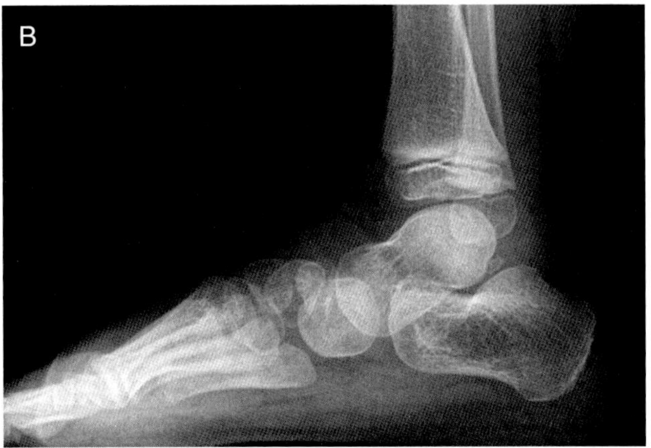

FIGURE 10-18 Radiographs of a skewfoot in a five-year-old girl. **A.** Anteroposterior image suggests eversion of subtalar joint, i.e. flat hindfoot, due to lateral subluxation of the navicular on the head of the talus. **B.** However, the expected plantar flexion of the talus, low calcaneal pitch, and midfoot sag are not seen on the lateral view, though the child has apparent severe clinical hindfoot valgus. (From the private collection of Vincent S. Mosca, MD.)

severe adductus of the forefoot will appear overall to be less deformed than either an isolated moderate flatfoot or a moderate case of metatarsus adductus, when they are assessed clinically and radiographically.

The anteroposterior radiograph of a skewfoot in an infant and young child shows the classic skew deformity, whereas the lateral radiograph usually appears fairly normal (Figure 10-18), without the plantar flexion of the talus and calcaneus that is seen in the older individual with a skewfoot (see Figures 10-15, 10-16, 10-17). The medial cuneiform is kidney-shaped in the young child with a skewfoot and assumes a trapezoidal-shape toward skeletal maturity (91,92,93,94). The proximal and distal articular surfaces of this bone converge medially.

Treatment

The incidence and natural history of skewfoot deformitise are unknown. One would assume that some skewfeet, like most isolated cases of metatarsus adductus and flexible flatfoot, correct spontaneously through normal growth and development. It is also evident that some skewfeet persist into adulthood and are a cause of disability (see Figure 10-16).

"Corrective shoes" are ineffective in correcting skewfoot deformities, just as they are ineffective in correcting other congenital foot deformities. It is reasonable to use serial long-leg casting to treat infant feet with partly flexible and rigid metatarsus adductus, whether they are isolated cases of metatarsus adductus or skewfoot deformities. Several authors have reported success with this approach, noting that it takes longer to correct the metatarsus adductus component of a skewfoot, and that additional care must be exercised to avoid valgus stress on the already deformed hindfoot (9,13,65,66,84,113). Berg (9) cautioned against the use of reverse last shoes and the Denis-Browne bar at the completion of casting, stating that their use increases valgus deformity of the hindfoot.

One must recognize that cast application is technically demanding and is only capable of correcting or improving the metatarsus adductus component of a skewfoot deformity. Casting will not correct valgus deformity of the hindfoot, whether it is an isolated deformity in a flatfoot or the valgus hindfoot deformity in a skewfoot. Duration of casting will be extensive and partial recurrence is likely, but that can be diminished by using a holding device, such as a straight last shoe or a molded night splint, after the casting is completed (83). Treatment should begin between ages four and twelve months when the foot has shown persistent deformity and rigidity, and there is sufficient foot length to allow appropriate molding. Casting may be initiated as late as age 18 to 24 months, but the chances for significant correction are diminished. No clinical problems are anticipated if a flatfoot is revealed following full correction of the forefoot adduction, but it is best not to increase the hindfoot valgus deformity by improper casting or bracing.

There are no large series reporting routinely successful surgical procedures for the symptomatic skewfoot in the young child that has either failed conservative treatment or for which there is no reasonable conservative treatment possible. Most operations have been described in case reports with limited length of follow up. The majority of authors have indicated that the surgical approach should be aggressive, and that incomplete correction and recurrence should be anticipated (10,23,54,64,109,113). Some authors recommended staged surgical treatment (10,54).

For the young child, plantar-medial soft tissue releases including midtarsal and tarsometatarsal capsulotomies have been utilized in concert with alignment, plication, and temporary pin fixation of the talonavicular joint, and wedge resection of the cuboid (23,54,55,64,109,141). At long-term follow up, Stark et al. (137) reported significant degenerative arthritis in tarsometatarsal joints that had undergone capsulotomies. This approach is, therefore, not recommended.

Rarely, a child in the middle of the first decade of life will present with pain and callus formation at the base of the fifth metatarsal or the medial side of the hallux, due to a severe and rigid adductus component of a skewfoot deformity. The arch is elevated, despite valgus angulation of the heel, and the tendo-Achilles is not contracted. If shoe modifications cannot relieve the symptoms, surgical correction is indicated. Recommendations in the literature for correction of the forefoot adduction component of skewfoot in this age group include: tarsometatarsal capsulotomies (55), metatarsal base osteotomies (10), and medial cuneiform opening wedge osteotomy (23,37,72), possibly combined with closing cuboid wedge osteotomy (85,141). Considering the reported risks and complications of the procedures, a closing wedge osteotomy of the cuboid with an opening wedge osteotomy of the medial cuneiform produces the best clinical results with the least morbidity. The hindfoot can usually be ignored at this age. The lengthening of the medial bone column of the foot, which results from the medial cuneiform opening wedge osteotomy, generally causes the soft tissues to pull the navicular somewhat medially to improve its alignment at the talonavicular joint. This occurs because of a windlass-type effect of the abductor hallucis and the medial skin of the foot.

Some older children, adolescents, and adults with skewfoot deformity will report pain and callus formation under the medial midfoot. Symptoms seem to shift with age from the forefoot/midfoot to the hindfoot/midfoot. From my personal experience, I have identified that these older individuals have developed a contracture of the tendo-Achilles and symptomatically resemble patients with FFF with a short tendo-Achilles. The clinical appearance is also similar. Radiographs will confirm the true diagnosis (see Figure 10-15 C,D).

Conservative management holds little promise for the symptomatic skewfoot with a short tendo-Achillis. Heel-cord stretching exercises are rarely successful when a hindfoot has severe valgus deformity. As with FFF-STA, arch supports in this situation place increased pressure under the arch and exacerbate the symptoms.

I feel that surgery is indicated for the adolescent with a skewfoot deformity and tendo-Achilles contracture who manifests intractable pain under the medial midfoot, in the sinus tarsi, and/or at the base of the fifth metatarsal despite prolonged attempts at conservative management. The deformities to treat include: severe forefoot adduction, trapezoid-shaped deformity of the medial cuneiform, midfoot/forefoot cavus, dorsolateral subluxation of the talonavicular joint with plantar flexed talus, subtalar joint eversion with external rotation of the acetabulum pedis, and, in many cases, shortening of the tendo-Achilles.

The Koutsogiannis-type oblique calcaneal slide osteotomy (67) and the Dwyer lateral opening wedge calcaneal osteotomy (34) have been recommended to correct the valgus hindfoot deformity in the older child with skewfoot. These osteotomies do not, however, correct the malalignment at the talonavicular joint. Subtalar and triple arthrodeses have been recommended for the adolescent with significant valgus hindfoot deformity and have been reported in combination with, or staged with, metatarsal osteotomies or a cuneiform osteotomy for the forefoot deformity (10,54,109). Tendo-Achilles lengthening has been added as needed.

Partial success in correcting the many deformities of the skewfoot has been reported with all of these procedures. Talonavicular (75), subtalar (48), and triple (1,3) arthrodeses may improve the surgeon's ability to correct the hindfoot deformity, but they shift stress to the ankle and mid-tarsal joints, leading to premature degenerative arthrosis at those sites and making them undesirable choices (1,3,29,82,120,123,127,129,132,134).

Mosca (93) proposed correction of the symptomatic skewfoot in the adolescent by combining the best and safest methods for correcting the individual deformities of the hindfoot and the forefoot. The technique consists of a calcaneal lengthening osteotomy, conceptualized by Evans (36) and elaborated by Mosca (94,98); a medial cuneiform opening wedge osteotomy, according to Fowler et al. (37); and lengthening of the tendo-Achilles (Figure 10-17). In 1993 (93), he reported the short-term results of the largest series of operatively treated skewfoot deformities using a single technique. Nine of the ten severe skewfoot deformities achieved satisfactory clinical and radiographic outcomes while maintaining subtalar joint mobility. Long-term follow up is clearly needed.

The advantages of this combination of procedures over its predecessors include complete correction of all deformities at the individual sites of deformity, preservation of subtalar joint motion, and low morbidity. The improved foot alignment will make arthrodesis technically easier if fusion is necessary to treat degenerative joint changes in the future. The optimum age for this procedure is unknown, but when significant symptoms persist despite appropriate conservative management, there may be an advantage to pursuing surgery without further delay. Theoretically, the joints should have a better ability to remodel when this combination of procedures is performed in an older child or adolescent than in an adult.

REFERENCES

1. Adelaar RS, Dannelly EA, Meunier PA et al. A long term study of triple arthrodesis in children. *Orthop Clin North Am* 7:895–908, 1976.
2. Anderson AF, Fowler SB. Anterior calcaneal osteotomy for symptomatic juvenile pes planus. *Foot Ankle* 4:274–283, 1984.
3. Angus PD, Cowell HR. Triple arthrodesis: A critical long-term review. *J Bone Joint Surg [Am]* 68:260–265, 1986
4. Arangio GA, Chopra V, Voloshin A, et al. A biomechanical analysis of the effect of lateral column lengthening calcaneal osteotomy on the flat foot. *Clin Biomech* 22:472–477, 2007.
5. Armstrong G, Carruthers CC. Evans elongation of lateral column of the foot for valgus deformity. *J Bone Joint Surg [Br]* 57:530, 1975.
6. Basmajian JV, Stecko G. The role of muscles in arch support of the foot. An electromyographic study. *J Bone Joint Surg [Am]* 45:1184–1190, 1963.
7. Basta NW, Mital MA, Bonadio O, et al. A comparative study of the role of shoes, arch supports, and navicular cookies in the management of symptomatic mobile flat feet in children. *Int Orthop* 1:143–148, 1977.
8. Benthien RA, Parks BG, Guyton GP, et al. Lateral column calcaneal lengthening, flexor digitorum longus transfer, and opening wedge medial cuneiform osteotomy for flexible flatfoot: A biomechanical study. *Foot Ankle Int* 28:70–77, 2007.
9. Berg EE. A reappraisal of metatarsus adductus and skewfoot. *J Bone Joint Surg [Am]* 68:1185–1196, 1986.
10. Berman A, Gartland JJ. Metatarsal osteotomy for the correction of adduction of the fore part of the foot in children. *J Bone Joint Surg [Am]* 53:498–505, 1971.
11. Bettmann E. The treatment of flat-foot by means of exercise. *J Bone Joint Surg* 19:821–825, 1937.
12. Bleck EE. The shoeing of children: sham or science? *Dev Med Child Neurol* 13:188–195, 1971.
13. Bleck EE, Berzins UJ. Conservative management of pes valgus with planter flexed talus, flexible. *Clin Orthop* 122:85–94, 1977.
14. Blount WP. *Fractures in children.* Huntington, NY: Kreiger, p. 185, 1977.
15. Bonnet WL, Baker DR. Diagnosis of pes planus by x-ray. *Radiology* 46:36–45, 1946.
16. Bordelon RL. Correction of hypermobile flatfoot in children by molded inserts. *Foot Ankle* 1:143–150, 1980.
17. Butte FL. Navicular-cuneiform arthrodesis for flatfoot: an end-result study. *J Bone Joint Surg* 19:496–502, 1937.
18. Caldwell GD. Surgical correction of relaxed flat foot by the Durham flat foot plasty. *Clin Orthop* 2:221–226, 1953.
19. Cappello T, Mosca VS. Metatarsus Adductus and Skewfoot. *Foot Ankle Clin* 3:683–700, 1998.
20. Chambers EFS. An operation for the correction of flexible flat feet of adolescents. *West J Surg Obstet Gynecol* 54:77–86, 1946.
21. Close JR, Inman VT. The action of the subtalar joint. *California Prosthetic Devices Research Report* Series 11 (24), 1953.
22. Close JR, Inman VT, Poor PM. et al. The function of the subtalar joint. *Clin Orthop* 50:159–179, 1967.
23. Coleman SS. *Complex foot deformities in children.* Philadelphia: Lea & Febiger, 193–222, 1983.
24. Cook D, Breed A, Cook T, et al. Observer variability in the radiographic measurement and classification of metatarsus adductus. *J Pediatr Orthop* 12:86–89, 1992.
25. Crego CH, Ford LT. An end-result study of various operative procedures for correcting flat feet in children. *J Bone Joint Surg [Am]* 34:183–195, 1952.
26. Davy R. On excision of the scaphoid bone for the relief of confirmed flatfoot. *Lancet* 1:675, 1889.
27. Doğan A, Albayrak M, Akman YE, et al. The results of calcaneal lengthening osteotomy for the treatment of flexible pes planovalgus and evaluation of alignment of the foot. *Acta Orthop Traumatol Turc* 40:356–366, 2006.
28. Dollard MD, Marcinko DE, Lazerson A, et al. The Evans calcaneal osteotomy for correction of flexible flatfoot syndrome. *J Foot Surg* 23:291–301, 1984.
29. Drew AJ. The late results of arthrodesis of the foot. *J Bone Joint Surg [Br]* 33:496–502, 1951.
30. Driano AN, Staheli L, Staheli LT. Psychosocial development and corrective shoewear use in childhood. *J Pediatr Orthop* 18:346–349, 1998.
31. Duchenne GB. *Physiology of motion.* Philadelphia: WB Saunders, 337, 1959.
32. DuMontier TA, Falicov A, Mosca V, et al. Calcaneal lengthening: Investigation of deformity correction in a flatfoot model. *Foot Ankle Int* 26:166–170, 2005.
33. Duncan JW, Lovell WW. Modified Hoke-Miller flatfoot procedure. *Clin Orthop* 181:24–27, 1983.
34. Dwyer FC. Osteotomy of the calcaneum for pes cavus. *J Bone Joint Surg [Br]* 41:80–86, 1959.
35. Elftman H. The transverse tarsal joint and its control. *Clin Orthop* 16:41–46, 1960.
36. Evans D. Calcaneo-valgus deformity. *J Bone Joint Surg [Br]* 57:270–278, 1975.
37. Fowler SB, Brooks AL, Parrish TF. The cavo-varus foot. *J Bone Joint Surg [Am]* 41:757, 1959.
38. Gamble FO, Yale I. *Clinical foot roentgenology.* Baltimore: Williams & Wilkins, 153, 1966.
39. Giannestrus NJ. Flexible valgus flatfoot resulting from naviculocuneiform and talonavicular sag. Surgical correction in the adolescent. In: Bateman, J. E., ed.: *Foot science.* Philadelphia: WB Saunders, 67–105, 1976.
40. Giannini S, Ceccarelli F, Benedetti MG, et al. Surgical treatment of flexible flatfoot in children: A four-year follow-up study. *J Bone Joint Surg [Am]* 83(Suppl 2, Pt 2):73–79, 2001.
41. Giannini S, Girolami M, Ceccarelli F. The surgical treatment of infantile flat foot: A new expanding orthotic implant. *J Orthop Traum* 11:315–322, 1985.
42. Giladi M, Milgrom C, Stein M, et al. The low arch, a protective factor in stress fractures. *Orthop Rev* 14:81–84, 1985.
43. Gleich A. Beitrag Zur Operativen Plattfussbehandlung. *Arch Klin Chir* 46:358, 1893.
44. Gocht H. Schenenoperation beim pes Plano-valgus. *Z Orthop Chir* 14:693–697, 1905.
45. Golding-Bird CH. Operations on the tarsus in confirmed flatfoot. *Lancet* 1:677, 1889.
46. Gould N, Moreland M, Alvarez R, et al. Development of the child's arch. *Foot Ankle* 9:241–245, 1989.
47. Gray E G, Basmajian JV. Electromyography and cinematography of the leg and foot ("normal" and flat) during walking. *Anat Rec* 161:1–16, 1968.
48. Grice DS. An extra-articular arthrodesis of the subastragalar joint for correction of paralytic flat feet in children. *J Bone Joint Surg [Am]* 34:927–940, 1952.
49. Gutierrez PR, Lara MH. Giannini prosthesis for flatfoot. *Foot Ankle Int* 26:918–926, 2005.
50. Haraldsson S. Pes plano-valgus staticus juvenilis and its operative treatment. Acta *Orthop Scand* 35:234–256, 1965.
51. Harris RI, Beath T. *Army foot survey, vol 1.* Ottawa: National Research Council of Canada, 1–268, 1947.

52. Harris RI, Beath T. Hypermobile flat-foot with short tendo Achillis. *J Bone Joint Surg [Am]* 30:116–138, 1948.
53. Helfet AJ. A new way of treating flatfeet in children. *Lancet* 1:262–264, 1956.
54. Herndon CH. Discussion of Berman, A., Gartland, J. J.: Metatarsal osteotomy for the correction of adduction of the fore part of the foot in children. *J Bone Joint Surg [Am]* 53:505–506, 1971.
55. Heyman CH, Herndon CH, Strong JM. Mobilization of the tarsometatarsal and intermetatarsal joints for the correction of resistant adduction of the fore part of the foot in congenital club-foot or congenital metatarsus varus. *J Bone Joint Surg [Am]* 40:299–310, 1958.
56. Hicks JH. The mechanics of the foot. I. The joints. *J Anat* 87:345–357, 1953.
57. Hicks JH. The mechanics of the foot. II. The plantar aponeurosis and the arch. *J Anat* 88:25–35, 1954.
58. Hoke M. An operation for the correction of extremely relaxed flatfeet. *J Bone Joint Surg* 13:773–783, 1931.
59. Husain ZS, Fallat LM. Biomechanical analysis of Maxwell-Brancheau Arthroereisis implants. *J Foot Ankle Surg* 41:352–358, 2002.
60. Inman VT. *The joints of the ankle.* Baltimore: Williams & Wilkins, 1976.
61. Jack EA. Naviculo-cuneiform fusion in the treatment of flat foot. *J Bone Joint Surg [Br]* 35:75–82, 1953.
62. Jones BS. Flat foot. A preliminary report of an operation for severe cases. *J Bone Joint Surg [Br]* 57:279–282, 1975.
63. Jones RL. The human foot. An experimental study of its mechanics and the role of its muscles and ligaments in support of the arch. *Am J Anat* 68:1–10, 1941.
64. Kendrick RE, Sharma NK, Hassler WL, et al. Tarsometatarsal mobilization for resistant adduction of the fore part of the foot. *J Bone Joint Surg [Am]* 52:61–70, 1970.
65. Kite JH. Congenital metatarsus varus: report of 300 cases. *J Bone Joint Surg [Am]* 32:500–506, 1950.
66. Kite JH. Congenital metatarsus varus. *J Bone Joint Surg [Am]* 49:388–397, 1967.
67. Koutsogiannis E. Treatment of mobile flatfoot by displacement osteotomy of the calcaneous. *J Bone Joint Surg[Br]* 53:96–100, 1971.
68. Kumar SJ, MacEwen GD. The incidence of hip dysplasia with metatarsus adductus. *Clin Orthop* 164:234–235, 1982.
69. Lanham RH Jr. Indications and complications of arthroeresis in hypermobile flatfoot. *J Am Podiatr Med Assoc* 69:178–185, 1979.
70. Legg AT. The treatment of congenital flatfoot by tendon transplantation. *Am J Orthop Surg* 10:584, 1912.
71. LeLievre J. Current concepts and correction in the valgus foot. *Clin Orthop* 70:43–55, 1970.
72. Lincoln CR, Wood KE, Bugg EI Jr. Metatarsus varus corrected by open wedge osteotomy of the first cuneiform bone. *Orthop Clin North Am* 7:795–798, 1976.
73. Lloyd-Roberts GC, Clark RC. Ball and socket ankle joint in metatarsus adductus varus (S-shaped or serpentine foot). *J Bone Joint Surg [Br]* 55:193–196, 1973.
74. Lord JP. Correction of extreme flat foot. *JAMA* 81:1502, 1923.
75. Lowman CL. An operative method for correction of certain forms of flat foot. *JAMA* 81:1500–1502, 1923.
76. Mann RA. Biomechanics of the foot and ankle. In: Mann, R. A., ed.: *Surgery of the foot.* St. Louis: CV Mosby, 1–30, 1986.
77. Mann RA. Miscellaneous afflictions of the foot. In: Mann, R. A., ed.: *Surgery of the foot.* St. Louis: CV Mosby, 230–238, 1986.
78. Mann R, Inman VT. Phasic activity of intrinsic muscles of the foot. *J Bone Joint Surg [Am]* 46:469–481, 1969.
79. Manter JT. Movements of the subtalar and transverse tarsal joints. *Anat Rec* 80:397–410, 1941.
80. Maxwell JR, Carro A, Sun C. Use of the Maxwell-Brancheau arthroereisis implant for the correction of posterior tibial tendon dysfunction. *Clin Podiatr Med Surg* 16:479–489, 1999.
81. Maxwell JR, Knudson W, Cerniglia M. The MBA arthroereisis implant: early prospective results. In: Vickers NS, Miller SJ, Mahan KT, eds.: *Reconstructive Surgery of the Foot and Leg.* Tucker, GA: Podiatry Institute, 256–264, 1997.
82. McCall R, Lillich J, Harris J, et al. The Grice extraarticular subtalar arthrodesis: A clinical review. *J Pediatr Orthop* 5:442–445, 1985.
83. McCauley J Jr, Lusskin R, Bromley J. Recurrence in congenital metatarsus varus. *J Bone Joint Surg [Am]* 46:525–532, 1964.
84. McCormick DW, Blount WP. Metatarsus adductovarus: "skewfoot." *JAMA* 141:449–453, 1949.
85. McHale KA, Lenhart MK. Treatment of residual clubfoot deformity – the "bean-shaped" foot – by open wedge medial cuneiform osteotomy and closing wedge cuboid osteotomy: clinical review and cadaver correlations. *J Pediatr Orthop* 11:374–381, 1991.
86. Meary R. On the measurement of the angle between the talus and the first metatarsal. Symposium: Le Pied Creux Essential. *Rev Chir Orthop* 53:389, 1967.
87. Mereday C, Dolan CM, Lusskin R. Evaluation of the University of California Biomechanics Laboratory shoe insert in "flexible" pes planus. *Clin Orthop* 82:45–58, 1972.
88. Miller GR. The operative treatment of hypermobile flatfeet in the young child. *Clin Orthop* 122:95–101, 1977.
89. Miller OL. A plastic flat foot operation. *J Bone Joint Surg* 9:84–91, 1927.
90. Morley AM. Knock-knee in children. *Br Med J* 11:978–979, 1957.
91. Morcuende J, Ponseti I. Congenital metatarsus adductus in early human fetal development: a histologic study. *Clin Orthop* 333:261–266, 1996.
92. Mosca VS. Flexible Flatfoot and Skewfoot. In: Drennan, J. C., ed.: *The Child's Foot and Ankle.* New York: Raven Press, 355–376, 1992.
93. Mosca VS. Skewfoot deformity in children: Correction by calcaneal neck lengthening and medial cuneiform opening wedge osteotomies. *J Pediatr Orthop* 13:807, 1993.
94. Mosca VS. Calcaneal lengthening for valgus deformity of the hindfoot: Results in children who had severe, symptomatic flatfoot and skewfoot. *J Bone Joint Surg [Am]* 77:500–512, 1995.
95. Mosca VS. Flexible flatfoot and skewfoot. An Instructional Course Lecture, The American Academy of Orthopaedic Surgeons. *J Bone Joint Surg [Am]* 77:1937–1945, 1995.
96. Mosca VS. The Child's Foot: Principles of Management [editorial]. *J Pediatr Orthop* 18:281–282, 1998.
97. Mosca VS. The Foot. In: Morrissy, R. T., Weinstein, S. L., eds.: *Lovell and Winter's Pediatric Orthopaedics.* 5th ed. Philadelphia: Lippincott Williams & Wilkins, 1151–1215, 2001.
98. Mosca VS. Calcaneal lengthening osteotomy for valgus deformity of the hindfoot. In: Skaggs DL, Tolo VT, eds.: *Master Techniques in Orthopaedic Surgery: Pediatrics.* Philadelphia: Lippincott Williams & Wilkins, 263–276, 2008.
98A. Mosca, V. S.: Letter to the JPO editors re: article by Ragab AA, et al. entitled "Implications of subtalar joint anatomic variation in calcaneal lengthening osteotomy." (*J Pediatr Orthop* 29:315–316, 2009.
99. Needleman RL. Current topic review: Subtalar arthroereisis for the correction of flexible flatfoot. *Foot Ankle Int* 26:336–346, 2005.
100. Nelson SC, Haycock DM, Little ER. Flexible flatfoot treatment with arthroereisis: Radiographic improvement and child health survey analysis. *J Foot Ankle Surg* 43:144–155, 2004.
101. Niederecker K. Operationsverfahren zur behandlung des plattfusses. *Chir Pediatr* 4:182–183, 1932.
102. Oeffinger DJ, Pectol RW, Tylkowski CM. Foot pressure and radiographic outcome measures of lateral column lengthening

for pes planovalgus deformity. *Gait & Posture* 12:189–195, 2000.

103. Oloff LM, Naylor BL, Jacobs AM. Complications of subtalar arthroereisis. *J Foot Ankle Surg* 26:136–140, 1987.
104. Ozonoff MB. *Pediatric orthopedic radiology.* Philadelphia: WB Saunders, 300, 1979.
105. Paley D. *Principles of Deformity Correction.* Berlin: Springer-Verlag, 2002.
106. Park KB, Park HW, Lee KS, et al. Changes in dynamic foot pressure after surgical treatment of valgus deformity of the hindfoot in cerebral palsy. *J Bone Joint Surg [Am]* 90:1712–1721, 2008.
107. Peabody CW, Muro F. Congenital metatarsus varus. *J Bone Joint Surg [Am]* 15:171–189, 1933.
108. Penneau K, Lutter LD, Winter RD. Pes planus: Radiographic changes with foot orthoses and shoes. *Foot Ankle* 2:299–303, 1982.
109. Peterson HA. Skewfoot (forefoot adduction with heel valgus). *J Pediatr Orthop* 6:24–30, 1986.
110. Peterson H. Growing pains. *Pediatr Clin North Am* 33:1365–1372, 1986.
111. Phelps AM. The etiology, pathology, and treatment of flat-foot. *Post Grad Med* 7: 104, 1892.
112. Phillips GE. A review of elongation of os calcis for flat feet. *J Bone Joint Surg [Br]* 65:15–18, 1983.
113. Ponseti IV, Becker JR. Congenital metatarsus adductus: The results of treatment. *J Bone Joint Surg [Am]* 48:702–711, 1966.
113A. Ragab AA, Stewart SL, Cooperman DR. Implications of subtalar joint anatomic variation in calcaneal lengthening osteotomy. *J Pediatr Orthop* 23:79–83, 2003.
114. Rao U, Joseph B. The influence of footwear on the prevalence of flat foot: A survey of 2300 children. *J Bone Joint Surg [Br]* 74:525–527, 1992.
115. Rathjen K, Mubarak S. Calcaneo-cuboid-cuneiform osteotomy for the correction of valgus foot deformities in children. *J Pediatr Orthop* 18:775–782, 1998.
116. Reiman I, Werner HH. Congenital metatarsus varus. A suggestion for a possible mechanism and relation to other foot deformities. *Clin Orthop* 110:223–226, 1975.
117. Roberts PW. An operation for valgus feet. *JAMA* 77: 1571, 1921.
118. Rose GK. Correction of the pronated foot. *J Bone Joint Surg [Br]* 40:674–683, 1958.
119. Rose GK. Correction of the pronated foot. *J Bone Joint Surg [Br]* 44:642–647, 1962.
120. Ross P, Lyne D. The Grice procedure: Indications and evaluation of long-term results. *Clin Orthop* 153:194–200, 1980.
121. Rushforth GF. The natural history of hooked forefoot. *J Bone Joint Surg [Br]* 60:530–532, 1978.
122. Ryerson EW. Tendon transplantation in flatfoot. *Am J Orthop Surg* 7: 505, 1909.
123. Saltzman CL, Fehrle MJ, Cooper RR. et al. Triple arthrodesis: Twenty-five and forty-four-year average follow-up of the same patients. *J Bone Joint Surg [Am]* 81:1391–1402, 1999.
124. Sangeorzan BJ, Mosca V, Hansen ST Jr. The effect of calcaneal lengthening on relationships among the hindfoot, midfoot, and forefoot. *Foot Ankle* 14:136–141, 1993.
125. Saxena A, Nguyen A. Preliminary radiographic findings and sizing implications on patients undergoing bioabsorbable subtalar arthroereisis. *J Foot Ankle Surg* 46:175–180, 2007.
126. Scarpa A. A memoir on the congenital club feet of children, and of the mode of correcting that deformity. Edinburgh: Archibald Constable, 8–15, 1818. (Translated by Wishart JH, *Clin Orthop* 308:4–7, 1994).
127. Scott S, Janes P, Stevens P. Grice subtalar arthrodesis followed to skeletal maturity. *J Pediatr Orthop* 8:176–183, 1988.
128. Scranton PE, Goldner JL, Lutter LD, Staheli LT. Management of hypermobile flatfoot in the child. *Contemp Orthop* 3:645–663, 1981.
129. Seymour N. The late results of naviculo-cuneiform fusion. *J Bone Joint Surg [Br]* 49:558–559, 1967.
130. Silver CM, Simon SD, Litchman HM. Long term follow-up observations on calcaneal osteotomy. *Clin Orthop* 99:181–187, 1974.
131. Sim-Fook L, Hodgson AR. A comparison of foot forms among the non-shoe and shoe-wearing Chinese population. *J Bone Joint Surg [Am]* 40:1058–1062, 1958.
132. Smith J, Westin G. Subtalar extra-articular arthrodesis. *J Bone Joint Surg [Am]* 50:1027–1035, 1968.
133. Smith SD, Millar EA. Arthrorereisis by means of a subtalar polyethylene peg implant for correction of hindfoot pronation in children. *Clin Orthop* 181:15–23, 1983.
134. Southwell R, Sherman F. Triple arthrodesis: A long-term study with force plate analysis. *Foot Ankle* 2:15–24, 1981.
135. Staheli LT, Chew DE, Corbett M. The longitudinal arch. A survey of eight hundred and eighty-two feet in normal children and adults. *J Bone Joint Surg [Am]* 69:426–428, 1987.
136. Staheli LT, Giffin L. Corrective shoes for children: a survey of current practice. *Pediatrics* 65:13–17, 1980.
137. Stark JG, Johanson JE, Winter RB. The Heyman-Herndon tarsometatarsal capsulotomy for metatarsus adductus: Results in 48 feet. *J Pediatr Orthop* 7:305–310, 1987.
138. Steel MW III, Johnson KA, DeWitz MA, et al. Radiographic measurements of the normal adult foot. *Foot Ankle* 1:151–158, 1980.
139. Stewart SF. Human gait and the human foot: an ethnological study of flatfoot. *Clin Orthop* 70:111–123, 1970.
140. Stokes W. Astragaloid osteotomy in the treatment of flatfoot. *Trans Acad Med Ireland* III: 141, 1885.
141. Tachdjian MO. *The child's foot.* Philadelphia: WB Saunders, 556–597, 1985.
142. Templeton AW, McAlister WH, Zim ID. Standardization of terminology and evaluation of osseous relationships in congenitally abnormal feet. *Am J Roentgenol* 93:374–381, 1965.
143. Theologis T, Gordon C, Benson M. Heel seats and shoe wear. *J Pediatr Orthop* 14:760–762, 1994.
144. Vanderwilde R, Staheli LT, Chew DE, et al. Measurements on radiographs of the foot in normal infants and children. *J Bone Joint Surg [Am]* 70:407–415, 1988.
145. Viegas GV. Reconstruction of the pediatric flexible planovalgus foot by using an Evans calcaneal osteotomy and augmentative medial split tibialis anterior tendon transfer. *J Foot Ankle Surg* 42:199–207, 2003.
146. Warme WJ, Mosca VS, Conrad EU. Comparison of structural bone allografts and autografts in pediatric foot surgery. *Orthop Trans* 21:651–652, 1997.
147. Wenger DR, Mauldin D, Speck G, et al. Corrective shoes and inserts as treatment for flexible flatfoot in infants and children. *J Bone Joint Surg [Am]* 71:800–810, 1989.
148. Yoo WJ, Chung CY, Choi IH, et al. Calcaneal lengthening for the planovalgus foot deformity in children with cerebral palsy. *J Pediatr Orthop* 25:781–785, 2005.
149. Young C. Operative treatment of pes planus. *Surg Gynecol Obstet* 68:1099–1101, 1939.
150. Zadek I. Transverse-wedge arthrodesis for the relief of pain in rigid flatfoot. *J Bone Joint Surg* 17:453–467, 1935.
151. Zaret DI, Myerson MS. Arthroerisis of the subtalar joint. *Foot Ankle Clin N Am* 8:605–617, 2003.
152. Zeifang F, Breusch SJ, Döderlein L. Evans calcaneal lengthening procedure for spastic flexible flatfoot in 32 patients (46 feet) with a followup of 3 to 9 years. *Foot Ankle Int* 27:500–507, 2006.

CHAPTER 11

Tarsal Coalition

Brad W. Olney

INTRODUCTION

A tarsal coalition is a congenital bony, cartilaginous, or fibrous connection between two or more tarsal bones. Bussine first described the condition in 1750 (8). Kirmission demonstrated radiographically a tarsal coalition in 1898 (35). Calcaneonavicular and talocalcaneal forms are the most common types. These two types were first described by Cruveillier in 1829 and Zuckerhanel in 1877, respectively (8,35). Bilateral talocalcaneal tarsal coalitions have been described in a pre-Columbian Indian skeleton dating from approximately 1000 AD (18).

Recognition of the clinical significance of a tarsal coalition was not described until 1880 when Holl proposed a possible connection with flatfeet (27). Peroneal spastic flatfeet were described by Sir Robert Jones in 1897 and this condition was later linked to cases of calcaneonavicular coalition by Slomann (35). Harris and Beath reported a correlation between talocalcaneal coalition and peroneal spastic flatfeet in 1948 (16). With the advent of improved radiographic imaging, such as computerized tomography (CT) and magnetic resonance imaging (MRI) scans, we are now better able to describe the anatomy, incidence, and clinical significance of tarsal coalitions.

ETIOLOGY AND HEREDITY

Pfitzner first studied the etiology of tarsal coalition (27). He hypothesized that this condition resulted from the incorporation of accessory ossicles with adjacent tarsal bones. He based his theory on extensive cadaver studies in which he noted that tarsal coalitions occurred in areas where sesamoid bones and accessory ossicles were known to exist. Harris' demonstration of six cases of talocalcaneal tarsal coalitions in 20 feet of human embryos disproved Pfitzner's theory (15). A fetal calcaneonavicular coalition was also reported by O'Rahilly et al. (39). Based on the work of Harris and O'Rahilly, it would appear that the tarsal coalition results from failure of differentiation and segmentation of primary mesenchyme in the developing fetus.

Tarsal coalitions are usually isolated findings but may occasionally be associated with generalized syndromes such as the Apert or Nievergelt-Pearlman syndromes (54). Apert syndrome includes synostosis of the tarsal and cranial bones, mid-face hypoplasia, and cutaneous or osseous syndactyly of the digits. The Nievergelt-Pearlman syndrome consists of multiple congenital anomalies including tarsal and radioulnar synostosis, dysplasia of the tibia and fibula, and multiple hand anomalies. Tarsal coalitions may also be associated with other congenital limb anomalies, such as proximal focal femoral deficiency, phocomelia, fibular hemimelia, adactylia, and ball-and-socket ankle. There is evidence the congenital ball-and-socket ankle may represent an adaptive change of the ankle mortise secondary to decreased subtalar motion in some cases of tarsal coalitions (55).

There are several reports of tarsal coalitions occurring in members of the same family, suggesting a genetic pattern. Wray et al. reported the occurrence of calcaneonavicular coalitions in three generations of the same family (61). They proposed that calcaneonavicular coalitions were transmitted in an autosomal dominant pattern with probable reduced penetrance. The most complete inheritance study of tarsal coalition was done by Leonard (27) who conducted family surveys in 31 patients with tarsal coalitions. He studied 98 first-degree relatives and found tarsal coalitions in 39% (33% of parents and 46.5% of siblings). Leonard concluded that tarsal coalition was a multifactorial disorder of autosomal dominant inheritance, very nearly of full penetrance. He further concluded there did not seem to be any genetic difference in the inheritance of the different forms of coalition, because 14% of the family members had a different type of coalition than the index patient. Another interesting fact from Leonard's study is that all the first-degree relatives with tarsal coalitions were asymptomatic.

Incidence and Classification

The overall incidence of tarsal coalition in the general population is unknown because many studies are based on a selected patient population (20). The current best estimate indicates that the incidence in the general population is probably less than 1% (27,51,53). The exact incidence may change as radiographic techniques improve. Although there is some disagreement between studies, it appears there is a male preponderance in the sex distribution. Leonard and Scranton showed an equal sex distribution in their studies of patients with calcaneonavicular and talocalcaneal coalitions (27,48). However, most studies show a male to female preponderance of patients with tarsal coalitions from 60% to 80% (13,20,34,37,51,53). When these studies are evaluated, it appears there is approximately a 2 to 1 male to female distribution.

The most common tarsal anomalies occur between the calcaneus and talus and between the calcaneus and navicular. These two types account for the vast majority of all tarsal coalitions and account for virtually all of the symptomatic feet with this condition. Studies differ regarding which is more common. Because talocalcaneal coalitions are not well visualized on plain radiographs, many older studies stated that the incidence of the calcaneonavicular condition was higher. With the advent and current use of computerized tomography and MRI scans, more talocalcaneal anomalies are being diagnosed (18). It now appears that talocalcaneal coalitions may be slightly more prevalent (8,35). Approximately 60% of the calcaneonavicular variety are bilateral compared to 50% of talocalcaneal coalitions (7). The coexistence of these two common types of coalitions occurring in the same foot is infrequent, but can occur (3,59). Numerous other coalitions have been recorded, but are extremely rare. Approximately 40 cases of talonavicular anomalies have been reported, although Schreiber (47) suggests that this form may be more common. Talonavicular coalitions are rarely associated with peroneal spastic flatfeet (35,42). Isolated cases of the calcaneocuboid coalitions have been reported, but are considered extremely uncommon and usually asymptomatic (1,28). Sporadic cases of naviculocuneiform (14,32) and cubonavicular coalitions (56) have been reported and are a rare cause of peroneal spastic flatfeet. Multiple tarsal coalitions in the same foot are more common than was once thought. One study showed that CT of 30 patients with tarsal coalitions demonstrated multiple coalitions in the same foot in six patients (3).

Tarsal coalitions may be fibrous, cartilaginous, or osseous. Coalitions are fibrous or cartilaginous during the first years of life and only later start to ossify. It is hypothesized that the non-ossified anomaly may allow some joint motion, which explains why tarsal coalitions rarely become symptomatic until the start of ossification. It has been suggested the mechanical stress across a tarsal coalition produces strain in the periosteum that is dissipated over a larger area when the coalition is still elastic such as a fibrous coalition. Once ossification occurs, the strain is concentrated in a smaller area of the periosteum and may account for the development of symptoms (22). This theory is supported in a histopathologic study that looked at 55 feet in 48 patients with non-osseous tarsal coalitions. The histologic findings of the coalitions showed no nerve elements in the fibrocollagenous tissue of the coalition but nerve elements were present in the periosteum and articular capsule surrounding the coalition. The stress across an incomplete coalition can therefore produce microfractures and remodeling that can result in pain from the nerve endings in the periosteum and capsule surrounding the coalition (23). The different types of tarsal coalition ossify at different times: talonavicular between 3 and 5 years; calcaneonavicular between 8 and 12 years; and talocalcaneal between 12 and 16 years (7). These seem to correlate with the times these different types of coalitions often become symptomatic.

The subtalar joint involves three facet joints between the calcaneus and talus (Figure 11-1). The largest is the posterior facet through which most of the body weight is born across the subtalar joint. The middle facet is supported by the sustentaculum tali on the medial aspect of the calcaneus. The small anterior facet of the calcaneus can be confluent with the middle facet. The most common bridge between the talus and calcaneus involves the middle facet. This condition can occasionally involve part of the anterior facet or rarely the posterior facet. Harris describes four types of medial talocalcaneal coalitions (17). The complete type involves a continuous bony bridge connecting the talus and calcaneus while the incomplete type has bony projections from the medial talus and sustentaculum tali separated by a thin plate of cartilage or fibrous tissue. This incomplete type may be a coalition that is in the final stage of ossification, although it may persist into adult life. Harris also describes two rudimentary forms of middle facet talocalcaneal coalitions in which either the talar or sustentaculum tali portion of the bridge is present. These rudimentary types have a bony projection extending from either the medial talus or calcaneus which allows limited subtalar motion, but blocks inversion. The rudimentary coalitions may present symptomatically like a complete bridge and are more consistent with an anomalous middle facet. All four of these types of middle facet coalitions were found in the computerized tomography evaluation of 20 symptomatic talocalcaneal coalitions by Herzenberg et al (19).

Another variation of the middle facet coalition has recently been described by Rassi (45). This study described 19 patients that had 23 feet that were clinically very similar to the findings of a middle facet coalition. In these patients, the CT scan and MRI scan were normal but a bone scan showed slight uptake in the area of the middle facet. The study concluded this was a form of arthrofibrosis involving the middle facet of the talocalcaneal joint. At the time of surgery, a hypervascular capsule and synovium was found and resection of this tissue resulted in resolution of symptoms.

RADIOGRAPHY

The radiographic evaluation for a suspected tarsal coalition should begin with plain AP, lateral, and oblique

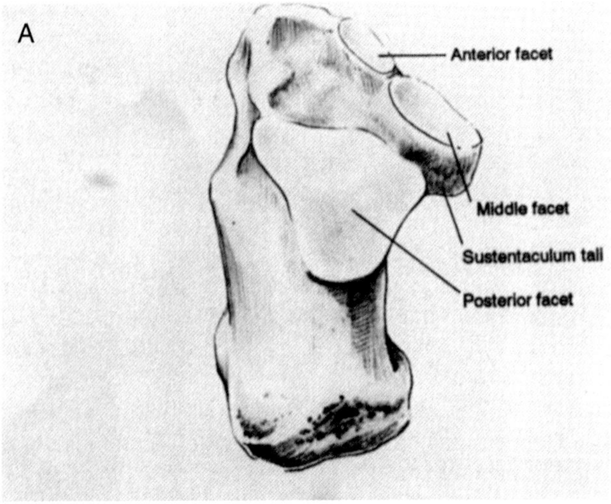

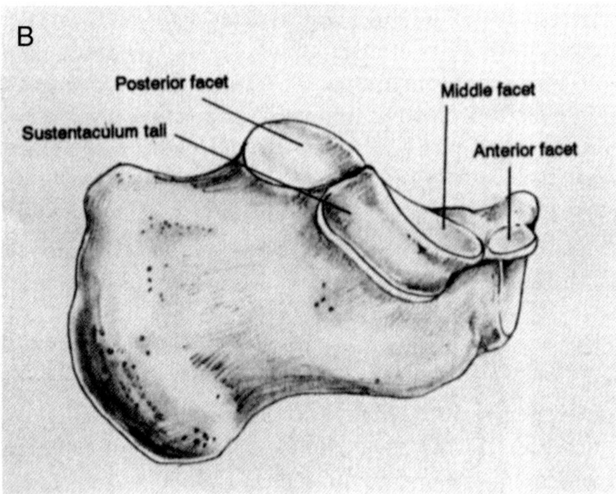

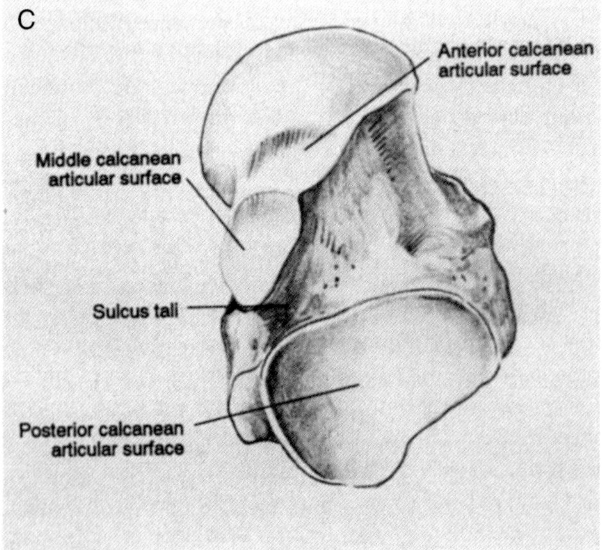

FIGURE 11-1 Dorsal view (**A**) and medial view (**B**) of the calcaneus demonstrating the arrangement of the articular facets. Plantar view (**C**) of the talus demonstrating the articular surfaces that articulate with their respective facets on the calcaneus.

radiographs of the foot. The diagnosis of calcaneonavicular, talonavicular, and calcaneocuboid coalitions can usually be made on plain radiographs, while the talocalcaneal variety cannot. The calcaneonavicular anomaly is best seen on the 45-degree oblique view where the space between the bones is totally obliterated in a complete ossified coalition (Figure 11-2). When the calcaneonavicular coalition is non-osseous the oblique radiograph demonstrated an elongation of either the calcaneus or navicular, and irregular juxtaposed cortical bone between them (Figure 11-3). The calcaneus and navicular do not normally articulate, so any apparent connection on the oblique radiograph is suggestive of a coalition. Other secondary signs of an incomplete calcaneonavicular bridge on the oblique radiograph are hypoplasia of the talar head and flattening of the navicular as it approaches the calcaneus. Occasionally, the overlapping structures of the foot may stimulate a calcaneonavicular coalition on the oblique view. The lateral x-ray of the foot in patients with a calcaneonavicular bridge will usually demonstrate the so-called "anteater nose sign" (36). This is a tubular elongation of the anterior superior aspect of the calcaneus directed toward or overlapping the middle portion of the navicular (Figure 11-4). The anterior superior aspect of the calcaneus may approach the mid-navicular region in feet without coalitions, but will lack the tubular protrusion noted in calcaneonavicular coalitions.

Even though the diagnosis of a calcaneonavicular coalition can usually be made on plain x-rays, a CT scan or MRI scan is usually recommended for complete evaluation. This is done for two primary reasons. The first is to rule out a second coalition in the same foot which can occasionally occur. The second indication for further radiographic evaluation of calcaneonavicular coalitions is the marked variability of this coalition. Cooperman et al. showed that the anatomy of calcaneonavicular coalitions is quite variable and often involves part of the subtalar or transverse tarsal joints (6). This study showed that in some cases the calcaneonavicular coalition partially or completely replaced the anterior calcaneal facet. This information may be helpful when planning surgical excision of this type of coalition. This possible extension of the calcaneonavicular coalition into the subtalar or transverse tarsal joints may also explain why some patients have less than satisfactory results after coalition excision.

Unlike the calcaneonavicular coalition, the talocalcaneal coalition cannot be seen on AP, lateral, and oblique radiographs of the foot. This is due largely to the fact that the obliquely orientated middle and posterior facets of the subtalar joint are obscured by overlapping bony shadows in most plain radiographs. The only plain radiograph that may demonstrate a subtalar coalition is an axial view of the calcaneus often called a Harris view. The Harris view, which is a 45-degree axial view of the hindfoot, was first described by Korvin in 1934 (21). This axial view can demonstrate a talocalcaneal coalition of the middle facet or posterior facet (Figure 11-5), but is often hard to interpret. The x-ray is taken with the patient

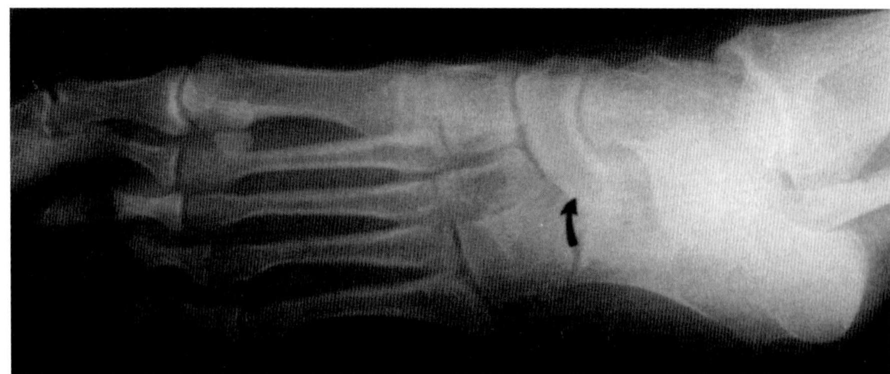

FIGURE 11-2 Oblique radiograph of the left foot of a 14-year-old girl with a completely ossified calcaneonavicular coalition.

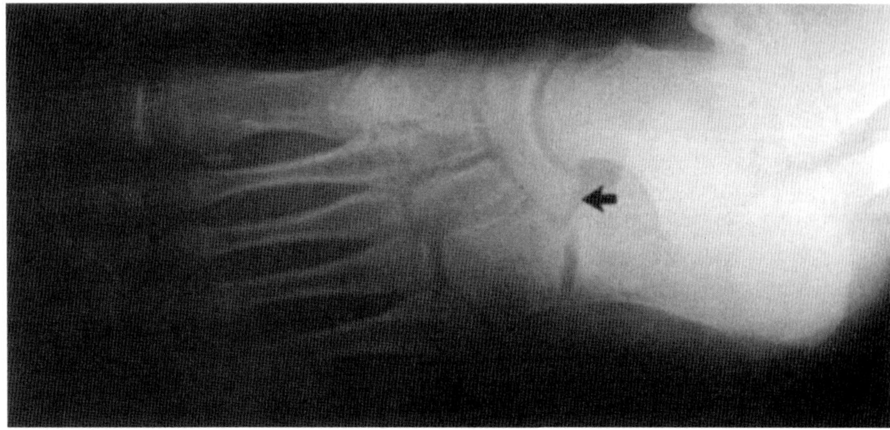

FIGURE 11-3 Oblique radiograph of the right foot of a 15-year-old boy with a cartilaginous calcaneonavicular coalition. Note the elongation of the navicular and the irregular juxtaposed cortical bone between the calcaneus and navicular.

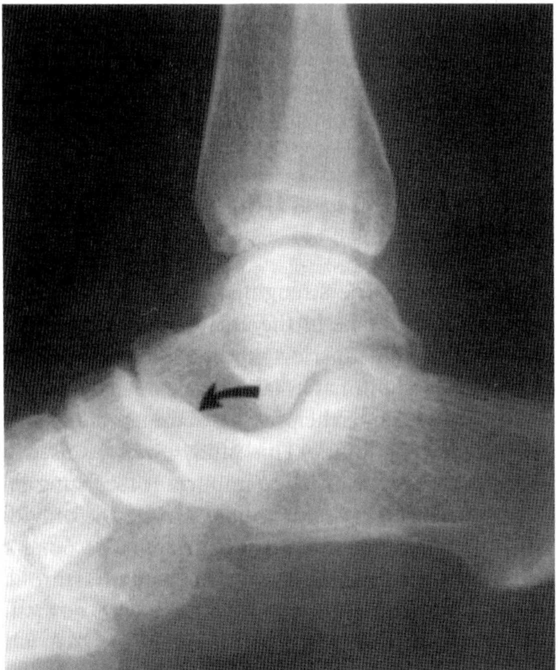

FIGURE 11-4 Lateral radiograph of the foot of a 14-year-old girl with a calcaneonavicular coalition demonstrating the "anteater sign."

standing on the film cassette and bending forward at the ankle at an angle of approximately 10 degrees. The x-ray tube is then positioned to shoot through the subtalar joint at an angle of 45 degrees to the horizontal. This is usually the angle of the middle and posterior facet, but final x-ray tube position may have to be adjusted for variations in the human foot. When the 45-degree axial view does not demonstrate the middle and posterior facets, then the angle these form with the horizontal can be measured on the lateral radiograph and the x-ray tube adjusted accordingly (7). On the axial view, the posterior and middle facets are horizontal and parallel to each other. In a completely ossified coalition, the middle facet will be obliterated and hypertrophic bone may be present. An oblique plane of the middle facet or hypertrophy of the sustentaculum tali are suggestive of a fibrous or cartilaginous coalition (41). The anterior facet cannot be visualized on the Harris view. The axial view is often difficult to interpret and treatment should not be based on this view alone. Computerized tomography and MRI scans have almost completely replaced the axial view in the diagnosis of talocalcaneal coalitions.

Like the calcaneonavicular coalitions, the talocalcaneal coalitions also have secondary radiographic signs that are sometimes seen on the lateral radiograph of the foot. The findings include: (i) talar beaking; (ii) posterior facet narrowing; and (iii) flattening or broadening of the lateral talar process (7) (Figure 11-6). Additional signs include a concave under-surface of the talar neck and failure to visualize the middle subtalar facet (10). While these findings are more common in talocalcaneal coalitions, they can sometimes be present in calcaneonavicular bridges or any condition that restricts subtalar motion. The talar beaking

should look closely at the area posterior to the sustentaculum tali for signs of non-osseous coalition.

Although CT has long been considered a gold standard for diagnosis of middle facet coalition, it is being replaced in some institutions by the MRI scan. Studies have shown that both a CT scan and MRI scan are very good at diagnosing most types of middle facet coalitions. The CT scan is more cost effective while the MRI scan is considered better at diagnosing fibrous coalitions (57). Another advantage of the MRI scan over CT scan is the MRI scan's ability to demonstrate osteochondral lesions of the ankle or subtalar joint, if this condition is suspected in addition to a middle facet coalition (11).

PATHOMECHANICS

At birth the tarsal coalitions are usually fibrous or cartilaginous and allow some motion across the affected joint. This explains why young children are usually asymptomatic and why plain radiographs are usually normal. The various forms start to ossify at different times: talonavicular forms at 3 to 5 years; calcaneonavicular at 8 to 12 years; and talocalcaneal at 12 to 16 years. When the coalition ossifies, it limits subtalar motion and can lead to the onset of symptoms. Subtalar motion is restricted in talonavicular and calcaneonavicular coalitions while usually absent in talocalcaneal coalitions. Even with complete absence of subtalar motion secondary to a tarsal coalition, there may be increase secondary motion at the ankle joint which can be misinterrupted as subtalar motion on physical exam. Why some coalitions become symptomatic and others do not is not yet known. One histopathology study by Kumai et al. looked at 55 feet in 48 patients with non-osseous tarsal coalitions (23). The histologic findings were similar to those observed in sites of Osgood-Schlatter disease or accessory navicular. Nerve elements were present only in the periosteum and surrounding capsule of the coalition. It was suggested from this study that incomplete coalitions produce micro fractures and mechanical stress across the tarsal coalition. This led to degenerative changes that seemed to induce pain from nerve endings in the periosteum and in the capsule surrounding the coalition. A case report by Katayama et al. showed the association of the onset of symptoms in a patient with a talocalcaneal coalition when progressive ossification was seen on diagnostic imaging. This case study also suggested that the potential pain with tarsal coalition was caused by mechanical stress (22).

The development of a significant valgus deformity of the foot with tarsal coalitions may also be related to the development of symptoms. During walking, the normal subtalar joint has a rotatory and gliding motion. The gliding movement has been demonstrated by cineradiography (40). There is a forward sliding of the calcaneus on the talus during dorsiflexion. During initial stance phase, there is an average of 4 degrees of external rotation/valgus of the calcaneus. As stance continues, the subtalar rotation returns to neutral and then proceeds to approximately 16 degrees of internal rotation/varus at the end of stance phase (35). When subtalar motion is restricted by a tarsal coalition the calcaneus is forced into valgus and the navicular starts to override the head of the talus. The overriding of the navicular on the talus leads to the talar beaking often seen in patients with tarsal coalitions. The talar beaking is felt to be the result of traction on the joint capsule and dorsal talonavicular ligament by the abnormal motion of the navicular (40). The valgus tilt of the calcaneus ranges from very slight without loss of the longitudinal arch, to very severe with associated mid-foot valgus and complete loss of the longitude arch. There does not seem to be a direct correlation between the amount of deformity and severity of symptoms although two recent studies have demonstrated a poorer prognosis for coalition resections in patients with significant valgus (26,60). The valgus tilt of the calcaneus can also lead to narrowing of the posterior talocalcaneal facet and impingement of the talus on the lateral aspect of the calcaneus, causing broadening and flattening of the lateral talar process. Both of these signs can often be seen on the lateral radiograph of patients with tarsal coalitions.

Although peroneal spasms once thought to be common in patients with a tarsal coalition, is now in fact, an uncommon finding in this condition. There is some question whether this represents true muscle spasm or whether the clinical findings are a response to adaptive contracture of the peronei secondary to the rigid valgus of the hindfoot. Some patients have constant spasm of the peroneal muscles while others may demonstrate a reflex spasm only when an attempt is made to invert the foot. Reflex peroneal muscle spasm can result from the foot being forced into inversion, for example, with trauma such as an ankle sprain. This may explain why many patients with symptomatic tarsal coalitions relate a history of mild trauma or change in activity associated with the onset of symptoms. A second explanation includes the fact the valgus tilt of the subtalar joint is the "relaxed" position which allows for the least amount of intra-articular pressure (21). Any mechanism, for example, an ossifying talocalcaneal coalition that causes irritation of the subtalar joint can lead to reflex spasm as the peronei try to stabilize the joint. It should be noted there are additional causes of subtalar irritation which can lead to a similar clinical picture (8).

Although tarsal coalition is the most common cause of symptomatic decreased subtalar motion accompanied by peroneal spasm, other causes must be considered. A complete list of the differential diagnosis of peroneal spastic flatfeet (Table 11-1) was published by Mosier et al. and includes various types of systemic arthritis, infection, osteochondral injury, as well as iatrogenic causes (35). These rare causes of peroneal spastic flatfeet can usually be ruled out by a thorough history and physical examination.

CLINICAL FINDINGS

Tarsal coalitions may be totally asymptomatic and merely be an incidental radiographic finding. Pain is the

TABLE 11-1

Differential Diagnosis of Peroneal Spastic Flatfoot

1. Coalitions
   - Calcaneonavicular (common)
   - Talocalcaneal
     - anterior facet (rare)
     - middle facet (common)
     - Posterior facet (rare)
2. Arthritis of the tarsus
   - Rheumatoid
   - Gout with subtalar urate deposits
   - Osteoarthritis
   - Post-traumatic
   - Tuberculous, in which an early stage may be limited to part of a joint.
3. Inflammation of the tarsus
4. Infection of the tarsus, which may lead to bone ankylosis
5. Large bone-mass malformation of the sustentaculum leading to a block in motion; this may be difficult to diagnose radiographically.
6. Acromegaly
7. Fibrosarcoma
8. Osteochondral fracture of the undersurface of the talar head
9. Osteitis deformans
10. Osteochondritis dissecans
11. Osteochondrodystrophy (Morquio's disease)
12. Latrogenic, usually causing only secondary radiographic sings.[a]
    - Overzealous cast correction of clubfoot
    - Grice procedure
    - Gallie subtalar arthrodesis
    - Postoperative subtalar arthrodesis
13. Occupational strain leading to spasm
14. Rigid flatfoot, which is the same as peroneal spastic flatfoot but without the spasm.
15. Reflaxed or flexible flatfoot. This deformity exists in childhood: the mid-tarsal joint is hypermobile, and pain may develop in adolescent or later, caused by excessive ligament strain and traumatic arthritis.

[a] It is important to remember that these secondary radiographic signs are not specific for tarsal coalition. They are associated with limited subtalar motion, and any condition that decreases subtalar motion may result in similar radiographic signs. From Mosier KM, Asher MA. Tarsal coalition and peroneal spastic flatfoot. *J Bone Joint Surg [Am]* 66:976–983, 1984.

principal presenting symptom and usually develops during the second decade of life when ossification of the bar starts to occur. The pain is usually insidious in onset, although at times the onset is associated with a specific injury or change in activity. The discomfort is frequently aggravated by activity and relieved by rest. The pain in a talocalcaneal coalition is usually vague and located deep within the subtalar joint. At times, tenderness can be localized to the middle facet by palpation distal to the medial malleolus. Symptoms in talocalcaneal coalitions have also been reported in the area of the talonavicular joint. The pain in a calcaneonavicular coalition is usually located laterally over the area of the coalition and may also have tenderness to direct palpation of the area of fusion. Symptomatic talonavicular coalitions usually present as a hard prominence over the medial aspect of the foot with pain being less of a problem. Talonavicular coalitions may predispose adjacent joints to degenerative changes in adult life.

Subtalar motion is usually restricted when the coalition begins to ossify. Subtalar motion is obliterated in the talocalcaneal variety while in calcaneonavicular and talonavicular coalitions, subtalar and mid-foot motion is only moderately limited. Recurrent ankle sprains can occur with coalitions and can lead to ligamentous laxity. This laxity can give a false impression of subtalar motion on physical exam. The subtalar motion may appear normal in some cases of calcaneonavicular coalition with ligamentous laxity, whereas there is always some clinical restriction in talocalcaneal coalitions.

The appearance of the hindfoot is often in valgus and may progresses as the coalitions ossify. The amount of deformity can vary from minimal to marked valgus with talocalcaneal coalitions causing more valgus than other types of coalitions. Although the degree of symptoms does not necessarily correlate with the amount of deformity, it does appear that patients with a more neutral alignment of the heel have fewer symptoms than patients with marked hindfoot and mid-foot valgus (7). As stated previously, often the area of discomfort is over the coalition in talocalcaneal and calcaneonavicular coalitions. If there is a marked amount of valgus with loss of the longitudinal arch some symptoms may be related to the valgus position of the foot. In these particular patients the discomfort may be located laterally from impingement of the calcaneus on the tip of the fibula or pain in the medial aspect of the longitudinal arch. It is important to try to determine where the area of discomfort is most noted by the patient because it may make a difference in treatment of the coalition and/or valgus position of the foot.

Peroneal spasms are rarely encountered but can occur presenting as a fixed valgus of the hindfoot and eversion of the midfoot. Patients in this situation often complain of pain extending up the lateral aspect of the calf when spasm is present. Any attempts to invert the foot causes marked increase in pain. A varus deformity of the hindfoot secondary to spasm of the posterior and anterior tibial tendons has been reported with calcaneonavicular coalitions but it is extremely rare (49, 50). One study by Comfort and Johnson reported four patients with the uncommon varus deformity secondary to talocalcaneal coalition that had undergone resection of the coalition (5). Overall, this varus subgroup had a poor outcome from resection treatment.

TREATMENT

The treatment of symptomatic tarsal coalition consists of three basic types: conservative, coalition excision, and hindfoot arthrodesis. The initial treatment of any symptomatic tarsal coalition should be conservative and include activity modification and introduction of a custom plastizote insert. A four- to six-week period of immobilization in a short leg cast can be tried should these conservative measures fail. The trial of immobilization can be repeated, but if conservative methods continue to fail, then surgery is indicated. Resection can be considered with mild to moderate symptoms in calcaneonavicular coalitions since there is a higher likelihood of a good result. Resection is performed with the idea of obtaining as normal foot motion as possible (7). Because excision of talocalcaneal coalition has a less predictable outcome, resection should probably not be performed in the minimally symptomatic foot.

Most studies have reported good results with excision of calcaneonavicular coalitions (13,20,33,34). Gonzales et al. (13) reported a 77% good or excellent result with this procedure. They stated their best results were found in patients less than 16 years of age and that this group showed no deterioration in results in 10 years of follow up. Even though this study suggested the results were better in younger patients, Cohen et al. reported 13 calcaneonavicular coalition excisions in 12 adult patients (4). Subjective relief of preoperative symptoms was achieved in all but two of these adult patients suggesting that resection of a calcaneonavicular coalition can be considered in the older patient. Swiontkowski et al. (53) reported successful excision in 35 out of 39 patients with calcaneonavicular coalitions. The four patients with no improvement had degenerative changes of the talonavicular joint noted on radiographs at the time of the procedure. Inglis et al. (20) reported eleven patients with 16 calcaneonavicular coalition excisions followed an average of 23 years and found the good results continued with time. Chambers et al. (2) showed that patients with good subtalar motion after calcaneonavicular coalition resections developed a symmetrical gait pattern with functional testing.

Surgical excision of talocalcaneal coalitions is more controversial. Earlier studies favored triple arthrodesis while more recent studies report encouraging success with talocalcaneal coalition excisions. Olney et al. (38) reported eight out of ten patients with excellent or good result with talocalcaneal coalition excisions. The functional results of these patients were comparable to the results of patients with calcaneonavicular coalition excision. Scranton (48) had 13 of 14 good results of talocalcaneal coalition excision. His indications included a coalition involving less than half the subtalar joint and no associated radiographic talonavicular arthritis. Swiontkowski et al. (53) and Danielsson (9) also reported successful resection of talocalcaneal coalitions in small groups of patients. Since the results of resection talocalcaneal coalition is less predictable several recent studies have tried to identify subgroups of patients with poor outcomes. Two factors that seem to point to a poorer outcome after talocalcaneal coalition resection is an increase in the valgus deformity of the foot and a large coalition greater than 50% of the area of the posterior facet. (5,26,60). Luhmann and Schoenecker reported the results of talocalcaneal coalition resection in 25 feet (26). They found a better outcome from coalition resection if heel valgus was less than 21 degrees and the coalition was less than 50% of the size of the posterior facet. They recommended that if the hindfoot valgus was greater than 21 degrees then an orthosis was needed postoperatively to stabilize the hindfoot or a secondary calcaneal procedure was necessary to correct the hindfoot valgus. Wilde et al. looked at 20 feet with persistent symptomatic talocalcaneal coalitions treated with bar resection (60). They found a poorer outcome if the coalition was greater than 50% of the subtalar joint or the hindfoot valgus was greater than 16 degrees. Comfort and Johnson looked at talocalcaneal coalition resection in 20 persistently symptomatic feet. They found good or excellent clinical results in 77% of the patients if the size of the tarsal coalition was less than one-third of the surface area of the total subtalar joint (5).

From these more recent studies, it appears the size of the talocalcaneal coalition as well as the preoperative valgus deformity of the calcaneus both affect the possible outcome of coalition resection. Excision of the talocalcaneal coalition does not result in correction of the posture of the foot, a factor which needs to be discussed with the patient prior to surgery. It seems reasonable to attempt resection of talocalcaneal coalitions unless the coalition is unusually large or there are associated degenerative changes in adjacent joints. If the hindfoot valgus is significant, the patient needs to understand that orthotics may be necessary post resection to help support the foot or that secondary procedures such as calcaneal osteotomies or lateral column lengthenings may be necessary to correct the valgus deformity of the foot.

Most authors recommend hindfoot arthrodesis when excision of calcaneonavicular coalitions or talocalcaneal coalitions fail or if there are degenerative changes of the hindfoot present initially (3,29,30). This can be a triple arthrodesis if there are degenerative changes extensively in the hindfoot or possibly a subtalar fusion in some selective cases. The fusion is performed as an "*in situ*" arthrodesis when the hindfoot is in a satisfactory position or may include a corrective component when the hindfoot or mid-foot are in valgus. The presence of talar beaking is not a contraindication to coalition excision because it does not represent degenerative changes (25,53).

TECHNIQUE OF CALCANEONAVICULAR COALITION

The technique of excising a calcaneonavicular coalition (Figure 11-10) includes resection of the bony bar and the interposition of the extensor digitorum brevis muscle between the separated bones to act as a soft tissue barrier to recurrent bar formation (7,13). Under tourniquet control an oblique

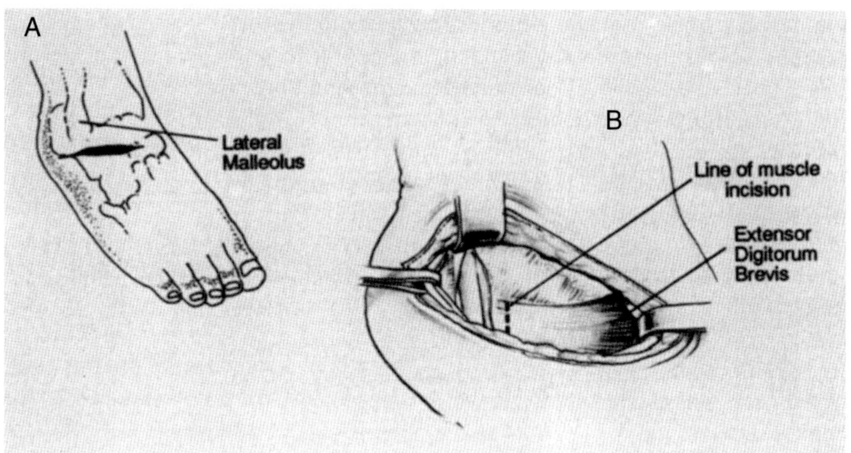

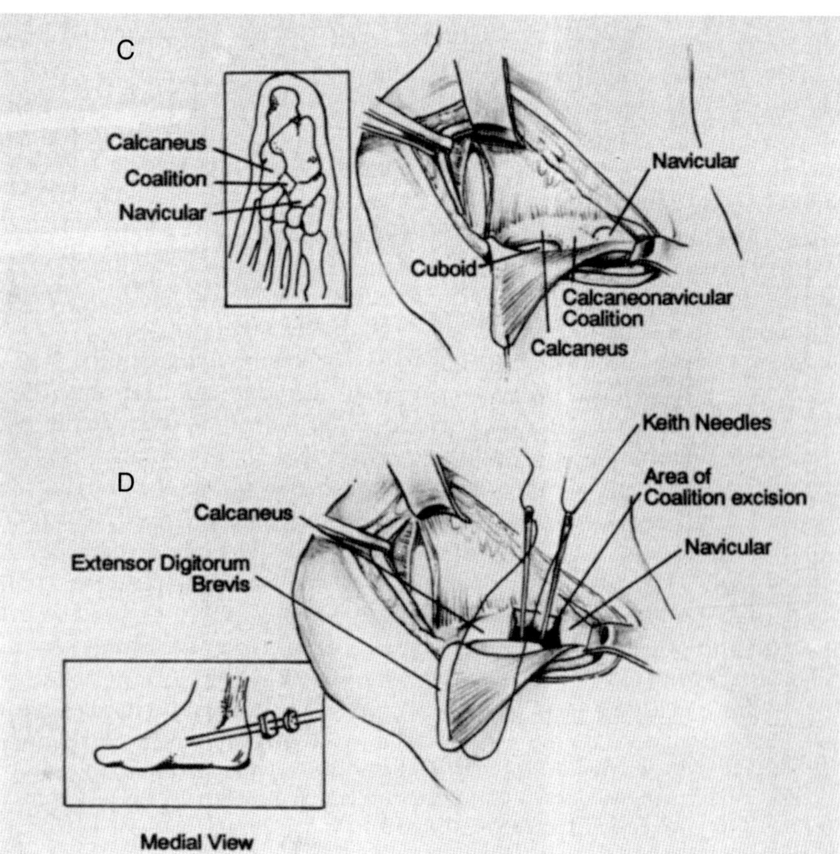

FIGURE 11-10 Technique of excision of calcaneonavicular coalition (see text). **A.** An oblique incision is made over the lateral aspect of the dorsal hindfoot. **B.** The peroneal tendons and sural nerve are retracted in the lower aspect of the incision. **C.** The extensor digitorum brevis is sharply elevated off the calcaneus to expose the coalition. The coalition is resected with two parallel cuts in the bone. **D.** Absorbable sutures are attached to the extensor digitorum brevis muscle and passed through the coalition reception to the medial aspect of the foot on Keith needles. When the sutures are tied over a button, the muscle is pulled into the void left by the coalition resections.

incision is made on the dorsolateral aspect of the hindfoot, centered over the coalition. The coalition can usually be palpated as fullness in the area of the sinus tarsi. The extensor digitorum brevis muscle is identified and sharply elevated from its origin on the calcaneus. Care should be taken to protect the peroneal tendons and sural nerve in the lower part of the incision. After elevating the extensor digitorum brevis muscle, the calcaneonavicular coalition can be identified. It is wise to demarcate the talonavicular, talocalcaneal, and calcaneocuboid joints after the coalition has been isolated. The surgeon must bear in mind that occasionally the calcaneonavicular coalition may involve all or part of the anterior facet of the subtalar joint (6). This will help prevent an iatrogenic insult to these joints which could result in decreased motion or eventual development of degenerative arthritis. The coalition is removed as a rectangle of bone by placing two parallel osteotome cuts perpendicular to the cortex. The piece of bone excised should be rectangular instead of a triangle to ensure that bony impingement will not occur in the depth of the resected area. Any bone remaining in the depth of the excision can be removed with a rongeur until only soft tissue is visible. There should now be demonstrable unrestricted motion between the calcaneus and navicular and between the talus and calcaneus. Bone wax is pressed onto the cut surfaces of the bone to control bleeding and to help prevent recurrence of the bar. Absorbable suture is placed through the origin of the extensor digitorum brevis muscle. The sutures are passed through the area of the coalition excision with a Keith needle and brought out through the non–weightbearing medial aspect of the mid-foot. The extensor digitorum brevis is pulled into the space that was created by the resection and the sutures are snugly tied over a felt pad and button. A free-fat graft can be placed into the area of coalition resection as an alternative spacer. Postoperatively the patient is placed in a short leg non–weight-bearing cast for three to four weeks. The cast and button are then removed. Non–weight-bearing active range of motion is begun and gradually increasing weight bearing is started at six weeks postoperatively when satisfactory motion has been achieved. An orthotic is used if there is significant hindfoot valgus and a secondary surgical procedure (medial shift or lengthening calcaneal osteotomy) is considered for persistent symptoms related to the valgus posture.

TECHNIQUE OF TALOCALCANEAL COALITION EXCISION

Excision of talocalcaneal coalitions (Figure 11-11) involves a medial approach to the middle facet approximately 6 cm in

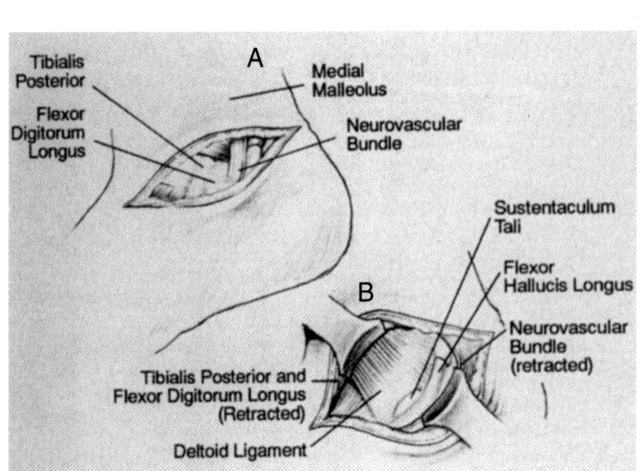

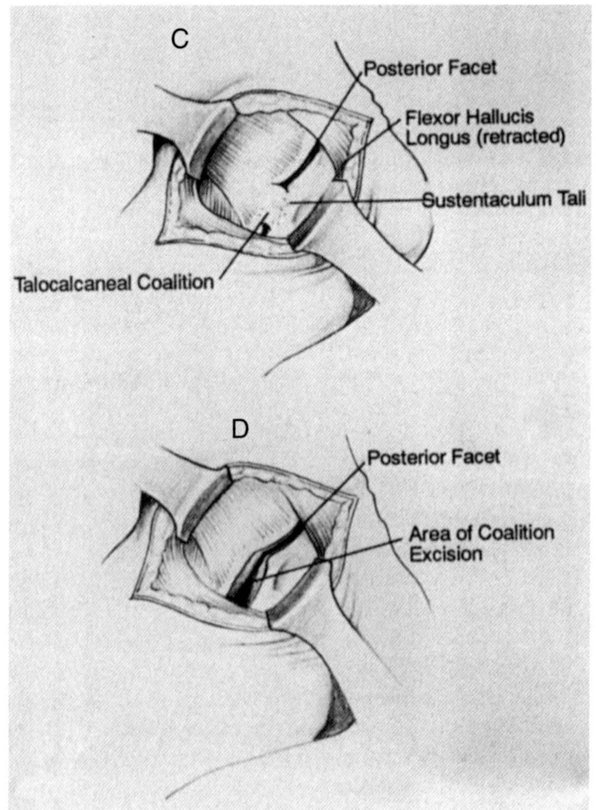

FIGURE 11-11 Technique of excision of talocalcaneal middle facet coalition (see text). **A.** An incision is made over the middle aspect of the hindfoot, centered over the sustentaculum tali. **B.** The tibialis posterior and flexor digitorum longus tendons are dissected off the coalition and retracted dorsally. The neurovascular bundle is retracted plantarward. **C.** The middle facet coalitions is identified just above the sustentaculum tali. **D.** The coalition is resected until there is free motion across the subtalar joint.

length and centered over the sustentaculum tali (37,38). The abductor hallucis muscle is reflected plantarward if necessary. The tendons and neurovascular structures behind the medial malleolus usually overlie the coalition and need to be dissected free in order to determine the anterior and posterior extent of the coalition. The exact location and size of the coalition should be determined preoperatively by coronal plane computerized tomography. The flexor digitorum longus, flexor hallucis longus, and neurovascular bundle (tibial nerve, posterior tibial artery, and vein) are dissected off the coalition and retracted plantarward. It is often easier to identify the posterior facet and trace it distally to find the posterior edge of the coalition. The anterior aspect of the coalition can be found anterior to the sustentaculum tali which can be identified by the flexor hallucis longus tendon running directly beneath it. Once the extent of the coalition is determined, it is removed with osteotomes, rongeurs, or a power burr. Care is taken not to injure the anterior and posterior facets and to leave enough of the sustentaculum tali to support the flexor hallucis longus tendon. The coalition must be completely resected until there is demonstrated motion across the subtalar joint without any accompanying crepitus or impingement. When the coalition involves only part of the middle facet, then resection is carried back to normal articular cartilage. The facet must be removed in its entirety when the coalition involves the whole facet. Bone wax is pressed onto the resected surfaces and a free fat graft is placed into the resultant space. The fat may be taken from the retrocalcaneal adipose tissue in the posterior aspect of the incision or through a separate incision along the medial border of the Achilles tendon. The fat is held in place by the closure of the overlying soft tissues which may include either the periosteum or tendon sheaths. The flexor retinaculum is repaired as well. The postoperative protocol is similar to that for calcaneonavicular coalition excision, including the possible use of orthotics and secondary valgus-correcting osteotomies.

The interposition of fat graft seems to be the most popular surgical technique following excision of talocalcaneal middle facet coalition, however several studies have reported alternatives to this surgical technique in isolated studies. Westberry reported the treatment of talocalcaneal middle facet coalitions by resection of the sustentaculum tali in 12 feet with excellent results in 8, good results in 3, and 1 patient with a poor result (58). Raikin reported middle facet coalition excision in 14 feet but interposed a split portion of the flexor hallucis longus tendon (44). This study showed excellent results in 11 patients, good results in 1, and 2 patients having fair or poor results. Takakura reported good results of talocalcaneal middle facet coalition excision but did not use a fat graft or other interposition material (55).

Since resection of talocalcaneal coalitions has shown favorable outcomes, it seems reasonable to attempt resection in most cases. The main contraindications are associated degenerative changes of the subtalar or adjacent joints, severe valgus, or large coalition which include a large surface area compared to the rest of the subtalar joint. The entire middle facet of the subtalar joint can be resected when the anterior and posterior facets are intact and uninvolved with the coalition (20). When these contraindications are present or when primary resection fails to relieve the symptoms, hindfoot arthrodesis is the treatment of choice. Triple arthrodesis has long been an accepted treatment for talocalcaneal coalitions. Indications for a triple arthrodesis should include correction of any moderate to severe valgus deformity of the foot. Several studies have reported that isolated subtalar fusion can relieve the pain associated with talocalcaneal coalitions (29,30,54), and this may represent an option when there is no associated arthritis in the talonavicular or calcaneocuboid joints.

KEY POINTS

1. The radiographic diagnosis of a calcaneonavicular coalition can be made on the oblique plain radiograph while the diagnosis of talocalcaneal coalitions requires a CT or MRI scan.
2. Even if the diagnosis of a tarsal coalition is made on plain radiographs, a CT scan or MRI scan should be obtained to rule out other anomalies such as a second coalition, as well as determine the exact size and location of the coalition.
3. Surgical excision of a persistently symptomatic coalition should be attempted prior to arthrodesis unless there are specific contraindications to surgical excision.
4. Surgical excision of a tarsal coalition does not alter the preoperative posture of the hindfoot or mid-foot.
5. Patients with a significant valgus deformity of the hindfoot are less likely to have a good result from surgical excision of a coalition alone and may require postoperative orthotic use or a secondary surgical procedure to correct the valgus deformity.

SUMMARY

A tarsal coalition is a congenital connection between two or more tarsal bones that may become symptomatic when it begins to ossify. The two most common types of tarsal coalition are the calcaneonavicular and talocalcaneal varieties. Physical examination may show a decrease in subtalar motion and the patient can complain of either vague hindfoot pain or specific pain over the coalition. Some feet with a tarsal coalition may assume a significant valgus posture that can contribute to the symptomatology. The calcaneonavicular coalitions can usually be seen on an oblique radiograph while the talocalcaneal coalitions require a CT or MRI scan. A CT or MRI scan should still be considered in all patients with a tarsal coalition to rule out a second coalition or other anomalies of the hindfoot or mid-foot. Conservative treatment with activity limitation, orthotics, or immobilization should be attempted in all patients with tarsal coalitions before surgical treatment is considered. Surgical excision of the tarsal coalition is indicated for persistently symptomatic feet and is preferable to an arthrodesis unless there is a contra indication to coalition excision such as associated arthritic changes in the subtalar or adjacent joints. Another relative contraindication of surgical excision is a large subtalar coalition that involves over 50% of the total subtalar joint. Patients with significant valgus deformities of the hindfoot also seem to have a less chance of a satisfactory outcome from surgical excision of the coalition. Because the excision of the coalition does not change the position of the foot, then a significant valgus deformity may require postoperative orthotics or possibly a secondary procedure to correct the valgus deformity of the foot. If the patient has contraindications to coalition excision or has a poor result after excision, then a subtalar or triple arthrodesis should be considered.

REFERENCES

1. Brobeck O. Cogenital bilateral synostosis of the calcaneus and cuboid and the triquetral and hamate bones. *Acta Orthop Scand* 1957;26:217.
2. Chambers RB, Cook TM, Cowell HR. Surgical reconstruction for calcaneonavicular coalition. *J Bone Joint Surg [Am]* 64:829–836, 1982.
3. Clarke DM. Multiple tarsal coalitions in the same foot. *J Pediatr Orthop* 17:777–780, 1997.
4. Cohen BE, Davis WH, Anderson RB. Success of calcaneonavicular coalition resection in the adult population. *Foot Ankle Int* 17(9):569–572, Sept 1996.
5. Comfort TK, Johnson LO. Resection for symptomatic talocalcaneal coalition. *J Pediatr Orthop* 18:283–288, 1998.
6. Cooperman DR, Janke BE, Gilmore A, Latimer BM, Brinker MR, Thompson GH. A three-dimensional study of calcaneonavicular tarsal coalitions. *J Pediatr Orthop* 21:648–651, Sep–Oct 2001.
7. Cowell HR. Diagnosis and management of peroneal spastic flatfoot. *Instr Course Lect* 1975;24:94–103.
8. Cowell HR. Talocalcaneal coalition and new causes of peroneal spastic flatfoot. *Clin Orthop* 85:16–22, 1972.
9. Danielsson LG. Talocalcaneal coalition treated with resection. *J Pediatr Orthop* 7:513–517, 1987.
10. Deutsch AL, Resnick D, Campbell G. Computed tomography and bone scintigraphy in the evaluation of tarsal coalitions. *Radiology* 144:137–140, 1982.
11. Emery KH, Bisset III GS, Johnson ND, Nunan PJ. Tarsal coalition: a blinded comparison of MRI and CT. *Pediatr Radiol* 28:612–616, 1998.
12. Goldman AB, Pavlov H, Schneider R. Radionuclide bone scanning in subtalar conditions: differential considerations. *Am J Radiology* 138:427–432, 1982.
13. Gonzalez P, Kumar SJ. Calcaneonavicular coalition treated by resection and interposition of the extensor digitorum brevis muscle. *J Bone Joint Surg* [Am] 72:71–77, 1990.
14. Gregersen HN. Naviculocuneiform coalition. *J Bone Joint Surg [Am]* 59:128–130, 1977.
15. Harris BJ. Anomalous structures in the developing human foot. *Anat Rec* 121:399 (abst), 1955.
16. Harris RI. Retrospect-peroneal spastic flatfoot (rigid valgus foot). *J Bone Joint Surg [Am]* 47:1657–1667, 1965.
17. Harris RI, Beath T. Etiology of peroneal spastic flatfoot. *J Bone Joint Surg [Br]* 30:624–634, 1948.
18. Heiple KG, Lovejoy CO. The antiquity of tarsal coalition: bilateral deformity in a pre-Columbian Indian skeleton. *J Bone Joint Surg [Am]* 51:979–983, 1969.
19. Herzenberg JE, Goldner JL, Martinez S, Silverman PM. Computerized tomography of talocalcaneal tarsal coalition: a clinical and anatomic study. *Foot Ankle* 6:273–288, 1986.
20. Inglis G, Buxton RA, Macnicol MF. Symptomatic calcaneonavicular bars: the results 20 years after surgical excision. *J Bone Joint Surg [Br]* 68:128–131, 1986.
21. Jayakumar S, Cowell HR. Rigid flatfoot. *Clin Orthop* 122:77–84, 1977.
22. Katayama T, Tanaka Y, Kadono K, Taniguchi A, Takakura Y. Talocalcaneal coalition: a case showing the ossification process. *Foot Ankle Int* 26:490–493, June 2005.
23. Kumai T, Takakura Y, Akiyama K, Higashiyama I, Tamai S. Histopathological study of nonosseous tarsal coalition. *Foot Ankle Int* 19:525–531, August 1998.
24. Lateur LM, VanHoe LR, VanGhillewe KV, Gryspeerdt SS, Baert AL, Dereymaeker GE. Subtalar coalition: diagnosis with the C sign on lateral radiographs of the ankle. *Radiology* 193:847–851, 1994.
25. Lee MS, Harcke HT, Kumer SJ, Bassett GS. Subtalar joint coalition in children: new observations. *Radiology* 172:635–639, 1989.
26. Luhmann SJ, Schoenecker PL. Symptomatic talocalcaneal coalition resection: indications and results. *J Pediatr Orthop* 18:748–754, 1998.
27. Ma L. The inheritance of tarsal coalition and its relationship to spastic flatfoot. *J Bone Joint Surg [Br]* 56:520–526, 1974.
28. Mahaffey HW. Bilateral congenital calcaneocuboid synostosis. Case report. *J Bone Joint Surg* 27:164, 1945.
29. Mann RA, Beaman DN, Horton GA. Isolated subtalar arthrodesis. *Foot Ankle Int* 19(8):511–519, 1998.
30. Marchisello PJ. The use of computerized axial tomography for the evolution of talocalcaneal coalition. *J Bone Joint Surg [Am]* 69:609–611, 1987.
31. Martinez S, Herzenberg JE, Apple JS. Computed tomography of hindfoot. *Orthop Clin North Am* 16:483–495, 1985.
32. Miki T, Yamamuro T, Iida H, Ohta S, Oka M. Naviculocuneiform coalition: a report of two cases. *Clin Orthop* 196:256–259, 1985.
33. Mitchell GP, Gibson JMC. Exicision of calcaneonavicular bar for painful spasmodic flatfoot. *J Bone Joint Surg [Br]* 49:281–287, 1967.
34. Morgan RC, Crawford AH. Surgical management of tarsal coalition in adolescent athletes. *Foot Ankle* 7(3):183–193, 1986.
35. Mosier KM, Asher MA. Tarsal coalition and peroneal spastic flatfoot. *J Bone Joint Surg [Am]* 66:976–983, 1984.
36. Oestereich AE, Mize WA, Crawford AH, Morgan RC. The 'anteater nose": a direct sign of calcaneonavicular coalition on the lateral radiograph. *J Pediatr Orthop* 7:709–711,1987.
37. Olney BW. Foot and ankle. In: Reckling FW, Reckling JB, Mohn PP, eds. *Orthopaedic anatomy and surgical approaches.* St. Louis: Mosby Year Book, 1990;421–478.
38. Olney BW, Asher MA. Excision of symptomatic coalition of the middle facet of the talocalcaneal joint. *J Bone Joint Surg [Am]* 69:539–544, 1987.
39. O'Rahilly R, Gardner E, Gray DJ. The skeletal development of the foot. *Clin Orthop* 16:7–14, 1960.
40. Outland T, Murphy ID. The pathomechanics of peroneal spastic flatfoot. *Clin Orthop* 16:64–73, 1960.
41. Ozonoff MB. *Pediatric orthopaedic radiology.* Philadelphia: WB Saunders, 1979.
42. Percy EC, Mann DL. Tarsal coalition: a review of the literature and presentation of 13 cases. *Foot Ankle* 9:40–44, 1988.
43. Pineda C, Resnick D, Greenway G. Diagnosis of tarsal coalition with computed tomography. *Clin Orthop* 208:282–288, 1986.
44. Raikin S, Cooperman DR, Thompson GH. Interposition of the split flexor hallucis longus tendon after resection of a coalition of the middle facet of the talocalcaneal joint. *J Bone Joint Surg [Am]* 81:11–19, 1999.
45. Rassi GE, Riddle EC, Kumar SJ. Arthrofibrosis involving the middle facet of the talocalcaneal joint in children and adolescents. *J Bone Joint Surg [Am]* 87:2227–2231, 2005.
46. Resnick D. Talar ridges, osteophytes, and beaks: a radiology commentary. *Radiology* 151:329–332, 1984.

47. Schreiber RR. Talonavicular synostosis. *J Bone Joint Surg [Am]* 45:170–172, 1963.
48. Scranton PE. Treatment of symptomatic talocalcaneal coalition. *J Bone Joint Surg [Am]* 69:533–538, 1987.
49. Simmons EH. Tibialis spastic varus foot with tarsal coalition. *J Bone Joint Surg [Br]* 47:533–536, 1965.
50. Stuecker RD, Bennett JT. Tarsal coalition presenting as a pes cavo-varus deformity: report of three cases and review of the literature. *Foot Ankle* 14(9):540–544, Nov–Dec 1993.
51. Stormont DM, Peterson HA. The relative incidence of tarsal coalition. *Clin Orthop* 181:28–36, 1983.
52. Stoskopf CA, Hernandez RJ, Kelikian A, Tachdjian MO, Dias LS. Evaluation of tarsal coalition by computed tomography. *J Pediatr Orthop* 4:365–369, 1984.
53. Swiontkowski MF, Scranton PE, Hansen S. Tarsal coalition: long-term results of surgical treatment. *J Pediatr Orthop* 3:287–292, 1983.
54. Tachdjian MO. *Pediatric orthopaedics, 2nd ed.* Philadelphia: WB Saunders, 1990.
55. Takakura Y, Tamai S, Mosuhara K. Genesis of the ball-and-socket ankle. *J Bone Joint Surg [Br]* 68:834–837, 1986.
56. Waugh W. Partial cubo-navicular coalition as a cause of peroneal spastic flatfoot. *J Bone Joint Surg [Br]* 39:520–523, 1957.
57. Wechsler RJ, Schweitzer ME, Deely DM, Horn BD, Pizzutillo PD. Tarsal coalition: depiction and characterization with CT and MR imaging. *Radiology* 193:447–452, 1994.
58. Westberry DE, Davids JR, Oros W. Surgical management of symptomatic talocalcaneal coalitions by resection of the sustentaculum tali. *J Pediatr Orthop* 23:493–497, 2003.
59. Wheeler R, Guevera A, Bleck EE. Tarsal coalitions. *Clin Orthop* 156:175–177, 1981.
60. Wilde PH, Torode IP, Dickens DR, Cole WG. Resection for symptomatic talocalcaneal coalition. *J Bone Joint Surg [Br]* 76:797–801, 1994.
61. Wray JB, Herndon CN. Hereditary transmission of congenital coalition of the calcaneus to the navicular. *J Bone Joint Surg [Am]* 45:365–372, 1963.

CHAPTER 12

Cavus Deformity

S. Jay Kumar, Durga N. Kowtharapu and Kenneth J. Rogers

INTRODUCTION

Definition and Epidemiology

The cavovarus foot is an enigmatic deformity which is usually not present at birth but becomes manifest as the child grows (25). The first description of pes cavus was made by Andrey in 1743 (4). Pes cavus refers to a fixed equinus deformity of the forefoot in relation to the hindfoot, resulting in an abnormally high arch (Figure 12-1). The apex may be located at the level of the metatarsocuneiform joints. The first metatarsal alone or all five metatarsals may be depressed. The apex can also occur more proximally in the mid-tarsus. The heel may be in neutral, varus, valgus, calcaneus. The forefoot equinus is often accompanied by clawing of the toes.

The deformity is typically progressive and results from imbalance between the antagonist muscles of the foot as well as weakness of the intrinsic muscles (Figure 12-2). The etiology is not always certain, the pathology complex, and the treatment varied. In the past, a large number of feet were classified as idiopathic (53). As testing methods have become more sophisticated, only a small percentage of children fall into this category.

The treatment of pes cavus continues to challenge the orthopedic surgeon due to the multiple combinations of clinical deformities, the varying patterns of muscle imbalance, the diverse theories regarding etiology and pathogenesis, and the myriad surgical procedures which have been proposed, not only to correct the deformity, but also to prevent its recurrence.

ETIOLOGY

Over the years many theories, some contradictory, have been proposed. It is possible that a combination of mechanisms may account for the deformity. Brewerton has compiled a list of 22 processes which could lead to cavus deformity (13). Mills' comments on the etiology of "claw foot" in 1923 still apply today: "So far, none of the various suggestions as to the cause of claw foot has received general acceptance … the impression left in my mind from reading the list [of causes of the cavus foot] was one of surprise that anyone managed to escape the disease."(56)

Theories include primary contracture of the plantar fascia (65), along with various combinations of underactivity or overactivity of the intrinsic and extrinsic muscles of the foot (57).

Lesions of the spinal cord such as diastomatomyelia, hydromyelia, poliomyelitis, sequelae of compartment syndrome of the foot, tethered cord, and tumors in the spinal cord often cause unilateral cavovarus feet. Bilateral cavovarus feet are characteristically secondary to a peripheral neuropathy like Charcot-Marie-Tooth disease, Freidreich's ataxia, Roussy-Levy syndrome, polyneuritis, Guillain-Barré syndrome, and cerebral palsy (70).

Approximately half the patients who present with a cavovarus foot deformity present as a result of a progressive neuropathy (13). A thorough family history is required. Examination of the parents' feet may reveal evidence of a previously unsuspected mild neuropathy. Dyck and Lambert have included under the general classification of the hereditary motor and sensory neuropathies (HMSN) several subtypes, including neuropathies previously called Charcot-Marie-Tooth, Dejerine-Sottas, and Refsum disease (26,27). Type I, the hypertrophic form of Charcot-Marie-Tooth, presents most commonly in the second decade of life, although it may be noted earlier. The most prevalent type is CMT-1A, which is an autosomal dominant form due to duplication of PMP-22 gene (60). In the type I disease, atrophy of the intrinsic muscles occurs early as does the development of a cavovarus foot. Nerve biopsy reveals typical hypertrophic changes consistent with repetitive cycles of demyelination and remyelination. With HMSN type I, all the muscles in the calf progressively atrophy. Drennan and Price (62) conducted a computed tomography (CT) analysis of the muscles in this group and found that intrinsic atrophy was the primary focus of muscle deterioration. Extrinsic

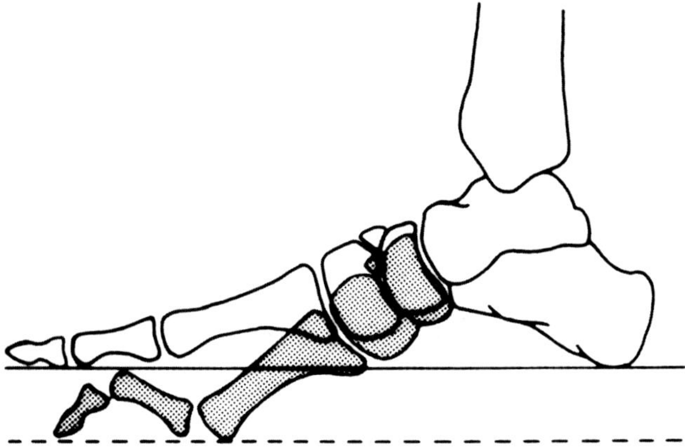

FIGURE 12-1 Fixed forefoot equinus. (From Home G. Pes cavovarus following ankle fracture. *Clin Orthop* 1984;184: 249, with permission.)

muscle involvement initially follows either the peroneal or tibial nerve distribution, but eventually all calf muscles were involved in the progressive deterioration (32,62).

Type II, the neuronal form of Charcot-Marie-Tooth, presents later, generally in the third decade, and demonstrates early involvement of all muscles distal to the knee and results in a calcaneovarus foot. The pathological changes in the peripheral nerves in type II show little evidence of hypertrophy but primarily neuronal degeneration. The progressive hereditary motor and sensory neuropathies should be distinguished from Friedreich's ataxia as the prognosis in the latter is much worse.

There may be a history of trauma (burns, tibial fracture) (48); gluteal injections (9); spinal cord injury (63); ankle fractures (39); tendon laceration (21); congenital deformities (talipes equinovarus) (69,71); or neuromuscular disease (polio, cerebral palsy, spina bifida, HMSN).

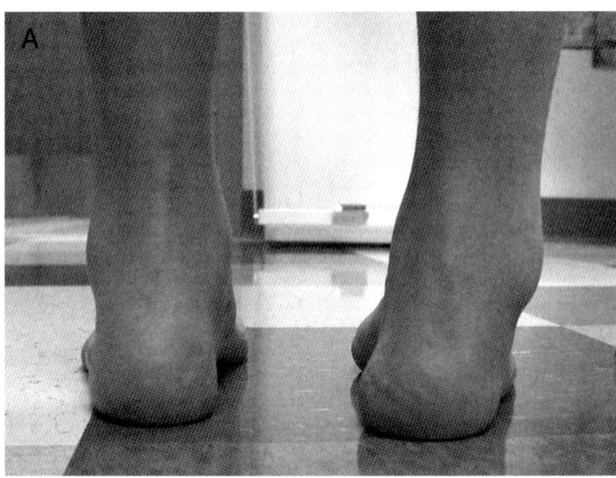

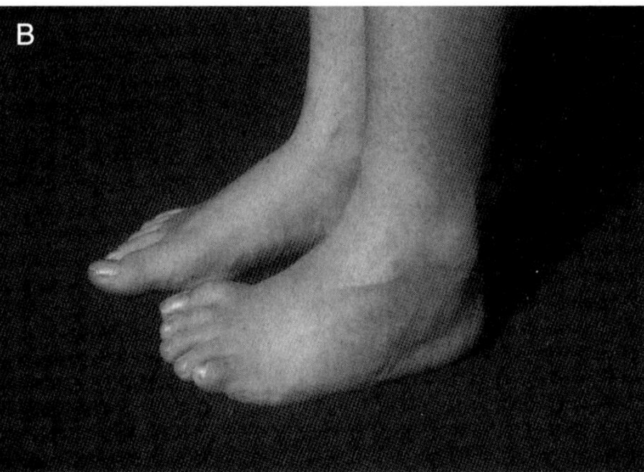

FIGURE 12-2 (**A**) Posterior view of the foot demonstrating a varus deformity of the hind foot. (*Right* > *Left*) (**B**) Medial view of the foot showing exaggerated medial longitudinal arch in the right foot. The left foot shows supination of the forefoot with clawing of the toes and entire weight bearing on the lateral aspect of the foot.

PATHOLOGY

The evolution of the cavus deformity has been studied in patients with Friedreich's ataxia (3) and Charcot-Marie-Tooth disease (14,66). One study found that initially only the first metatarsal is plantar flexed and pronated (Figure.12-3). Later, all the metatarsals assume an equinus position. In the third stage, the calcaneus develops a varus inclination. Sabir noted that in HMSN type I, the intrinsics are innervated by the longest axons of the sciatic nerve and are the first muscles affected by

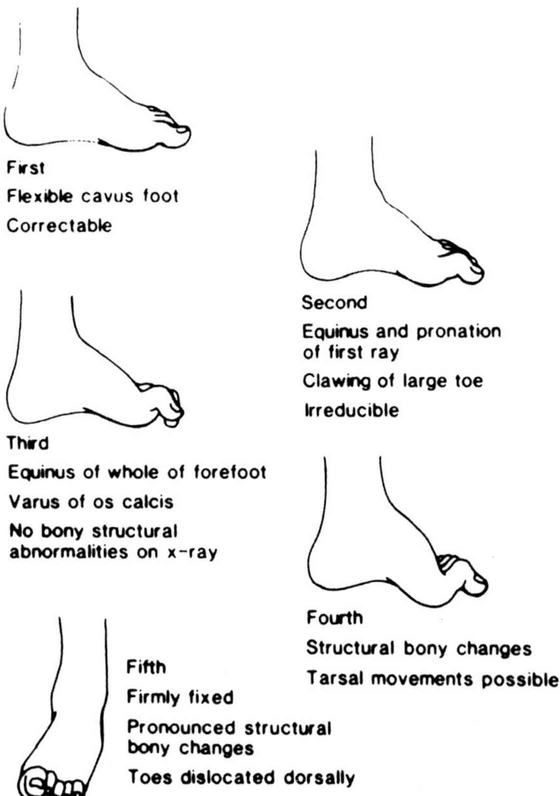

FIGURE 12-3 Evolution of the cavus foot: first, flexible; second, fixed equinus of first ray with clawing of hallux; third, fixed equinus of entire forefoot with heel varus; fourth, fixed bony changes; fifth, marked structural changes with no flexibility. (From Home G. Pes cavovarus following ankle fracture. *Clin Orthop* 1984;184: 249, with permission.)

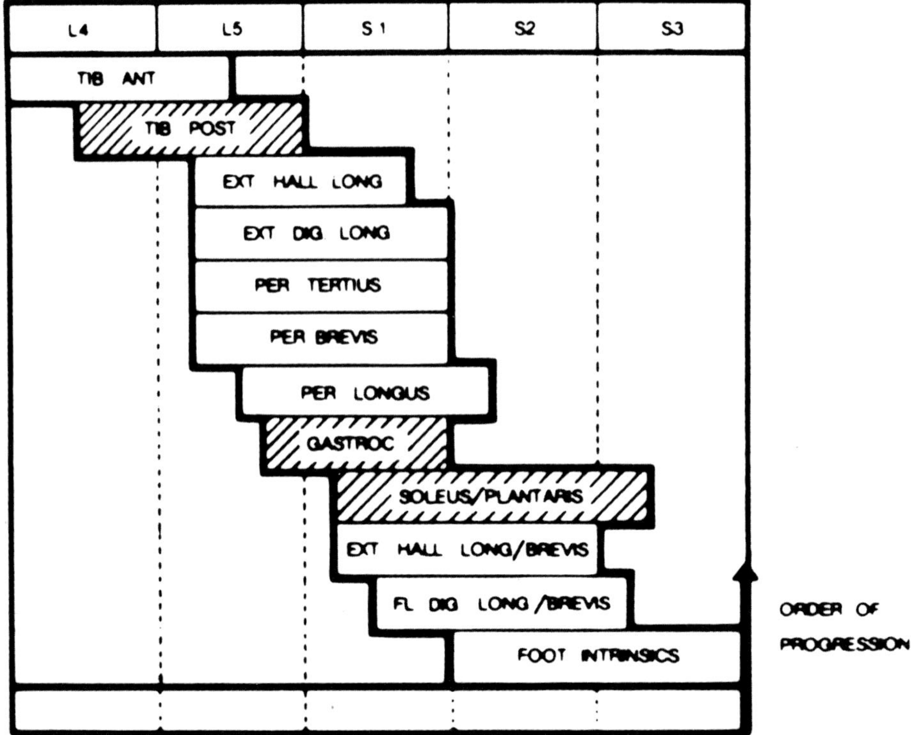

FIGURE 12-4 Pattern of denervation in Charcot-Marie-Tooth disease. The muscles with large bulk (tibialis posterior, gastrocsoleus) show atrophy at the late stage. (From Home G. Pes cavovarus following ankle fracture. *Clin Orthop* 1984;184: 249, with permission.)

neuronal degeneration (Figure 12-4). The atrophy leads first to weakness. The intrinsics lose their ability to stabilize the metatarsophalangeal joints, and this allows unopposed extension at the metatarsophalangeal joint and flexion of interphalangeal joints. With time, the muscles undergo fibrosis and shortening, leading to further elevation of the medial arch.

In Charcot-Marie-Tooth disease, both motor and sensory components of the peripheral nerve are involved. The pathology also involves the muscles, tendons, and fascia. Sensory loss is not apparent during the early phases of the disease. Because the tendons lose their elasticity, the heel cord does not stretch and appears to be tight, but the os calcis is in a position of calcaneus. Varying degrees of tibialis anterior muscle weakness are apparent. When the patient tries to dorsiflex the foot, the long toe extensor compensates for this weakness by elevating the proximal phalanx, resulting in a cocked-up big toe and a depressed first metatarsal. The weak tibialis anterior muscle contributes to the plantar flexion of the first metatarsal and if present a relatively strong peroneus longus accentuates the deformity. With the os calcis in calcaneus along with a drop in the first metatarsal, the plantar fascia gets contracted and acts like a bowstring and leads to varus of the hindfoot. Intrinsic muscle weakness contributes to the clawing of the great toe, as well as the lesser toes. The peroneals eventually get weaker but the tibialis posterior stays relatively strong. The presence of a contracted plantar fascia, weak peroneals and tibialis anterior, and a strong tibialis posterior muscle leads to varus at the hindfoot and supination at the forefoot and finally the foot assumes a cavovarus deformity. The clawing of the toes further compounds the problem by causing pressure over the dorsum of the toes when the patient wears shoes. At a later stage in the disease, upper extremity weakness may be apparent by wasting of the thenar and hypothenar muscles. Some degree of mild intrinsic muscle weakness in the hand manifests clinically by the child exhibiting poor writing skills. The ankle and knee reflexes may be weak or absent. In the early stages of the disease, the deformity is flexible; but if the cavovarus foot is left uncorrected, the bones adapt to the changes and a fixed deformity develops (10,76). Paulos et al (61) felt that initially when the patient walks, the pressure is distributed between the heel, the base of the fifth metatarsal, and the lateral metatarsal heads. However, recent pedobarographic studies reveal that most of the weight and foot pressure is distributed at the base of the fifth metatarsal and the heel and less pressure at the first metatarsal head (bipod effect) (16) (Figure 12-5).

The natural history of most children with cavovarus deformity is gradual progression, and certainly this is true for those with an underlying neurologic disorder. Yet the rate of progression may vary greatly from one patient to another, and some patients do remarkably well with little or no treatment. Many of those with Charcot-Marie-Tooth disease may have family members with the same disorder, but often the severity of the disease differs greatly from one family member to another (59).

The presence of cavovarus deformity along with a weak gastrocsoleus complex leads to increased pressure on

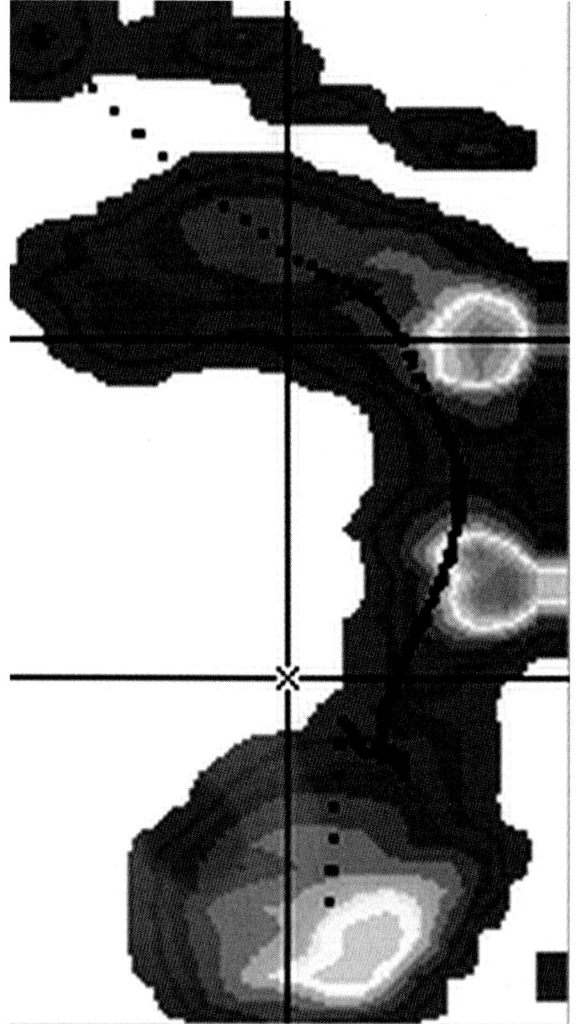

FIGURE 12-5 Pedobarograph of a child with cavus foot showing increased pressure distribution at the heel and lateral border of the foot.

the heel, base of the fifth metatarsal, and the first metatarsal head. This causes callosities and pain in these areas and leads to difficulties in wearing shoes. In addition, if the child has claw toes, the shoe rubs on the dorsum of the interphalangeal joints and causes pain and ulcerations.

The patients may complain of problems with shoe wear, frequent falling, or feeling that their ankles "give out." Pain may occur beneath the metatarsal heads or at the base of the fifth metatarsal.

PHYSICAL EXAM

To understand the principles of treatment, one should look at the foot as being made up of four components. The hindfoot is composed of the talus, os calcis, and the ankle joint and the mid-foot is composed of the calcaneocuboid, talonavicular, and mid-tarsal joints. The forefoot comprises the metatarsal complex and the toes comprise the fourth component. In the evolution of the disease, forefoot and mid-foot are involved before the hindfoot. If only the forefoot and mid-foot are involved, treatment is directed only to this part of the foot. As the disease progresses, the hindfoot may get involved and surgical correction of the hindfoot may be necessary at a later date.

When examining the foot, it is necessary to carefully examine each component of the deformity: the forefoot, mid-foot, and hindfoot. The flexibility of each component must then be determined. The toes should be inspected for the presence of flexible or fixed clawing, because not all cavus feet have evidence of clawing. If the toe deformity passively corrects when the forefoot and ankle are dorsiflexed, then surgical correction of the forefoot deformity will be followed by spontaneous correction of the clawing. After many years, fixed contractures will develop in the capsule, collateral ligaments, and intrinsics; then the toe deformities will also have to be surgically addressed.

The flexibility of all metatarsals must be checked. Only the first ray may be fixed in plantar flexion, or all five metatarsals. As Jahss noted, an apparent forefoot varus is often the result of "pseudo supinatory" motion (43). This is explained anatomically by the fact that the tarsometatarsal joints are on an oblique axis which slants medially. Equinus and adductus at the level of this joint, therefore, can falsely appear as a rotatory deformity at the midfoot, particularly because the lateral two metatarsals are the most mobile. The cavus deformity becomes symptomatic when the sole of the foot cannot dorsiflex to neutral position in relation to the long axis of the tibia, the so-called tibioplantar angle of Jahss (7,43).

To determine if the hindfoot is involved, Coleman devised the block test, which is a simple clinical test (19). To perform this test, the patient stands with the feet plantigrade on a level floor. The examiner stands behind the patient and observes the position of the heel to see if it is in varus, neutral, or valgus. In a normal foot, the heel will assume a slightly valgus position. The patient then stands on a rectangular block 1-1/2″ to 2″ in height to accommodate the entire length and width of the foot. The first and second metatarsals are allowed to overhang on the medial side of the block. The examiner stands behind the patient and observes the heel. If the varus heel of a cavus foot corrects to neutral or valgus, it means the hindfoot is supple and treatment should be directed only to the forefoot (Figure 12-6). Radiographically this can be documented by performing a lateral radiograph with the patient standing on the block with the first and second metatarsals hanging free on the medial side of the block. While Dr. Coleman initially described this radiographic view, the changes seen were not well documented. In 2005, Dr. Azmaipairashvili clearly explained the changes in this radiographic view (5). In a patient with cavus feet, the standing lateral radiograph demonstrates that the ankle joint appears to be seen in the anteroposterior (AP) projection, whereas the foot appears to be seen in the lateral projection and the head of the talus appears to be flat topped (Figure 12-7A). In the Coleman block test lateral view, if the hindfoot is flexible, the ankle joint assumes a normal lateral configuration and the head of the talus appears to be normal (Figure 12-7B).

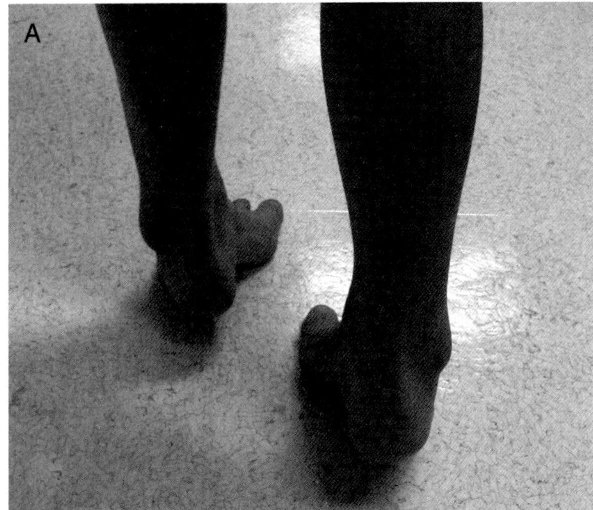

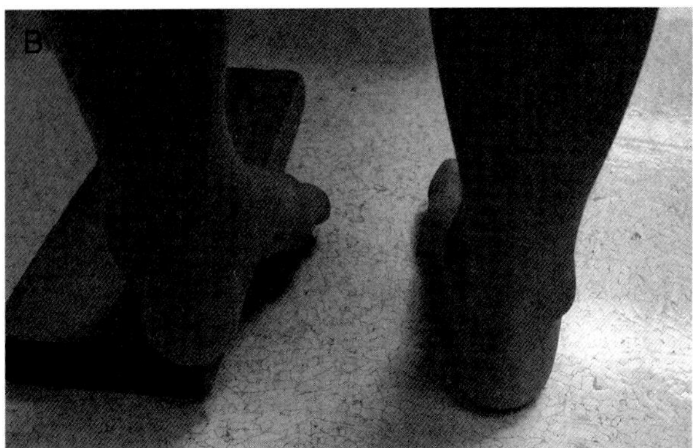

FIGURE 12-6 (**A**) There is varus at the hindfoot and supination of the forefoot more pronounced on the left. (**B**) Coleman block test showing correction of hindfoot varus, which indicates flexibility of the hindfoot.

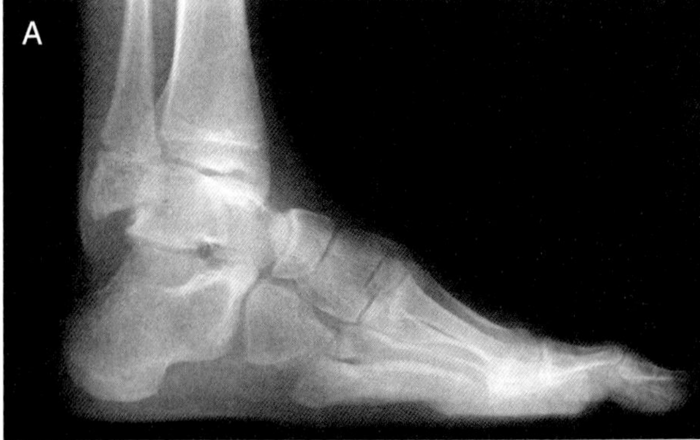

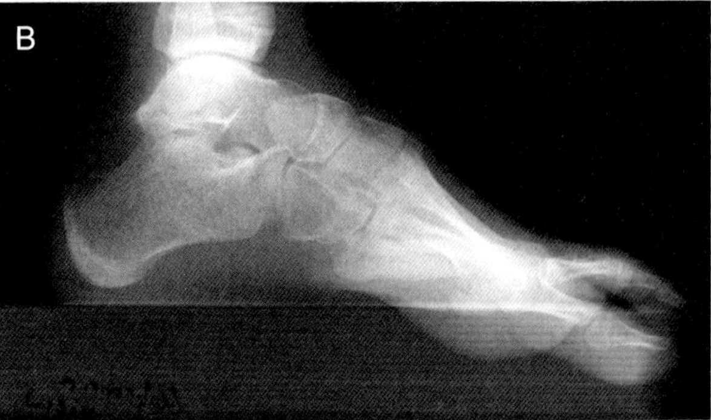

FIGURE 12-7 (**A**) Standing lateral radiographic view of the ankle showing that the ankle joint appears to be in an anteroposterior projection, whereas the foot appears to be in lateral projection with a flat-topped dome of the talus. (**B**) Coleman block lateral radiographic view of the ankle showing a normal lateral view of the ankle joint with a normal dome of the talus, which indicates that the hindfoot is flexible.

A careful neurologic exam should be performed. The back should be carefully visualized for scoliosis, kyphoscoliosis, dimpling, or an abnormal hairy patch. These may suggest an underlying spinal dysraphism which will require further investigation. James et al (44) noted that if the cause of the spinal dysraphism can be identified and corrected early in the course of the deformity, the cavus may resolve spontaneously (44). Deep tendon reflexes, motor strength, balance, and sensation should be fully evaluated and any deficits recorded. An examination by a pediatric neurologist is always recommended. An evaluation by a geneticist may also be helpful to determine if there is an underlying genetic condition, for children with a particularly difficult diagnosis.

IMAGING

Radiographic Studies

We suggest that the following tests to be performed prior to treatment (3):

1. The following radiographs should be performed for all children with cavovarus foot deformity.
   a. Standing AP and lateral view of the foot
   b. Standing AP and lateral of the ankle
   c. The lateral Coleman block view
   d. Harris view (35)
   e. Spine radiographs

On the standing lateral radiograph, if the base of the fifth metatarsal is at a lower level than the heel, it indicates supination of the forefoot. The amount of this displacement is documented by drawing a horizontal line from the heel to the head of the fifth metatarsal and measuring the distance between the base of the fifth metatarsal and this horizontal line (5). The severity of pes cavus can be measured by the methods of Meary or Hibbs. The angle of Meary is determined by lines drawn through the long axis of the first metatarsal and the talus; these lines should be parallel (normal 0–5°) (55). The angle of Hibbs is determined by lines drawn along the axis of the calcaneus and the axis of the first metatarsal. The angle of Hibbs should not be less than 150° degrees (64). The calcaneal pitch can be assessed by the angle formed between a line on the plantar surface of the calcaneus and the weight-bearing surface. Calcaneal pitch angle more than 30° indicates calcaneus of the os calcis (47) (Figure 12-8).

Paulo et al devised a method for radiographically quantifying heel varus (61). With the advent of digital

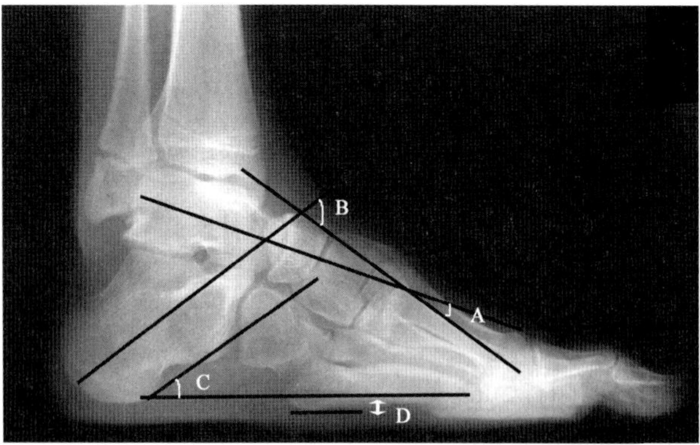

FIGURE 12-8 Illustration of the radiological parameters. Meary angle (A); Hibbs angle (B); calcaneal pitch angle (C); and supination of the forefoot (D).

radiography, this method is rarely performed. The Harris Radiograph will accomplish the same result.

Radiographs of the entire spine are needed to rule out evidence of spinal cord tumor, spinal dysraphism, scoliosis, or other abnormalities. If there are any abnormalities noted, a magnetic resonance (MRI) scan is the appropriate test to further evaluate the spine in most circumstances.

An MRI is useful especially if the cavus foot is unilateral to rule out intraspinal pathology (70,80). The number of genes involved in some of the peripheral neuropathies like Charcot-Marie-Tooth disease is changing frequently and it is beyond the scope of this chapter to discuss these in detail (6,46).

Additional Investigation

The following additional tests should be considered in selected patients as needed:

1. An MRI of the entire spinal cord including the brain
2. Electrodiagnostic testing (EDT)
3. Muscle biopsy
4. Pedobarographic studies
5. Gait analysis
6. Gene Mapping

Electrodiagnostic Testing (EDT)

The neurological assessment of the cavus foot may include electrodiagnostic testing (EDT) which includes an electromyogram (EMG), and a nerve conduction velocity study (NCV). This may reveal evidence of either a myopathy or neuropathy. Axonal degeneration will cause a prolonged latency, and demyelination will slow conduction. Denervation may show positive sharp waves or fibrillations on the EMG (15,26).

Muscle Biopsy

Even after the spinal radiographs, MRI, and EDT the diagnosis may be in doubt, and a muscle biopsy may be required. Careful coordination is needed between the neurologist, pathologist, and surgeon to ensure that the appropriate biopsy location, size, and preparation is obtained.

Pedobarographic Studies

Pedobarographic studies are valuable to help establish the diagnosis, identify areas of high pressure, before and after treatment of cavovarus feet to document changes in the weight-bearing patterns of the foot (16).

Gait Analysis

Abnormalities in the child's gait will be determined by the pattern of muscle weakness. Gait analysis has been performed on patients with Charcot-Marie-Tooth (66). During normal stance phase, the heel strikes first, followed by the lateral border of the foot, and last the metatarsal heads; at the end of the stance phase, the weight has been shifted to the medial three rays.

In HMSN, there is weakness both of the anterior tibialis leading to dropfoot and weakness of the gastrocsoleus. Classically, the gait pattern has been described as "steppage" (increased flexion of the hip and knee in swing phase to allow for clearance of the foot). Sabir's studies noted abnormal pelvic elevation during swing phase to allow for clearance of the foot, along with increased external rotation and circumduction of the extremity. This abnormal pelvic elevation would cause a loss of balance, but the elevation is compensated by the upper trunk deviating toward the side of the pelvic elevation. Sabir calls this the "marionette gait." Video motion analysis may be helpful in analyzing the components of the pathologic gait; dynamic electromyography may be used to assess abnormal patterns of muscle activity; and forced plate analysis can quantify the abnormal pressure distribution resulting from the deformed foot.

Inman has carefully studied the events of the gait cycle, specifically those mechanisms occurring within the foot which allow the events of the gait cycle to proceed smoothly (41).

TREATMENT

Non-surgical Care

Orthotics do not correct the cavovarus deformity, but have some role in the management of dynamic foot deformities and also help in unloading the pressure areas in rigid feet. Some authors have suggested nonoperative management as an option in the management of mild or non-progressive deformity of the foot (2). Dwyer thought that a bar under the metatarsal heads along with passive stretching of the plantar fascia was more effective than a shoe insert, in controlling dynamic foot deformities (25,68). Alexander and Johnson (12) have suggested that the use of extra-depth shoes with support to unload the metatarsal heads is often helpful. For runners, activity adjustment, pain management, stretching, quadriceps muscle strengthening, shoe modification, use of flexible orthotics, and replacement of worn jogging shoes are helpful (52).

The use of ankle-foot orthoses (AFOs) as night splints to diminish any progressive tendency towards cavus has questionable merit; AFOs may help in preventing progression of an equinus contracture. Muscle strengthening and stretching exercises may delay progression in neuromuscular pes cavus, but it is doubtful that these exercises significantly alter the natural history of the deformity. Nonoperative measures generally do not stop progression or prevent deformity; therefore, their role is extremely limited.

Surgical Options

Surgical options include soft-tissue surgery, such as tendon transfers, lengthenings, and soft-tissue releases. Bony procedures include osteotomies and joint fusions (57,68). In all of these children, the plantar fascia is contracted and acts like a bowstring. Lengthening of the tight plantar fascia is an essential first step in the correction of this deformity. The tibialis posterior stays as a viable muscle long after all the other muscles have become weak and, hence, acts as a deforming force in all children and this muscle has to be transferred through the interosseous membrane to the dorsal aspect of the foot to compensate for the weak tibialis anterior and to help in dorsiflexion of the foot. In the presence of a functioning tibialis anterior, the tibialis posterior is transferred to the lateral cuneiform. If the tibialis anterior is non-functional, then the tibialis posterior tendon is transferred to the middle cuneiform.

In young children between eight and twelve years of age, if both the forefoot and hindfoot are flexible, then a successful outcome can be achieved with soft-tissue surgery alone, which consists of releasing the plantar fascia and transferring the tendon of the tibialis posterior through the intraosseous membrane to the dorsum of the foot (5).

Plantar Release

Techniques of open and percutaneous plantar release have been described since 1898. Steindler in 1920 described a more thorough procedure to strip the plantar muscles from the calcaneus (74)(Figure 12-9). Both medial and lateral incisions have been utilized. The plantar fascia must be released (72). Serial casting then provides satisfactory correction for younger children.

Mid-foot osteotomy (Author's preferred technique)

This surgical technique includes five important steps to correct the deformity:

Step 1. Plantar fascia release: Through a 1-cm longitudinal incision over the medial side of the plantar fascia the middle third is exposed. After careful separation of the plantar fascia from the medial plantar nerve the fascia is released. This helps in releasing the tether at the medial side of the foot.

Step 2. Under fluoroscopic guidance, the centre of the medial cuneiform is identified. Through a 3-cm medial longitudinal incision centered over the medial cuneiform the medial aspect of the bone is exposed. A guide wire is passed from the medial aspect of the medial cuneiform toward the center of the lateral cuneiform to define the imaginary plane of the mid-foot osteotomy. After marking the plane, a transverse osteotomy through the middle of the medial and middle cuneiform is performed. Through the same incision, the tibialis posterior is detached from the navicular bone and a Bunnell suture is placed through the distal end of the cut tendon.

Step 3. The center of the cuboid is identified with flouroscopy. Through a 3-cm longitudinal incision centered over the cuboid, the lateral aspect of the bone is exposed A guide wire is passed from the lateral aspect of the cuboid toward the center of the lateral cuneiform to define the plane of the mid-foot osteotomy and a transverse osteotomy through the middle of the cuboid performed.

Step 4. The center of the lateral cuneiform is identified with fluoroscopy. Through a 3-cm longitudinal incision centered over the lateral cuneiform, the bone is exposed. A transverse osteotomy through the middle of the lateral cuneiform that connects the medial and lateral osteotomy lines is performed. Now, the whole mid-foot is completely mobile. A controlled dorsolateral wedge of the bone is removed from the three cuneiform bones and cuboid to correct the deformity. After achieving satisfactory correction, the cuboid osteotomy is stabilized with two staples and the medial cuneiform osteotomy is stabilized with two Steinmann pins.

Step 5. Depending on the strength of the tibialis anterior, the tibialis posterior muscle that was detached from the navicular is transferred through the interosseous membrane to the lateral or middle cuneiform.

Because the forefoot is shortened by this wedge osteotomy, the flexor tendons are relatively lengthened and clawing of the toes improves. Following surgery, these patients are casted for six weeks. After the cast removal, an articulating ankle foot orthosis, with 90-degree plantar flexion stop is worn for six months. Long-term follow up in our cases shows maintenance of good correction of the deformity (Figure 12-10).

If the deformity at the hindfoot is also rigid, a Dwyer's calcaneal osteotomy (25) should be performed in addition to the other midfoot procedures already described.

Tendon Transfers

Tendon transfers are indicated to maintain correction and prevent recurrent deformities. Subclinical weakness can lead to significant clinical deformity over time, and in those cases, decision making on transfers can be difficult. It is important to realize that the tendon transfer will not

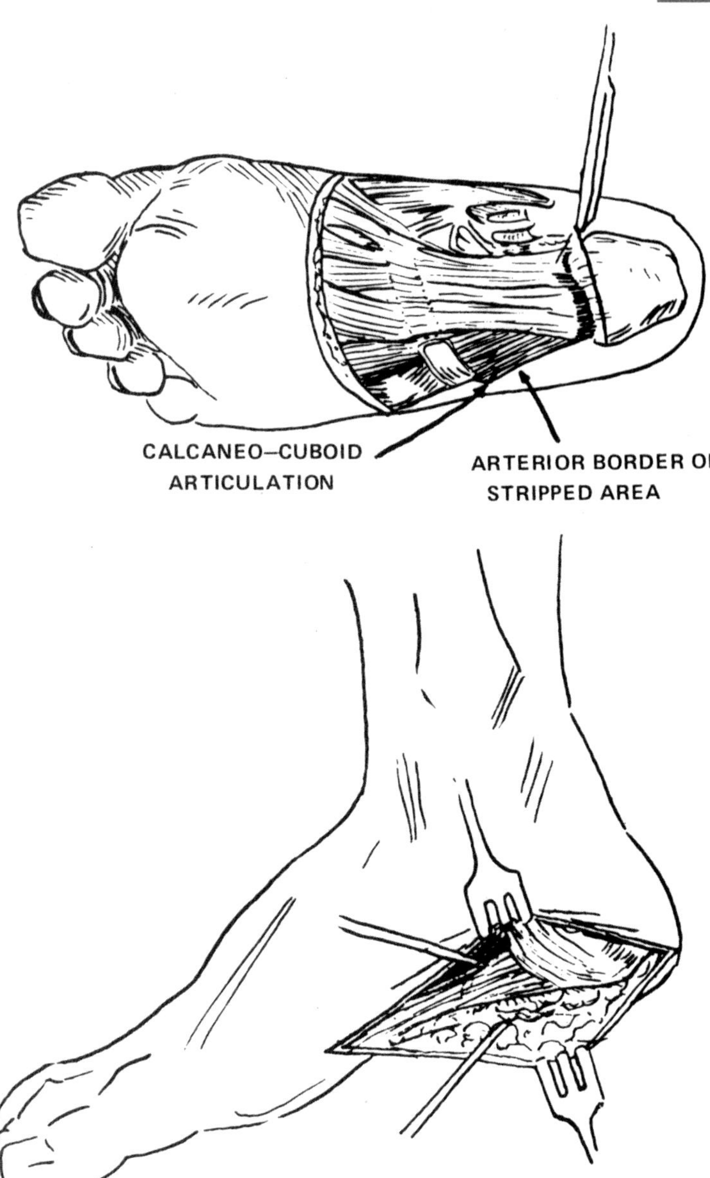

FIGURE 12-9 Steindler's plantar release. (From *Archives of Surgery,* 1921, Vol. 2, with permission.)

correct even minor degrees of fixed deformity. Muscles to be transferred should be at least grade IV in strength. Occasionally when there is diffuse muscle weakness, transfer of more than one muscle can be considered. One must remember that assessment of muscle strength about the foot cannot be performed after triple or subtalar arthrodesis (43). Transfers described by Bentzon (8), Chuinard and Baskin (17), Cole (18), Farill (28), Fowler et al (30), Frank and Johnson (31), Hallgrimson (34), Hibbs (37), and Hsu and Inbus(40) are rarely performed,

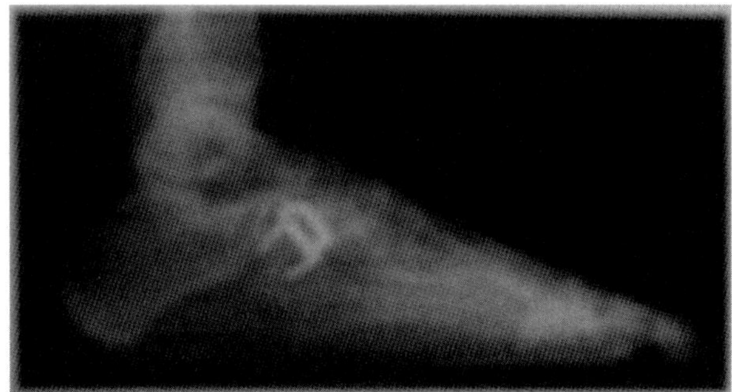

FIGURE 12-10 Lateral radiograph of the ankle and foot showing the long-term results of mid-foot osteotomy and tibialis posterior transfer.

Posterior tibial tendon transfer through the interosseous membrane or subcutaneously is frequently utilized in progressive cavus deformities such as HSMN I where there may be weakness of the anterior tibialis and peroneals. Coleman lengthened the posterior tibial tendon as part of his plantar medial release, which he performed in the presence of fixed hindfoot varus (61). Coleman had 85% acceptable results in his series, but there were few cases of progressive neuromuscular disease. In situations of progressive neuromuscular imbalance, it is best to preserve the posterior tibial tendon to be transferred anteriorly. The transferred tendon should be fixed through a drill hole in bone and stabilized with a button on the plantar surface of the foot.

Other Osseous Procedures

In children older than 12 years, the foot is less flexible. The Coleman block test is used to assess the flexibility of the hindfoot. In patients with a flexible hindfoot and a rigid forefoot, a number of procedures have been described. These include:

1. Dorsal closing wedge osteotomy at the base of first metatarsal with a Jones procedure (12,22)
2. Medial cuneiform plantar opening wedge osteotomy (30)
3. Triple arthrodesis (29)

In children with CMT who underwent a first metatarsal osteotomy with a Jones procedure, the supination of the forefoot was not fully corrected because this procedure addresses only the first metatarsal drop (Figure 12-11). The medial cuneiform opening wedge osteotomy also corrects the metatarsal drop but does not correct the forefoot equinus and supination (Figure 12-12). Triple arthrodesis in the past was the standard operation for these patients. But long-term follow-up studies showed development of ankle arthritis secondary to fusion of the subtalar and mid-tarsal joints (87) (Figure 12-13). In our hands, a properly performed dorsal closing wedge midfoot osteotomy, which consists of an osteotomy of the cuboid and the three cuneiforms with a dorsolateral wedge, corrects the supination as well as the plantar flexed forefoot (5) (Figure 12-14A,B&C).

Correction of the fixed cavus deformity can be performed by utilizing osteotomies or arthrodesis. Osteotomies have the advantage of preserving mobility of the foot; this will allow better function of the foot and avoid destructive changes in unfused joints. In the past, an approach of benign neglect in the child until the foot was close to skeletal maturity was common, at which point a triple arthrodesis and tendon transfer would be performed. The advocates of triple arthrodesis claim better correction and better maintenance of correction. However, several recent studies (85,87) have shown that the long-term results of the triple arthrodesis are often unsatisfactory. The authors advocate joint preserving procedures whenever possible. One must always remember when planning a surgical correction of the mid-foot deformity that an additional procedure is often required to correct the fixed heel deformity.

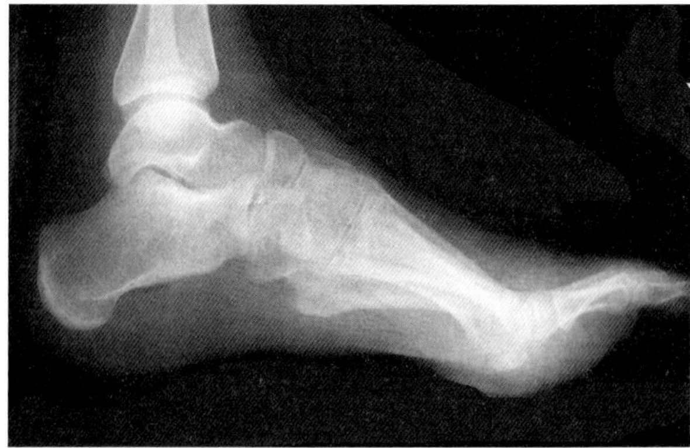

FIGURE 12-12 Lateral radiograph of the ankle and foot showing persistence of forefoot drop, supination, and claw toes after medial cuneiform opening wedge osteotomy.

Procedures that are Rarely Performed

Jahss has recommended a closing wedge dorsal arthrodesis at the level of the tarsometatarsal joint (42). In his opinion, this arthrodesis offers several advantages over multiple osteotomies: (i) internal fixation is not required; (ii) a greater surface area of bone for arthrodesis is available, therefore, union is more likely; and (iii) improved correction as the location of the arthrodesis is closer to the apex of the deformity. A plantar release is also generally required with all these bony procedures. In addition to the wide resection of bone dorsally, several millimeters of bone are also resected on the plantar aspect of the osteotomy or arthrodesis; the use of a truncated wedge relaxes the plantar structures and allows additional forefoot correction (Figure 12-15). This principle applies also to the other mid-foot osteotomies. The rocker bottom tendency can also occur following this procedure, in addition, overcorrection of the adduction of the forefoot will lead to a noticeable medial prominence just proximal to the osteotomy at the level of the medial aspect of the first cuneiform.

Both Saunders (69) and Cole (18) recommended a mid-tarsal dorsal wedge resection for the correction of the pes cavus deformity. The disadvantage of the dorsal closing wedge of Cole is that an already shortened foot is

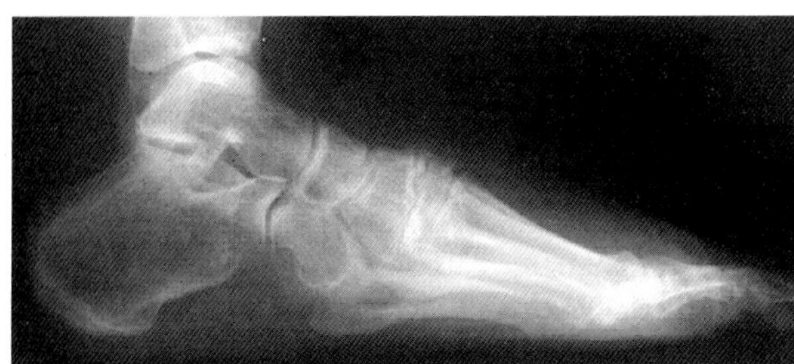

FIGURE 12-11 Lateral radiograph of the ankle and foot showing persistence of supination after first metatarsal osteotomy and Jones procedure.

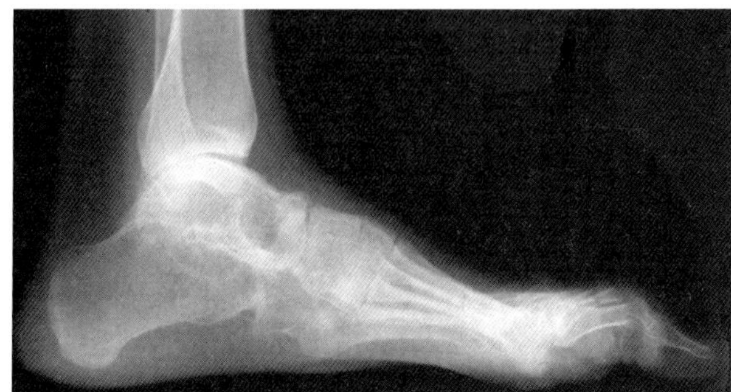

FIGURE 12-13 Lateral radiograph of the ankle and foot showing early degenerative arthritis at the ankle and persistence of claw toes after triple arthrodesis.

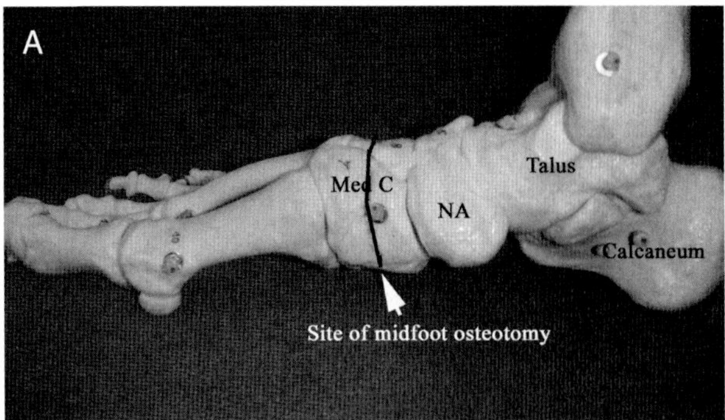

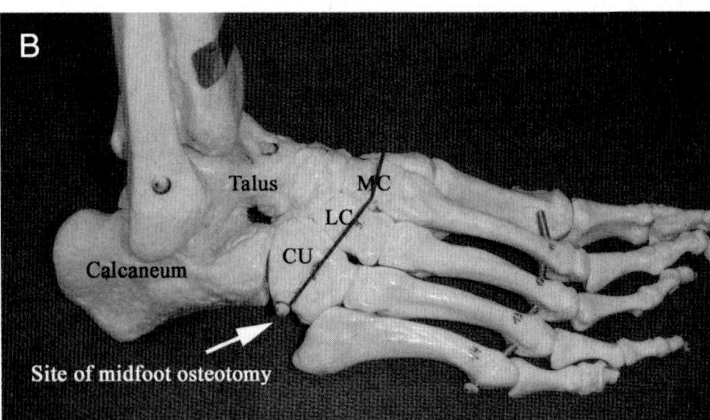

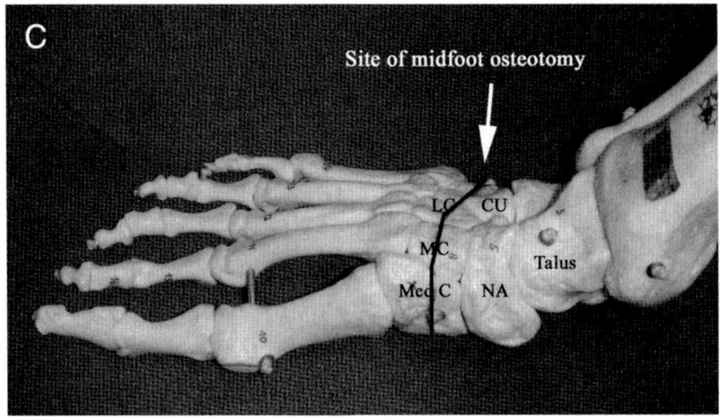

FIGURE 12-14 (A, B, and C) Bone model showing the site of midfoot osteotomy. MC- Middle cuneiform; LC- Lateral cuneiform; Med C- Medial cuneiform; CU-Cuboid; NA- Navicular.

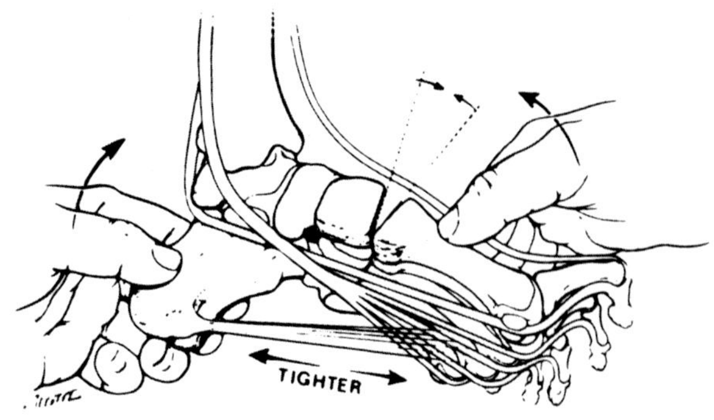

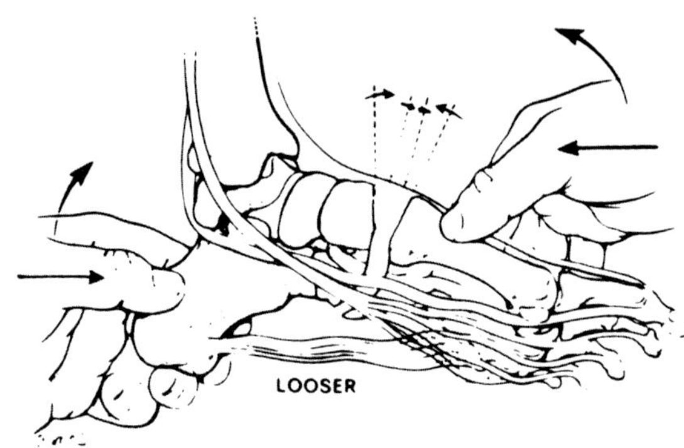

FIGURE 12-15 Truncated closing wedge osteotomy allows easier closure of osteotomy site. (From Jahss MH. Evaluation of the cavus foot for orthopaedic treatment. *Clin Orthop* 1983;181: 52, with permission.)

Other osteotomies and fusions have been advocated at an even more proximal level to correct the forefoot cavus which are of interest from a historical standpoint only. Steindler recommended removal of the dorsal wedge from the talar neck in order to correct the forefoot equinus (74). Stuart (75) used this procedure but also in combination of correction at the level of the midtarsal joint. Other shortened further. In order to avoid this, Japas (45) devised a V-osteotomy which is located at the apex of the cavus deformity. When the osteotomy is completed, traction is applied to the foot, and the metatarsal heads are elevated as the base of the distal fragment is pressed in a plantar direction. However, with the V-shape, this minimized the ability to correct forefoot varus, valgus, or rotatory problems. In order to provide the ability to correct these latter problems, the so-called Akron midtarsal "dome" osteotomy was devised (Figure 12-16). Weiner et al. advocated this procedure, as they felt this osteotomy optimally corrected all the components of the forefoot deformity (86). The osteotomy is located at the apex of the deformity, allows for excellent osseous contact for the arthrodesis, and postoperatively still maintains good motion of the foot. Their results were good except for those patients who were less than eight years of age at the time of the osteotomy. The authors' do not prefer a transverse skin incision.

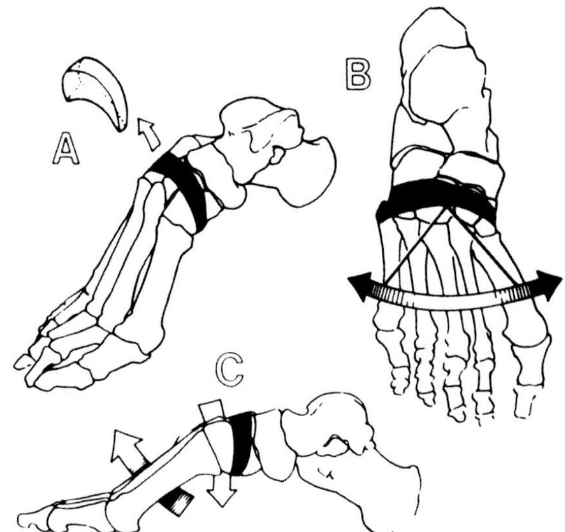

FIGURE 12-16 Akron midtarsal "dome" osteotomy. (From Wilcox P, Weiner D. The Akron midtarsal dome osteotomy in the treatment of rigid pes cavus: a preliminary review. *J Pediatr Orthop* 1985;5: 330–338, with permission.)

fusions which have been recommended include fusion of the metatarsal-cuneiform and cuneiform-navicular joint, described by McElvenny and Caldwell (33,54). It is difficult to balance the foot with metatarsal osteotomies alone (77,8182)

Osteotomy of the Os Calcis for Varus Deformity

In 1959, Dwyer described an osteotomy in the calcaneus for the correction of the cavus foot (25). In his opinion, when the heel varus was corrected primarily, the correction of the forefoot would often follow with time. Dwyer initially described a lateral closing wedge osteotomy for the correction of the heel varus (Figure 12-17). When the calcaneus was somewhat small, he also described an opening wedge osteotomy of the medial aspect of the calcaneus. However, the opening wedge osteotomy runs the risk of significant skin slough and is rarely utilized. The closing wedge osteotomy provides very satisfactory correction of the heel varus (20,21), but it can shorten the heel. This is rarely a problem. A third alternative for the correction of heel varus is the sliding osteotomy, which was initially described for pes valgus. Providing the varus deformity is not excessively severe, a sliding osteotomy will provide excellent correction of the heel varus without shortening the heel. In children, if the osteotomy is attempted from the lateral aspect, the calcaneal periosteum may prevent significant displacement at the osteotomy site, therefore more correction can be achieved from a medial approach. The displacement can be easily 50% of the width of the osteotomy, and it is held in the corrected position with a large Steinmann pin.

Calcaneocavus Foot

The calcaneocavus foot is commonly seen in children with spina bifida and poliomyelitis. The deformity is also encountered in other neurological conditions like cerebral palsy, CMT, Friedrich's ataxia, Roussy-Levy syndrome, diastomatomyelia, and also secondary to over-lengthening of the calf musculature for equinus deformities (83). In these children who are ambulators, the gastrocsoleus muscle is

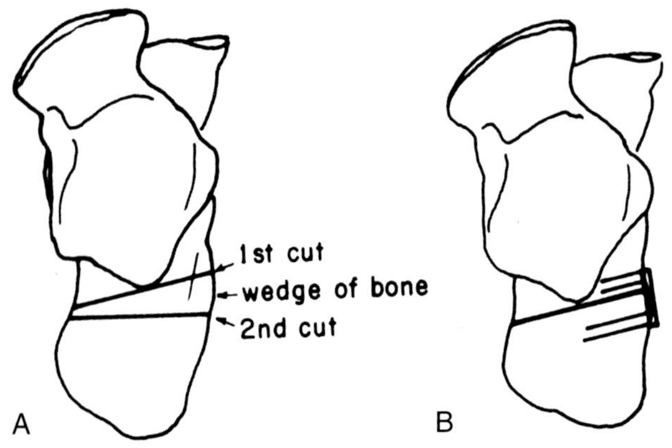

FIGURE 12-17 (**A, B**) Dwyer closing wedge osteotomy of the os calcis. (From *Foot and Ankle,* Vol. 4, No. 5, p. 270, with permission.)

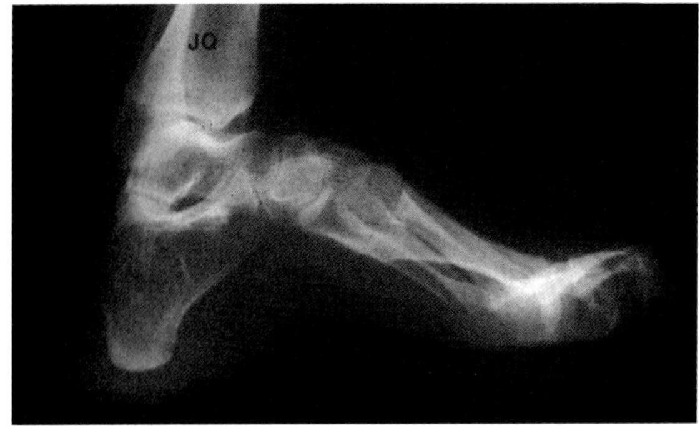

FIGURE 12-18 Lateral radiograph of the ankle and foot illustrating the calcaneo cavus deformity. The os calcis is in a dorsiflexed position with an increased calcaneal pitch angle.

weak and leads to a calcaneus deformity. The tibialis anterior acts as a deforming force and pulls the first metatarsal and ankle dorsally. The deformity that results is often termed a "pistol grip" deformity with the calcaneus forming the butt and the metatarsals forming the barrel of the pistol (Figure 12-18). Clinical examination reveals calcaneus at the hindfoot, plantar flexion of the forefoot, high arch at the mid-foot and claw toes. A lateral view radiograph of the foot shows a dorsiflexed os calcis with an increased calcaneal pitch angle (> 30°). Presence of a weak peroneal longus muscle leads to a dorsal bunion deformity at the first metatarsophalangeal joint.

To correct this deformity, the os calcis has to be pulled cephalad from the calcaneus position. If the deformity is supple, this can be achieved by transferring the tibialis anterior tendon through the interosseous membrane to the superior surface of the os calcis after plicating the tendon through the tendo Achilles. If the deformity is fixed, then a Mitchell (58) calcaneal osteotomy has to be performed. This has to be supplemented with a transfer of any available anterior muscles to the tendo Achilles. In children who do not have any muscles to transfer, then the tendo Achilles is tenodesed to the fibula as described by Westin et al (84).

Triple Arthrodesis

As the child with forefoot and hindfoot deformities reaches skeletal maturity, triple arthrodesis may be best utilized to correct the deformity (1,53,87). In patients with severe cavus deformities, in order to achieve correction, it may be necessary to remove a large wedge of the talar head and neck. This can lead to avascular necrosis of the talus. In order to avoid this, Siffert designed the "beak" triple arthrodesis; with this technique, only the plantar two-thirds of the talar head are excised, leaving an intact dorsal ledge to preserve the blood supply (73)(Figure 12-19). However, this may leave the patient with a dorsal prominence. Care must be taken not to place the forefoot in excessive pronation. The Lambrinudi (50) triple arthrodesis may be utilized for fixed equinocavus.

The long-term follow-up studies for triple arthrodesis in patients with polio are generally satisfactory. However, recent reports on the results of triple arthrodesis in

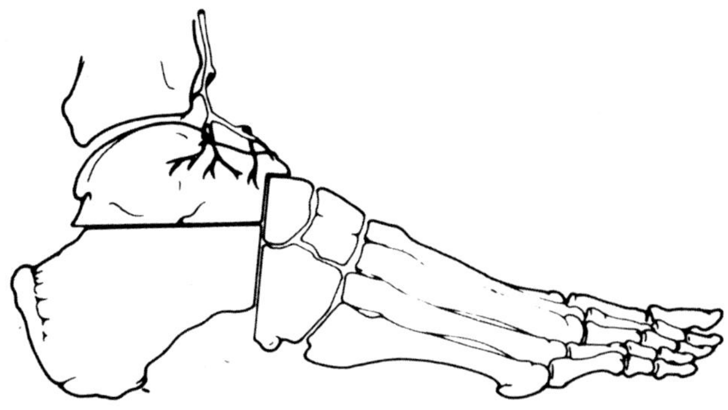

FIGURE 12-19 Beak triple arthrodesis. (From Fert RS, del Torto U. "Beak" triple arthrodesis for severe cavus deformity. *Clin Orthop Relat Res* 1983;181: 64–67, with permission.)

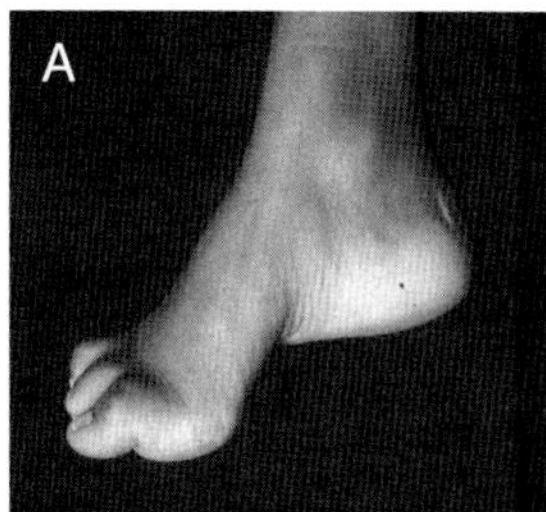

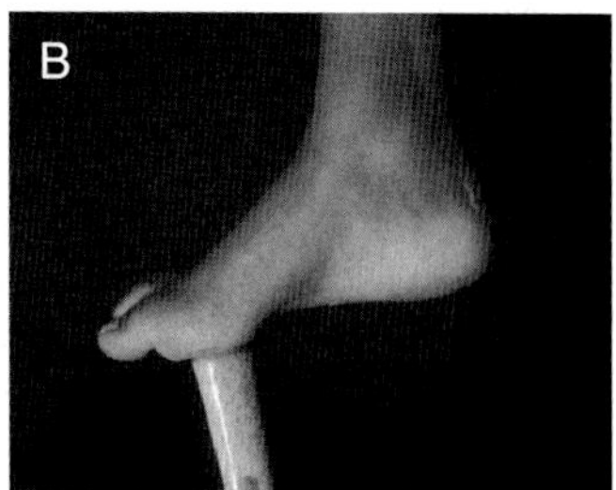

FIGURE 12-20 (**A**) Clinical picture showing claw toes in a cavovarus foot. (**B**) Kelikian test: If the deformity corrects by applying pressure at the base of first metataro-phalangeal joint, it indicates that the deformity is flexible. Persistence of the clawing indicates the deformity is rigid and will need an interphalangeal joint fusion.

patients with progressive neuromuscular disorders have not been as favorable. Similarly, the long-term results of triples in patients with spina bifida have been poor. Wetmore and Drennan found only 24% satisfactory result in a 20-year follow up of patients with HMSN type I (85). The poor results may be due to degenerative arthritis of the ankle or mid-tarsal joints, pseudoarthrosis, residual deformity, or pain. On the other hand, Levitt et al., with a shorter follow up, found that both osseous procedures (excluding triple arthrodesis) and soft-tissue surgery in peripheral neuropathies tended to deteriorate with time (51). Therefore, there still may be some controversy as to whether to proceed with combined mid-foot and hindfoot osteotomies versus the triple arthrodesis.

The authors feel that, in light of the poor results which have been reported with the use of triple arthrodesis in the progressive neuromuscular disorders, one should attempt to use joint-preserving procedures unless degenerative changes or the severity of the deformity mandate otherwise. Osteotomies and soft-tissue procedures are recommended for the skeletally immature foot. When there is residual or recurrent deformity requiring triple arthrodesis at a later date, the procedures will be much easier to perform. A plantigrade foot must be obtained by the end of growth, or persistent cavus deformity will become progressively disabling in adulthood.

Toe Deformities (Claw Toes)

Claw toes are frequently associated with the cavus foot. When the mid-foot is corrected, the claw toes improve significantly and rarely need surgical intervention. Initially, the claw toe deformity is flexible and passive dorsiflexion of the forefoot and ankle corrects the deformity. In this case, no surgical procedures on the toes are required. A fixed extension contracture at the metatarsophalangeal joint, as proven by the Kelikian test (49) (Figure 12-20) will require a dorsal capsulotomy. The Girdlestone-Taylor procedure (79) (transfer of the long-toe flexors to the extensor mechanism) is a rather extensive procedure for toe-clawing with somewhat unpredictable results, and the authors do not recommend its use. Soft-tissue procedures like flexor tenotomies and flexor to extensor muscle transfers have not worked very well in our hands; the toes can be better addressed by an interphalangeal joint fusion (78).

SUMMARY

The cavovarus foot deformity is usually progressive and most commonly associated with an underlying neurologic disorder. Careful evaluation should be performed to evaluate for interspinal pathology, especially in the setting of a unilateral cavus foot. Pes cavus refers to a fixed equinus deformity of the forefoot in relation to the hindfoot resulting in an abnormally high arch (see Figure.12-1). The heel may be in neutral, varus, valgus, or calcaneus, and often becomes fixed in the older child and young adult. The forefoot equinus is often accompanied by clawing of the toes.

The treatment of pes cavus continues to challenge the orthopedic surgeon. Treatment should be focused on correcting the muscle imbalance early in flexible feet and bony deformities later when the deformities become fixed. Triple arthrodesis should only be considered as a salvage procedure.

The authors wish to thank Dr. John G. Thometz, MD for his valuable suggestions and contributions.

REFERENCES

1. Adelaar RS, Dannely EA, Meunier PA. A long term study of triple arthrodesis in children. *Orthop Clin North Am* 1976;7: 895.
2. Alexander IJ, Johnson KA. Assessment and management of pes cavus in Charcot-Marie Tooth disease. *Clin Orthop Relat Res* 1989;246:273–281.
3. Allard P, Sirois JP, Thiry PS, Geoffroy G, Duhaime M. Roentgenographic study of cavus foot deformity in Friedreich's ataxia patients. Preliminary report. *Can J Neurol Sci* 1982;9(2):113.
4. Andrey N. *Orthopaedia,* London: A. Millar, 1743.
5. Azmaipairashvili Z, Riddle EC, Kumar SJ, et al. Correction of cavovarus foot deformity in Charcot-Marie-Tooth disease. *J Pediatr Orthop* 2005;25(3):360–365.

6. Barisic N, Claeys KG, Sirotkovic-Skerlev M., et al. Charcot-Marie-Tooth Disease: A Clinico-genetic Confrontation. *Ann Hum Genet* 2008. [Epub ahead of print]
7. Barwell R. Pes planus and pes cavus: an anatomical and clinical study. *Edinburgh Med J* 1898;3:113.
8. Bentzon PGK. Pes cavus and the m. peroneus longus. *Acta Orthop Scand* 1933;4:50.
9. Bigos SJ, Coleman SS. Foot deformities secondary to gluteal injection in infancy. *J Pediatr Orthop* 1984;4:560.
10. Bowden RE, Guttman ME. Denervation and reinnervation of human voluntary muscle. *Brain* 1944;67:273.
11. Bradley GW, Coleman SS. Treatment of the calcaneocavus foot deformity. *J Bone Joint Surg (Am)* 1981;63:1159.
12. Breusch SJ, Wenz W, Doderlein L. Function after correction of a clawed great toe by a modified Robert Jones transfer. *J Bone Joint Surg B.* 2000;82(2):250–254.
13. Brewerton DA, Sandifer PH, Sweetman DR. "Idiopathic" pes cavus, and investigation of its etiology. *Br Med J* 1963;358:659.
14. Brewster SH, Larson CB. Cavus feet. *J Bone Joint Surg* 1940;22:361.
15. Buchthal F, Behse F. Peroneal muscular atrophy (PMA) and related disorders. I. Clinical manifestations as related to biopsy findings, nerve conduction and electromyography. *Brain* 1977;Mar;100 Pt 1:41–66.
16. Chan G, Sampath J, Miller F, et al. The role of the dynamic pedobarographs in assessing treatment of cavovarus feet in children with Charcot-Marie-Tooth disease. *J Pediatr Orthop* 2007;27(5):510–516.
17. Chuinard EG, Baskin M. Claw foot deformity. Treatment by transferring the long extensors into the metatarsals and fusion of the interphalangeal joints. *J Bone Joint Surg [Am]* 1973;55:351.
18. Cole WH. The treatment of claw foot. *J Bone Joint Surg Am* 1940;22: 895.
19. Coleman SS, Chesnut WJ. *A simple test for hindfoot flexibility in the cavovarus foot. Clin Orthop Relat Res* 1977;123:60–62.
20. Dekel S, Weissman SL. Osteotomy of the calcaneus and concomitant plantar stripping in children with talipes equinovarus. *J Bone Joint Surg (Br)* 1973;55:802.
21. Deluca PA, Panta S. Pes cavovarus as a late consequence of peroneus longus tendon laceration. *J Pediatr Orthop* 1985;5:582.
22. De Palma L, Colonna E, Travasi M. The modified Jones procedure for pes cavovarus with claw hallux. *J Foot Ankle Surg* 1997;36(4): 279–283.
23. Drennan JC. *Orthopaedic management of neuromuscular disorders.* Philadelphia: JB Lippincott, 1983.
24. Duchenne BG. In: Kaplan EB, translator and ed. *Physiology of motion.* Philadelphia: WB Saunders, 1959;384.
25. Dwyer FC. The present status of the problem of pes cavus. *Clin Orthop Relat Res* 1975;106:254–275.
26. Dyck PJ, Chance PF, Lebo RV, et al. Hereditary motor and sensory neuropathies. In: Dyck PJ, Thomas JW, Griffin PA, Ed. *Peripheral Neuropathy,* 3rd ed. Philadelphia: WB Saunders. 1094, 1992.
27. Dyck P, Lambert E. Lower motor and primary sensory neuron diseases with peroneal muscular atrophy. Part I. Neurologic, genetic, and electrophysiologic findings in hereditary polyneuropathies. Part II. Neurologic, genetic, and electrophysiologic findings in various neuronae degenerations. *Arch Neurol* 1968;18: 603–619.
28. Farill J. A tendon transfer for the treatment of certain cases of cavus deformity of the foot. *J Bone Joint Surg (Am)* 1963;45:1779.
29. Fert RS, del Torto U. "Beak" triple arthrodesis for severe cavus deformity. *Clin Orthop Relat Res* 1983;181:64–67.
30. Fowler B, Brooks AL, Parrish TF. *The cavo varus foot. J Bone Joint Surg* 1959; 41(A): 757.
31. Frank GR, Johnson WM. The extensor shift procedure in the correction of claw-toe deformities in children. *South Med J* 1966;59:889.
32. Garceau GJ, Brahms MA. A preliminary study of selective plantar-muscle denervation of pes cavus. *J Bone Joint Surg (Am)* 1956;38:553.
33. Gould N. Surgery in advanced Charcot-Marie-Tooth disease. *Foot Ankle* 1984;4:267.
34. Hallgrimson S. Pes cavus, seine behandlung and einige bemerkungen uber seine atiologie. *Acta Orthop Scand* 1939; 10:73.
35. Harris RJ, Beath T. Etiology of peroneal spastic flat foot. *J Bone Joint Surg* 1948;30(B):624–634.
36. Heron JR. Neurological syndromes associated with pes cavus. *Proc R Soc Med* 1969;62:270.
37. Hibbs RA. An operation for "claw foot." *JAMA* 1919;73:1583.
38. Holmes JR, Hansen ST Jr. Foot and ankle manifestations of Charcot-Marie-Tooth disease. *Foot Ankle* 1993;14(8):476–486.
39. Home G. Pes cavovarus following ankle fracture. *Clin Orthop* 1984;184:249.
40. Hsu JD, Inbus CE. Pes cavus. In: Jahss MH, ed. *Disorders of the foot.* Philadelphia: WB Saunders, 1982;463–485.
41. Inman. *Human walking.* Baltimore: Williams & Wilkins, 1981.
42. Jahss MH. Tarsometatarsal truncated-wedge arthrodesis for pes cavus and equinovarus deformity of the forepart of the foot. *J Bone Joint Surg (Am)* 1980;62:713.
43. Jahss MH. Evaluation of the cavus foot for orthopaedic treatment. *Clin Orthop* 1983;181:52.
44. James HE, McLaurin RL, Watkins WT. Remission of pes cavus in surgically treated spinal dysraphism. Report of a case. *J Bone Joint Surg (Am)* 1979;61:1096.
45. Japas LM. Surgical treatment of pes cavus by tarsal V-osteotomy. Preliminary report. *J Bone Joint Surg Am* 1968;50(5): 927–944.
46. Kabzinska D, Hausmanowa-Petrusewicz I, Kochanski A. Charcot-Marie-Tooth disorders with an autosomal recessive mode of inheritance. *Clin Neuropathol* 2008;27(1):1–12.
47. Kanatli U, Yetkin H, Cila E. Footprint and radiographic analysis of the feet. *J Pediatr Ortho* 2001;21(2):225–228.
48. Karlstrom G, Lonnerholm T, Olerud S. Cavus deformity of the foot after fracture of the tibial shaft. *J Bone Joint Surg (Am)* 1975;57:893.
49. Kelikian H. *Hallux valgus, allied deformities of the forefoot and metatarsalgia.* Philadelphia: WB Saunders. 305, 1965.
50. Lambrinudi C. New operation on drop foot. *Br J Surg* 1927;15:193–200.
51. Levitt RL, Canale ST, Cooke AJ.Jr, Gartland JJ. The role of foot surgery in progressive neuromuscular disorders in children. *J Bone Joint Surg (Am)* 1973;55:1396.
52. Lutter LD. Cavus foot in runners. *Foot Ankle* 1981;1(4):225–228.
53. McCluskey WP, Lovell WW, Cummings RJ. The cavovarus foot deformity: Etiology and management. *Clin Orthop* 1989; 247:27.
54. McElvenny RT, Caldwell GD. A new operation for correction of cavus foot. *Clin Orthop* 1958;11:58.
55. Meary R. On the measurement of the angle between the talus and the first metatarsal. *Rev Chir Orthop* 1967;53:389.
56. Mills GP. The etiology and treatment of claw foot. *J Bone Joint Surg* 1924;6:142.
57. Missirian J, Mann RA. Pathophysiology of Charcot-Marie-Tooth disease. Paper presented at Foot Society, Anaheim, CA, March, 1983.
58. Mitchell GP. Posterior displacement osteotomy of the calcaneus. *J Bone Joint Surg (Am)* 1977;59:233.
59. Nagai MK, Chan G, Guille JT, et al. Prevalence of Charcot-Marie-Tooth disease in patients who have bilateral cavovarus feet. *J Pediatr Orthop* 2006;26(4):438–443.
60. Nelis E, Timmerman V, De Jonghe P, et al. Linkage and mutation analysis in an extended family with Charcot-Marie-Tooth disease type 1B. *J Med Genet* 1994;31(10): 811–815.

61. Paulos L, Coleman SS, Samuelson KM. Pes cavovarus. Review of a surgical approach using selective soft-tissue procedures. *J Bone Joint Surg Am* 1980;62(6):942–953.
62. Price A, Drennan JC. Computed tomographic analysis of pes cavus in patients with peripheral neuropathies. *J Pediatr Orthop* 1988;8:233.
63. Rivera-Dominguez M, DiBenedetto M, Frisbie JH, Rossier AB. Pes cavus and claw toe deformity in patients with spinal cord injury and multiple sclerosis. *Paraplegia* 1978;16:375.
64. Robinow M, Johnston M, Anderson M. Feet of normal children. *J Pediatr* 1943;23:141–149.
65. Rugh JT. An operation for the correction of plantar and adduction contraction of the foot arch. *J Bone Joint Surg* 1924;6:664.
66. Sabir M, Lyttie D. Pathogenesis of pes cavus in Charcot-Marie-Tooth disease. *Clin Orthop* 1983;175:173.
67. Samilson RL. Calcaneocavus feet—a plan of management in children. *Orthop Rev* 1981;10:121.
68. Samilson RL, Dillin W. Cavus, cavovarus, and calcaneocavus. An update. *Clin Orthop Relat Res* 1983;177:125–132.
69. Saunders JT. The etiology and treatment of clubfoot. *Arch Surg* 1935;30:179.
70. Schwend RM, Drennan JC. Cavus foot deformity in children. *J Am Acad Orthop Surg* 2003;11(3):201–211.
71. Shaffer NM. Non-deforming clubfoot. With remarks on its pathology. *Med Rec* 1885;27:561.
72. Sherman FC, Westin GW. Plantar release in the correction of deformity of the foot in childhood. *J Bone Joint Surg (Am)* 1981;63:1382.
73. Siffert RS, DelTorco U. "Beak" triple arthrodesis for severe cavus deformity. *Clin Orthop* 1983;181:64.
74. Steindler A. Stripping of the os calcis. *J Orthop Surg* 1920;2:8.
75. Stuart W. Claw foot—its treatment. *J Bone Joint Surg* 1924;6:360–367.
76. Sunderland SS. *Nerves and nerve injuries.* London: Churchill Livingstone, 1978.
77. Swanson AB, Braune HS, Coleman JA. The cavus foot concept of production and treatment by metatarsal osteotomy. *J Bone Joint Surg (Am)* 1966;48:1019.
78. Taylor R. An operative note for the treatment of hammer toe and claw toe. *J Bone Joint Surg* 1940;22:608–609.
79. Taylor RG. The treatment of claw toes by multiple transfer of flexors into extensor tendons. *J Bone Joint Surg (Br)* 1951;33: 539.
80. Tynan MC, Klenerman L, Helliwell TR, et al. Investigation of muscle imbalance in the leg in symptomatic forefoot pes cavus: a multidisciplinary study. *Foot Ankle* 1992;13(9): 489–501.
81. Wang G, Shaffer LW. Osteotomy of the metatarsals for pes cavus. *South Med J* 1977;79:77.
82. Watanabe RS. Metatarsal osteotomy for the cavus foot. *Clin Orthop* 1990;252:217.
83. Weinstein SL, Morrissey RT, Winter RB, et al. *Lovell and Winter's Paediatric orthopedic,*. 5th ed. Philadelphia: Lippincott Williams & Wilkins, 942–943, 2001.
84. Westin GW, Dingeman RD, Gausewitz SH. The results of tenodesis of the tendo achilles to the fibula for paralytic pes calcaneus. *J Bone Joint Surg Am* 1988;70:320–328.
85. Wetmore RS, Drennan JC. Long-term results in triple arthrodesis in Charcot-Marie-Tooth. *J Bone Joint Surg (Am)* 1989;71: 417–422.
86. Wilcox P, Weiner D. The Akron midtarsal dome osteotomy in the treatment of rigid pes cavus: a preliminary review. *J Pediatr Orthop* 1985;5:330–338.
87. Wukic, DK, Bowen JR. A long-term study of triple arthrodesis for correction of pes cavovarus in Charcot-Marie-Tooth disease. *J Pediatr Orthop* 1989;9(4):433–437.

CHAPTER 13

Cerebral Palsy

H. Kerr Graham

INTRODUCTION

Cerebral palsy (CP) was first described in 1861 by William Little, an English physician, in an address to the Obstetrical Society of London. He proposed a link between abnormal parturition, difficult labor, premature birth, asphyxia neonatorum, and physical deformities (59). The term "cerebral palsy" was also used by Sir William Osler in 1889 in a book titled "The Cerebral Palsies of Children" (74). In 1893, Freud considered cerebral palsy to be caused not just at parturition but also earlier in pregnancy because of "deeper effects that influenced the development of the foetus" (33). Since the contributions of these pioneers, cerebral palsy has continued to be the subject of intense investigation, in areas including epidemiology, etiology, pathology, and management. This is because cerebral palsy is common, affecting approximately 2 children per 1,000 live births in most developed countries (51). This makes it, by a considerable margin, the most common cause of physical disability in childhood. It is also very expensive to care for individuals with cerebral palsy. The economic burden of CP in the United States was recently estimated at $1.18 billion in direct medical costs, $1.05 billion in direct non-medical costs and an additional $9.24 billion in indirect costs, for a total cost of $11.5 billion or $921,000 average cost per person (62).

Disorders of the foot and ankle are very common in children with cerebral palsy and demand careful assessment, monitoring, and management from early childhood through adolescence and into adult life. In individuals with cerebral palsy, foot and ankle deformities may be a relatively isolated issue such as equinovarus in a child with spastic hemiplegia. At the other end of the complexity spectrum, a child with spastic quadriplegia may have pes valgus, in the setting of severe crouch gait and multiple deformities in the proximal limb segments. In this chapter we will try to outline a systematic approach to the management of disorders of the foot and ankle across the cerebral palsy spectrum.

Cerebral Palsy: Definition

The definition of cerebral palsy has been evolving over many years, since the first description by William Little. This is because cerebral palsy is not a single entity but rather a collection of heterogeneous clinical syndromes, linked by the common themes that the cerebral lesion is non-progressive and must have occurred in the womb, at birth, or soon afterward. Even though the cerebral lesion is by definition a static encephalopathy, many authorities have emphasized the variable nature of the motor disorder and the progressive nature of the associated musculoskeletal pathology. Mercer Rang's classic 1990 definition was succinct and accurate:

"Cerebral palsy is the result of an insult to the developing brain that produces a disorder of movement and posture that is permanent but not unchanging"(79).

Both the definition and the classification of cerebral palsy have been revised by an international committee. The new definition is:

Cerebral palsy (CP) describes a group of permanent disorders of the development of movement and posture, causing activity limitation, that are attributed to non-progressive disturbances that occurred in the developing fetal or infant brain. The motor disorders of cerebral palsy are often accompanied by disturbances of sensation, perception, cognition, communication, and behaviour, by epilepsy, and by secondary musculoskeletal problems" (85).

Cerebral Palsy: Classification

The International Committee that developed the definition of cerebral palsy also developed proposals in respect of classification, based on motor abnormalities, associated impairments, anatomic and radiological findings, causation, and timing.

From a musculoskeletal perspective, it is useful to classify cerebral palsy in three principal domains: motor type, topographical distribution, and gross motor function (39). All three components of the classification are important.

1. **Classification by Movement Disorder:**
   - Spastic 60% to 80%
   - Dyskinetic 10% to 25%
   - Mixed 10% to 25%
   - Ataxic 2% to 5%
   - Hypotonic 2% to 5%

   Many terms are used to describe the movement disorders associated with cerebral palsy and neither the terms nor their definitions have been fully agreed. Different classifications are used in North America, Europe, and Australasia, making communication difficult. In addition, classification by movement disorder is neither reliable nor stable (9). However, despite the difficulties, classification by movement disorder is important in determining prognosis and is highly relevant to management. The system we prefer is spastic, dyskinetic, mixed, ataxic, and hypotonic (39,51).

   Spasticity has been defined as a velocity-dependant resistance to movement and is characterized by exaggerated deep tendon reflexes and co-contraction. It is usually attributed to pyramidal tract lesions and is associated with weakness and loss of selective motor control. The spastic motor type is the most common (60% to 85%) and predictable in terms of surgical outcomes (51).

   Dyskinetic cerebral palsy is associated with lesions of the extrapyramidal system and is characterized by involuntary movements of the limbs, including dystonia, athetosis, chorea, and ballismus. Compared to spastic motor types, there is usually less fixed deformity, and many more unpredictable surgical outcomes.

   Mixed movement disorders are very common because many children have diffuse brain involvement, including lesions in both the pyramidal and extrapyramidal systems. The child with what seems to be spastic quadriplegia almost always is found to have spastic-dystonia as an adolescent. Surgical outcomes are less predictable in mixed movement disorders.

   Ataxia and hypotonic types are uncommon. Children with ataxia have cerebellar dysfunction and difficulties with balance and coordination, best observed during walking. They rarely develop fixed contractures and hardly ever require surgery. Hypotonia is quite common in infancy but many children develop hypertonia with time. Contractures are uncommon during the hypotonic phase but hip displacement may develop (95).
2. **Classification by Topographical Distribution**

   Unilateral CP:
   - Monoplegia
   - Hemiplegia

   Bilateral CP:
   - Diplegia
   - Triplegia
   - Quadriplegia

   Classification by topographical distribution is important and useful because it identifies which limb segments are involved and is a surrogate for gross motor function. The terms which are used include monoplegia (one limb); hemiplegia (one side of the body); diplegia (both lower limbs); triplegia (three limb involvement); and quadriplegia, also known as whole body involvement. Hemiplegia, diplegia, and quadriplegia each make up about one-third of cerebral palsy in large population-based studies. (51) Monoplegia and triplegia are uncommon. Classification by topographical distribution is more robust and reliable than classification by motor type. However, reliability is still relatively poor especially the differentiation between diplegia and quadriplegia. Bilateral cerebral palsy is a continuum and the differentiation between diplegia and quadriplegia is purely arbitrary. These terms are much less reliable and less useful than classification based on gross motor function.
3. **Classification by Gross Motor Function: GMFCS**

   The key element in classifying cerebral palsy by gross motor function is the Gross Motor Function Classification System (GMFCS). This is a five-level ordinal grading system in which there are descriptors according to four distinct age bands (75). The descriptors and illustrations for children aged 6–12 are found in Figure 13-1. This is a highly relevant age when most surgical procedures for foot and ankle problems in children with cerebral palsy are performed. At GMFCS Level I, children have mild limitations of higher functions such as running. At GMFCS Level II, children walk independently in the community but have difficulty running. At GMFCS Level III, children can walk only with an assistive device such as a walker or crutches. At GMFCS Level IV, children have very limited ability to step but can stand for transfers and at GMFCS Level V children lack head control and sitting balance. They are unable to stand or walk and are transported by wheel chairs in the community.

   It can be readily appreciated that most children with spastic hemiplegia function at GMFCS Levels I and II. Children with spastic diplegia are usually GMFCS Levels II and III. Children with spastic quadriplegia are usually GMFCS Levels IV and V (51). However, for the first time the GMFCS provides a simple, universal language to describe physical function in cerebral palsy, which is valid, reliable, and useful (68) (Figure 13-1).

   In general, deformities of the foot and ankle are more severe and are more subject to complications and relapse following surgical intervention the higher the GMFCS level.

Epidemiology of Cerebral Palsy

As noted above, cerebral palsy is not a disease entity but a heterogeneous collection of clinical syndromes (96). There is no single cause for CP but multiple associations have been identified including prematurity, low birth weight, multiple pregnancy, maternal infections, and genetically determined congenital malformations of the central nervous system (6). Despite prevailing legal opinion, few cases are the result of obstetrical errors. Many children who are diagnosed with cerebral palsy have multiple antecedents and it is much more appropriate to consider causal pathways which lead to cerebral palsy, than discrete causes (96).

The prevalence of cerebral palsy is about 2 per 1,000 live births in most developed countries and shows little change

GMFCS for children aged 6-12 years: Descriptors and illustrations

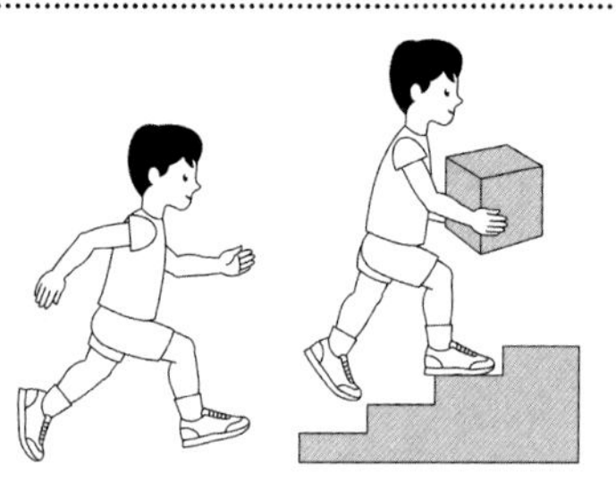

GMFCS Level I

Children walk indoors and outdoors and climb stairs without limitation. Children perform gross motor skills including running and jumping, but speed, balance and coordination are impaired.

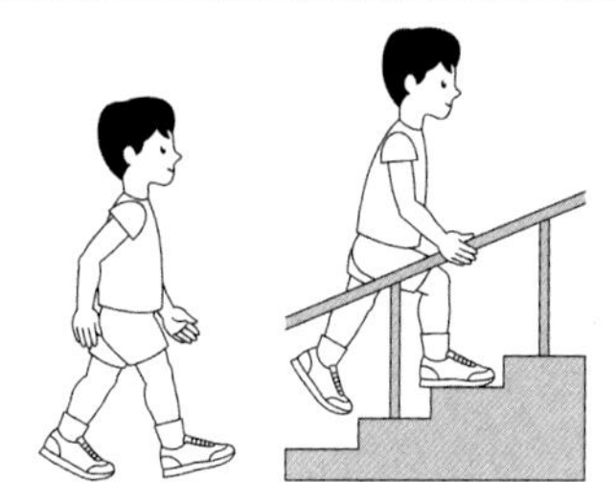

GMFCS Level II

Children walk indoors and outdoors and climb stairs holding onto a railing but experience limitations walking on uneven surfaces and inclines and walking in crowds or confined spaces and with long distances.

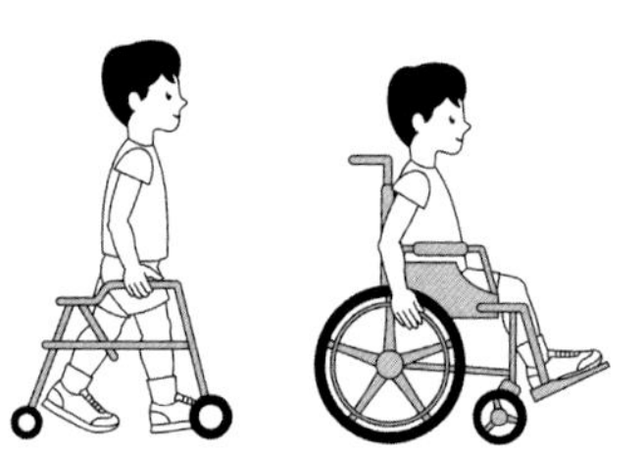

GMFCS Level III

Children walk indoors or outdoors on a level surface with an assistive mobility device and may climb stairs holding onto a railing. Children may use wheelchair mobility when traveling for long distances or outdoors on uneven terrain.

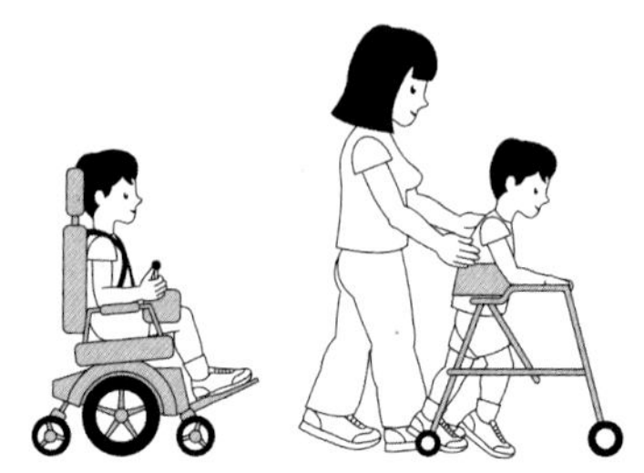

GMFCS Level IV

Children use methods of mobility that usually require adult assistance. They may continue to walk for short distances with physical assistance at home but rely more on wheeled mobility (pushed by an adult or operate a powered chair) outdoors, at school and in the community.

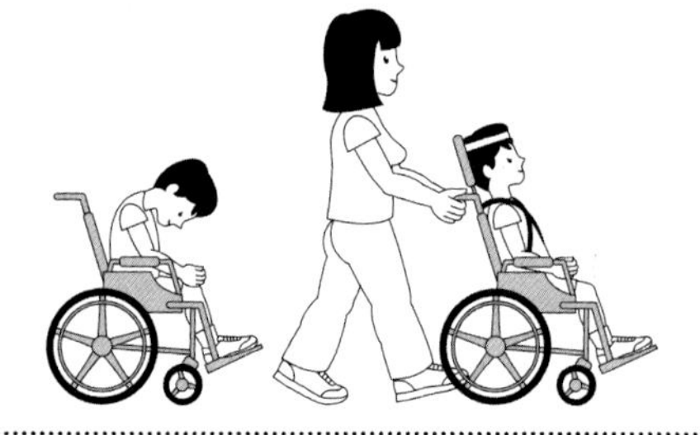

GMFCS Level V

Physical impairment restricts voluntary control of movement and the ability to maintain antigravity head and trunk postures. All areas of motor function are limited. Children have no means of independent mobility and are transported by an adult.

FIGURE 13-1 Gross Motor Classification System (GMFCS) for children with cerebral palsy ages 6–12 years (From Palisano R, Rosenbaum P, Walter S, Russell D, Wood E, Galuppi B. Development and reliability of a system to classify gross motor function in children with cerebral palsy. *Dev Med Child Neurol* 39:214–223, 1997, with permission.)

with time (51). However, the type of cerebral palsy has changed considerably even though the prevalence has not. Athetoid cerebral palsy has been almost eliminated by improved management of Rhesus factor incompatibility and reducing kernicterus in newborns. Diplegia has become more common because of increased survival of premature and very low birth weight babies. Many opportunities exist for the prevention of cerebral palsy by careful epidemiological work which identifies causal pathways and influences public policy in the development of preventative measures (96).

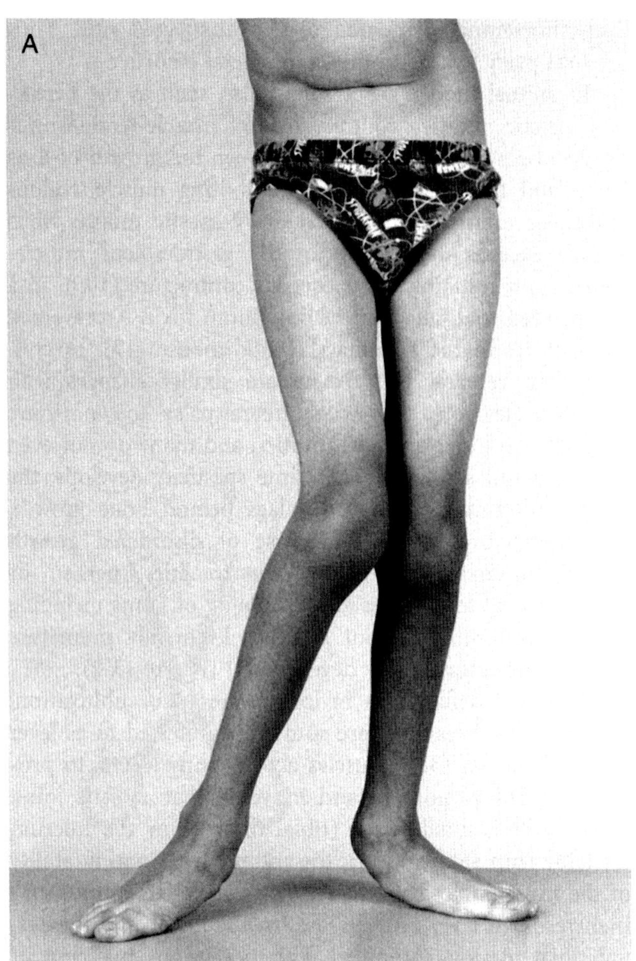

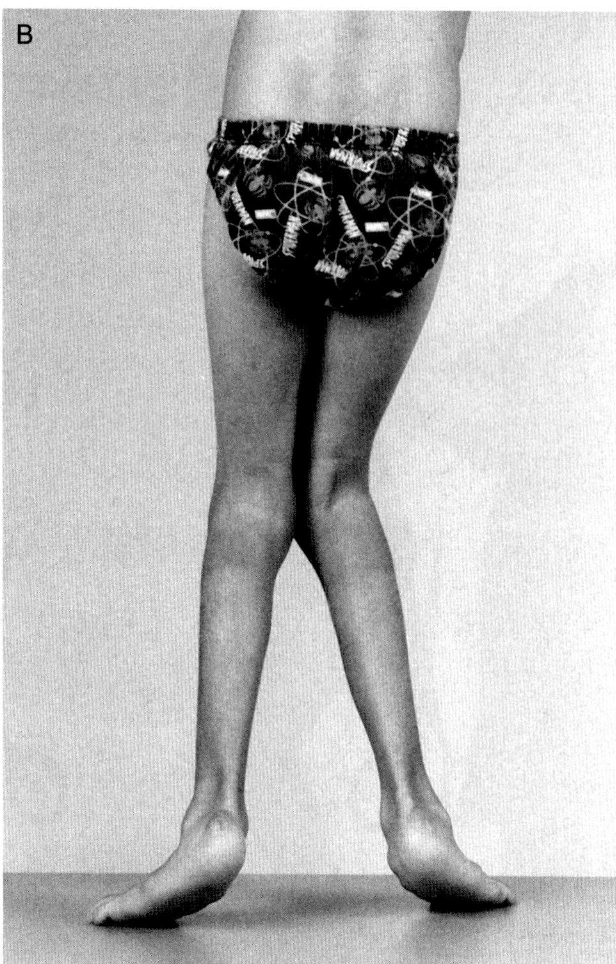

FIGURE 13-2 **A,B.** This 10-year-old boy has spastic diplegia (GMFCS level III) and pes equinovalgus. However in addition to the obvious deformities of his feet, he has contractures of his hamstrings and iliopsoas as well as medial femoral torsion and lateral tibial torsion. All deformities were corrected during multilevel surgery which included bilateral Strayer calf-lengthening procedures for his equinus and subtalar fusions for his severe foot deformities.

Pathology of Cerebral Palsy: A Neuromusculoskeletal Disorder

The pathology of cerebral palsy can be considered in two principal domains, the nervous system and the musculoskeletal system. Cerebral palsy was formerly described as a "neuromuscular disease," but the term "neuromusculoskeletal" is a much better term. With the development of cerebral palsy registers and advances in brain imaging, a large amount of information has become available as to the causal pathways, which result in cerebral palsy, in individual patients and in populations. Brain imaging includes ultrasound, computed tomography (CT) magnetic resonance imaging (MRI), positron emission tomography, and proton spectroscopy. Cerebral palsy was formerly a clinical diagnosis with occasional confirmation by imaging. With the availability of MRI and safer anesthesia for children, the majority of children suspected of having a cerebral palsy will have some form of brain imaging (6). A recent practice parameter from the American Neurological Association recommended that the diagnosis of cerebral palsy be confirmed by imaging (1).

In a large recently published multicenter study (6), the brain lesions identified by MRI were:

- white matter damage of prematurity: 43%
- basal ganglia damage: 13%
- cortical/subcortical damage: 9%
- central nervous system (CNS) malformations: 9%
- focal infarcts: 7%
- miscellaneous lesions: 7%
- normal MRI: 12%

On the basis of their MRI scans, only 20% of cases of cerebral palsy were considered as possibly being secondary to some type of obstetric mishap. A minority of cases, with a clinical diagnosis of cerebral palsy, had a normal MRI scan.

Despite the fact that by definition, cerebral palsy is a static encephalopathy, the musculoskeletal pathology is frequently progressive (40). In simple terms, chronic neurologic impairment from early childhood affects the development of muscles and the skeleton. In spastic hemiplegia, the affected side demonstrates muscle atrophy and

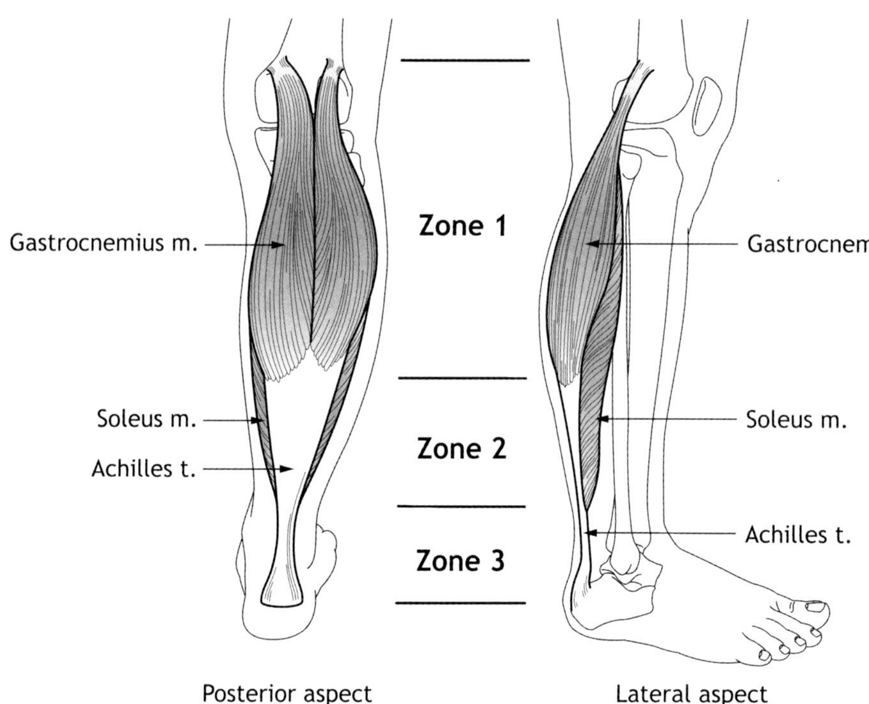

FIGURE 13-6 The anatomy of the gastrocsoleus can be considered in three distinct zones as illustrated. Zone 1 is from the gastrocnemius origin, on the popliteal surface of the femur to the most distal fibers of the medial gastrocnemius belly. Zone 2 is from the distal extent of the gastrocnemius muscle to the end of the soleus muscle fibers. Zone 3 is the Achilles tendon. Operations for lengthening of the gastrocsoleus muscle-tendon-unit can be considered in each anatomical zone.

A B C

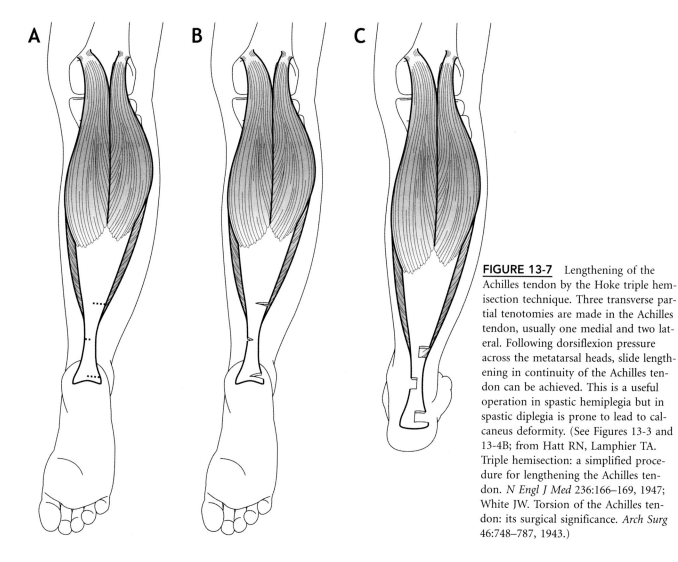

FIGURE 13-7 Lengthening of the Achilles tendon by the Hoke triple hemisection technique. Three transverse partial tenotomies are made in the Achilles tendon, usually one medial and two lateral. Following dorsiflexion pressure across the metatarsal heads, slide lengthening in continuity of the Achilles tendon can be achieved. This is a useful operation in spastic hemiplegia but in spastic diplegia is prone to lead to calcaneus deformity. (See Figures 13-3 and 13-4B; from Hatt RN, Lamphier TA. Triple hemisection: a simplified procedure for lengthening the Achilles tendon. *N Engl J Med* 236:166–169, 1947; White JW. Torsion of the Achilles tendon: its surgical significance. *Arch Surg* 46:748–787, 1943.)

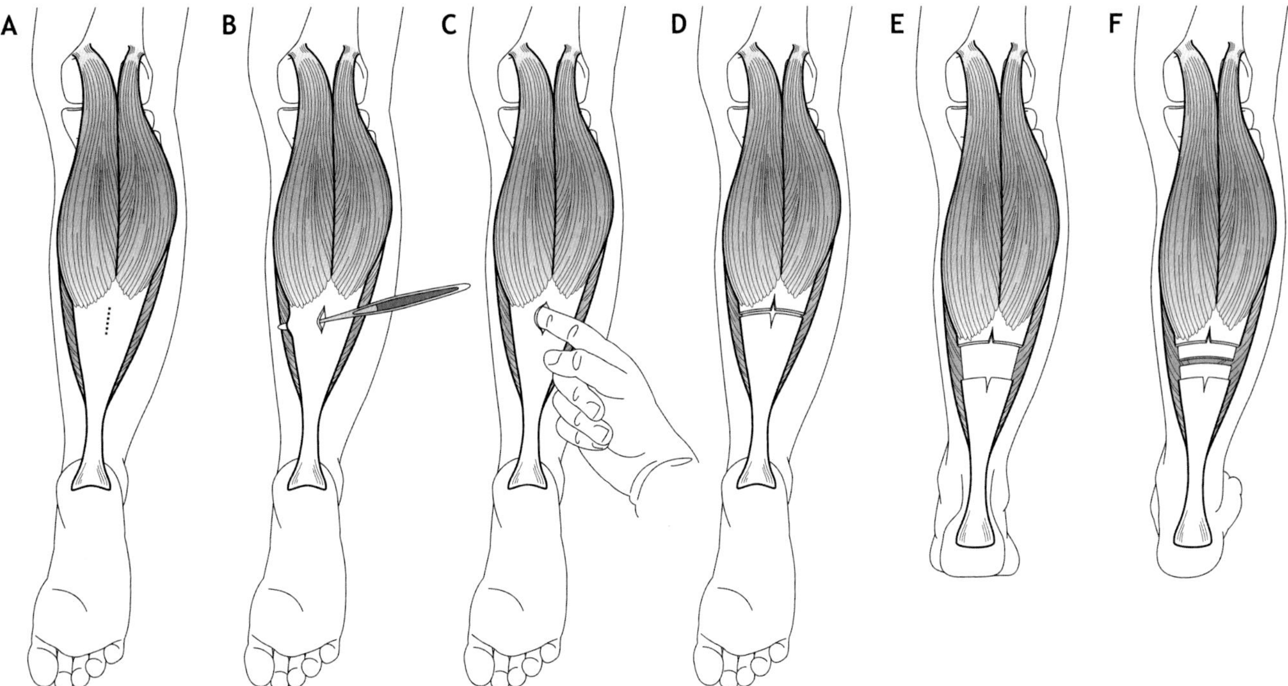

FIGURE 13-8 The distal gastrocnemius recession described by Strayer consists of isolated transverse section of the gastrocnemius aponeurosis. The gastrocnemius aponeurosis must be first isolated and separated from the underlying soleus fascia as shown in **A, B,** and **C.** Following division of the gastrocnemius aponeurosis, the ankle is dorsiflexed and the two ends of the gastrocnemius aponeurosis separate by up to 2 cm. In the gap is seen the soleus fascia but no muscle fibers should be visible (**E**). However if there is still an equinus deformity present, the soleus fascia may also be divided by a transverse cut and the foot and ankle dorsiflexed again. Note that this is not part of the original procedure as described by Strayer but was added subsequently by Dr. Jim Gage. (From Gage JR. *The treatment of gait problems in cerebral palsy.* Clinics in Developmental Medicine No 164–165. London: Mac Keith Press, 2004; and Strayer LM. Recession of the gastrocnemius An operation to relieve spastic contracture of the calf muscles. *J Bone Joint Surg* 32-A:671–676, 1950.)

In type I hemiplegia, there is drop foot in the swing phase of gait. In type II, there is an equinus deformity which is obvious in both stance and swing phases of gait. In type III, as well as the equinus deformity there is involvement at the knee level. In type IV, there is equinus deformity, involvement at the knee with co-contraction of the hamstrings and rectus femoris and involvement at the hip. This system has limitations in that not all children with hemiplegia can be assigned to one of the four groups. In addition the system does not take into account involvement in the coronal and transverse planes. In addition, children with type II hemiplegia may have an equinus deformity, equinovalgus or equinovarus.

In children with spastic diplegia, sagittal gait patterns may be classified into four broad groups. These are true equinus, jump gait, apparent equinus, and crouch (83). In true equinus, the ankle is in equinus and the hips and knees are in extension. In jump gait, the ankle is in equinus but the hips and knees show variable degrees of flexion. In apparent equinus, the ankle is relatively plantargrade with respect to the tibia but the hips and knees are excessively flexed. In crouch gait, the ankle is in a functionally calcaneus range with excessive flexion at the hip and knee (Figure 13-3). This system is also useful in identifying broad surgical strategies as well as defining appropriate orthotic intervention.

Diagnostic Procedures in Cerebral Palsy

It is important to have the diagnosis of children with neuromuscular disease established as firmly as possible. In the majority of children with cerebral palsy this will involve a careful history, including a birth history and developmental history. Physical examination and brain imaging are also very important (1,6). In the past, the diagnosis of cerebral palsy was mainly established on clinical grounds. The American Neurological Association has recommended in a practice parameter that brain imaging be considered as part of the diagnostic work-up (6).

Differential diagnoses include other causes of developmental delay, such as mental retardation, spinal cord lesions, muscular dystrophies, idiopathic toe walking, dopa-sensitive dystonia, and mitochondrial disorders. The majority of diagnostic dilemmas can be resolved by assessing the history, performing a careful physical examination, and obtaining an MRI scan of the brain and spinal cord. In a few cases, additional investigations such as muscle and nerve biopsies and chromosomal analysis will be helpful.

The question of clinical progression is important. When a child is noted to have a functional deterioration, the question may be raised, is this related to neurological deterioration (in which case, the condition is not cerebral

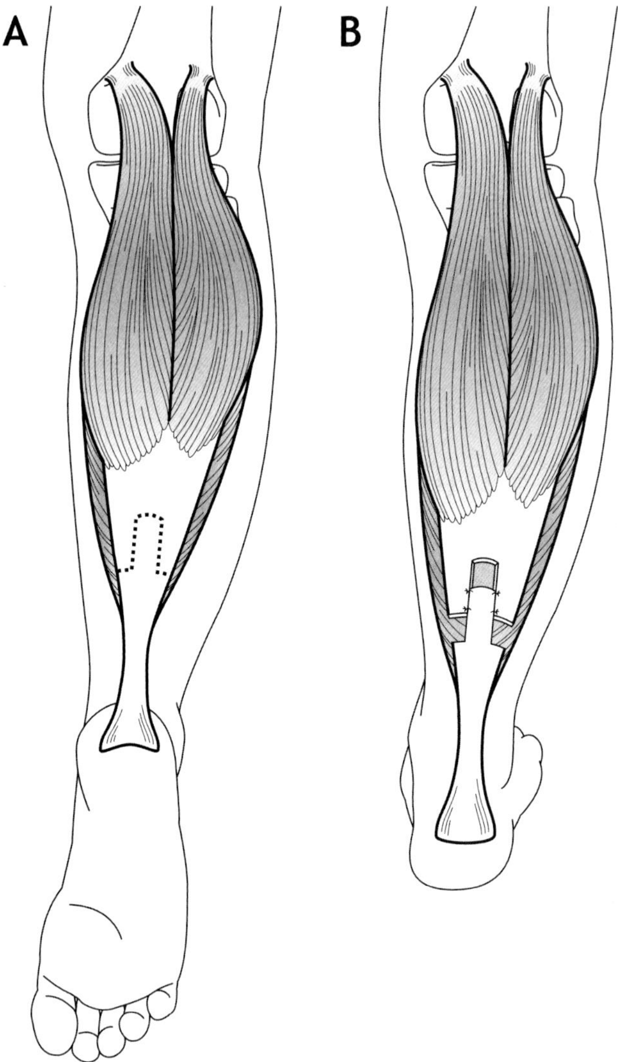

FIGURE 13-9 The Baker "tongue in groove" lengthening in Zone 2 consists of an inverted U shaped cut in both the gastrocnemius aponeurosis and the soleus fascia. Following dorsiflexion at the ankle separation of the fascia occurs as shown. Suturing of the lengthened fascia is optional. (From Baker LD. Triceps surae syndrome in cerebral palsy. *Arch Surg* 63:216, 1954.)

palsy), or is there some other explanation? Rapid deterioration in a younger child is always suspicious. Deterioration in the older child is often the result of progressive musculoskeletal pathology, e.g., progressive contractures or a subluxated hip.

In children with cerebral palsy, much additional information can be obtained from instrumented gait analysis which is highly relevant to the management of disorders of the foot and ankle (35,36,90). Instrumented gait analysis consists of a number of components including standardized physical examination, two-dimensional video recording of gait, three dimensional kinematics and kinetics, dynamic electromyography, pedabarography, and radiology. Not every child with cerebral palsy and a disorder of the foot and ankle requires instrumented gait analysis. The child with the type II hemiplegia and a simple equinus deformity at the ankle can be confidently managed without access to instrumented gait analysis. At the other end of the spectrum, children with type IV hemiplegia and children with spastic diplegia can benefit greatly from the additional information provided by instrumented gait analysis (25).

With respect to disorders of the foot and ankle, pedabarography is being used in some centers with increasing benefits (13,14). However it is not yet widely available and problems remain regarding standardization of the graphical output. Weight-bearing radiographs of the foot and ankle are extremely useful in serial assessment of disorders of the foot and ankle (Figures 13-4 and 13-18). Davids and colleagues performed quantitative segmental analysis on weight-bearing radiographs of 60 normal subjects (19). They identified 10 key radiographic parameters which fully characterize segmental alignment in the normal foot and reported normal values and ranges. The parameters had excellent intra-observer and inter-observer reliability and will be of great value in analyzing deformities of the foot and ankle in children with cerebral palsy.

Function of the Foot and Ankle in Normal Gait

This has been covered elsewhere in this text and will be discussed only briefly here. Understanding normal gait and the role of the foot and ankle is a very helpful basis for the discussion of the impact of fixed deformities in CP. The statements of the pre-requisites for normal gait by Gage, emphasize specific issues at the foot and ankle level, including stability in stance, clearance in swing and appropriate prepositioning in terminal swing, ready for the next foot contact (35).

Perry's description of ankle and foot rockers is also very useful to the understanding of normal gait and the impact of fixed deformities (76).

First rocker is the period from initial contact until foot flat. Initial contact is made by the heel and the foot is lowered to the ground, controlled by eccentric contraction of tibialis anterior. First rocker is disrupted in the majority of individuals with CP.

Second rocker begins at foot flat and ends at heel rise. During second rocker the foot is flat on the ground and tibial progression over the planted foot is controlled by eccentric contraction of the gastrocsoleus. Second rocker is disrupted in both spastic equinus and spastic crouch.

Third rocker is from heel rise to toe-off. It is controlled by concentric contraction of the gastrocsoleus, which generates the power for push-off, elevation of the body center of mass, and adds the energy to the gait cycle for forward progression.

The normal foot and ankle rockers may be disrupted by two main deficits in individuals with CP. These are disorders of motor control and contractures of muscle tendon units. The control of first rocker by tibialis anterior is exquisitely precise in normal gait but frequently absent in even the mildest cases of hemiplegia. Impaired selective motor control also contributes to swing phase problems such as drop foot and poor clearance. Spasticity or contracture of the gastrocsoleus prevents eccentric

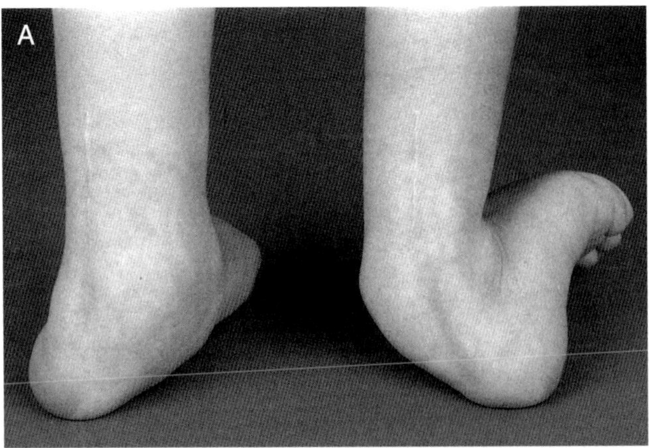

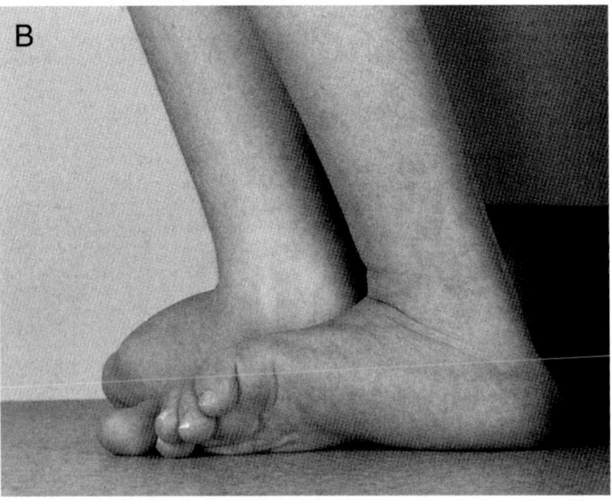

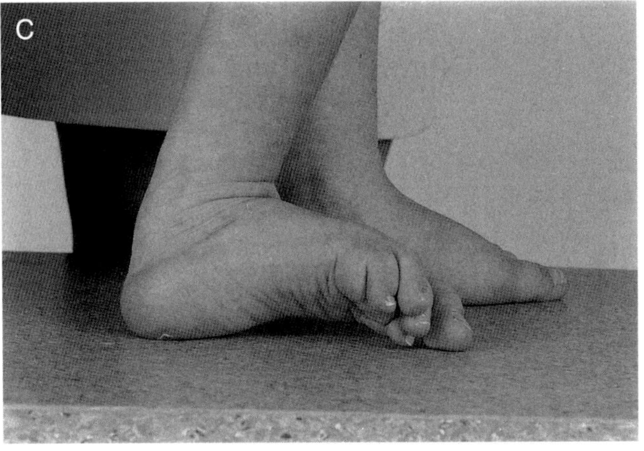

FIGURE 13-10 **A.** Twelve-year-old girl GMFCS level IV who has lost her ability to stand for transfers following bilateral Baker calf lengthening procedures at the age of four years. Both feet have collapsed into severe calcaneo-cavo-valgus deformities as seen in the posterior (**A**) and lateral views (**B,C**). This patient had spastic dystonia affecting tibialis anterior and the peronei which was responsible for the progressive deformities occurring in the eight years following the bilateral Baker's procedures. (Figure 13-10A reproduced by permission of the Journal of Pediatric Orthopaedics).

lengthening of the gastrocsoleus during second rocker with impairment of second and third rocker.

The function of the distal limb segments is coupled with the function of the proximal limb segments in both normal and pathological gait. The plantar flexion, knee extension (PF-KE) couple is a vital concept in understanding gait deviations in CP (35). Normal PF-KE coupling ensures smooth progression in normal gait and contributes to energy conservation. An overactive PF-KE couple results in recurvatum at the knee and deficient PF-KE coupling results in crouch gait (35,82).

For a fuller discussion of normal gait, see Chapter 4 in this text and the suggested further reading, at the end of this chapter.

FIGURE 13-11 Following tibio-talocalcaneal fusion most of the deformities have been corrected and standing transfer ability was regained. (Figure 13-11 reproduced by permission of the Journal of Pediatric Orthopaedics).

CLASSIFICATION OF FOOT AND ANKLE DISORDERS IN CEREBRAL PALSY

1. Sagittal plane ankle deformities: equinus and calcaneus
2. Coronal plane deformities of the foot: pes varus and pes valgus
3. Transverse plane deformities of the foot: abduction and adduction
4. Transverse plane deformities of the tibia: medial torsion, lateral torsion
5. Forefoot deformities: hallux valgus, dorsal bunion, toe flexion deformities.

At first the number of possible combinations would seem to be overwhelming. However because of the phenomenon of kinematic coupling, deformities are also coupled into common combinations. In cerebral palsy, the common combinations are equinovarus, equinovalgus, and calcaneovalgus. Equinovarus is usually coupled with

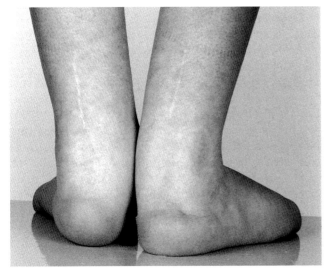

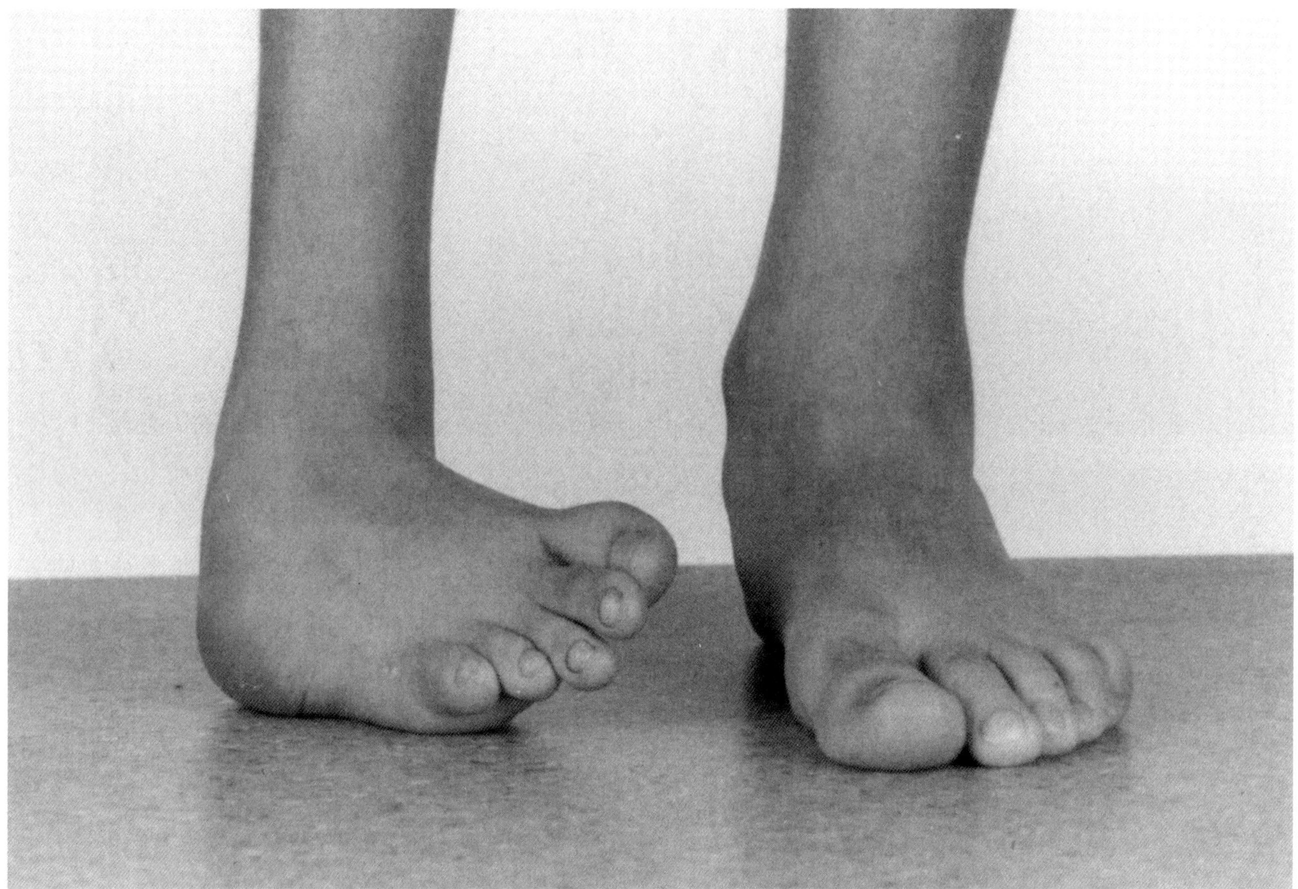

FIGURE 13-12 Severe varus deformity in a seven-year-old with right spastic hemiplegia. All the weight-bearing stresses are concentrated on the lateral border of the foot which is excessively supinated. The foot is painful and cannot be braced.

some degree of forefoot adduction and equinovalgus with forefoot abduction. Other deformities such as cavus are less common in untreated cerebral palsy and when encountered should provoke a search for other etiologies such as tethered cord.

Treatment: Non-surgical Care

In younger children with cerebral palsy, gross motor function is constantly changing and the final prognosis, gait pattern, and functional level are not easily established. Fortunately during this early phase, from two to six years, most deformities of the foot and ankle are the result of spasticity and fixed deformity is less common. During this phase, non-operative management using a combination of interventions for spasticity and orthotic support can be very useful. This is not because the functional gains from injections of Botulinum toxin A are large (they are very small) but because the long-term impact of surgical mistakes can be very high. In the younger child with CP, as in every branch of medicine, the primary rule should be "*primum non nocere*", *first do no harm.*

Spastic Hemiplegia: Age 1–6 years

In children with spastic hemiplegia, spastic equinus is common with approximately 40% of children demonstrating equinovarus, 30% equinovalgus, and 30% a relatively pure equinus. Before the onset of fixed shortening of the gastrocsoleus, spastic deformities can be safely and effectively managed by intramuscular injection of Botulinum neurotoxin A (BoNT-A) combined with the provision of an appropriate orthosis (18,57). The Tardieu and Silfverskiold tests are useful for determining the amount of spasticity and the relative contribution of the gastrocnemius and soleus respectively (32). Intramuscular injection of the gastrocnemius, soleus, and when indicated, tibialis posterior can improve foot and ankle alignment, allowing the provision of a suitable ankle-foot-orthosis (AFO) and improving gait and function. The principal disadvantage is that injections may need to be repeated every six to nine months and eventually most children develop fixed contracture and stop responding to injection treatment. However, given that the results of surgical management are much more predictable after the age of six years, most parents, physical therapists, and some orthopedic surgeons consider it advantageous to recommend focal spasticity management and orthoses for the younger child (12).

The transition from dynamic equinus (spasticity) to fixed equinus (contracture) is gradual. When spastic equinus stops responding to injections of BoNT-A, serial casting may augment and prolong the response to injection. A recent randomized trial found no benefit from the addition of BoNT-A in the management of

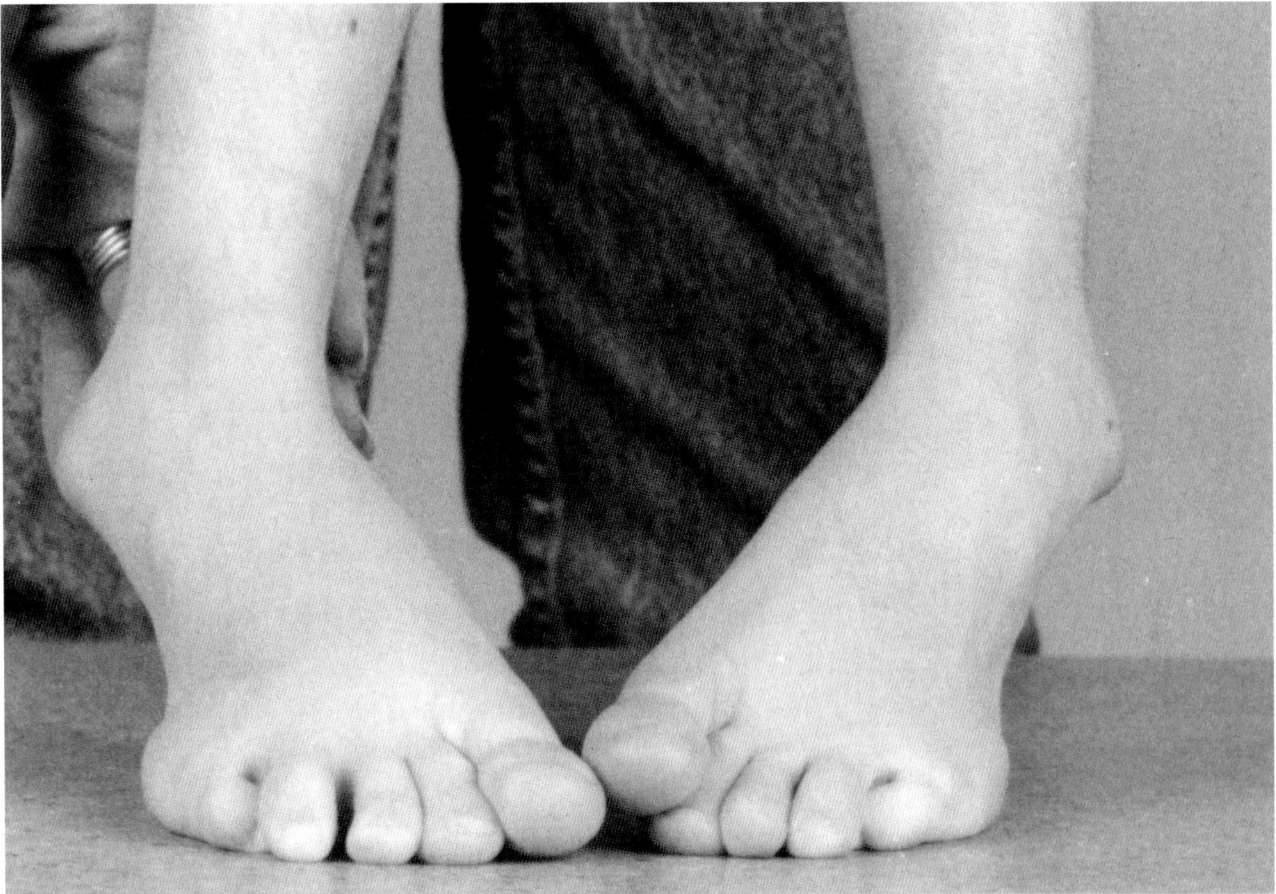

FIGURE 13-13 Equinovarus deformities in a 10-year-old boy with spastic diplegia. Varus is less common in spastic diplegia and following surgery, over correction into calcaneo-valgus is a real risk, particularly in patients GMFCS levels III and IV with spastic dystonia.

equinus contracture (55). However, a more recent study suggests that serial casting after injection of BoNT-A is beneficial but should not start until at least two weeks after injection (72).

Spastic Diplegia: Non-operative Management

In children with spastic diplegia, spastic equinus may prevent the child from gaining a suitable base of support and progressing to independent ambulation. Again, non-operative management with serial injections of Botulinum toxin A to the gastrocsoleus combined with provision of ankle-foot-orthoses and a program of physical therapy will allow many children to progress in gaining the ability to walk either independently or with an assistive device. The majority of children eventually will develop fixed contractures and require multilevel surgery. Delaying surgery until aged six to eight years is advantageous for the majority (12).

One important difference between spastic hemiplegia and spastic diplegia in terms of orthotic prescription is the incidence of spastic equinus versus spastic crouch. For practical purposes, children with hemiplegia never develop crouch gait because the unaffected side provides enough support moment to maintain the lower limbs extended. Hinged AFOs are suitable for the majority of children with spastic hemiplegia because restriction of second rocker is not critical to effective PF-KE coupling and upright gait. The majority of children with spastic diplegia have spastic equinus when they learn to walk but many gradually develop crouch gait, as part of the natural history or because the gastrocsoleus has been excessively weakened by injection of BoNT-A or surgical lengthening. Restriction of excessive dorsiflexion during second rocker then becomes critical to preventing progressive crouch gait. This requires a solid or ground reaction AFO.

Botulinum neurotoxin A is approved in many countries for the management of spasticity in children with cerebral palsy but not in the United States. Technical issues regarding appropriate doses, dilution, and target muscle localization have been fully covered in previous publications (16,42). It should be noted that injection guided only by palpation and surface anatomy is not accurate and should be supplemented by electromyography, muscle stimulation, or ultrasound. In addition, there are three commercially available preparations of type A toxin currently available and one preparation of type B. All have different dose requirements, diffusion properties, and safety profiles.

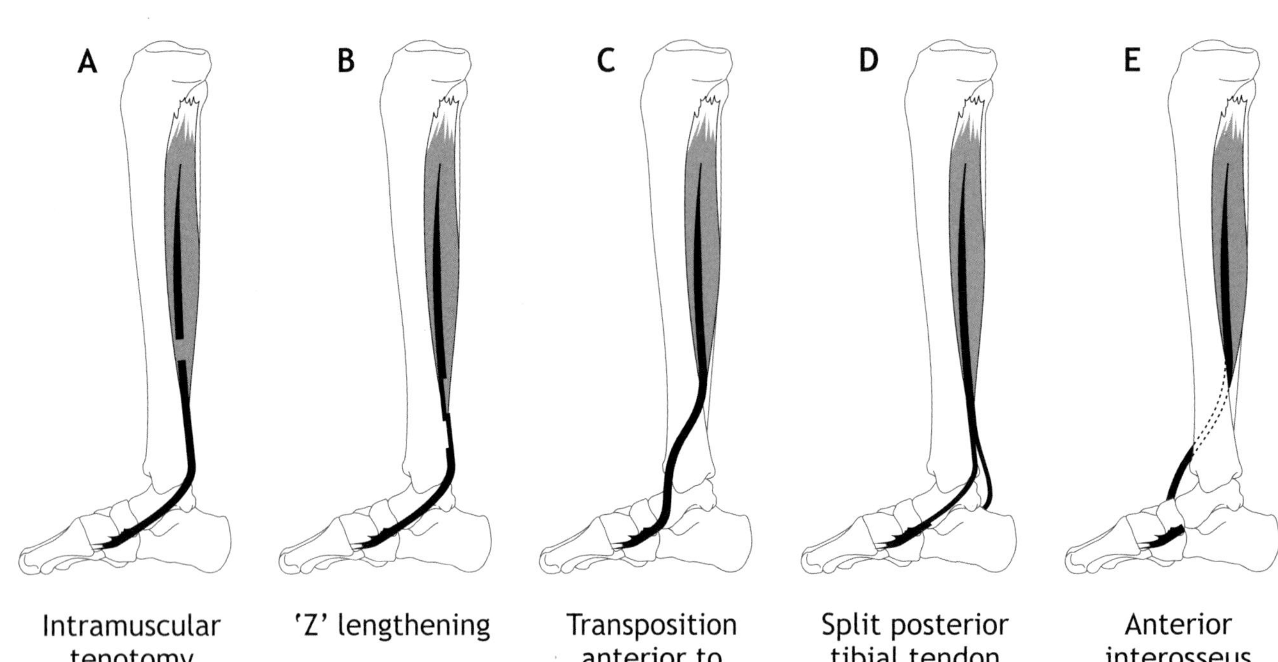

FIGURE 13-14 Tibialis posterior surgery for pes varus. Many operations have been described on the posterior tibial tendon for the correction of pes varus some of which are illustrated here. **A.** Intramuscular tenotomy is a very simple and effective procedure for mild pes varus in the younger patient. (From Ruda R, Frost HM. Cerebral palsy: spastic varus and forefoot adductus treated by intramuscular posterior tibialis tendon lengthening. *Clin Orthop* 79:61–70, 1971.) **B.** Z lengthening above medial malleolus is probably more effective than intramuscular lengthening and is therefore more liable to result in valgus deformity in the longer term. (From Chang CH, Albarracin JP, Lipton GE, Miller F. Long-term follow-up of surgery for equinovarus foot deformity in children with cerebral palsy. *J Pediatr Orthop* 22:792–799, 2002.) **C.** Transposition of the posterior tibial tendon from its normal location behind the medial malleolus to a subcutaneous location in front of the medial malleolus is no longer practiced because of unpredictable results. (From Johnson WL, Lester EL. Transposition of the posterior tibial tendon. *Clin Orthop* 245:223–227,1989.) **D.** The split posterior tibial tendon transfer (SPOTT) involves splitting of the tendon from the insertion on the navicular up to the musculotendinous junction and transferring the medial half of the tendon to the peroneus brevis on the lateral side of the foot to the peroneus brevis. This transfer is very predictable in spastic hemiplegia and there are many reports with good medium term results. Sometimes an intramuscular lengthening above the transfer is required. (From Green NE, Griffin PP, Shiavi R. Split posterior tibial tendon transfer in spastic cerebral palsy. *J Bone Joint Surg* 65-A:748–754, 1983.) **E.** Anterior transfer of the whole tendon through the interosseus membrane to the dorsum of the foot used to be popular. Long-term follow up in many studies shows a very high incidence of severe calcaneovalgus deformity and this procedure has rightfully been abandoned by most surgeons. (From Root L, Miller SR, Kirz P. Posterior tibial-tendon transfer in patients with cerebral palsy. *J Bone Joint Surg* 69:1133–1139, 1987.) Summary: When simple lengthening of tibialis posterior is required the intramuscular tenotomy **(A)** is ideal. In spastic hemiplegia with more severe deformities and when recurrence is likely, the split posterior tibial tendon transfer is the best choice **(D)**.

Orthoses in the Management of Cerebral Palsy

The principal orthosis used in children with cerebral palsy is the ankle-foot-orthosis which comes in a variety of types including posterior leaf spring, hinged, solid, and ground reaction (69). Bracing above the knee level is too cumbersome and does not work. For children with mild involvement, in shoe orthoses such as the UCBL or the dynamic ankle-foot-orthosis can be useful. Ankle-foot-orthoses have two principal actions: control of foot and ankle alignment and improving the alignment at proximal levels especially the knee and hip.

In children with hemiplegia, and children with diplegia who have a true equinus or jump gait, hinged ankle-foot-orthoses are most commonly prescribed. These allow for a variable degree of ankle dorsiflexion during stance

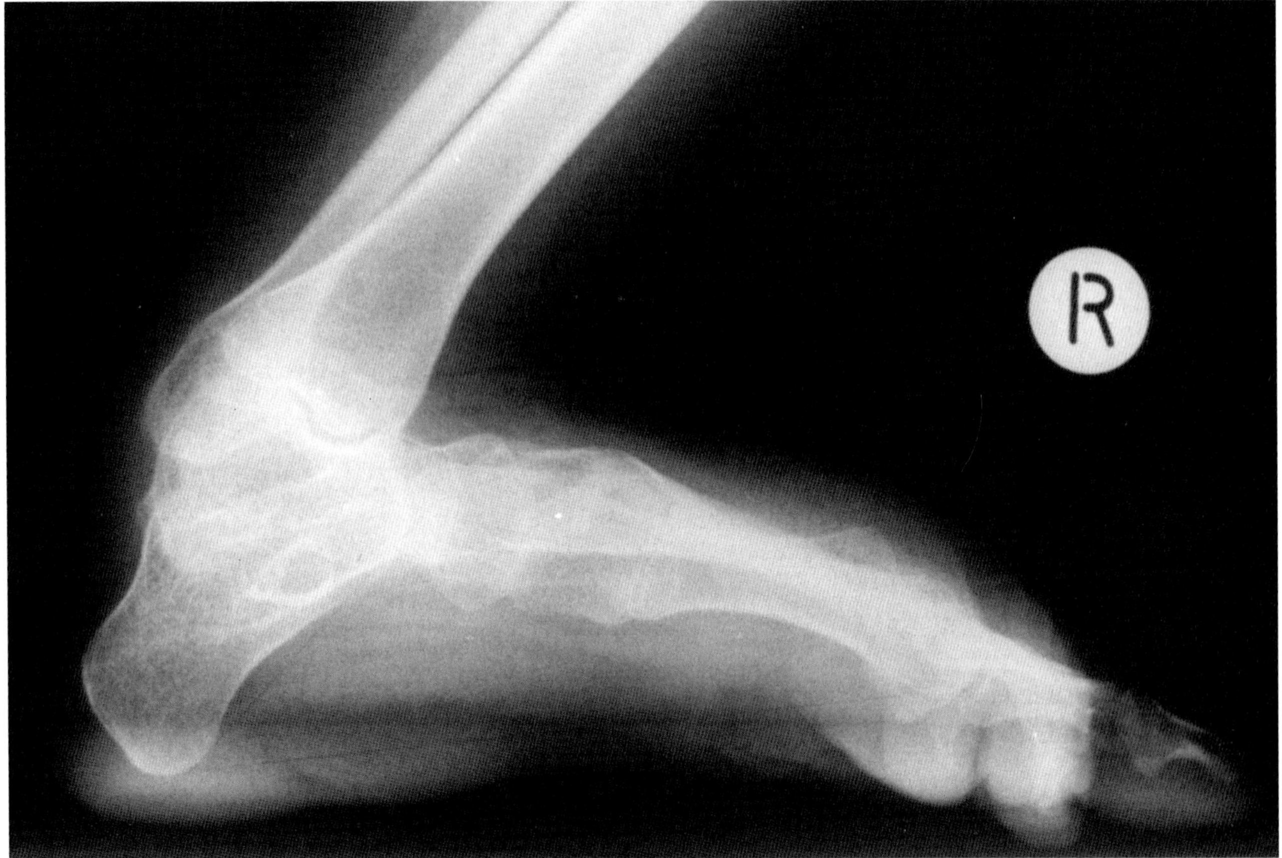

FIGURE 13-15 Severe calcaneo-cavo-valgus deformity following Baker gastrocsoleus lengthening in a 12-year-old girl with spastic dystonia. (Same patient as 13-10A, B, and C.)

phase of gait. In children who exhibit excessive knee and hip flexion, solid ankle-foot-orthoses or ground reaction ankle-foot-orthoses are more useful as these not only support the foot and ankle but also improve extension at the knee and hip, reducing the demand on the quadriceps and improving the efficiency of the gait pattern (83). Ankle-foot-orthoses are useful both in the younger child during the non-operative phase of management when Botox and physical therapy are important adjuncts. In addition, ankle-foot-orthoses are extremely important during the rehabilitation after single level or multilevel orthopaedic surgery (25,83).

Ankle-foot-orthoses are overused in CP. They are unable to correct fixed deformities and are poorly tolerated when deformities are rigid or severe. (101) They should be considered to be a holding measure until the child and the foot is at an appropriate age for reconstructive surgery.

Surgical Management of Equinus Deformity in Cerebral Palsy

Equinus is the most common deformity in cerebral palsy and although it may occur in isolation, in bilateral cerebral palsy it most often occurs as part of a complex constellation of deformities leading to gait dysfunction. Surgery for equinus deformity may be indicated when there is fixed shortening of the gastrocsoleus preventing dorsiflexion of the foot and ankle during stance. In some children, for example type II hemiplegia, equinus deformity may occur in isolation. However in the majority of children with spastic diplegia, equinus is part of multilevel deformity. These deformities must be identified by instrumented gait analysis and dealt with appropriately. Surgical correction of equinus in type II hemiplegia is simple and predictable. Isolated correction of equinus in spastic diplegia will result in iatrogenic crouch gait if proximal problems are not recognized and dealt with simultaneously (12).

The most commonly stated myth about equinus, perpetuated in many texts, is the suggestion that equinus is the result of muscle imbalance, specifically that the spastic gastrocsoleus overpowers a weaker tibialis anterior (94). This concept is not only wrong, but the implication that the gastrocsoleus should be weakened is dangerous. Tibialis anterior is a relatively small anterior compartment muscle which is active at initial contact (to control first rocker) and in swing phase (to provide clearance and prepositioning). The gastrocsoleus (triceps surae) is a very large muscle complex, which contracts eccentrically in stance to control second rocker and contracts concentrically at push-off (third rocker) to lift the entire body center of mass. Tibialis anterior and the gastrocsoleus are active during different phases of the gait cycle and they have different biomechanical functions. In CP they are not

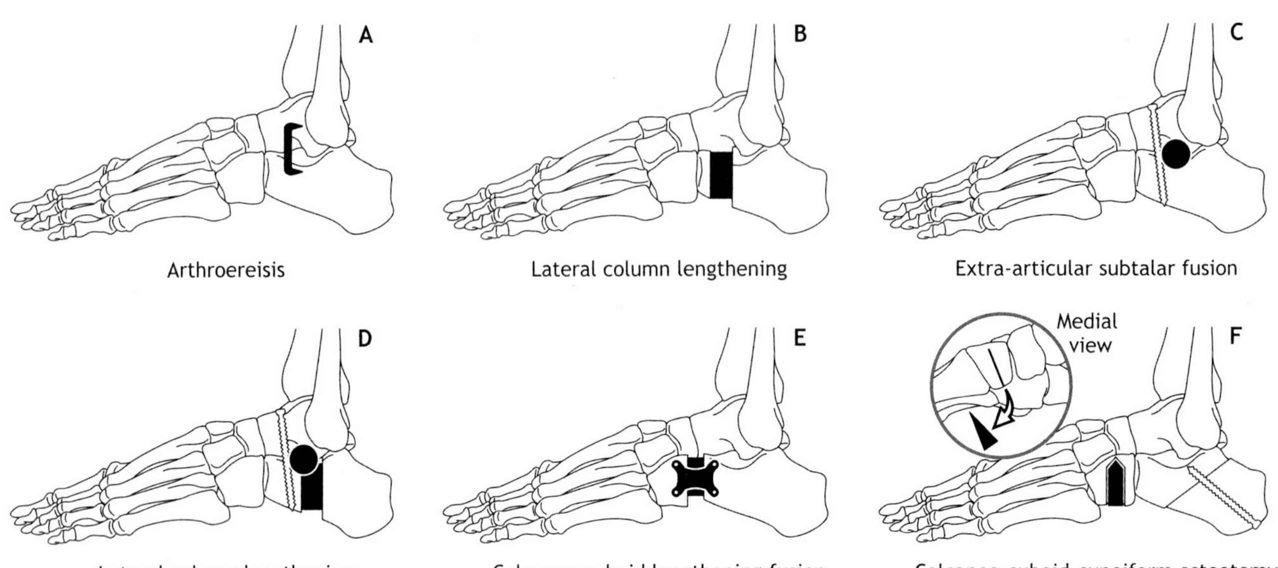

FIGURE 13-16 Surgical procedures for the management of pes valgus in cerebral palsy
In pes valgus, the sinus tarsi is closed as the talus becomes more vertical in the lateral radiograph and as the talocalcaneal axes separate on the anteroposterior radiograph. Surgical procedures for the correction of pes valgus all have in common opening of the sinus tarsi and realignment of the talo-calcaneal axes. **A.** Arthroereisis is a term applied to mechanically blocking the subtalar joint with the sinus tarsi open. A variety of devices have been described, and a staple is shown in the illustration. Arthoreresis works best in mild deformities which may not in the long term require any surgery. In children with more severe cerebral palsy, the failure rate is so high that the procedure cannot be recommended. (From Sanchez AA, Rathjen K, Mubarak S. Subtalar staple arthroereisis for planovalgus foot deformity in children with neuromuscular disease. *J Pediatr Orthop* 19:34–38, 1999.) **B.** Lateral column lengthening as described by Evans and popularized by Mosca has become the most widely used current procedure for pes valgus in cerebral palsy. The lengthening of the lateral column has a profound corrective action on the segmental malalignment of the foot. (From Evans D. Calcaneo-valgus deformity. *J Bone Joint Surg* 57-B:270–278, 1975; and Mosca VS. Calcaneal lengthening for valgus deformity of the hindfoot. Results in children who had severe, symptomatic flatfoot and skewfoot. *J Bone Joint Surg* 77-A:500–512, 1995.) **C.** Extra-articular subtalar fusion using screw fixation and a bone graft in the sinus tarsi is probably more effective than lateral column lengthening, for more severe deformities and GMFCS levels III and IV. (From Dennyson WG, Fulford GE. Subtalar arthrodesis by cancellous grafts and metallic internal fixation. *J Bone Joint Surg* 58-B:507–510, 1976.) **D.** Several authors refer to combining lateral column lengthening and subtalar fusion for severe deformities in which there is a combination of severe abduction (corrected by the lateral column lengthening) and a very vertical orientation of the talus (corrected by the subtalar fusion). No results of the combined procedure have been published to date. **E.** In the adolescent with a stiff abduction deformity as part of pes valgus, excision and lengthening-fusion of the calcaneal cuboid joint using an interposed graft and small fixation plate is a useful option. (From Hansen ST. *Functional reconstruction of the foot and ankle.* Philadelphia: Lippincott Williams & Wilkins, 2000.) **F.** Calcaneal-cuboid-cuneiform osteotomy as described by Mubarak and colleagues is an anatomically sound combination of osteotomies addressing multiple segmental malalignments in the pes valgus complex. The oblique osteotomy of the calcaneum allows a medial shift of the weight bearing surface of the heel under the ankle joint. This procedure is sometimes performed in isolation. The opening medial wedge osteotomy of the cuboid reduces the segmental malalignment much as the lateral column lengthening of Evans and Mosca. The plantar closing wedge osteotomy of the medial cuneiform corrects any supination deformity present in the first ray. (From Rathjen KE. Calcaneal-cuboid-cuneiform osteotomy for correction of valgus foot deformities in children. *J Pediatr Orthop* 18: 775–782, 1998.)

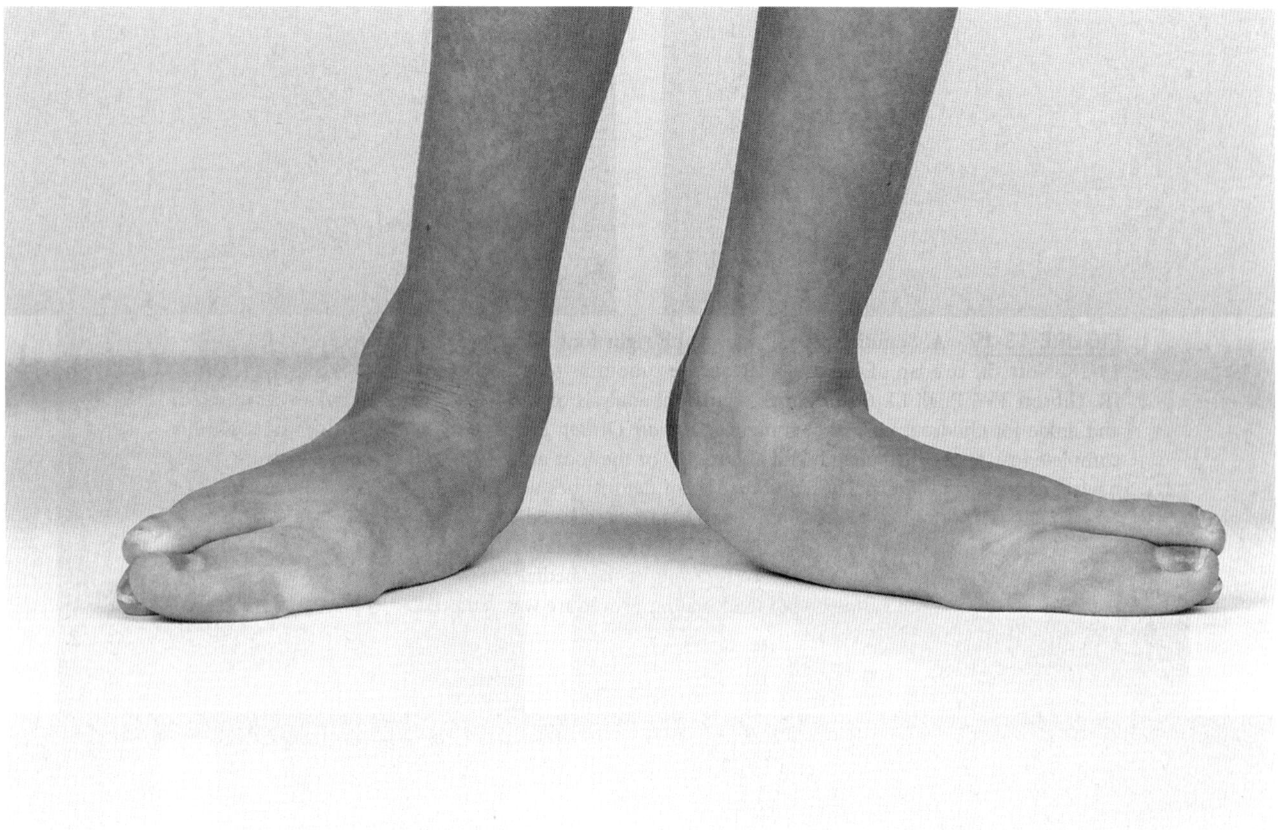

FIGURE 13-17 Multiple segmental malalignments are present in the typical pes planovalgus deformity including hindfoot valgus, pronation of the mid-foot and forefoot, abduction of the forefoot, and hallux valgus.

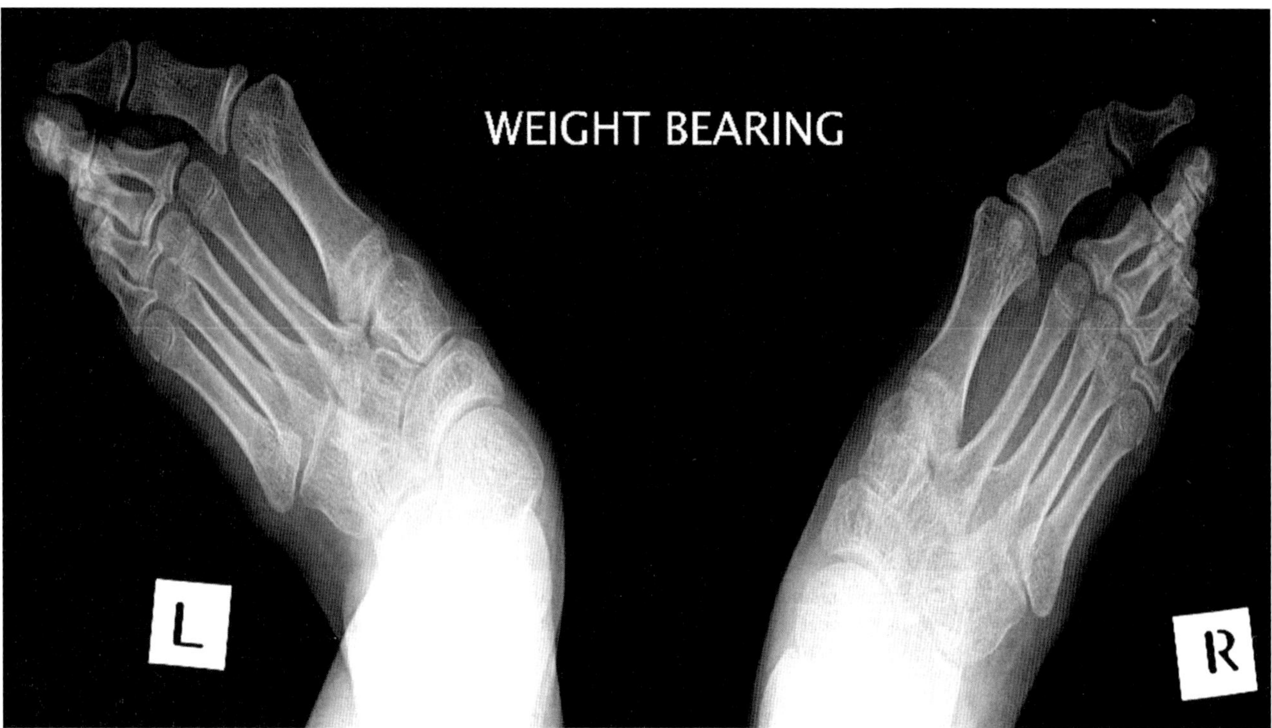

FIGURE 13-18 Standing weight-bearing views of the patient whose photographs are seen in Figure 13-17. Note the hallux valgus, abduction of the mid-foot and uncovering of the talar head by the navicular.

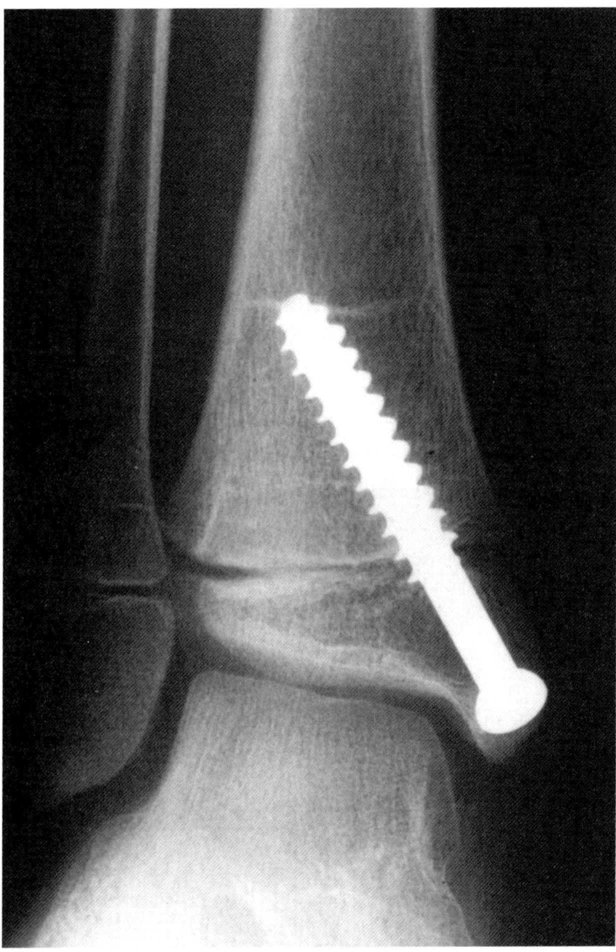

FIGURE 13-23 A mortise view of the ankle should be obtained in all cases of pes valgus otherwise significant ankle valgus as seen in this radiograph may be missed. Correction of ankle valgus can be achieved at the time of supramalleolar osteotomy by tilting the vertical limb of the T plate. However screw epiphysiodesis of the medial malleolus is also valuable if a supramalleolar osteotomy is not required. The head of the screw can be counter sunk to avoid irritation by an AFO or shoe. NB: Children and adolescents with cerebral palsy may have advanced or delayed skeletal maturation and growth plate surgery must be closely monitored to avoid under-correction or over-correction.

child sinks into crouch. This is why crouch gait is part of the natural history in spastic diplegic CP and why interventions for equinus need to be applied very carefully.

Equinus gait may impair function, lead to pain, difficulties with shoe wear, and contribute to associated deformities such as mid-foot breaching. The degree of functional impairment is not always easily quantified because equinus interacts with other factors such as selective motor control. The child with idiopathic toe walking (and some children with mild spastic diplegia), may walk quickly and confidently in high equinus, with little obvious discomfort or functional limitation. The child with severe CP, impaired selective motor control, and impaired balance may be unable to stand or walk until equinus is corrected and plantigrade alignment of the foot and ankle is achieved. The indication to proceed with surgical correction of equinus is usually failure to respond to non-operative measures, such as injection of BoNT-A, serial casting, and the use of AFOs. This is often when spastic equinus has gradually progressed to fixed equinus, between the ages of four and eight years. This seems to occur earlier in hemiplegia than in diplegia (42).

Evaluation of the degree of dynamic and fixed contracture is best evaluated by the Tardieu test, which has been described in detail elsewhere (32). In the Tardieu test, the range of passive ankle dorsiflexion is recorded slowly, to assess fixed contracture (R2) and quickly, to assess dynamic or spastic contracture (R1). Both tests are recorded with the knee flexed (for soleus) and with the knee extended (for gastrocnemius) as in the Silfverskiold test. Understanding the degree of fixed versus dynamic contracture and the relative contributions of gastrocnemius versus soleus, is critical in the selection of surgical procedures.

The triceps surae consists of the soleus and the medial and lateral gastrocnemius muscles which connect via the soleus fascia and the gastrocnemius aponeurosis to form the Achilles tendon. White reported the 90-degree rotation of the fibres which make up the Achilles tendon. This is the anatomical basis for slide lengthening of the Achilles tendon by double hemi-section (102). Surgical procedures for equinus deformity are best classified by dividing the triceps surae muscle-tendon unit into three distinct anatomical zones (Figure 13-6).

Zone I is from the origin of the gastrocnemius bellies, on the popliteal surface of the femur, to the distal end of the medial belly of the gastrocnemius. Zone I operations are selective lengthening of the gastrocnemius by proximal recession (93) or distal recession (98) or differential lengthening of the gastrocnemius and soleus (88).

Zone II is from the end of the medial gastrocnemius belly to the distal end of the soleus muscle belly. Zone II operations include lengthening of the combined gastrocnemius aponeurosis and soleus fascia as described by Vulpius (100) and Baker (3).

Zone III is the Achilles tendon. Zone III operations include lengthening or translocation of the Achilles tendon (77).

Many procedures are of historical interest and have no role in contemporary practice. These include Silfverskiold's proximal recession, combined with neurectomy of the soleus (93). The dissection is too extensive and neurectomy too unpredictable. Translocation of the Achilles tendon is flawed on both theoretical and practical grounds, as outlined by Dr. Freeman Miller (65,77).

The evidence base for the choice of surgical procedure for equinus deformity is poor. There have been no randomized trials and only a few comparative trials. Most studies are retrospective cohort studies with short periods of follow up and subjective outcome measures. The most valuable studies are those with standardized selection criteria, long term follow up and objective outcome measure, preferably instrumented gait analysis. For example, studies utilizing ankle kinematics permit objective classification of outcome as over-correction, appropriate correction, and under-correction, by reference to normal ankle range of motion. Studies utilizing gait analysis report a high incidence of calcaneal gait which may go undetected by observational gait analysis (65,91). Ankle kinetics provide another important outcome measure by showing whether push off power has been preserved. Precise correction of equinus deformity results in increased power generation in late stance, which is highly desirable. Over-correction or under-correction may impair push-off power.

Every surgical procedure described for the correction of equinus deformity is capable of achieving the correct degree of correction, but may also result in recurrent equinus or calcaneus. However, the proportions of over correction and under correction vary according to the type of cerebral palsy, the age of the patient at index surgery, the length of follow up, and the operative procedure (12,43,50,65). Children with hemiplegia are prone to recurrent equinus and children with diplegia to calcaneus, because this is their natural history. Surgical outcomes are much more predictable after age six to eight years than under age six years. Long-term follow up using gait analysis reveals far more cases of recurrent equinus and calcaneus gait than studies which stop before the pubertal growth spurt or skeletal maturity (12,65).

In general, proximal procedures in the gastrocsoleus muscle-tendon-unit produce the least lengthening and preserve the most push off power. The more distal procedures result in more lengthening, more weakening, and a greater reduction in push off. An important corollary is that proximal procedures are more likely to result in recurrent equinus and distal procedures are more likely to result in over-correction, calcaneus, and crouch. Given that recurrent equinus is easily treated by repeat surgery and over-lengthening is impossible to salvage, it is better to err on the side of caution (65).

In cerebral palsy, a range of procedures are required. In spastic hemiplegia there is often a contracture of both the gastrocnemius and soleus and a lengthening of both muscles may be required (43). When the deformity is severe this is most easily accomplished by tendo Achilles lengthening (TAL). Slide lengthening by double (White) or triple (Hoke) hemisection are equally effective techniques (47,102) (Figure 13-7). Slide lengthening is simple and effective, the surgical scars are small and early weight bearing in a below-knee cast is feasible. The long-term results of TAL in spastic hemiplegia are very good but it is liable to cause calcaneus gait in diplegia (12,43).

In diplegia, the contracture affects mainly the gastrocnemius (12,36). A distal recession of the gastrocnemius aponeurosis by the method described by Strayer is then the safest and most effective procedure (98) (Figure 13-8). The surgical scar is more prominent than the scar for a slide lengthening of the Achilles tendon and is in a more prominent area of the leg. Lengthening of the gastrocsoleus aponeurosis-soleus fascia by the method of Vulpius or Baker is effective for intermediate level contractures of the gastrocnemius and soleus, especially in spastic diplegia (Figure 13-9).

In children with cerebral palsy, stable surgery permits early weight bearing and faster rehabilitation. It is therefore important to choose methods which are inherently stable and allow early weight bearing. Distal gastrocnemius recession (Strayer), Baker, and Vulpius lengthenings and slide lengthenings of the Achilles tendon are all amenable to early weight bearing, in a below-knee cast. Open Z lengthening of the Achilles tendon and suture repair is not a stable surgery and therefore may dictate non–weight bearing for up to six weeks.

An ankle-foot-orthosis (AFO) is usually required after cast removal, especially in children with spastic diplegia who have multilevel surgery. We routinely use an AFO with hinges closed after surgery for equinus, until the return of gastrocsoleus strength is confirmed by clinical examination and a video recording of gait. If there is satisfactory plantar flexion, knee extension (PF-KE) coupling, the hinges in the AFO are opened. The duration of AFO use after surgery for equinus has not been tested in clinical trials. In children and adolescents with diplegia who are considered to be at risk of crouch gait, it may be best to continue the use of solid AFOs until skeletal maturity. Alternatively, kinematic and kinetic analysis of barefoot gait compared to braced walking may indicate which children need and those who do not need long term bracing.

Practice pearl: Use gastrocnemius recession for equinus deformity in spastic diplegia and reserve slide lengthening of the Achilles tendon for equinus deformity in spastic hemiplegia.

Calcaneus Deformity in Cerebral Palsy

Calcaneus deformity is a fixed dorsiflexion deformity of the ankle and may be defined as inability to plantar flex the ankle past neutral (24). Calcaneus deformity is seen in severe CP, GMFCS Levels IV and V. These individuals usually have spastic dystonia with a mass withdrawal reflex, consisting of hip flexion, knee flexion, and ankle dorsiflexion. Surgery for equinus in these children tends to result in calcaneus deformity after a few years and most are more safely managed by injections of BoNT-A and an AFO (Figures 13-10 and 13-15).

Calcaneus gait may be defined as ankle dorsiflexion greater than the normal range during stance phase. It is commonly seen in ambulant children with spastic diplegia, GMFCS Levels II and III but is much less common in spastic hemiplegia. Calcaneus gait is part of the natural history in spastic diplegia but is also very common after surgical correction of equinus, especially lengthening of the Achilles tendon (12,65).

At first presentation calcaneus gait may be mild and asymptomatic. However, insidious progression is very common, with rapid deterioration in gait and function, at the time of the pubertal growth spurt. Calcaneus gait then becomes part of symptomatic crouch gait with high stress failure of the knee extensor mechanism and lever arm deformities. Equinus deformity is easy to over correct and calcaneus deformity is very difficult to manage and is best avoided (12) (Figure 13-13).

Complete correction of proximal flexion deformity at the knee and hip and support of the weak or over-lengthened gastrocsoleus in a solid or ground reaction AFO may alleviate the problems to some degree (82). Surgical shortening of the gastrocsoleus has been attempted without success. We have occasionally resorted to tibiotalocalcaneal fusion for disabling calcaneus with some benefits (71). Full-blown crouch gait may require correction of knee flexion deformity by supracondylar extension osteotomy of the distal femur combined with surgical shortening of the patellar tendon. This is a high price for Achilles tendon lengthening in early childhood. Anterior interosseous transfer of tibialis posterior is also a major risk factor for calcaneus. In a recent report of crouch gait surgery, 11 of 12 subjects had previous bilateral tendo-Achilles lengthening (82).

Practice pearl: Avoid calcaneus gait in spastic diplegia by delaying surgery for equinus until age six to eight years. Never perform surgical lengthening of the gastrocsoleus as an isolated procedure, in spastic diplegia. Combine surgery for equinus with complete correction of all proximal flexion deformities and bony deformities, by multilevel surgery.

Equinovarus Deformity in Cerebral Palsy

Adduction of the forefoot, combined with supination of the mid-foot and varus of the heel are kinematically coupled movements, principally caused by activity in tibialis posterior and tibialis anterior, with smaller contributions from other muscles. If the evertors of the foot and ankle are constantly over powered by the invertors, fixed deformity may result. The deformities are also usually coupled with the usual pattern consisting of adduction of the forefoot, supination of the mid-foot, and varus of the heel. However, this complex of deformities is often simply referred to as "varus foot." Symptoms include pain, cosmesis, difficulties with bracing and shoe wear, and difficulties in walking. The equinovarus foot has lost its flexibility and has impaired shock absorption. The deformities can progress from dynamic to fixed and result in concentration of shear forces and weight-bearing stress on the lateral border of the foot. This may lead to painful callus formation and in severe cases, stress fractures in the lateral metatarsals (65).

The relative contributions of tibialis anterior and tibialis posterior to varus deformities of the foot has been studied and debated for many years. Previous studies have been inconclusive because of small numbers and inconsistent use of objective assessments such as electromyography. A recent large study by Michlitsch and colleagues has gone a long way to resolve the controversies associated with the cause of the varus foot in CP (64). They studied 88 feet in 78 individuals with cerebral palsy using instrumented gait analysis, including surface and fine wire electromyography of the tibialis anterior and tibialis posterior, respectively. They found that the main cause of varus was overactivity in tibialis anterior in 30 feet, overactivity of tibialis posterior in 29 feet, and overactivity in both muscles in 27 feet. Importantly, the timing of varus (stance phase, swing phase, or stance and swing phases) was not predictive of the contributing muscle or muscles. This landmark study has important implications for management. Firstly, management of the varus foot may require surgery to the tibialis anterior, tibialis posterior, or to both muscles. Secondly, informed decision making requires gait analysis. However, although surgical series to date have not had the benefit of consistent use of instrumented gait analysis, there are valuable lessons from these studies which form the basis of current surgical recommendations.

Equinovarus is a much more common problem in spastic hemiplegia (Figure 13-12) than in spastic diplegia (50,65) (Figure 13-13). In spastic diplegia, varus is often imposed by proximal transverse plane deformities including medial femoral torsion. If the first ray of the foot is inside the line of progression because of medial femoral torsion, then the foot tends to roll over into a varus position with little or no fixed varus deformity or evidence of over-activity in tibialis posterior. This is known as "roll over varus." Correction of the femoral torsion almost always results in correction of the foot alignment which may quickly revert to plantargrade or even valgus. Lengthening of tibialis posterior may result in severe valgus. However in spastic hemiplegia, true equinovarus is very common. Because of kinematic coupling, the usual alignment of the foot and ankle is a combination of equinus, varus of the heel, with supination and adduction of the forefoot.

The surgical options include surgery to tibialis posterior, surgery to tibialis anterior, or to both. Dynamic deformities are managed by soft tissue surgery, tendon lengthening, or transfers. Fixed deformities may require bony procedures in addition to soft tissue procedures. The literature is difficult to summarize because many studies contain heterogeneous patient populations, rely on subjective outcome measures, and have relatively short-term follow up. The most useful studies are those with long-term follow up and with well defined indications and outcome measures.

Tibialis Posterior Surgery

1. Intramuscular lengthening (86)
2. Z lengthening (15)
3. Transposition of the tendon, anterior to the medial malleolus (54)
4. Split posterior tibial tendon transfer (SPOTT) (44)
5. Anterior interosseous transfer (84)

Intramuscular lengthening is the simplest procedure and was first reported by Ruda and Frost in 1971 (86). It has been used widely since then and seems to be a good choice for mild varus deformities, in younger children with hemiplegia (65). Z lengthening has also been widely used and is probably more effective if the tibialis posterior has developed a substantial contracture (15,50,65). It may be both more effective and more likely to result in overcorrection than intramuscular lengthening. Scarring within the confines of the tendon sheath prevents excursion and leads to recurrent contracture in some cases.

There are three main types of posterior tibial tendon transfer. Transposition of the PT tendon from behind the medial malleolus to a subcutaneous site in front of the medial malleolus was described by Baker and Hill. It has fallen out of favor because of unpredictable results (50,54). Split tendon transfers have a sound theoretical and biomechanical basis. When dynamic imbalance exists in the foot and ankle because of muscle imbalance, caused by over-pull of a single muscle-tendon unit with an eccentric insertion, splitting the tendon insertion, to equalize the pull on the forefoot would seem logical. There is a general impression from the literature that split transfers improve the long-term reliability of surgical correction with a reduced incidence of over-correction and under-correction. The split transfer of tibialis posterior was first reported by Green and colleagues in 1983 and several studies have reported good short- to medium-term results (44,56,99). It is important to note that a shortened posterior tibial tendon may require a proximal intramuscular lengthening, to give enough length for the split transfer distally.

Transfer of tibialis posterior through the interosseous membrane to the dorsum of the foot has a long and interesting history (50,65,84,103). This is an "out of phase" transfer in which the expectation is that the transfer will remove a deforming (varus) force and provide a corrective force, i.e., dorsiflexion and eversion. It works very well in lower motor neuron disorders such as poliomyelitis where the transfer can change phase and be "re-educated" to work in the swing phase of gait. However, in upper motor neuron disorders such as CP, there is no evidence that a muscle can change phase, limiting the theoretical use of the transfer to individuals in which tibialis posterior is active only in swing phase. Although some series have reported reasonable short-term results, the long-term results are very poor and this transfer has no role in the contemporary management of the varus foot in CP (89).

Tibialis Anterior Surgery

1. Lateral transfer (78)
2. Split lateral transfer (SPLATT) (48)

Transfer of the whole tibialis anterior tendon laterally in the foot has been and continues to be used in the management of talipes equinovarus with good results (48,49). It is difficult to achieve precise rebalancing in the spastic foot and it has been completely superseded by split transfer (5,48,49,73,78). The split transfer of tibialis anterior was first described by Hoffer and colleagues in 1974. Several studies report good short- to medium-term results in the hemiplegic foot (5,48,49). The lateral half of tibialis anterior is transferred to the cuboid and secured by insertion into a bony tunnel, sometimes with a pull-out suture over a button in the sole of the foot. Bony tunnels and plantar buttons are associated with significant complications. Direct suture to a turn-up of half of the peroneus brevis or the use of an interference screw in the cuboid may provide a more secure fixation and less morbidity (34).

All of the procedures listed can deliver good short-term results in some feet. However, all procedures can result in both over-correction and under-correction (50,65). Crucially, results deteriorate with time and only studies with long-term follow up are authoritative in their conclusions. The study by Chang et al. is the benchmark (15). They reported the outcome of 108 children with CP who had a variety of tendon transfers and lengthening after a mean of 7.3 years. The procedures included intramuscular lengthening, Z lengthening, and split transfer of tibialis posterior. They used a variety of outcome measures and looked for evidence of both over- and under-correction. Children with hemiplegia had the best results, regardless of age or surgical procedure. Children with spastic diplegia and spastic quadriplegia had very poor results, with the worst results in children under the age of eight years and those who could not walk. The authors advised against tibialis posterior surgery in these patients, but did not suggest viable alternatives.

The varus foot is usually an equinovarus foot but the degree of equinus is variable. If the principal deformity is varus, it is easy to overestimate the degree of equinus and to perform too much gastrocsoleus lengthening. In one study which utilized instrumented gait analysis, sagittal ankle kinematics showed substantial overcorrection when lengthening of Achilles tendon was performed routinely, with split transfer of tibialis posterior (73).

Practice pearl: When correcting the varus foot in CP, perform a careful assessment of gastrocsoleus length, after correction of the varus deformity. Lengthen the gastrocsoleus only by the amount required to achieve 5 degrees of dorsiflexion. Often a gastrocsoleus recession is preferable to a TAL.

The natural history, varus in hemiplegia, and valgus in diplegia and quadriplegia tends to re-assert itself. Children should be managed non-operatively until the pattern of deformity is clear and surgery more predictable. Conservative procedures should be employed and careful long term-follow up instituted to detect failures. Parents should be counselled about the high incidence of failure, the need for long-term follow up and the likelihood of further surgery.

Summary: Surgical Management of Pes Varus in Cerebral Palsy

1. Isolated tibialis posterior (TP) overactivity: intramuscular lengthening or split posterior tibial tendon transfer (SPOTT)
2. Isolated tibialis anterior (TA) overactivity: split transfer of tibialis anterior (SPLATT)
3. Combined overactivity in TP and TA: intramuscular lengthening of TP combined with SPLATT

Bony Surgery for the Varus Foot in Cerebral Palsy

Bony surgery is only necessary for fixed deformity and is rarely required, if appropriate soft tissue surgery is performed at the right time. However, late presenting cases are not uncommon and relapse after seemingly successful soft tissue surgery is also common. A careful analysis of muscle balance is important because bony correction will fail if muscle balance is not established. The outcome of previous surgery must be carefully evaluated. For example, some feet show evidence of tibialis posterior contracture after previous intramuscular lengthening or Z lengthening. Revision surgery will then be necessary. Many feet will require a combination of tibialis posterior lengthening and a split transfer of tibialis anterior.

The principal issues to be addressed are fixed heel varus and an imbalance in the length of the medial and lateral columns of the feet. This can be analyzed by careful clinical examination and weight-bearing radiographs of the feet. The most useful procedures are a closing lateral wedge osteotomy of the calcaneum for fixed heel varus and a calcaneocuboid shortening-fusion to equalize column lengths (27). Few long-term studies have been reported.

The ultimate salvage for recurrent varus deformity is a triple arthrodesis (50). Careful muscle balancing, combined with excision of appropriate wedges from the triple joint and internal fixation, make this a reliable and successful salvage procedure, when required.

Cavus Foot in Cerebral Palsy

Cavus is not a common deformity in CP but occasionally may be encountered and is always coupled with more common deformity patterns. These are:

1. Equino-cavo-varus, in spastic hemiplegia (28)
2. Calcaneo-cavo-valgus in hypotonia/ataxia (65) and
3. Calcaneo-cavo-valgus after over-lengthened heel cords in spastic-dystonia (71) (Figure 13-15)

Evaluation and management is guided by the movement disorder, topographical distribution, and functional demands of the individual.

In the first group, equino-cavovarus in spastic hemiplegia, the cavus is a result of forefoot equinus and can be confused with pure ankle equinus. The area available for weight bearing is reduced to a small tripod and the concentration of weight-bearing forces and shear stresses may result in pain and plantar callosities.

Spasticity in the intrinsic muscles of the foot, especially the abductor hallucis and imbalance in the extrinsic muscles are the probable causative factors. The standing lateral radiograph is very helpful to separate the degree of ankle equinus from forefoot plantaris. Relying on assessing the equinus by testing only passive ankle dorsiflexion will lead to missing the plantaris deformity and excessive lengthening of the gastrocsoleus. The next task is to assess how fixed the hind-foot varus is by the Coleman block test, described in Chapter xx.

Management should then address all components of this complex segmental malalignment. In mild, flexible deformities this usually includes lengthening of tibialis posterior, abductor hallucis, and the plantar fascia, via a medial incision. The degree of residual equinus should then be corrected but over-lengthening should be avoided. There may be value in serial cast correction after these soft tissue procedures and long-term use of an appropriate AFO postoperatively. When the deformities are fixed, the Dwyer osteotomy can be very effective (27,28). Correction of symptomatic deformities of the toes should not be forgotten. The principles are similar to those discussed in Chapter xx.

Mild calcaneo-cavo-valgus in hypotonia/ataxia can usually be managed without surgery. A custom-molded AFO is usually all that is required (77).

There is no effective answer to severe calcaneo-cavo-valgus in spastic-dystonia after over-lengthened heel cords. Tibio-talo-calcaneal fusion can restore the ability to stand for transfers in some individuals (71). This is an extreme form of salvage surgery and best avoided by avoiding the cause, isolated TAL in the younger child with spastic-dystonia (Figures 13-10 and 13-11).

Surgical Management of the Valgus Foot in Cerebral Palsy

"Valgus foot" is a casual term widely used to describe a range of foot deformities in children with cerebral palsy. These constitute by far the largest group, and although they are more common in children with bilateral cerebral palsy (spastic diplegia and spastic quadriplegia) than unilateral cerebral palsy (spastic hemiplegia), they may be found in any topographical type and movement disorder (2,77). The variation in foot posturing alignment is wide and the clinical effects equally varied. In the ambulant child (GMFCS I, II, and III), the valgus foot is primarily the result of tibialis posterior deficiency, not spasticity in the peronei (2,8). In some non-ambulant children (GMFCS IV and V), particularly those with dystonia, peroneal over-activity may be the major factor. This important difference is the key to understanding pathogenesis and management. Genetic influences on underlying foot posture and ligamentous laxity may also be important (77).

The anatomy of the normal subtalar joint is complex and the subject of ongoing study. The concept of the acetabulum pedis is particularly helpful because concepts are drawn from the more familiar hip joint. The head of the talus is the "ball," which articulates with an "acetabulum pedis," composed of the calcaneus inferiorly and the navicular anteriorly (29). This construct allows free motion in the unloaded state, such as in swing phase of gait. In the loaded state, the construct is much more constrained and can be effectively stabilized by interplay between the invertors and evertors of the foot, during the stance phase of gait.

Abnormal foot and ankle biomechanics is also a major contributory factor to pes valgus (Figure 13-2). Long-standing equinus deformity results in weight bearing on the forefoot. This causes excessive loading and bending through the mid-foot, with progressive dissociation and separation of the talo-calcaneal axes (2). The AP and lateral talo-calcaneal angles both increase until the head of the talus is not supported by the sustentaculum and more rapid plantar flexion of the talus occurs. The talus gradually assumes a more and more vertical orientation on weight-bearing lateral radiographs of the foot. The uncovered head of the talus and the navicular present as a bony prominence in the medial aspect of the mid-foot. This makes bracing difficult and often leads to skin callosities and pain (2,41) (Figure 13-17).

Valgus foot usually refers to a group of foot and ankle deformities which consist to varying degrees of heel valgus, mid-foot breaching, and forefoot abduction with pronation. As with all foot and ankle deformities in cerebral palsy, there are frequently associated deformities which are very important to recognize. Isolated management of the valgus foot is rarely indicated. All associated deformities must be carefully evaluated and consideration given to establishing a management plan encompassing the correction of the majority of deformities in one sitting. The most common associations with pes valgus are crouch gait with flexion deformities at the hips and knees, external tibial torsion, overt or occult equinus, hallux valgus, and deformities of the toes (35,41).

Pes valgus constitutes an important part of the spectrum of skeletal deformities sometimes referred to as "lever arm deformities." The important concept, articulated by Gage, is that the breakdown of the foot, associated with external tibial torsion and the long gastrocsoleus, contributes to deficiency in plantar flexion/knee extension coupling, and inability to generate an appropriate extensor moment and sinking into "crouch gait." As with other deformities of the foot and ankle, assessment may involve combinations of careful history taking, physical examination and evaluations which must include radiology, and for ambulant patients instrumented gait analysis (36).

Despite the variety of associated deformities in the pes valgus spectrum, because of the phenomenon of kinematic coupling, there is almost always a degree of "deformity coupling." (Figure 13-5) As the normal talocalcaneal relationship is lost in the standing lateral radiograph, the talus rotates medially and plantar flexes, the os calcis everts and rotates laterally, there is inevitably a widening of the AP talocalcaneal angle with subluxation of the navicular on the head of the talus and progressive abduction through the mid-foot with excessive loading of the forefoot and a tendency to hallux valgus and deformities of the lesser toes. In this collapsed position, the sinus tarsi closes. Most of this deformity spectrum is probably related to passive biomechanical issues, not active muscle imbalance as with the equinovarus foot (8). Hence bony stabilization procedures are the keystone for the correction of the valgus foot. Tendon transfers and muscle-balancing procedures, apart from the correction of occult equinus, are much less important. There may be adaptive shortening of the gastrocnemius and peroneus brevis to the characteristic pes abductovalgus posture, meaning that gastrocnemius recession and lengthening of the peroneus brevis, may be necessary strategies in the overall correction. However this is to accommodate improved joint alignment, not because these are the primary deforming forces (2,41). Given that the unifying concept of foot collapse is closure of the sinus tarsi, the principal procedures used for correction of pes valgus involve opening the sinus tarsi by bony realignment.

Surgical Procedures for Pes Valgus in Cerebral Palsy

1. Staple arthroeresis: Mubarak (87)
2. Lateral column lengthening: Evans (30), Mosca (70)
3. Subtalar fusion: Dennyson and Fulford (22)
4. Combined subtalar fusion-lateral column lengthening
5. Calcaneocuboid lengthening fusion: Hansen (46)
6. Calcaneo-cuboid-cuneiform osteotomy: Mubarak (80)
7. Heel shift: extra-articular osteotomy of the calcaneus
8. Triple arthrodesis (52)

The list of surgical options is extensive, and many other options and combinations have been reported. However, only a few options have gained widespread acceptance and will be discussed here. The most frequently used options are lateral column lengthening as described by Evans (30) and popularized by Mosca (70), and subtalar fusion or combinations of the two.

1. Arthroeresis for Pes Valgus in Cerebral Palsy

Opening of the sinus tarsi and stabilization in the opened position can be accomplished by a variety of implants, including staples, silastic plugs, and screws (55,81). These procedures work best for mild, flexible deformities in younger children However, in these children, as Miller points out, the natural history is not well known and many can be managed nonoperatively (77). The literature to date includes multiple diagnoses and short-term follow-up. It is clear that the failure rate and need for revision surgery is high and cumulative with long-term follow up. At this time, this is not a recommended procedure for pes valgus in cerebral palsy (50,65).

2. Calcaneal Lengthening for Pes Valgus in Cerebral Palsy

Osteotomy of the anterior process of the os calcis and insertion of a bone graft as described by Evans and popularized by Mosca, has become the most widely used procedure for flexible flat foot in children with cerebral palsy (30,70). Despite the conceptual simplicity of the procedure, the effects on the alignment of the hindfoot and mid-foot are profound with most of the components of the pes abductovalgus deformity being corrected simultaneously by lengthening of the lateral column. Evans reported that he discovered the principle linking the length of the medial and lateral columns of the foot, in a discussion of clubfoot management in 1961. He then developed a reliable surgical method for the correction of a short lateral column in valgus foot deformity. In 1975, he described the technique and reported the results of his procedure in 56 valgus feet (30). The majority of valgus feet were described as overcorrected club feet or idiopathic pes valgus. None had cerebral palsy and Evans stated that neurological disorders, including spasticity, were a contraindication.

The procedure described by Evans was refined by Mosca and applied to a range of valgus foot deformities, including skewfoot and valgus deformities in children with cerebral palsy (70). Since then, lengthening of the calcaneum has become widely used in cerebral palsy and has largely replaced subtalar fusion (77). The procedure has been fully described by both Evans and Mosca (30,70). Unresolved questions include the type of bone graft, the need for internal fixation, and the postoperative management.

Following the popularization of os calcis lengthening by Mosca, we utilized this procedure almost exclusively for a number of years in our cerebral palsy population. Longer term follow-up has demonstrated a substantial failure rate, and this was particularly noticeable in the more severely involved child, GMFCS levels III and IV. Mild deformities in independent ambulators (GMFCS levels I and II) in contrast did much better. We therefore now tend to reserve os calcis lengthening for mild deformities in independent ambulators. The avoidance of a fusion is most valuable in this group and less important in the more involved group. Children at GMFCS Level IV spend little time on their feet each day and many require life-long bracing.

We think that allograft has significant advantages over autograft and has in our hands been very successful. The advantages of allograft are the avoidance of an additional incision to harvest iliac crest autograft, the availability of strong cortico-cancellous grafts which do not collapse under loading, the ability to secure a stable "press fit" in the os calcis osteotomy, the confidence not to use internal fixation, and to permit early weight bearing. The disadvantages of allograft include cost and the potential for graft-transmitted infection.

We routinely use iliac crest allograft and prepare a series of trapezoidal wedges cut from the crest. These can be shaped and trimmed to fit the distraction gap once the os calcis osteotomy has been completed. They can be impacted ensuring a stable "press fit." In the majority of cases, we think that internal fixation with K wires is not required. Early healing of the soft tissues occurs allowing us to commence unrestricted weight bearing at three to six weeks after surgery. Incorporation of the graft occurs gradually over 6–12 months. During this time, we encourage no unprotected weight bearing, i.e., the use of a well molded ankle-foot-orthosis at all times.

Our indications for os calcis lengthening are a flexible mild to moderate pes abductovalgus deformity in a child with cerebral palsy aged six to ten years, GMFCS Levels I and II. In general these are children who have started to exhibit signs of brace intolerance and are usually candidates for multilevel surgery (2).

Practice Pearl: Following correction of the foot by os calcis lengthening, it is essential to examine the passive ankle dorsiflexion. Even when there has been no fixed equinus before stabilization of the foot, correction of the midfoot and hindfoot "re-tensions" the gastrocnemius and a gastrocnemius recession is often required at the end of the procedure. If this is not recognized and appropriate calf lengthening performed, the forefoot and mid-foot will be excessively loaded and recurrent deformity is certain.

Following satisfactory correction of the foot by os calcis lengthening, it is important to check once again the tibial alignment. Failure to correct external tibial torsion or ankle valgus will result in failure to correct the overall lever arm and the gait pattern may not be fully corrected. Correction of external tibial torsion by supramalleolar osteotomy of the tibia and consideration of ankle valgus by medial malleolar screw epiphysiodesis are therefore always important considerations.

3. Subtalar Fusion for Pes Valgus in Cerebral Palsy

Extra-articular fusion of the subtalar joint by bone grafting and more recently by bone grafting combined with internal fixation has been widely used in children with cerebral palsy (22). The procedure dates from the poliomyelitis era when a variety of autografts were used without internal fixation (45). The introduction of screw fixation combined with bone grafting of the sinus tarsi has made the procedure much more reliable in spastic disorders (22,77).

The indications in our hands for subtalar fusion in cerebral palsy are a moderate to severe abductovalgus deformity of the foot which remains fully correctable in equinus and inversion. In general we reserve subtalar fusion for children who walk with assistance or have transfer abilities (GMFCS Levels III and IV) and who have moderate to severe deformities which are still passively correctible. As noted above, associated deformities must be carefully considered and the majority will require correction at the same time.

Having tried a wide range of both fixation devices and graft materials, our preference is now to use cannulated screw fixation and cylindrical iliac crest allograft Figure 13-19.

As with os calcis lengthening, the principle of the operation is to open the collapsed or closed sinus tarsi in a permanent manner. The screw fixation achieves the immediate stability to hold the sinus tarsi open and the sinus tarsi bone graft achieves this in the longer term once the graft is fully incorporated. As the sinus tarsi is opened, the talus is lifted on top of the os calcis and immediate stability achieved by screw fixation.

The entry point for the screw should be dorsomedial avoiding encroachment on the talonavicular joint and counter sinking the screw head into the dip on the superior surface of the talus to avoid impingement on the ankle joint during dorsiflexion.

There is a tendency to insert both the guide wire and screw obliquely looking for the longest possible screw fixation within the os calcis. However, this screw alignment may inadvertently find the axis of rotation of the subtalar joint and is much less stable than a screw placed anteriorly, almost parallel to the reduced talonavicular and calcaneocuboid joints. By concentrating on more anterior positioning of this screw, we have improved the stability of fixation and avoided loss of reduction which sometimes occurred with more obliquely orientated screws.

Preparing the sinus tarsi for fusion can be time consuming and difficult. This is particularly so toward the end of multilevel surgery when a bloodless field with a tourniquet is not always achievable and surgeon fatigue may be a factor. We have recently used hemispherical reamers from a set usually used for preparation of the first metatarsophalangeal (MTP) joint in arthrodesis surgery (Figure 13-20). This allows rapid removal of soft tissue and decortication of the appropriate under surface of the talus and superior aspect of the os calcis to receive a hemispherical corticocancellous graft.

A wide variety of graft material can be used both autograft and allograft. Our current preference is for a circular corticocancellous graft, cut a with a barrel reamer from an iliac crest allograft. This is inserted with a press fit into the prepared sinus tarsi.

As noted above, the gastrocsoleus length must be examined carefully at the end of the procedure and in many cases, a gastrocnemius recession is required as well as lengthening of the peroneus brevis but never the peroneus longus. Correction of external tibial torsion and ankle valgus should also be considered when appropriate.

Practice Pearl: As in calcaneal lengthening, forefoot supination must be carefully evaluated, following correction of the hindfoot and midfoot. In many feet, correction of the first ray supination is not required because it is mild and flexible. However, when more severe and not easily corrigible, a plantar flexion osteotomy of the first ray must be considered. Failure to correct fixed supination after calcaneal lengthening or subtalar fusion, will lead to relapse and recurrent deformity. The combined stability of screw fixation and press fit allograft is such that weight bearing as tolerated is permitted from three weeks after surgery. A well molded AFO is recommended for all weight-bearing activities for at a least a year after surgery. Allograft may take longer to incorporate than autograft. (28)

4. Combined Subtalar Fusion-Lateral Column Lengthening

In pes valgus deformities are coupled. Valgus is always accompanied by forefoot abduction and is usually well corrected by lateral column lengthening or subtalar fusion. However, there is a subgroup of deformed feet, where the lateral column is so short and the talus so vertical, that a combination of lateral column lengthening and subtalar fusion is required to fully correct all the components of the deformity. Two grafts are used, one for the lateral column and one for the sinus tarsi. For bilateral surgery, this means a total of four grafts. Iliac crest allograft is a more attractive option than harvesting four autogenous grafts from the patient's iliac crest. Internal fixation is required because the construct is less stable than isolated lateral column lengthening. No series have been published describing the outcome of the combined procedure.

5. Calcaneocuboid Lengthening-fusion in Cerebral Palsy

In the adolescent with abductus deformity as the main symptomatic component of the pes valgus deformity complex, lengthening of the lateral column may not be successful if the deformity is severe and stiff. A graft is forced into the lateral column of a stiff foot, is liable to cause displacement and excessive compression of the articular cartilage of the calcaneocuboid joint. In this situation, a lengthening-fusion through the calcaneocuboid joint can be very useful. The joint surfaces are excised; a trapezoidal graft of corticocancellous bone is inserted. A small plate which bridges the graft and secures it to both the anterior process of the calcaneus and the cuboid completes the construct (46). Graft incorporation can be slow. This is why plate fixation is mandatory, combined with protection by a well moulded AFO for at least one year. No long term-results have been published.

6. The Calcaneocuboid-Cuneiform Osteotomy for Pes Valgus in Cerebral Palsy

Mubarak and colleagues have reported an innovative calcaneo-cuboid-cuneiform combination of osteotomies to address multiple components of pes valgus in cerebral palsy (80). The medial sliding osteotomy of the calcaneum corrects the valgus heel. The opening lateral wedge osteotomy of the cuboid lengthens the lateral column and corrects multiple components of the deformity, especially the forefoot abductus. Finally, the closing plantar wedge osteotomy of the medial cuneiform allows pronation and plantar flexion of the forefoot. This combination addresses multiple components of the pes planoabductovalgus deformity and results in good clinical and radiological improvement in the majority of feet. Further studies and long-term studies are necessary but the short-term results are promising and the combination seems biomechanically sound.

7. Medial Heel Shift: Extra-articular Osteotomy of the Calcaneus

This simple procedure does not address the primary lateral peritalar subluxation but simply shifts the weight-bearing surface of the heel medially under the foot and ankle. It may have a small role in pes valgus in cerebral palsy but the indications are difficult to define and few reports are available in the literature (65).

8. Triple Arthrodesis

Triple arthrodesis can be used as a primary procedure for severe pes valgus in non-ambulators (GMFCS IV and V). It should be avoided in ambulant patients (GMFCS I, II and III) because of the well publicized deleterious effects of fusion on contiguous joints. It is sometimes required as a salvage procedure after failure of previous procedures. The valgus triple is technically demanding because joint excision further reduces bone stock and corrective wedges are difficult to excise from the lateral side of the foot. Supplemental bone grafting to the sinus tarsi or lateral column may help correct hindfoot valgus and forefoot abduction respectively. Internal fixation with small plates and screws is required, followed by 6–12 weeks in cast and protection in an AFO until sound fusion has been confirmed on radiographs. Few long term results have been reported in the cerebral palsy population (65).

Surgical Correction of Hallux Valgus Deformity in Cerebral Palsy

Hallux valgus is a common deformity in adolescents with cerebral palsy and often results in significant pain and functional limitations. In adolescents with idiopathic juvenile hallux valgus, the concerns are primarily cosmetic, with pain and functional limitations secondary concerns. The hallux valgus deformity in cerebral palsy is usually severe because it is the most distal segment in a foot with significant proximal segmental malalignment, invariably pes abductovalgus.

The first study which addressed the natural history and management of hallux valgus in cerebral palsy was by Renshaw, Sirkin, and Drennan in 1979, who reported that the majority of affected individuals were teenagers with spastic diplegia (81). They reported the results of McBride soft tissue reconstruction to be poor, the results of the Mitchell osteotomy to be fair, and the most reliable results were achieved following the McKeever arthrodesis of the first metatarsophalangeal joint (first MTPJ) (60,61,67). Failures of the McBride and Mitchell procedures were salvaged by first MTPJ fusion.

The pathomechanics of hallux valgus deformity in cerebral palsy must take into account the following facts. The majority of affected teenagers have pes abductovalgus and poor clearance during the swing phase of gait. The majority have mild equinus deformity and stiff-knee gait because of rectus femoris dysfunction. This leads to constant "toe drag" in which the medial border of the first ray is the leading edge of the foot at initial contact. Each step results in an abduction force across the first MTPJ which becomes progressively deformed in the typical hallux valgus deformity.

The pathomechanics and natural history outlined by Renshaw and colleagues is relevant to management. First the proximal segmental malalignments should be clearly identified and may require correction. Second, in the face of such abnormal biomechanics, first MTPJ fusion may be the only procedure which can resist the deforming forces.

The definitive study of first MTPJ fusion in cerebral palsy was published by Davids et al. in 2001. They reported a comprehensive outcome analysis of 26 first MTPJ fusions in 16 adolescents with CP and hallux valgus (20). They emphasized the segmental malalignment in the proximal limb segments and in the feet affected by hallux valgus and the need to correct these deformities by multilevel surgery. Their outcome evaluation was comprehensive including technical domains as well as function, satisfaction, and quality of life. The one weakness in their study was the variety of methods used for fixation of the MTPJ, ranging from cross K wires to single screw fixation (McKeever technique). However, the technical results were good with only one non-union.

Our experience is similar to that of Davids and colleagues. When an adolescent with cerebral palsy presents with a painful bunion, the feet, proximal limb segments, and gait should be fully evaluated, even if there has been previous multilevel surgery. Factors leading to poor clearance and toe scuffing should be identified and correction carefully considered. In general, orthopaedic surgery for adolescents with cerebral palsy is demanding of the surgeon and the patient. Healing and rehabilitation are slower than in childhood and dissatisfaction with surgical outcomes is high. In this context, first MTPJ fusion has a very high success rate in terms of patient satisfaction. However, the technical aspects of surgery are very important.

Preparation of the first MTPJ with hemispherical, cup, and cone reamers is very useful because it allows the joint to be aligned carefully in all three planes. Fixation with a small dorsal plate adds to the reliability of the procedure and permits earlier weight bearing, important considerations for the adolescent patient (Figure 13-21).

Practice Pearl: Preparation of the first MTPJ for fusion by cup and cone reamers permits precise correction of deformity in all three planes without further bone resection (Figure 13-20).

Surgical Management of the Dorsal Bunion in Cerebral Palsy

Dorsal bunion is less common than hallux valgus in cerebral palsy and there are few reports of surgical correction (10,37). It is characterized by elevation of the first ray and plantar flexion at the first MTPJ. It results from imbalance in the intrinsic and extrinsic muscles including the gastrocsoleus-tibialis anterior, the flexor hallucis longus-extensor hallucis longus, and the flexor brevis. It occurs in two main groups of adolescents with cerebral palsy, ambulant patients after correction of pes valgus and non-ambulant teenagers with spastic dystonia.

The ambulant patients have usually had a correction of pes valgus deformity which has resulted in unrecognized forefoot supination. In this deformity the first ray remains elevated and the dorsal bunion gradually develops.

The non-ambulant group have severe symptomatic deformities which are painful and interfere with activities of daily living, including bathing, dressing, and wearing shoes. The adolescents all have spastic-dystonia and exhibit an involuntary, mass flexor-withdrawal response. The hips and knees flex and the tibialis anterior contracts, overcoming a weak gastrocsoleus and pulling the foot and ankle into calcaneus. The calcaneus alignment may be spontaneous or precipitated by gastrocsoleus lengthening.

Soft tissue rebalancing procedures for dorsal bunion have been reported, with good results (10,37). We prefer lengthening of the tibialis anterior, combined with fusion of the first MTPJ. The FHL then acts as a correcting force, depressing the first ray.

Practice Pearl: In long-standing dorsal bunion, the articular cartilage of the first MTPJ is usually severely eroded, necessitating first MTPJ fusion for salvage.

Toe Flexion Deformities in Cerebral Palsy

In younger children, toe flexion deformities are usually flexible and asymptomatic (10,50,65). In severe equinus, the long toe flexors adaptively shorten and become much tighter after surgical correction of equinus. This is much more pronounced after TAL in spastic hemiplegia,than gastrocnemius recession in spastic diplegia. If the toes will not passively correct after equinus correction, intramuscular lengthening of the flexor digitorum longus and flexor hallucis longus should be considered at the time of the surgery for equinus. The short flexors can then be stretched out by a long toe plate in the cast and in the AFO.

It is preferable to correct toe flexion deformities before they become excessively stiff. Simple tenotomy of the long and short flexors through a small plantar incision is very effective (65). There seems to be little advantage to the more complex flexor to extensor transfer (4,10).

Practice Pearl: Avoid the need for interphalangeal fusions of the lesser toes, in cerebral palsy by simple flexor tenotomies, when the deformities are still flexible.

Torsional Malalignment of the Tibia in Cerebral Palsy

Torsional deformities of the femur and tibia are common in cerebral palsy and may be overt or occult. The fetal alignment is medial femoral torsion and medial tibial torsion. In children with normal development, both tend to resolve spontaneously under the influence of normal muscle forces and normal weight bearing forces. In CP, delayed gross motor milestones and abnormal biomechanics conspire to delay the resolution of the normal fetal alignment and in many children cause acquired torsional deformities later in childhood (1,35,41) (Figure 13-2).

If a child does not walk independently until age 4–5 years, the opportunity to remodel medial tibial torsion may be missed. However, acquired lateral tibial torsion is much more common than medial tibial torsion. It seems to develop in ambulant children with poor clearance. The distal tibial physis is sensitive to external torque imposed under walking with poor clearance and external toe drag. These are the same conditions discussed earlier, which favour the development of pes valgus and hallux valgus. Once again, it is necessary to look for all segmental malalignments in the lower limbs to formulate a rational surgical plan. The need to correct tibial torsion in isolation is rare. It is almost always performed as part of multilevel surgery.

External tibial torsion is difficult to evaluate clinically and is the least reliable clinical measure in the standardized gait laboratory assessment. Clinical assessment by measurement of thigh-foot angle and bimalleolar axis in the prone position may be supplemented by radiological measurement (35). Neither ultrasound nor CT is entirely satisfactory.

Increased external tibial torsion is part of the spectrum of bony deformities labelled as "lever arm deformities" by Gage and may contribute to ineffective plantarflexion-knee extension coupling and crouch gait (35). We are prepared to observe individuals with torsional deformities of the tibia who walk with full knee extension. However, if symptomatic crouch gait develops, correction should be considered, in the context of a full gait laboratory evaluation and multilevel surgery (83).

Three large surgical series have been reported with broadly similar results (26,31,92). In all three series, the supramalleolar region of the tibia and fibula was chosen as the optimum site for surgical correction. Rotational osteotomy in the proximal tibia carries increased risks of serious neurovascular complications and is contraindicated, unless there is a concomitant varus or valgus malalignment at the knee. The method of fixation in the three series was different, ranging from cross K wires (26), pins-in-plaster (31) to the AO-ASIF T plate (92) (Figure 13-22). Each has advantages and disadvantages. Plate fixation is the most precise, allows the earliest weight bearing but requires another operation for the removal of implants. It is particularly valuable in teenagers and young adults, where stable fixation and early weight bearing are advantageous. Percutaneous osteotomy and fixation with an interlocking nail is an alternative for the skeletally mature individual when a purely rotational correction is required (31).

Practice Pearl: The cross-sectional profile of the distal tibia is elliptical. During rotational correction, there is a tendency for the distal fragment to move medially and tilt into varus during internal rotation of the distal fragment. This may be advantageous if the ankle is mildly valgus. External rotation of the distal fragment tends to cause lateral translation and valgus tilt. This is always unwise and should be avoided by careful attention to detail.

Ankle Valgus in Cerebral Palsy

In the assessment of pes valgus, the coronal alignment of the ankle should be evaluated clinically and radiologically. A standing mortise view radiograph is required. This is not always easy in the presence of severe torsional deformity. Ankle valgus is never an isolated deformity and is usually accompanied by external tibial torsion and pes valgus.

In the skeletally immature patient, correction may be achieved by growth plate surgery. In the skeletally mature patient, an osteotomy will be required, usually a supramalleolar osteotomy of the tibia and fibula, in which rotational correction and valgus correction are combined. Internal fixation with a T plate is particularly useful for the correction of valgus and external rotation. The vertical limb of the T plate is used to fine tune the coronal plane alignment, after distal fixation.

Correction of ankle valgus in the immature patient can be achieved using a screw, staple, or "8" plate, placed across the medial aspect of the distal tibial growth plate (21, 97) (Figure 13-23). The rate of correction varies according to the child's bone age and rate of growth. Growth plate surgery in cerebral palsy is unpredictable because of both premature and delayed skeletal maturation, which may be seen in these children.

Practice Pearl: Epiphysiodesis for the correction of ankle valgus can be achieved using a screw in the medial malleolus which can be countersunk to avoid irritation. Use of the "8" plate may be indicated in the younger

pediatric orthopaedic surgery. Philadelphia: JB Lippincott Company. 1995:498–500.

67. Mitchell CL, Fleming JL, Allen R, Glenney C, Sanford GA. Osteotomy-bunionectomy hallux valgus. *J Bone Joint Surg* 40-A:41–60, 1958.
68. Morris C, Bartlett D. Gross Motor Function Classification System: impact and utility. *Dev Med Child Neurol* 46:60–65, 2004.
69. Morris C. Cerebral Palsy. In: *Pediatric Orthotics* Morris C, (Ed) Dias LS, (Ortho Ed). London: Mac Keith Press, 2007.
70. Mosca VS. Calcaneal lengthening for valgus deformity of the hindfoot. Results in children who had severe, symptomatic flatfoot and skewfoot. *J Bone Joint Surg* 77–A:500–512, 1995.
71. Muir D, Angliss RD, Nattrass GR, Graham HK. Tibiotalocalcaneal arthrodesis for severe calcaneovalgus deformity in cerebral palsy. *J Pediatr Orthop* 25:651–656, 2005.
72. Newman C, Kennedy A, Walsh M, O'Brien T, Lynch B, Hensey O. A pilot study of delayed versus immediate serial casting after Botulinum toxin injection for partially reducible spastic equinus. *J Pediatr Orthoped* 27:882–885, 2007.
73. O'Byrne JM, Kennedy A, Jenkinson A, et al. Split tibialis posterior tendon transfer in the treatment of spastic equinovarus foot. *J Pediatr Orthop* 17:481–485, 1997.
74. Osler W. *The cerebral palsies of children.* A Clinical Study for the Infirmary for Nervous Diseases. Philadelphia: Blakiston, 1889.
75. Palisano R, Rosenbaum P, Walter S, Russell D, Wood E, Galuppi B. Development and reliability of a system to classify gross motor function in children with cerebral palsy. *Dev Med Child Neurol* 39:214–223, 1997.
76. Perry J. *Gait Analysis. Normal and Pathological Function.* Thorofare, NJ: Slack Inc., 1992.
77. Pierrot AH, Murphy OB. Heel cord advancement: a new approach to the spastic equinus deformity. *Orthop Clin North Am* 5:117–126, 1974.
78. Ponsetti IV. *Congenital Clubfoot. Fundamentals of treatment.* Oxford: Oxford University Press, 1996.
79. Rang M. Cerebral Palsy. In: Morrissey R.T., ed.: *Lovell and Winter's Paediatric Orthopaedics*, 3rd ed. vol. 1. Philadelphia: J. B. Lippincott, 1990, 465–506.
80. Rathjen KE. Calcaneal-cuboid-cuneiform osteotomy for correction of valgus foot deformities in children. *J Pediatr Orthop* 18: 775–782, 1998.
81. Renshaw TS, Sirkin RB, Drennan JC. The management of hallux valgus in cerebral palsy. *Dev Med Child Neurol* 21:202–208, 1979.
82. Rodda JM, Graham HK, Galea MP, Baker R, Nattrass GR, Wolfe R. Correction of severe crouch gait in spastic diplegia by multilevel orthopaedic surgery: Outcome at one and five years. *J Bone Joint Surg* 88-A:2653–2664, 2006.
83. Rodda JM, Graham HK, Carson L, Galea MP, Wolfe R. Sagittal gait patterns in spastic diplegia. *J Bone Joint Surg* 86-B:251–258, 2004.
84. Root L, Miller SR, Kirz P. Posterior tibial-tendon transfer in patients with cerebral palsy. *J Bone Joint Surg* 69:1133–1139, 1987.
85. Rosenbaum P, Paneth N, Leviton A, Goldstein M, Bax M. A report: the definition and classification of cerebral palsy, April 2006. *Dev Med Child Neurol* 49 (Suppl 109):1–44, 2007.
86. Ruda R, Frost HM. Cerebral palsy: spastic varus and forefoot adductus treated by intramuscular posterior tibialis tendon lengthening. *Clin Orthop* 79:61–70, 1971.
87. Sanchez AA, Rathjen K, Mubarak S. Subtalar staple arthroereisis for planovalgus foot deformity in children with neuromuscular disease. *J Pediatr Orthop* 19:34–38, 1999.
88. Saraph V, Zwick EB, Uitz C, Linhart W, Steinwender G. The Baumann procedure for fixed contracture of the gastrocsoleus in cerebral palsy. Evaluation of function of the ankle after multilevel surgery. *J Bone Joint Surg* 82-B:535–540, 2000.
89. Schneider M, Balon K. Deformity of the foot following anterior transfer of the posterior tibial tendon and lengthening of the Achilles tendon for spastic equinovarus. *Clin Orthop* 125:113–118, 1977.
90. Schwartz MH, Viehweger E, Stout J, Novacheck TF, Gage J. Comprehensive treatment of ambulatory children with cerebral palsy. An outcome assessment. *J Pediatr Orthop* 24:45–53, 2004.
91. Segal LS, Thomas SE, Mazur JM, Mauterer M. Calcaneal gait in spastic diplegia after heel cord lengthening: a study with gait analysis. *J Pediatr Orthop* 9:697–701, 1989.
92. Selber P, Filho ER, Dallalana R, Pirpiris M, Nattrass GR, Graham HK. Supramalleolar derotation osteotomy of the tibia, with T plate fixation: Technique and Results. *J Bone Joint Surg* 86-B:1170–1175, 2004.
93. Silfverskiold N. Reduction of the uncrossed two-joints muscles of the leg to one-joint muscles in spastic conditions. *Acta Chir Scand* 56:315–330, 1923–1924.
94. Silver RL, de la Garza J, Rang M. The myth of muscle balance. *J Bone Joint Surg* 67-B:432–437, 1985.
95. Soo B, Howard J, Boyd RN, Reid S, Lanigan A, Wolfe R, Reddihough D, Graham HK. Hip displacement in cerebral palsy: A population based study of incidence in relation to motor type, topographical distribution and gross motor function. *J Bone Joint Surgery* 88–A:121–129, 2006.
96. Stanley FJ, Blair E, Alberman E. What are the cerebral palsies? In Bax M, Hart HM, eds. *Cerebral Palsies: Epidemiology and Causal Pathways.* London: Mac Keith Press, 8–13, 2000.
97. Stevens PM. Guided growth for angular correction. A preliminary series using a tension band plate. *J Pediatr Orthop* 27:253–259, 2007.
98. Strayer LM. Recession of the gastrocnemius An operation to relieve spastic contracture of the calf muscles. *J Bone Joint Surg* 32-A:671–676, 1950.
99. Synder M, Jay Kumar S, Stecyk MD. Split tibialis posterior tendon transfer and tendo-Achilles lengthening for spastic equinovarus feet. *J Pediatr Orthop* 13:20–23, 1993.
100. Vulpius O, Stoffel A. Tenotomie der end schen der mm. Gastrocnemius el soleus mittels rutschenlassens nach Vulpius. In: *Orthopaedische Operationslehre* Ferdinand Enke, 1920:29–31.
101. Westberry DE, Davids JR, Shaver JC, Tanner SL, Blackhurst DW, Davis RB. Impact of ankle-foot orthoses on static foot alignment in children with cerebral palsy. *J Bone Joint Surg* 89:806–813, 2007.
102. White JW. Torsion of the Achilles tendon: its surgical significance. *Arch Surg* 46:748–787, 1943.
103. Williams PF. Restoration of muscle balance of the foot by transfer of the tibialis posterior. *J Bone Joint Surg* 58-B:217–219, 1976.
104. Winters T, Gage J, Hicks R. Gait patterns in spastic hemiplegia in children and adults. *J Bone Joint Surg* 69-A:437–441, 1987.
105. Ziv I, Blackburn N, Rang M, Koreska J. Muscle growth in the normal and spastic mouse. *Dev Med Child Neurol* 26:94–99, 1984.

RECOMMENDED READING

1. Gage JR. *The treatment of gait problems in cerebral palsy.* Clinics in Developmental Medicine No 164–165. London: Mac Keith Press, 2004.
2. Miller F. *Cerebral Palsy.* Springer. New York 2005.
3. Horstmann HM, Bleck EE. *Orthopaedic Management in Cerebral Palsy.* Clinics in Developmental Medicine. No 173–174. London: Mac Keith Press, 2007.

CHAPTER 14

Myelomeningocele

Gaia Georgopoulos

INTRODUCTION

Myelomeningocele is a congenital malformation of the spinal column and neural elements in which absence of the posterior vertebral elements is associated with a cystic expansion of the meninges, which contains the spinal cord and/or nerve roots. The incidence is approximately 1 in 1,000, and the risk is significantly reduced by supplementation with folic acid during pregnancy. Both the maternal serum alpha fetoprotein level and ultrasound are used for prenatal screening, and an elective caesarean section is utilized for delivery (17). The diverse needs of children with myelomeningocele are best addressed in a multidisciplinary clinic. Myelomeningocele is a dynamic disease, and changes in neurologic function are common and may be associated with worsening of musculoskeletal deformities. A standardized clinical assessment (including manual muscle testing) should be performed at 6–12 month intervals to identify such changes. Chronic pain is common, can occur in a variety of locations, and is often unrecognized; one study found that pain was experienced more than once per week in greater than 50% of patients.

While orthopedic treatment aims to maximize function, the overall goal of treatment is to facilitate the transition into adulthood. Most adolescents with myelomeningocele are able to perform activities of daily living; however, many adults are unemployed and unable to live independently. More than 80% of patients will live beyond 16 years, and survival into the fourth decade is reduced in patients who require shunting.

The child with myelomeningocele presents a unique set of challenges to the treating physician. Foot deformities are extremely common in the myelomeningocele population. With the exception of children with low sacral level lesions, most children have or will develop foot deformities. Deformities can be present at birth, such as clubfeet or vertical talus, or can develop during childhood. The etiology of the deformities can be secondary to muscle imbalance (such as calcaneus deformity in low lumbar or sacral level), teratologic factors, forces placed on the foot by weight bearing or gravity, or changes in neurological function. These children may also have spasticity of their muscles, which complicates the evaluation.

Patients with myelodysplasia have increased wound dehiscence and ulcer formation compared with the normal population. Sun et al. (33) reported that patients with myelodysplasia had a lower ABI but similar TcO2 compared with the control group, suggesting that that patients with myelodysplasia may have decreased peripheral circulation compared with normal controls. This may play a role in healing complications and ulcer formation in these patients.

Nearly all children will require treatment of their foot deformities. Even non-ambulatory patients require treatment of their feet to permit satisfactory shoe wear, positioning of their feet on the wheelchair rests, and to prevent pressure sores. Ambulatory children require accurate correction of their foot deformities. Even small residual deformities can lead to functional difficulties or skin issues due to weakness of the hips and knees and the inability to compensate for malposition of their feet.

The vast majority of ambulatory children require bracing for ambulation. Therefore, the general goal of treatment is to provide the child with a braceable, plantigrade and supple foot. This is usually accomplished by correction of the bony deformity and muscle imbalance. Correcting muscle imbalance can be accomplished by tendon lengthening, tenotomy, tendon excision, or tendon transfer. Most practitioners favor excision of a section of the tendon, particularly when a brace will be required for ambulation. When the child is able to ambulate without orthotics, then the deforming muscle must be strong enough to consider a tendon transfer as the procedure of choice.

In addition to pedal deformity and muscle imbalance, these children also have compromised sensation and proprioception. Stiffness and residual deformity will often lead to callus formation and pressure sores. Whenever possible, arthrodesis to correct deformity should be avoided. Stiffness of the foot results in limitation of shock absorption, which in turn can result in the development of Charcot joints. Even if the deformity is corrected, callus and ulceration can still develop in a foot with limited motion. Therefore, obtaining alignment and preservation of motion are the goals of treatment regardless of the specific deformity.

Children with myelomeningocele undergo numerous surgical procedures throughout their lives, not only orthopedic procedures, but also urologic and neurosurgical operations. For this reason, multiple procedures should be done under one anesthetic to limit the number of trips to the operating room.

In evaluating these patients to determine a treatment plan, it is important to have an accurate assessment of the type and degree of deformity, an accurate neurological evaluation, and documentation of hip and knee deformity and muscle strength. Determination of the child's overall level of development is necessary to help determine the timing of surgical intervention. A child with poor head and trunk control is not ready to begin standing, and surgical correction of the foot, perhaps, should be delayed until they are ready to stand. Other treatments, such as casting, bracing, and physical therapy can be instituted instead as temporizing measures.

CLASSIFICATION

Children with myleodysplasia are typically classified by their neurological level, which in turn is related to the ability to ambulate. Patients with thoracic and upper lumbar myelomeningocele often achieve standing or limited ambulation with orthotic support during childhood, but ultimately rely on a wheelchair for mobility in adolescence and adulthood. Patients with mid-lumbar involvement (functional quadriceps) are usually household or community-level ambulators, with or without an assistive device. Lower lumbar and sacral level mylomeningocele patients may be community ambulators with orthotics.

The goal in non-ambulators is a stable seating posture, which includes a straight spine, symmetrical lower extremities, level pelvis, and adequate lower extremity motion. Foot deformities are treated when there are issues with brace wear, shoe wear, or positioning for standing, transfers, and position on wheelchair footrest. For the ambulatory patient, treatment focuses on maximizing ambulatory potential by maintaining or restoring range of motion, correcting malalignment, and providing the most appropriate orthosis.

CLUBFOOT

Talipes equinovarus deformity of the foot is the most common deformity associated with myelomeningocele. Clubfoot is seen in at least 30% of children with myelomeningocele and accounts for 50% of all the foot deformities seen (6). It is present from birth, and varying degrees of severity are encountered. The feet may range from extremely stiff, arthrogrypotic in nature, to less severe and similar to the typical idiopathic clubfoot (Figure 14-1).

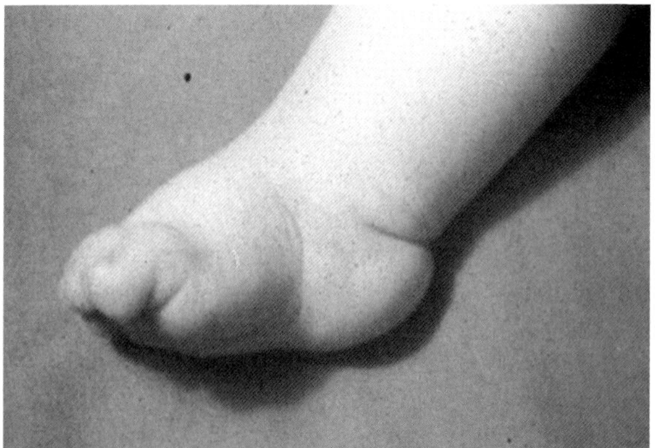

FIGURE 14-1 Clubfoot deformity associated with myelomeningocele. Note the shortness of the foot and the deep posterior and medial creases. The cock-up great toe deformity is usually indicative of a cavus component to the foot.

As with idiopathic clubfeet, manipulation and serial casting are the first line of treatment and should be started as soon as possible. These children undergo closure of their defect soon after birth and are often in a newborn ICU. Their feet are often used for vascular access, and casting may delayed until the child is more stable. While some of these feet respond to casting, a large percentage of them are extremely rigid and do not correct. Serial casting, however, should be attempted. With improvements gained by using the Ponseti technique, serial casting may be more successful than in the past (23,24). In my hands, I have had some success with serial casting and Achilles tenotomy in this population (Figure 14-2). It is minimally invasive, does not breech the joints, and does not limit any future treatment. The tenotomy can be done in the clinic setting without anesthetic, as these children are insensate. Long-term bracing is required to help prevent recurrence, but the deformity may still recur.

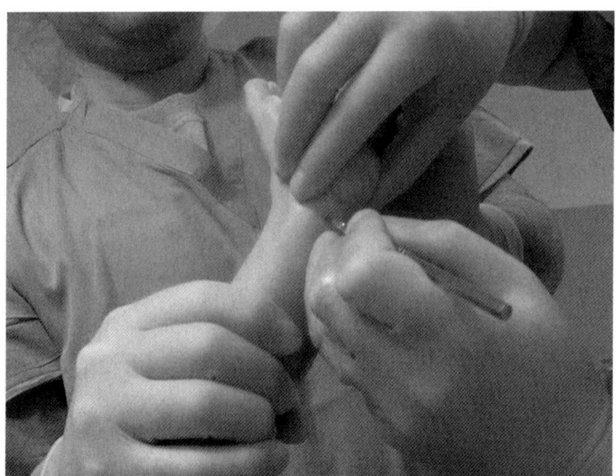

FIGURE 14-2 Achilles tenotomy can be done in the clinic setting as these children lack sensation and tolerate the procedure very well.

Surgery is required for those feet that do not respond to serial casting, The initial surgical procedure is a posteromedial soft-tissue release. Tendons should be resected instead of performing a tenotomy. This includes the posterior tibial, anterior tibial, flexor digitorum longus, and flexor hallucis longus tendons. There is some controversy regarding the Achilles tendon. While some recommend resection, others recommend lengthening. Diaz et al. recommend a radical posterior medial lateral release, using a Cincinnati incision (6,20). They recommended excising one to two centimeters of all tendons. The release involves the subtalar joint including the interosseous ligament. The talus is derotated using a K-wire and then the talonavicular joint is pinned. Lindseth recommends a complete subtalar release as well as release of the talonavicular and calcaneo-cuboid joints and a plantar release. Recently Flynn et al. (14) reviewed 72 clubfeet treated by an extensive posteromedial release including tenotomies, without internal fixation. At eight years' follow up, results were graded as good (62.5%), fair (25%), and poor (12.5%). No relationship was found between outcome and functional motor level or age.

Postoperatively, the patients are casted in a foam-padded cast, which is changed at 10 to 14 days to a long leg cast. Total casting time is 4–6 weeks. After four weeks, the long leg cast is removed, the patient is molded for an ankle-foot-orthosis (AFO), and is then replaced into a short leg cast for an additional two weeks. Long-term bracing is again required to prevent recurrence.

The timing of surgery is also important. When the patient is still crawling, there will be a high risk of recurrence. Waiting until the child is about a year of age allows the patient to begin walking and weight bearing, which helps in maintaining correction.

Despite our best efforts, these deformities do recur, and at a higher rate than idiopathic clubfeet. There are a number of options available for the recurrent deformity. Occasionally, a repeat soft-tissue release is possible. A lateral column shortening can be added to help correct recurrent forefoot deformity (Figure 14-3). Additional procedures include cuboid decancellation, closing wedge osteotomy of the cuboid, or occasionally calcaneocuboid fusion.

When soft-tissue surgery is unsuccessful, bony procedures can be performed. Calcaneal osteotomies can correct hindfoot varus (34). Forefoot and mid-foot deformities are corrected by metatarsal osteotomies or opening wedge medial cuneiform osteotomy combined with closing wedge cuboid osteotomy. Talectomy has been proposed as both an initial and salvage procedure for clubfoot deformity in the child with myelomeningocele (7). Unfortunately, even after talectomy the deformity has a tendency to recur. The malleoli are closer to the floor after talectomy, making bracing more difficult. Finally, ground reaction forces are poorly distributed, leading to recurrent pressure sores (28). For these reasons, I do not recommend talectomy as the first-line treatment for clubfoot associated with myelomeningocele. It can be a salvage procedure when no other options are available. Similarly, triple arthrodesis may be

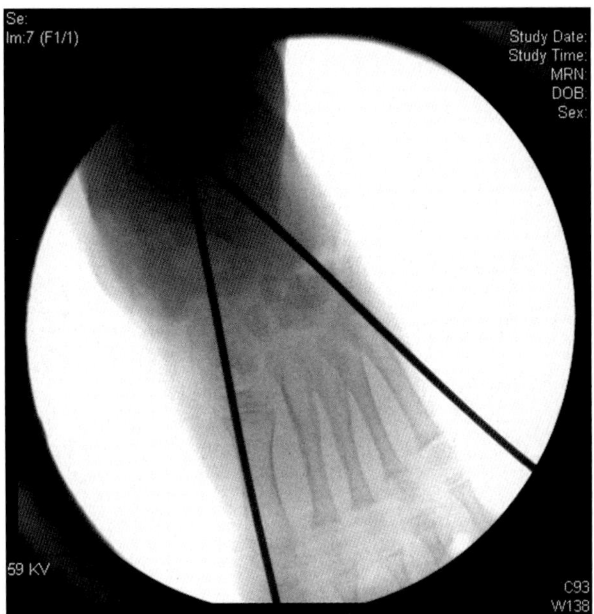

FIGURE 14-3 The radiograph shows a lateral closing wedge cuboid osteotomy done in conjunction with a repeat soft-tissue release.

considered to correct residual or recurrent deformity, following soft tissue release; insensate feet do poorly with triple arthrodesis (11,15,21). However, stiffness of the foot results in limited shock absorption, which can lead to Charcot joints. Even with a corrected deformity, the limited motion leads to callus and ulceration. Triple arthrodesis should be considered a salvage procedure. Finally, a distal tibial osteotomy can reposition the foot in a plantigrade position. This preserves motion of the foot (Figure 14-4).

CALCANEUS DEFORMITY

Calcaneus deformity is caused by unopposed function of the tibialis anterior, toe extensors, or peroneals, or spastic muscles, and is most commonly seen in the L4 level myelomeningocele (Figure 14-5). The heel may be in either varus or valgus. This is a progressive deformity, and it leads to difficulty with brace and shoe wear, pressure sores, and gait impairment. Initially, there is no fixed bony deformity. Over time the calcaneus becomes more vertically positioned under the talus. In stance the heel contacts the floor and the forefoot remains elevated. This results in poor balance, and in order to get the forefoot to contact the floor, the knees flex, resulting in a crouched gait. Over time the heel pad becomes hypertrophic and can easily break down and ulcerate. As the forefoot attempts to contact the ground, a severe midfoot cavus deformity can also develop in addition to the hindfoot deformity.

Early treatment consists of passive stretching done by the parents, followed by bracing to control dorsiflexion. These treatments are only temporizing, as the deformity is not controlled by either. Once the child is old enough,

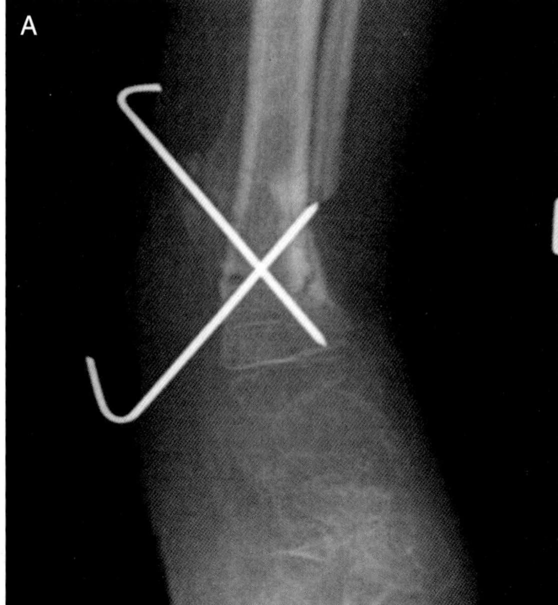

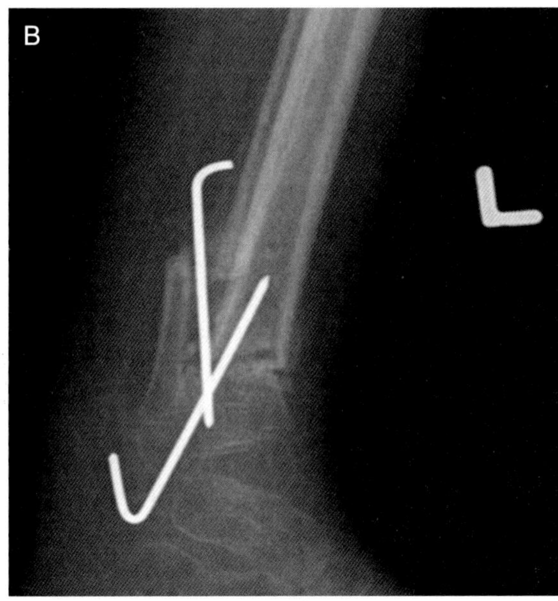

FIGURE 14-4 A and B. These x-rays show a supramalleolar osteotomy utilized to correct equinus and varus.

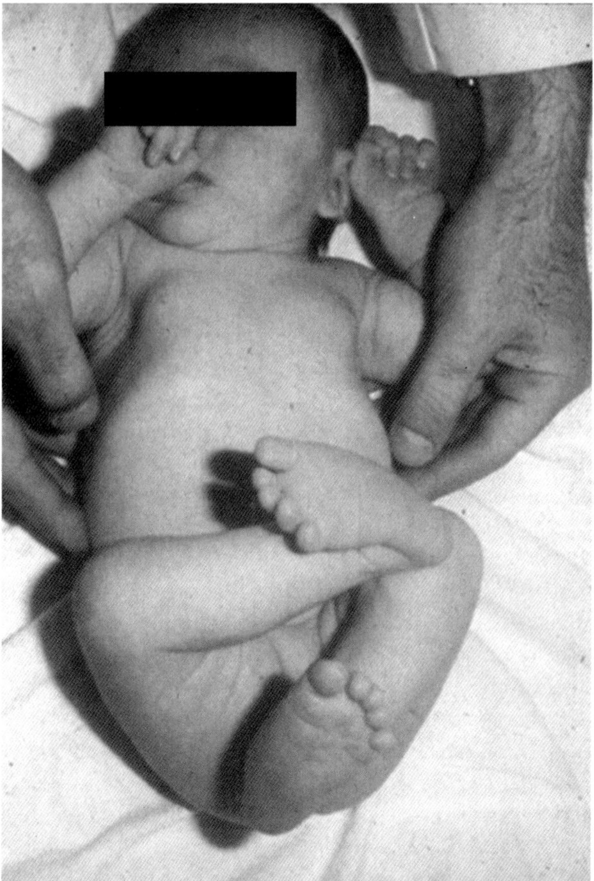

FIGURE 14-5 Clinical illustration of an infant with L4 level myelomeningocele and bilateral calcaneovalgus foot deformities.

surgical treatment can be undertaken. There are two types of procedures, releases or tendon transfer. The release has been described by Rodrigues et al (25). Through an anterior transverse incision, the tibialis anterior, extensor hallucis longus, extensor digitorum, and peroneus tertius tendons are excised. If needed, an anterior ankle capsulotomy can also be carried out. When there is an associated valgus deformity the peroneal tendons can also be divided through an incision posterior to the fibula. A short leg cast is applied for two weeks, followed by an AFO to prevent dorsiflexion. The benefit of this procedure is the short time of immobilization, the fact that it can be done even in the face of weak tibialis anterior function, and is probably the best option when the muscles are spastic. If the tibialis anterior strength is at least a grade IV, transfer of the tendon through the interosseus membrane to the calcaneus, may be a better option (3,32). It is important to remember that with transfer the muscle will lose up to a grade of strength. The primary goal of this transfer is to prevent progressive deformity, and provide a supple braceable foot. Occasionally, the transfer is strong enough to work as an active transfer, but in the great majority of cases it seems to act primarily as a tenodesis. Gait studies by Stott showed that after the transfer, gait was improved with a brace. Their conclusion was that this procedure was not meant to make the child brace free, but rather to make him or her a better brace wearer (32). Poor results in this study occurred when the tibialis anterior muscle was spastic or when it was done at too young an age. The recommended age for surgery is two years old. This is a much more extensive surgical procedure compared to the anterolateral release. The anterior tibial tendon is exposed through a small medial incision. A second incision is made anteorlaterally in the leg, where the interosseous membrane is exposed. A window is made in the interosseous ligament, and the tendon is passed from the anterior incision to the second incision. It is then passed through the interosseous ligament to the posterolateral aspect of the calcaneus. A drill hole is made in the calcaneus, and the tendon is passed through the drill hole and the sutures are passed through the heel and tied over felt and a button. When the tibialis anterior tendon is too short, it can be attached to the stump of the tendoachillis. The child is then casted in plantar flexion for six weeks. Afterward, the child is placed in an AFO that restricts dorsiflexion.

Once the calcaneus assumes a vertical position under the talus, soft tissue procedures alone are no longer successful. Calcaneal osteotomy can improve the calcaneal pitch and any varus or valgus that may be present (Figures 14-6A and 14-6B). If the forefoot has dropped into plantarflexion, a primary radical plantar release must be done before a second stage calcaneal osteotomy. The hindfoot must be fixed to permit the forefoot to be dorsiflexed to avoid 'pseudo-correction' (4,19). If there is still plantar flexion of the forefoot, a plantar opening wedge osteotomy of the medial cuneiform can also be done. If there is still unopposed anterior tibial tendon function, tenotomy or transfer can also be added to the procedure, either at the same sitting or at a later date. This may prevent recurrent deformity in the growing child.

An uncorrected deformity leads to ulceration of the hypertrophic heel pad. Occasionally, correction of the deformity with excision of the ulcer and prominent calcaneus can be successful. Often there is recurrent ulceration with the development of chronic osteomyelitis. This may require below-knee amputation.

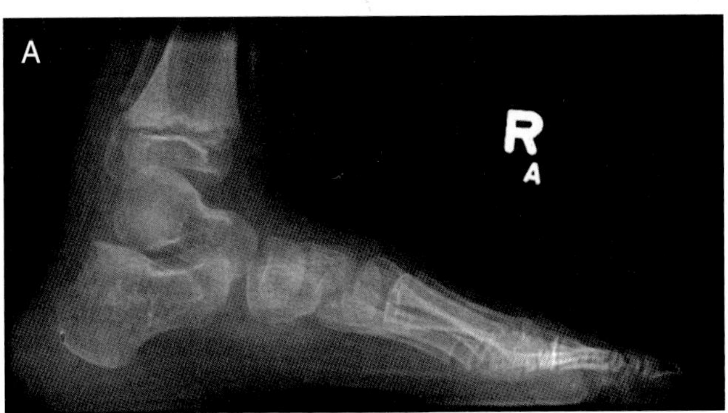

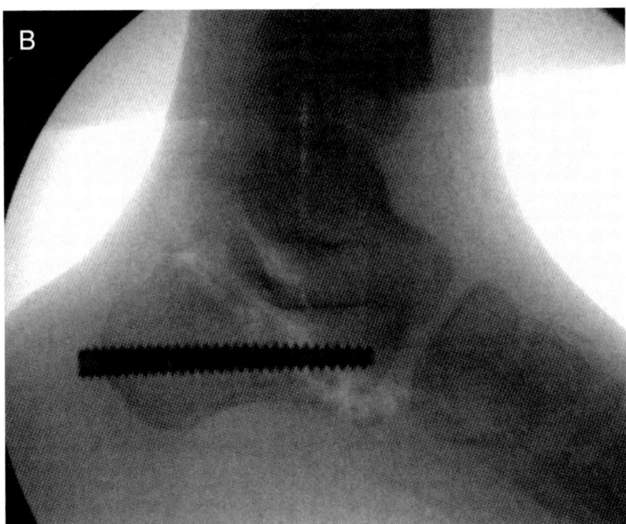

FIGURE 14-6 **A** demonstrates the x-ray of a calcaneus deformity. Notice the abnormal pitch of the calcaneus and the increased size of the heel pad. **B** shows improved position after calcaneal slide osteotomy.

CONGENITAL VERTICAL TALUS

Congenital convex pes valgus represents the most complex foot deformity in the myelomeningocele population. Congenital vertical talus combines rigid hindfoot equinus with mid- and fore-foot dorsiflexion and eversion (Fig 14-7). The major problem with the medial longitudinal column is the dorsal dislocation of the navicular onto the anterior talar head and neck. The more severe form also involves the lateral longitudinal column with dorsal subluxation or dislocation at the calcaneo-cuboid joint (Fig 14-8).

Weakness of the tibialis posterior has been proposed as the major muscle factor (8). The dislocation through the transverse tarsal articulation (talo-navicular and calcaneo-cuboid joints) occurs in line with the anterior surface of the tibia.

Surgical Technique (9,10) Following preliminary soft tissue casting, operative correction is performed at nine months of age. The one-stage open reduction is undertaken through the Cincinnati incision in children under 2 years of age. Surgery include open reduction of all dislocated joints and lengthening of tendo-Achillis and shortening of tibialis posterior. Tenotomy of the peronei, long and short toe extensors and reduction of the calcaneo-cuboid joint is accomplished through an auxiliary dorsolateral incision. Muscle balance is achieved by transferring tibialis anterior to the talar neck and peroneus longus to the navicular, and reattaching its distal stump to peroneus brevis.

Reduction of the talo-navicular dislocation and correction of hindfoot equinus is enhanced by using a retrograde Kirschner wire that exits the posterior talus and

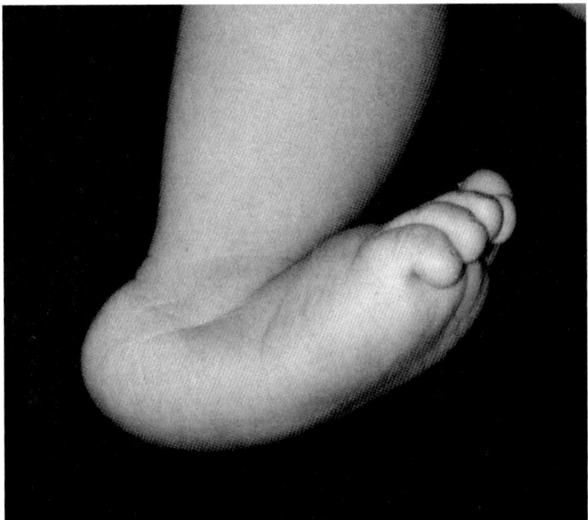

FIGURE 14-7 The infant has a vertical talus. The hindfoot is in equinus and the forefoot is dorsiflexed, giving the foot a rocker bottom appearance.

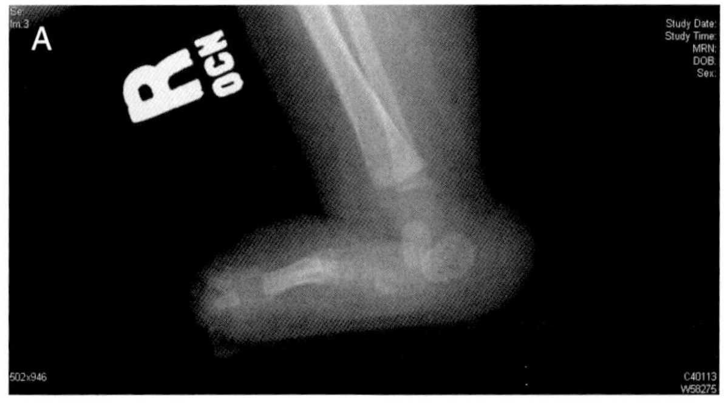

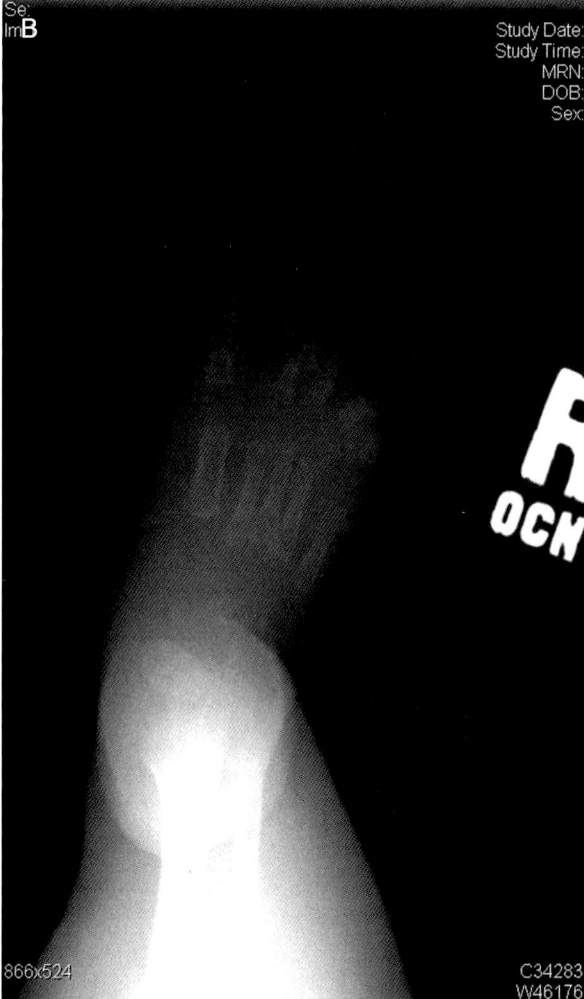

FIGURE 14-8 AP and lateral x-rays of the vertical talus show the long axis of the talus parallel with the tibia. The first metatarsal does not line up with the long axis of the talus on either view.

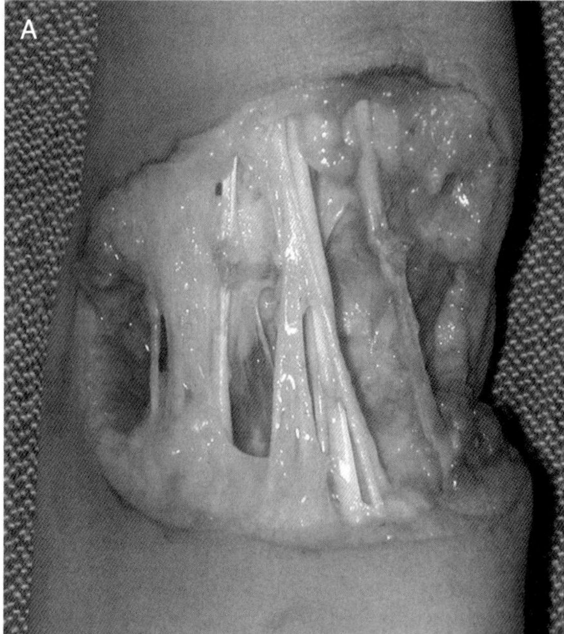

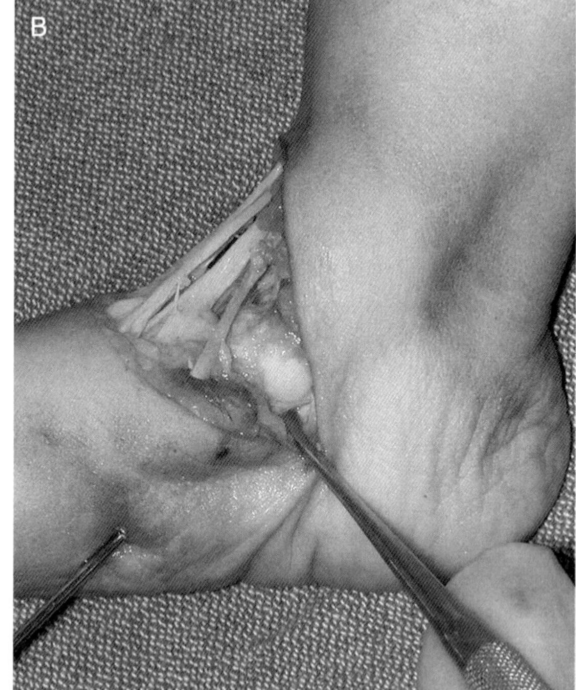

FIGURE 14-9 **A** and **B.** The dorsal approach for the correction of a vertical talus deformity allows for direct access to the tight structures and the talonavicular joint. The freer is holding the talus elevated while a K-wire is advanced across the joint.

acts as a joystick. The talar dorsal articular cartilage extends up the talar neck and may confuse the surgeon attempting to reduce the talo-navicular dislocation. This underlines the need to obtain intra-operative radiographs. Two or three Kirschner wire fixation is obligatory. Long leg casting is continued for 2 months followed by utilization of ankle foot orthotics.

There is a small subset of patients with a vertical talus with more limited rigidity. Seimon (27) used a single dorso-lateral incision. Mazzocca (16) reported on comparison of two techniques, and concluded that the dorsal approach resulted in better correction with fewer complications (13). It seemed to be a simpler procedure with shorter tourniquet time. The posterior approach had a significant incidence of avascular necrosis of the talus, most likely secondary to the extensive release that was done (16). My preferred treatment is to correct the deformity through a dorsal incision (Fig 14-9). The surgery is simple and the pathoanatomy can be directly approached.

I prefer to either lengthen or tenotomize the anterior tibial tendon. In terms of surgical timing, I approach this deformity like a clubfoot. Most of these corrections are done at about a year of age, so that weight bearing and ambulation may prevent recurrent deformity. This procedure can be successful if done before the two- to three-year age range.

In the older child, soft-tissue release alone is rarely successful. Often some combination of soft-tissue release with medial column shortening +/- lateral column lengthening is required for correction. Other options for treatment in older child include: subtalar arthrodesis; lateral column lengthening combined with peroneal lengthening; and triple arthrodesis. Again, in this population, procedures which stiffen the foot should be avoided it at all possible. Early detection and treatment result in a foot which functions well.

VALGUS DEFORMITY

Valgus deformity occurs commonly in the ambulatory patient with myelomeningocele. It is often associated with external rotation of the foot (Figure 14-10). The valgus may be from the ankle joint, the subtalar joint, or both. Determining the level of the deformity cannot be done on clinical exam therefore standing radiographs of the foot and ankle are necessary (Figures 14-11A,14-11B, and 14-11C).

As long as the child is functioning well and is not having problems with brace or shoe wear, no treatment is required. More often, these patients will develop severe callus formation and skin breakdown over their prominent talar head medially. Indications for treatment are progressive valgus greater than ten degrees which causes difficulty with shoe or brace wear, and callus formation and breakdown over the prominent talar head and medial malleolus. Conservative treatment at this point is usually ineffective. Occasionally, there is an associated contracture of the gastrocsoleus, which results in obligatory valgus of the hindfoot. Stretching with serial casting or a lengthening procedure (tendo Achilles lengthening [TAL] or Strayer) does not correct the deformity, but can make the child a better brace wearer.

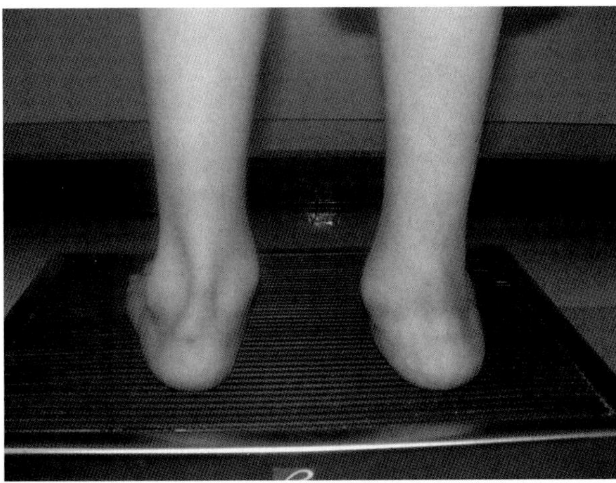

FIGURE 14-10 Severe valgus deformity in an ambulatory child with a low lumbar level myelomeningocele.

When surgical treatment is required, it is first important to determine the level of the deformity. There are a number of procedures to correct valgus of the ankle joint (1,2,5,30,31). When there is a significant associated external torsion of the tibia, then a supramalleolar osteotomy can correct both of these deformities. This surgery can be done through a small incision with or without internal fixation. If no fixation is used, a long leg cast with knee flexed is required to maintain the rotational correction. I prefer to use cannulated screws to hold the osteotomy, as this allows the child to be placed in a short leg cast. This also avoids exposed hardware, which is common when using K-wires. The hardware usually does not need to be removed. A corrective osteotomy through the physis has also been described by Lubicky and Altiok. The benefits of this location for correction include: the osteotomy is closer to the level of the deformity, therefore allowing for greater correction with less iatrogenic secondary deformity; the metaphyseal location heals more rapidly; and by doing the osteotomy through the physis there is no recurrence. In Lubicky's study, leg length discrepancy was not a problem as these children tended to be older and closer to physeal closure.

If the ankle valgus does not have an associated external rotation deformity, the valgus can be corrected with a medial malleolar hemiepiphyseodesis (Figure 14-12). Both Davids et al. and Stevens et al. use a transphyseal medial malleolar screw to correct the deformity (5,30). The parents must be made aware that this is a slow correction that occurs with growth. Once the deformity is corrected, the screws can be removed with resumption of growth. Stevens has recommended using an eight plate and screws on either side of the physis. The benefit of this device is that the tether is more medial, allowing for more and quicker correction. It does require a larger incision and may be uncomfortable because it is subcutaneous.

Finally, ankle valgus can also be corrected with a fibular-Achilles tenodesis (31). Indications for this procedure include: an ambulatory patient with a flail calf, symptomatic ankle valgus, talar tilt greater than 5 degrees, and fibular station grade I–III. The ideal age is four to ten years of age. In this procedure, 80% of the medial portion of the Achilles tendon is harvested, leaving the distal end attached to the calcaneus. The free end is then passed posterior to the peroneal tendons and sutured to the shaft of the fibula through two drill holes. The site of attachment is approximately 4 cm proximal to the epiphysis, which gives it a relatively vertical line of pull.

As mentioned above, the valgus deformity may also occur in the subtalar joint. This deformity may be corrected with a varus producing calcaneal slide osteotomy. (34) In addition, Mosca has suggested using the Evans calcaneal lengthening osteotomy for correction of the hindfoot valgus (12,18). This procedure, like the calcaneal slide osteotomy, corrects the deformity while preserving motion. The Evans procedure does not correct any forefoot deformity, so if the foot is supinated after the

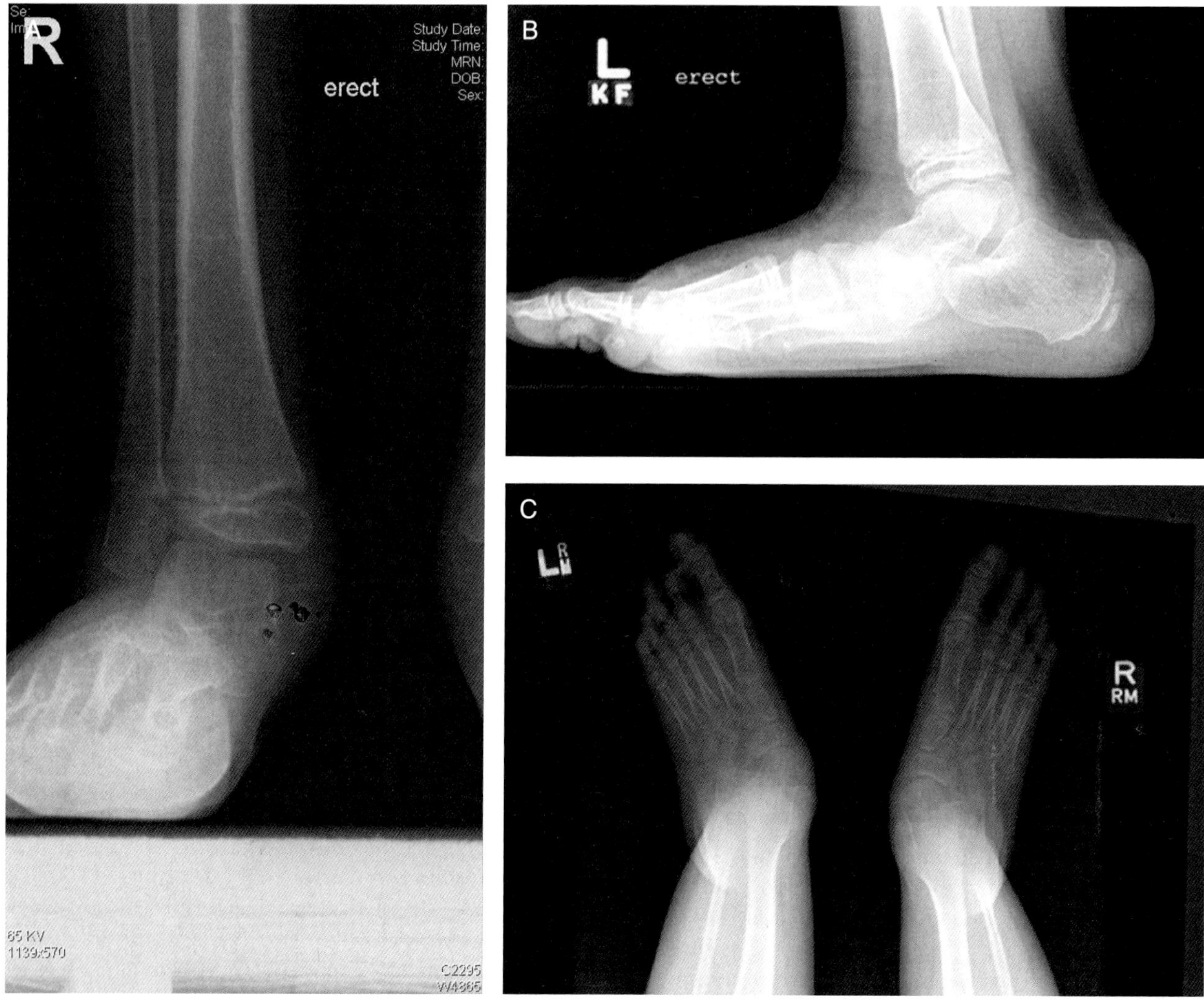

FIGURE 14-11 A. Standing AP radiograph shows valgus in the ankle joint. **B** and **C.** Standing AP and lateral views of the feet will often show a sag through the midfoot (the talus is oblique and does not line up with the first metatarsal) and abduction of the forefoot with uncovering of the talar head.

lengthening, a plantar closing wedge osteotomy through the medial cuneiform needs to be included. It is also important to remember that the Achilles tendon is often contracted, so a lengthening procedure, either a TAL or a Strayer, needs to be done as well.

Subtalar fusions or triple arthrodesis can also successfully correct the subtalar valgus deformity. (15,21) However; these feet are stiff, and are more likely to develop pressure sores or ulceration as well as Charcot changes. These procedures should be considered last resort salvage procedures, and every effort should be made to avoid them.

CAVUS DEFORMITY

Cavus deformity is commonly seen in the patient with myelomeningocele. Most often it is seen in the sacral level patients. The deformity in this group is secondary to absent intrinsic function. The tibialis anterior and toe extensors elevate the midfoot. A functioning peroneus longus plantar flexes the first metatarsal, and functioning toe flexors in the absence of functioning intrinsics, results in hyperextension of the MTP joints with flexion of the PIP joints, or claw toes. These children may also have some relative weakness of the gastrocsoleus which results in a mild hindfoot calcaneus deformity.

This deformity can also occur as the result of a tethered cord. When the deformity has a delayed onset, especially in a patient with a level of paralysis where cavus deformity is not generally seen, a neurosurgical evaluation should be obtained.

In the evaluation, it is important to do a thorough motor test to determine which muscles are functioning. It is also important to determine the flexibility of the deformity. Early on, the cavus deformity is flexible, but can become rigid over time. The Coleman block test determines the flexibility of the hind foot, varus deformity (Figure 14-14).

Brace treatment may occasionally be beneficial with a flexible deformity. However, most of these patients are independently ambulatory, and it is often difficult to get

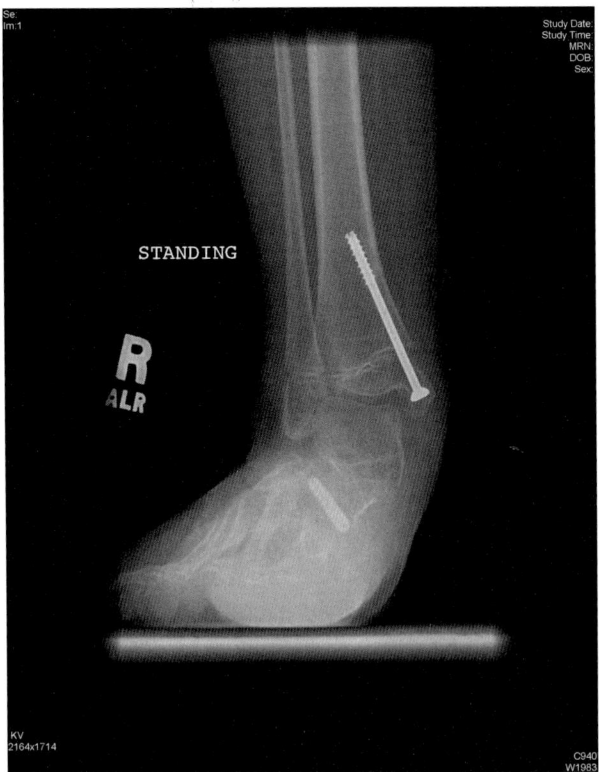

FIGURE 14-12 This patient has undergone a medial malleolar screw hemiepiphyseodesis. This procedure can be done with a small incision using a cannulated screw.

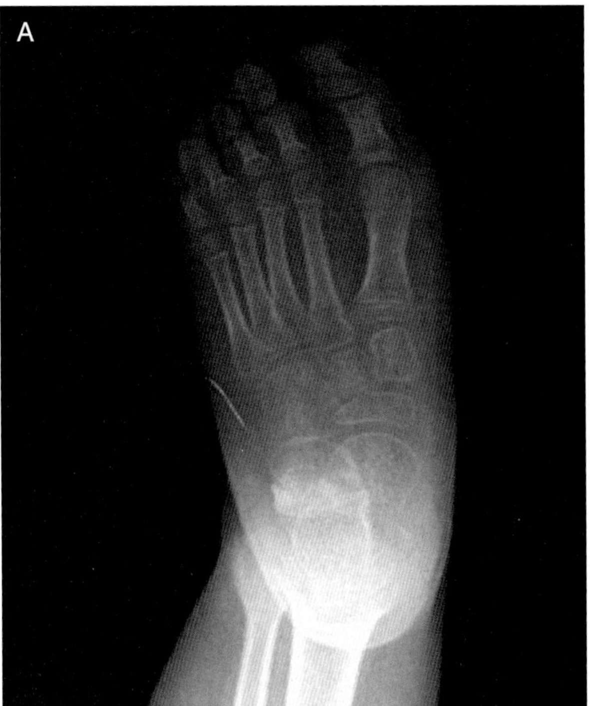

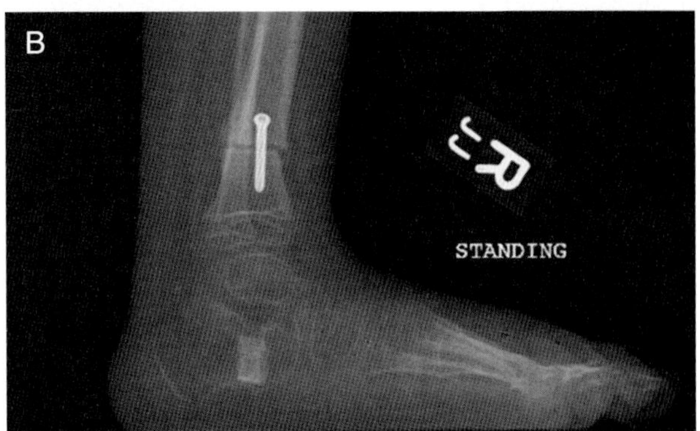

FIGURE 14-13 AP and lateral views of the foot show correction of the valgus deformity following an Evans calcaneal lengthening. On the lateral view, the talus is no longer oblique and lines up with the first metatarsal. On the AP view, the abduction of the forefoot is corrected and the navicular now covers the talar head.

them to comply with brace wear. Surgical correction should be undertaken when there is progressive deformity, painful callosities or ulceration, or ankle instability. When pressure sores are present, every effort should be made to heal the ulcers prior to undertaking operative correction.

Surgical correction should be undertaken in a stepwise fashion (Figure 14-15). All components of the cavus deformity need to be corrected and if possible muscle balance should be restored. A radical plantar lateral release, in which the remnants of abductor hallucis, quadratus plantae, flexor digitorum, plantar fascia, and occasionally the long toe flexors are released, is the initial procedure (4,19,22,26,29). The correction of the deformity is assessed to determine whether additional surgery is required. When the Coleman block test demonstrates a rigid hindfoot deformity, or if the calcaneus is still in varus or calcaneus, then a calcaneal osteotomy can be undertaken. Hindfoot varus correction is performed through a lateral approach and can be either a displacement osteotomy or a Dwyer lateral closing wedge osteotomy. I prefer to use a buried headless screw to hold the osteotomy in place. The foot is reevaluated again, and if there is still plantar flexion of the first metatarsal, I prefer to do a plantar opening wedge medial cuneiform osteotomy using a tricortical iliac allograft. For cock-up deformities of the toes, Jones procedure for the hallux and transfers of the extensors around the metatarsal neck with PIP joint fusions will correct the lesser toes' position. Postoperatively, there can be significant swelling of the feet; therefore, I use a foam padded cast for the first week to 10 days. Correcting both feet at the same sitting should be considered, as it limits the number of surgical procedures for these children. If the deformity is a calcaneocavus deformity secondary to an unopposed tibialis anterior, I will usually add an anterior tibial tendon transfer to the calcaneus at four to six weeks postoperatively. Alternatively, the tendon can be lengthened to weaken its unopposed function.

SUMMARY

The child with myelomeningocele presents a unique set of challenges to the treating physician. Children with myelomeningocele undergo numerous surgical procedures

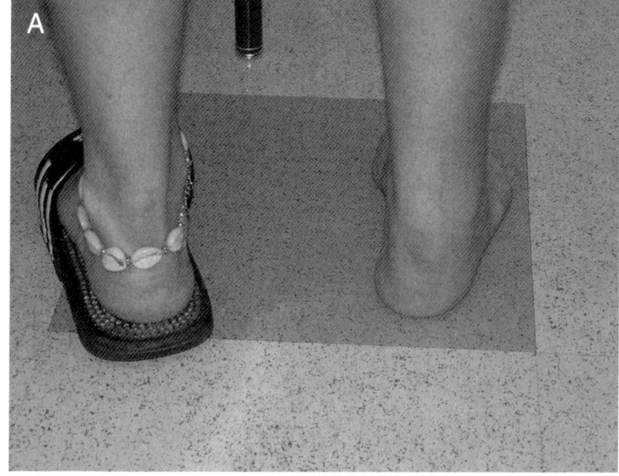

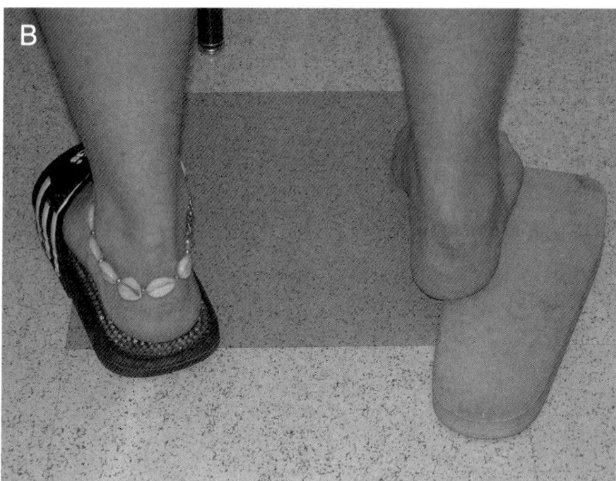

FIGURE 14-14 **A** and **B.** The Coleman block test demonstrates the flexibility of the hindfoot. This patient's foot partially corrects but does not go into valgus at the hindfoot.

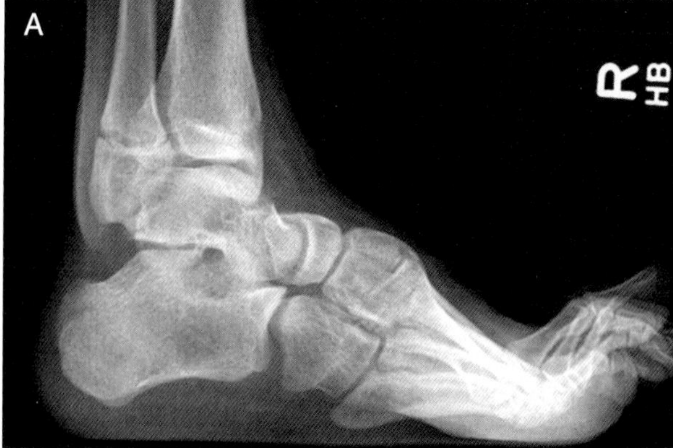

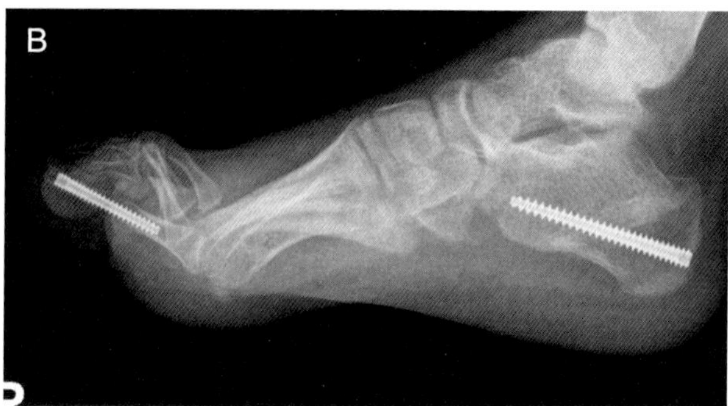

FIGURE 14-15 Pre- and post-operative x-rays of a cavus foot deformity. Preoperatively, the hindfoot varus is evident by the absence of overlapping of the talus and calcaneus (see-through subtalar joint). Postoperatively, the position of the foot is markedly improved.

throughout their lives; therefore, multiple procedures should be done under one anesthetic when possible, and careful evaluation of the patient their goals are needed to determine the best operative course. Treatment options include casting and bracing, which must performed with great care and close follow up, given the patients' lack of sensation. Surgical intervention is often needed, to allow for brace wear or improve foot positioning. Foot deformities are less flexible than idiopathic fort deformities, and complications and recurrence rates are higher.

REFERENCES

1. Abraham E, Lubicky, JP, Songer MS, Miller EA. Supramalleolar osteotomy for ankle valgus in myelomeningocele. *J Pediatr Orthop* 16:774, 1996.
2. Beals RK. Treatment of ankle valgus by surface epiphyseodesis. *Clin Orthop* 266:162, 1991.
3. Bliss DG, Menelaus MB. The results of transfer of the tibialis anterior to the heel in patients who have a myelomeningocele. *J Bone Joint Surg (Am)* 68:1258, 1986.
4. Bradley GW, Coleman SS. The treatment of the calcaneocavus foot deformity. *J Bone Joint Surg (Am)* 63:1159, 1981.
5. Davids JR, Valandie AL, Ferguson RL, Bray EW III, Allen BL. Surgical management of ankle valgus in children: Use of a trans-epiphyseal medial malleolar screw. *J Pediatr Orthop* 17:3, 1997.
6. Dias LS. Surgical management of acquired foot and ankle deformities. In Sarwark JF, Lubicky JP, eds. *Caring for the child with spina bifida, 1st ed.* Rosemont, IL American Academy of Orthopaedic Surgeons, 161–169, 2001.
7. Dias LS, Stern LS. Talectomy in the treatment of resistant Talipes equinovarus deformity in myelomeningocele and arthrogryposis. *J Pediatr Orthop* 7:39, 1987.
8. Drennan JC, Sharrard WJW. The pathologic anatomy of convex pes valgus. *J Bone Joint Surg (Br)* 5455, 1971.
9. Drennan JC. Foot deformities in myelomeningocele. *Instruc Course Lect* 40:287, 1991.
10. Drennan JC. Current concepts in myelomeningocele. *Instruc Course Lect* 48:543, 1999.
11. Duncan JW, Lovell WW. Hoke triple arthrodesis. *J Bone Joint Surg (Am)* 60:795, 1978.
12. Evans D. Calcaneo-valgus deformity. *J Bone Joint Surg (Br)* 57:270, 1975.
13. Fitton JM, Nevelos AB. The treatment of congenital vertical talus. *J Bone Joint Surg (Br)* 61:481, 1979.
14. Flynn JM, Herrera-Soto JA, Ramirez NF, Fernandez-Feliberti R, Vilella F, Guzman J. Clubfoot release in myelodysplasia. *J Pediatr Orthop (Br)* 2004;13(4):259–262.
15. Gallien R, Morin F, Marquis F. Subtalar arthrodesis in children. *J Pediatr Orthop* 9:59, 1989.
16. Mazzocca AD, Thompson JD, Deluca PA, Romness MJ. Comparison of the posterior approach versus the dorsal approach in the treatment of congenital vertical talus. *J Pediatr Orthop* 21:212, 2001.

17. Morrow JD, Kelsey K. Folic acid for prevention of neural tube defects: pediatric anticipatory guidance. *J Pediatr Health Care* 1998 Mar-Apr;12(2):55–59.
18. Mosca VS. Calcaneal lengthening for valgus of the hindfoot: Results in children who had severe symptomatic flatfoot and skewfoot. *J Bone Joint Surg (Am)* 77:500, 1995.
19. Mosca VS. The cavus foot. *J Pediatr Orthop* 21: 423, 2001.
20. Neto J, Diaz LS, Gabrieli AP. Congenital talipes equinovarus in spina bifida: Treatment and results. *J Pediatr Orthop* 16:782, 1996.
21. Olney BW, Menelaus MB. Triple arthrodesis of the foot in spina bifida patients. *J Bone Joint Surg (Br)* 70:234, 1988.
22. Paulos L, Coleman SS, Samuelson KM. Pes cavovarus. Review of a surgical approach using selective soft tissue procedures. *J Bone Joint Surg (Am)* 62:942, 1980.
23. Ponseti IV. *Congenital clubfoot: Fundamentals of treatment.* Oxford: Oxford University Press, 1996.
24. Ponseti IV, Smoley EN. Congenital clubfoot: The results of Treatment. *J Bone Joint Surg (Am)* 45:261, 1963.
25. Rodrigues RC, Dias LS. Calcaneus deformity in spina bifida: results of anterolateral release. *J Pediatr Orthop* 12:461, 1992.
26. Schwend RM, Drennan JC. Cavus foot deformity in children. *J Am Acad Orthop Surg* 11:201, 2001.
27. Seimon LE. Surgical correction of congenital vertical talus under the age of 2 years. *J Pediatr Orthop* 7:405, 1987.
28. Sherk HH, Marchinski JL, Clancy M, Melchonnie J. Ground reaction forces on the plantar surface of the foot after talectomy in the myelomeningocele. *J Pediatr Orthop* 9:269, 1989.
29. Sherman FC, Westin GW. Plantar release in the correction of deformities of the foot in childhood. *J Bone Joint Surg (Am)* 63:1382, 1981.
30. Stevens PM. Screw epiphyseodesis for ankle valgus. *J Pediatr Orthop* 17:9 1997.
31. Stevens PM, Toomey E. Fibular-Achilles tenodesis for paralytic ankle valgus. *J Pediatr Orthop* 8:169, 1988.
32. Stott NS, Zionts LE, Gronlay JK, Perry J. Tibialis anterior tendon transfer for calcaneal deformity: A postoperative gait analysis. *J Pediatr Orthop* 16:792, 1996.
33. Sun EC, Yen YM, Ip T, Otsuka NY. Peripheral circulation in patients with myelodysplasia. *J Pediatr Orthop* 2003 Nov-Dec;23(6):714–717.
34. Trishmann H, Millis M, Hall J, Watts H. Sliding calcaneal osteotomy for treatment of hindfoot deformity. *Orthop Trans* 4:305, 1980.

CHAPTER 15

Poliomyelitis

James C. Drennan

Acute anterior poliomyelitis results from an acute viral infection which localizes its neurotropic effects on the anterior horn cells of the spinal cord and certain brain stem motor ncuclei. These motor cells undergo necrosis with subsequent loss of innervation of their motor units. While the acquired asymmetric flaccid paralysis is usually caused by one of the three types of poliomyelitis virus, a similar clinical picture can develop from infections caused by other members of the enteroviral group including coxsackie and echo viruses. Each type of polio virus has strains of varying virulence, and individual types do not offer cross immunity to the other types.

Over 20,000 cases of polio were reported in the United States as recently as 1960. Currently, less than 10 paralytic cases are documented annually in this country and these most commonly result from the use of active oral polio vaccine (59). Outbreaks relating to wild strains or active oral polio virus have been reported in a number of North American and European countries (36,79,90,60,61). The World Health Organization reported more than 35,000 cases in 1987, and as recently as 1989, Robertson concluded that there were more than 200,000 cases annually. There has been a dramatic decrease in the incidence since that time. Currently, ten countries have been identified as having paralytic polio (3) India reported 1,600 cases during 2002 (86). Social issues in Nigeria have led to a recrudescence of the disease which has MW spread to neighboring West Africa, nations (58). Outbreaks relating to mild strains have been reported in North America and Europe. In the past decade, polio outbreaks associated with circulatory vaccine derived polio (cVPDVs) have been identified (44). Children with primary immunodeficiencies are also a vulnerable category (89).

The average age of onset in third world countries has recently diminished from 20 to 11 months, underlining the appropriateness of the term "infantile poliomyelitis." The age shift supports the current international strategy of focusing vaccination at the infant population. Two-thirds of the world's infants are currently being immunized. Kohler found an increased risk factor of developing paralytic poliomyelitis in patients who had received oral polio virus Type 3 and who had received any injection in the 30 days of incubation of the virus (45).

The debate on the use of active (OPV) versus inactive (IPV) oral vaccine remains unsettled (49,69). The active form offers the advantage of "herd immunity" by which immunization of a sufficient proportion of the population creates a barrier to the introduction and spread of the virus and thus indirectly protects susceptible nonvaccinated persons. The inactive form offers an equal degree of protection to the individual and avoids the potential complication of the immunized individual developing poliomyelitis from the active vaccine (66). In addition, there are reports from third world countries where the incidence of failure of protection from active oral vaccine is as high as 15% (75,84). Sen compared patients who developed polio who developed polio who had received properly spaced doses of active polio vaccine with patients who had not been vaccinated. At the time of presentation, the vaccinated patients retained better average muscle power and also had been subjected to a much higher incidence of provocative injection.

PATHOLOGY

The oropharyngeal route is the most common route by which the poliomyelitis virus invades the body. The virus multiplies in the alimentary tract lymph nodes before spreading to the central nervous system by the hematogenous route. The anterior horn cells, especially in the lumber and cervical spinal cord enlargements, as well as the medulla, cerebellum, and midbrain, are acutely attacked.

It has long been recognized that peripheral trauma, such as an intramuscular injection or surgery within the fortnight preceding the onset of the disease can affect the localization of the paralysis to anatomically related segments of the cord. There is recent evidence to suggest that polio virus may reach the central nervous system via peripheral nerve endings with passage along the nerve pathways (96). The entry of polio virus from many sites at nerve endings and muscles is consistent with the clinical, experimental, and pathologic data and provides an explanation for the polioclastic incubation times. Third world country infants with fevers of unknown etiology who lack polio immunization and who receive intramuscular injections during the preparalytic phase, particularly in the gluteal area, have a greatly increased risk factor and this may contribute to the phenomenon of paralysis in the injected muscle within a few hours after the injection (54). Tonsillectomy can lead to the development of bulbar poliomyelitis within 7 to 14 days following surgery, and this is also thought to be related to the entry of the virus from the peripheral nerve endings in the tonsillar bed. A severe paralysis following exercise may be explained as an effect of increased blood supply to the areas of the central nervous system that have already been invaded by the virus.

The resultant asymmetric flaccid paralysis varies greatly both in the number and severity of individual muscles involved. The clinical weakness is proportional to the number of lost motor units. Sharrard (77) reports that weakness is clinically detectible when more than 60% of the motor nerve cells supplying a muscle have been destroyed. He demonstrated histologically and clinically that muscles with short motor nerve cell columns are often severely paralyzed, whereas those with long anterior horn cell columns are more frequently paretic (75,76). The tibialis anterior is the most frerquently involved extrinsic muscle to the foot. Sacral nerve roots are spared (46), resulting in retained function of intrinsic muscles of the foot.

Clinical recovery begins during the first month following the acute illness and is nearly complete by the sixth month, although limited potential for additional recovery persists through the second year. An individual muscle with a particular motor grade is less likely to demonstrate significant recovery when surrounded by severely paretic muscles.

MANAGEMENT

The responsibility of the orthopedist changes during the different phases of the disease. Skill as a rehabilitation physician based on a thorough understanding of the disease and a variety of therapy modalities as well as surgical judgment and skill, are necessary for appropriate management of the patient. The severity and extent of paralysis as well as the age of the patient form important variables in the equation of care.

Acute phase

The acute phase generally lasts 9 to 10 days. Treatment during the acute febrile stage is primarily managed by the pediatrician because there may be medical problems, particularly respiratory, that may be life threatening. The role of the orthopedist is limited to the musculoskeletal system with emphasis on prevention of deformity and patient comfort. Sharrard has stressed the rapid occurrence of loss of elasticity coupled with shortening in tendons, fascia, and ligaments (77), while secondary postural contractures tend to develop over a longer period of time. These acute contractures include the tendocalcaneus and the fascia on the plantar surface of the foot, and therefore, proper positioning of the foot and ankle is essential. A padded foot board is employed to maintain the feet and ankles in a neutral position when the patient is supine. The end of the mattress must be separated from the foot board to provide an innerspace for neutral positioning of the foot when the patient is in the prone position. These two positions are alternated on a regular basis. Strong muscle spasms can lead to rapid shortening and do respond favorably to the use of moist heat, both to relieve the muscle sensitivity as well as relieve of discomfort. Should passive stretching and proper positioning not lead to control of the ankle and foot deformity, there is a strong likelihood that an underlying muscle imbalance is present that will require later surgical management. Despite the fact that the patient is irritable and apprehensive, it is important that the joints be put through a full range of motion several times a day.

Convalescent Phase

Prophylactic rehabilitation becomes the focus once the patient has been afebrile for 24 hours. The goals during this period include continuation of efforts to prevent unnecessary deformity, restoration and maintenance of a normal range of joint motion, and assisting in the individual muscles achieving maximum recovery. Lack of adequate immobilization and passive range of motion can lead to a fixed equinus at the ankle unless proper protected positioning and passive range of motion are continued on a daily basis. In the majority of individual muscles, power improvement is noted during the beginning of the convalescent stage which continues for two years. Muscle assessment on a quarterly basis offers a satisfactory guide to potential recovery. Muscles showing evidence of more than 80% return of strength returning spontaneously will require no specific therapy for that muscle (41). Physical therapy is directed toward making individual muscles assume maximum capability within their normal pattern of motor activity and not permitting adaptive substitute patterns of associated muscles to persist. Management of a paretic anterior tibial muscle requires that the ankle joint be passively dorsiflexed through its full arc of motion, thereby overcoming any contracture of the antagonistic triceps surae. The patient can then be placed in a side-lying position to eliminate the force of gravity and the ankle can then be passively dorsiflexed and inverted to assist the patient with biofeedback to localize the action of the anterior tibial muscle and avoid substituting the dorsiflexor power of the toe extensors. The patient can then attempt a sustained active contracture of the muscle with an without assistance. With returning strength, the limb can be placed in a supine position to add the effects of gravity and eventually manual resistance can be applied. The use of bivalved casts or ankle-foot orthotics are required at all times when the patient is not receiving the active therapy program. Hydrotherapy is an important adjunct to the return of ankle dorsiflexors and may include ambulation in a therapy pool. Ambulatory orthotics are restricted to those needed to make a significant major contribution to ambulation.

Chronic Phase

The orthopedist is confronted with managing the long-term consequences of muscle imbalanace, and no further clinical improvement can be expected. Focus shifts to the achievement of maximal functional activity. Goals include preventing or correcting soft tissue contracture and its subsequent bony deformation and achieving muscle balance. Physical therapy continues with active hypertrophy exercises and a passive stretching program, and now makes functional objectives its highest priority. Orthotics become more important particularly in controlling flaccid paralysis where static joint instability permits effective orthotic control. Orthotic management becomes more difficult when there is a dynamic component added to the joint instability. Surgical correction of both muscle imbalance and the associated soft tissue or bony deformity may be a prerequisite to successful orthotic control.

SURGICAL MANAGEMENT

Careful preoperative assessment and postoperative management are essential in polio patients with muscle imbalance about the foot and ankle (Figure 15-1). The ability to achieve muscle balance in the child with dynamic instability will halt progression of the paralytic deformity (72). Tendon transfers are indicated when dynamic muscle imbalance is sufficient to produce deformity and when orthotic control is required. The timing of the individual tendon transfer has to be considered in relation to the total rehabilitation program.

The objectives of tendon transfer include: (i) provision of active motor power to replace function of a paralyzed muscle of muscles, (ii) the elimination of the deforming effect of a muscle when its antagonist is paralyzed, and (iii) the production of stability through better muscle balance. The prerequisites for successful tendon transfer must be carefully observed (31,56).

1. The muscle to be transferred should rate good or normal before transfer and must have sufficient motor strength to actively carry out the desired function. Subnormal-strength muscles may be transferred if they are a factor in dynamic instability. On the average, one grade of motor power is lost after muscle transfer.
2. The strength, range of motion, and phase of the transferred muscle and that of the muscle being replaced must be similar.
3. Loss of original function resulting from tendon transfers must be balanced against potential gain. Removal of a muscle without consideration of its strength or its antagonist leads to a secondary iatrogenic deformity.
4. Free passive range of motion is essential in the absence of deformity at the joint to be moved by the tendon.
5. Osseous deformity must be corrected prior to tendon transfer. A transplant is an adjunct to bony stabilization and cannot be expected to overcome a fixed bony deformity (48).
6. Smooth gliding channel for the tendon transfer is essential. The tendon should be passed through the subcutaneous tissue because tendons pass beneath the ankle and frequently become adherent and function only as a passive tenodesis.
7. The neurovascular supply to the transferred muscle should be ensured by atraumatic handling of muscle tissue.
8. The tendon should be routed in a straight line between its origin and its new insertion.

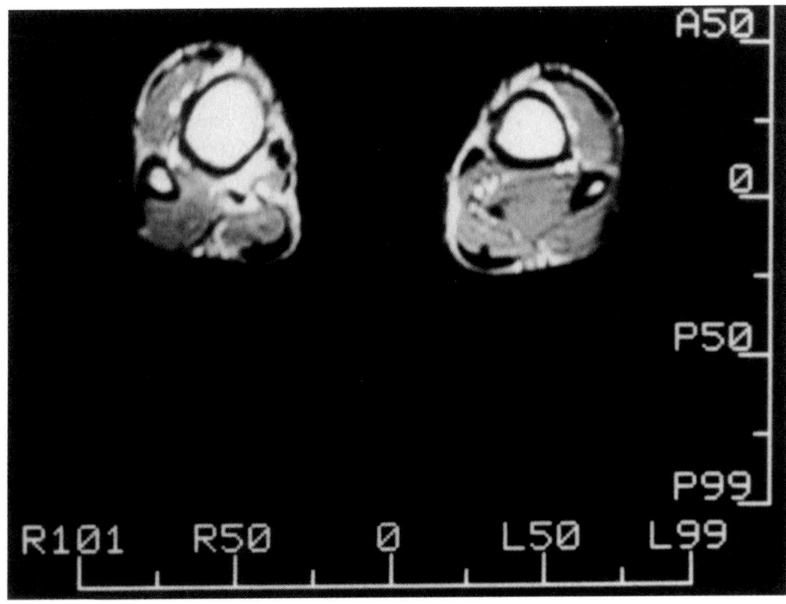

FIGURE 15-1 Magnetic resonance imaging of the middle portion of the right calf demonstrates atrophy of the flexor digitorum longus and flexor hallucis longus.

9. The tendon transfer should be attached under sufficient tension to correspond to normal physiologic conditions and should be attached to bone.

SOFT TISSUE SURGERY

Dorsiflexor Paralysis

In poliomyelitis, most tendon transfers are performed for drop-foot deformity. The pull of gravity and the weight and length of the forefoot allow the unsupported foot to fall into plantar flexion and permit anterior ankle soft tissue structures to gradually stretch. Transfers that allow the toes to clear the ground obviate the need for AFOs.

Paralysis of the anterior tribial muscle is common and the resultant loss of dorsiflexor and invertor power leads to the development of equinovalgus deformity which is initially noted in swing-phase and later can be demonstrated in both phases of gait. The long-toe extensors which act as auxiliary dorsiflexors become overactive during swing-phase and attempt to replace the paralyzed tibialis anterior. This results in secondary hyperextension of the proximal phalanges and depression of the metatarsal heads (Figure 15-2). Hindfoot equinus and valgus develop as the functioning triceps surae contracts. Management includes a transfer of the peroneus longus to the base of the second metatarsal with the distal stump of the peroneus longus being sutured to the peroneus brevis to avoid the development of a secondary dorsal bunion (39). Another surgical option would include the recession of the extensor digitorum longus to the dorsum of the mid-foot. Claw-toe deformities are managed by transferring the long-toe extensors into the metatarsal necks.

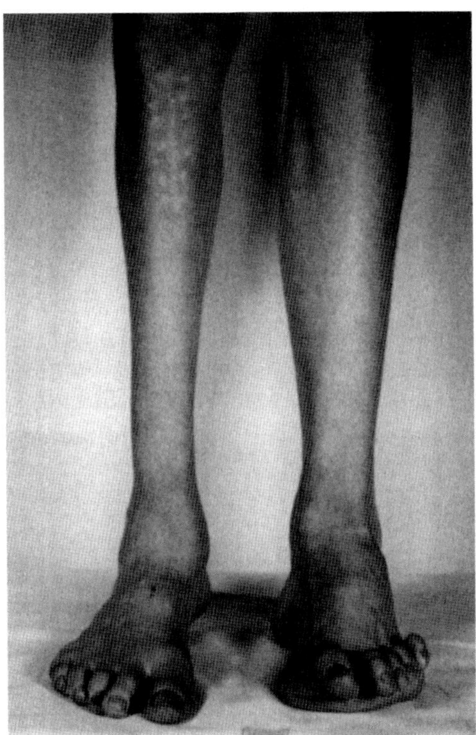

FIGURE 15-2 Claw toes associated with cavus deformity are corrected by transfer of the long extensor tendons into the necks of the metatarsal combined with interphalangeal fusion. (From Patterson RI, Parrish FF, Hathaway EN. Stabilizing Operations on the foot. A study of the indications, techniques used, and end results. *J Bone Joint Surg* [*Am*] 1950;32:1, with permission.)

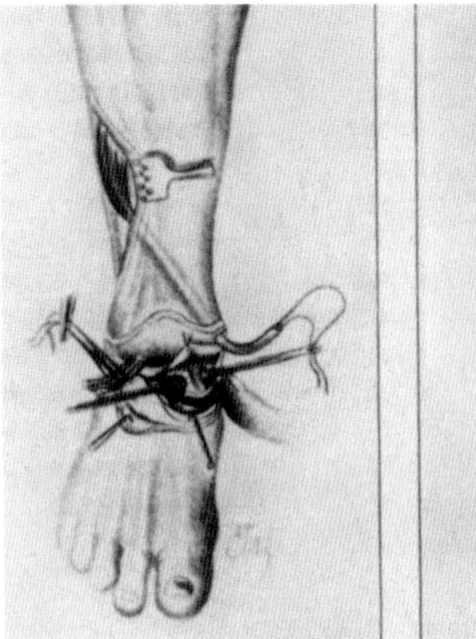

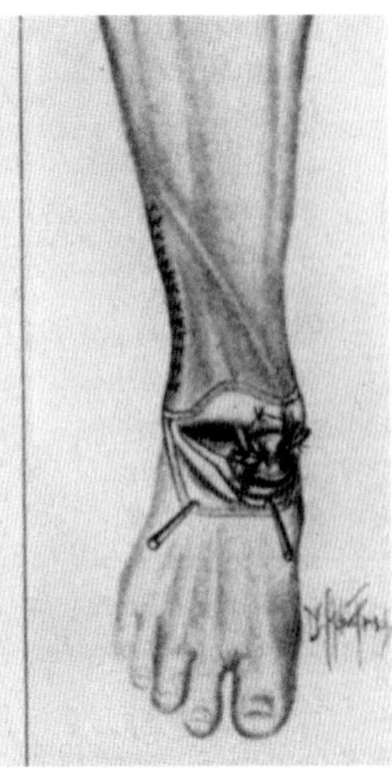

FIGURE 15-3 An active midline dorsiflexor is created by inserting the cojoined tendon through the medial talar neck. (From Axer A. Intro-talus transposition of tendons for correction of paralytic valgus foot after poliomyelitis in children. *J Bone Joint Surg* 1960;42:1119, with permission.)

Paralysis of both the tibialis anterior and tibialis posterior causes a more rapid development of hindfoot and forefoot equinovalgus. Secondary shortening of the heelcord and peroneal muscles occur and the unsupported talar head assumes a vertical position in weight bearing.

Management includes serial casting of the contracting heelcord to avoid weakening of the triceps surae (27) coupled with a transfer of the peroneus longus to the base of the second metatarsal and one of the long-toe flexors to substitute for the paretic tibialis posterior.

Paralysis of the tibialis posterior is uncommon and leads to hindfoot and forefoot eversion (23). Both the flexor hallucis longus and flexor digitorum longus have been used successfully as tendon transfers.

Axer recommends that children ages three to six years who have a moderate paralytic valgus deformity be managed by transferring the conjoined tendon of the extensor digitorum longus and peroneus tertius through a transverse talar neck tunnel (Figure 15-3). More severe valgus will require transfer of the peroneus longus to the medial aspect of the peroneus brevis and the lateral aspect of the talar neck.

Paralysis of the tibialis anterior, toe extensors, and peronei leads to progressive severe equinovarus deformity because of the unopposed activity of the tibialis posterior and triceps surae (Figure 15-4). Dynamic contracture of the tibialis posterior increases forefoot equinus and cavus deformities by depressing the metatarsal heads and shortening the medial arch of the foot. The triceps surae causes equinus and secondary varus deformity. The plantar fascia is shortened and the cavus deformity becomes fixed. Serial corrective casts are recommended to correct the hindfoot equinus, but a heelcord lengthening may be required. Soft

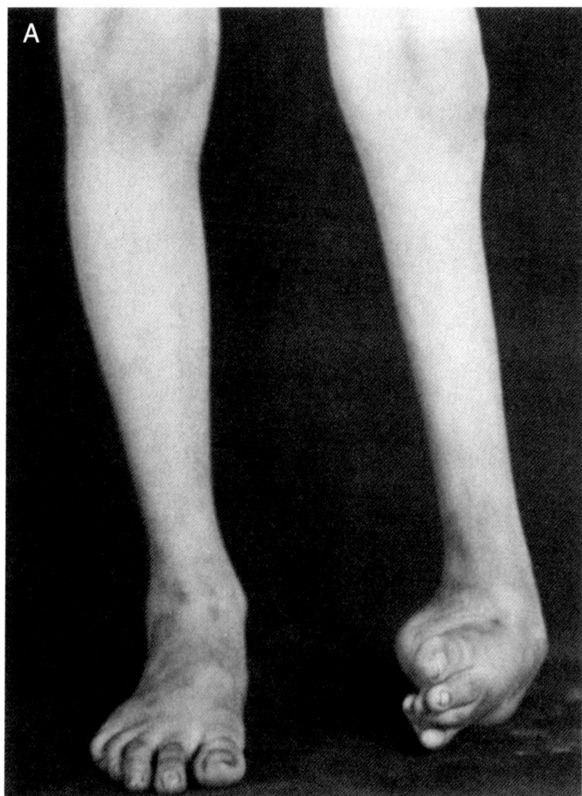

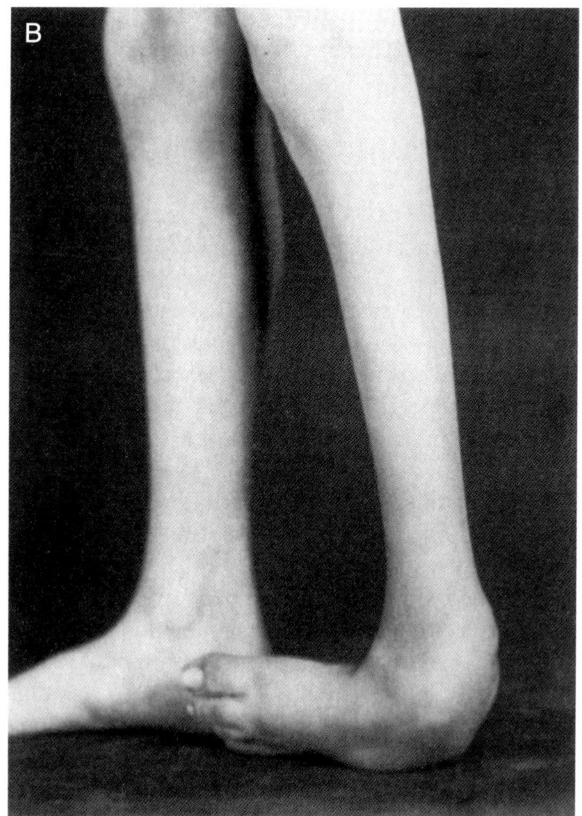

FIGURE 15-4 **A,B.** Unopposed tibialis anterior and tibialis posterior activity produces severe per varus.

tissue release of the cavus deformity through a lateral heel incision may also be necessary. Anterior transfer of the tibialis posterior through the interosseous membrane to the base of the third metatarsal is the procedure of choice and may be supplemented by a similar anterior transfer of the long-toe flexors (28). This transplantation without joint stabilization is usually sufficient, and the deformity can be controlled through physical therapy and bracing. This author's preferred method includes a creating a bony tunnel through the second cuneiform and suturing the transfer to a button over a felt pad placed on the non–weight-bearing aspect of the plantar surface of the foot. Suture can be tied over the plantar fascia, but the viability of the plantar skin is questionable.

Isolated paralysis of the peronei is rare in poliomyelitis and results in severe hindfoot varus deformity caused by the unopposed tiabilis posterior (Figure 15-5). The entire foot is inverted and the varus deformities increased by the dynamic activity of the invertor muscles in gait, particularly the tibialis anterior. The first metatarsal may become dorsiflexed and a dorsal bunion results (Figure 15-6). Muscle balance is restored by the lateral transfer of the tibialis anterior to the base of the second metatarsal bone with only loss of a one-half grade of muscle power (52). It may be necessary to lengthen the extensor hallucis longus to prevent hyperextension of the great toe. Older children may benefit from having this muscle transferred to the first metatarsal head. The tibialis anterior is transferred to the base of the third metatarsal bone when peroneal and long-toe extensors are paralyzed and the equinovarus deformity is less severe.

Paralysis of the Triceps Surae

Paralysis of the triceps surae leads to a rapidly progressive calcaneal deformity of the foot which increases as a result of unopposed dorsiflexor function, coupled with the attenuation of the triceps surae tendon. The patient cannot stabilize the calcaneus or transfer body weight distally to the metatarsal head and thus loses push-off power in walking.

An increase in the range of ankle dorsiflexion is the earliest clinical sign and occurs as the talus is displaced upward and the os calcis rotates under and into a more vertical position (26). This reduces the posterior lever arm and the insertion of the triceps surae migrates upward on the tuber. The stimulus to be normal longitudinal development of the tuber is diminished and a shortened os calcis results. The foot further shortens as the os calcis rotates into an increasingly more vertical position. The remaining active muscles force the forefoot into equinus, thus creating a cavus deformity (Figure 15-7).

The triceps surae is the strongest muscle group of the body and must be able to lift the entire body weight with each step. Adequate tension of the tendo-Achillis is important in the normal function of the long-toe flexors and extensors as well as the intrinsics (Figure 15-8). When the triceps surae is weak, the associated tibialis posterior, peronei, and long-toe flexors become ineffective hindfoot plantar flexors but are still capable of depressing the metatarsal head, thus causing forefoot equinus. The vertical position of the os calcis allows the intrinsics and

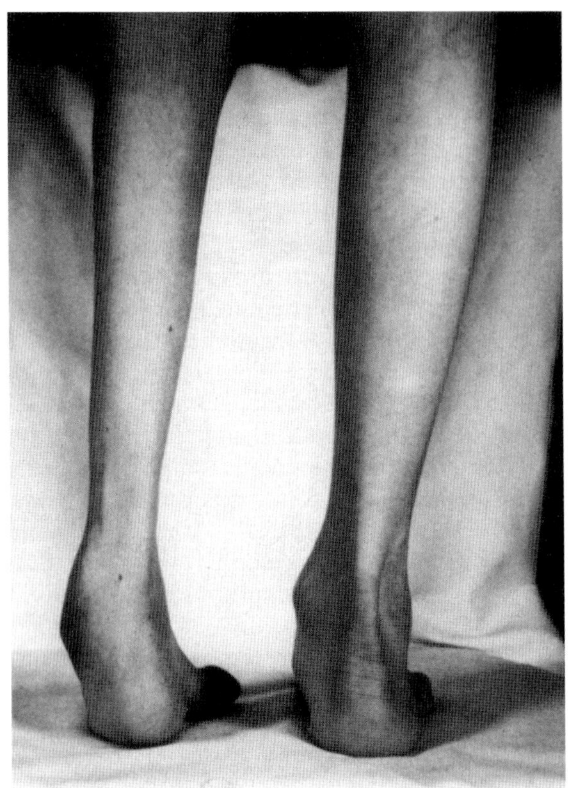

FIGURE 15-5 Unopposed tibialis posterior activity causes hindfoot varus and medial translation of triceps surae.

plantar fascia to shorten the distance between the metatarsal heads and the os calcis. Eventually, the long axis of the tibia and os calcis coincide and any residual triceps surae power is lost.

Management

During the acute phase of poliomyelitis, the paretic triceps surae is managed by keeping the foot in a position of slight equinus. Early walking in the convalescent phase is discouraged and the position of slight equinus is maintained. The rapid development of his deformity requires taking serial standing radiographs especially in children younger than five years of age (25,31). Operative correction is performed to prevent the development of calcaneal deformity and to restore functional hindfoot plantar flexion. Gait is improved by preventing retrograde displacement of the tibia, providing a more stable base for stance and gait, and creating a counter-thrust against which the remaining intact muscle can function. The calcaneocavus recurs if the deforming tendons are not transferred and if muscle balance and lateral stability are not achieved. This foot deformity represents the only absolute indication for tendon transfers about the foot and ankle in children younger than five years of age.

The amount and combination of muscles requiring posterior transfer are determined by the residual triceps surae strength and the pattern of remaining muscle function (Figure 15-9). When the retained motor strength of the triceps surae rates fair, the posterior transfer of two or

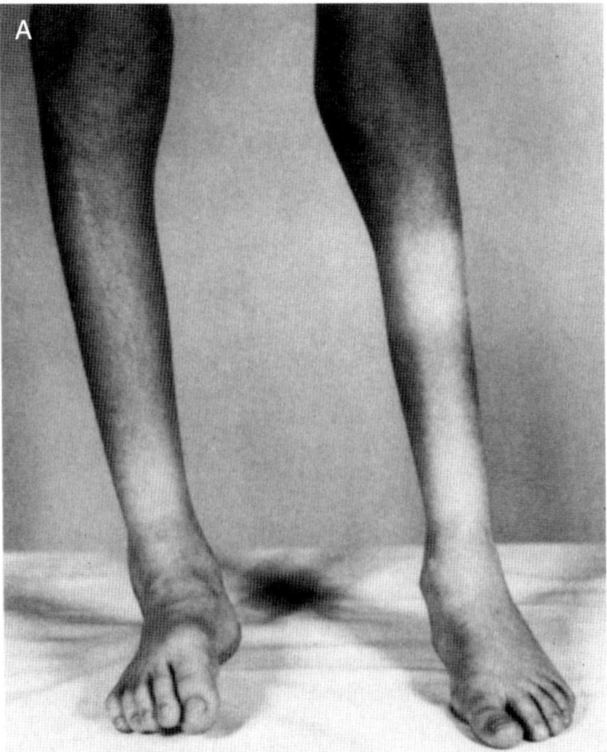

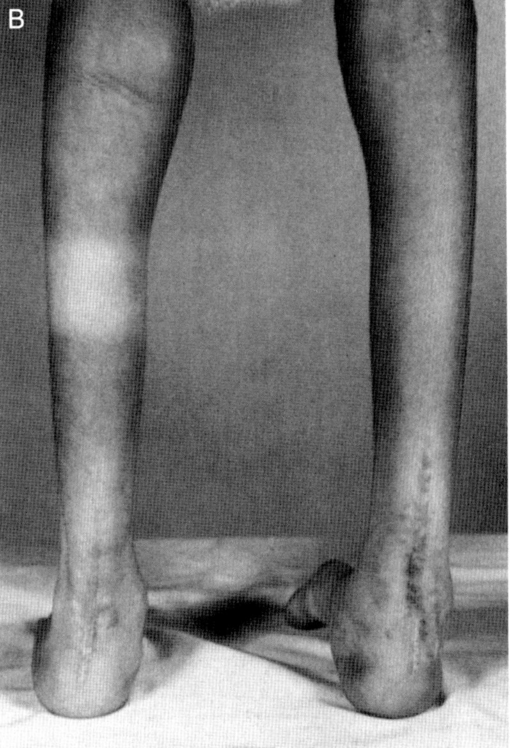

FIGURE 15-6 **A,B.** The first metatarsus is dorsiflexed by a strong tibialis anterior combined with weak perneus longus. Active secondary great toe plantar flexion permits first ray weight bearing and assists in terminal stance gait.

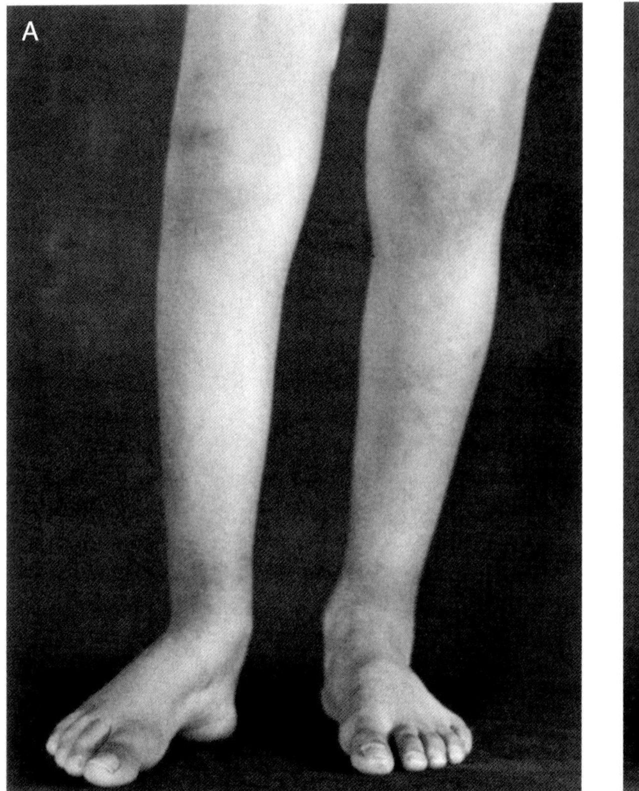

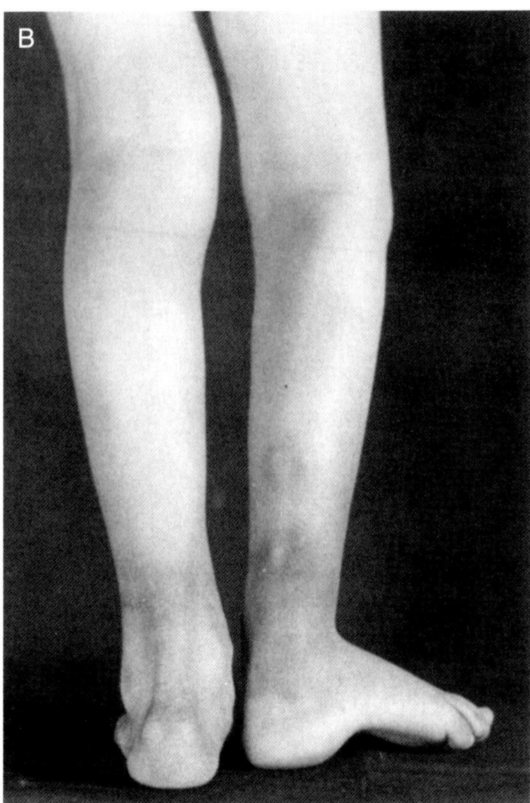

FIGURE 15-7 **A,B.** Calcaneocavus deformity results from triceps surae paralysis. Note the loss of the prominence of the os tuber.

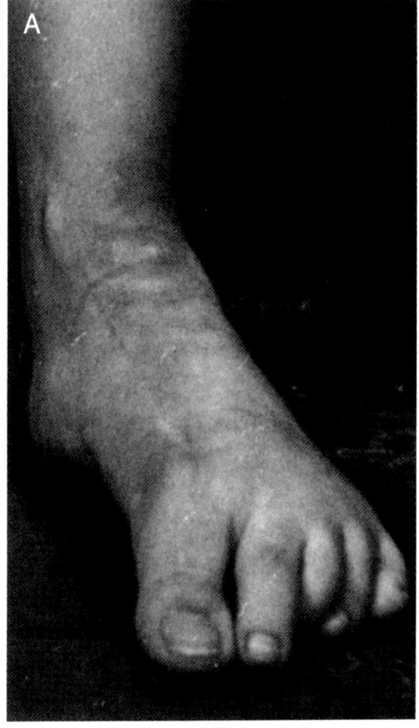

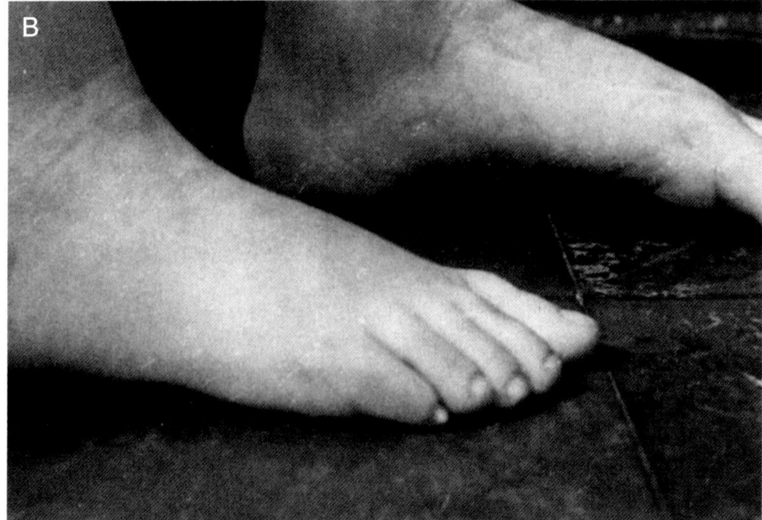

FIGURE 15-8 **A,B.** Dorsal bunion resulting from active plantar flexion of great toe and secondary dorsiflexion of first metatarsus. Long-toe flexors are assisting weakened triceps surae at the end of stance phase of gait.

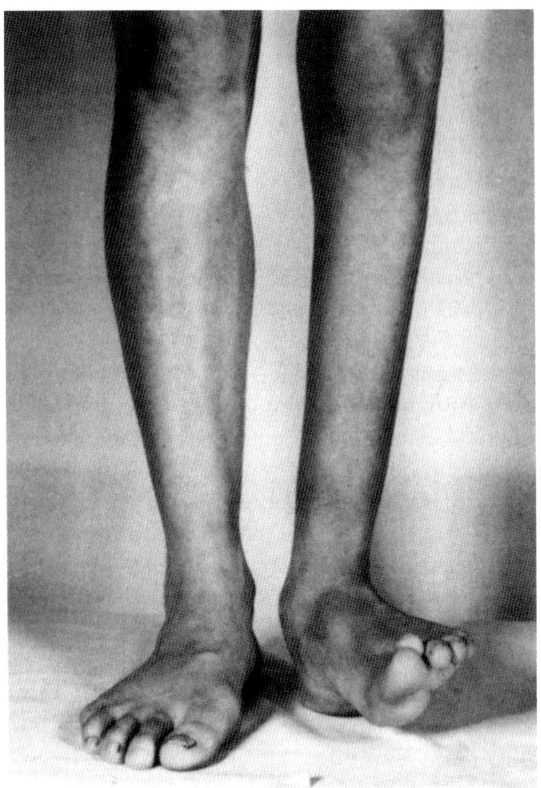

FIGURE 15-9 Retained function in long-toe extensors and peronei coupled with weak triceps surae leads to calcaneovalgus deformity.

three muscles may lead to normal gift. Complete triceps surae paralysis is managed by posterior transfer of as many muscles as are available with the exception of the tibialis anterior, which may be utilized for a secondary procedure, or alternatively, moved to the dorsum of the midfoot. A fixed cavus deformity a plantar soft tissue release before tendon transfers can be performed.

Tendon Transfers for Calcaneal Deformity

The tibialis anterior is the strongest muscle when compared with the triceps surae and it may be transferred to the os tuber as early as 18 months after the acute stage of poliomyelitis or when no further return of the triceps function is apparent (31). This can be accomplished as an isolated procedure when the lateral stabilizers are balanced and the strong toe extensors can be used for dorsiflexion. Claw-toe deformities may develop in the latter situation and require transfer of the toe extensors to the metatarsal heads together with proximal interphalangeal fusions.

Maximum length of the tibialis anterior tendon is necessary because the muscle may have shortened as a result of the calcaneal deformity. The transfer is taken through the interosseous membrane and attached to the os tuber. The foot is placed in a position of maximum plantar flexion to ensure the transfer is attached under sufficient tension. Additional soft tissue structures including the ankle joint capsule may require release and the long-toe extensors may need to be lengthened. The attenuated tendo-Achillis may need to be shortened, which can be accomplished by a Z-plasty and the transferred tibialis anterior attached both directly to the tuber and to the distal stump of the tendo-Achillis. Postoperative management includes long-leg casts for five weeks, followed by an ankle-foot orthosis.

Pure calcaneal cavus develops when the inverters and everters are balanced and the posterior transfer of only one set of these muscles would result in instability and secondary deformity. The peroneus brevis and tibialis posterior are antagonists and transfer of these two muscles to the heel controls the calcaneus deformity and provides the additional power to a triceps surae that has retained fair strength to permit the patient to regain a normal gait pattern. Cavus deformity with hindfoot imbalance requires transportation of the acting inverter or everter to the heel. Calcaneocavovalgus deformity is managed by transferring both peronei to the heel, whereas the tibialis posterior and flexor hallucis longus are the preferred muscles for cavovarus.

Westin and Dias (15,93) advocate tenodesis of the tendo-Achillis to the fibula for patients with paralytic pes calcaneus. The development of an equinus deformity following this procedure was common and occurred most often in patients who had a procedure at a younger age or when the calcaneal tibial angel measured more than 70 degrees at the time of tenodesis. Residual cavovarus deformity was managed by a plantar release.

Makin (55) preferred translocation of the peroneus longus in the presence of mobile calcaneal deformity. The tendon was translocated into a groove cut into the posterior calcaneus with no change in its origin or insertion. It was necessary to free the tendon both proximal to the lateral malleolus and at the cuboid groove. The foot is then maximally plantar flexed and the peroneus longus can be displaced posteriorly into the calcaneal groove where it will eventually become scarified with the bone (5). An extra-articular subtler arthrodesis is occasionally necessary as a second procedure.

Hamstrings have been used to replace the triceps surae when there are no inverters or everters present for transfer (20). Prerequisites for this rare operation include: complete paralysis of the triceps surae, strong medical hamstrings or biceps femoris muscle, and strong ankle dorsiflexors and quadriceps. The insertions of the semitendinosus and gracilis and occasionally semimembranosus are freed, passed subcutaneously, and are attached to the sagittally cut tendo-Achillis. It is important to use a mattress suture at the proximal end of the tendo-Achillis to prevent this cut from further extending proximally. Tendon apposition is accomplished with the knee flexed to 25 degrees and the foot in plantar flexion.

Flail Foot

Equinus deformity develops when all muscles distal to the knee are paralyzed. Because sacral sparing is common in poliomyelitis, the intrinsic muscles generally retain function. This may result in forefoot equinus or cavo equinus deformity which can be controlled by a plantar soft tissue release sometimes combined with a plantar neurectomy. Older patients may require a second stage mid-foot wedge resection for forefoot equinus deformity in order to be able to utilize an ankle-foot orthosis (12,83).

ARTHRODESIS OF THE FOOT AND ANKLE

It is necessary to correct structural bony deformity before tendon transfers can be performed in patients with poliomyelitis residual. The type of procedure is determined by the age of the patient and the rate of progression of the deformity. The cartilage of the small bones of the foot are responsible for growth as well as articulation, and therefore, arthrodesis affecting the longitudinal growth of the foot must be delayed until the patient is older than 10 years in order to avoid producing an excessively short foot. Bony deformity found in younger children may be corrected by osteotomies or capsulotomies.

The list of stabilizing procedures for the foot and ankle include: extra-articular subtler arthrodesis, triple arthrodesis, anterior or posterior bone blocks to limit motion at the ankle joint, and ankle arthrodesis. These can be performed as separate operations or in combination.

Extra-Articular Subtler Arthrodesis

Paralysis of the tibialis anterior and posterior combined with unopposed action of the peronei and triceps surae will produce a paralytic equinovalgus deformity. The os calcis is everted and displaced laterally and posteriorly. The sustentaculum tali, the calcaneal buttress for the talar head, is lost and the anterior talus shifts medially and into equinus. Hindfoot equinovalgus and forefoot pronation rapidly develop and with growth, the deformity becomes fixed.

Initial management includes an ankle-foot orthosis which imcorporates a varus-producing window and a Gillette UCBL heel. Surgical correction is frequently necessary (16). Grice developed an extra-articular subtler fusion for patients between three and eight years which restored the height of the medial longitudinal arch (27). The technique of Dennyson and Fulfort which incorporates metallic internal fixation with cancellous grafts is now recommended (13). The valgus deformity of the subtler joint can be corrected and the calcaneus manipulated into its normal position beneath the talus which sometimes requires a lateral release of the anterior and posterior subtler joint capsules. Preoperative assessment includes weight-bearing radiographs of the foot and ankle to ascertain whether the valgus deformity is primarily located in the subtler joint or the ankle joint. When the hindfoot is corrected and the forefoot is left with residual supination, it is necessary to perform an opening-wedge medial cuneiform osteotomy in order to make the first metatarsal assume a weight-bearing position. Failure to accomplish this results in a development of a painful callus over the fifth metatarsal head. A staged tendon transfer may be necessary to achieve dynamic hindfoot balance and to prevent recurrence of the primary deformity which may occur in spite of an extra-articular subtler arthrodesis (37).

Smith and Westin found that most of these procedures performed for poliomyelitis produced a satisfactory long-term result (80). However, additional tendon transfers were frequently required. The small number of unsatisfactory results were identified early in the postoperative course. Overcorrection resulting in varus deformity and increased ankle joint valgus were most frequently found in calcaneovalgus feet (62). They also reported pseudoarthrosis, graft resorption, and degenerative arthritis of the metatarsal joints as complications. Cast immobilization should be maintained until there is radiographic evidence of trabecular union on both the talar and calcaneal side of the graft. This sign is best appreciated on an oblique of the hindfoot.

A Grice procedure resulting in hindfoot varus can be corrected by realigning the original graft or by inserting a new graft. Most of these secondary procedures were successful.

Seymour and Evans obtained extra-articular fusion by inserting a fibular graft through the talar neck into the calcenus (73). This approach is not currently recommended because of the high rate of fatigue fracture and resorption of the fibular graft. A second complication is the proximal migration of the distal fibula from nonunion at the fibular donor site, which may result in an unacceptable ankle valgus.

Makin noted that patients who contracted poliomyelitis before reaching the age of two years frequently had fibular underdevelopment leading to ankle valgus deformity (55). The distal tibial growth plate remained intact and horizontal but the tibial epiphysis became deformed. The distal fibular epiphysis is delayed in ossification, whereas the tibia ossified appropriately. By the time the distal fibula is visualized radiographically, the majority of fibular shortening had already occurred. Initial management is attempted with an ankle-foot orthosis. A stapling type of epiphysiodesis of the medial distal tibial growth plate can be performed in patients over the age of eight years. Eventual correction of a marked ankle valgus deformity can be accomplished by a supramalleolar closing-wedge osteotomy and should be reserved for the patient nearing skeletal maturation.

Calcaneal Osteotomy

Hindfoot varus or valgus deformity can be corrected by calcaneal osteotomy in the skeletally immature child (18). Release of the intrinsic muscles and plantar fascia may also be necessary in the management of cavovarus deformity. A posterior calcaneal displacement osteotomy can be utilized for calcaneocavus deformity (Figure 15-10) (57). Heel varuS is most frequently managed by means of a closing-wedge resection based laterally when the heel is of adequate height and size (Figure 15-11). Fixed subtalar valgus deformity may require a medial displacement osteotomy made in a plane parallel with the peroneal tendons (47).

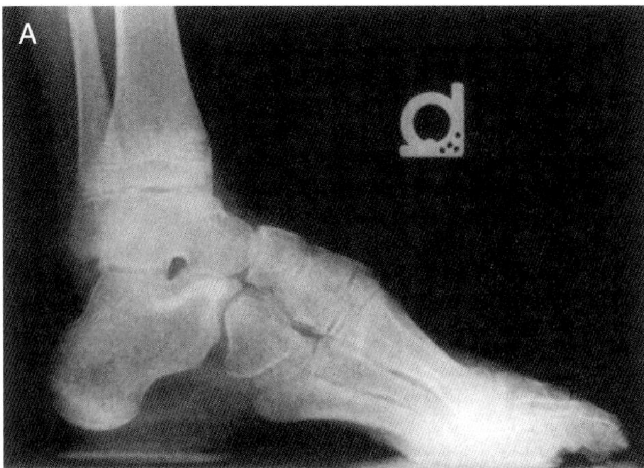

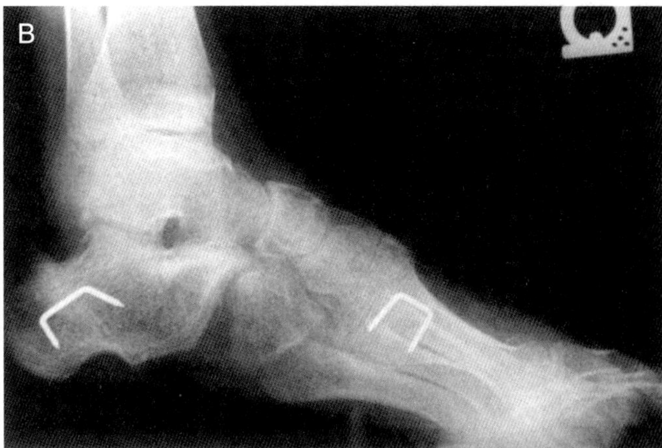

FIGURE 15-10 Posterior displacement calcaneal osteotomy decrease cavus deformity and enhances triceps surae function by lengthening the posterior lever arm. **A:** preoperative deformity. **B:** Postoperative correction.

Triple Arthodesis

Triple arthrodesis includes a fusion of the subtalar, calcaneocuboid, and talonavicular joints and is the most effective stabilizing procedure of the hind- and mid-foot. Ryerson considered the three joints as a physiologic unit that is critical to the development of hindfoot lateral stability (68). He noted that the talar body is held securely in position by the malleoli. The arthrodesis is designed to fasten the remaining hindfoot bones to the talus, thereby controlling lateral stability. Triple arthrodesis restricts motion of the foot and ankle to plantar flexion and dorsiflexion and is indicated when most of the weakness and deformity occurs at the subtalar and midtarsal joints (77).

The objectives of triple arthrodesis include:

1. Stable and static realignment of the foot
2. Removal of deforming forces

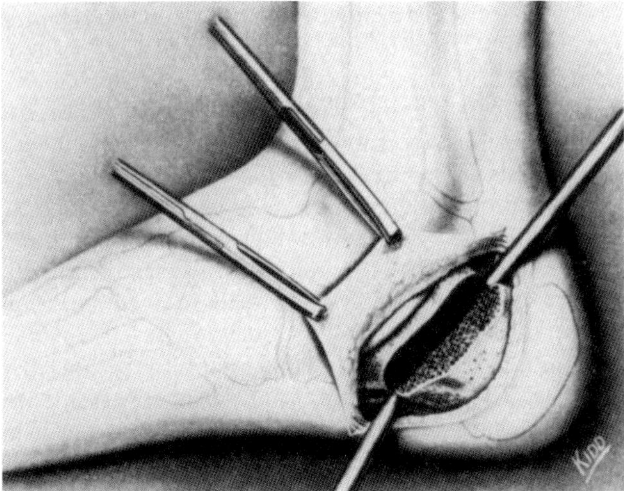

FIGURE 15-11 The ideal time for a closing wedge calcaneal osteotomy is 3 or 4 years of age. The procedure translates the insertion of triceps surae laterally. (From Dias LS. Ankle valgus in children with myelomeningocele. *Dev Med Child Neurol* 1978;20:627, with permission.)

3. Arrest of progression of deformity
4. Elimination of pain and decrease of limp
5. Elimination of the need for a short-leg brace or to realign the foot to permit application of a long-leg brace
6. A normal-appearing foot

The age of the patient has significant influence on the expected outcome. In one series, 47% of triple arthrodeses failed in children younger than nine years of age, whereas the failure rate was only 9% in children over ten years of age. Failure was due primarily to undercorrection. No major growth disturbances were noted in the older group.

Talar stability in the ankle mortise is essential for a favorable result in polio patients. Failure to recognize ankle instability may result in an unstable foot in weight bearing and possibly a recurrence of the deformity. Preoperative radiographic evaluation is needed to complement the clinical assessment. Careful tracings of the tibiotalar and calcaneal components should be made on a lateral radiographic image of the ankle and then reassembled with the foot in the corrected position to allow accurate measurement of the size and shape of the wedges to be removed.

The Ryerson form of triple arthrodesis is most effective when poliomyelitis patients retain dorsiflexion and plantar flexion strength (Figure 15-12). This procedure does not permit posterior displacement of the foot, sometimes needed to assist in correction of muscle imbalance, particularly weakness of the triceps surae. Posterior displacement effectively lengthens the posterior lever arm of the foot. This can be accomplished by the Dunn technique which accomplishes displacement by excising the navicular and a portion of the talar head and neck (17).

The Hoke method combined subtalar arthrodesis with resection, reshaping, and reinsertion of the talar head and neck and achieved less posterior displacement (34). The latter technique is generally selected because it can be adapted successfully to the correction of any of the combination of foot deformities.

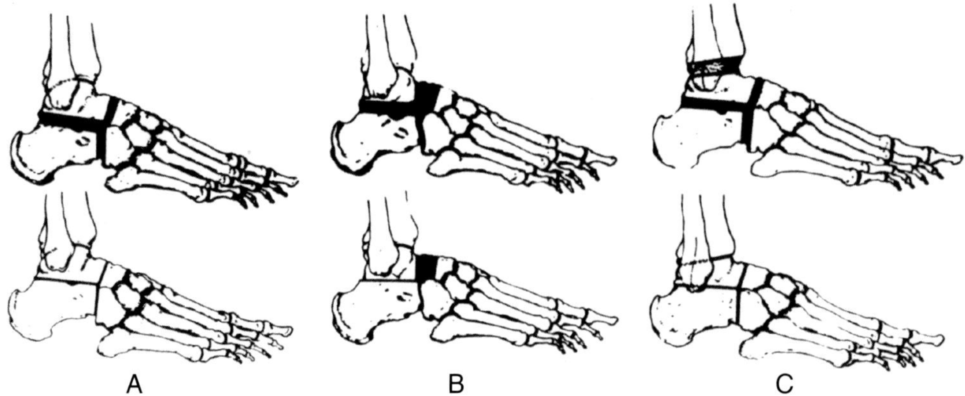

FIGURE 15-12 **A,B,C.** The shaded areas indicate the amoun of bone removed during different types of triple and pantalar arthrodeses. (From Patterson RI, Parrish FF, Hathaway EN. Stabilizing Operations on the foot. A study of the indications, techniques used, and end results. *J Bone Joint Surg* [*Am*] 1950;32:1, with permission.)

Specific operative technique varies with the type of deformity. Talipes equinovalgus includes medial longitudinal arch depression, talar head plantar flexion, and forefoot abduction. The arch may be restored by raising the talar head and shifting the sustentaculum tali medially beneath the talar head and neck. The surgery is performed through and Ollier approach with excision of a subtalar joint wedge based medially, including portion of the talar head and neck (Figure 15-13). There is a tendency toward forefoot supination with correction of the hindfoot valgus and this must be controlled at the time of triple arthrodesis by midtarsal joint resection with a wedge based medially. An additional medial incision for resection of the talonavicular joint may be required. The enlarged talar head in talipes equinovarus blocks dorsiflexion and lies lateral to the midline axis of the foot. This must be reduced to a position slightly medial to the midline axis of the foot and can be accomplished by a subtalar wedge based laterally, coupled with a mid-tarsal joint resection with the wedge based laterally. It is important to align the foot with the ankle mortise and not with the knee. Any associated rotation or angular deformity in the remainder of the extremity should be corrected by a separate procedure (2).

Fixed equinus deformity can be corrected through the subtalar joint by the Lambrinudi dropfoot arthrodesis (Figure 15-14) (50). The deformity develops as a result of retained activity of the triceps surae combined with inactive dorsiflexors and peronei (4,22,30). The posterior talus abuts the tibia and the posterior ankle joint capsule contracts creating a physiologic bone block. The procedure utilizes the fixed plantar flexed position of the talus against which the rest of the foot can be brought up to the desired degree of dorsiflexion. Poliomyelitis patients who lack this extreme degree of equinus gradually stretch the dorsal capsules and tendon and a recurrence of the deformity can be expected. The procedure is limited to patients older than nine years of age. Residual active muscle power requires either a tendon resection or transfer to prevent development of varus or valgus deformity (63). This dropfoot arthrodesis is not recommended for a fail foot and is

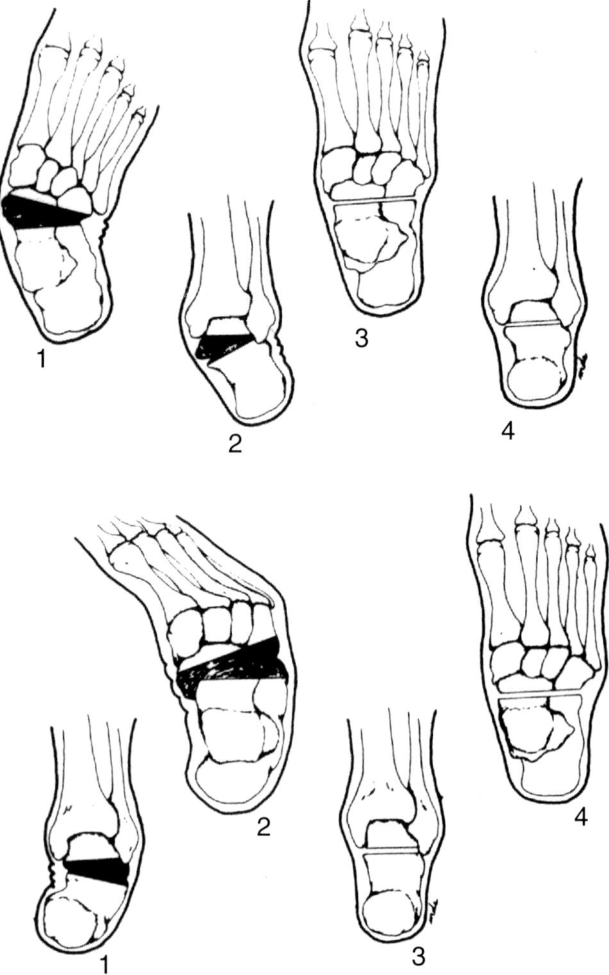

FIGURE 15-13 *Top*: Triple arthrodesis for rigid valgus deformity. Wedge resections necessary for correction of forefoot abduction and heel valgus are indicated by shaded areas (1 and 2). Position of bones after surgery is illustrated (*3 and 4*). *Bottom*: Triple arthrodesis for rigid varus deformity. Wedge resection necessary for correction of forefoot adduction and hindfoot varus are indicated by shaded areas (*1 and 2*). Position of bone after surgery (*3 and 4*). (From Dennyson WG, Fulford GE, Subtalar arthrodesis by cancellous grafts and metallic internal fixation. *J Bone Joint Surg (Br)* 1940;58:507, with permission.)

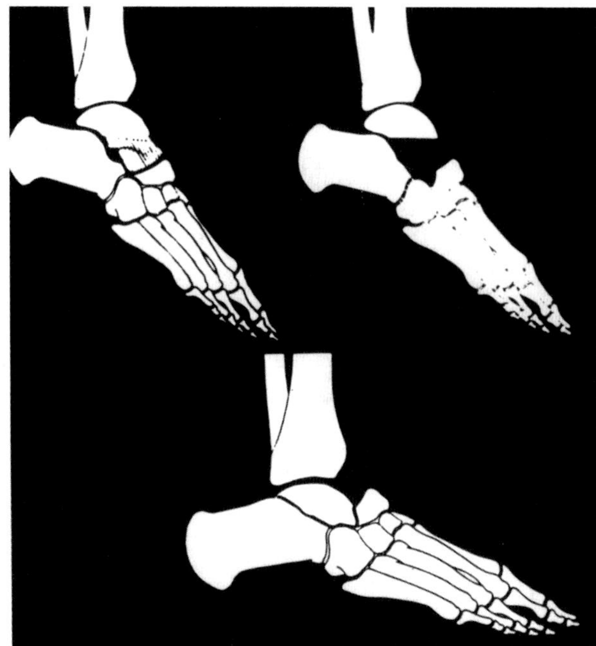

FIGURE 15-14 Lambrinudi triple arthrodesis. The talar beak is wedged into the navicular trough, and the remaining osseous structures are opposed. (From Dias LS. Ankle valgus in children with myelomeningocele. *Dev Med Child Neurol* 1978;20:627, with permission.)

less successful when done to relieve pain and hindfoot instability or to free a patient from a brace (53). It is not indicated when paralysis in the rest of the limb will require the ongoing use of a brace because of hip or knee instability. The strength of the dorsal ligaments of the ankle joint determine the success of the operation. Anterior talar subluxation noted on a weight-bearing lateral radiograph indicates the need for two-stage pantalar arthrodesis.

Complications

Pseudoarthrosis is the most common complication of triple arthrodesis, particularly in the talonavicular joint. The limitations of mobility of the hindfoot place additional stress on the ankle joint and may lead to the development of degenerative arthritis. Progressive ankle joint ligamentous laxity following triple arthrodesis may require an ankle fusion. Excessive resection of the talus may result in avascular necrosis, particularly in the skeletally immature adolescent, and can be demonstrated by radiographs obtained three to four weeks after triple arthrodesis. This latter complication is treated with non-weight bearing until vascular healing is evident. The persistence of muscle imbalance following hindfoot stabilization may lead to forefoot deformity with an unopposed tibialis anterior or peronei being the most common cause for this secondary deformity. Pseudoarthrosis of the talonavicular joint is the most common complication of the Lambrinudi dropfoot arthrodesis, particularly in patients over 20 years of age. This is the result of inadequate contact of the talar beak and the navicular bone. Other complications include ankle instability and residual varus or valgus deformity secondary to muscle imbalance.

Talipes Calceneus

Talipes calcenus is a rapidly progressive deformity resulting from triceps insufficiency combined with unopposed dorsiflexor activity. Paralysis of the triceps surae results in a fatiguing calcaneal gait. Tension on the tendo-Achillis is also essential for stabilizing the os calcis and for permitting normal function of the dorsiflexors and plantar flexors, as well as the intrinsic foot muscles.

Peabody recommended redistribution of muscle power in the early post-paralytic stages in order to prevent progressive calcaneus (64). Triceps surae paralysis and subsequent progressive calcaneal deformity serve as the only absolute indication from tendon transfer in children younger than five years with poliomyelitis.

Astragalectomy can be performed for calceneus or calcaneovalgus deformity and provide stability and posterior displacement of the foot and is the preferred treatment for children between the ages of five and twelve when hindfoot arthrodesis cannot be performed (35,51,94). Talectomy creates a physiologic tibiotarsal bone block or ankylosis and limits motion between the leg and foot, especially in dorsiflexion. The procedure produces even weight distribution and good lateral stability of the hindfoot and places the lower tibia over the center of the weight-bearing area by displacing the foot posteriorly. The outcome is a pain-free foot with a satisfactory appearance that does not require special shoes or external support.

Thompson reported that muscle imbalance is the most common cause of failure of talectomy with the presence of a strong tibialis anterior or tibialis posterior the most frequent cause (87). Forefoot equinus deformity can also develop from intrinsic muscle activity with a secondary contracture of the plantar fascia. Surgery performed on children younger than five years of age have a higher incidence of recurrence of the deformity and pain has been noted in patients over 15 years of age at the time of surgery. The only alternative to an unsuccessful talectomy is a tibial calcaneal arthrodesis. Carmack and Hallock recommended an anterior approach with the foot left in slight equinus position and found that the procedure was most frequently performed for residual pain at an average of seven years after talectomy (8). Staples has recommended a posterior arthrodesis which included an iliac graft being slotted into the os calcis and fixed to the tibia by a screw (82).

This deformity in poliomyelitis patients over 10 years of age can be effectively managed by the Elmslie double tarsal wedge osteotomy (Figure 15-15) (10,19). Other forms of triple arthrodesis require substantial resection of bone from both the calcaneus and talus. The first stage of the Elmslie procedure includes the release of the plantar soft tissue through a lateral hindfoot incision coupled with a dorsal wedge excision arthrodesis of the talonavicular and calcaneocuboid joint. Correction of the cavus deformity results. The cast is applied in a position of marked dorsiflexion and requires sufficient soft padding between the leg and foot to prevent maceration. Six weeks later a second-stage procedure is done through a vertical

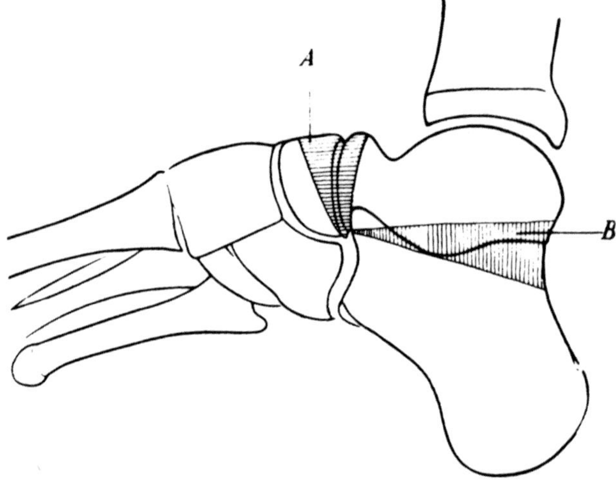

FIGURE 15-15 Elmslie double tarsal wedge osteotomy with shaded areas indicating the two-stage wedge resections (From Carmack JC, Hallock H. Tibiotarsal arthodesis after astragalectomy, a report of eight cases. *J Bone Joint Surg* 1947;29:476, with permission.)

incision along the medial border of the tendo-Achillis. The long-toe flexors are divided distally and a posterior wedge excision arthrodesis of the subtalar joint is performed with the wedge extending distally to the point of the previous osteotomy. The foot is then plantar flexed to bring the bony surfaces together. The now redundant tendo-Achillis is surgically shortened and the posterior surface of the tibia is exposed to permit anchoring of the strip of the distal tendo-Achillis to the tibia when the foot is plantar flexed. The long-toe flexors are also inserted into the tendo-Achillis.

Ankle Fusion

Ankle fusion has been most commonly performed for dangle foot or flail foot (57) but may also be indicated when ankle deformity recurs following triple arthrodesis. The Charnley or Calandruccio compression arthrodesis has been widely accepted for use in these patients (9). Chuinard and Peterson have described an ankle fusion for skeletally immature patients with flail feet which is recommended for children because it does not disturb the distal tibial growth plate (11).

Pantalar Arthrodesis

Pantalar arthrodesis benefits the polio patient whose flail foot is coupled with paralyzed quadriceps and may result in the elimination of a long leg brace (32). A strong gluteus maximus is a prerequisite to initiate toe-off at the end of stance phase with a normally aligned knee that has full extension or few degrees of hyperextension. The ankle should be fused at 10 degrees of equinus to produce the backward thrust on the knee joint necessary for stable weight bearing during stance (51). Lateral radiographs obtained at surgery permit accurate determination of plantar flexion because excessive equinus position may result in pain and increased pressure under the metatarsal heads. Waugh identified a compensatory increase in forefoot motion that assists in the stance gait pattern (92). The younger the patient, the greater the compensatory motion achieved.

Complications of pantalar arthrodesis include pseudoarthrosis, painful plantar callosities secondary to unequal weight distribution, and excessive heel equinus deformity which leads to increased pressure on the forefoot.

Claw-Toe Deformity

Claw-toe deformity is characterized by hyperextension of the metatarsophalangela joints coupled with flexion of the interphalangeal joints and may develop in the poliomyelitis patient when long-toe extensors are needed during the swing-phase to substitute for a severely weakened ankle dorsiflexor. Generally, the deformity is noted only during the swing-phase. However, marked deformity may occur when the tendo-Achillis is contracted. Treatment includes correction of any fixed ankle equinus deformity and appropriate tendon transfers to restore active ankle dorsiflexion.

Clawing may also develop when the long-toe flexors are used to substitute for a paretic triceps surae in the toe-off phase of stance. Appropriate tendon transfers to restore active ankle plantar flexion generally eliminate the need for corrective toe surgery. Claw toes associated with cavus deformity can be corrected by appropriate soft-tissue or osseous surgery for the cavus and usually results in spontaneous resolution of the toe deformity. Clawing of the lateral toes caused by long-toe flexor over activity can be corrected by a Girdlestone-Taylor transfer of the long-toe flexor into the dorsal hood of the extensor tendon (85).

Residual clawing of the great toe may be noted following corrective surgery for ankle dorsiflexor insufficiency and can be corrected by a Jones transfer of the extensor hallucis longus tendon to the neck of the first metatarsal (43). Arthrodesis of the hallucal interphalangeal joint and suturing the distal stump of the extensor hallucis longus to the extensor hallucis brevis are also parts of the procedure. Great-toe clawing resulting from ankle plantar flexion insufficiency can be treated by the Dickson-Diveley procedure. The extensor hallucis longus tendon is tenotomized, routed medially, and inserted into the flexor hallucis longus tendon at the plantar aspect of the first metatarsal head. Fusion of the interphalangeal joint is requited.

Cavus Deformity

Pes cavus is usually associated with an underlying neuromuscular disease and an established diagnosis is necessary before treatment should be undertaken. The differential diagnosis includes anterior horn cell involvement with poliomyelitis; spinal cord lesions (myelomeningocele); spinocerebellar tract (Friedreich's ataxis); peripheral nerves (hereditary sensory and motor neuropathies); and skeletal muscle (myopathies). Pes cavus describes a forefoot drop on a fixed hindfoot with the triceps surae either of normal length or slightly contracted (Figure 15-16). In poliomyelitis, the development of cavus commonly follows this pattern or may represent a calcaneocavus deformity caused by weakness or overstretching of the triceps surae. Lateral radiographs with the foot stressed in maximum dorsiflexion can be used to determine the degree of forefoot mobility on the fixed hindfoot.

The pathogenesis of pes cavus is discussed in Chapter 12. The deformity can develop because of weakness or imbalance between both intrinsic and extrinsic muscle groups. The foot dynamics involved have influenced the choice of management of several of the authors.

Soft-tissue procedures for fixed cavus are indicated before adaptive bony changes have occurred. The Steindler stripping is generally considered the procedure of choice because it lengthens the medial longitudinal arch, but the result is excessive skin tension following the traditional medial Steindler incision. This author prefers an Elmslie lateral heel incision which is carried forward from the os tuber to the calcaneocuboid joint. Osseous procedures are generally preceded by plantar release and are reserved for more severe cavus deformity. Cole described a closing dorsal tarsal wedge osteotomy for cavus without varus deformity of the calcaneus or gross muscle imbalance (12). This permits corrections without loss of motion in the subtalar joint. Severe cavovarus deformity is best managed by a triple arthrodesis.

Posterior bone block eliminates ankle plantar flexion while retaining a functional range of dorsiflexion and may rarely be indicated when the procedure would eliminate the need for dropfoot brace (91). It has its greatest use in patients with the completely flail foot and weak quadriceps muscle who can be made brace free by a combination of triple arthrodesis and posterior bone block. Best results are reported in patients between the ages of 10 to 20 years in whom a discrepancy of less than two grades between plantar flexion and dorsiflexion muscles and in whom plantar flexion of at least a grade 3 is retained (42). The procedure is contraindicated in full-time brace wearers.

Campbell constructed a bone buttress on the posterior aspect of the talus and superior surface of the calcaneus that impinged on the distal tibia to prevent ankle plantar flexion (5). Inclan performed a first-stage Hoke triple arthrodesis and used the resected talar head to create a staged posterior bone block (38). An osteochondral flap was raised from the posterior superior talus and the graft wedge beneath this, thus widening the posterior talus while retaining a congruous cartilaginous join surface. Ingram and Huntley reviewed the long-term results in 90 poliomyelitis patients treated with a Campbell posterior bone block (40). Degenerative ankle arthritis developed in more than half the patients, with avascular necrosis of the talus in one-fourth of the patients. Performing the

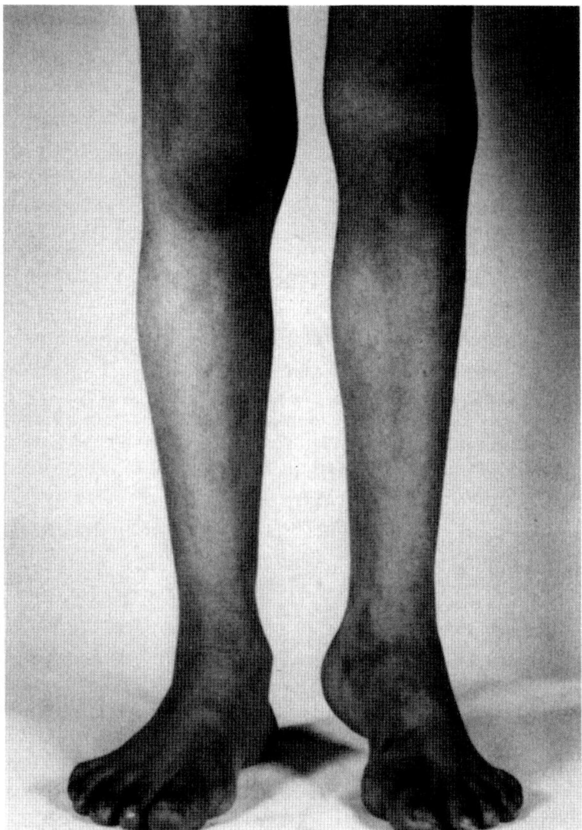
A

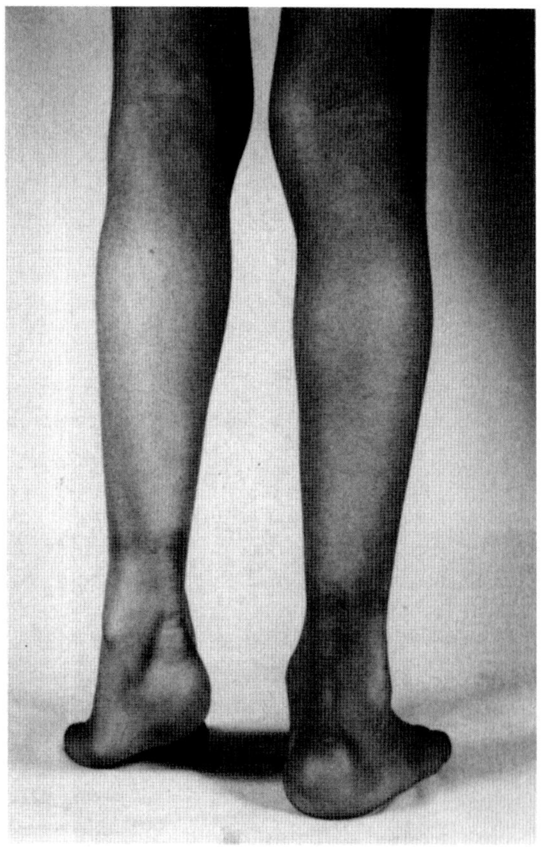
B

FIGURE 15-16 **A,B:** Patient whose forefoot equinus compensates for limb length inequality resulting from unilateral calf paralysis during infancy.

procedure in patients with a flat foot may lead to ankle joint ankylosis.

POST-POLIO SYNDROME

The diagnosis is based on five criteria and is essentially a diagnosis by exclusion. The criteria include: (i) a confirmed history of poliomyelitis; (ii) partial to failry complete neurologic and functional recovery; (iii) a period of neurologic and functional stability of at least 15 years' duration; (iv) onset of two or more of the following medical problems since achieving a period of stability: muscle or joint pain or both; unaccustomed fatigue, new weakness in muscles previously affected or unaffected, functional loss, cold intolerance and new atrophy; (v) no other explanation for the development of these medical issues. The median age of onset of acute polio in these patients was seven years. Post-polio syndrome is more likely to develop in patients whose onset was later than 10 years of age as older children are more likely to have severe clinical involvement of poliomyelitis. Two-thirds of post-polio syndrome patients are female, with onset generally 30 years after the acute onset. Nearly half of Halsted's patients had acute involvement of all four extremities and required hospitalization (29).

The fatigue in post-polio syndrome may be reported in previously affected muscles, particularly those used during free ambulation or walking with a cane. The location of pain is generally related to use. Management of these patients is conservative and includes reducing the activity level, changing the time and duration of exercise, and possibly using a wheelchair on a part-time basis (78). It may be necessary to reassess and modify sitting and sleeping postures and activities. Nonsteroidal anti-inflammatory drugs (NSAIDs) have been effective. Orthotics may need to be introduced. Surgery employs the same technique and indications as those utilized in the chronic phase (14,21,72,81,97).

Twenty percent of these patients have definite post-poliomyelitis muscle atrophy. Pathologic investigation indicated that their spinal cords had smoldering ongoing activity for many years after the acute onset in contradistinction to the generally accepted dictum that acute poliomyelitis is a monophasic disease (65). Patients with post-polio muscular atrophy have perivacular and parenchymal inflammatory cells that continue many years after the acute viral insult, particularly in the anterior horn area of the cord.

The etiology of the post-polio syndrome has not been established. Recovery from the acute episodes may take up to seven years due to a process of reinervation by terminal axon sprouting, with a single terminal axon sprout innervating a group of previously denervated muscle fibers. The uninvolved motor neurons take on as many fibers as possible, even though the neuron cannot supply each with normal transmission. The sequelae of polio may leave the motor neuron permanently scarred and metabolically unable to provide normal transmission and may lead to the neuron undergoing premature degeneration (6). Tomlinson's research suggests that normal motor units begin to lose function after a person reaches 60 years of age and perhaps polio causes this process to begin prematurely (88).

REFERENCES

1. Arcy LB. *Developmental anatomy: A textbook and laboratory manual of embryology,* 7th ed. Philadelphia: WB Saunders, 1974.
2. Asirvatham R, Watts HG, Rooney RJ. Rotation Osteotomy of the tibia after poliomyelitis. A review of 51 patients. *J Bone Joint Surg (Br)* 1990;72:409–411.
3. Basu RN. Challenges in the final stage of polio eradication. *Indian J Pediatr* 2004; 71:339–340.
4. Bernau A. Long term results following Lambrinudi arthrodesis. *J Bone Joint Surg (Am)* 1977;59:473.
5. Bickel WH, Moe JH. Translocation of the peroneus longus tendon for paralytic calcaneus deformity of the foot. *Surg Gynecol Obstet* 1944;78:627.
6. Bradley WG, Tandan R, Robinson SH. Clinical subtypes, DNA repair efficiency and therapeutic trails in the post-polio syndrome. *Birth Defects* 1987;23:343.
7. Campbell WC. An operation for the correction "drop-foot." *J Bone Joint Surg* 1923;5:815.
8. Carmack JC, Hallock H. Tibiotarsal arthrodesis after astragalectomy, a report of eight cases. *J Bone Joint Surg* 1947;29:476.
9. Charnley J. Compression arthrodesis of the ankle and shoulder, *J Bone Joint Surg (Br)* 1951;33:180.
10. Cholmeley JA. Elmslies operation for the calcenus foot. *J Bone Joint Surg (Br)* 1953;35:46.
11. Chuinard EG, Peterson RE. Distraction-compression bone graft arthrodeses of the ankle. A method especially applicable for children. *J Bone Joint Surg (Am)* 1963;45:481.
12. Cole WH The treatment of claw foot. *J Bone Joint Surg* 1940;22:895.
13. Dennyson WG, Fulford GE. Subtalar arthodesis by cancellous grafts and metallic internal fixation. *J Bone Joint Surg (Br)* 1940;58:507.
14. Dhillon MS, Sandhu HS. Surgical options in the management of residual foot problems in poliomyelitis. *Foot Ankle Clinic* 2000:327–347.
15. Dias LS. Ankle valgus in children with myelomeningocele. *Dev Med Child Neurol* 1978;20:627.
16. Drennan JC. *Othopaedoc management of neuromuscular disorders.* Philadelphia: JB Lippincott, 1983.
17. Dunn J. Stabilizing operations in the treatment of paralytic deformity of the foot. *Proc R Soc Med (Orthopaedics)* 1922;15:15.
18. Dwyer FE. Osteotomy of the calcaneum for pes cavus. *J Bone Joint Surg (Br)* 1959:41:80.
19. Elmslie RI. In: Turner 00, ed. *Modern operative surgery,* 2nd ed. London: Cassell, 1934.
20. Emmel HE, LeCocq JF. Hamstring transplant for the prevention of calcaneocavus foot in poliomyelitis. *J Bone Joint Surg (Am)* 1958;40:911.
21. Faraj AA. Modified Jones Procedure for post-polio claw hallux deformity. *J Foot Ankle Surg* 1997,36:356–359.
22. Fitzgerald FP, Seddon HJ. Lambrinudi's operation for drop-foof. *Br J Surg* 1937;25:283.
23. Fried A, Hendel C. Paralytic valgus deformity of the ankle. Replacement of the paralyzed tibiablis posterior by the preoneus longus. *J Bone joint Surg (Am)* 1957;39:921.
24. Gaebler JW, Kleiman MD, French ML, Chastain G, Barrett C, Griffin C. Neurologic complilcations in oral polio vaccine recipients. *J Pediatr* 1986; 108:878.

25. Goldner JI, Irwin CE. Paralytic deformities of the foot. *Instr Course Lect* 1948;5:1990.
26. Green WT, Grice OS. The management of calcaneus deformity. *Instr Course Lect* 1956;13:135.
27. Grice DS. The role of subtalar fusion in the treatment of valgus deformities of the feet. *Instr Course Lect* 1959;16:127.
28. Gunn DR, Molesworth BD. The use of tibialis posterior as a dorsiflexor. *J Bone Joint Surg (Am)* 1957;39:674.
29. Halstead LS. Post-polio syndrome. *Aci Am* 1998, 278:42–47.
30. Hart VL. Corrective cast for flexion contracture defotmity of the knee. *J Bone Joint Surg* 1934:16:970.
31. Herndon CR, Tendon transplantation at the knee and foot. *Instr Course Lect* 1961;18:145.
32. Heyman CH. A method of the correction of paralytic genu recurvatum. Report of a biliateral case. *J Bone Joint Surg* 1924;6:689.
33. Hoffman J. Uber chroniscbe spinale Muskelatrophie im Kinder. salter, auf familiarer Basis. Deutsche. *Z Nervenheilk* 1893;3:427.
34. Hoke M. An operation for stabilizing paralytic feet. *Am J Orthop Surg* 1921;3:494.
35. Holmdahl HE. Astraga Ectomy as a stabilizing operation for foot paralysis following poliomyelitis: results of a follow-up investigation of 153 cases. *Acta Orthop Scand* 1956;25:207.
36. Houvilainen A, Kinnunen L, Ferguson M, Hovi T. Antigenic variation among 173 strains of type 3 poliovirus isolated in Finland during the 1984 to 1985 outbreak. *J Gen Virol* 1988;69: 1941–1948.
37. Hunt JC, Brooks AI. Subtalar extraarticular arthrodesis for correction of paralytic valgus deformity of the foot. Evaluation of forty-four procedures with particular reference to associated tendon transference. *J Bone Joint Surg (Am)* 1965;47:1310.
38. Inclan A. End results in physiological blocking of flail Joints. *J Bone Joint Surg* (Am) 1949;31:748.
39. Ingersoll RE. Transplantation of peroneus longus to anterior tibial insertion in poliomyelitis. *Surg Gynecol Obstet.* 1948;86:717.
40. Ingram AJ, Hundley JM. Posterior bone block of the ankle for paralytic equinus. An end-result study. *J Bone! Joint Surg (Am)* 1951;33:679.
41. Johnson EW Jr. Results of modern methods of treatment of poliomyelitis. *J Bone Joint Surg* 1945;27:223.
42. Jones GB. Paralytic dislocation of the hip. *J Bone Joint Surg (Br) J* 1962;44:573.
43. Jones R. The soldier's foot and the treatment of common deformities of the foot. *Br Med J* 1916;1(2891):749.
44. Kew (BWHO), Kew OM, Wright PF, Agolvi, Delpeyroux F, Shimizu H, Nathanson N, Pallansch MA. Circulating vaccine-derived polioviruses: Current state of knowledge. *Bull Who,* 2003, 81(4):312.
45. Kohler KA, Hlady WG, Banerjee K, Sutter RW. Outbreak of poliomyelitis due to type 3 poliovirus, northern India, 1999–2000: Injections: a major contributing factor. *Int J Epidemiol* 2003, Apr;32(2):272–277.
46. Kojima H, Fujita Y, Fujioka M, Nagashima K. Onuf's motoneuron is resistant to poliovirus. *J Neurol Sci* 1989; 93:85–92.
47. Koutsomiannis E. Treatment of mobile flatfeet by displacement of osteotomy. *J Bone Joint Surg [Br]* 1971; 53:96.
48. Kuhlmann RF. Bell JF. A clinical evaluation of tendon transplantations for poliomyelitis affecting the lower extremities. *J Bone Joint Surg (Am)* 1952;34:915.
49. LaForce FM. Poliomyelitis vaccines. Success and controversy. *Infect Dis Clin North Am* 1990;4:75–83.
50. Lambrinudi C. New operation on drop-foot. *Br J Surg* 1927;15:193.
51. Liebolt FL. Pantalar arthrodesis in poliomyelitis. *Surgery* 1939;6:31.
52. Lipscomb PR. Sanchez JJ. Anterior transplantation of the posterior tibial tendon for persistent palsy of the common peroneal nerve. *J Bone Joint Surg (Am)* 1961; 43:60.
53. MacKenzie G. Lambrinudi's arthrodesis. *J Bone Joint Surg (Br)* 1959;41:738.
54. Mahadevan S. Ananthakrisbnan S. Srinivasan S, et al. Poliomyelitis: 20 years-the Pondicherry experience. *J Trop Med Hyg* 1989,92:416421.
55. Makin M, Yossipovitch A. Translocation of the peroneus longus in the treatment of paralytic pes calcaneus. A follow-up study of thirty-three cases. *J Bone Joint Surg (Am)* 1966;48:1541.
56. Mayer L. The physiologic method of tendon transplants. Review after forty year. *Instr Course Lect* 1956; 13: 116.
57. Mitchell GP. Posterior displacement osteotomy of the calcaneus *J Bone Joint Surg (Br)* 1977;59:233.
58. *MMWR Morb.* Progress toward poliomyelitis eradication – Nigeria, Jan 2003–March 2004, 53(16): 343–346.
59. *MMWR Morb.* Poliovirus infections in four unvaccinated children. Minnesota, August–October 2005, 2005;54(41):1053–1055.
60. *MMWR Mord.* Seroprevalence of poliovirus antibodies among children in Dominican Community – Puerto Rico, 2002–2005; 54(24):608.
61. *MMWR Morb.* Distribution of insecticide-treated bednets during a polio immunization campaign – Niger, 2005–2006;55(33): 913–916.
62. Paluska DJ, Blount WP. Ankle valgus after the Grice subtalar stablization: the late evaluation of a personal series with a modified technic. *Clin Orthop* 1968;59:137.
63. Patterson RI, Patrish FF, Hathaway EN. Stabilizing operations on the foot. A study of the indications, techniques used. and end results. *J Bone Joint Surg (Am)* 1950;32:1.
64. Peabody CW. Tendon transposition in the paralytic foot. *Instr Course Led* 1949;6:179.
65. Pezeshk Pour GH, Dalakas MC. Long-term changes in the spinal cord of patients with old poliomyelitis. Signs of continuous disease activity. *Arch Neurol* 1988; 45:505.
66. Querfurth H, Swanson PD. Vaccine-associated paralytic poliomyelitis. Regional case series and review. *Arch Neurol* 1990;47:541–544.
67. Robertson SE, Chao C, Kim-Farley R, Ward N. Worldwide status of poliomyelitis in 1986, 1987 and 1988, and plans for its global eradication by the year 2000. *World Health Stat Q* 1990;43:80–90.
68. Ryerson EW. Arthrodesing operations on the feet. *J Bone Joint Surg* 1923;5:453.
69. Salk D. Polio immunization policy in the United States: a new challenge for a new generation. *Am J Pub Health* 1988;78:296–300.
70. Schaap EJ, Huy J, Tonino AJ. Long-term results of arthrodesis of the ankle. *Int Orthop* 1990;14:9–12.
71. Schottsdaedt ER. Larsen IJ. Bost FC. Complete muscle transposition. *J Bone Joint Surg (Am)* 1955;37:897.
72. Scott SM, Janes PC, Stevens PM. Grice subtalar arthrodesis followed to skeletal maturity. *J Ped Orthop* 1988; 8:176–183.
73. Seymour N, Evans K. A modification of the Grice subtalar arthrodesis. *J Bone Joint Surg (Br)* 1968;50:371.
74. Sharma M, Sen S, Ahuja B, Dhamija K. Paralytic poliomyelitis 1976–1988: report from a Sentinel Centre. *Indian Pediatr* 1990;27:143–150.
75. Sharrard WJW. The segmental innervation of the lower limb muscles in man. *Ann R Coil Surg Engl* 1964;35:106.
76. Sharrard WJW. Posterior iliopsoas transplantation in the treatment of paralytic dislocation of the hip. *J Bone Joint Surg (Br)* 1964;46:426.
77. Sharrard WJW. Muscle recovery in poliomyelitis. *J Bone Joint Surg (Br)* 1955;37:63.
78. Sheth NP, Keenan ME. Orthopaedic surgery considerations in post-polio syndrome. *Am J Orthop* 2007: 36:348–353.
79. Slater PE, Orenstein W A, Morag A, et al. Poliomyelitis outbreak in Israel in 1988; a report with two commentaries. *Lancet* 1990;335:1192–1195.
80. Smith JB, Westin GW. Subtalar extraarticular arthrodesis. *J Bone Joint Surg (Am)* 1968;50:1027.
81. Song HR, Mybroh V, Ohcu CW, Leest Lee SH. Tibial lengthening and concomitant foot deformity correction in 14 patients with permanent deformity after poliomyelitis. *Acta Orthop* 2005; 76:261–269.

82. Staples OS. Posterior arthrodesis of the ankle and subtalar joints. *J Bone Joint Surg (Am)* 1956;38:50.
83. Steindler A. Stripping of the os calcis. *J Or/hop Surg* 1920;2:8.
84. Suielcha C. Sujamol S, Suguna Bai NS, Cherian T, John TJ. An epidemic of poliomyelitis in southern Kenya. *Int J Epidemiol* 1990;19:177–181.
85. Taylor RG. The treatment of claw toes by multiple transfers of flexors into extensor tendons. *J Bone Joint Surg (Br)* 1951;33:539.
86. Thacker N, Shendurnikar N. Current status of polio eradication and future prospects. *Indian J Pediatr* 2004; 71:1141–1142.
87. Thompson TC. Astragalectomy and the treatment of calcaneovalgus. *J Bone Joint Surg* 1939;21:627.
88. Tomlinson BE, Irving D. Changes in spinal cord motor neurons of possible relevance to the late effects of poliomyelitis. In Halsted LF, Weicher DO, eds. *Late effects of poliomyelitis.* Miami: Symposia Foundation, 1985:51.
89. Triki H, Barbouche MR, Bahri O, Bejaoui M, Dellagi K. Community acquired poliovirus infection in children with primary immunodeficiencies in Tunisia. *J Clin Microbiol* 2003; 41:1203–1211.
90. Varughese PV, Charter AO, Acres SE, Furesz J. Eradication of indigenous poliomyelitis in Canada: impact of immunization strategies. *Can J Pub Health* 1989;80:363–368.
91. Wagner LC. Modified bone block(Campbell of ankle for paralytic drop foot with report of twenty-seven cases. *J Bone Joint Surg* 1931; 13:142.
92. Waugh TR, Wagner J, Stinchfield FE. An evaluation of pantalar arthrodesis. A follow-up study of one hundred and sixteen operations. *J Bone Joint Surg (Am)* 1965;47:1315.
93. Westin GW. Dingeman RD, Gausewitz SH. The results of tenodesis of the tendo-Achillis to the fibula for paralytic pes calcaneus. *J Bone Joint Surg [Am)* 1988;70:320–328.
94. Whitman A. Astragalectomy and backward displacement of the foot. An investigation of its practical results. *J Bone Joint Surg* 1922;4:266.
95. Wilson FC Jr, Fay GF, Lamotte P, Williams JC. Triple arthrodesis. A study of the factors affecting fusion after three hundred and one procedures. *J Bone Joint Surg [Am)* 1965;47:340.
96. Wyatt HV. Incubation of poliomyelitis as calculated from the time of entry into the central nervous system via the peripheral nerve pathways. *Rev Infect Dis* 1990;12:547–556.
97. Zorer G, Bagatur AE, Dogan A, Unlu T. Dennyson-Fulford subtalar extra-articular arthrodesis in the treatment of paralytic pes planovalgus and its value in the alignment of the foot. *Acta Orthop Traumatol Turc* 2003;37(2):162–169.

CHAPTER 16

Arthrogryposis

William F. Schrantz

INTRODUCTION

Foot and ankle deformities in children with arthrogryposis present a spectrum of disorders including clubfoot, vertical talus, cavus, metatarsus adductus, and equinus. Unlike the idiopathic forms, the child with arthrogryposis often has a much more rigid and severe deformity, making traditional treatments more difficult and recurrence more likely. Additionally, other lower extremity deformities and upper extremity involvement may alter postoperative rehabilitation as well as surgical indications.

DEFINITION

Arthrogryposis is from the Greek meaning crooked or stiff joint. The term has evolved and is used both as a description and a diagnosis. Arthrogryposis is a heterogeneous group of non-progressive disorders characterized multiple joint contractures. It typically does not affect sensation or intellect. Children with arthrogryposis have extraordinary adaptive capabilities and become surprisingly functional. The initial description of arthrogryposis was reported by Otto in 1848 (45), although the condition had been recognized earlier, as depicted in the picture of La Pied Bot (The Club Foot) by Jose de Ribera in 1642 (Figure 16-1). Stern first introduced the term arthrogryposis multiplex congenita in 1923 (57). Specific terminology for the multitude of different clinical groups with an arthrogrypotic component has continued to evolve. Recently, Hall has used the term amyoplasia to identify the most common clinical form of arthrogryposis (26). It was not until the classic descriptions of arthrogryposis by Lloyd-Roberts (40), Mead (43), and Friedlander (19) in the 1950s and 1960s that treatments specific to the arthrogrypotic foot were separated from treatments of the idiopathic clubfoot. Management of the arthrogrypotic foot (15,22,24,34,61) takes its precedent from the classical forms of treatment used for the most difficult clubfeet including the multiply operated idiopathic talipes equinovarus (ITEV) (1,17,23,32,33); the neglected ITEV (35,54); and other multifactoral or teratologic club feet including those associated with myelodysplasia (12,39,54). These subgroups of severe clubfeet have been typically grouped together because of their common characteristics of high recurrence and complications.

EPIDEMIOLOGY

Multiple congenital pathologic contractures (arthrogryposis) occur in about 1 of every 3,000 live births. Amyoplasia occurs in 1 of every 10,000 live births (28).

PATHOLOGY

The pathoanatomy of arthrogryposis includes both the spinal cord and muscle with their secondary effects on the growing bony structures. The spinal cord is small in size. There is dysgenesis of the spinal anterior horn cells as well as the motor nuclei of the brain stem with decreased neurons and loss of nuclear group patterns. Abnormalities in the muscle fibers includes smaller than normal cross section diameter, with fibrosis suggesting that maturation was impaired because of the lack of neuronal influences (2,14). The pathologic changes of the clubfoot are well described (33,52). It has been noted that the only difference between the classic idiopathic clubfoot and the arthrogrypotic clubfoot is the thickness of the talonavicular capsule medially (11). However, the severity of bony deformity is at the extreme end of the pathologic changes present in all clubfeet. This may be the result of the onset of deformity early in fetal development in conjunction with the continued neuromuscular deficit. It is the severity of the deformity and the remodeling potential of each patient that determines whether soft-tissue release or bony realignment is appropriate. In my opinion, the arthrogrypotic deformity occurring early in gestation and present in a severe form at birth is similar in many ways to a neglected ITEV foot presenting at age four. Scarpa pointed out, the "descriptions of bones of the tarsus in

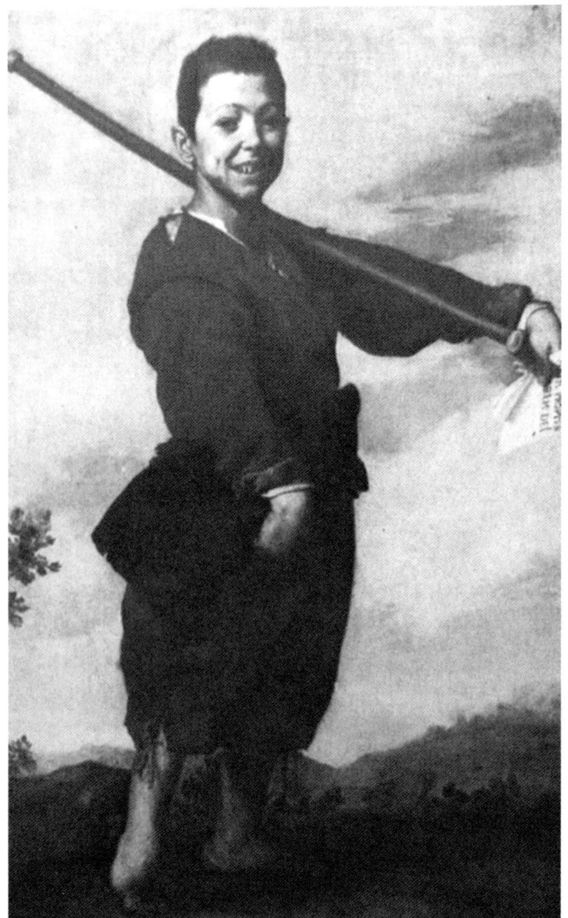

FIGURE 16-1 La Pied Bot (The Club Foot) by Jose de Ribera, 1642.

congenital club foot will always differ from one to another according to the degree of the deformity and ages from which the description is taken" (17) (Wishart 1818). Different degrees of deformity demand distinct types of management, with the longer standing and severe deformity requiring more aggressive treatment to achieve a satisfactory result.

Stage 1 No soft-tissue contractures. Easy reduction without manipulation.

Stage 2 Soft-tissue contracture without bony remodeling. Manipulation is required to achieve reduction. (Typical ITEV at birth.)

Stage 3 Soft-tissue contracture with bony remodeling. Time is required after reduction to allow for remodeling to correct the deformity back toward more normal alignment. (The more severe ITEV or a mild arthrogrypotic foot.)

Stage 4 Soft-tissue contracture and bony deformity. Articular surfaces that, even if reduced, do not have enough remaining growth to permit adequate remodeling to achieve an acceptable physiologic position. Bony correction is required as close to the deformity as possible. (ITEV untreated over age four or the typical arthrogrypotic clubfoot at birth.)

Stage 5 Soft-tissue contracture and bony deformity present long enough to result in irreversible degenerative joint changes. Salvage joint arthroplasty or fusion required. (The failure to achieve a physiologically acceptable foot by foot maturity.)

ETIOLOGY

The etiology of arthrogryposis is varied and not completely understood, but the consensus indicates the inability of the developing fetus to have intrauterine movement (14). Research models supporting the theory of reduced fetal movement, genetic components (40), and mechanical factors are well described (20,28,30). Recognition of the dominance of either a neurogenic or a primary muscular etiology remains helpful clinically, especially in reminding one that the balancing of motor forces acting on a joint may need to be addressed (5).

NATURAL HISTORY

A wide variety of deformity patterns and severity exist. A history of exposure to teratologic agents or the presence of oligohydramnios may be noted. The distal arthrogryposis form has mild muscular involvement and may respond to serial casting and not require surgery. In classic arthrogryposis the joints are characterized by symmetric rigid deformity with fibrous replacement of muscle. Vigorous physical therapy may restore motion to stiff joints and is usually more successful proximally than distally. Foot deformity in arthrogryposis is present in 70% to 80% of cases and is the most common deformity (Figure 16-2). Talipes equinovarus is the most common foot problem but vertical talus, cavus, metatarsus adductus, and equinus may also occur (11,15,19,25,56). The various

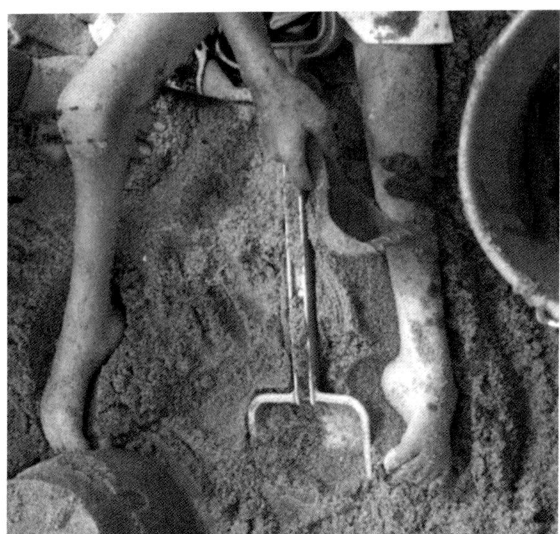

FIGURE 16-2 Bilateral clubfeet in a five-year-old patient with arthrogryposis.

TABLE 16-1

1. Disorders with mainly limb involvement (amyoplasia, distal forms of arthrogryposis).
2. Disorders with limb involvement and involvement of some other body parts.
3. Disorders with limb involvement and central nervous system dysfunction.

conditions are not progressive but persistent deformity is common from under-correction or recurrence due to scarring from surgery.

CLASSIFICATION

Classification systems by Hall and Goldberg have attempted to place some order in the differential diagnosis of the multiple disorders with arthrogrypotic characteristics (20,27,28) (Tables 16-1 and 16-2). There are over 150 distinct entities with characteristics of arthrogryposis, thus the continued confusion with terminology is understandable. Amyoplasia (26) or arthrogryposis multiplex congenita (57) are both terms frequently used to describe the most common form of the disease. What has been accepted as "typical arthrogryposis" or "amyoplasia" is the patient normal or high intelligence who is small in stature, has symmetric nonprogressive large joint deformities, and has no other associated major system abnormalities (11) (Figures 16-3 and 16-4).

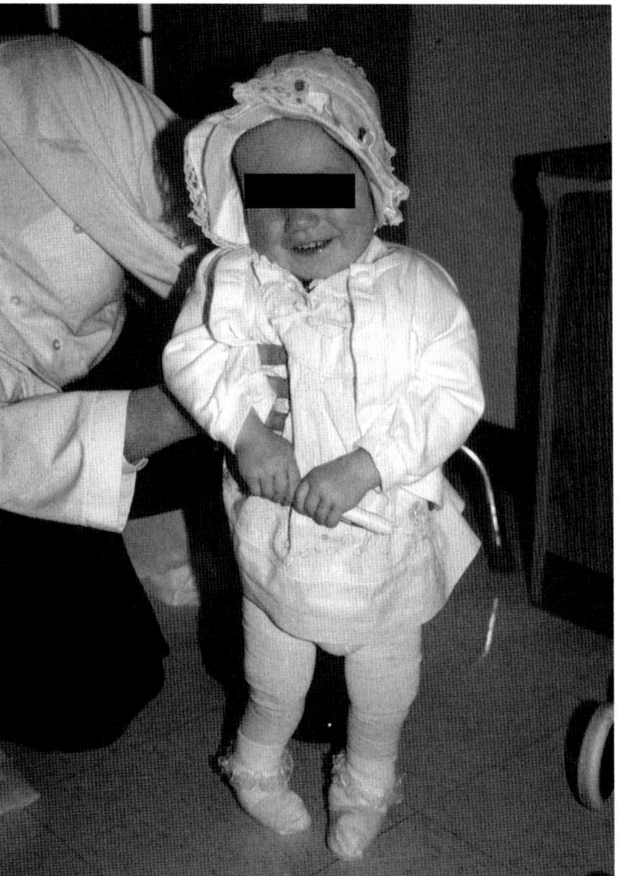

FIGURE 16-3 Two year old with arthrogryposis and bilateral club feet and dislocated hips.

PHYSICAL EXAM

The clinical presentation of arthrogryposis is obvious at birth. The classic findings of multiple large joint dislocations, limited joint motion, atrophy of the muscles affecting those joints, shiny skin, and webbing of the affected joints usually leaves little doubt of the diagnosis (5,6,7).

Examination of the patient starts with the upper extremity, important because of its potential effect on the patient's ability to use ambulatory aids both post-operatively and perhaps permanently. Adducted internally rotated shoulders, stiff elbows, and restricted motion in the wrist and fingers are variably present.

Spinal involvement has been described (Figure 16-5) and with pelvic obliquity there may be issues affecting apparent leg length and the management of the lower extremity deformities (10,60). Hip dislocation does not prohibit ambulation but limb length discrepancy, rotational deformity, and restricted hip range of motion can affect ultimate ambulatory potential, thereby influencing decisions regarding correction of foot deformity (Figure 16-6).

Both the position and motor control of the knee are critical factors in determining the ambulatory potential allowing the foot to obtain a plantigrade position. Rotational and flexion deformities may need correction as part of the overall management plan (5,11,19,21,40) (Figure 16-7). In my experience, attaining some hyperextension of the knee can allow ambulation even if there is no quadriceps function by allowing the stiff foot in slight equinus, to stabilize the extremity in the "back knee" position, a

TABLE 16-2

An Orthopedic Surgeon's Clinical Classification of Arthrogryposis

1. Generalized arthrogryposis (all four limbs are involved).
2. The more common syndromes.
   a. Classic arthrogryposis multiplex congenita.
   b. Larsen syndrome.
3. Syndromes that are rare, lethal, or both.
   a. Potter syndrome (oligohydramnios syndrome).
4. Arthrogryposis involving the ends (hands, feet, and face).
5. Distal arthrogryposis syndrome
6. Freeman-Sheldon, or "whistling face" syndrome
7. Pterygia syndromes (it's the web)
8. Generalized webs
   a. Multiple pterygium syndrome
9. Synostosis syndromes (the joints and bone)

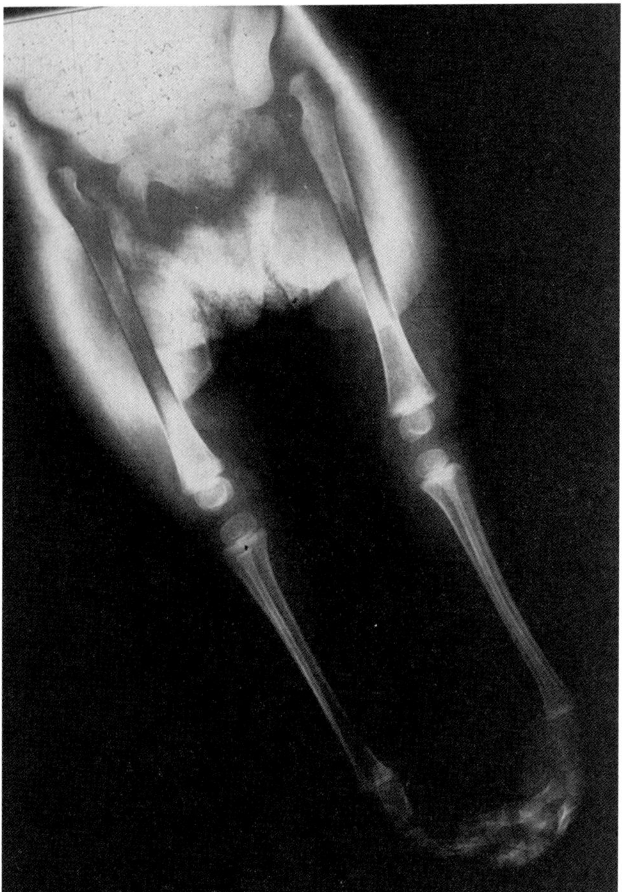

FIGURE 16-4 Same patient as in Figure 16-3. The dislocated hips were not operated, but the clubfeet were surgically corrected.

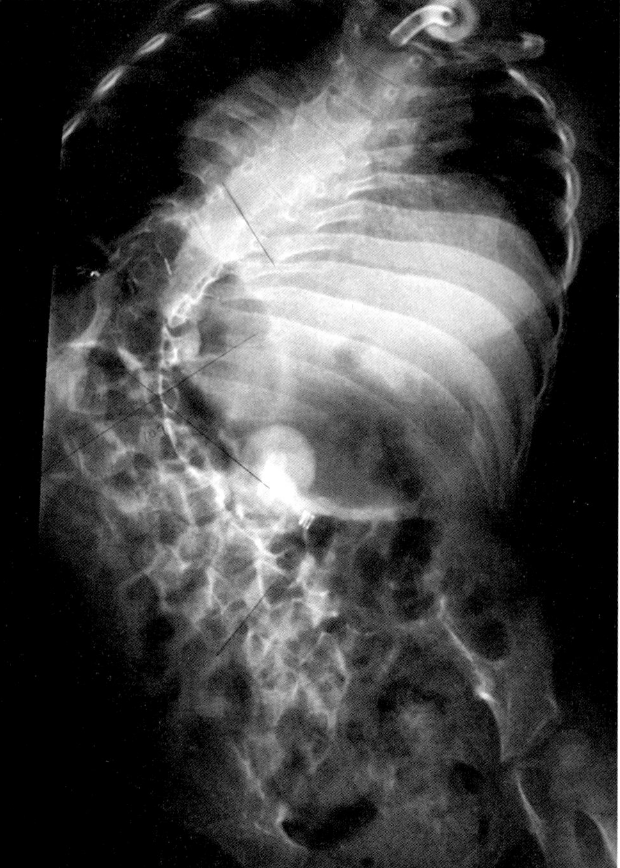

FIGURE 16-5 Paralytic C-shaped neuromuscular type curve in a seven-year-old patient with arthrogryposis. Treated subsequently with an instrumented posterior spinal fusion.

lesson well learned in management of the polio patient with no quadriceps function.

Neurologic examination should include sensory, motor, and deep tendon reflexes. Grading motor strength is particularly important in evaluating the balance of the foot. Detailed examination of the foot itself is critical. Evaluation of hindfoot, midfoot, and forefoot alignment and range of motion must be used both in pre-surgical planning and in evaluation of results after treatment. The exam should also document calf size, ankle range of motion, assessment of the skin, joint stiffness at each level, and finally, assessment of the motor patterns of gait in the ambulatory child.

DIAGNOSTICS

The diagnosis is primarily based on clinical examination. Magnetic resonance imaging (MRI) of the head, neck, or if upper extremities are spared, thoraco-lumbar portions of the spine may be helpful in distinguishing arthrogryposis from traumatic or congenital/developmental disorders of the spine. Muscle biopsy, electromyelogram (EMG), and nerve conduction studies can sometimes separate neurogenic from primary muscle disease. Once advanced changes in the muscle have occurred, differentiating the dominant component as neurogenic or muscular is impossible (2). All other laboratory tests are normal in the patient with arthrogryposis. Neurologic and genetic consults are certainly appropriate if there is any question of the diagnosis, especially if there is multisystem involvement.

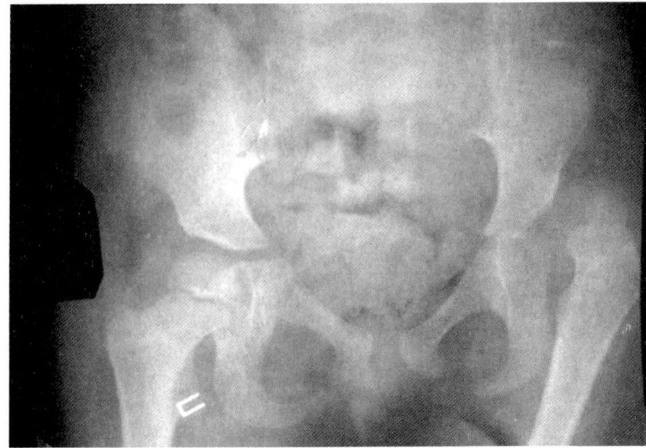

FIGURE 16-6 Unilateral dislocated hip in a seven-year-old patient with arthrogryposis. The hip was painless but contributed to a short leg/Trendelenberg-type limp. Surgical reduction and varization of the femur and an acetabuloplasty was tried but the hip re-dislocated within a year of the surgery.

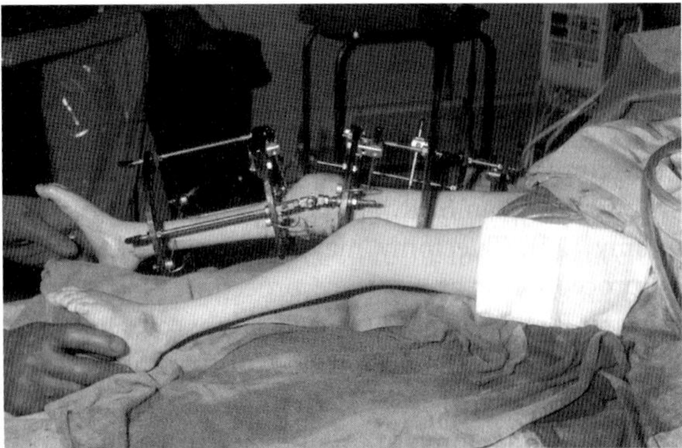

FIGURE 16-7 35-degree knee flexion contractures with webbing in the patient noted in Figure 16-2 corrected with the Ilizarov method.

IMAGING

X-rays of the foot and ankle are helpful in planning surgery and assessing results. Antero-posterior (AP) and lateral views of the foot as well as the ankle are helpful. Specific AP measurements include (Kite angle) talo-calcaneal angle (nl > 20 degrees (4); the lateral (Turco angle); talo-calcaneal angle (nl > 20 degrees) (Figure 16-8); and the combination of both measurements, known as the talo-calcaneal index (nl range of 44–69 degrees) (3). These three measurements have been the most consistently used and helpful in planning surgery and assessing results. Also referred to in various studies using the AP view of the foot are the navicular-first cuneiform angle, the talus-first metatarsal angle, the percentage of cuboid coverage of the calcanocuboid joint, and the percentage of navicular coverage of the talonavicular joint. The lateral radiograph of the foot allows measurement of the talar-first metatarsal angle (Meary's angle) as well as assessment of forefoot supination with metatarsal height measurements (31,42).

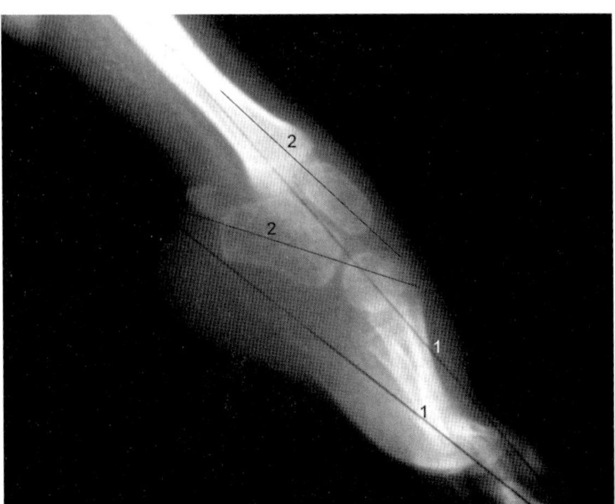

FIGURE 16-8 Lateral radiograph of the foot of the patient in Figure 16-2 patient illustrating the severe equinus of the foot to the tibia (*1*) and the parallelism of the talus and calcaneus (*2*).

DIFFERENTIAL DIAGNOSIS

The differential diagnosis should include disorders that result in diminished motion of the extremities as well as disorders associated with major joint deformity and dislocation. This includes disorders of the brain (hypotonic cerebral palsy); cervical spine (Arnold-Chiari malformations, cervical spine instabilities, or cervical trauma); thoracic or lumbar spine (spinal dysraphism, myelodysplasia, or spinal cord tumor); anterior horn cell disease (spinal muscular atrophy or polio); disease of the neuromuscular junction (myasthenia gravis); congenital or acquired primary peripheral nerve disease; or myopathies.

TREATMENT

The goal of treatment is a plantigrade foot. Even when there is no potential for ambulation, a plantigrade foot is important for stable placement on a wheelchair platform, shoe wear, or physiologic standing activities.

While the success in the typical idiopathic clubfoot treated with manipulation and casting approaches 90%, subgroups, such as the arthrogrypotic clubfoot (15,25,34,44,61); the failed and multiply operated idiopathic clubfoot (1,17,23,32,33); the neglected clubfoot (35,54); and other multifactoral or teratologic clubfeet (12,39,54) became recognized for their unique characteristics, especially recurrence and poor functional results (19,40,43). Treatment algorithms are based on the surgeries classically used for the ITEV and vary according to the degree of the deformity being treated.

Treatment protocols may be compared based on functional, anatomic, and radiographic outcomes. A large variety of criteria has been suggested. Studying groups with similar degrees of deformity is ideal but cannot always be accomplished because of the relatively small numbers of patients fitting into the appropriate categories. The most popular criteria have been those of Goldner, Catterrall, Ponseti, and more recently Demiglio and Pirani (4,8,13,16,18,21,36,38,50).

The amount of deformity of the bony structures of the hind, mid- and forefoot, and the patient's age, dictates the surgery selected. Review of the surgical literature identifies a tendency to select one operation and apply it universally. However, because of the wide variability in the soft tissues as well as the varied bony abnormalities needing to be addressed, applying the rules of the management of bony deformity in childhood is particularly important. When the soft tissues are too stiff to permit manipulation that over time will result in joint reduction, then surgical soft-tissue release is indicated. In cases where bony remodeling has occurred and there is sufficient growth potential remaining and the joint is properly reduced, deformity may be corrected by further remodeling, then soft-tissue release alone is satisfactory. When bony deformity has progressed to a degree of severity that there is insufficient growth remaining for adequate

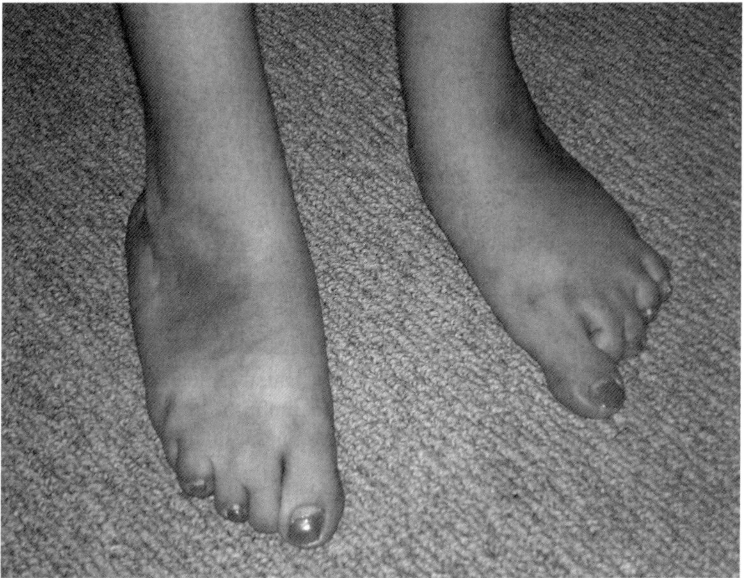

FIGURE 16-11 Nine-year postoperative picture of the patient in Figure 16-2. Lesser toe deformities are present but asymptomatic with full weight bearing.

1. The correction can be purely through soft tissues or combined with bony procedures.
2. Decompress the tarsal tunnel for corrections over 20°, especially when associated with varus correction.
3. Overcorrect with the fixator for six weeks and then hold in a cast for four weeks with bracing.
4. Correction can be with a hinge (constrained) for one plane deformity correction, or no hinge (unconstrained) for multiplane reconstructions.
5. The ankle fixator should be constructed to allow ankle distraction during the correction.
6. Fixation can be applied to the talus and calcaneus to prevent over distraction of the subtalar joint.
7. The younger the child, generally less than eight years old, the more tendency to just do soft-tissue distraction only for ITEV. However, with arthrogryposis, even in the younger child, the severity of the stiffness usually dictates combining soft tissue distraction with osteotomies and/or joint arthrodesis.
8. Overcorrect 5–10 degrees in the plane of deformity to avoid recurrence.
9. Toe contractures may occur during the correction and may be controlled with therapy and toe splints.
10. Consider percutaneous flexor tendon releases.
11. Beware that distraction of the distal tibial physis can occur. Control this with a transepiphyseal wire.
12. Correction can be in the Ponseti sequence of clubfoot correction. First correct adduction and varus before equinus. A lateral olive in the talar neck mimics the orthopedist's thumb on the talus. After normal talo-calcaneal relationship is restored, the ankle can then be dorsiflexed.

Even more than with traditional surgeries the complexity of these, multiplane deformity corrections require medical centers and surgeons versed in the use of the Ilizarov technologies.

Choi reported 12 cases of recurrent arthrogryposis clubfoot deformities to which he applied a modified Ilizarov technique. The mean age was 5.3 years old. The posterior tibial tendon was released, if present, as well as the talonavicular capsule and scar. A two-ring Ilizarov frame was placed on tibia. The fibula was not fixed. A half ring was placed on the midfoot and a half ring on the hindfoot. A lateral talar neck olive wire with a small washer allowed some acute derotation of the talus, improving the talocalcaneal angle. As the orientation of the frame changed, the talar wire was changed on the calcaneal ring, so the talus was able to move in an arc. In three cases a 2-mm Steinman pin was inserted into the tibial epiphysis to avoid epiphyseolysis. In one patient a medial pin was placed into the base of the first metatarsal also to prevent first metatarsal epiphysolysis. The ankle was over distracted 3–4 mm during the procedure. Correction was obtained in a mean of three weeks, and held in the fixator for another one and a half weeks. Pins were then placed across the talonavicular and calcanocuboid joints and immobilized for a mean of 14 weeks. The correction of the talocalcaneal angle is successful only when there is some motion at subtalar joint. He points out this soft-tissue procedure is not successful when bony fusion is present in mid or hind foot or when equivalent stiffness from multiple prior operations is present. Complications were epiphyseolysis and recurrence (9).

Huerta reported seven cases (12 feet) of neglected club foot deformities with no prior surgery. The average age was 27 years. Distraction was 1 mm per day in four .25-mm increments. Five to eight months were used for the distraction. Three patients had recurrent adductus deformity. Average ankle motion at one year was 10 degrees and all patients achieved a plantigrade foot (35) (Figures 16-12, 16-13, 16-14, 16-15, and 16-16).

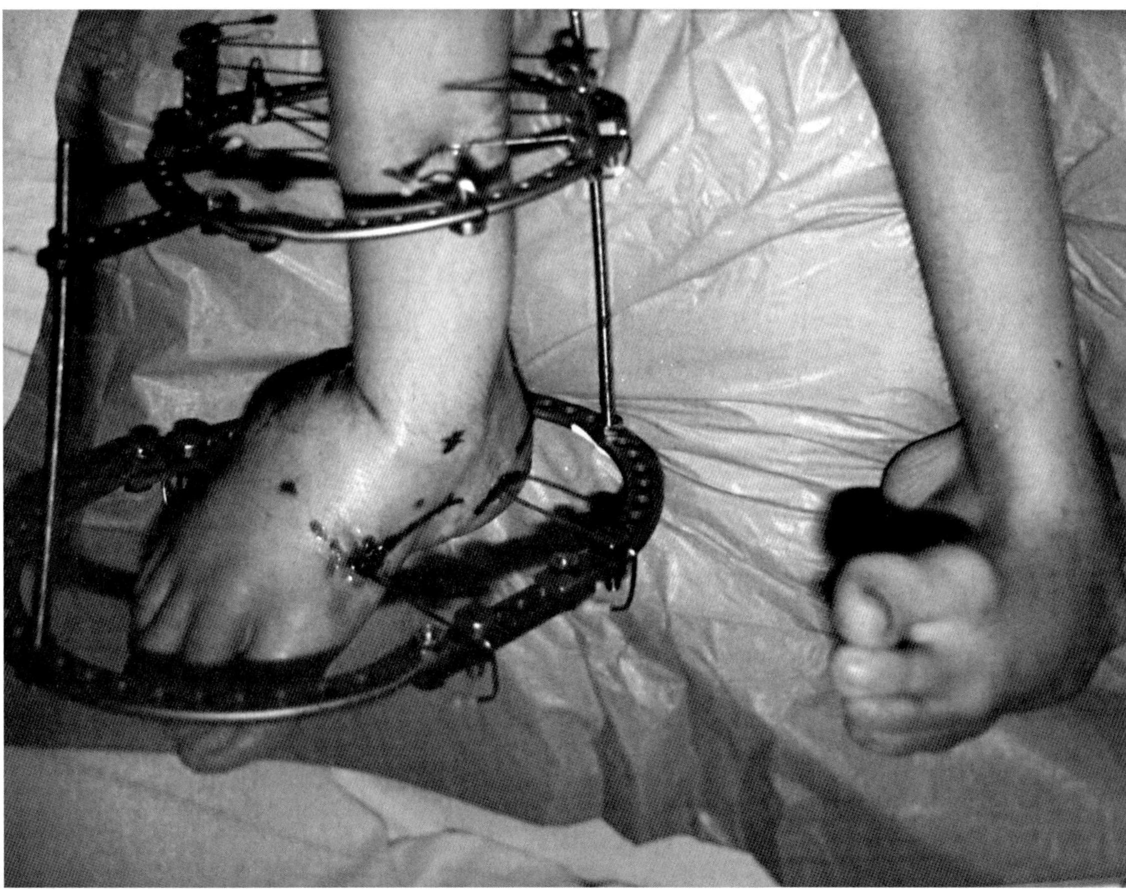

FIGURE 16-12 Typical Ilizarov construct for soft tissue correction of a four year old with recurrence of club foot deformity after cast correction. Both feet had identical deformities. More forefoot dorsiflexion is planned before completing the active correction.

Supramalleolar Osteotomy

Indications for this procedure include associated limb length problems and/or deformity of the ankle requiring correction. This may also be useful in the multiply operated foot where hind- and mid-foot bony procedure have already been performed but a plantigrade foot has not been achieved. However, it is always preferable, where adequate pedal bone remains, to do corrective osteotomies as close to the deformity as possible.

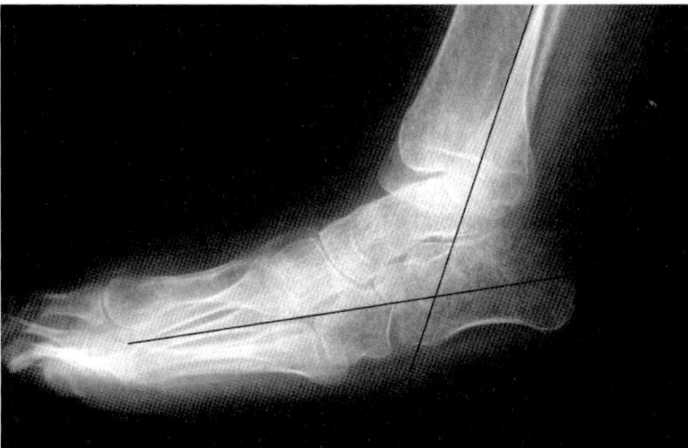

FIGURE 16-13 Eleven year old with recurrent arthrogrypotic clubfoot deformity. Lateral radiograph preoperatively demonstrating 35 degrees of equinus.

Osteotomy Through the Calcaneus and Talus (Figure 16-17A)

Indications include deformity of the talus, such as a flat top talus. The osteotomy begins posteriorally in the calcaneus, proceeds anterior beneath the subtalar joint, and finally across the sinus tarsi and through the neck of the

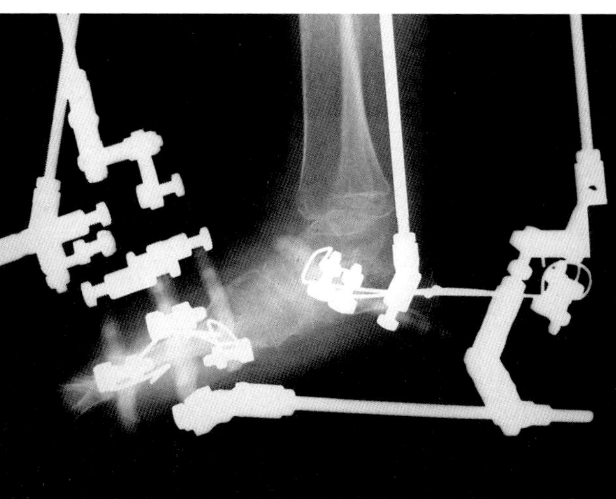

FIGURE 16-14 Soft-tissue Illzarov correction using calcaneal and metatarsal fixation linked to tibial fixation.

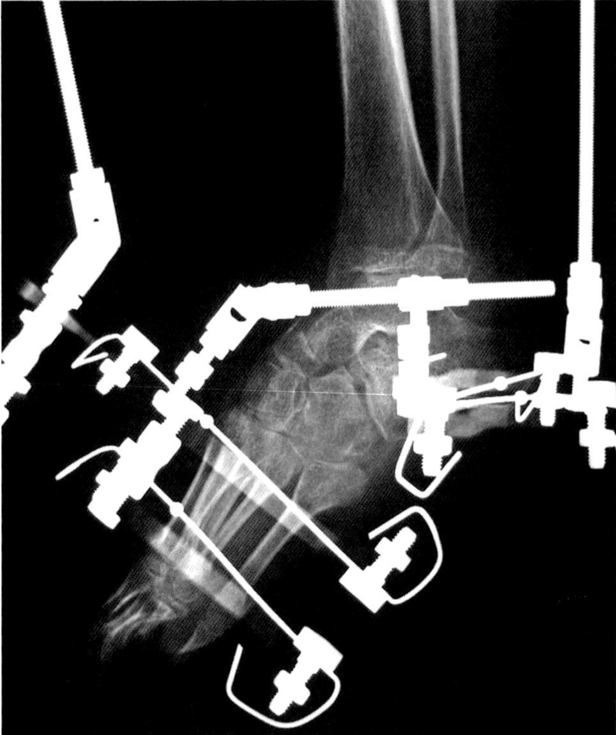

FIGURE 16-15 Ten year old with recurrent clubfoot deformity. Lateral radiograph demonstrating significant mid- and forefoot equinus and supination the day the Ilizarov was applied.

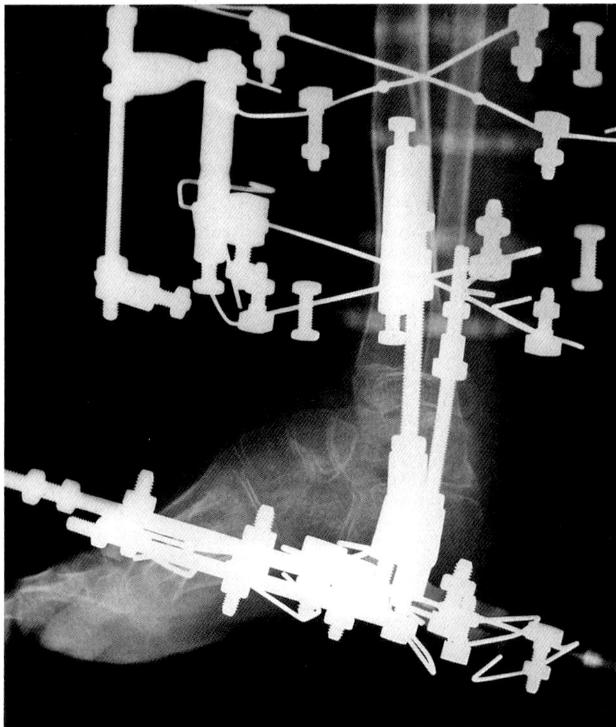

FIGURE 16-16 Lateral radiograph of the same patient demonstrating significant improvement in forefoot position. As the forefoot was corrected, the Illizarov was modified for hindfoot correction.

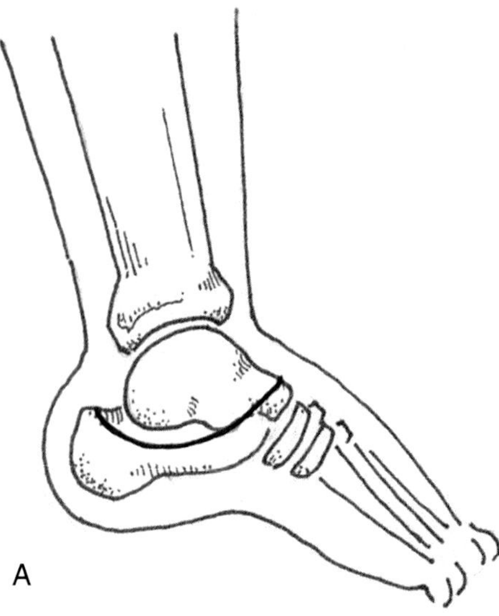

FIGURE 16-17A U osteotomy through the calcaneus and the neck of the talus. V osteotomy through the calcaneus into the midfoot.

talus. This osteotomy can correct hindfoot height, as well as equinus, calcaneus, varus, or valgus deformities of the talus. It does block subtalar motion and should not be used when there is normal subtalar motion. The U osteotomy does not correct mid-foot deformities (40,47,48).

Osteotomy Through the Calcaneus and Talus (Figure 16-17B)

Indications include deformity of the mid-foot in addition to the hindfoot. The posterior arm of the osteotomy begins posterior to the subtalar joint. The anterior arm of the osteotomy should be through the mid-foot bones when there is functional subtalar motion present. The anterior arm may be directed through the cubo-navicular row or cubo-cuneiform row, to correct mid-foot

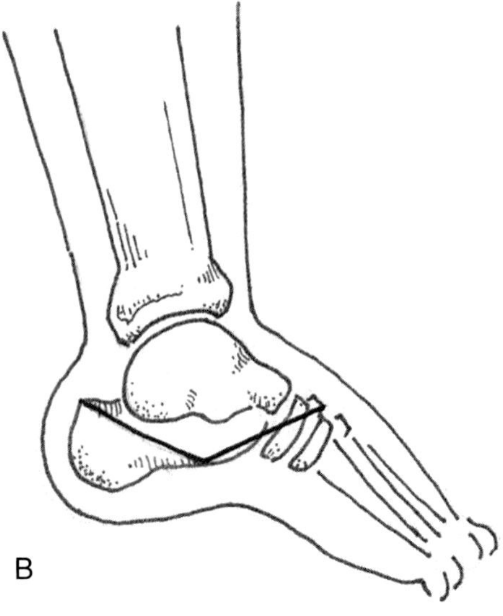

FIGURE 16-17B V osteotomy through the calcaneus into the midfoot.

deformity. The osteotomy meets on the plantar surface of the calcaneus. The triangular subtalar portion of calcaneus should be fixed to the talus during the correction. The anterior portion of the osteotomy should be performed through the mid-foot bones when there is functional subtalar motion present calcaneus should be fixed to the talus during the correction. The anterior portion of the osteotomy should be performed through the mid-foot bones when there is functional subtalar motion present (39,46,47).

Other Pedal Osteotomies (Figure 16-18)

Other osteotomies of the pedal bones can be used for acute correction alone or as a supplement to the Ilizarov frame when more severe deformity requires gradual correction. They include osteotomy of the talar neck (30); wedge or sliding osteotomy of the calcaneus; opening wedge of the first cuneiform and closing wedge cuboid (32,41,42); midfoot osteotomies (15,48); and metatarsal osteotomies (11,15,56,61). Paley cautions that the use of metatarsal osteotomies with lengthening techniques should be reserved for specific metatarsal deformity and that the mid foot should be preferentially used if adequate bone remains (48). Guidera points out that metatarsal osteotomies can be a good adjunct to correct residual forefoot adductus remaining after correction of the hindfoot with a triple arthrodesis (25).

Arthrodesis

Calcaneocuboid fusion may be used as an isolated procedure (1,17) or combined with a talectomy (51). Triple arthrodesis may be successfully used as a salvage procedure in the patient over 10 years for correction of deformity or pain due to degenerative joint disease (15,40). Ankle arthrodesis, when deformity or pain is present in the ankle joint or pantalar arthrodesis when there is also significant deformity or pain in the subtalar joint may also be considered (15).

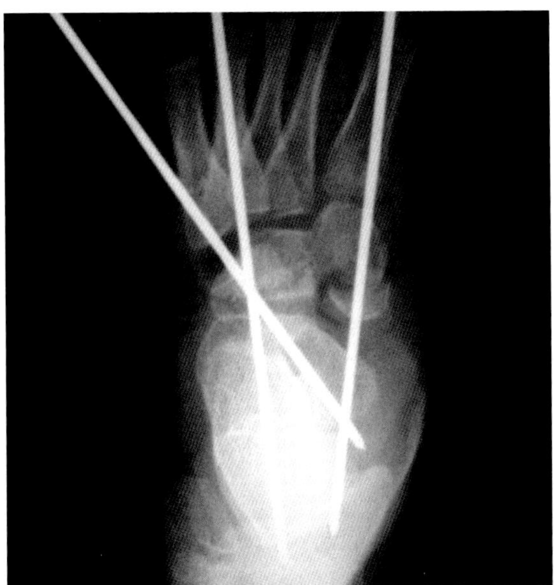

FIGURE 16-18 AP radiograph of an eight year old with arthrogryposis and recurrent mid- and forefoot deformity. The adducted, supinated forefoot has been corrected by a medial column lengthening of the first cuneiform and closing wedge osteotomy through the cuboid.

OTHER FOOT DEFORMITIES IN ARTHROGRYPOSIS

Vertical talus (congenital convex pes valgus, rocker-bottom foot). Although this is the second most common foot deformity associated with arthrogryposis, the number of patients is small and even the largest series have only a few patients (11,25,40). As with management of the arthrogrypotic clubfoot, a general philosophy of casting early and surgical releases when the size of the foot allows (between three and six months) applies. Even more rare are the isolated cases of metatarsus adductus, cavus, or equinus. Treatment of these must be individualized.

COMPLICATIONS

Higher complication rates are noted in the arthrogrypotic foot than with idiopathic clubfoot management (15,19,25,43,56,61). With multiple different surgeries advocated, complications specific to each particular surgery can be expected, plus the added problems caused by additional soft tissue deficit (25). The recurrence rate is higher, as one would expect, because of the greater severity and more advanced stage at which treatment starts in the arthrogrypotic patient. The hindfoot has received the most attention as the primary deformity, but neglected residual mid- and forefoot deformities are the most common reason for reoperation. Lesser toe deformities may develop secondary to repositioning the foot either acutely or dynamically, and can be managed with therapy or, if necessary, release of toe flexors or surgical procedures specific to each individual toe deformity (48,50). Using distraction techniques there is the possibility of epiphyseolysis of the distal tibial and proximal first metatarsal physes. To avoid these complications when distraction occurs across these areas, a transfixing pin is recommended at the time of placing the apparatus (9,39).

PEARLS/KEY POINTS

1. Staging and timing – In patients with multiple lower extremity joint involvement, start with the feet and then address the hip and knee joints. Correction that coincides with the child being able to stand will allow the forces of weight bearing to help maintain the corrected position of the foot and lessen the likelihood of recurrence. Upper extremity management can usually be delayed until the patient can cooperate with the required rehabilitation.
2. Capsule stiffness – The limited motion of the foot and ankle is unlikely to improve even with aggressive

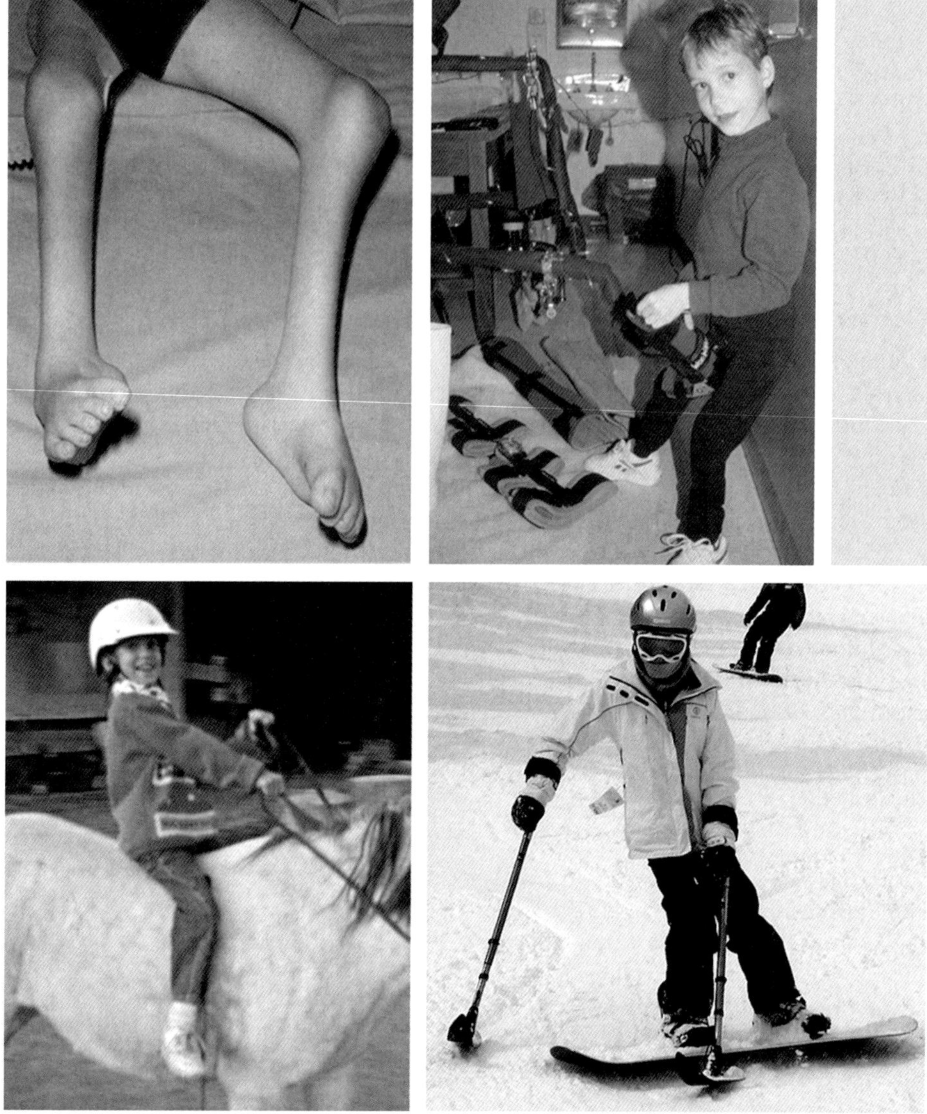

FIGURE 16-19 In spite of an early life of surgeries and bracing, G. C. Lloyd-Roberts noted, "The intelligence, adaptability and determination of these children flatters even modest surgical success."

manipulation and surgical release. However, the limited arc can be placed in a more functional position.

3. Location of surgical correction – Focus the primary surgery at the joint most responsible for the deformity, usually in the hindfoot. Mid- and forefoot deformity significant enough to prevent attaining a plantigrade foot, even with good hindfoot correction, should be addressed at the initial surgery whenever possible. Staging procedures or using the gradual correction of each deformity level separately with the Ilizarov techniques can be part of the initial surgical plan.
4. Muscle balancing – Rarely is there a grade 4 motor group with satisfactory excursion that would function in a transferred position. In all other cases tendon resection removes a potentially deforming force and, therefore, is usually preferred.
5. Avoiding recurrence – Maximum correction at all levels of deformity at the time of the first surgery and prolonged immobilization (three to six months) and orthotic support (until the completion of growth) post-operatively can be useful in controlling the reported high recurrence rates (19,24,44,61). Post-operative serial casting to correct residual deformity is unlikely to be successful. Correction must be obtained at the time of surgery, unless one of the dynamic external fixator techniques is used. Resection of the posterior tibial, toe flexors, or Achilles tendons should be considered whenever they are potentially contributing to the deformity, especially when they have no function.

SUMMARY

The number of disorders identified with the characteristic of stiff joints remains numerous, with multifactoral etiology and identifying terminology. Whether the most typical case is referred to as amyoplasia or arthrogryposis multiplex congenita, the difficulties and management challenges remain. Establishing a cohesive plan addressing the multiple joints involved and establishing reasonable and attainable goals with the child's family remains at the center of the surgeon's relationship with the family. The goal of surgery in the arthrogrypotic foot is usually to convert a deformed rigid structure to a plantigrade platform. While admitting normal gait and lower extremity function is usually not an option, G. C. Lloyd-Roberts eloquently noted, "The intelligence, adaptability and determination of these children flatters even modest surgical success" (Figure 16-19).

REFERENCES

1. Abrams RC. Relapsed club foot. *The Journal of Bone and Joint Surgery* 1969;51–A:270–282.
2. Adams C, Becker LE, Murphy EG. Neurogenic arthrogryposis multiplex congenital: Clinical and muscle biopsy findings. *Pediatr Neurosci* 1988;14:97–102.
3. Aronson J, Puskarich CL. Deformity and disability from treated clubfoot. *Journal of Pediatric Orthopaedics* 1990;10:109–119.
4. Beatson TR, Pearson JR. A method of assessing correction in club feet. *The Journal of Bone and Joint Surger.* 1966;48–B:40–50.
5. Benjamin A, Michael G. Syndromes of orthopaedic importance. In: Morrissy R, Weinstein S, ed.: *Pediatric orthopaedics*, 6th ed. Philadelphia: Lippincott Williams & Wilkins, 293–303, 2006.
6. Bernstein, R. Arthrogryposis and amyoplasia. *J Am Acad Orthop Surg* 2002;Vol 10, No 6, November/December:417–424.
7. Bevan W, Hall JG, Bamshad M, et al. Arthrogryposis multiplex congenita (amyoplasis): An orthopaedic perspective. *J Pediatr Orthop* 2007 July–Aug;27(5):594–599.
8. Catterall A. A method of assessment of the clubfoot deformity. *Clinical Orthopaedics and Related Research* 1991;March (264): 48–53.
9. Choi IH, Yang MS, Chung CY, et al. The treatment of recurrent arthrogrypotic club foot in children by the Ilizarov method. *The Journal of Bone and Joint Surgery* 2001;83–B:731–737.
10. Daher YH, Lonstein JE, Winter RB, et al. Spinal deformities in patients with arthrogryposis. *Spine* 1985;10(7):609–613.
11. Davidson RS, Drummond, DS: Arthrogryposis foot. In: Drennan JC. *The child's foot and ankle. New York:* Raven Press Ltd., 1992:253–266.
12. Dias LS, Stern LS. Talectomy in the treatment of resistant talipes equinovarus deformity in myelomeningocele and arthrogryposis. *Journal of Pediatric Orthopedics* 1987;7:39–41.
13. Dimeglio A, Bensahel H, Souchet P, et al. Classification of clubfoot. *J Pediatr Orthop* 1995;4:129–136.
14. Drachman DB, Coulombre AJ. Experimental clubfoot and arthrogryposis multiplex congenita. *Lancet* 1962;2:523.
15. Drummond DS, Cruess RL. The management of the foot and ankle in arthrogryposis multiplex congenita. *The Journal of Bone and Joint Surgery* 1978;60–B:96–99.
16. Dyer PJ, Davis N. The role of the Pirani scoring system in the management of clubfoot by the Ponseti method. *The Journal of Bone and Joint Surgery* 2006;88–B:1082–1084.
17. Evans D, Cardiff, Wales. Relapsed club foot. *The Journal of Bone and Joint Surgery* 1961;43–B:722–733.
18. Flynn JM, Donohoe M, Mackenzie WG. An independent assessment of two clubfoot-classification systems. *J Pediatr Orthop* 1998;18(3):323–327.
19. Friedlander HL, Westin WG, Wood WL. Arthrogryposis multiplex congenita (A review of forty-five cases). *The Journal of Bone and Joint Surgery* 1968;50–A:89–112.
20. Goldberg MJ. Arthrogryposis multiplex congenita and arthrogryposis syndromes. *The dysmorphic child an orthopedic perspective.* New York: Raven Press, 1987:1–50.
21. Goldner LJ, Durham. Clubfoot: Changing concepts of pathology, diagnosis, and treatment. *Journal of the Southern Orthopaedic Association* 1992;1:26–50.
22. Green ADL, Fixsen JA, Lloyd-Roberts GC. Talectomy for arthrogryposis multiplex congenita. *The Journal of Bone and Joint Surgery (Br)* 1984;66:697–699.
23. Grill F, Franke J. The Ilizarov distractor for the correction of relapsed or neglected clubfoot. *The Journal of Bone and Joint Surgery* 1987;69–B:593–597.
24. Gross, RH. The Role of the Verebelyi-Ogston procedure in the management of the arthrogrypotic foot. *Clinical Orthopaedics and Related Research* 1985;194:99–103.
25. Guidera KJ, Drennan JC. Foot and ankle deformities in arthrogryposis multiplex congenita. *Clinical Orthopaedics and Related Research* 1985;194:93–98.
26. Hall JG, Reed SD, Driscoll EP: Part 1. Amyoplasia: A common, sporadic condition with congenital contractures. *Am J Med Genet* 1983;15:571–590.
27. Hall JG, Reed SD, Green G. The distal arthrogryposes: Delineation of new entities. Review and nosologic discussion. *Am J Med Genet* 1982;11:185–239
28. Hall JG. Arthrogryposis multiplex congenita: Etiology, genetics, classification, diagnostic approach, and general aspects. *J Pediatr Orthop B* 1997;6(3):159–166.
29. Herzenberg JE, Paley D. Ilizarov applications in foot and ankle surgery. *Adv Orthop Surg* 1992;16(3):162–174.
30. Hillman JW, Johnson JT. Arthrogryposis multiplex congenita in twins. *The Journal of Bone and Joint Surgery* 1952;34:211–214.
31. Hjelmstedt A, Sahlstedt B. Talo-calcaneal osteotomy and soft tissue procedures in the treatment of clubfeet: Indications, principles and technique. *Orthop Scand* 1980;51:335–347.
32. Hofman AA, Constine RM, McBride,GG, Coleman SS. Osteotomy of the first cuneiform as treatment of residual adduction of the fore part of the foot in club foot. *The Journal of Bone and Joint Surgery* 1984;66–A:985–990.
33. Howard CB, Benson. Clubfoot: Its pathological anatomy. *Journal of Pediatric Orthopaedics* 1993;13:654–659.
34. Hsu LES, Jaffray D, Leong JC. Talectomy for club foot in arthrogryposis. *The Journal of Bone and Joint Surgery (Br)* 1984;66:694–696.
35. Huerta FD. Correction of the neglected clubfoot by the Ilizarov method. *Clinical Orthopaedics and Related Research* 1994;301: 89–93.
36. Ippolito E, Farsetti P, Caterini R, et al. Long-term comparative results in patients with congenital clubfoot treated with two different protocols. *The Journal of Bone and Joint Surgery* 2003; 85–A:1286–1294.
37. Kopits S. Orthopaedic management. In: Freeman J, *ed. Practical management of meningomyelocele.* Baltimore: University Park Press, 1974:139–145.
38. Laaveg SJ, Ponseti IV. Long-term result of treatment of congenital club foot. *The Journal of Bone and Joint Surgery Am* 1980;62:23–31.
39. Lamm BM, Standard SC, Galley IJ, et al. Externalfixation for the foot and ankle in children. *Clinics in Podiatric Medicine and Surgery* 2006;23:137–166.
40. Lloyd-Roberts GC, Lettin LWF. Arthrogryposis multiplex congenita. *The Journal of Bone and Joint Surgery* 1970;52B:494–508.
41. Lourenco AF, Dias LS, Zoellick DM, et al. Treatment of residual adduction deformity in clubfoot: The double osteotomy. *Journal of Pediatric Orthopaedics* 2001;21:713–718.
42. McHale KA, Lenhart MK. Treatment of residual clubfoot deformity – the "bean-shaped" Foot – by opening wedge medial cuneiform osteotomy and closing wedge cuboid osteotomy. Clinical review and cadaver correlations. *Journal of Pediatric Orthopaedics* 1991;11:374–381.

43. Mead NG, Lithgow WC, Sweeney HJ. Arthrogryposis multiplex congenita. *The Journal of Bone and Joint Surgery* 1958;40–A: 1285–1309.
44. Niki H, Staheli L, Mosca V. Management of clubfoot deformity in amyoplasia. *J Pediatr Orthop* 1997;17:803–807.
45. Otto AG. *Monstrorum sec centorum description anatomica in uratislavae museum, Anatomico-Pathologicum Uratislaviense*, 1841.
46. Paley D, Herzenberg JE. Applications of external fixation to foot and ankle reconstruction. In: Myerson MS, ed. *Foot and ankle disorders, vol. 2.* Philadelphia: WB Saunders; 2000: 1135–1138.
47. Paley D. Principals of foot deformity correction: Ilizarov technique. In: Gould JS, editor. Operative foot surgery. Philadelphia: WB Saunders; 1994. p. 476–514.
48. Paley D. The correction of complex foot deformities using Ilizarov's distraction osteotomies. *Clin Orthop* 1993;293:97–111.
49. Palmer PM, MacEwen DG, Bowen RJ. Passive motion therapy for infants with arthrogryposis. *Clinical Orthopaedics* April, 1985;184:54–59.
50. Pirani S, Outerbridge H, Moran M, et al. A method of evaluating the virgin clubfoot with substantial inter-observer reliability. *POSNA* 1995; Miami, FL.
51. Pirpiris M, Ching DE, Kuhns CA. Calcaneocuboid fusion in children undergoing talectomy. *J Pediatr Orthop* 2005;25:777–780.
52. Ponseti IV. *Congenital clubfoot. Fundamentals of treatment.* Oxford, Oxford University Press, 1996.
53. Prem H, Zenios M, Farrell R, et al. Soft tissue Ilizarov correction of congenital talipes equinovarus—5 to 10 years postsurgery. *J Pediatr Orthop* 2007;27:220–224.
54. Reinker KA, Carpenter CT. Ilizarov applications in the pediatric foot. *Journal of Pediatric Orthopaedics* 1997;17:796–802.
55. Segal LS, Mann DC, Feiwell E. Equinovarus deformity in arthrogryposis and myelomeningocele. *Foot and Ankle* 1989;10: 12–16.
56. Södergård J, Ryöppy S. Foot deformities in arthrogryposis multiplex congenita. *Journal of Pediatric Orthopaedics* 1994;14:768–772.
57. Stern WG. Arthrogyryposis multiple congenita. *JAMA* 1923;81:1507.
58. vanBosse JPH, Marangoz S, Lehman WB, Sala DA. Correction of arthrogrypotic clubfoot with a modified Ponseti technique. POSNA presentation May 2008, Albuquerque, NM.
59. Wilkins, Kaye. Horizontal osteotomy of the talus. *Personal communication.* Unpublished data.
60. Yingsakmongkol W, Kumar SJ. Scoliosis in arthrogryposis multiplex congenita: Results after nonsurgical and surgical treatment. *J Pediatr Orthop* 2000 Sep–Oct;20(5):656–61.
61. Zimbler S, Craig CL. The arthrogrypotic foot plan of management and results of treatment. *Foot and Ankle* 1983;3:211–218.

CHAPTER 17

Ankle Injuries

Richard Miller

INTRODUCTION

Ankle injuries in children encompass a wide spectrum of clinical problems. This chapter will discuss both pediatric patients, defined as those who are skeletally immature and adolescent patients who have already reached skeletal maturity.

Ankle injuries in children range from sports related and overuse injuries to severe open trauma with tissue loss (e.g., lawnmower accidents). The former group generally heal with little or no long-term sequelae, while the latter group may have lifelong difficulties and problems that change over time due to growth disturbances, muscle imbalance, and changes in body habitus and activity patterns (Figure 17-1A, 1B). In addition, congenital anomalies including tarsal coalition and accessory navicular may predispose children to ankle and hindfoot injury and pain.

This chapter will review common injuries to the ankle and hindfoot which are seen in the pediatric and adolescent population. Some of the aforementioned congenital anomalies, severe injuries, and fractures are covered in other chapters. Sports injuries are also discussed in chapter 25.

EPIDEMIOLOGY AND PREVENTION

Athletic participation among children is at an all-time high and is the cause of many foot and ankle injuries. Sports-related injuries represent 41% of all childhood musculoskeletal injuries presenting to the emergency department (5). Damore found that foot and ankle injuries accounted for 20% of all musculoskeletal injuries and were the most commonly injured area in basketball and also were frequently injured in soccer and multiple other sports.

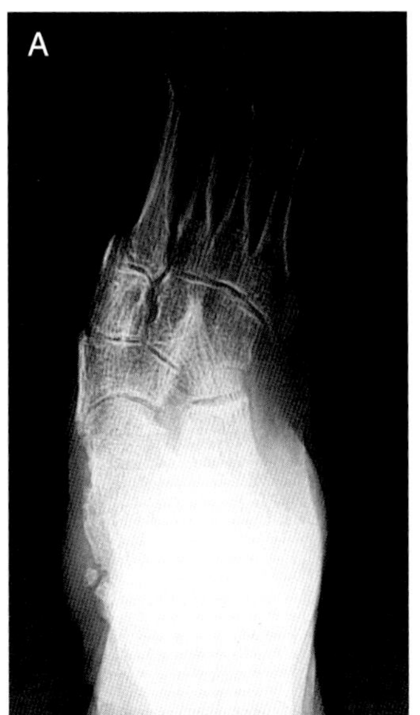

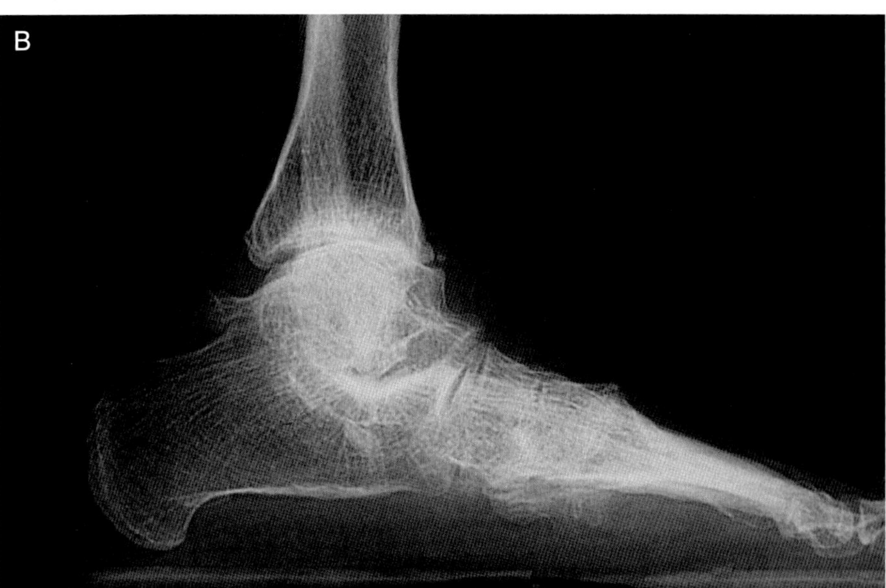

FIGURE 17-1 **A, B.** AP and lateral radiographs of a 40-year-old woman who sustained a lawnmower accident at age eight. First ray and second toe amputations were performed along with skin grafting at that time. As an adult, she has painful ankle and hindfoot arthritis.

Overuse may also be the source of foot and ankle disorders. Participation in multiple sports, on multiple teams during a season, yearlong training, improper training techniques, and inadequate shoewear or equipment may lead to pain from overuse in this age group. These issues should be addressed when treating the young athlete.

Prophylactic ankle bracing has been shown to decrease the incidence of sports-related ankle injuries (11). It is more commonly utilized when there has been a previous ankle injury. Appropriate warm up and training may also decrease injury rates. Breakaway baseball and softball bases have also been shown to decrease the number of injuries from sliding in these sports (15).

DIAGNOSIS OF ANKLE INJURIES

History, physical exam, and appropriate imaging are the key components to the diagnosis of ankle injuries. In general, the location of the pain and tenderness narrows the differential diagnosis. The anatomic structures present in the area of pain (i.e., bone, joint, tendon, ligament, nerve) may be the damaged tissue. Some causes of ankle pain may present with symptoms in more than one location. For instance, tarsal coalition may present with medial and/or lateral pain. Osteochondral lesions of the talus usually present with ankle pain on the side of the lesion.

Skeletally mature patients tend to have similar injury patterns as adults. Certain injuries seen in skeletally mature patients have only very rarely been reported in pediatric patients. These include Achilles tendon rupture, subtalar dislocation, and lateral process of talus fractures, commonly referred to as snowboarder's fracture (7,10,19).

There may not be a specific history of injury for some causes of ankle pain. For instance, patients with symptomatic tarsal coalition may present with a complaint of an ankle sprain or recurrent sprains without a history of a twisting injury. Pain from Haglund's deformity or an accessory navicular might be associated with new shoewear or increased activity. In these conditions, the pain may be due to the rubbing of the bony prominence or secondary to surrounding inflammation and not from a specific injury.

IMAGING

Radiographs of the ankle are routinely required after an ankle injury. Radiographs of the foot may be necessary to visualize fractures distal to the ankle which can mimic ankle sprains. These would include fifth metatarsal base fractures, cuboid fractures, anterior process of calcaneus fractures (Figure 17-2), and tarsometatarsal or Lisfranc joint injuries. Calcaneonavicular tarsal coalition is best seen on the standard forty-five degree internal oblique view of the foot, whereas an accessory navicular or navicular tuberosity fracture is best visualized on an external rotation oblique view of the foot.

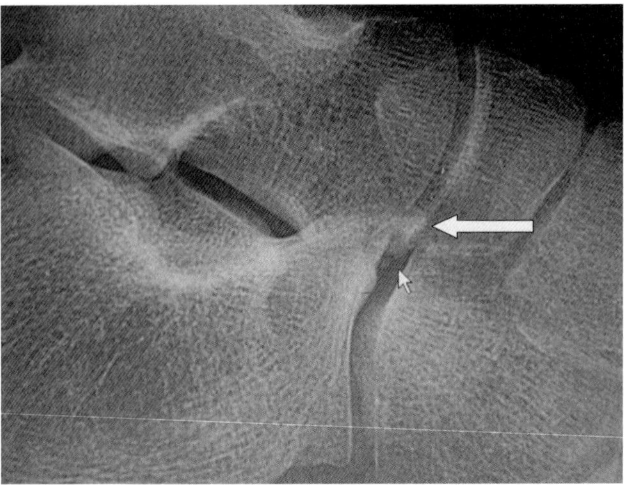

FIGURE 17-2 An anterior process of calcaneus fracture in a 14-year-old boy (*arrow*). He was originally felt to have an ankle sprain. The correct diagnosis was made six months after his injury. Excision of the fracture nonunion resulted in relief of his symptoms.

Computerized tomography (CT) and magnetic resonance imaging (MRI) scans may at times be necessary to better evaluate and diagnose ankle injuries.

ANKLE SPRAINS

Ankle sprains are ligamentous injuries most commonly due to ankle inversion affecting the lateral ankle ligaments. Syndesmosis and deltoid ligament injury can occur as well and are usually the result of eversion, dorsiflexion, or external rotation injury.

The anterior talofibular and calcaneofibular ligaments are most commonly injured. Lateral pain, swelling, and ecchymosis occur to varying degrees depending on the severity of the injury. Physical exam reveals tenderness over the ligaments, whereas a distal fibular fracture or growth plate injury would have well-localized pain over the fibula itself. Instability of the ankle is difficult to assess in the acutely injured period due to guarding by the patient. Inversion stress and anterior drawer tests help assess the laxity present once acute pain has subsided. Dislocating peroneal tendons can also present with lateral ankle pain and examination for this should be included.

Radiographs should be taken to assess for possible malleolar and physeal fractures and to rule out other fractures included in the differential diagnosis of lateral ankle pain.

Occasionally, an os fibulare may be present (Figure 17-3). Excision of this structure should be considered if lateral pain persists or if ankle ligament reconstruction is to be performed because of recurrent sprains and instability. Osteochondral lesions of the talar body can also result from an inversion ankle injury and should be treated as outlined in the section on this disorder.

Ankle sprains are common in skeletally mature adolescent patients; however, it is assumed, and often stated, that lateral ligament injury is less common than distal fibular epiphyseal injury in the skeletally immature patient.

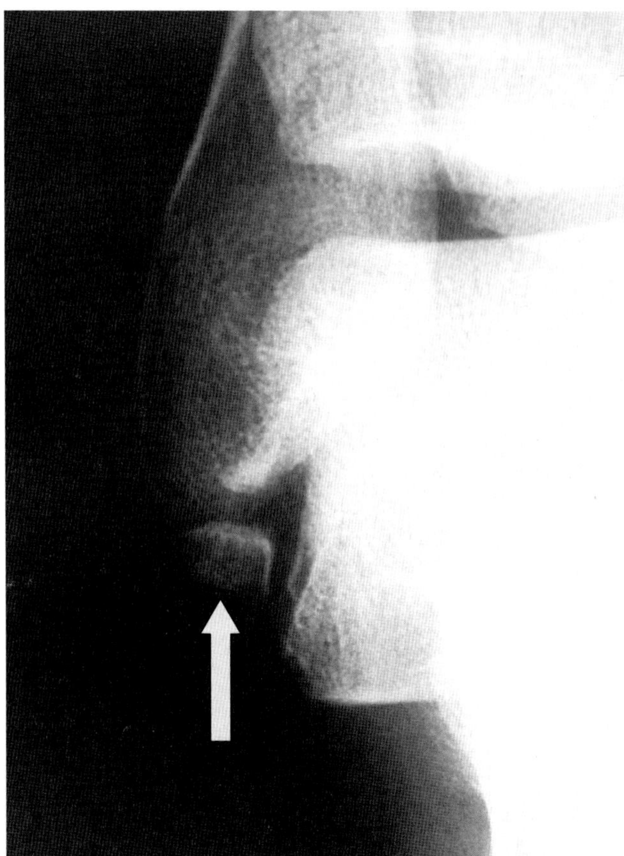

FIGURE 17-3 Ankle radiograph in a patient with lateral ligament laxity and on os fibulare (*arrow*). Excision of the ossicle and a modified Brostrom reconstruction was performed.

Nevertheless, ankle sprains do occur in the pediatric patient population. The true incidence of sprains may be underreported, because patients are more apt to seek medical care after fractures than after less severe sprains. Marsh also proposed that if the severity of the inversion stress is less than that required to damage the physis, ligament and capsular injury can occur. Repetitive submaximal trauma leads to instability and recurrent sprains in this age group (21).

Acute ankle sprains are treated conservatively, and the majority of patients obtain a good result. Rest, ice, and soft tissue protection with a functional brace or cast is performed. A removeable cast boot allows for early weight bearing and range of motion in children with more severe sprains. Once acute symptoms subside, physical therapy emphasizing proprioception and eversion strength is helpful. Prophylactic bracing before the initiation of a sports activity may be desired to protect a child's ankle from recurrent sprains.

Vahvanen reported on primary surgical treatment for children with lateral ankle ligament sprains (32,33). He found that there was a high rate of avulsion of the ligaments associated with an attached cartilaginous or bony fragment. Although they achieved excellent results with primary surgery, this approach has not gained wide acceptance, and nonoperative treatment remains the treatment of choice for most ankle sprains.

Surgical treatment for lateral ankle sprains is indicated for recurrent instability and persistent laxity. A number of techniques have been described. Anatomic repairs for pediatric and adolescent patients include the modififed Brostrom procedure in which the anterolateral capsuloligamentous structures are tightened and then reinforced with the extensor retinaculum. Bell reported excellent long-term results with an average of 26-year follow up after this procedure (1).

Augmented procedures utilize tendon grafts, usually the peroneal tendons, to reconstruct the lateral ankle stabilizers. Marsh reported on the modified Chrisman-Snook augmented reconstruction in children with ankle instability (21). In this technique, one-half of the peroneus brevis tendon is used to reconstruct the ligaments through drill holes in the fibula and calcaneus. In skeletally immature patients, the fibular drill hole is made distal to the growth plate to avoid injury to this structure. Excellent stability and function were restored in the majority of patients. Coughlin and Schenck anatomically reconstructed the ankle ligaments in skeletally mature patients with a hamstring graft taken from the ipsilateral knee. This approach spares the peroneal tendons which are important functional stabilizers of the lateral ankle. They obtained excellent or good results in all 28 patients studied (4).

The history and physical exam of the patient with recurrent ankle sprains should also consider the possibility of generalized ligamentous laxity or a neurologic disorder. For instance, Charcot-Marie-Tooth disease may result in weak hindfoot eversion and fixed heel varus which will predispose a patient to inversion sprains. If surgical correction is to be performed in the presence of fixed hindfoot varus, a lateral closing wedge calcaneal osteotomy should be included in the surgical procedure.

SYNDESMOSIS LIGAMENT SPRAIN

Syndesmosis ligament sprains, often referred to as high ankle sprains, are less common than lateral ankle sprains (13). The mechanism of injury is eversion, dorsiflexion, or external rotation of the foot. The injury varies from ligament sprain without instability to more severe injuries with displacement characterized by radiographic widening of the medial ankle clear space and loss of the distal tibiofibular overlap.

High ankle sprains should be considered in patients with pain, swelling, and tenderness at the syndesmosis. The squeeze test may be positive. This is performed by squeezing the fibula toward the tibia at the midcalf level and noting pain in the syndesmosis region. The external rotation stress test may also be positive with syndesmosis injury. This test is performed by stabilizing the leg and externally rotating the foot with the knee in ninety degrees of flexion. The squeeze test is more sensitive than the external rotation stress test (9).

Radiographs should be obtained to look for displacement and fractures. A stress radiograph may reveal instability requiring open reduction and internal fixation if displacement occurs. The normal tibiofibular clear space is less than 6 millimeters in both the anteroposterior (AP) and mortise views. The tibiofibular overlap should be greater than 6 millimeters or 42% of the width of the fibula on the AP view and greater than 1 millimeter on the mortise view (37). Radiographic evaluation of the syndesmosis is different for children than for adults. Bozic showed that the tibiofibular overlap begins at a mean age of five years on the AP view. On the mortise view, the overlap begins at age 10 years for girls and 16 years for boys (3). Contralateral radiographs may be of benefit when trying to determine if displacement exists in skeletally immature individuals suspected of having a syndesmosis injury. MRI scanning can also reveal the ligament injury.

Syndesmosis sprains without displacement should be treated with a non–weight-bearing cast for 2 to 4 weeks depending on the severity of the symptoms. This is followed by a walking boot and ankle rehabilitation. Surgery should be considered when displacement exists. Usually syndesmosis screw fixation is performed (37).

Although most studies concerning high ankle sprains have demonstrated a prolonged recovery time when compared with lateral ankle sprains, most patients recover without residual symptoms (13). Ossification of the syndesmosis is frequently seen after these injuries but is rarely symptomatic. When symptoms develop, excision of the ossification may be beneficial (1,17).

OSTEOCHONDRAL LESIONS OF THE TALUS

Osteochondral lesions of the talar dome are often the result of a twisting injury. Although more common in skeletally mature patients, they can occur in skeletally immature patients as well.

Osteochondral lesions often present as persistent pain after an ankle sprain. Swelling, tenderness, stiffness, and catching may be present. The lesion may not be visible on initial radiographs; therefore, follow-up radiographs, MRI, or CT scanning may be required to make the diagnosis. Other entities such as tarsal coalition, fifth metatarsal base fractures, lateral process of talus fracture, anterior process of calcaneus fracture, and tendon injury are included in the differential diagnosis when a patient presents with persistent pain after an ankle sprain.

The Berndt and Harty classification of osteochondral lesions of the talus has four stages (2). In stage 1, there is compression of the articular surface. Stage 2 represents a partially attached fragment. In stage 3, there is a completely detached fragment remaining within its bed, and stage 4 is when the completely detached fragment is displaced. CT, MRI, and arthroscopic classifications have been developed to take into account the presence of subchondral cysts, bone marrow signal change, and the status of the articular surface (6,12).

An MRI scan is useful in suspected osteochondral lesions not visible on Xrays. It can also better identify other periarticular injuries such as ligament and tendon pathology. A CT scan is more helpful in determining size, location, and displacement of the osteochondral lesion (Figure 17-4).

Nonoperative treatment with a short leg cast can be attempted for lesions without displacement. The outcome

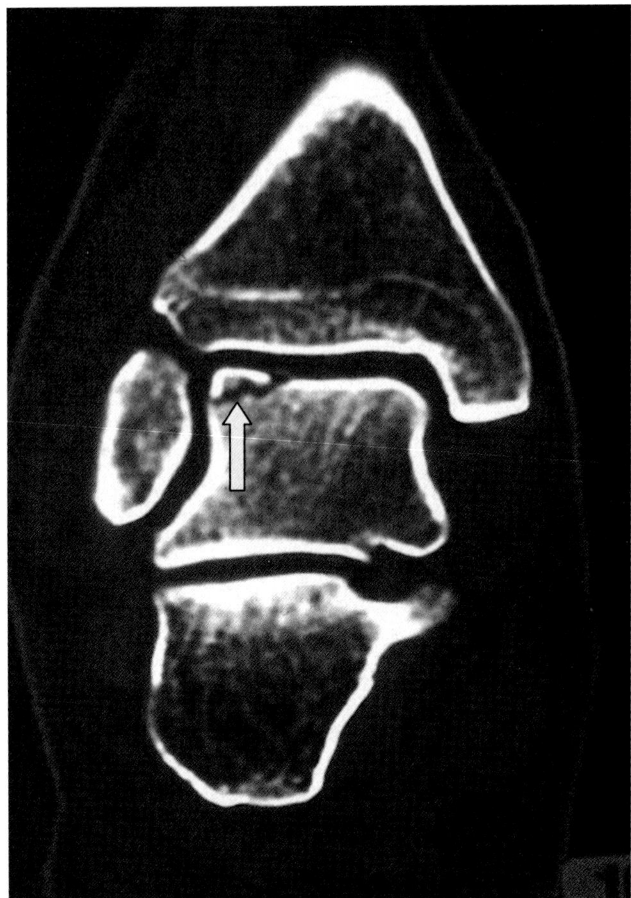

FIGURE 17-4 CT scan demonstrating a displaced osteochondral lesion of the lateral talar dome (*arrow*).

of this approach in the skeletally immature population has not been established.

Displaced osteochondral lesions and those which remain symptomatic in spite of prolonged nonoperative treatment may require operative intervention. Arthroscopy or arthrotomy permits debridement of the osteochondral lesion and drilling of the base with K-wires or an arthroscopic microfracture set (Figure 17-5). If arthroscopic examination demonstrates intact articular cartilage, retrograde drilling of the lesion is performed. Retrograde drilling through the talus avoids injury to intact articular cartilage (Figure 17-6). A success rate of 85% has been reported after debridement and drilling of osteochondral lesions (31). At the time of surgery, hypertrophic synovium and other intraarticular pathology can be debrided. Concomitant ligamentous injury resulting in laxity and instability can be addressed with a lateral ligament reconstruction described earlier in the chapter.

Large osteochondral lesions are amenable to open reduction and internal fixation. Headless screws or bioabsorbable pins are used for fixation. Preparation of the fracture bed accompanied by the occasional use of bone graft may be required.

A malleolar osteotomy may be necessary for adequate exposure of the lesion in the skeletally mature patient but should not be used in the pediatric patient. For osteochondral lesions which remain symptomatic after surgical

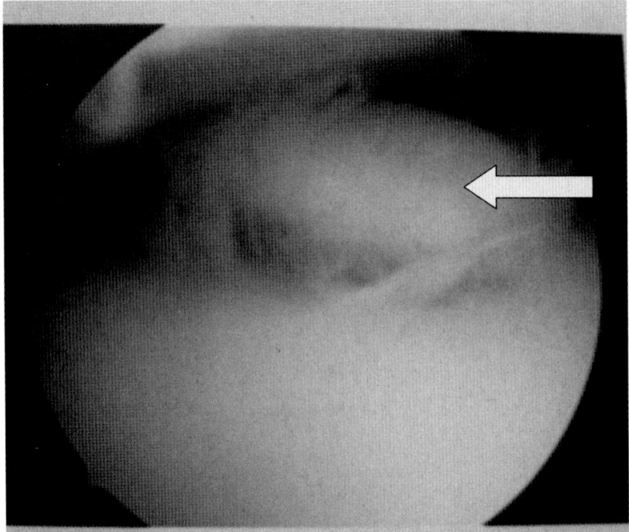

FIGURE 17-5 An arthroscopic view of a displaced osteochondral lesion of the talus (*arrow*). Excision of the fragment and microfracture of the base was performed.

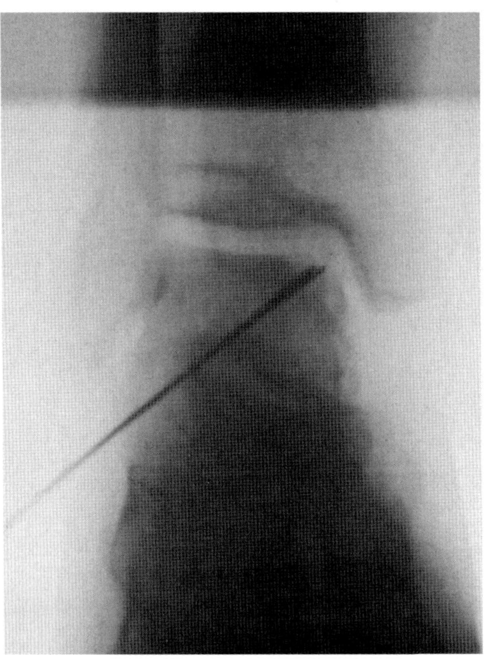

FIGURE 17-6 Retrograde drilling of a talar osteochondral lesion is demonstrated. This technique avoids puncturing the intact articular cartilage found during arthroscopy to be overlying the lesion. The tips of the pins are within the lesion.

treatment, osteoarticular autograft and chondrocyte transplantation have been utilized.

SELECT PEDIATRIC FOOT THAT MIMIC ANKLE INJURIES

Medial Ankle Injuries

This section will discuss disorders of the navicular which can present as medial ankle pain in a child. Pathologic conditions of this bone may not be visible on ankle radiographs; therefore, foot radiographs should also be obtained when navicular problems are suspected. Kohler's disease, symptomatic accessory navicular, and navicular stress fractures are three foot conditions found in children which may present with medial ankle pain. These are discussed in more detail in chapter 28.

Kohler's Disease

Kohler's disease is an osteochondrosis of the navicular that typically presents around the age of four or five years. No known injury may have occurred. Males are more commonly affected than females. Patients present with pain, swelling, and a limp. Radiographs show collapse of the navicular and areas of sclerosis. Rest, symptomatic treatment, and casting have been recommended. The navicular eventually regains its normal radiographic appearance, and residual symptoms are rare (14).

Accessory Navicular

Accessory navicular has been classified into three types (22). In type I, there is a sesamoid bone within the posterior tibial tendon adjacent to the navicular tuberosity. Type II represents a synchondrosis with a connection between the accessory navicular and the tubersosity. Type III accessory navicular is a prominent tuberosity without a separate bony fragment. An accessory navicular may become symptomatic from shoewear irritation. Medial pain over the navicular tuberosity can also be the result of injury to the synchondrosis between a type II accessory navicular and the body of the navicular. In that case, an MRI will often show bone marrow signal change. Pain, swelling, activity limitation, and a limp may be present. Nonoperative treatment for symptomatic accessory navicular consists of rest, soft insoles, and anti-inflammatory medications. A cast can be applied in patients who are not improving with the above measures or for whom rest of the foot is difficult to achieve. Excision of the accessory navicular with repair of the defect of the posterior tibial tendon can be performed if symptoms persist after nonoperative measures.

Navicular Stress Fracture

Navicular stress fracture is an overuse injury that may present with medial ankle pain in high school-aged athletes. Vague, activity-related pain about the navicular is reported. Point tenderness over the bone is common. This diagnosis must be considered in patients who present with medial ankle pain. The fracture typically occurs in the middle third of the navicular body but may not be easily identified on routine radiographs. A delay of diagnosis is common. MRI and CT scan should be considered to help make the diagnosis and assess the degree of injury. Navicular stress fractures have been classified into three types (27). In type I, there is a dorsal cortical break. Type II fractures extend into the navicular body, and type III fractures exit through the plantar cortex. A non–weight-bearing cast for six weeks can lead to healing in many cases. Open reduction and internal fixation may be required especially in type II and III injuries (27) (Figure 17-7A,B,C).

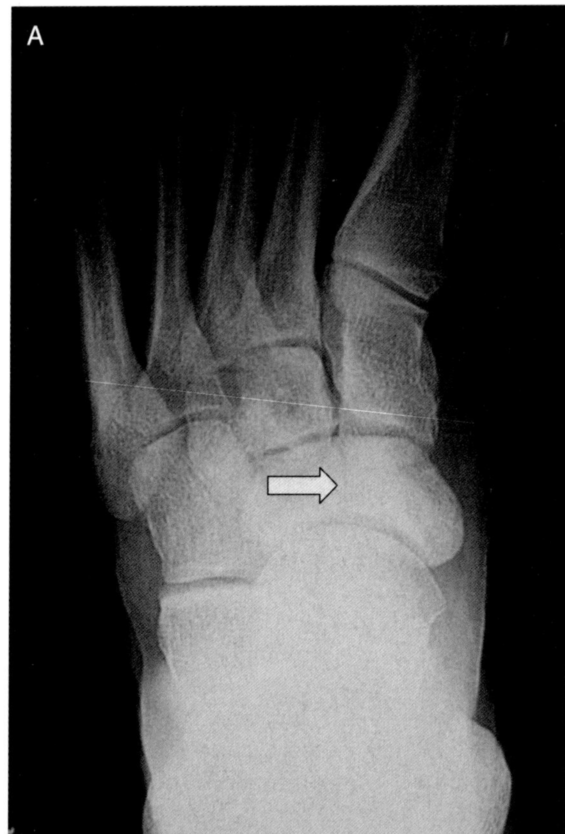

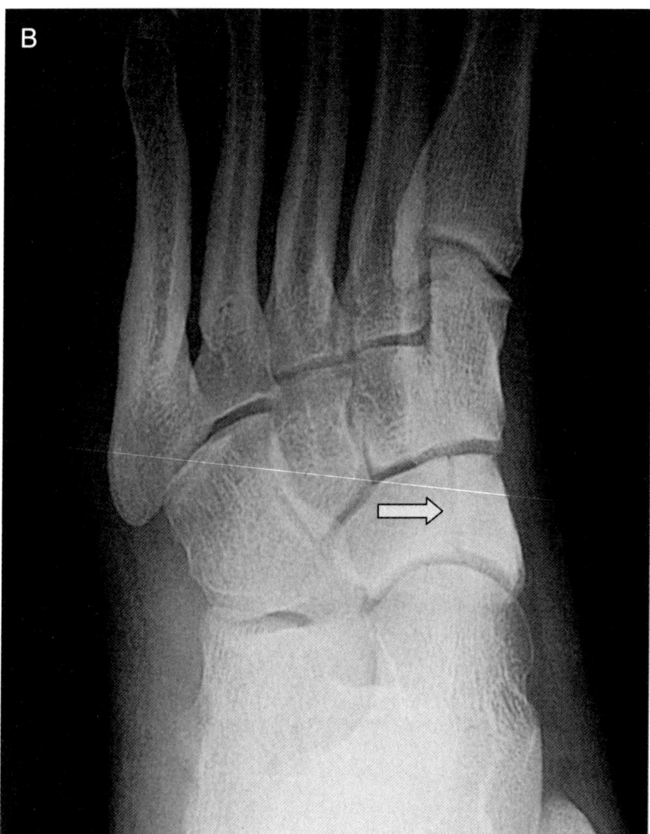

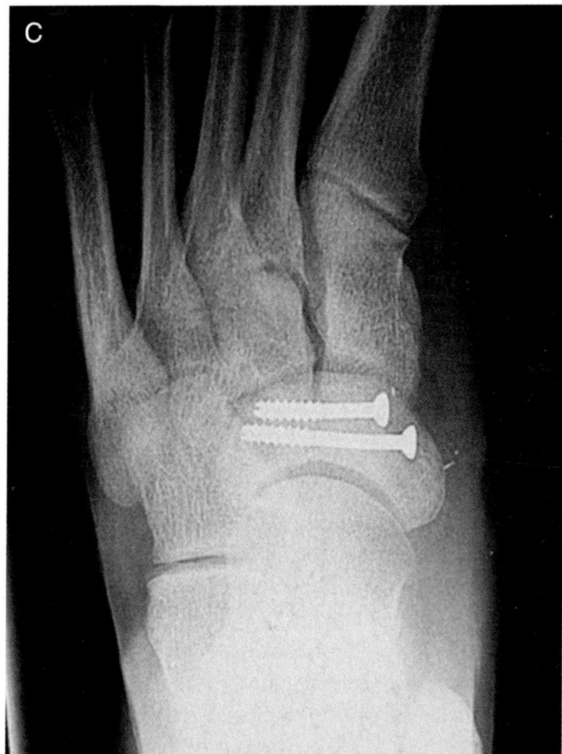

FIGURE 17-7 **A, B.** AP and oblique radiographs of a 17-year-old male who plays high school football, basketball, and baseball. He had complained of foot pain for 10 months. The arrows point to his navicular stress fracture. **C.** Screw fixation of the stress fracture resulted in healing and return to his activities.

POSTERIOR ANKLE INJURIES

A number of posterior ankle and foot disorders can result in posterior ankle pain. In this section, Haglund's deformity, Sever's apophysitis, os trigonum syndrome, tenosynovitis of the flexor hallucis longus tendon, and toddler's fracture of the calcaneus will be discussed.

Haglund's Deformity

Haglund's deformity is a bony prominence of the posterior superior portion of the calcaneal tuberosity anterior and adjacent to the Achilles tendon. Also referred to as a "pump bump," the bone prominence may be irritated by rubbing of the shoe counter leading to pain, callus formation, and blisters. Associated inflammation of the retrocalcaneal bursa may also occur (Figure 17-8A, B). This may be differentiated from Achilles tendonitis which typically presents with pain over the substance of the tendon. Nonoperative treatment includes shoewear selection to avoid rubbing of the area as well as cushioning the patient's heel with moleskin or large corn pads. Surgical treatment for Haglund's deformity includes open excision of the bony prominence and debridement of the retrocalcaneal bursa while either avoiding significant detachment of the Achilles tendon or reattaching the tendon (25). Endoscopic excision has also been described with good results (24).

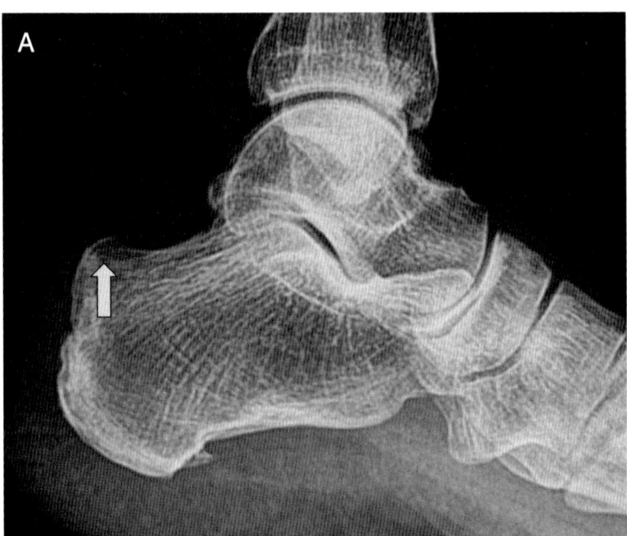

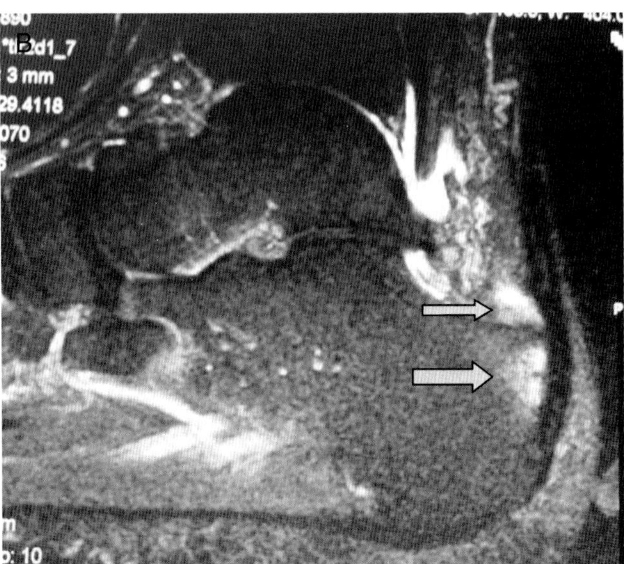

FIGURE 17-8 **A, B.** Lateral radiograph and MRI scan of a skeletally mature patient with Haglund's deformity demonstrating the superior bony prominence with associated bursitis and bone marrow edema (*arrows*).

Sever's Apophysitis

Sever's apophysitis presents with posterior or plantar heel pain. Patients are typically active children who complain of pain in the area of the apophysis with weight bearing and manual pressure. Sever's disease is an overuse injury, and the pain worsens with activity. Radiographs show the posterior calcaneal apophysis has not yet fused to the body of the calcaneus. Sclerosis and fragmentation may be present; however, these radiographic findings may also be seen in the asymptomatic individual. Ogden identified MRI signal changes in the calcaneal metaphysis and apophysis of patients with this disorder (23). They concluded that this was consistent with bone bruising or stress fracture.

The treatment for Sever's disease is always conservative. Rest, ice, activity modification, and anti-inflammatory medication can alleviate symptoms. A heel cushion or other orthotic device along with supportive shoewear can help. Consideration should be given to placing the patient in a cast or cast boot for persistent symptoms which interfere with activities.

Os Trigonum and Flexor Hallucis Longus Tenosynovitis

Additional causes of posterior ankle pain include posterior impingement from an os trigonum and tenosynovitis of the flexor hallucis longus tendon. Impingement of the os trigonum at the ankle or subtalar joint occurs in plantar flexion. The posterior ankle pain may also be due to injury of the synchondrosis between this bone and the talus or due to irritation of the adjacent flexor hallucis longus tendon (16). Nonoperative treatment options include a steroid injection as well as the measures described above for Sever's disease. Excision of the os trigonum through a medial or lateral incision can be done for resistant cases (20).

Tenosynovitis of the flexor hallucis longus tendon presents with posteromedial ankle pain. Swelling and tenderness over the tendon may be present. Nodule formation can lead to triggering of the great toe. This disorder has been described in ballet dancers. Operative release can be performed for patients who do not respond sufficiently to nonoperative measures (31).

Toddler's Calcaneus Fracture

Toddler's fracture of the calcaneus should be considered in children between the ages of one and four years who present with acute limping or refusal to walk. There may or may not be a history of trauma. Radiographs are often initially negative and the diagnosis can be made by bone scan

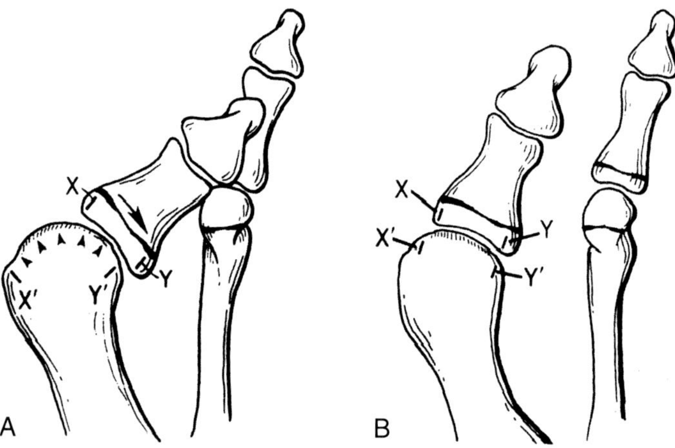

FIGURE 18-3 Subluxated (**A**) and congruous (**B**) first metatarsophalangeal joint. *X′* and *Y′*: extent of metatarsal articular surface *X* and *Y*: extent of proximal phalanx articular surface. (From Coughlin M. Juvenile hallux valgus. In Coughlin M, Mann R, eds. *Surgery of the foot and ankle, 7th ed.* St. Louis: Mosby, 1999:270, with permission.)

bowstring toward the lateral side, the sesamoids displace laterally from their normal location in the grooves on the plantar surface of the first metatarsal head.

The **first metatarsophalangeal joint** is clearly the critical articulation in the development of the deformity. This joint is considered to be a shallow ball-and-socket joint and, as such, it depends on the surrounding ligaments and capsule for its stability. As the other factors act on this joint, there is stretching and decompensation of these soft-tissue structures that allows the deformity to progress. Most authors (5,13,15) believe that ligamentous laxity plays a role in the development of hallux valgus, therefore suggesting that the native ligaments about the MTP joint are clearly not as competent as those in the normal population. The ultimate migration of the great toe may or may not leave the MTP joint congruent or incongruent. As mentioned, 45% of patients with juvenile bunions have or will develop incongruent MTP joints.

The **IP joint** tends to be normal in the juvenile bunion, unlike the adult patient who may have hallux interphalangeus and a deformity of this joint. As the hallux valgus progresses, it is not uncommon to see overlapping of the second toe (see Figure 18-1).

Often forgotten in the discussion of bunion deformity is the **MTC joint**. The obliquity of this joint has frequently been indicted as a significant factor in the development of juvenile bunions (5). As the plane of the MTC joint becomes more oblique to the transverse axis of the foot, the more unstable it becomes. The stability of the first metatarsal depends in large part on the stability of the joint at its base. If treatment ultimately is to be successful, this joint must be carefully assessed and appropriately aligned closer to the transverse axis of the foot. Additionally, a small articular facet may exist between the base of the first metatarsal and the base of the second metatarsal. Its presence generally signifies increased movement at the base of the first metatarsal. This fact should be considered in the planning of surgical treatment.

The role of the **soft tissues** of the foot in the development of hallus valgus deformity cannot be underestimated. Not only are the lax ligamentous supporting structures of the first MTP joint significant in the development of juvenile bunions, but also the overall ligamentous and fascial supporting structures of the entire foot are often viewed as contributing factors. These include the marginally competent plantar fascia as well as the ligaments of the midfoot and hindfoot. The significance of pronation remains somewhat of an open question. Many of these children have pronation, usually the result of congenital hypermobile flatfeet. The unanswered question remains to what degree pronation plays a role in the development of the bunion.

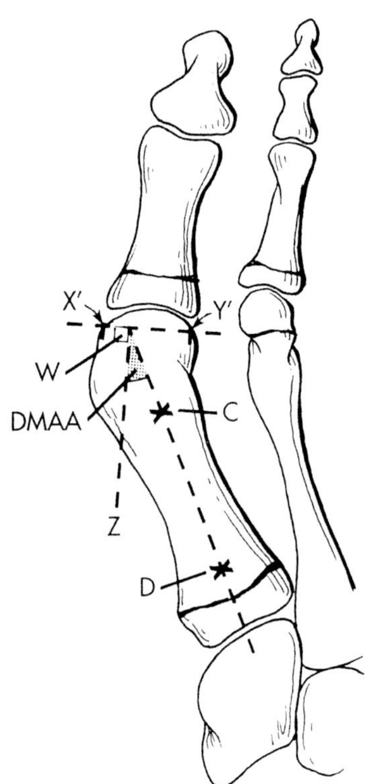

FIGURE 18-4 The distal metatarsal articular angle (DMAA) quantifies the angular relationship between the articular surface and the shaft of the metatarsal. The DMMA is the angle between the metatarsal shaft (*C-D*) and the line (*W-Z*) that is perpendicular to the articular surface (*X′-Y′*). (From Coughlin M. Juvenile hallux valgus. In Coughlin M, Mann R, eds. *Surgery of the foot and ankle, 7th ed.* St. Louis: Mosby, 1999:270, with permission.)

The tendinous structures surrounding the MTP joint, as mentioned earlier, also contribute to the deformity. Adduction contracture, abductor migration, plantar plate incompetence, sesamoid subluxation, hallux valgus, pronation of the hallux and second toe override occur as a continuum of deformity. Pronation of the hallux refers to the fact that the nail of hallux comes to face medially. The tendon imbalance resulting in this phenomenon is complex and not well described. Probably one of the most important factors is the progressive incompetence of the plantar plate permitting the MTP joint to rotate excessively. Correction of the pronation is usually accomplished at the time of medial imbrication of the capsule at the time of the distal soft tissue reconstruction.

CLINICAL EVALUATION

Physical Examination

It is extremely important when performing the **physical examination** of these children and adolescents to observe the foot both weight bearing and non-weight bearing. Assessing the child's gait will give the examiner a clue about the amount of pain that the bunion may be causing. Walking with an antalgic limp (shortened stance time on the affected limb) suggests that the patient is symptomatic and having discomfort. Observing the child standing allows evaluation of the degree of pronation of the foot (see Figure 18-1). Observed from the back, varying degrees of hindfoot valgus can be evaluated. It is also important to examine the entire child to evaluate for generalized conditions, such as ligamentous laxity or subtle neurological conditions. Observing the patient toe-standing will allow an appreciation of overall foot mobility. Specifically, if the foot is flat on weight bearing and the arch appears as the patient goes up on their toes, this suggests that the patient has a hypermobile flatfoot, which is the most common form of flatfoot. Any pronation of the great toe will also be accentuated with weight bearing.

Joint mobility is best assessed with the patient seated on the examining table. The MTC joint as well as the MTP joint can be evaluated by attempting to translate these joints both vertically and horizontally. Palpation of each joint will also permit assessment and localization of pain that the patient may be experiencing. An inflamed bursa may be present over the medial aspect of the first metatarsal head, resulting from pressure and chronic friction over this area. The remainder of the foot should be examined carefully. Range of motion of the joints of the hindfoot and mid-foot, contractures of any muscle groups, especially the triceps surae, and overall limb alignment should be assessed. Contractures of extrinsic muscles of the foot can force alterations in foot position and may be related to the progression of the deformity.

Radiology

Once the patient has been examined physically, **radiographic studies** are then performed. As it is important to clinically examine the foot weight bearing and non-weight bearing, it is also important to assess the foot radiographically (21) in both modes. The weight-bearing films are the more important, because they will amplify the deformity. In addition, the standard radiographic measurements are typically made using the weight-bearing films. Several specific angles are traditionally measured during the evaluation of the patient and during the process of surgical planning. The degree of pronation can be evaluated radiographically by noting the position of the calcaneus on the AP view and the calcaneal pitch angle on the lateral.

The three important angles to measure are:

Hallux valgus angle, which assesses the relationship between the long axis of the proximal phalanx and that of the first metatarsal. Normally, this angle should be less than 15 degrees.

Intermetatarsal angle, which measures the angle between the long axes of the first and second metatarsal. Normally, this angle should be 9 degrees or less. High angles indicate the degree of metatarsus primus varus (MPV).

Distal metatarsal articular angle (DMAA), which evaluates the relationship between the articular surface of the first metatarsal head and the long axis of the shaft of the bone. The larger this angle tends to be, the greater is the lateral orientation of the articular surface, hence contributing to a greater degree of hallux valgus.

The examiner should carefully compare the length of the first metatarsal in relation to the second (25) as well as the very important, although frequently overlooked, orientation of the first metatarsocuneiform articulation (Figure 18-5). The greater the obliquity of this joint relative to the long axis of the foot and/or first ray, the greater will be the instability of that joint with a greater tendency for the deformity to occur or recur following surgery.

TREATMENT

The psychological implications of the deformity should be considered during the initial assessment of these adolescents. Cosmesis is frequently downplayed or negated, but nonetheless is a critical factor in determining treatment. Many of these young people will complain bitterly of pain and/or difficulty with shoe wear merely in an effort to encourage the treating physician to move more rapidly to surgical correction. If one can determine that cosmesis is the sole motivation, it is probably best to postpone any surgery and encourage **non-surgical care** (10). Even though improving shoe wear is a well-recognized approach to delaying the development of deformity, it is almost impossible to encourage an adolescent to wear the "appropriate" shoe. In addition, the use of over-the-counter or custom-made orthotics to balance the arch has

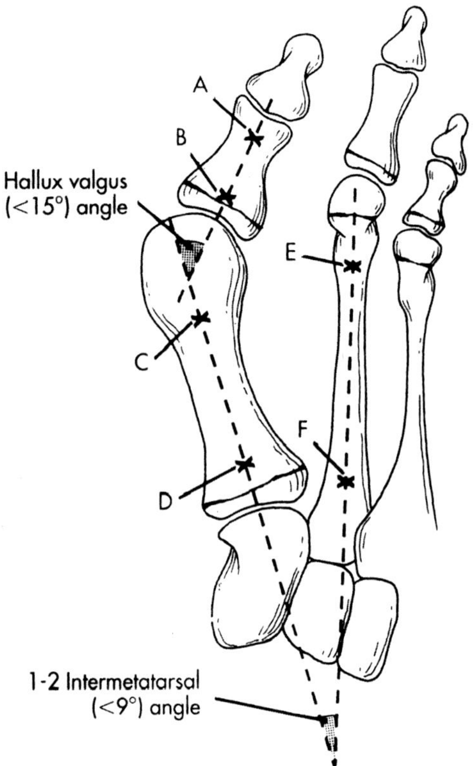

FIGURE 18-5 Hallux valgus and first, second intermetatarsal angle. *A-B*: axis of proximal phalanx; *C-D*: axis of first metatarsal; *D-F*; axis of second metatarsal. (From Coughlin M. Juvenile hallux valgus. In Coughlin M, Mann R, eds. *Surgery of the foot and ankle, 7th ed.* St. Louis: Mosby, 1999:270, with permission.)

been encouraged by some authors (4,10). Here again, the problem of noncompliance tends to override the recommendation to use such devices in most instances.

Sleeping with toe wedges between the first and second toe with the thought that they may delay progression, also is usually met with mixed feelings. Commercially available shoe stretchers that can be applied to the shoe in an effort to widen the toe box may help to relieve pressure over the first metatarsal head and, hence, decrease pain in this area. However, flip-flops or thong-type sandals are today's norm, making these devices an inappropriate recommendation.

Most authors tend to encourage the treating physician to both broach the issue of cosmesis and to suggest delaying surgical correction until such time as the foot has achieved a more adult configuration both skeletally and functionally. This age group is notorious for compliance failures for both non-surgical and surgical care.

SURGERY

Once the decision to proceed with surgical treatment has been made, the next challenge is to decide what type of procedure to employ. There are over 130 different types of surgical procedures described for the correction of bunion deformity (15). This makes the selection of the optimal procedure truly a daunting task (11). Several tenets must be followed. First and foremost, success with surgical intervention rests primarily on the **restoration of normal anatomy**. Specifically, this includes correction of the intermetatarsal angle, normalization of the distal metatarsal articular angle, and appropriate management of any abnormality of the metatarsocuneiform joint. Secondly, it is clear that no one procedure can accomplish all of these tasks and that **individualized selection** is the key. Some individuals may require only a soft-tissue procedure, some may require osteotomies, others may require a joint arthrodesis, and many will require a combination of two or more (29).

Soft-Tissue Procedures

For many years, **soft-tissue procedures** alone were relied on to deal with the unsightly bunion. Currently, the classic **McBride procedure** and its variations are most often used in combination with a concomitant bony procedure (20). Release of the adductor tendon in an effort to reduce the hallux valgus as well as capsulotomy on the lateral side of the MTP are relatively standard to most soft-tissue corrections. Medial capsular imbrication or advancement similarly are common techniques aimed at decreasing the hallux valgus and also correcting any pronation of the great toe. Although excision of the lateral sesamoid had been considered a standard part of the McBride procedure for many years, it can be complicated by incidental laceration of the flexor brevis and subsequent cock-up deformity of the toe. Most authors tend to discourage sesamoid excision, especially in adolescents, if not in all patients.

Osteotomies

The problem of inadequate correction by soft-tissue techniques has been more fully appreciated as poor long-term results have been reported (20,24). As a result, the need to perform **bony procedures** to gain full correction has been realized. Because most of the correction is needed through the first ray, it is logical that realignment procedures of that segment have gained in popularity. This realignment is typically accomplished by using an osteotomy of one or more of the bones of the first ray. The "keystone" of the deformity usually is considered to be the first metatarsal and its adjacent joints. Current discussion now centers on the level of the first metatarsal osteotomy, rather than on the need to perform it.

Distal metatarsal osteotomies such as the Mitchell procedure (3,7,22) and the Chevron osteotomy (32) have both been used extensively in the correction of modest hallux valgus deformity, typically defined as intermetatarsal angles less the 15 degrees. Many authors (5,9) report good and excellent results with distal osteotomies of the first metatarsal for these more modest deformities. When the intermetatarsal angle is greater than 15 degrees, these procedures alone are generally inadequate to achieve complete correction. Canale points out that the cause of fair and poor results was generally inadequate correction at

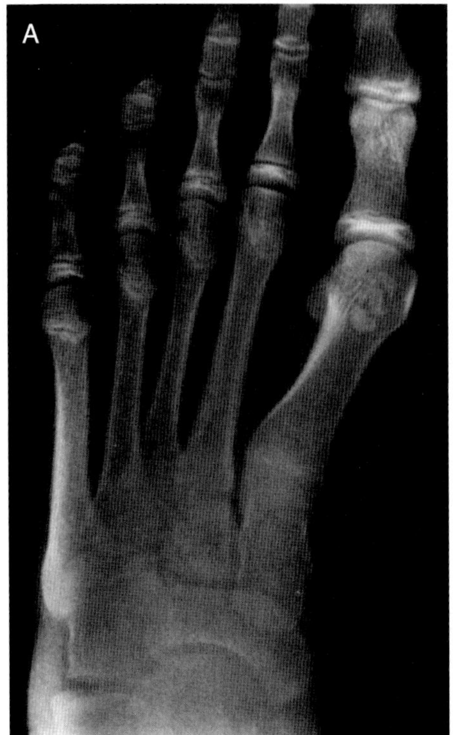

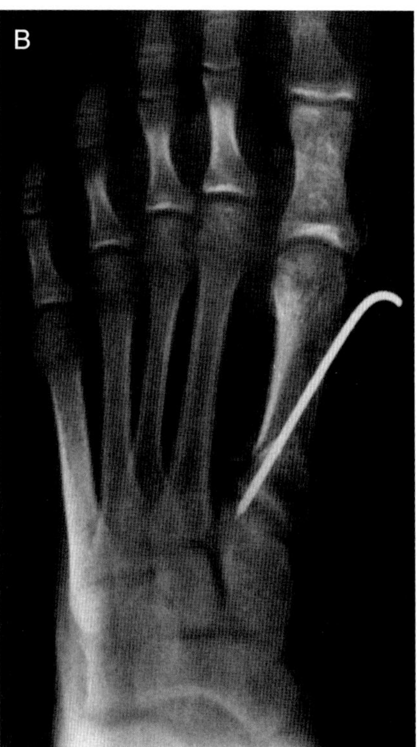

FIGURE 18-6 Anteroposterior view of the right foot of a 13-year, 2-month-old girl who had painful bunions secondary to metatarsus primus varus (**A**). Twenty months later, proximal metatarsal osteotomy and bunionectomy were performed because of the inability to provide relief by modification of the shoe wear that was acceptable to the patient. Six weeks after surgery (**B**), the correction of the metatarsus primus varus and removal of the bunion are seen. (From: Morrissy R, Weinstein S. *Atlas of pediatric orthopaedic surgery, 3rd ed.* Philadelphia: Lippincott Williams & Wilkins: 2001, with permission.)

the time of surgery (3). Because distal osteotomies are generally limited in their ability to correct large intermetatarsal angles, the proximal osteotomies have been recognized as providing that versatility. Proximal osteotomies "at the site of the deformity" are being employed more frequently.

Proximal metatarsal osteotomies (5,20) (Figure 18-6) usually are performed just distal to the physis of the first metatarsal. The configuration of the osteotomy depends on the specific procedure chosen. A medial opening wedge at the base can be done, with some authors using the excised exostosis as a graft to hold the wedge open. Also available are a closing lateral wedge and the crescentic osteotomy popularized by Roger Mann (20). All result in some degree of lateral deviation of the first metatarsal and coincident decrease in the intermetatarsal angle. With the realization that more severe bunions require more aggressive surgery, the need to correct the MPV and reduce the intermetatarsal angle is evident.

Double Osteotomies

Lastly, the **double osteotomy** popularized by Peterson (1,25) offers the unique opportunity to correct the deformity at multiple levels (Figure 18-7). It not only allows correction of the intermetatarsal angle through a proximal osteotomy, but it also permits normalization of the DMAA through the distal one. Several reports on this procedure acclaim its overall excellent results and unique versatility in the adolescent age group. The goal remains the same whatever procedure is chosen: Restore orthogonal alignment of the first ray.

With that goal in mind, surgical planning must consider all of the bones of the ray. Deformities of the proximal phalanx are generally uncommon in the adolescent age group; for that reason it is unlikely that an osteotomy of the **proximal phalanx,** such as that described by Akin (33), would be required. However, when the deformity does exist, then it is appropriate to add this procedure to osteotomies of the metatarsal in an effort to gain complete correction.

The abnormal obliquity of the **first MTC articulation** is one of the unique characteristics of juvenile bunion deformity. Successful surgery depends on correcting this deformity and stabilizing this joint. Mosca (23) has recommended that virtually all juvenile bunions should include an opening wedge osteotomy of the medial cuneiform, when the obliquity of the joint is excessive. Failure to do so leaves the MTC joint unstable, resulting in higher recurrence rates after surgery. Arthrodesis of the

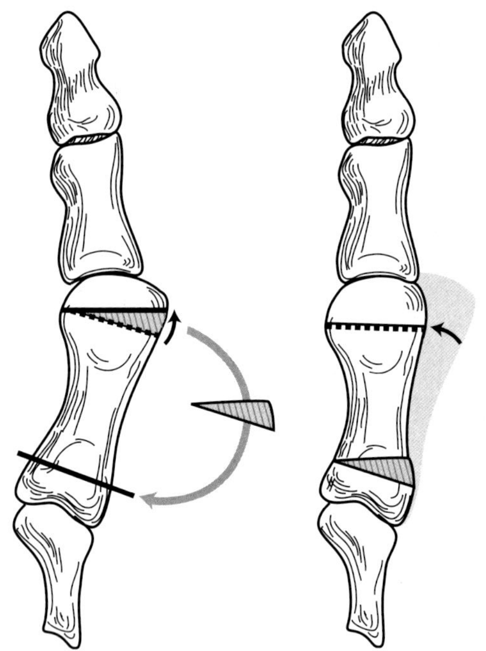

FIGURE 18-7 Peterson double metatarsal osteotomy. Location of osteotomies. (Adapted from Peterson H. Adolescent bunion. *JPO* 1993;13(1):81.)

MTC joint, popularized by Lapidus is an alternative approach. This may be the preferred approach when there is an accompanying unstable facet between the bases of the first and second metatarsals.

Arthrodesis of the first MTP joint is an option in the skeletally mature patient, when there are degenerative changes (hallux rigidus) or rheumatoid changes of the joint. However fusion in the skeletally immature group is rarely applicable. One clear exception to this dictum is spastic hallux valgus. Children with cerebral palsy and other neuromuscular diseases characterized by muscle imbalance are subject to the deforming forces about the first MTP joint (27). Severe hallux valgus commonly follows. The more traditional procedures mentioned above are not applicable to this subset of patients, since the recurrence rates are extremely high.

The open physis at the base of the first metatarsal has been the source of concern for some surgeons. Potential damage to this structure has been the rationale stated for avoiding certain procedures proximate to the growth plate. These include proximal osteotomies of the first metatarsal, osteotomy of the medial cuneiform, and fusion of the MTC joint. Currently, there is very little literature to support this concern.

There are numerous procedures that the treating physician may select for a specific type of bunion. For a modest deformity that is primarily distal, a soft-tissue balancing procedure alone or in combination with a distal osteotomy may be all that is required. On the other hand, extensive deformities which are present at multiple levels may require combinations of a distal soft-tissue balance, a proximal or double osteotomy of the metatarsal, and a procedure to realign the MTC joint, whether the latter be osteotomy or fusion. However, in keeping with the overarching principle of restoring the anatomy, the more severe the bunion, the more aggressive the surgical procedure needs to be, to ensure that the long-term results are acceptable.

COMPLICATIONS OF TREATMENT

Non-union in the adolescent age group is uncommon, but has been reported (15,20). The distal Mitchell osteotomy and opening wedge osteotomies at the base seem to be particularly prone to this infrequent complication. If non-union occurs, then revision surgery will be required to achieve union and a stable first ray, thereby eliminating the associated pain and risk of recurrence of deformity.

Avascular necrosis of the first metatarsal head, although uncommon, presents a therapeutic challenge should it occur. Typically it is a complication of distal first metatarsal osteotomies, especially when combined with a distal soft tissue procedure. The primary blood supply to the head enters distally from the lateral side. Therefore, incisions placed on the medial and lateral sides of the first metatarsal head place the vascularity of the head at risk. For example, performing a Mitchell procedure or a Chevron osteotomy in conjunction with adductor tendon release and lateral capsulotomy may well disrupt flow to the head. Salvage usually requires arthrodesis of the MTP joint.

Transfer metatarsalgia occurs if there is a disruption of the normal force distribution across the metatarsal heads. Typically these patients develop a painful callous under the head of the second metatarsal (13). Normally, the head of the first metatarsal carries about 50% of the load across the forefoot. The remaining 50% is roughly distributed evenly over the other four. Because many of these patients have a short first metatarsal, despite literature to the contrary (28), osteotomies of the first metatarsal, which either further shorten the metatarsal relative to the second or allow for dorsal displacement of the first metatarsal head (especially the Mitchell procedure), can be complicated by transfer metatarsalgia. Modest symptoms can be controlled with simple metatarsal pads or metatarsal bars. However, in the younger population, osteotomy of the second metatarsal to unload the painful metatarsal head may be required. Several different techniques have been described (15). Dorsal wedge osteotomy of the neck or shortening through the neck both carry a risk of avascular necrosis of the head or non-union of the osteotomy. Oblique osteotomy of the shaft with fixation seems to produce more reproducible results with fewer complications.

Hallus varus follows overly aggressive correction of the hallux valgus deformity. The great toe then deviates toward the medial side, which in many ways is more problematic and symptomatic than the original deformity.

Excision of the medial exostosis when overly generous is of particular concern, especially in juvenile bunions. These patients typically do not have a large medial exostosis. Unfortunately, there has been a tendency over the years to try and correct the deformity by sacrificing too large a segment of the medial metatarsal head. This destabilizes the first MTP and results in hallux varus, as the proximal phalanx "falls off of the metatarsal head" medially. Revision surgery to correct this problem is complex and usually results in less than optimal results. Arthrodesis of the MTP joint in adults generally produces better long-term results than some of the soft-tissue rebalancing procedures that have been described (20,24). There is very little information available regarding this complication in the adolescent age group.

Physeal damage is a concern unique to the adolescent age group. Proximal osteotomies, performed too close to the physis or damaging the physis during the course of the procedure, have been reported to cause premature arrest of the plate. Potentially this can result in subsequent shortening or angular deformity of the metatarsal. This complication is rare and reports tend to be anecdotal.

Joint stiffness is more common in adults following bunion surgery. The MTP joint, especially in adults and to a lesser degree in adolescents, is vulnerable to delayed arthrofibrosis. This is more of a problem with distal metatarsal osteotomies than with those performed in the proximal portion of the metatarsal. Early physical therapy, occasional use of intraarticular steroids, and encouraging early motion of the joint will lessen the risk of this complication.

"The problem of recurrence" is without a doubt the major concern of most surgeons caring for adolescent bunion deformity. Conventional wisdom (2) surrounding the adolescent bunion is that many of them recur. Scranton (29) in his classic article reports recurrence rates of 20% to 25%. Current authors have tended to reduce this number to 10% to 12% (9). There is general agreement that recurrence of deformity in the younger age group represents a more significant problem than it is in the adult. Whether the recurrence is due to ongoing growth of the first metatarsal and the foot in general; or whether it is due to the overall tendency of the surgeon to be less aggressive in the adolescent foot remains an open question. The older literature tends to suggest the use of more limited procedures in the younger patient. The modest procedures failed to completely correct the deformity, thus resulting in a reported "recurrence." Today more aggressive procedures are the norm and the more recent literature reports lower recurrence rates (6,9).

Cosmesis is oftentimes the overriding indication for surgical intervention both on the part of the patient as well as their parents. Postoperatively, dissatisfaction with the appearance of the foot continues to be a significant problem in some patients and their families. It behooves the surgeon to candidly discuss the realistic expectations to be achieved from any of these surgical procedures, because frequently the quest for perfection by the family and the patient is grossly unrealistic.

CONTROVERSIES

The **timing of surgery** still generates significant discussion. Traditional teaching (2,10,15) encouraged delay in the surgical treatment of adolescent bunion deformity. Many individuals felt that the extensive ligamentous laxity in conjunction with an open growth plate inordinately increased the risks of recurrence. More current literature has shown reliable results with standard surgical techniques. There still exist, however, issues related to the timing of surgical procedures. Some surgeons often point to the problem of noncompliance in adolescents as a reason for delaying operative intervention. Many fear that cosmesis is the main reason driving the desire for surgery. Others are still uncomfortable with the thought of osteotomies performed proximate to an open growth plate.

Pronation and ligamentous laxity have for many years been implicated in the etiology of juvenile hallux valgus. There are several current publications which have debated this issue (17). Coughlin (5,6) and Kilmartin (18) were unable to correlate pronation deformity with that of juvenile bunions. Both reached the conclusion that the incidence of pronation in their patients with juvenile bunion deformity was no greater than that of the normal population. Kalen (14), however, published an article which, based on measurements of talar pitch, calcaneoplantar angle, and dorsoplantar talonavicular angles, suggested that the incidence of flatfeet in adolescents with bunions was 8 to 24 times greater than expected. Hence, the role of pronation and to a lesser degree the relationship with ligamentous laxity continues to be debated in the literature. It is fair to say, however, that the more current literature indicates that pronation is not a factor. While pronation is not likely a factor, ligamentous laxity is another story. Virtually all current literature alludes to it as a contributing factor in the development of the deformity.

The **length of the first metatarsal** has only recently been debated. For many years, most authors have believed that a relatively short first metatarsal contributed to the development of adolescent hallux valgus (20). Recently, some have suggested that they felt that the first metatarsal was uniquely long in children and adolescents with hallux valgus. Aronson (1) has summarized most current thinking when he concluded that the variation in metatarsal length in these patients was no different than that expected in the normal population. Peterson suggested that the variation in length may be more apparent than real by demonstrating the effect of the x-ray beam on length measurements (Figure 18-8). This leaves the question: "Is it better for the first metatarsal to be too long or too short?" The fact seems to be that it probably makes no difference, as long as it is considered in the surgical

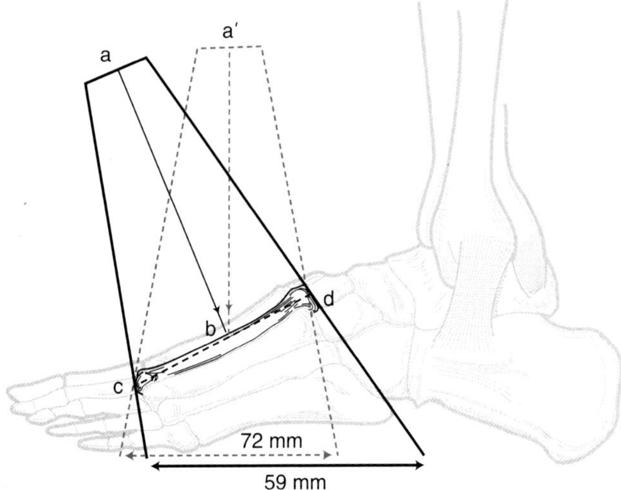

FIGURE 18-8 Length of the same first metatarsal varied considerably on radiographs (e.g., 59 mm versus 72 mm) because of the obliquity of metatarsals (line *c-d*); the angle of the x-ray (angle *b* formed by lines *a* and *a'*); and the focal distance (lines *a-b* and *a'-b*). (Adapted from: Peterson H. Adolescent bunion. *JPO* 1993;13(1):83.)

planning. For example, a Mitchell procedure, that arguably shortens the first metatarsal, is probably not the optimal procedure for a patient who already has a foreshortened first metatarsal.

Metatarsus adductus, whether dynamic or fixed, does increase the tendency of the forefoot to deviate medially (17). Many children, at an early age, also have an atavistic great toe. For many years, there was a controversy as over the role that metatarsus adductus and to a lesser degree, the atavistic great toe, played in the etiology and progression of adolescent bunion deformity. Lapidus (15,24) emphasized the prehensile nature of the metatarsus adductus and the atavistic great toe, concluding that the hallux valgus deformity was an expected consequence of them. Piggott (26) and subsequently Helal (11) did not embrace the direct relationship between these deformities. More recent articles, especially one by Coughlin (6), have indicated that indeed there is a relationship between the two. The controversy continues.

SUMMARY

Adolescent bunion deformity continues to cause concern for patients and their families. Although not a common foot problem in children, it can be a source of pain, and more importantly a source of unhappiness due to the unacceptable appearance of the forefoot. The genetic aspects of the deformity appear to be clear and because maternal transmission rates are high, many of these young people have benefited from their mother's advice regarding treatment. Careful evaluation and extensive discussion surrounding surgical expectations are important before embarking on an operative course. The results of surgery clearly depend on selecting procedures that best permit anatomic alignment of the first ray. Experience over the years has documented that minimal surgery for maximal deformity will most certainly yield poor results. With appropriate patient selection and procedure selection, the results have trended toward improvement.

REFERENCES

1. Aronson J. Early results of modified Peterson bunion procedure for adolescent hallux valgus. *JPO* 2001;21(1):65–69.
2. Bonney G, Macnab I. Hallux valgus and hallux rigidus. *JBJS (Br)* 1952;34:366.
3. Canale P, Aronsson DD. Mitchell procedure for the treatment of adolescent hallux valgus. A long term study. *JBJS* 1993;75A(11):1610–1618.
4. Coughlin M. Juvenile hallux valgus: Etiology and treatment. *Foot Ankle Int* 1995;16(11):682–697.
5. Coughlin M. Pathophysiology of juvenile bunion. *AAOS Instr Course Lect* 1987;36:123–136.
6. Coughlin M. Juvenile hallux valgus. In: Coughlin M, Mann R, eds. *Surgery of the foot and ankle 7th ed.* St. Louis: Mosby,1999:270.
7. Das, De S. Distal metatarsal osteotomy for adolescent hallux valgus. *JPO* 1984;4(1):32–38.
8. Davids JR, Mason TA. Surgical treatment of hallux valgus deformity in children with CP. *JPO* 2001;21(1):89–94.
9. Geissile AE, Stanton R. Surgical treatment of adolescent hallux valgus. *JPO* 1990;10:642.
10. Grosio JA. Juvenile hallux valgus. A conservative approach to treatment. *JBJS* 1992;74A(9):1367–1374.
11. Helal B. Surgery for adolescent hallux valgus. *CORR* 1981;157:50–63.
12. Houghton GR, Dickson RA. Hallux valgus in younger patients. The structural abnormality. *JBJS* 1979; 61B:!76–177.
13. Joplin RJ. Sling procedure for correction of splay foot, metatarus primus varus and hallux valgus. *JBJS* 1950:32;779.
14. Kalen V, Brecher A. Relationship between adolescent bunion and flatfeet. *Foot Ankle* 1988; 8(6):331–336.
15. Kelikian H. *Allied deformities of the forefoot and metatarsalgia.* Philadelphia: WB Saunders: 1965;241.
16. Kidner FC. The prehallux and its relation to flatfoot. *JAMA* 1933:101:1539.
17. Kilmartin TE, Barrington RL. Metatarsus primus varus: A statistical study. *JBJS (Br)* 1991;73:937.
18. Kilmartin TE, Wallace WA. Significance of pes planus in juvenile hallux valgus. *Foot Ankle* 1992;13(2):53–56.
19. Limbird TJ, DaSilva RM. Osteotomy of the first metatarsal base for metatarsus primus varus. *Foot Ankle* 1989;9(4):158–162.
20. Mann R, Rudicel S, Graves SC. Repair of hallux valgus with distal soft tissue procedure and proximal metatarsal osteotomy. A long term follow up. *JBJS (Am)* 1992;74:124.
21. McCluny JG, Tinley P. Radiographic measurements of patients with juvenile hallux valgus. *J Foot Ankle Surg* 2006;45(3):161–167.
22. McDonald MG. Modified Mitchell bunionectomy for the management of adolescent hallux valgus. *CORR* 1996;332:163–169.
23. Mosca V. The foot. In: *Lovell and Winter's pediatric orthopaedics, 7th ed.* Morrissy R, Weinstein S, eds. Philadelphia: Lippincott Williams & Wilkins:2003:1200.
24. Myerson M (ed.). *Foot and ankle clinics.* Philadelphia: WB Saunders, 2000.
25. Peterson HA, Newman SR. Adolescent bunion deformity treated with double osteotomy and longitudinal pin fixation of the first ray. *JPO* 1993;13(1):80–84.
26. Piggott H. The natural history of hallux valgus in adolescents. *JBJS* 1960;42B:749–760.
27. Renshaw TR, Sirkin R, Drennan J. Management of hallux valgus in cerebral palsy. *Dev Med Child Neurol* 1979;21:202.

1. Save the digit with the best axial alignment.
2. Resect the projecting, symptomatic toe.
3. Repair the capsule and balance the soft tissues.
4. Remove any metatarsal prominence.

Excision of the rudimentary digit, be it pre- or postaxial, is the treatment of choice for patients with the type B deformity. It may be difficult to decide whether the fifth or sixth toe should be amputated for patients with the postaxial type A deformity. While it is desirable to preserve the more functional toe, the inherent risk of removing the fifth toe is that the child may develop an angular deformity of the lateral toe or have an objectionable space between the fourth and fifth toes remaining. Meticulous repair of collateral ligaments or syndactylization will help prevent this. It is best to remove duplicated metatarsals in order to narrow the forefoot and avoid a prominent step-off on the lateral border of the foot. The resection is best accomplished through a laterally based, racket-shaped incision to avoid a plantar scar. Waiting until the child is walking facilitates functional and anatomic assessment and permits easier visualization of the associated neurovascular bundle at surgery.

Preaxial duplications may be compounded by hallux varus and have a higher rate of recurrent varus deformity following surgical treatment. It is important to repair the collateral ligaments to try to prevent this and to consider syndactylization of the first and second toes in more difficult cases.

Hallux Varus

There are several varieties of hallux varus, none of which respond to non-operative management. These types should be differentiated by obtaining weight-bearing radiographs, as the surgical treatment of each type is different.

Congenital hallux varus is an uncommon anomaly which may present as an idiopathic, isolated condition with a tethering medial band of tissue which pulls the toe into varus. Medial deviation of the proximal phalanx, relative to the first metatarsal is evident on radiographs. Surgical correction consists of division of the medial fibrous band, lengthening of the abductor hallucis and medial capsulotomy of the metatarsophalangeal (MTP) joint, with temporary K-wire fixation of the toe. Surgery should be undertaken at a young age as the deformity usually prohibits shoe wear.

Hallux varus may result from metatarsus primus varus, often in combination with an unusually broad forefoot. Typically there is a medial slope of the first metatarsal-cuneiform joint resulting in medial deviation of the entire first ray. In this situation, the metatarsophalangeal joint is best left alone; rather a crescentic osteotomy at the base of the first metatarsal may be warranted. The surgeon should be mindful of the proximal location of the physis and can wait until the child is older, as dictated by symptoms.

Hallux varus may be related to a longitudinal epiphyseal bracket, involving the first metatarsal, which is short and broad. Often there is an adjacent medial accessory bone which is thought to represent a form fruste of preaxial polydactyly and proves more difficult to treat. In addition to the medial contracture and muscle imbalance, the growth retardation of the first ray may contribute to recurrence despite surgery. Several soft-tissue reconstructive techniques have been described (Farmer, MacElvenny, Kelikian) with a common goal of realigning the toe, stabilizing the MTP joint and balancing the muscles, both the intrinsic and extrinsic. It may be necessary to syndactylize the hallux to the second toe in order to control its alignment and prevent recurrence.

Metatarsal osteotomy, with or without lengthening, may be necessary in order to address the deformity of the first ray; the need for revision procedures should be anticipated.

Acquired hallux varus is iatrogenic, following bunion surgery. Contributing causes include overzealous soft-issue procedures (McBride) (9,33) and/or resection of too much of the metatarsal head. Once this complication has occurred, the only predictable salvage procedure is an arthrodesis of the first MTP joint which can be done for the symptomatic patient expecting some shortening of the first ray.

Syndactyly

Syndactyly of the toes is a common, often inherited trait which may be classified into two types.

Type 1

Zygosyndactyly is a cutaneous complete or incomplete webbing, usually between the second and third toes. This is often bilateral and, contrary to many congenital toe problems, likely to remain asymptomatic throughout life. Because there are no shoe fitting or functional problems, surgical treatment is not warranted.

Type 2

Polysyndactyly represents a more complex sequela of failure of differentiation of the apical ectodermal ridge during the first trimester. The fourth and fifth toes are often connected; there is a duplication of the fifth toe and occasionally synostosis of the lateral metatarsals. It may occur as part of a syndrome, such as Apert's, or in isolation. This may be either uni- or bilateral and there may be similar involvement of the hands. As the child grows, pain and shoe-fitting problems often become manifest due to disproportionate widening of the forefoot. In addition, there may be recurrent episodes of inflammation related to synonychia (double nail).

The symptoms may present during the toddler phase and are best resolved surgically. Preoperative radiographs will demonstrate the need to pare down any divergent metatarsals as the condition is heterogeneous. It is best to ablate the duplicated toe without disturbing the syndactyly between the fourth and fifth toe because those toes, when separated, may subsequently spread and cause recurrent symptoms.

Varus Fifth Toe

Congenital varus of the fifth toe, or overlapping fifth toe, is frequently bilateral and is a hereditary deformity of

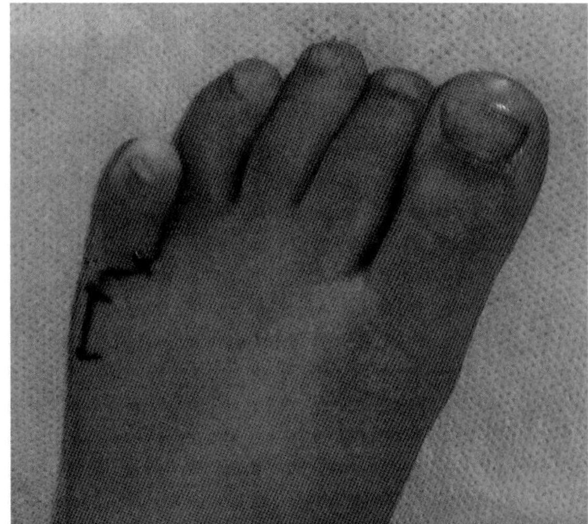

FIGURE 19-5 Varus (overlapping) fifth toe.

unknown cause. At birth the fifth toe is noted to cock-up and override the fourth toe (Figure 19-5). There is a dorsal contracture involving skin, extensor tendon and capsule of the MTP joint. In addition, the toe may rotate outward with the nail assuming a vertical position. The adjacent toes may manifest a flexible hammer toe deformity. The deformities will not correct with stretching exercises or taping and, while young children are usually asymptomatic, local irritation from shoes often causes painful calluses or nail problems during the teenage or adult years in about half of patients.

Several procedures have been described for correction of the deformity, ranging from soft-tissue reconstruction to bony resection with syndactylization (McFarland) or even ablation. The latter is cosmetically inferior and may be followed by tenderness over the fifth metatarsal head and is therefore not recommended. Phalangectomy may be reserved for patients who have scarring due to a previous procedure. The procedure which has gained favor is the Butler procedure which involves a circumferential incision at the base of the toe with plantar and dorsal extension. The incision permits release of the MTP capsule and extensor mechanism while protecting the neurovascular bundles. Complete release of the toe will permit the toe to lie in normal position without additional force. All of the procedures with dorsal incisions have a potential complication of exuberant scar formation (leading to recurrence, but the results from the Butler procedure are generally good (4,6). Regardless of the technique selected, it is mandatory to protect the neurovascular bundle from injury or excessive traction.

Undergrowth (Hypoplasia)

Brachymetatarsia

Brachymetatarsia is manifest by congenital hypoplasia of a metatarsal, usually the fourth. This condition, which is often bilateral and symmetrical, may represent a sequela of aberrant dissolution of the apical ectodermal ridge or premature closure of the metatarsal physis. Less commonly, multiple metatarsals may be foreshortened. Although it can be associated with numerous conditions and syndromes, such as hereditary multiple exostoses, it frequently is isolated. Most commonly, it is asymptomatic and the principal concern of the patient is the cosmetic appearance. In some cases, the involved toe resides on the dorsum of the forefoot, in extension at the MTP joint, where it is subject to pressure and trauma from shoe wear. Patients may also complain of metatarsalgia from the loss of the normal cascade of metatarsal heads.

Taping or splinting is futile, as are efforts at manipulative reduction of the toe. Accomodative shoes and inserts should be used to help manage symptoms. In patients with recalcitrant symptoms, surgery may be indicated. Extensor tenotomy and capsulotomy are unlikely to provide sufficient correction. The most direct solution is fusion of the toe at the metatarsophalangeal joint or resection of the toe or the involved ray; however, these have cosmetic drawbacks.

Metatarsal lengthening has been described in numerous articles by both gradual callotasis and acute lengthening procedures (Figures 19-6 and 19-7). The greatest complication is potential stiffness at the MTP joint and it is likely only appropriate in rare cases of symptomatic patients who fail extensive conservative care and are well prepared for the procedure and its potential problems (2,29,32).

Congenital Constriction Band Syndrome

Congenital constriction band syndrome, also known as Streeter's dysplasia, is thought to be due to amniotic bands which entrap the developing limb, causing partial or complete circumferential constriction bands. These are common in the lower extremities, frequently involving the calf

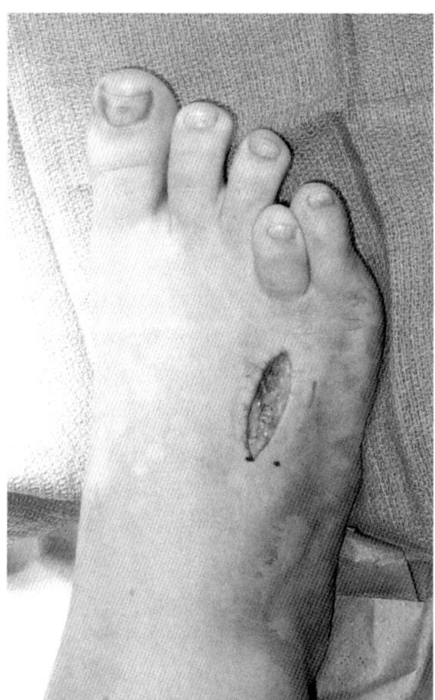

FIGURE 19-6 Inter-operative photograph of brachymetatarsia prior to acute lengthening.

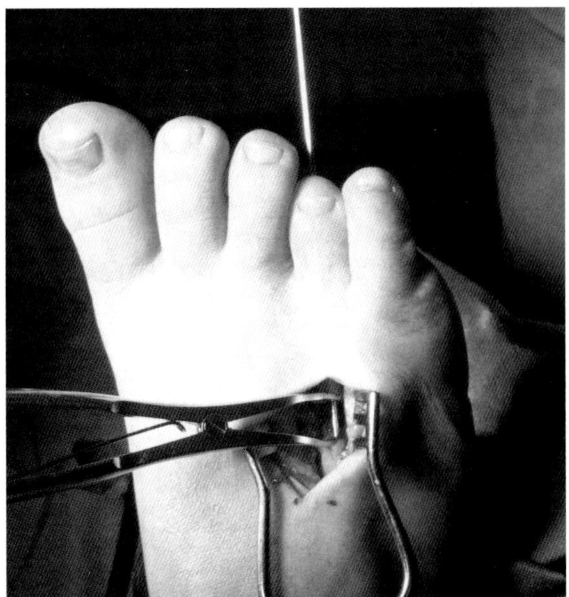

FIGURE 19-7 Inter-operative photograph of an acute lengthening for brachymetatarsia.

or ankle. Compression of the peroneal nerve may cause weakness of the peroneal muscles leading to equinovarus deformity of the foot. Toe problems range from reduction deformities with contractures to autoamputation.

The circumferential bands, which may affect circulation and lymphatic drainage, are best treated by means of Z-plasties, which may need to be done emergently to prevent loss of limb (11,13,23). The foot deformity, which may consist of a teratologic clubfoot, may require tendon lengthening and extensive capsulotomies in order to obtain a plantigrade foot (1,16). Having corrected the deformity, consider tendon transfers in order to prevent recurrence. The toe deformities are sometimes asymptomatic, requiring no treatment. Individual toes may be straightened, with or without syndactylization, as indicated. Recurrence and progression of deformities should be anticipated; therefore, these children should be followed to maturity.

Generalized Skeletal Abnormalities (Miscellaneous/ Developmental)

Curly Toe

Of the various dynamic sagittal toe deformities presenting in childhood, curly toes are the most common. These are inherited as a dominant trait, most often involving the third and/or fourth toes; typically with bilateral, symmetrical involvement (Figure 19-8). There is a flexion deformity of the proximal interphalangeal joint, with or without flexion deformity of the distal interphalangeal joint. The toe often rotates laterally and goes into varus; as a result it underrides the adjacent toe. While initially flexible and painless, the affected toes may eventually become stiff, developing painful corns and calluses, even on the dorsum of the adjacent, innocent overlapping toe. Taping and stretching exercises are ineffectual in managing this deformity and do not change the 25% rate of spontaneous improvement with time (39,40).

During childhood, the flexible nature of this deformity may be verified by flexing the MTP joint of the involved digit(s) and noting passive correction of the distal deformities. This indicates the foreshortened resting length of the toe flexors without capsular contractures. Operative treatment of the adjacent overriding medial toe by extensor tenotomy represents a therapeutic pitfall and is doomed to failure.

The type of deformity is best resolved by open tenotomy of the long and short flexors (15,27,30,40). This may be done through a transverse plantar incision, at the risk of skin tension and possible wound dehiscence. A longitudinal plantar incision avoids this problem, but it is important to not cross flexor creases in order to avoid recurrence due to scar contracture. No internal fixation is required, rather the involved toes are taped to adjacent normal toes for three to four weeks postoperatively. Eventually, the varus and rotational deformities, which were probably secondary to chronic flexion of the toe, tend to resolve spontaneously.

This procedure is optimally performed on preschool children, before the onset of stiffness or secondary deformities. More complex solutions, such as a flexor to extensor tendon transfer, the Girdlestone-Taylor procedure, have been described (3). However, the results are no better than simple tenotomy, and there is an inherent risk of producing a stiff or hyperextended toe.

Glomus Tumor

Glomus tumors are rare, markedly painful lesions which are apt to involve the distal phalanx and commonly occur under the nail plate. It is a sensitive hypertrophy of the glomus body and the pain is exacerbated by cold temperatures. The patient is able to localize the pain to an exact point, unlike Raynaud's phenomenon. Most often they occur as solitary tumors, although there is an uncommon entity known as multiple glomus tumors. Plain radiographs

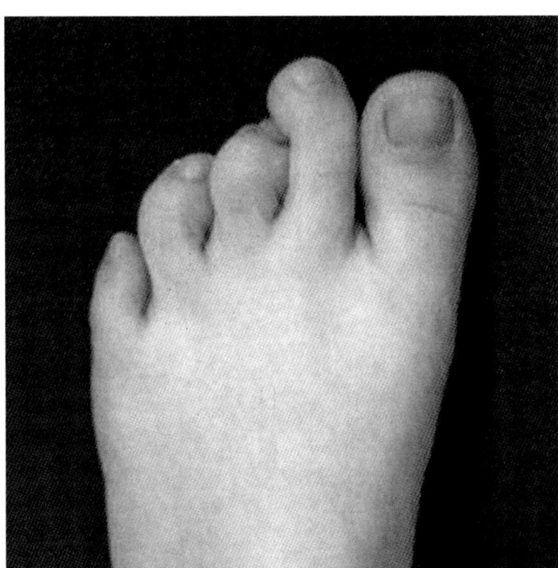

FIGURE 19-8 Third curly toe and, to a lesser extent, fourth curly toe.

may show a well circumscribed, round, radiolucent lesion within the distal phalanx. Doppler studies may demonstrate hyperemia with an arteriovenous malformation. While they resemble cavernous hemangiomas, they may be differentiated histologically by the presence of intraluminal glomus cells. The treatment of choice consists of complete surgical removal of the lesion (28,36).

Subungual Exostosis

A subungual exostosis is a benign bony lesion which protrudes from the dorsal surface of the distal phalanx, most commonly that of the great toe, distorting the overlying nail. It may be misdiagnosed as pyogenic disease, verrucae, mycoses, or even malignancy; mistaken ablation of the great toe has been reported. A lateral radiograph will demonstrate the osseous portion of the tumor. Historically, this was thought to be posttraumatic in origin, but recent genetic studies have demonstrated a consistent chromosome X:6 translocation which supports a neoplastic etiology (38,42).

The treatment of choice consists of total excision of the lesion in order to prevent local recurrence (19,25). Histologically, the specimen consists of a mature, trabecular bony base, formed by intramembranous or occasionally by endochondral ossification, capped with fibrocartilage. Adequate exposure requires removal of the overlying nail and longitudinal division of the underlying nail bed. The germinal matrix is preserved so that the nail will regrow postoperatively. After excising the exostosis, it is helpful to seal the cancellous base with bone wax. The matrix is repaired and a sterile compression dressing applied. Recurrence is likely when there is inadequate resection.

Ingrown Toenails

Ingrown toenails may present anytime during growth, typically involving one or both borders of the great toenail. An inflammatory reaction develops when the nail is permitted to grow into the surrounding paronychia. Hereditary factors, constrictive shoe wear, and personal care habits to include tearing of nails or improper trimming may each play a role in the development and progression of this common problem. Conservative treatment may suffice when diagnosed early in the course, before multiple inflammatory episodes have occurred. This includes cautious manipulation of the nail border from under the skin after soaking to permit placement of a cotton patch under the nail corner. The nail should be permitted to grow out slightly and then trimmed in a squared-off fashion.

The patient is advised to avoid high-heeled or pointed shoes, in order to minimize local friction. Proper hygiene is critical, including daily bathing and the use of clean, dry cotton socks. It is helpful for the patient to have two or more pair of shoes to allow the toe box to adequately dry out.

Periods of inflammation may require warm soaks and oral antibiotics. Persistent symptoms may indicate the need for surgical intervention; however, it is important to clear up any ongoing infection preoperatively. It is also wise to take preoperative radiographs if there is concern that the paronychial pain could be secondary to phalangeal fracture, subungual exostosis, or glomus tumor.

If symptoms are recurrent, the treatment of choice is surgical intervention. Simple nail avulsion is not considered a definitive treatment as recurrence is common once the nail grows back. Heifetz described wedge resection of one or both borders of the nail; this is a relatively simple procedure with a low recurrence rate, provided you are careful to remove, or cauterize with phenol, the corresponding germinal portion at the base of the nail (17,26). In severe and persistent cases, it may become necessary to remove the entire nail along with the germinal portion, as described by Zadek (41). If a subungual exostosis is identified, this should be excised at the time of the toenail procedure.

Freiberg's Disease

In 1914, Freiberg described six patients with a painful condition affecting the second metatarsal head (10). He recommended conservative management with an insole or a cast. A risk factor with strong correlation is that most afflicted patients are female and have a relatively long second metatarsal. Consideration of etiology includes osteochondrosis and repetitive trauma to the long metatarsal (12,35) Initial radiographs may be unrevealing; in such cases a technetium scan may yield an early diagnosis (22). Over the course of time and seemingly irrespective of conservative treatment, typical changes of osteonecrosis evolve (Figure 19-9). This may result in the painful

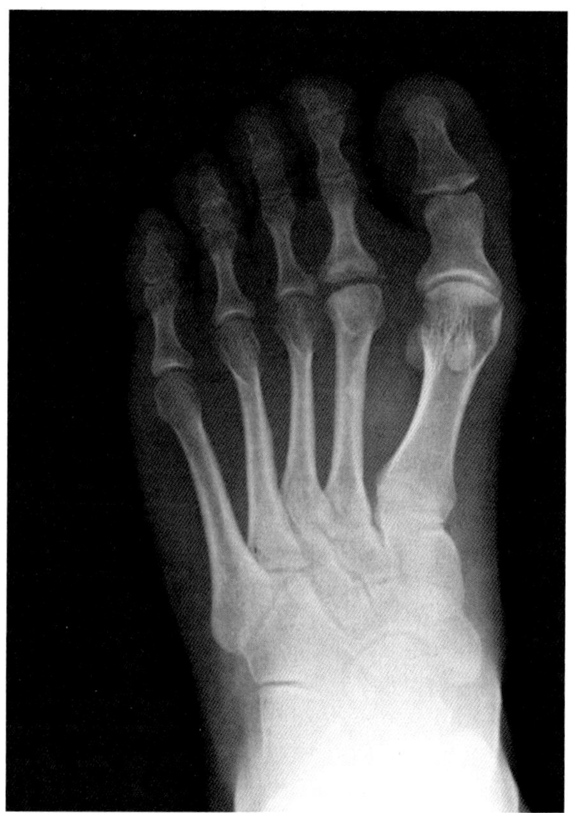

FIGURE 19-9 Radiograph of a Frieberg's Infraction.

collapse and shortening of the second metatarsal and painful plantar callosity. Conservative management consists of inserts to give more rigidity to the shoe and metatarsal pads to relieve the second metatarsal head.

With persistent symptoms and progressive radiographic changes, operative treatment is often warranted. While some authors have advocated excision of the second metatarsal head, this may exacerbate "transfer lesions" consisting of painful callosities under the first and third metatarsal heads and should be done only in extenuating circumstances. Curettage and bone grafting, core decompression, osteochondral plug transplantation and debridement of the joint and drilling of the epiphysis have also been reported. Good results have been reported with dorsiflexion osteotomy of the metatarsal neck, with 2–4 mm of shortening. The fragments are fixed with a mini-plate and screws (18). Theoretically, this helps to unload the overstressed metatarsal head while preserving it as a weight-bearing structure. Care must be taken to not to extend the metatarsal too far and give transfer lesions to the first and third metatarsals. Whether the effect is secondary to the dorsiflexion, shortening, or the osteotomy of the bone is unclear, as studies where shortening alone was done also have had a good result (34).

Hammertoe

A hammertoe is, in many respects, similar to a curly toe to the extent that initially there are no discernible capsular contractures and no deformity of the MTP joint. Usually, however, there is no medial deviation or malrotation of the involved toe. The toe fully extends as the MTP joint is plantar flexed. Any or all of the lesser toes may be involved and the family history is variable. In the presence of other foot deformities, in particular cavus or hindfoot varus, neurogenic causes should be sought.

During childhood, the flexible toes are rarely symptomatic. However, the involved toes may become more stiff and sometimes painful as the child grows. Once again, non-operative treatment is an exercise in futility. Between the ages of four and ten, flexor tenotomy is likely to suffice, whereas in the teenage years this may have to be supplemented with arthrodesis of the proximal interphalangeal joint secondary to acquired contracture.

Mallet Toe

In mallet toe, the flexion deformity is isolated to the distal interphalangeal joint (Figures 19-10 and 19-11). Treatment indications are similar to those of the curly and hammer toe.

Provided this is a flexible deformity, a long flexor tenotomy will suffice. After maturity, if the deformity is rigid, fusion of the distal interphalangeal joint is necessary.

Clawtoes

A clawtoe is characterized by extension contracture or dorsal subluxation of the metatarsophalangeal (MTP) joint, combined with flexion deformity of the proximal and distal interphalangeal joints. Typically all of the toes, including the great toe, are involved. These deformities prove more difficult to manage than hammertoes. As the deformities become more rigid, the patient develops painful dorsal calluses over the proximal interphalangeal joints and plantar calluses under the MTP joints; shoe fitting becomes progressively more difficult. There may be concomitant foot deformities such as cavus or cavovarus, suggesting a possible underlying neurogenic cause.

The family history may be helpful in considering or ruling out Charcot-Marie-Tooth or other inheritable diseases. When there is a high index of suspicion, a neurologic workup, including spine x-rays, magnetic resonance

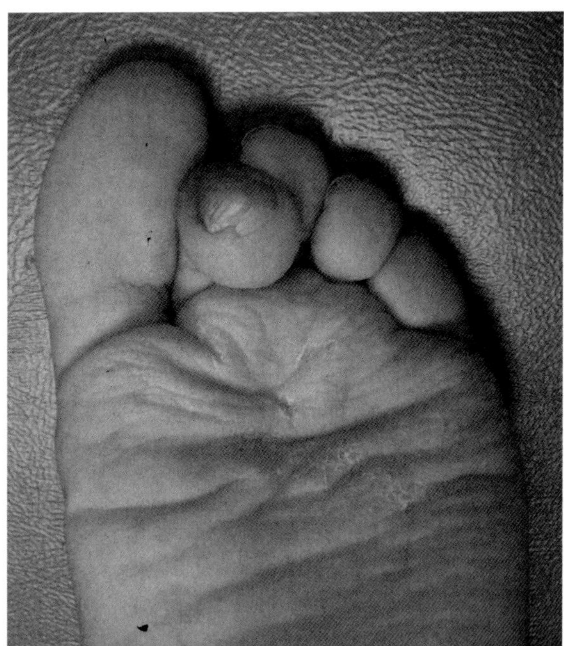

FIGURE 19-10 Mallet Toe with extreme plantar prominence.

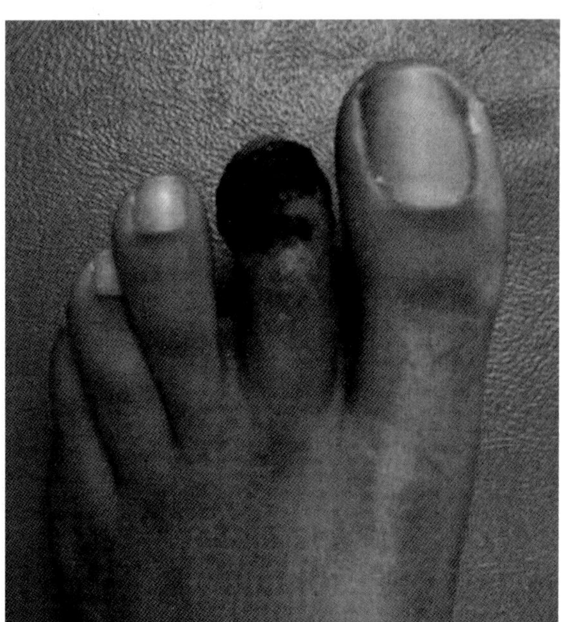

FIGURE 19-11 Necrosis of the same toe after flexor tendon release emphasizing the importance of being vigilant of the neurovascular bundles during release.

imaging (MRI), electromyelogram (EMG), and nerve conduction studies, may be indicated. Having first ruled out neuromyopathies, spinal dysraphism, or other causes, it is appropriate to treat the symptomatic toes. When the deformity is flexible and corrects with passive elevation of the metatarsal heads, one may temporize with a metatarsal bar beneath the metatarsal necks. With respect to surgery, a long extensor tendon transfer to the metatarsal neck, with or without flexor tenotomy, may provide satisfactory correction.

Over time, the juxta-articular soft tissues, including tine dorsal skin, the capsule, and the collateral ligaments become further contracted. The intrinsic toe flexors weaken and may subluxate dorsally as the contracture worsens. Once the deformed toes become rigid, it is likely that an arthrodesis of the proximal interphalangeal joint will be necessary, often combined with a dorsal capsulotomy of the MTP joint, in order to correct the clawtoe. This is best accomplished through a longitudinal dorsal incision in order to avoid excessive wound tension. Because all of the juxta-articular soft tissues may be contracted, it may be necessary to divide the dorsal portion of the collateral ligaments and the interossei as well.

A clawtoe deformity of the great toe may be resolved using the Jones procedure. The extensor hallucis longus is transferred from the base of the distal phalanx to the neck of the first metatarsal. This can be accomplished either through a drill hole or with a suture anchor, converting the muscle from an indirect plantar flexor of the first metatarsal to an active elevator of the first metatarsal. The interphalangeal joint is simultaneously fused, with a small AO cancellous screw or K-wire fixation, in order to prevent a subsequent flexion deformity.

Post-Ablation Hallux Valgus

Loss of the second toe, either due to trauma or amputation, will predictably result in hallux valgus. Therefore, when ablation is contemplated, regardless of the etiology of a second toe problem, ray resection is preferable to disarticulation at the MTP joint. Ultimately, arthrodesis of the first MTP joint of the great toe may be required for long lasting correction of this complex problem. Ray resection to close the distance between the file and third rays should also be considered and will provide the lateral strut of support to the Hallux.

Hallux Rigidus

Hallux rigidus is rare in childhood but may present during adolescence. It is manifested by pain and stiffness of the first MTP joint secondary to degenerative change, accompanied by progressive radiographic changes which include narrowing of the joint space and dorsal osteophyte formation. In adolescents, the condition may be noticed during sports participation. Since first described by Davies-Colley in 1887, several theories have been advanced regarding the etiology of the degeneration. These include repetitive trauma to the hypermobile or overlong first ray, osteochondritis dissecans, and idiopathic change. The hallux is obstructed from dorsiflexion by the dorsal osteophytes, and the associated pain is from this obstruction and the underlying synovitis.

Initial management consists of stiff-soled shoes to prevent dorsiflexion, activity restrictions, and non-steroidal medication; however, treatment must be individualized. When activity restrictions and shoe modifications do not suffice, particularly in the presence of radiographic degeneration, surgery may be considered. Surgical options include cheilectomy and/or osteotomy of the metatarsal or proximal phalanx. The uncommon nature of the condition in adolescents results in little literature on which to draw conclusions for the younger patients (7,8).

CONCLUSION

Most congenital toe deformities evolve from problems that originate between the fifth and eighth week of gestation. During that period of rapid limb bud development, errors of formation or of separation of the digits result in deformities that are usually evident at birth. Continued growth and pressure from shoe wear may combine to produce significant symptoms during childhood. Armed with an understanding of the natural history of various deformities and with adequate radiographs, one can accurately project the problems that lie ahead. When indicated, well-timed, carefully executed surgery can have lasting benefit.

REFERENCES

1. Allington NJ, Kumar SJ, Guille JT. Clubfeet associated with congenital constriction bands of the ipsilateral lower extremity. *J Pediatr Orthop* 15:599–603, 1995.
2. Baek GH, Chung MS. The treatment of congenital brachymetatarsia by one-stage lengthening. *J Bone Joint Surg* 80:1040–1044, 1998.
3. Biyani A, Jones DA, Murray JM. Flexor to extensor tendon transfer for curly toes: 43 children reviewed after 8 (1–25) years. *Acta Orthop Scand* 63(4):451–454, 1992.
4. Black GB, Groganj DP, Bobechko WP. Butler arthroplasty for correction of the adducted fifth toe: A retrospective study of 36 operations between 1968 and 1982. *J Pediatr Orthop* 5:539–441, 1985.
5. Blauth W, Borisch NC. Cleft feet: Proposals for a new classification based on roentgenographic morphology. *Clin Orthop* 258:41–48, 1990.
6. Cockin J. Butler's operation for an over-riding fifth toe. *Br J Bone Joint Surg* 50:78–81, 1968.
7. Coughlin MJ, Shurnas PS. Hallux rigidus: Demographics, etiology and radiographic assessment. *Foot Ankle* 24:731–743, 2003.
8. Coughlin MJ, Shurnas PS. Hallux rigidus: Grading and long-term results of operative treatment. *J Bone Joint Surg* 85:2072–2088, 2003.
9. Donley BG. Acquired hallux varus. *Foot Ankle Int* 18(9):586–592, 1997.
10. Freiberg A. Infraction of the second metatarsal bone. *Surg Gynecol Obstet*, 19:191–193, 1914.
11. Gabos PG. Modified technique for the surgical treatment of congenital constriction bands of the arms and legs of infants and children. *Orthopedics* 5:401–404, 2006.
12. Gauthier G, Elbaz R. Freiberg's infraction: A subchondral bone fatigue fracture, *Clin Orthop* 142:93–96, 1979.

13. Greene WB. One-stage release of congenital circumferential constriction bands. *J Bone Joint Surg* 75:650–655, 1993.
14. Gurnet CA, Dobbs MB, Nordsieck EJ, et al. *Am J Med Genetics* 140:1744–1748, 2006.
15. Hamer AJ, Stanley D, Smith TWD. Surgery for curly-toe deformity: A double-blind, randomized, prospective trial. *J Bone Joint Surg* 75:662–663, 1993.
16. Hennigan SP, Kuo KN. Resistant talipes equinovarus associated with congenital constriction band syndrome. *J Pediatr Orthop* 20:240–245, 2000.
17. Islan S, Lin EM, Drongowski R, et al.: The effect of phenol on ingrown toenail excision in children. *J Pediatr Surg*, 40:290–292, 2005.
18. Kinnard P, Lirette R. Dorsiflexion osteotomy in Freiberg's disease. *Foot Ankle* 9:226–231, 1989.
19. Letts M, Davidson D, Nizalik E. Subungual exostosis: Diagnosis and treatment in children. *J Trauma* 44:346–349, 1998.
20. Light TR, Ogden JA. The longitudinal epiphyseal bracket: Implications for surgical correction. *J Pediatr Orthop* 3:299–305, 1981.
21. Lokiec F, Ezra E, Krasin E, et al. A simple and efficient surgical technique for subungual exostosis. *J Pediatr Orthop* 21:76–79, 2001.
22. Mandell G, Harcke H. Scintigraphic manifestations of infarction of the second metatarsal (Freiberg's disease). *J Nucl Med* 28: 249–251, 1987.
23. Moses JM, Flatt AE, Cooper RR. Annular constricting bands. *J Bone Joint Surg* 61:562–562, 1979.
24. Mubarak SJ, O'Brien TJ, Davids JR. Metatarsal epiphyseal bracket: Treatment by central physiolysis. *J Pediatr Orthop* 13: 5–8, 1993.
25. Multhoop-Stephens H, Walling AK. Subungual (Dupuytren's) exostosis. *J Pediatr Orthop* 15:582–584, 1995.
26. Pettine KA, Cofield RH, Johnson KA, et al. Ingrown toenail: Results of surgical treatment. *Foot Ankle* 9:130–134, 1988.
27. Pollard JP, Morrison PJ. Flexor tenotomy in the treatment of curly toes. *Proc R Soc Med* 68:480–481, 1975.
28. Rettig AC, Strickland JW. Glomus tumor of the digits. *J Hand Surg* 4:261–265, 1977.
29. Robinsonf JF, Ouzounian TJ. Brachymetatarsia: Congenitally short third and fourth metatarsals treated by distraction lengthening—A case report and literature summary. *Foot & Ankle Intern* 19:713–718, 1998.
30. Ross ERS, Menelaus MB. Open flexor tenotomy for hammer toes and curly toes in childhood. *J Bone Joint Surg* 5:770–771, 1984.
31. Shea KG, Mubarak SJ, Alamin T. Preossified longitudinal epiphyseal bracket of the foot: Treatment by partial bracket excision before ossification. *J Pediatr Orthop* 21:360–365, 2001.
32. Shimi JS, Park SJ. Treatment of brachymetatarsia by distraction osteogenesis. *J Pediatr Orthop* 26:250–254, 2006.
33. Skalley TC, Myerson MS. The operative treatment of acquired hallux varus. *Clin Orthop Rel Res* 306:183–191, 1994.
34. Smith TWD, Stanley D, Rowley DI. Treatment of Freiberg's disease. *J Bone Joint Surg* 1:129–133, 1991.
35. Stanley D, Betts R, Rowley D, et al. Assessment of etiologic factors in the development of Freiberg's disease. *J Foot Sung*, 29:444–447, 1990.
36. Stansbury NA, Weber JB. Glomus tumor. *Orthopedics* 5: 636–637, 1993.
37. Stevens PM, Arms D. Postaxial hypoplasia of the lower extremity. *J Pediatr Orthop* 20:166–172, 2000.
38. Storlazzi CT, Wozniak A, Panagopoulos I, et al. Rearrangement of the COL12A1 and COL4A5 genes in subungual exostosis: Molecular cytogenetic delineation of the tumor-specific translocation t(X;6)(ql3–14;q22). *Int J Cancer* 118:1972–1976, 2006.
39. Sweetham R. Congenital curly toes: An investigation into the value of treatment. *Lancet* 398–400, 1958.
40. Turner PL. Strapping of curly toes in children. *Aust NZ J Surg* 57:467–470, 1987.
41. Zadek I, Cohen HG. Epidermoid cyst of the terminal phalanx of a finger; with a review of the literature. *Am J Surg* Jun; 85(6):771–774, 1953.
42. Zambrano E, Nose V, Perez-Atayde AR, et al. Distinct chromosomal rearrangements in subungual (Dupuytren) exostosis and bizarre parosteal osteochondromatous proliferation (nora lesion). *Am J Surg Pathol* 8:1033–1039, 2004.

CHAPTER 20

Limb Deficiencies and Reconstruction

John G. Birch

INTRODUCTION

The major lower extremity congenital limb deficiencies include congenital fibular deficiency, congenital tibial deficiency, and congenital femoral deficiency. Congenital fibular and tibial deficiencies (or hemimelia) almost always manifest associated foot and/or ankle deformities that play significant roles in the function of the extremity and the selection of various reconstructive strategies. Foot deformities are not a component of congenital femoral deficiency per se. However, fibular or tibial deficiencies are commonly associated with congenital femoral deficiency, and foot deformities attendant to those conditions may impact reconstructive strategies for congenital femoral deficiency. Interestingly, relatively little attention has been given in the literature to the management of foot deformities associated with congenital limb deficiencies. In this chapter, we will review the nature of foot and ankle deformities in the major congenital limb deficiencies, their influence on the overall management of these deformities, and specific treatment options for the foot deformities themselves.

CONGENITAL FIBULAR DEFICIENCY

Classification of Fibular Deficiency

Fibular deficiency is considered the most common congenital long bone deficiency. While syndromic and familial forms of the condition exist, by far the most frequently encountered forms are sporadic in nature, and not thought to be inheritable or transmissible (1,20,43,57,67,83,96,98). In these cases, the etiology and pathogenesis of fibular deficiency remains elusive.

The morphological features of congenital fibular deficiency are readily recognizable to the initiated (Figure 20-1A,B). They present with a longitudinal lateral deficiency of the entire lower leg, characterized by slight hypoplasia of the femur including mild femoral neck valgus and shortening, external rotational deformity, hypoplastic distal femoral lateral condyle which causes mild to moderate genu valgum, tibial shortening (often with an apex anteromedial bow), fibular deficiency, and lateral ray deficiency. The disorder represents a spectrum in each of these aspects, and each component can vary from barely detectable to severe (Figure 20-2). Specifically, femoral shortening can be minimal or more severe than associated tibial shortening (causing confusion in defining a limb deficiency as "congenital femoral deficiency with associated fibular deficiency" or as "congenital fibular deficiency with associated severe femoral shortening"), dominating the associated limb length discrepancy. Tibial shortening can be sufficiently mild to escape detection until adolescence, or striking at birth. Some patients will demonstrate typical morphological and radiographic features of fibular deficiency, but with a normal appearing, five-rayed foot, or the foot can in the severest forms be so rudimentary that there are no actual rays or digits present. Occasionally, the limb will have the typical morphological features of congenital fibular deficiency, but radiographically, the fibula appears to be normal (5,79).

Several classifications exist for this condition (1,7,15, 20,54,83). The most commonly referenced are those of Coventry and Johnson (2) (Table 20-1) and Achterman and Kalamchi (1) (Table 20-2). Each of these schemes classifies congenital fibular deficiency primarily on the state of preservation of the fibula itself (as hypoplastic, or rudimentary/absent), with the implication that the presence of only a rudimentary fibula or its complete absence is indicative of more severe lower leg dysplasia. Both of these reviews and others (4,8,10,22,32,33,43,51,60,65,69,96,98) recommended Syme or Boyd amputation for fibular deficiency associated with a rudimentary or absent fibula, unless there is bilateral limb involvement. The implication of bilateral fibular deficiency, even if severe, is that limb length inequality is negligible, and reconstructive procedures to render the foot plantigrade should be considered.

Unfortunately, documentation of successful reconstructive foot and ankle procedures for severe deformities in large or long-term studies are currently lacking (15,34,45,60,62,69,99). Furthermore, in a review of

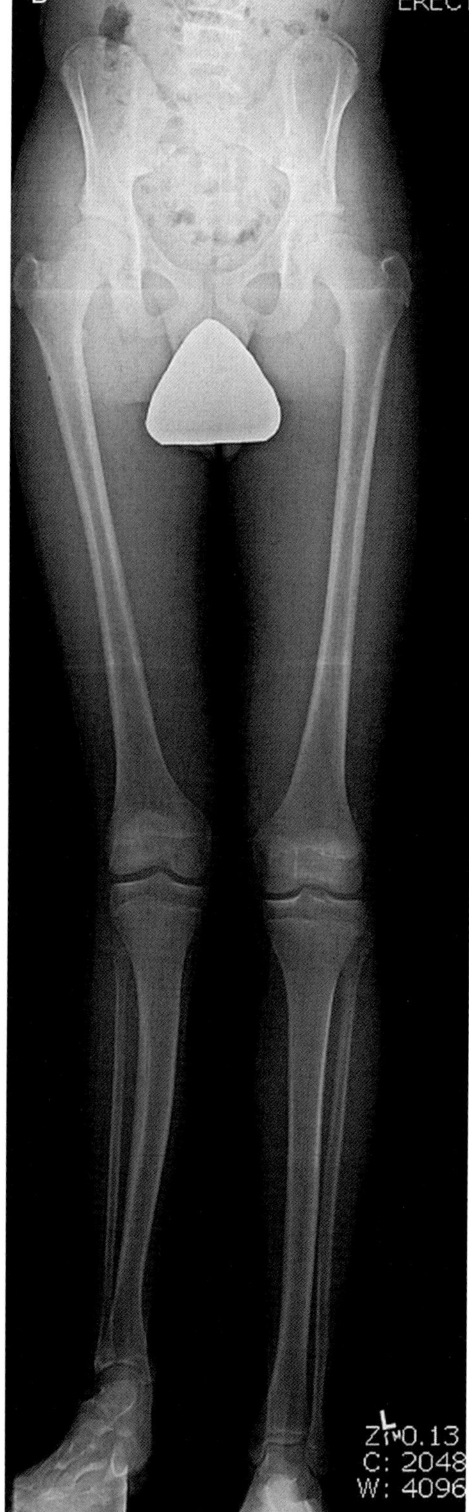

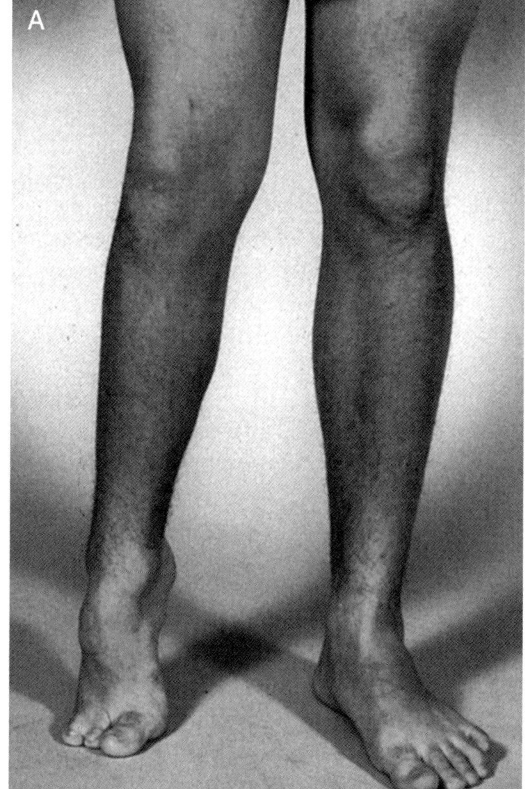

FIGURE 20-1 **A.** Clinical features of congenital fibular deficiency in a 12-year-old boy. There is shortening of the affected leg, with valgus deformity and absent lateral rays of the foot. **B.** Radiographic features of congenital fibular deficiency. There is shortening of the femur with valgus, shortening of the tibia, hypoplasia of the fibula and in this case, a ball-and-socket ankle mortise.

patients with fibular deficiency at our institution, we noted that there was not always a direct correlation between the extent of fibular reduction and the severity of the overall dyplasia of the lower leg (8). As a consequence of this experience, we prefer to use a "functional classification" taking into account the status of the foot and the associated shortening in determining reconstruction requirements. Ironically, few classifications specifically

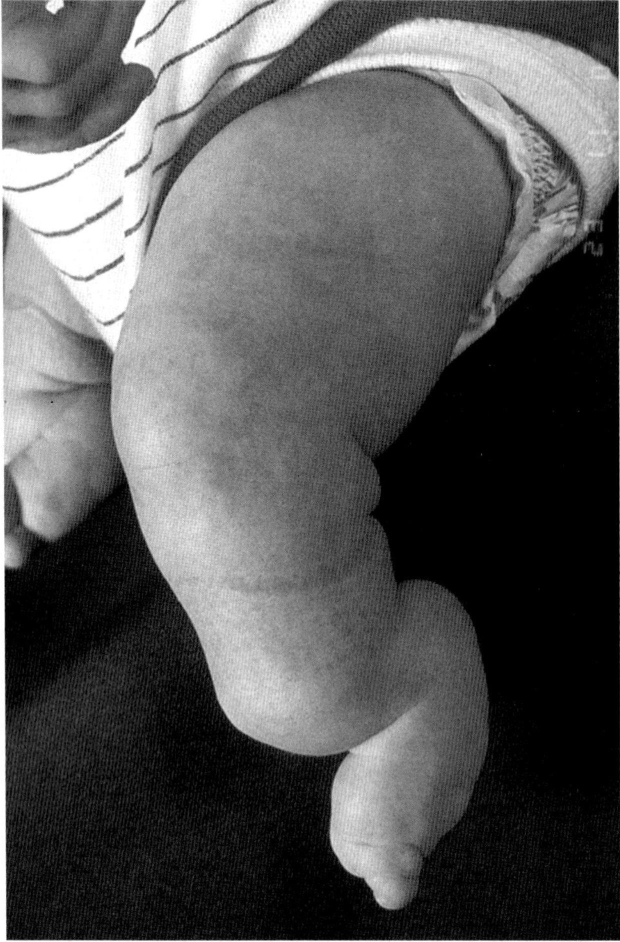

FIGURE 20-2 Severe fibular deficiency in an infant. The lower leg is very short, and there is only a rudimentary foot in equinovalgus.

address associated foot and ankle deformity (83), although the various manifestations and significance of these deformities are recognized (38,57,79,83,86,89,90).

Ankle and Foot Deformities Associated with Congenital Fibular Deficiency

There are several foot and ankle deformities associated with congenital fibular deficiency, and, typical for this limb deficiency, they vary in presence and severity (Table 20-3).

TABLE 20-1

Coventry Classification of Fibular Deficiency

Type	*Characteristics*	*Treatment Recommended*
I	Hypoplastic fibula	Epiphysiodesis or lengthening as needed
II	Fibula rudimentary or absent	Syme or Boyd amputation
III	Bilateral or associated anomalies	No procedures anticipated

TABLE 20-2

Achterman and Kalamchi Classification of Fibular Deficiency

Type	*Characteristics*	*Treatment Recommended*
IA	Hypoplastic fibula (proximal to talar dome)	Epiphysiodesis or lengthening as needed
IB	Fibula does not support talus	Epiphysiodesis or lengthening as needed
II	Fibula rudimentary or absent	Syme or Boyd amputation

TABLE 20-3

Foot and Ankle Deformities Associated with Fibular Deficiency

Ankle	*Foot*
Ball-and-socket	Equinovalgus
Planar	Equinovarus
Incompetent fibula	Tarsal coalition
	Lateral ray reduction

Ankle Deformity

Two types of ankle deformity are commonly seen in congenital fibular deficiency, a planar ankle mortise (Figure 20-3), or a so-called ball-and-socket ankle (6,16,17,52,67, 71,97) (Figure 20-4). Most frequently, planar ankle deformity is noted in patients with a rudimentary or completely absent fibula. A ball-and-socket ankle mortise is more commonly seen in patients with less severe fibular deficiency, i.e., when the fibula is hypoplastic, but contributes to the ankle mortise. Traditionally, ball-and-socket ankle deformity has been thought to be a mobility adaptation to the frequently associated tarsal coalition (6,17,42,67,71,88,89). However, most planar ankle joints have feet with obvious coalition, so the presence of tarsal coalition alone does not fully explain the pathogenesis of ball-and-socket ankle deformity in congenital fibular deficiency (18). As perhaps typical of any effort to qualify the morphological features of congenital fibular deficiency, exceptions to these generalizations are regularly noted.

Reconstructive procedures to correct planar ankle deformity have been described, specifically the "Gruca procedure"(80,90) fashioning some form of lateral malleolus by transfer of bone to the lateral malleolar area with cross-union of the graft to the distal tibia or by splitting the distal tibia into two components to form a more traditional-appearing ankle mortise radiographically, or performing a "bending osteotomy" of the distal tibial metaphysis to create a semblance of competent posterolateral mortise (29). These reports are mostly anecdotal with

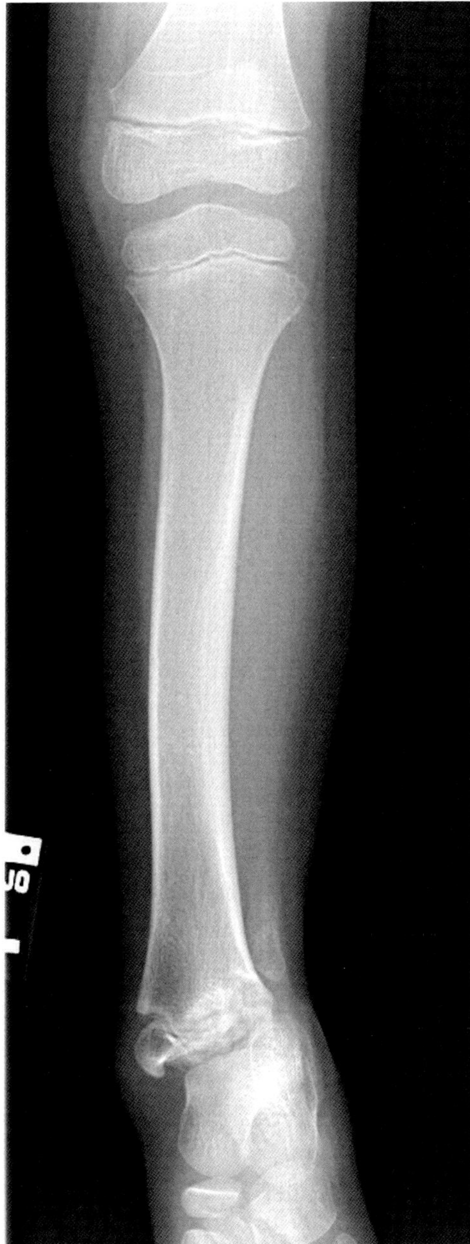

FIGURE 20-3 Planar ankle mortise. This type of ankle deformity is most commonly associated with rudimentary or completely absent fibula.

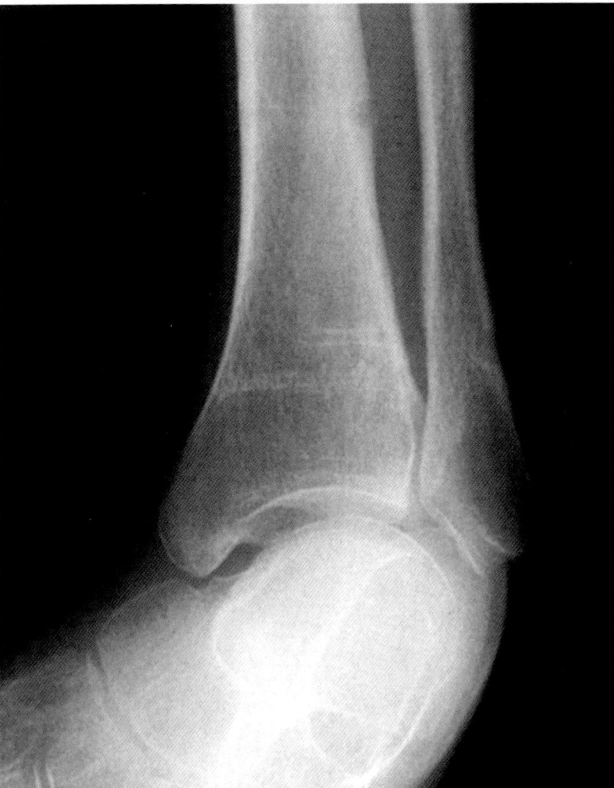

FIGURE 20-4 Ball-and-socket ankle joint. This type of ankle deformity is usually seen with a fibula that contributes to the ankle mortise. Tarsal coalition is frequently present as well.

limited or no longitudinal follow up. At our institution, the planar ankle joint itself is not treated unless pain and stiffness, or symptomatic subluxation associated with staged reconstructions require ankle fusion. There may be an associated apex anterior or anteromedial deformity of the distal tibia causing or compounding the typical equinovalgus position of the foot in fibular deficiency. If sufficiently severe, this deformity may be treated by distal tibial osteotomy either by an acute opening or closing wedge technique, or by gradual correction using an external fixator. When correcting severe deformity gradually with an external fixator, use of a circular fixation with fixation of the foot is advantageous, particularly with associated planar ankle joint to prevent subluxation during deformity correction (Figure 20-5).

Ball-and-Socket Ankle

A stereotypical radiographic morphological feature of congenital fibular deficiency is the presence of a spherical, so-called ball-and-socket, ankle joint. The distal tibial mortise has a concave surface, and the talus will have a matching convex appearance on the anteroposterior radiograph (see Figure 20-4). Often this deformity is not obvious in infants or young children because of the cartilaginous nature of the distal tibia at this stage of development but will become more obvious with maturation (16,88,89). As a generality, this deformity is most commonly associated with milder forms of fibular deficiency, including relatively mild shortening, and with sufficient fibular preservation that a rudimentary lateral malleolus is present and contributes to the spherical appearance of the ankle mortise. Clinically, this deformity is often not recognized because the foot may be plantigrade with excellent motion.

The pathogenesis of the ball-and-socket ankle joint is not known but has been hypothesized to result because of the presence of tarsal coalition (6,17,42,67,71,88,89). The need for subtalar coronal and axial motion results in the adaptation of the ankle mortise into its spherical shape to compensate for hindfoot and/or mid-foot rigidity (42). While this may be true in some cases, it cannot be the

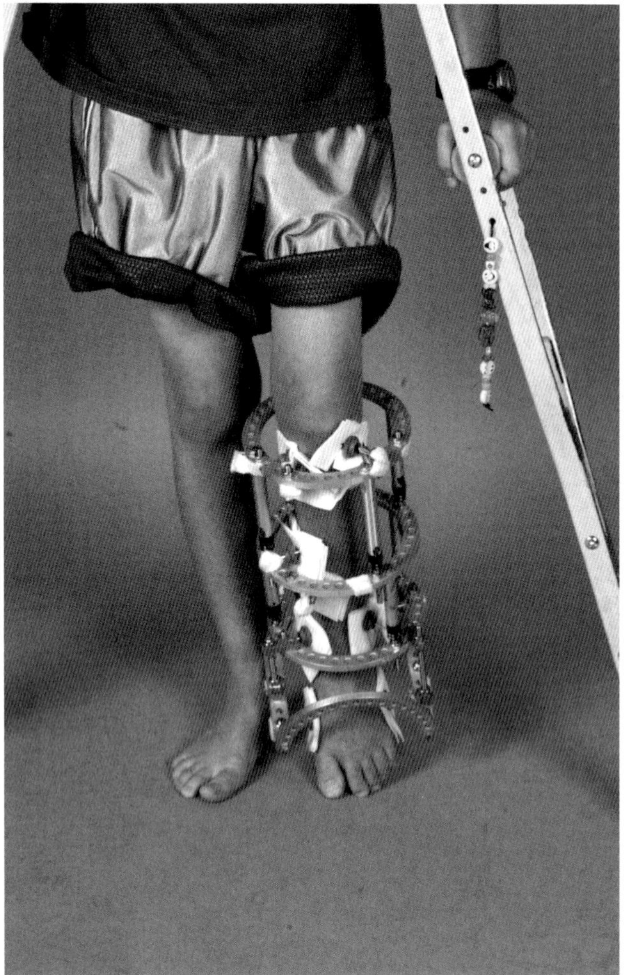

FIGURE 20-5 When distal valgus deformity is corrected gradually with an external fixator, incorporation of the foot to stabilize the ankle may be required. In-fixator photograph of a 10-year-old boy undergoing distal tibial angular deformity correction and simultaneous proximal tibial lengthening.

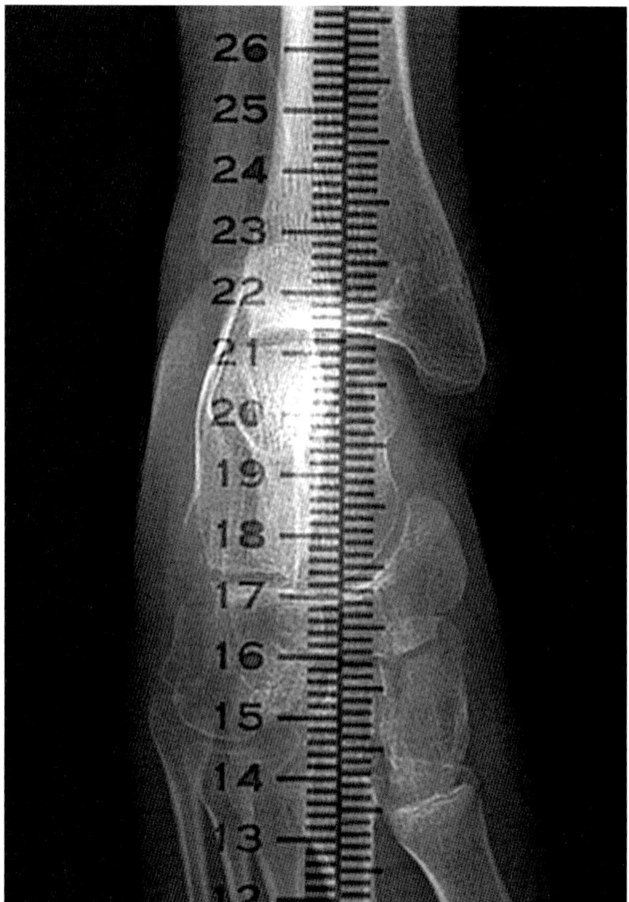

FIGURE 20-6 Ball-and-socket ankle mortise in a 12-year-old girl with only a rudimentary fibula.

sole explanation, as planar ankle joints described above frequently have feet with obvious tarsal coalition as. Nor can the presence of a rudimentary lateral malleous be required for the development of a ball-and-socket ankle joint, because on occasion, one will be present when the fibula is rudimentary or absent (Figure 20-6).

Paley (66) described gradual distal translation of a hypoplastic fibula to reconstruct a more normal distal fibular-ankle mortise relationship, but cautioned that only very young patients (under age four years) should be considered for this procedure, as ankle stiffness might result. Our experience is that few patients with ball-and-socket joints rarely manifest any signs or symptoms associated with such a joint, and these ankles tend to function virtually normally in the vast majority of cases (6,16,17,42,52,67,71,97). Valgus deformity of the ankle and foot may be present, and if symptomatic, supramalleolar osteotomy can be considered to correct it (66). Stevens (85) described correction of symptomatic valgus deformity in ten patients by medial distal tibial (screw) hemiepiphyseodesis. Rarely, complaints of "ankle sprain" or instability due to the excessive mobility of the joint may be present, and can be treated conservatively with orthotics if symptoms warrant. There is a single case report of late degenerative arthritis in a ball-and-socket ankle joint treated by arthrodesis (23). In the child's foot, this is an uncommon occurrence, except when significant or repeated lengthenings may result in stiffness, equinus contracture, or cartilage loss and arthrosis (15,34,45). In such cases, arthrodesis (with significant loss of total ankle/foot motion) may be required.

Foot Deformity

Equinovalgus Deformity

The most common attitude of the foot in congenital fibular deficiency is equinovalgus. The morphological features which result in this position are complex and usually multifactorial. In different individuals, each locus of deformity may or may not contribute significantly to this positional deformity. The major components include:

1. Apex anterior or anteromedial bowing of the tibia. This deformity may be diaphyseal, distal metaphyseal (18), or both (Figure 20-7A,B).
2. Associated soft tissue contracture of the lateral and posterior compartments of the leg pulling the foot into the equinus or equinovalgus position, with an associated

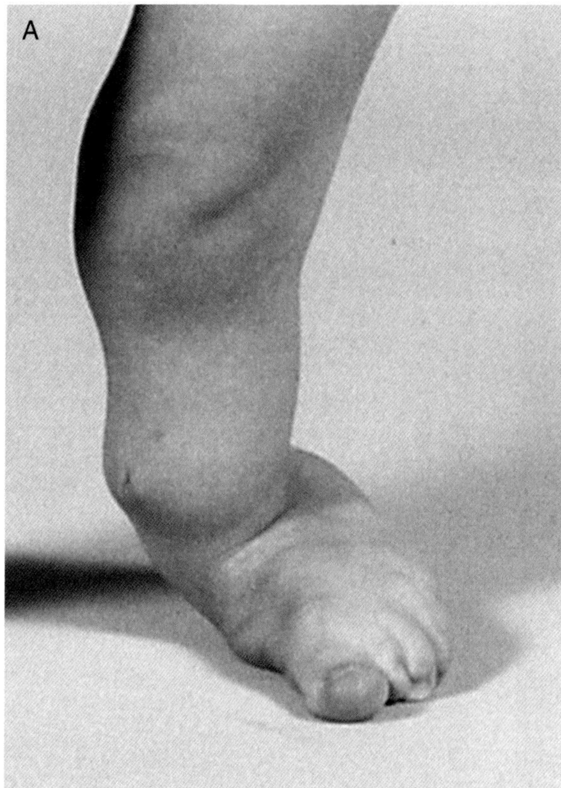

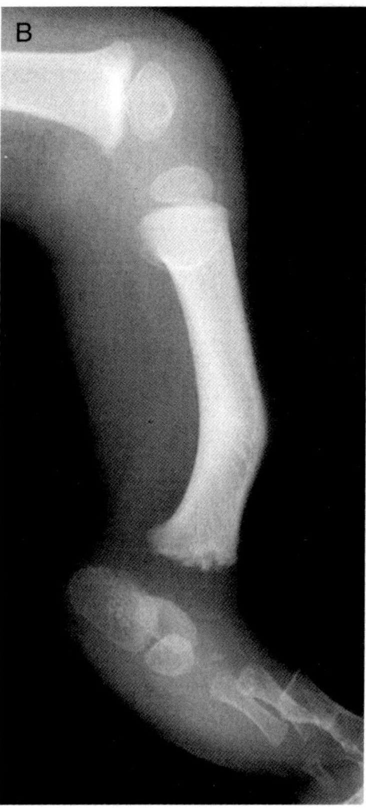

FIGURE 20-7 Apex anteromedial bowing of the tibia associated with congenital fibular deficiency in a one-year-old child. **A**. Clinical appearance. **B**. Radiographic appearance.

limitation of motion of both the ankle and the hindfoot. The presence of such contractures is logical in the context of the hypoplastic nature of the entire posterolateral lower leg as the defining morphological characteristic of congenital fibular deficiency. However, lengthening of the peroneal tendons and Achilles tendon alone, with or without ankle capsulotomy, will rarely resolve equinous or equinovalgus deformities associated with congenital fibular deficiency. There is invariably associated both bony deformity of the distal tibia and/or foot, and limited joint motion. Therefore, even if present, when repositioning of the foot into a plantigrade position is needed, soft tissue lengthening usually must be combined with osteotomy of the tibia to render the foot plantigrade (Figure 20-8).

3. Bony deformity of the hindfoot and the midfoot, causing both valgus and restricted motion of the hindfoot and midfoot. This is usually associated with tarsal coalition. The most common morphological appearance is that of subtalar coalition with a hypoplastic talus, talocalcaneal coalition, and lateral displacement of the calcaneus relative to the talus and lower leg (Figure 20-9). The consequence of this bony deformity is lateral translation of the hindfoot relative to the lower leg. Our experience is that the majority of such feet function asymptomatically and do not warrant intervention.

Clubfoot Deformity

An interesting, somewhat incongruous, foot anomaly associated with congenital fibular deficiency is that of true congenital equinovarus, or clubfoot. This deformity has been noted by several authors (1,7,14,54). It may occur with all the other clinical and radiographic morphological features of congenital fibular deficiency, including ray reduction and ball-and-socket ankle mortise (Figure 20-10). There are no reports of effective conservative management for congenital clubfoot associated with congenital fibular deficiency. Surgical correction has been described. It is possible that more effective conservative methods for clubfoot deformity correction such as that of Ponseti (64,72,73) or the French physical therapy method (25,27,50,75) may effect correction of this type of clubfoot deformity, but there are no reports of such successful treatment to date, nor have we experienced any.

The presence of a congenital clubfoot does not significantly influence decision making regarding the management of congenital fibular deficiency at our institution. We consider whether to recommend foot ablation based on the overall size of the foot, the severity of the limb shortening, and the family wishes, as described below. Based on our experience to date, however, we anticipate that surgical correction of the clubfoot will be required, prior to walking age. When such surgery is undertaken, it is very important for the surgeon to be cognizant of the cartilaginous structure of the ankle, hindfoot, and potentially midfoot. We perform a posteromedial release, but the surgeon must be aware of the abnormality of the ankle joint (either planar or ball-and-socket) and the almost certain presence of tarsal coalition, both talocalcaneal and potentially midfoot (talonavicular, calcaneocuboid, others, or combinations).

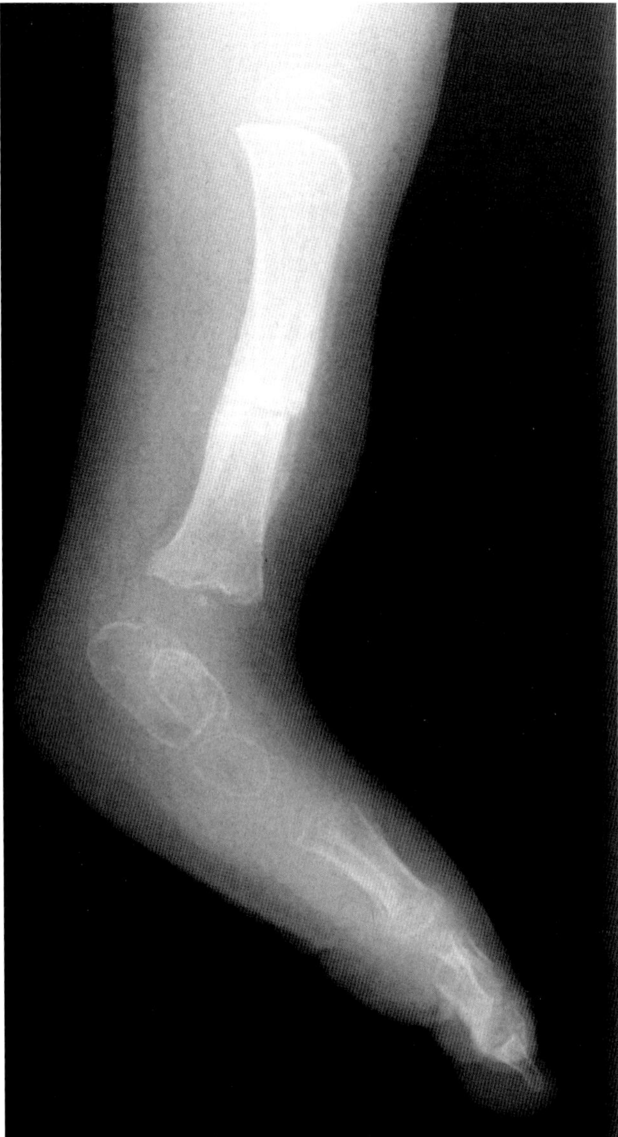

FIGURE 20-8 Correction of anteromedial bow of the foot and equinovalgus contracture at the age of fourteen months (same patient as Figure 20-7). Both osteotomy and soft tissue releases were required to render the foot plantigrade.

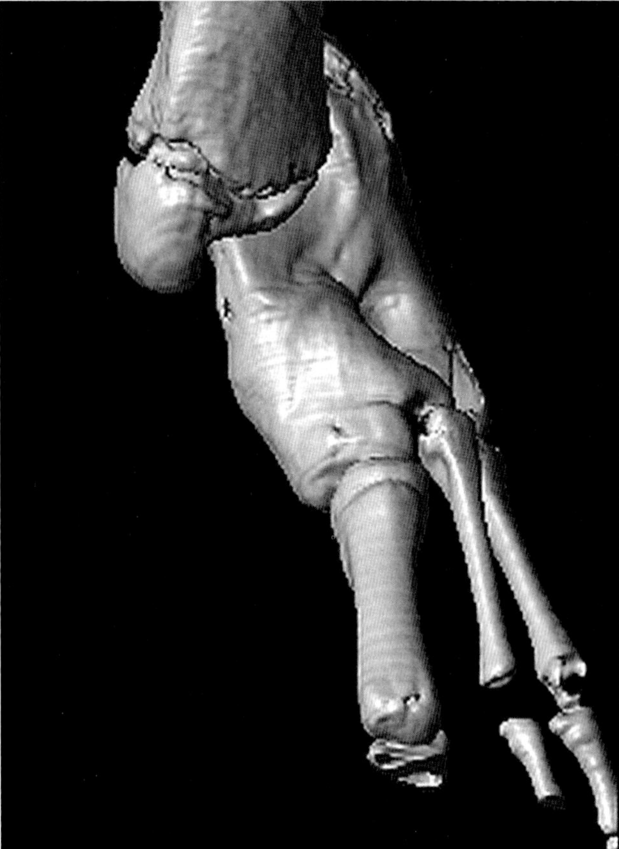

FIGURE 20-9 Fused talus and calcaneus identified on CT scan in a 14-year-old boy. Lateral translation of the calcaneus can be seen, creating an osseous valgus deformity of the hindfoot.

The foot will usually respond well to surgical release in that a stable, functionally plantigrade foot will be obtained and maintained. However, lateral displacement of the calcaneus relative to the talus may be present. We have not treated this last deformity by surgical separation of the talus and calcaneus. Typically, serviceable feet with mixed, off-setting deformities of distal tibial valgus, hindfoot lateral displacement, and forefoot supination, result (Figure 20-11A,B).

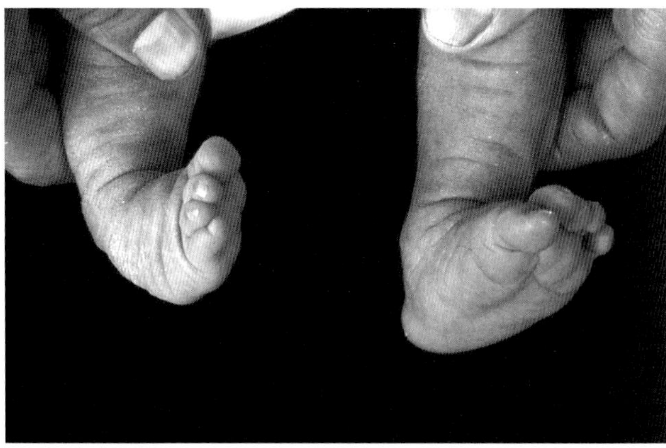

FIGURE 20-10 Congenital talipes equinovarus (clubfoot) in an infant with congenital fibular deficiency. Note the absent lateral ray.

Tarsal Coalition

One of the most common radiographic features of congenital fibular deficiency is that of tarsal coalition (1,14,20, 21,38,42,53,67,88,89). Talocalcaneal coalition is most common, but talonavicular, calcaneocuboid, others, combinations, or massive coalitions are all seen with congenital fibular deficiency (Figure 20-12). The coalitions rarely present problems of themselves but do contribute to the diminution of the foot both in length and in height. A relatively shortened hindfoot often contributes to the functional leg length discrepancy of the affected extremity; this results in reduced foot motion which may be partially offset by the presence of an associated ball-and-socket ankle mortise and may be a component of the valgus deformity secondary to the lateral displacement of the calcaneus to the talus. The most important aspect of tarsal coalition in congenital

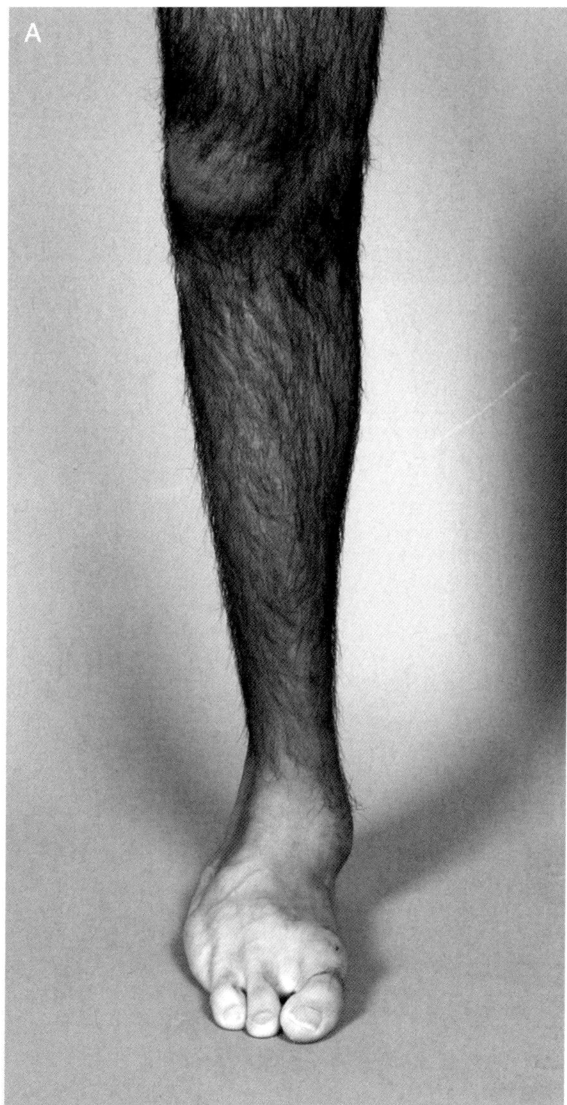

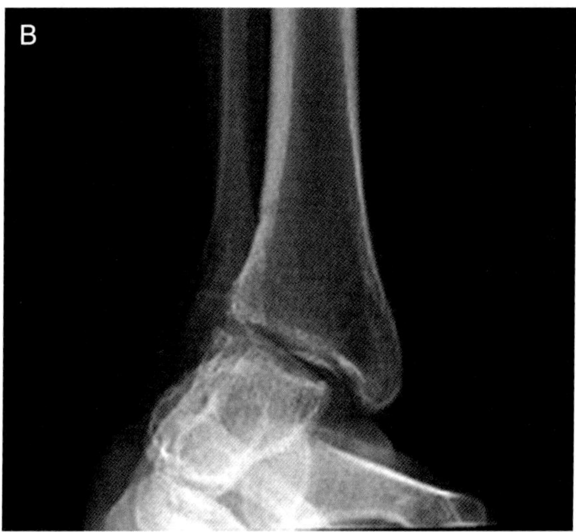

FIGURE 20-11 **A.** Clinical appearance of the foot of a 15-year-old boy with fibular deficiency treated by posteriomedial release at the age of one year. Patient is asymptomatic and active. **B.** Radiographic appearance of the ankle. Note the distal tibial valgus and planar ankle joint. Associated hindfoot valgus results in the functionally plantigrade foot noted in A. The options are surgical correction of both deformities, or no treatment (which was elected because the patient was asymptomatic).

fibular deficiency is the need for the surgeon to be aware of its presence when operating to render a foot plantigrade, particularly when associated clubfoot deformity requires surgical correction. Talocalcaneal coalitions tend to be formed such that the calcaneus is translated lateral to, rather than under, the talus (see Figure 20-9).

Ray Reduction

A hallmark of congenital fibular deficiency is some component of lateral ray reduction. The severity of this reduction varies from effectively none at all, to no true ray present, only some hindfoot and mid-foot remnant (Figure 20-13). In general, the severity of ray reduction is commensurate with the overall severity of the fibular deficiency, with respect to tibial shortening and deformity, fibular hypoplasia, and ankle deformity and stiffness.

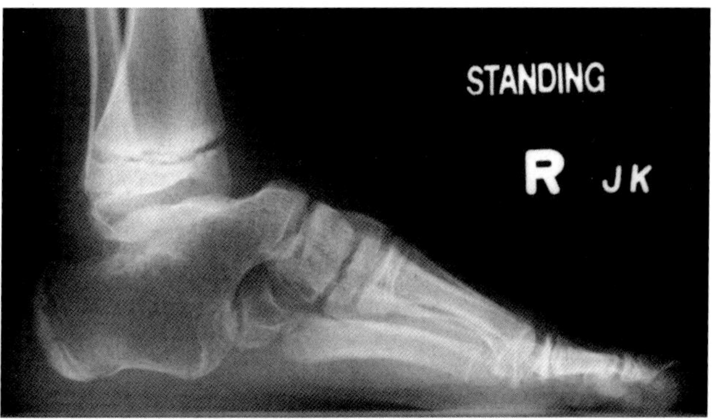

FIGURE 20-12 Tarsal coalition associated with congenital fibular deficiency in a 10-year-old boy. Note the solid bony mass of the fused talus and calcaneus.

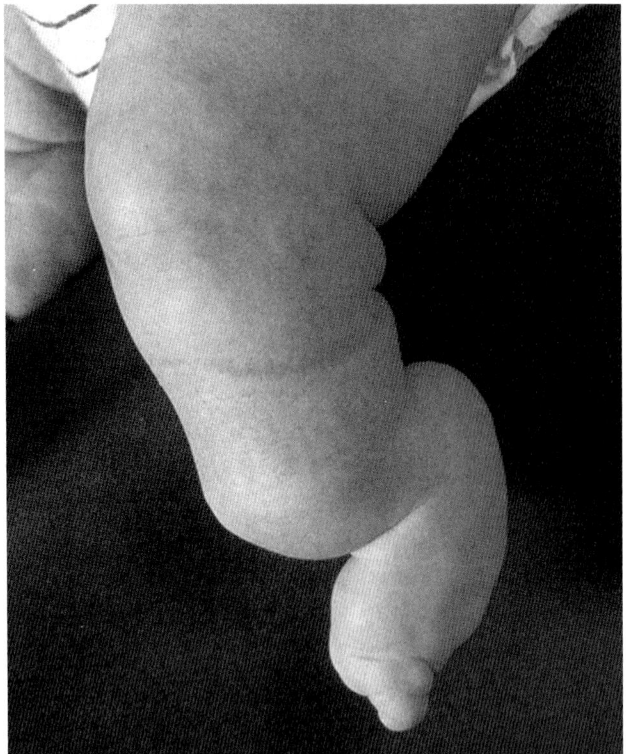

FIGURE 20-13 An infant with severe reduction of foot, with only a rudimentary hindfoot and solitary ray.

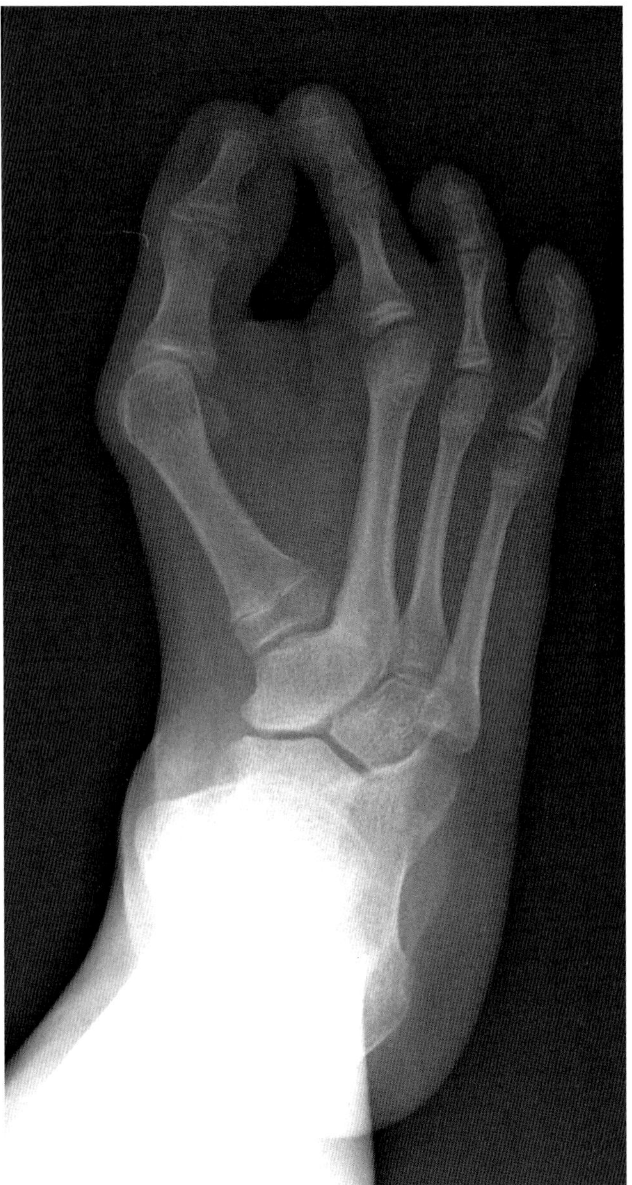

FIGURE 20-14 Twelve-year-old boy with fused, divergent residual rays associated with congenital fibular deficiency.

However, many exceptions to this generality exist, and each patient must have these components of the features of fibular deficiency assessed independently. Specifically, severe shortening and deformity of the lower leg may have a near-normal foot, or a relatively mild shortening may be associated with severe lateral ray reduction and ankle stiffness and deformity. The remaining rays are often normal in appearance, if reduced in size, but metatarsal fusions and toe syndactyly are occasionally seen in the residual rays (Figure 20-14). In our experience, the presence of these deformities have not required or specifically influenced treatment decisions.

The primary problem produced by ray reduction is the decreased volume of the foot, which may challenge the wearing of normal shoes. This issue may be overcome relatively easily by the fabrication of a "shoe filler" which can be formed to the existing foot and fit into a shoe of comparable size to the contralateral foot (Figure 20-15). In our experience, the severity of ray reduction correlates in most patients with the severity of associated shortening and ankle deformity, and in this context, at our institution, there is a correlation between number of residual rays and the likelihood that the surgeon and family elect SYME amputation as the primary definitive management of fibular deficiency.

Overview of the Primary Management of Congenital Fibular Deficiency

Treatment Alternatives

As we have noted above, the components of congenital fibular deficiency include limb shortening due to variable femoral and tibial shortening, distal femoral valgus and external rotation deformities, tibial angular deformity, ankle deformity, and foot deformity and lateral ray reduction. Controversy exists regarding indications for reconstructive limb salvage or primary foot ablation, as well as the appropriate extent and sequence of reconstructive surgeries (1,4,8,15,20,34,36, 41,43,45,54,60,62,81,86,92,98,99). It is a challenge to parents and surgeons alike to make a balanced, appropriate decision for the affected infant, particularly as reconstructive techniques continue to evolve and improve. No one can appropriately set "boundaries" of deformity severity beyond which amputation (only) is appropriate, or shy of which, reconstructive procedures including foot repositioning and limb lengthening (only) are indicated. As an example, not all patients or their parents are suited to tolerate the discomfort and discipline required to undergo limb lengthening with any reasonable hope of success. We have a number of

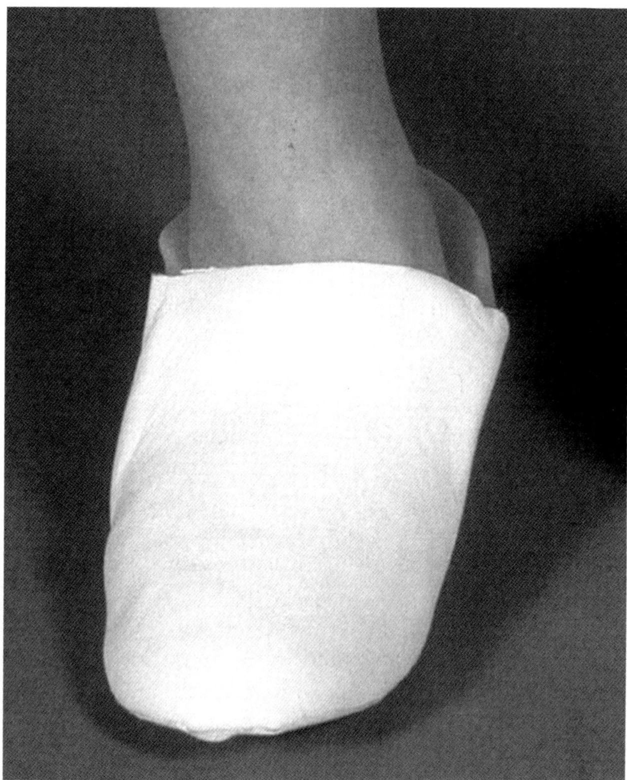

FIGURE 20-15 "Shoe filler" orthotic that may be custom fabricated to compensate for foot size reduction so that the patient may wear similar sized shoes.

patients who have declined both amputation and prosthetic fitting, or limb reconstruction, and who choose to function in an extension orthosis, or use no special aide whatsoever (Figure 20-16A,B).

In general, the primary decision parents and surgeons have to consider includes all the combined components of the deformity of congenital fibular deficiency. Their decision may vary from foot ablation and prosthetic fitting, to limb reconstruction including foot repositioning as needed or limb lengthening (repeated as needed, depending on the severity of deformity) representing the appropriate management course for the child. At our institution, we base that decision on a combination of a prediction of the extent of surgical treatment required (using our functional classification [8]), and we educate the parents by affording them the opportunity to interact with families who have chosen either amputation or limb salvage reconstruction for their children. In general, we encourage families to accept amputation as the definitive surgical management when we perceive that the foot will not function well (deformed, malpositioned, stiff, with three or fewer rays present) or when the extent of total limb shortening exceeds 30% of the contralateral limb, as surgical correction of such shortening will involve at least three separate stages of limb lengthening in our experience. We carefully counsel families with children with less severe deformities about the surgical treatments that will

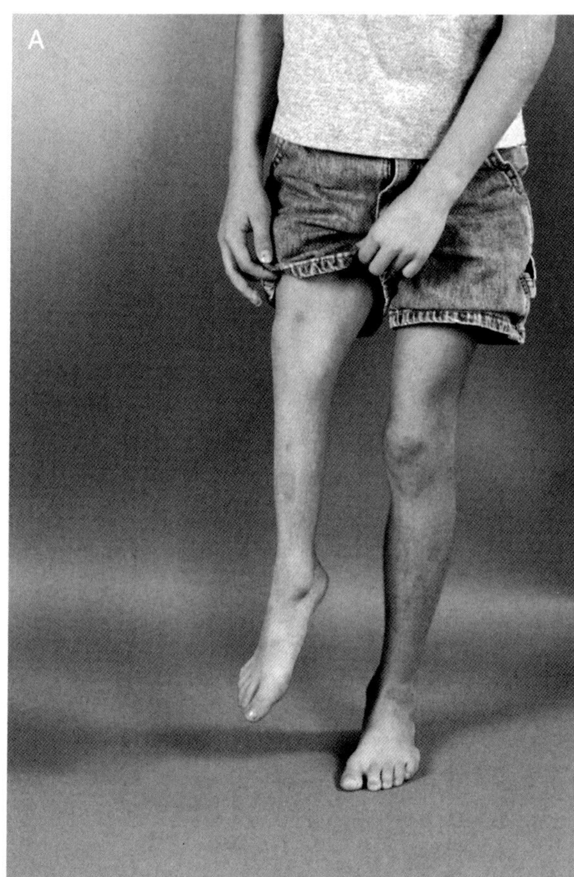

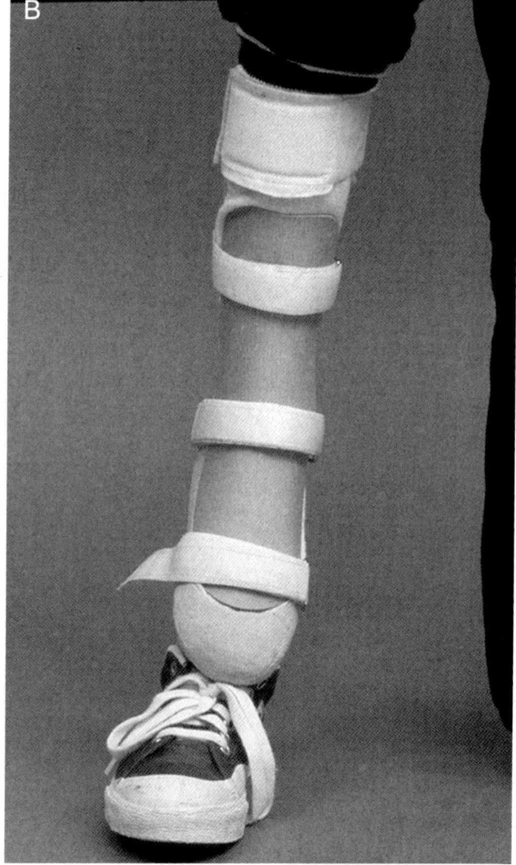

FIGURE 20-16 **A.** A 12-year-old girl with severe fibular deficiency and limb shortening who has declined amputation and limb salvage reconstruction surgery. **B.** Patient functions with a custom extension orthosis.

be required, because, once limb lengthening is involved, significant time and effort will be required of the families and their child. Based on current techniques, complications of limb lengthening requiring unplanned corrective surgeries occur with sufficient regularity as to be the norm (15,34,36,45,60,62,92,99). The major treatment alternatives, when the manifestations of congenital fibular deficiency are sufficiently severe that surgical treatment is required, are outlined below.

Syme Amputation

A mainstay of management of congenital fibular deficiency has long been Syme amputation (1,4,8,20,41,51,60,96,98). In children with congenital fibular deficiency, this procedure is effectively an ankle disarticulation. Because the fibula is by definition, hypoplastic, trimming or other reduction of the lateral malleolus is effectively never necessary (Figure 20-17). Several studies have documented the efficacy and long-term function of Syme amputation in the management of congenital fibular deficiency (7,60,96), and it remains an important surgical option for the more severe end of this spectrum. While Syme amputation may be performed at any age, our institution prefers to perform it just at the age when the child is learning to walk, as wound-healing and recovery occur relatively quickly. The child readily adapts to prosthetic fitting with effectively no training or education required.

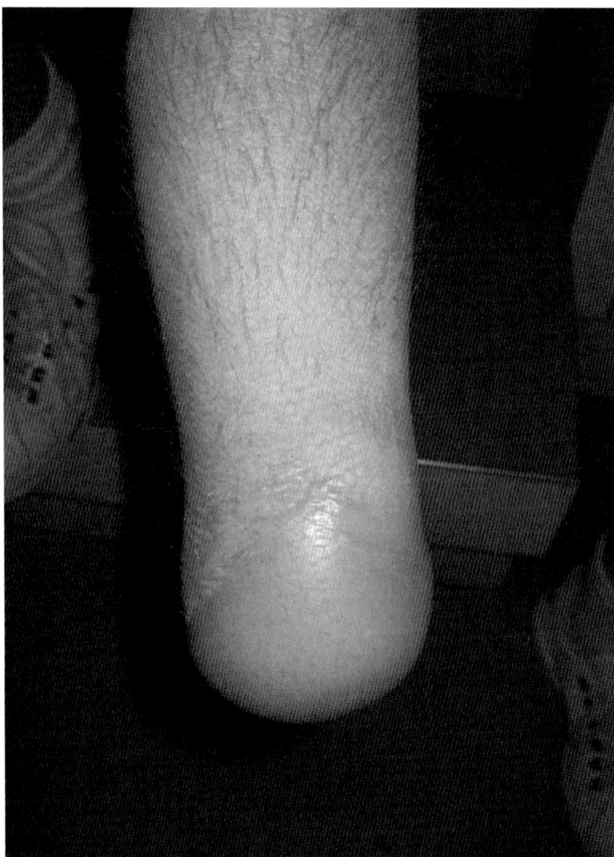

FIGURE 20-17 The hypoplasia or absence of the fibula and the associated hypoplasia of the distal tibia make malleolar "trimming" during Syme amputation unnecessary.

Boyd Amputation

The Boyd amputation is a variation of foot ablation preferred by some authors (10,60) (Figure 20-18). The procedure varies from Syme in that the calcaneus and heelpad are preserved and fused to the end of the tibia. The primary purpose is to avoid posterior slipping of the heelpad which can coour with Syme amputation (Figure 20-19) and may interfere with comfortable end-bearing on the residual limb either in or out of a prosthesis. The surgeon must manage two technical challenges: the talocalcaneal fusion if present, and the cartilaginous distal tibial epiphysis present when the procedure is performed in very young patients. Usually, the mass of talus and calcaneus are trimmed and afford a good fusion surface to the distal tibia. The distal tibial epiphysis including the physis is excised to provide good bone-to-bone contact between the distal tibia and the tarsal remnant. Otherwise, the indications for Boyd amputation in congenital fibular deficiency are similar to a Syme amputation.

Limb Salvage Reconstruction

Forms of fibular deficiency with relatively mild predicted final limb length inequality (less than eight centimeters)

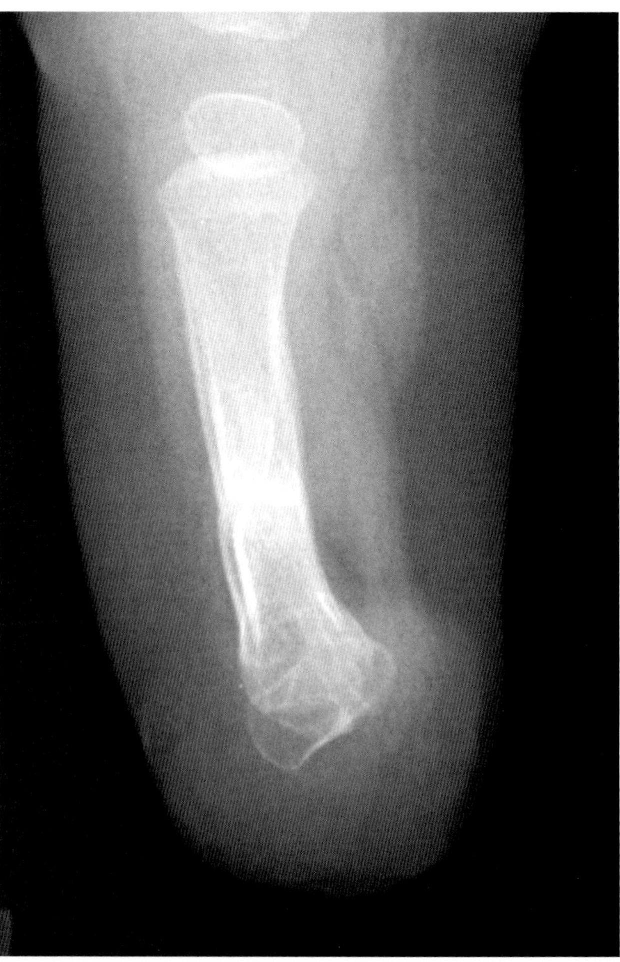

FIGURE 20-18 Boyd amputation consists of calcaneal (or talo-calcaneal mass) fusion to the distal tibia. This procedure helps prevent posterior displacement of the heelpad noted often after Syme amputation.

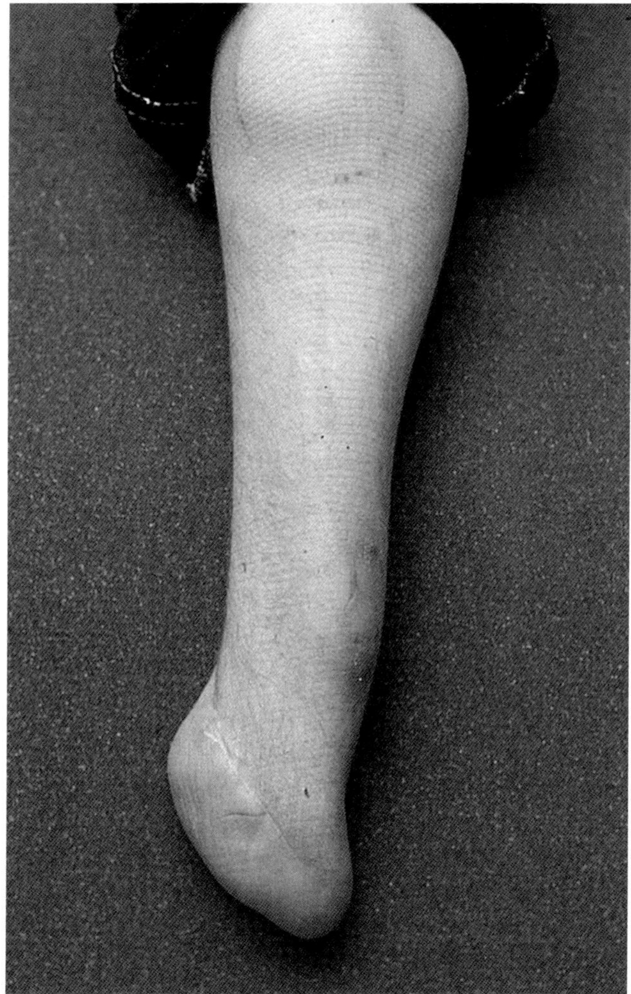

FIGURE 20-19 Posterior slipping of the heelpad after Syme amputation for congenital fibular deficiency. This patient was asymptomatic, as are most in our experience.

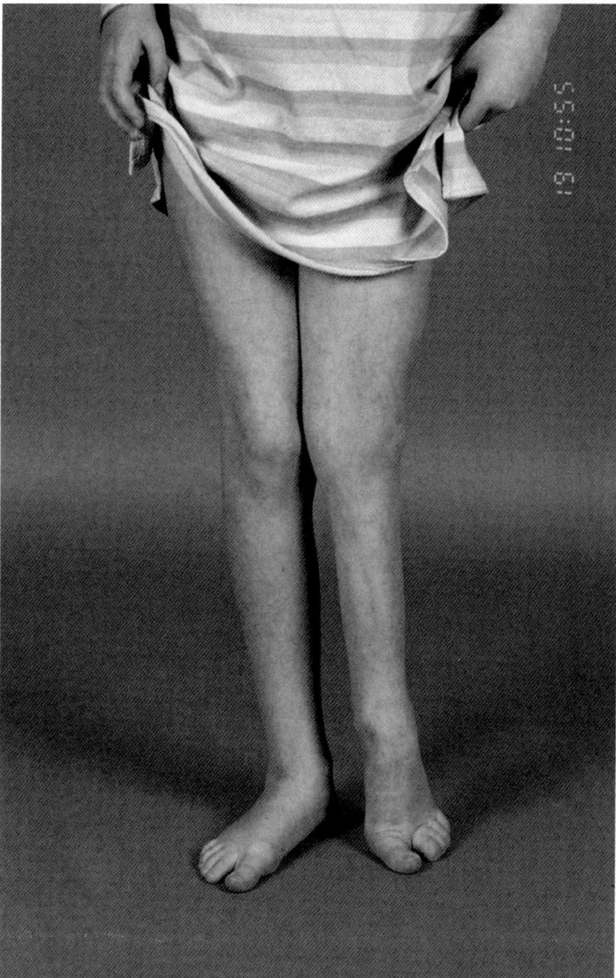

FIGURE 20-20 An 11-year-old girl with moderate shortening of the leg and severe equinus deformity. The patient walks unaided on the ball of the foot, and the stiffness of the hindfoot and ankle do not interfere with function. Limb lengthening and rendering the foot plantigrade risk the creation of stiffness-related foot symptoms.

can be managed by contralateral epiphysiodesis in the milder cases, or single-staged lengthening. Angular deformity correction of the ipsilateral distal femur, contralateral epiphysiodesis, or repositioning of the foot in a plantigrade position, may be combined with the primary surgical modalities of contralateral epiphysiodesis or ipsilateral limb lengthening, as dictated by the individual patient's deformity. In such cases, no specific foot deformity considerations are required, other than reposition for equinus or equinovalgus deformity, or associated clubfoot deformity, with the considerations described previously.

When more significant shortening is expected, and the surgeon and family have elected (staged) lengthening procedures, subsequent difficulty with the foot and ankle are frequent, as discussed previously. With relatively severe shortening, patients adopt a toe-toe gait to compensate for limb length inequality, with or without an associated fixed equinovalgus position of the foot. Most patients will adapt well to this position, either in or out of an extension orthosis (Figure 20-20), and the foot in this position is actually helpful in overcoming the limb length inequality. The lack of flexibility in the ankle due to associated deformity and contracture, and the foot itself due to tarsal coalition, may be overlooked when the patient is walking in such a fixed equinus position. The foot functions effectively as an extension post to compensate for the discrepancy, and the patient will weight-bear on the foot with relatively little complaint. Only the occasional patient develops symptomatic ankle instability that will require the use of an equinous ankle-foot-orthosis to stabilize the ankle (Figure 20-21). However, with successful lengthening, the foot will need to be brought into a plantigrade position, usually by a combination of soft tissue lengthening and/or distal tibial correcting osteotomy. At this point, the foot and ankle will frequently become symptomatic. Several factors may contribute to the development of such symptoms. The foot and ankle may be inherently stiff, which was immaterial and asymptomatic when the patient walked in a position of extreme equinus. Bony deformity previously considered minor when the weight-bearing surface of the foot was only the ball of the foot may become problematic because the

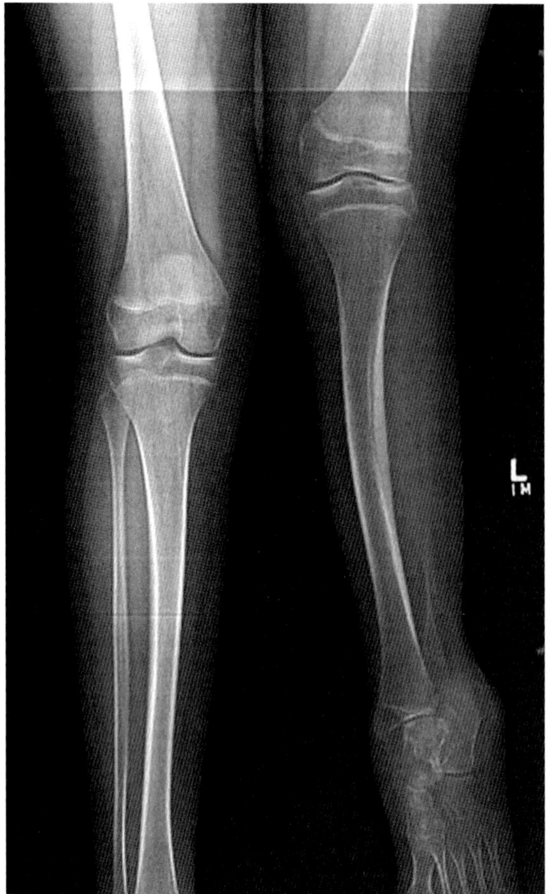

FIGURE 20-21 Radiographs of a 12-year-old girl with symptomatic ankle valgus. The patient walks with an equinous orthosis (similar to that depicted in Figure 20-16B) because of valgus ankle instability.

foot is neither truly plantigrade nor flexible. Finally, the tibio-talar joint may have become stiff or arthritic as a complication of limb lengthening. The currently limited literature and personal experience indicate that patients undergoing major limb lengthening reconstruction procedures for congenital fibular deficiency frequently ultimately require a tibio-talar fusion for symptomatic subluxation and/or arthritis (Figure 20-22A). Standard ankle arthrodesis procedures may be used to manage such symptoms (Figure 20-22B). The possible need for such fusion should be taken into account in deciding the best reconstructive options for each patient.

CONGENITAL TIBIAL DEFICIENCY

Classification of Tibial Deficiency

Congenital tibial deficiency is the least common of the three major lower limb congenital deficiencies. The condition is characterized by severe shortening of the lower leg due to the rudimentary or absent tibia, and the foot is typically in a position of extreme equninovarus due to the associated absence of a competent ankle mortise. Ironically, the medial rays of the foot may be duplicated. The condition may be unilateral or bilateral (30,48,49,70,76,78,82). Familial, autosomal dominant forms have been described (30,55,58, 59,61,63,74,76,77,84,87).

The most commonly used classification of congenital tibial deficiency is that of Jones (48) (Table 20-4), although other classification schemes have been described (49). Type I by definition has no ossified proximal tibial epiphysis at birth, and is subdivided into a Type IA and

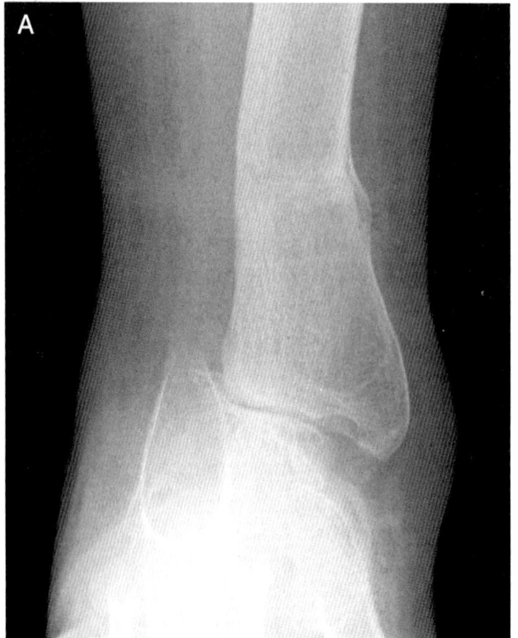

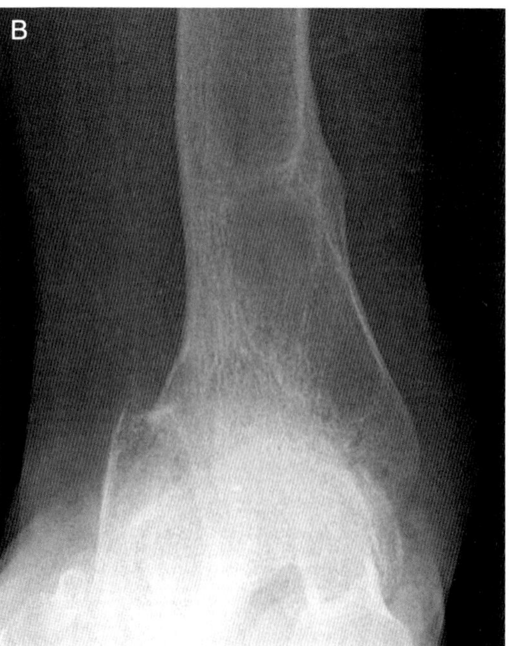

FIGURE 20-22 **A.** Lateral subluxation and degenerative changes in the planar ankle joint of a 15-year-old girl who has undergone two tibial lengthenings for shortening of the leg associated with congenital fibular deficiency. **B.** Tibio-talar arthrodesis was required after failure of conservative treatments.

TABLE 20-4

Jones Classification of Tibial Deficiency

Type	*Feature*	*Treatment Recommended*
IA	Proximal tibial epiphysis unossified at birth (tibia absent)	Brown procedure or knee disarticulation (recommended)
IB	Proximal tibial epiphysis unossified at birth (epiphysis present, ossifies later)	Similar to Type II
II	Proximal tibial epiphysis present, distal tibia absent	Fibular transfer to proximal tibial epiphysis, and foot ablation
III	Proximal tibial epiphysis absent, distal tibial epiphysis present	Knee disarticulation
IV	Tibio-fibular diastasis	Foot ablation OR Distal tibial-talar fusion and staged tibial lengthenings

Type IB. The distinction between these subtypes is crucial, in that Type IA has no proximal tibial epiphysis whereas type IB has a cartilaginous proximal tibial epiphysis which subsequently ossifies. Almost all type IA patients have effectively no knee, often no quadriceps, and therefore lack active knee extension. Brown (11) described a surgical procedure combining transposition of the fibular remnant to the femoral condylar notch and attempted reconstruction of the quadriceps mechanism into the transposed fibula. This procedure was most frequently combined with foot ablation, converting the limb into a functional below-knee or Syme amputation residual limb functionally. While some studies (19,47) have reported satisfactory outcome, others have demonstrated poor results with the Brown procedure, characterized by knee joint stiffness, poor extensor function, and flexion contracture (28,56,95)

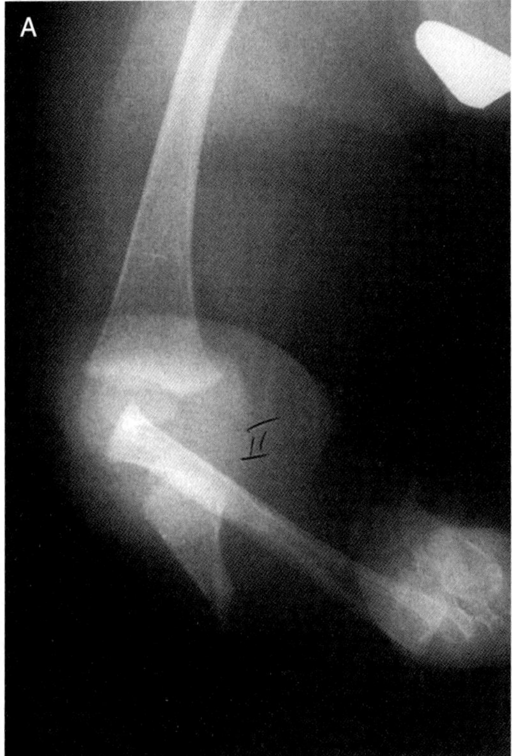

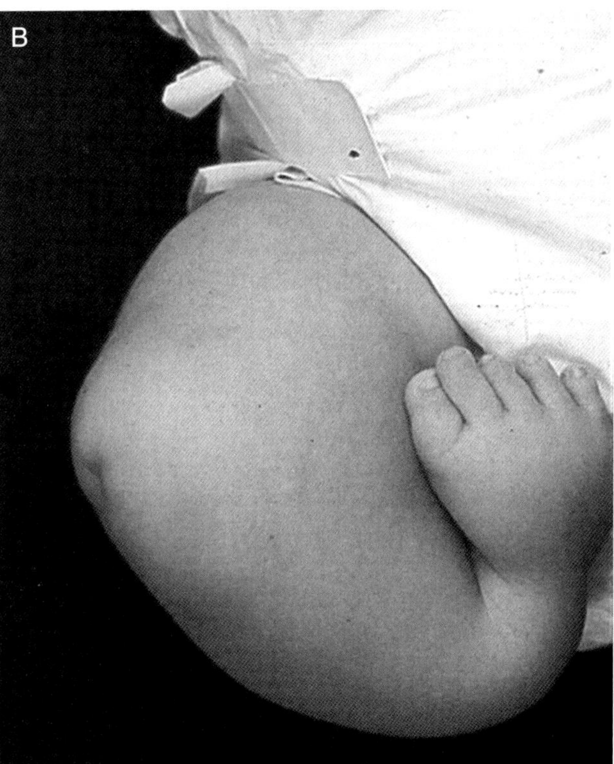

FIGURE 20-23 **A.** Radiographic appearance of congenital tibial deficiency, Jones Type II in an infant. There is preservation of the proximal tibia, but severe tibial shortening, no ankle mortise, and an unstable foot deformed in varus. **B.** Clinical appearance.

As a consequence, Type IA tibial deficiency patients are usually best served by knee disarticulation at walking age, and subsequent knee-disarticulation prosthetic fitting (30,49,55,56,70,78,82). Rarely, associated severe upper extremity deficiency requires preservation of the foot to serve as a prehensile grasp substitution. In such cases, amputation must be delayed until upper extremity substitution patterns have been clearly established.

Type IB is distinguished from Type IA by the (unossified at birth) presence of a cartilaginous upper tibial remnant, which appears on radiographs with subsequent growth and development. The distinction between the two types is important, because Type IB patients typically have preserved knee function, with both a congruent joint and intact quadriceps mechanism. Simple physical examination of the infant (palpation of the proximal tibial remnant and detection of active knee extension) will usually suffice to document the presence of the preserved proximal tibia. Ultrasonographic or MRI studies can confirm the presence of the unossified proximal tibia in unclear cases (26,37,53). Type IB deformity has the other characteristics of type IA tibial deficiency, which include severe shortening of the lower leg, no ankle mortise, and an unsupported foot in a varus position. Type IB patients may be treated similarly to type II tibial deficiency with transposition of the fibula to the tibial remnant to elongate the residual below-knee segment (described below). Theoretically, the foot may be stabilized on the distal end of the fibula, usually by tibio-talar arthrodesis (13,30,44,46,70,77,78,82,95). However, this obviously results in a very short lower limb with limited foot movement, generally in need of multiple lower leg lengthening procedures. Thus, amputation of the foot and below-knee prosthetic fitting is preferable in most cases.

Type II tibial deficiency is characterized by preservation of the proximal tibia (and with it, a functioning knee joint with competent quadriceps function). There is, however, severe lower leg shortening, no ankle mortise, and foot deformity as noted in type I deficiencies (Figure 20-23). These patients are usually best treated by a combination of Syme amputation and transfer of the fibular remnant to the residual tibia. The latter procedure results in a longer below-knee residual limb for easier prosthetic fitting and improved lever arm function. Preservation of the distal fibular epiphysis avoids symptomatic bony overgrowth which can be problematic with diaphyseal or metaphyseal amputations in children, requiring multiple revisions during growth. Often, the two procedures need to be staged (foot ablation at walking age to allow reasonable prosthetic fit, with fibular transfer deferred until the proximal tibial remnant and fibula have enlarged sufficiently to make the procedure technically feasible)(Figure 20-24).

Type III tibial deficiency is extremely rare (49,78). According to the Jones classification, the deformity is characterized by absence of the proximal tibia, with preservation of the distal tibia (and ankle mortise). Similar to Type IA, the absence of effective knee function in such deformity generally results in a limb deficiency best served by knee disarticulation and prosthetic fit at walking age. Occasionally, a patient's deformity is more aptly described as a global, central, severe shortening, with at least a rudimentary knee and ankle function (Figure 20-25A,B). In such patients, treatment must be individualized, and consideration given to knee disarticulation, Syme amputation, or an extension orthosis (49,78). Limb lengthening and reconstruction have not been described for this condition.

Type IV tibial deficiency is also referred to as "tibiofibular diastasis" (9,30,78,82,91,95), which aptly describes

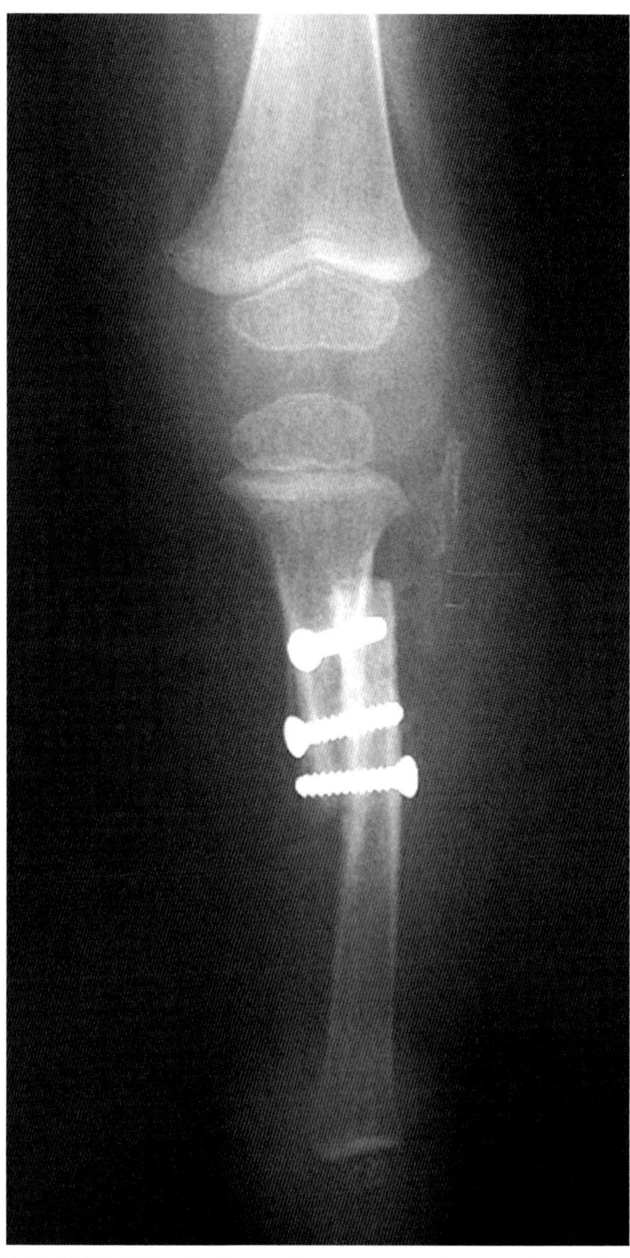

FIGURE 20-24 Radiographic appearance after transfer of the fibula to the proximal tibia in Type II tibial deficiency at the age of two years. This procedure creates a longer residual limb for below-knee prosthesis fitting. While this procedure may be combined with foot centralization and lengthening, it is more often combined with foot ablation.

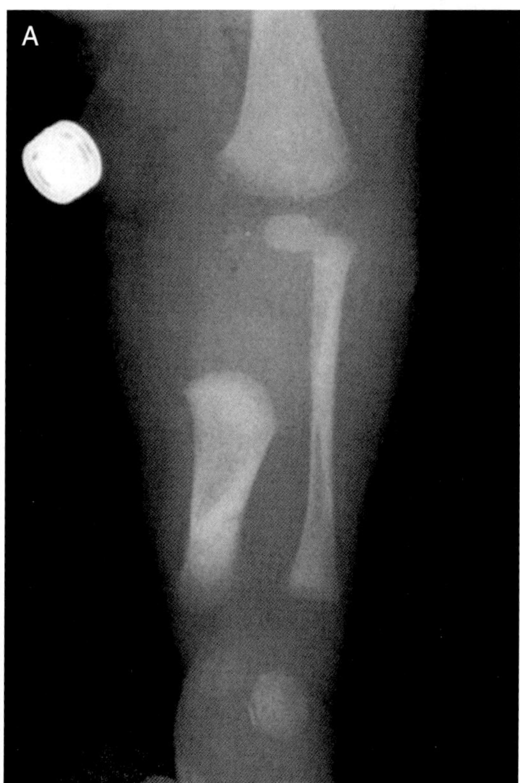

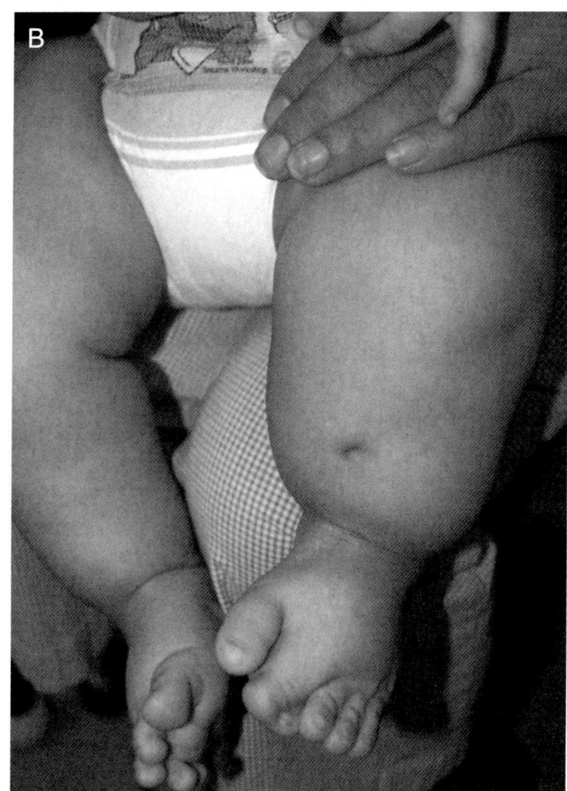

FIGURE 20-25 **A**. Radiographic appearance of Type III tibial deficiency in an infant. There is no true true proximal tibial articular surface, and the "knee" region is unstable. **B**. Clinical appearance at the age of 12 months.

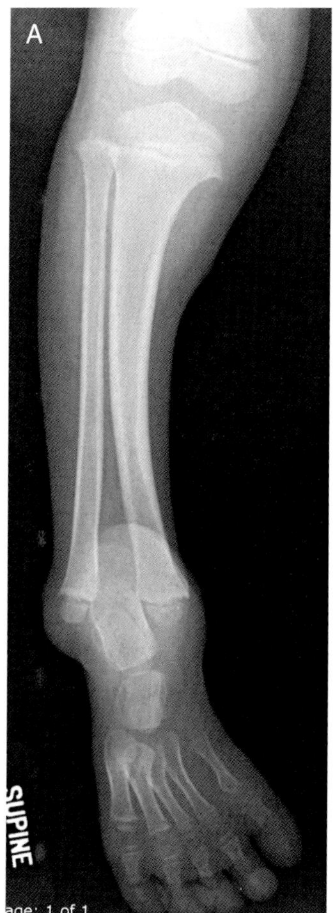

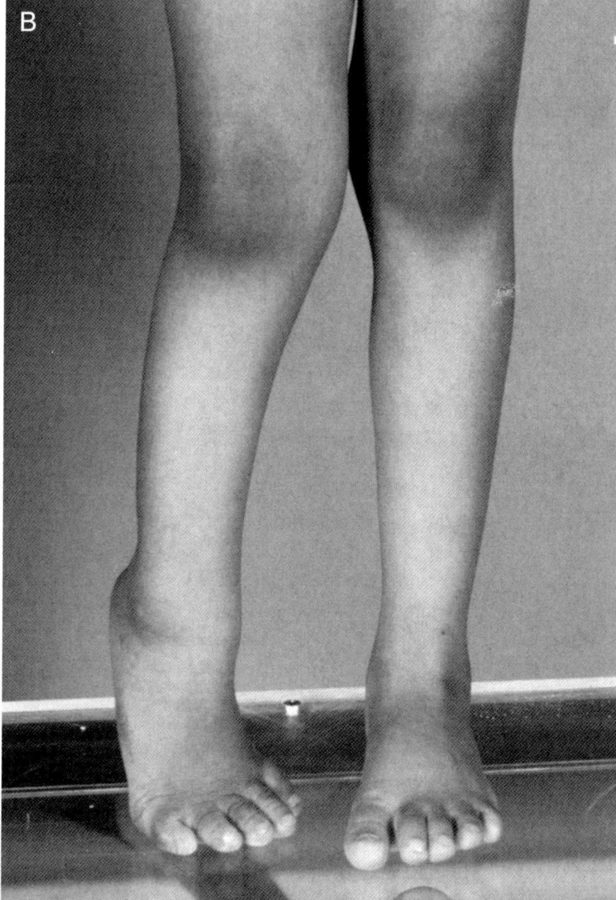

FIGURE 20-26 Type IV tibial deficiency, or "tibio-fibular diastasis." **A.** Radiographic appearance at the age of three years. Note distal divergence of the tibia and fibula, the absent ankle mortise, and the relative hypertrophy of the fibula. **B.** Clinical appearance at the age of three years. The foot is in a position of rigid equinous and internal rotation.

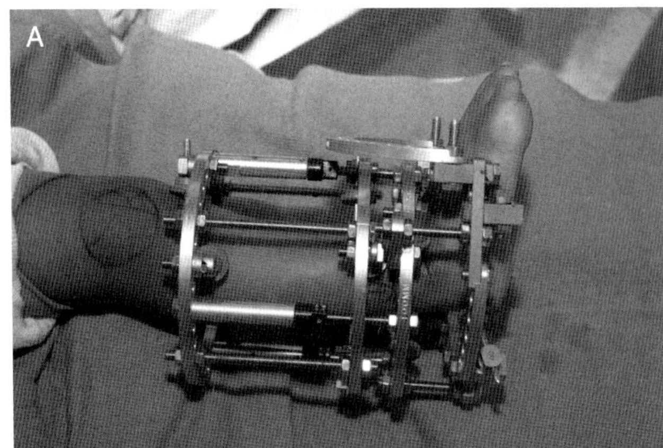

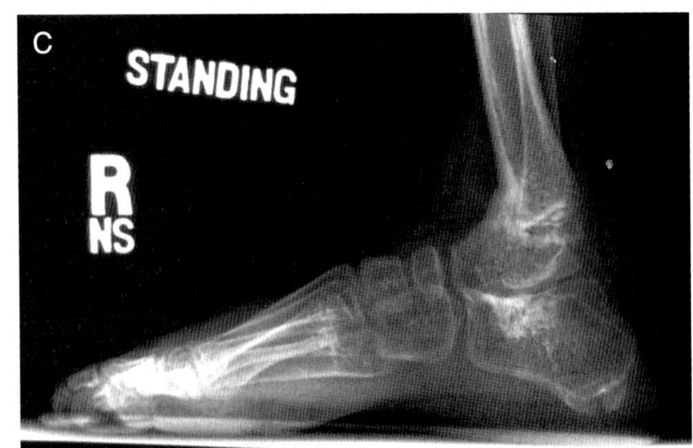

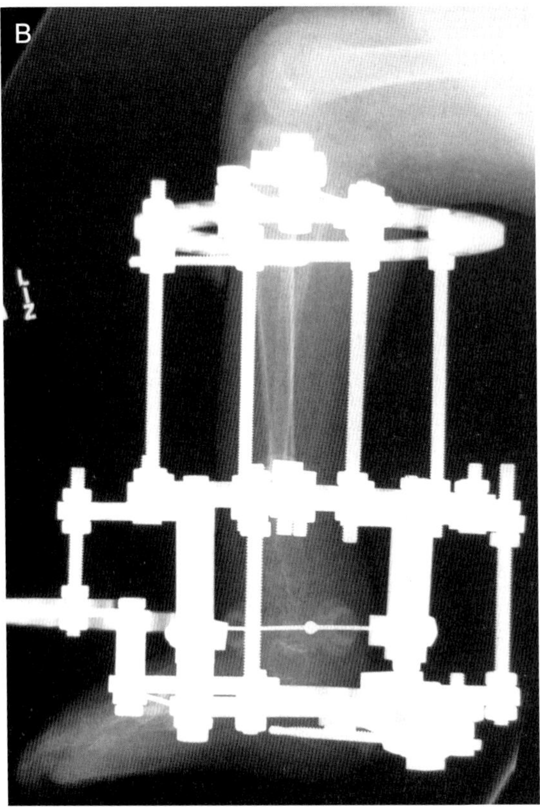

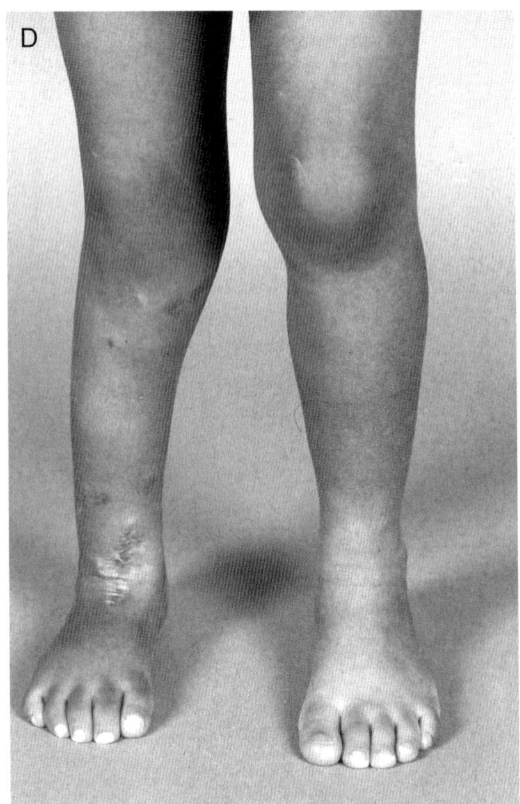

FIGURE 20-27 Staged reconstruction for Type IV tibial deficiency commenced at the age of five years. (Patient illustrated in Figure 20-26.) **A.** Clinical appearance after soft tissue release and application of Ilizarov circular fixator to translate foot distally to the level of the distal tibial epiphysis. **B.** Appearance after open tibio-talar fusion, and proximal tibial osteotomy for lengthening. **C.** Radiographic appearance after consolidation of the fusion and tibial lengthening site. The distal tibial physis has inadvertently incorporated into the fusion mass. **D.** Clinical appearance. Patient can now wear a shoe on the affected foot but requires a lift to compensate for residual leg length inequality. **E.** Radiographic appearance during second tibial lengthening at the age of 10 years. **F.** Clinical appearance after completion of second lengthening. A final lengthening (or contralateral epiphysiodesis) will be required to complete treatment of leg length inequality.

the clinical and radiographic features of this condition (Figure 20-26A,B). Similar to the other forms of tibial deficiency, there is usually pronounced lower leg shortening. Mildly affected children may have only modest lower leg shortening which may be overlooked in the neonatal period. The knee functions normally. There is a pronounced, clubfoot-like, equinovarus deformity of the foot, characterized by both extreme rigidity and significant internal rotation of the foot relative to the lower leg. The fibula will be noted to be longer than the tibia in most cases, and may be more substantial than the tibia (Figure 20-26A,B). Thus, the reconstructive challenges in type IV

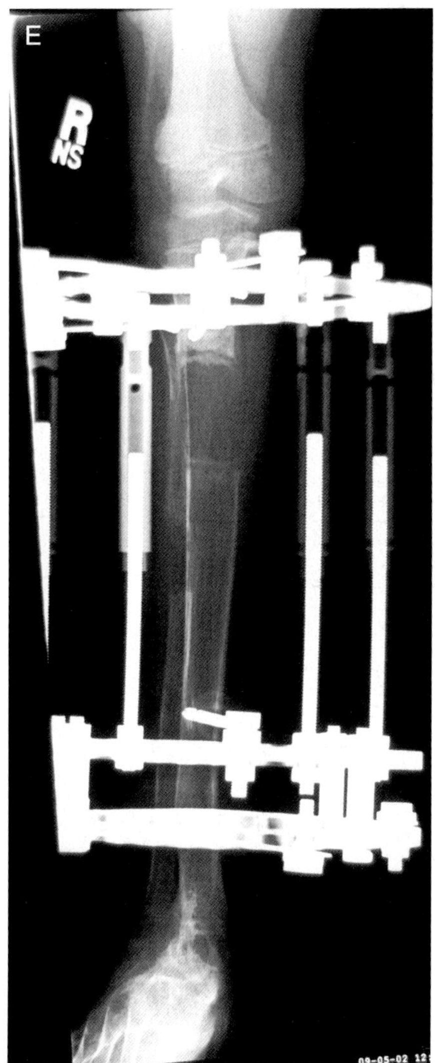

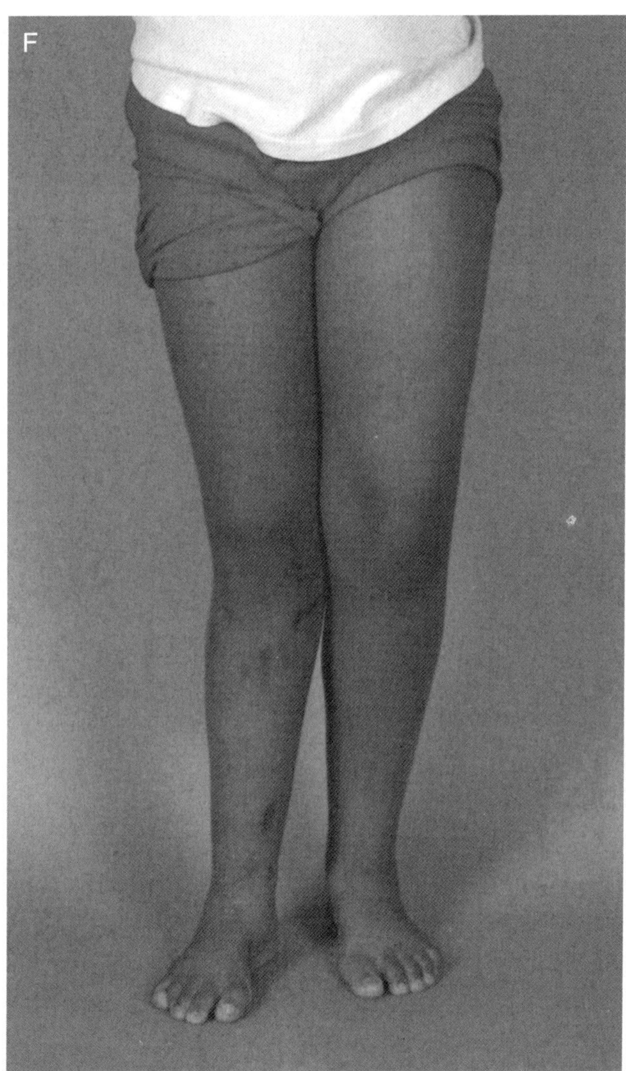

FIGURE 20-27 (*Continued*)

deficiency include significant tibial shortening, no ankle mortise to support the foot, and rigid equinovarus deformity of the foot. These challenges are effective resolved by Syme amputation, and this management is the most frequent accepted by children's families in our institution.

A limb salvage reconstructive option for Type IV tibial deficiency is to stabilize the foot on the distal tibia (i.e., by tibio-talar fusion) with staged lengthenings of the tibia (Figure 20-27). Significant proximal migration of the foot between the tibia and fibula as well as extreme plantar flexion and internal rotation are typical. As a consequence, either extensive shortening of the tibia to relax the soft tissues, or alternatively, surgical release, external fixation, and distal translation of the foot relative to the tibia are required to achieve a plantigrade foot.

An "unclassifiable" manifestation of congenital tibial dysplasia which does not fit within the Jones classification has been reported (24). This deformity is characterized by milder tibial shortening (often an apex anterolateral bow), relative fibular "overgrowth," and essentially normal knee and ankle morphology. There may be associated varus deformity of the foot and medial ray or digit duplications (Figure 20-28). Treatment consists of management of the limb length inequality as appropriate for the patient and reduction of the duplication.

CONGENITAL FEMORAL DEFICIENCY

Congenital femoral deficiency is of intermediate frequency, between congenital fibular deficiency and congenital tibial deficiency. The severity, complexity, and variability of the morphological characteristics of congenital femoral deficiency can confuse the inexperienced practitioner and thwart simple classification schemes. The range of associated joint abnormality adds further complexity to both classification systems and reconstructive strategies. Specifically, the hip may be stiff or unstable (to the extreme of

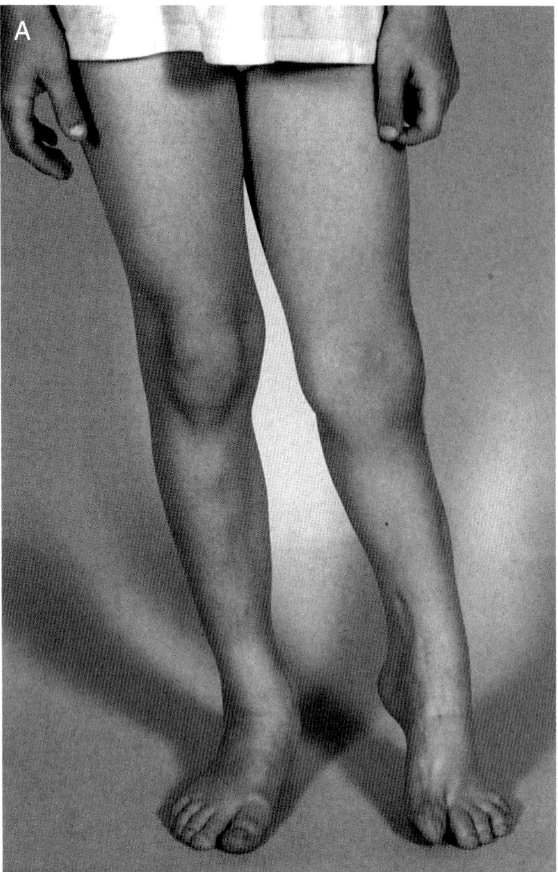

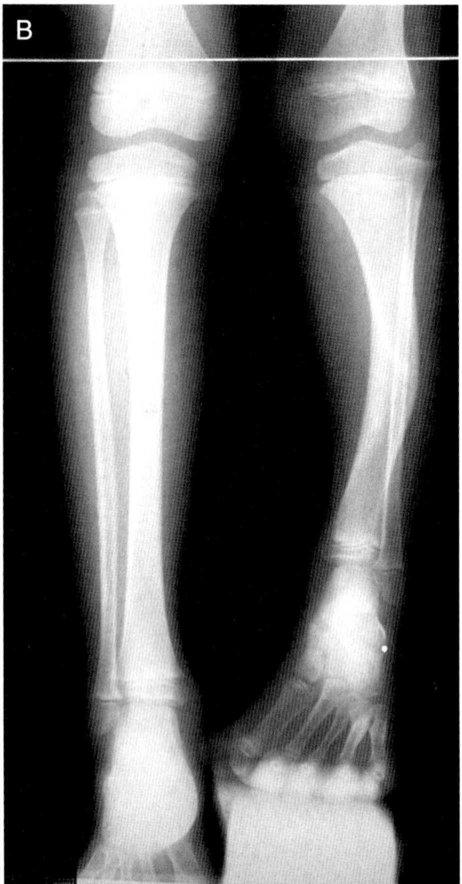

FIGURE 20-28 "Unclassifiable tibial deficiency". This congenital tibial deficiency is characterized by milder tibial shortening, occasional anterolateral bow, relative fibular overgrowth, comparatively normal knee and ankle joints, and pre-axial polydactyly or ray duplication. **A.** Clinical appearance in a patient aged eight years. **B.** Anteroposterior radiographic appearance prior to treatment.

complete absence), and while multiplanar knee instability is typical, flexion contracture and stiffness are sometimes present. The most important thing to appreciate regarding classification schemes for congenital femoral deficiency is that there are two schools of thought: those which separate "proximal femoral focal deficiency" (the most severe end of the spectrum) and congenital short femur (characterized by less severe femoral shortening and hip deficiency) and the "inclusive" classification schemes.

The most recognized classification scheme for proximal femoral focal deficiency (representing the most severe end of the spectrum of congenital femoral deficiency) is that of Aitken (2). Four "classes" are described: "A," where the upper femur is in severe varus with an apparent pseudarthrosis (which may ossify spontaneously); "B" where a true pseudarthrosis of the upper femur is present; "C" where the femoral head and acetabulum are severely dysplastic; and "D," where the femoral head and acetabulum are absent. All these groups look and function similarly: the thigh is extremely shortened and funnel-shaped, with a poorly-functioning hip in a position of flexion, abduction, and external rotation.

The congenital femoral deficiency classifications of Pappas (68) and Gillespie and Torode (35) include both the proximal femoral focal deficiency variants at the severe end of the spectrum, and less severe shortening and femoral deformity at the milder. Gillespie and Torode (35) classify all congenital femoral deficiencies into three types:

A. "Femur long enough" for lengthening. The foot of the affected leg, drawn to full length, reaches the mid-tibia level of the contralateral leg (Figure 20-29). These patients may be considered for (staged) femoral lengthening, depending on associated hip and knee deformities, family expectations, and patient tolerance. The milder forms share the morphologic characteristics noted in the femora of many patients with congenital fibular deficiency, specifically, femoral shortening, distal femoral valgus deformity, and increased external rotation of the limb. Proximal femoral varus or valgus and acetabular dysplasia may be present.
B. "Femur too short" for lengthening. When the affected limb is drawn to full length against the contralateral, the foot does not reach the level of the contralateral

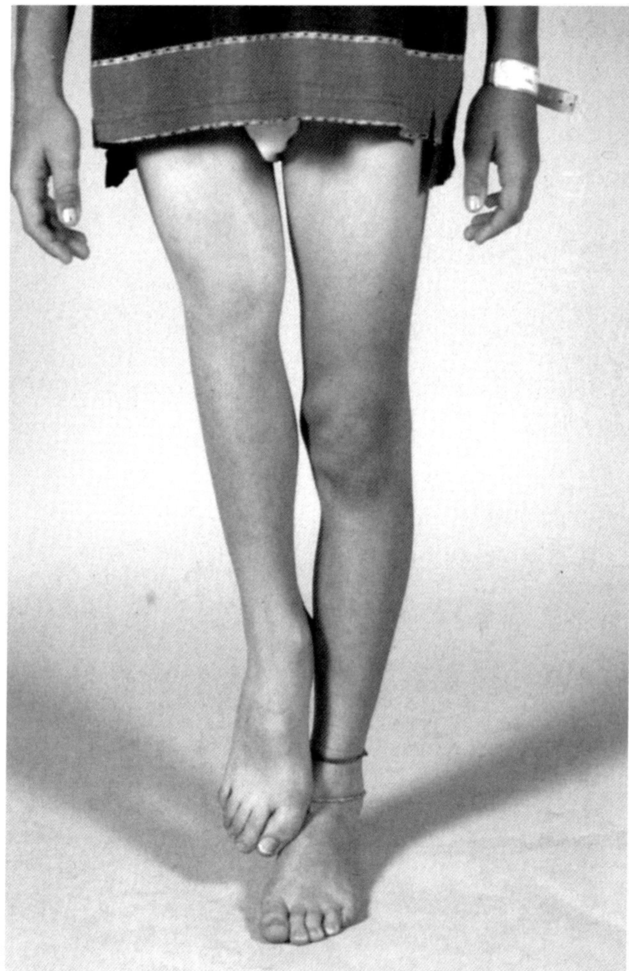

FIGURE 20-29 Congenital femoral deficiency, Gillespie and Torode Type "A" (femur long enough) as seen in a 10-year-old boy. The foot of the affected leg reaches the level of the contralateral mid-tibia. The patient is a potential candidate for (staged) lengthening procedures.

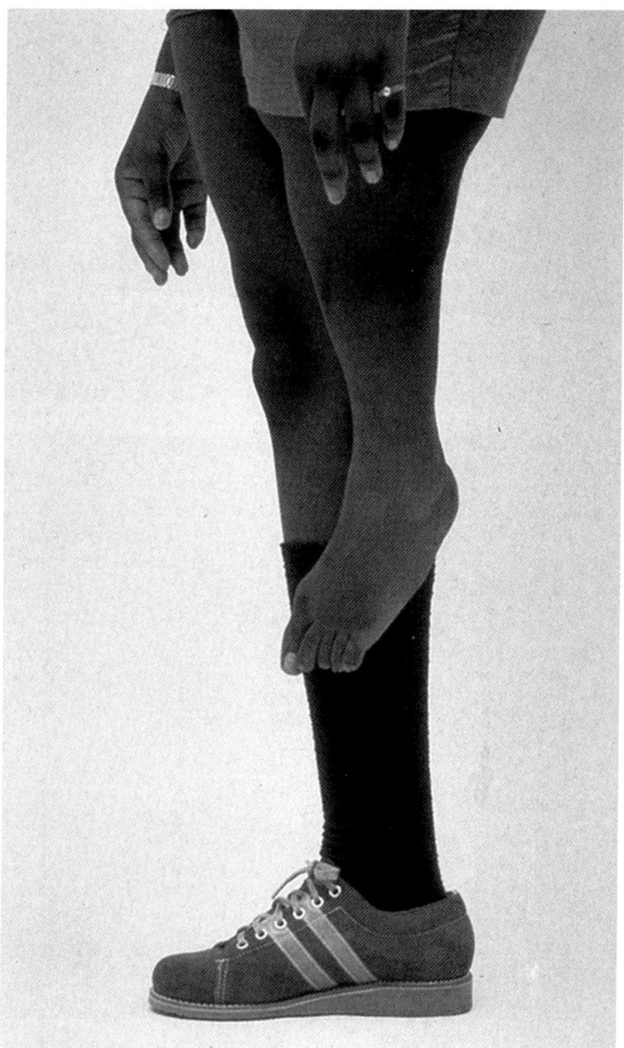

FIGURE 20-30 Congenital femoral deficiency, Gillespie and Torode Type "B" (femur too short) in a five-year-old girl who has refused reconstructive treatments. The foot of the affected leg does not reach the level of the contralateral mid-tibia. The patient will normally be a candidate for reconstruction to maximize function in a prosthesis.

mid-tibia (Figure 20-30). Amputation, rotationplasty (3,31,39,93), and other residual limb reconstructions to enhance function in a prosthesis or extension orthosis are usually recommended. The short, abducted and flexed, funnel-shaped thigh can make prosthetic fit challenging.

C. "Femur is too short." These patients are similar to "B," but have effectively no femur, and as such, may not have the flexed, abducted deformity that challenge prosthetic fitting in "B" patients.

In the severest forms of congenital femoral deficiencies, including Gillespie and Torode types "B" and "C", the challenges of limb salvage reconstruction required due to the marked limb shortening and associated hip and knee deformities are considered beyond the scope of limb salvage reconstruction by most centers. Reports of detailed evaluation of limb function after major staged reconstructions these severest forms of congenital femoral deficiency are currently lacking. As a consequence, reconstructive efforts usually aim to maximize limb function in a prosthesis or extension orthosis. One option to be considered for the severest forms of congenital femoral deficiency is rotationplasty, either as described by Van Nes (94) or Brown (12) (Figure 20-31A-C). In both of these reconstructive options, the strength and mobility of the foot must be taken into consideration (3,31,39,93). Associated congenital fibular deficiency with attendant ankle instability, stiffness, or deformity, or appreciable ray reduction, will usually make efforts (unrealistic) at rotationplasty with the goal of using the foot/ankle complex to serve as a knee. In such cases, prosthetic management with or without foot amputation and knee fusion

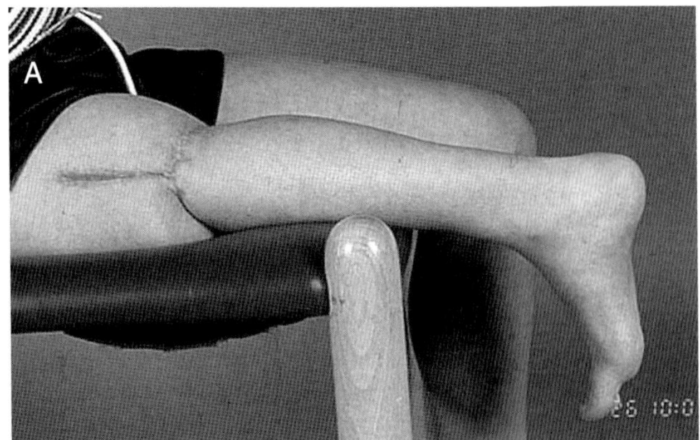

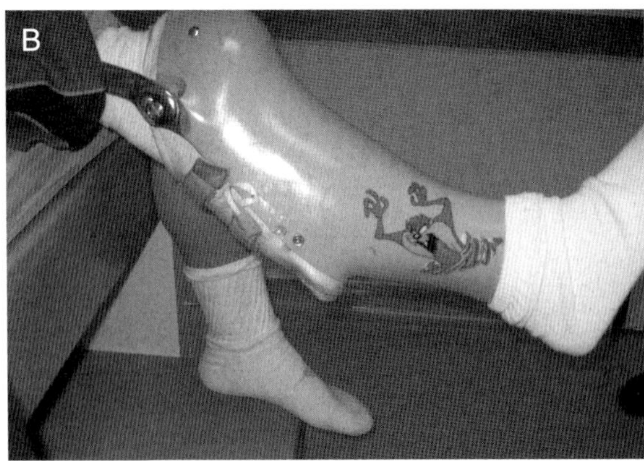

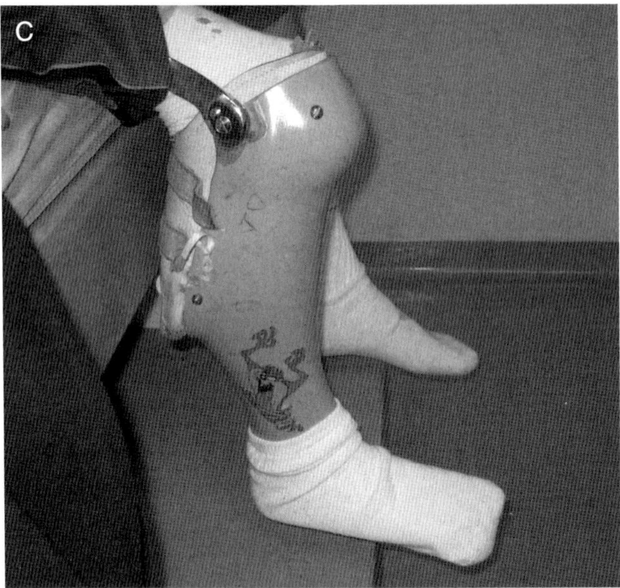

FIGURE 20-31 Rotationplasty for congenital femoral deficiency, Type "B". The patient has undergone a knee fusion, with external rotation of the leg through the fusion site and a second tibial osteotomy. **A.** Clinical appearance of the residual limb at the age of twelve years. Note the position of the foot. **B.** Prosthesis being held in extension by ankle plantarflexion. **C.** Prosthesis being held in flexion by ankle dorsiflexion.

typically provide the most expedient and functional outcome in management of children with this deformity.

REFERENCES

1. Achterman C, Kalamchi A. Congenital deficiency of the fibula. *J Bone Joint Surg Br* 1979; 61–B:133–137.
2. Aitken GT. Proximal femoral focal deficiency - definition, classification, and management. In: Aitken GT, ed. *Proximal Femoral Focal Deficiency. A Congenital Anomaly.* Washington D.C.: National Academy of Sciences, 1969:1–22.
3. Alman BA, Krajbich JI, Hubbard S. Proximal femoral focal deficiency: results of rotationplasty and Syme amputation. *J Bone Joint Surg Am* 1995; 77:1876–1882.
4. Anderson L, Westin GW, Oppenheim WL. Syme amputation in children: indications, results, and long-term follow-up. *J Pediatr Orthop* 1984; 4:550–554.
5. Baek GH, Kim JK, Chung MS, Lee SK. Terminal hemimelia of the lower extremity: absent lateral ray and a normal fibula. *Int Orthop* 2008; 32:263–267.
6. Bettin D, Karbowski A, Schwering L. Congenital ball-and-socket anomaly of the ankle. *J Pediatr Orthop* 1996; 16:492–496.
7. Birch JG, Lincoln TL, Mack PW. Chapter 14: Functional classification of fibular deficiency. In: Herring JA, Birch JG, eds. *The child with a limb deficiency.* Rosemont: American Academy of Orthopaedic Surgeons, 1998:161–170.
8. Birch JG, Walsh SJ, Small JM, et al. Syme amputation for the treatment of fibular deficiency. An evaluation of long-term physical and psychological functional status. *J Bone Joint Surg Am* 1999; 81:1511–1518.
9. Blauth W, Hippe P. The surgical treatment of partial tibial deficiency and ankle diastasis. *Prosthet Orthot Int* 1991; 15: 127–130.
10. Blum CE, Kalamchi A. Boyd amputations in children. *Clin Orthop Relat Res* 1982:138–143.
11. Brown FW. Construction of a knee joint in congenital total absence of the tibia (paraxial hemimelia tibia): A preliminary report. *J Bone Joint Surg Am* 1965; 47:695–704.
12. Brown KL. Resection, rotationplasty, and femoropelvic arthrodesis in severe congenital femoral deficiency. A report of the surgical technique and three cases. *J Bone Joint Surg Am* 2001; 83–A: 78–85.

13. Carranza-Bencano A, Gonzalez-Rodriguez E. Unilateral tibial hemimelia with leg length inequality and varus foot: external fixator treatment. *Foot Ankle Int* 1999; 20:392–396.
14. Caskey PM, Lester EL. Association of fibular hemimelia and clubfoot. *J Pediatr Orthop* 2002; 22:522–525.
15. Catagni MA, Bolano L, Cattaneo R. Management of fibular hemimelia using the Ilizarov method. *Orthop Clin North Am* 1991; 22:715–722.
16. Cetinus E, Uzel M, Bilgic E, Karaoguz A. [A case of ball-and-socket deformity of the ankle joint]. *Acta Orthop Traumatol Turc* 2003; 37:406–409.
17. Channon GM, Brotherton BJ. The ball and socket ankle joint. *J Bone Joint Surg Br* 1979; 61:85–89.
18. Choi IH, Lipton GE, Mackenzie W, Bowen JR, Kumar SJ. Wedge-shaped distal tibial epiphysis in the pathogenesis of equinovalgus deformity of the foot and ankle in tibial lengthening for fibular hemimelia. *J Pediatr Orthop* 2000; 20:428–436.
19. Christini D, Levy EJ, Facanha FA, Kumar SJ. Fibular transfer for congenital absence of the tibia. *J Pediatr Orthop* 1993; 13:378–381.
20. Coventry MB, Johnson EW. Congenital absence of the fibula. *J Bone Joint Surg* 1952; 34–A:941–955.
21. Cuervo M, Albinana J, Cebrian J, Juarez C. Congenital hypoplasia of the fibula: clinical manifestations. *J Pediatr Orthop B* 1996; 5:35–38.
22. Davidson WH, Bohne WH. The Syme amputation in children. *J Bone Joint Surg Am* 1975; 57:905–909.
23. Dennis DA, Clayton ML, Ferlic DC. Osteoarthritis associated with a ball-and-socket ankle joint. A case report. *Clin Orthop Relat Res* 1987:196–200.
24. Devitt AT, O'Donnell T, Fogarty EE, Dowling FE, Moore DP. Tibial hemimelia of a different class. *J Pediatr Orthop* 2000; 20:616–622.
25. Dimeglio A, Bonnet F, Mazeau P, De Rosa V. Orthopaedic treatment and passive motion machine: consequences for the surgical treatment of clubfoot. *J Pediatr Orthop B* 1996; 5:173–180.
26. Dreyfus M, Baldauf JJ, Rigaut E, Clavert JM, Gasser B, Ritter J. Prenatal diagnosis of unilateral tibial hemimelia. *Ultrasound Obstet Gynecol* 1996; 7:205–207.
27. El-Hawary R, Karol LA, Jeans KA, Richards BS. Gait analysis of children treated for clubfoot with physical therapy or the Ponseti cast technique. *J Bone Joint Surg Am* 2008; 90:1508–1516.
28. Epps CH, Jr., Tooms RE, Edholm CD, Kruger LM, Bryant DD, 3rd. Failure of centralization of the fibula for congenital longitudinal deficiency of the tibia. *J Bone Joint Surg Am* 1991; 73:858–867.
29. Exner GU. Bending osteotomy through the distal tibial physis in fibular hemimelia for stable reduction of the hindfoot. *J Pediatr Orthop B* 2003; 12:27–32.
30. Fernandez-Palazzi F, Bendahan J, Rivas S. Congenital deficiency of the tibia: a report on 22 cases. *J Pediatr Orthop B* 1998; 7:298–302.
31. Fowler EG, Hester DM, Oppenheim WL, Setoguchi Y, Zernicke RF. Contrasts in gait mechanics of individuals with proximal femoral focal deficiency: Syme amputation versus Van Nes rotational osteotomy. *J Pediatr Orthop* 1999; 19:720–731.
32. Fulp T, Davids JR, Meyer LC, Blackhurst DW. Longitudinal deficiency of the fibula. Operative treatment. *J Bone Joint Surg Am* 1996; 78:674–682.
33. Gaine WJ, McCreath SW. Syme's amputation revisited: a review of 46 cases. *J Bone Joint Surg Br* 1996; 78:461–467.
34. Gibbons PJ, Bradish CF. Fibular hemimelia: a preliminary report on management of the severe abnormality. *J Pediatr Orthop B* 1996; 5:20–26.
35. Gillespie R, Torode IP. Classification and management of congenital abnormalities of the femur. *J Bone Joint Surg Br* 1983; 65:557–568.
36. Griffith SI, McCarthy JJ, Davidson RS. Comparison of the complication rates between first and second (repeated) lengthening in the same limb segment. *J Pediatr Orthop* 2006; 26:534–536.
37. Grissom LE, Harcke HT, Kumar SJ. Sonography in the management of tibial hemimelia. *Clin Orthop Relat Res* 1990:266–270.
38. Grogan DP, Holt GR, Ogden JA. Talocalcaneal coalition in patients who have fibular hemimelia or proximal femoral focal deficiency. A comparison of the radiographic and pathological findings. *J Bone Joint Surg Am* 1994; 76:1363–1370.
39. Hamel J, Winkelmann W, Becker W. A new modification of rotationplasty in a patient with proximal femoral focal deficiency Pappas type II. *J Pediatr Orthop B* 1999; 8:200–202.
40. Herring JA, Barnhill B, Gaffney C. Syme amputation. An evaluation of the physical and psychological function in young patients. *J Bone Joint Surg Am* 1986; 68:573–578.
41. Herring JA. Symes amputation for fibular hemimelia: a second look in the Ilizarov era. *Instr Course Lect* 1992; 41:435–436.
42. Hiroshima K, Kurata Y, Nakamura M, Ono K. Ball-and-socket ankle joint: anatomical and kinematic analysis of the hindfoot. *J Pediatr Orthop* 1984; 4:564–568.
43. Hootnick D, Boyd NA, Fixsen JA, Lloyd-Roberts GC. The natural history and management of congenital short tibia with dysplasia or absence of the fibula. *J Bone Joint Surg Br* 1977; 59:267–271.
44. Hosny GA. Treatment of tibial hemimelia without amputation: preliminary report. *J Pediatr Orthop B* 2005; 14:250–255.
45. Jasiewicz B, Kacki W, Koniarski A, Kasprzyk M, Zarzycka M, Tesiorowski M. Leg lengthening in patients with congenital fibular hemimelia. *Ortop Traumatol Rehabil* 2002; 4:413–420.
46. Javid M, Shahcheraghi GH, Nooraie H. Ilizarov lengthening in centralized fibula. *J Pediatr Orthop* 2000; 20:160–162.
47. Jayakumar SS, Eilert RE. Fibular transfer for congenital absence of the tibia. *Clin Orthop Relat Res* 1979:97–101.
48. Jones D, Barnes J, Lloyd-Roberts GC. Congenital aplasia and dysplasia of the tibia with intact fibula. Classification and management. *J Bone Joint Surg Br* 1978; 60:31–39.
49. Kalamchi A, Dawe RV. Congenital deficiency of the tibia. *J Bone Joint Surg Br* 1985; 67:581–584.
50. Karol LA, O'Brien SE, Wilson H, Johnston CE, Richards BS. Gait analysis in children with severe clubfeet: early results of physiotherapy versus surgical release. *J Pediatr Orthop* 2005; 25:236–240.
51. Kruger LM, Talbott RD. Amputation and prosthesis as definitive treatment in congenital absence of the fibula. *J Bone Joint Surg Am* 1961; 43-A:625–642.
52. Lamb D. The ball and socket ankle joint; a congenital abnormality. *J Bone Joint Surg Br* 1958; 40–B:240–243.
53. Laor T, Jaramillo D, Hoffer FA, Kasser JR. MR imaging in congenital lower limb deformities. *Pediatr Radiol* 1996; 26:381–387.
54. Letts M, Vincent N. Congenital longitudinal deficiency of the fibula (fibular hemimelia). Parental refusal of amputation. *Clin Orthop Relat Res* 1993:160–166.
55. Lezirovitz K, Maestrelli SR, Cotrim NH, Otto PA, Pearson PL, Mingroni-Netto RC. A novel locus for split-hand/foot malformation associated with tibial hemimelia (SHFLD syndrome) maps to chromosome region 17p13.1–17p13.3. *Hum Genet* 2008; 123:625–631.
56. Loder RT, Herring JA. Fibular transfer for congenital absence of the tibia: a reassessment. *J Pediatr Orthop* 1987; 7:8–13.
57. Maffulli N, Fixsen JA. Fibular hypoplasia with absent lateral rays of the foot. *J Bone Joint Surg Br* 1991; 73:1002–1004.
58. Managoli SS, Chaturvedi P. Tibial hemimelia-split hand/foot syndrome with rare anomalies. *Indian Pediatr* 2005; 42:190–191.
59. Matsuyama J, Mabuchi A, Zhang J, et al. A pair of sibs with tibial hemimelia born to phenotypically normal parents. *J Hum Genet* 2003; 48:173–176.
60. McCarthy JJ, Glancy GL, Chnag FM, Eilert RE. Fibular hemimelia: comparison of outcome measurments after amputation and lengthening. *J Bone Joint Surg Am* 2000; 82-A:1732–1735.
61. McKay M, Clarren SK, Zorn R. Isolated tibial hemimelia in sibs: an autosomal-recessive disorder? Am *J Med Genet* 1984; 17:603–607.

the more severe congenital malformations. The feet of children are in constant motion from dawn to dusk and frequent prosthetic repairs are necessary as well as modifications to accommodate for rapid growth spurts. The interaction between the prosthetic and medical staffs in specialized juvenile amputee clinics is essential (3,131,235).

Where the foot has been lost through trauma, many of these anxieties and fears can be discussed through doll play, even after the foot or a portion of it has been removed. In particular, postoperative fears and anxieties that are present in these children, along with guilt feelings that the child has been naughty to have been playing around the machinery or in the road, can be worked out satisfactorily. Other aspects of the treatment can be dealt with such as casts, traction, internal fixation, and prosthetic devices that may be required.

The non-threatening role of this technique not only minimizes guilt feelings and provides an outlet for hostility for the child but also helps to alleviate fears and concerns in parents as well. It is recommended that for children under seven years of age this technique be considered in the preoperative psychological preparation prior to amputation or a major ablation of a portion of the foot.

The use of doll play in quiet discussions in which children act out and ventilate their anxieties about their bodies often relieves them of unrealistic and unwarranted anger at the surgeon and the rest of the medical team. Doll play and puppetry utilized by a trained therapist or other appropriate pediatric support staff has two major objectives: (i) to allay the anxiety of the hospitalization by explaining the hospital routine through doll play; and (ii) to explain through the medium of the dolls the reasons for procedures and the course that the impending surgery will follow. Doll play is a supportive one-on-one explanation of the child's fears and fantasies and is supplemental to other standard techniques of preparation of the child for surgery, such as preoperative visits to the hospital and night-before visits to the operating and recovery rooms (151)(Figure 21-1).

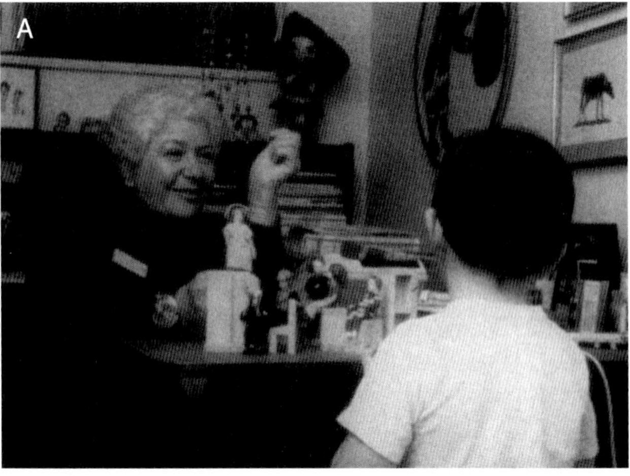

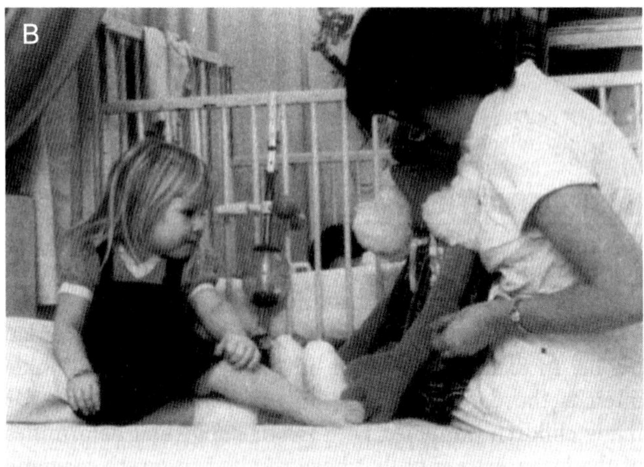

FIGURE 21-1 **A.** Doll play helps the child cope with the complete or partial loss of a foot and assists in avoiding psychological trauma as a result of loss of a part of the body image. **B.** Puppets are useful to explain hospital procedures, surgical operations, including amputations and to allay anxiety in the hospitalized child. (From Letts M, Stevens L, Coleman J, Kettner R. Puppetry and doll play as an adjunct to pediatric orthopaedics. *J Pediatr Orthop* 1983;3:605. with permission.)

Although it is difficult to be dogmatic about the overall numbers of congenital or acquired amputations of the foot in childhood, it is generally accepted that about 60% of the childhood amputations are congenital in origin and 40% are acquired. This figure may vary depending on the locale of the juvenile amputee clinic that is surveyed. Some clinics may refer complicated congenital abnormalities to more major centers, and other clinics may be located in an area such as a farming community where the incidence of trauma to the lower extremity in children is much higher than in more urban settings.

CONGENITAL AMPUTATIONS

There is a wide diversity of congenital malformations of the lower extremity that result either in failure of development of a portion of the foot or a severely misshapen foot that is non-functional and will require a reconstructive procedure to facilitate amputation. The orthopedic surgeon should be involved early in such cases in order to reassure distraught parents that the outlook need not be bleak and that a functional weight-bearing limb is usually possible with today's surgical techniques and prosthetic technology. Where the deformity affects only the foot or ankle, assurance of a near-normal gait can be much more optimistic.

The presence or absence of other congenital malformations should always be carefully assessed. This may well influence the decision-making process regarding what type of reconstruction will be necessary at the level of the foot and ankle. Associated limb length inequality is frequently an accompaniment of an abnormality in the lower extremity and this aspect should always be considered in treatment planning and reconstructive procedures involving the foot and ankle (64). When there is an associated proximal focal femoral deficiency with considerable limb length inequality it may be more appropriate to preserve the ankle and use it ultimately in a Van Nes rotational osteotomy to function as

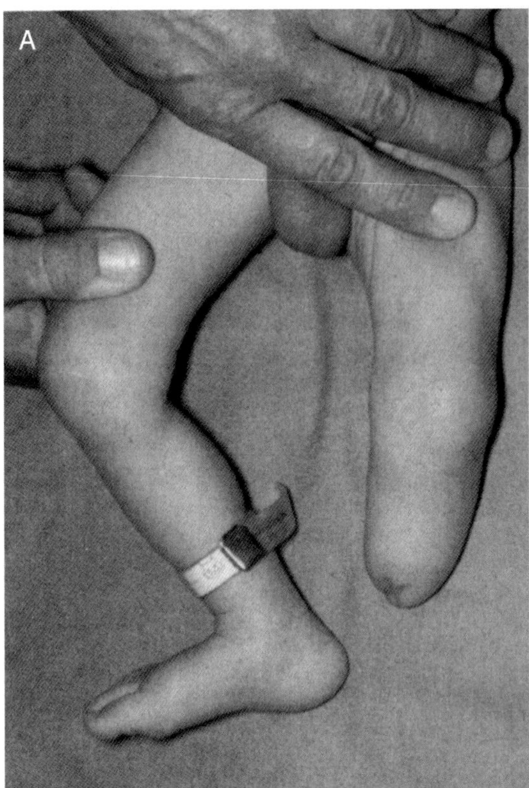

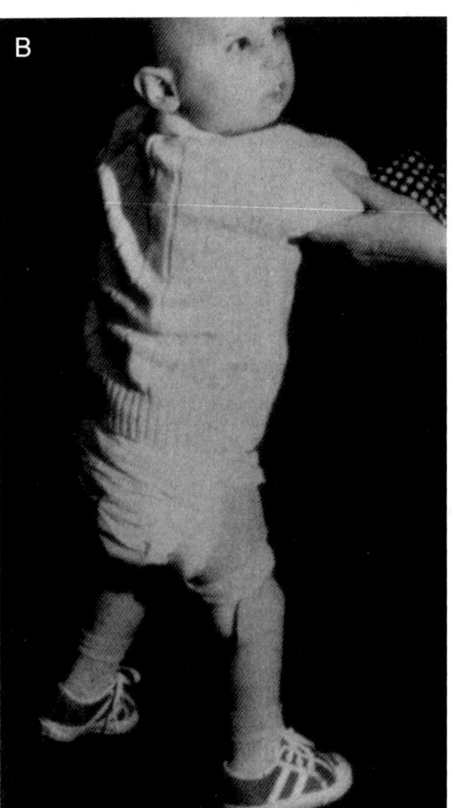

FIGURE 21-2 **A.** An infant with Möbius' syndrome and congenital amputation of the ankle of the foot. **B.** At months of age using a Syme's type prosthesis for ambulation.

a knee joint at a later age (72). The surgeon and treatment team should avoid stereotyping a child with a particular congenital malformation into requiring a certain course of treatment. Each child should be individualized depending on the type of congenital malformation, the association of other malformations, the amount of limb length discrepancy, and the feeling of the family. Where possible, maximal limb growth should always be ensured by growth plate preservation. Surgical modification of the extremity is directed primarily toward facilitation of the prosthetic adaptation as well as improved cosmesis of the limb. Reconstructive procedures for congenital malformation of the lower limb involving the foot and ankle should be performed by a knowledgeable surgeon who is experienced in the limb-deficient child and well aware of the natural history of the deficiency. Most children with congenital deficiencies in the lower extremity limited to the foot and ankle region will be able to walk without prosthetic assistance. Early limb fitting is recommended once the child starts to stand in those patients who have an ankle level amputation. Early prosthetic fitting in these children will allow asymmetry of limb activities and allow the child to learn to use the prosthetic much more effectively, as well as incorporate it into the body image (Figure 21-2). It is important that the clinic team provide an explanation of the treatment plan to the parents and the family's general practitioner or pediatrician so that everyone fully understands the temporal sequence of events that may follow to ensure a functional limb for the child. It is essential that the limb be used as much as possible as this ensures good muscle tone and development which will be necessary for the child to effectively use a prosthesis. This can be accomplished through early prosthetic fitting as well as the involvement of a therapist at the time the child becomes ambulatory (22). Function of the proximal knee joint must be ensured and the presence of other deformities must be ascertained, such as tibial kyphosis that may require a corrective osteotomy either at the time of the amputation or shortly thereafter.

Genetics and Foot Deficiencies

Hereditary malformations of the foot are not common, but similar deformities have been noted in some families and population groups. The presence of some familial patterns of foot deformities indicate that further careful documentation and critical analysis is necessary in order to identify syndrome complexes that may have genetic etiology.

Transverse Defects

The vast majority of congenital foot deficiencies and partial congenital amputations are sporadic and not inherited. Bilateral transverse defects of the lower extremities, transverse defects of the feet associated with microglossia or aglossia, and transverse defects of the foot secondary to annular rings are usually not a risk for future children. However, some rare varieties have been demonstrated to have an autosomal dominant or recessive inheritance pattern in some families (229,244). Acheirpody, an autosomal recessive condition which may involve both arms and legs, has been described in 22 Brazilian families with 82% consanguinity (142). Another autosomal recessive syndrome, Tetramilic terminal defects with ectodermal dysplasia, has been identified (68). These individuals have transverse defects of the lower limbs or feet as well as hands and are associated with hypotrichosis, hypodontia, hypoplastic nails, small stature, mental deficiency, and hypogonadism.

Fibular hemimelia usually is a sporadic entity. However, some rare genetic syndromes involving fibular defects have been described (227). Roberts syndrome or pseudothalidimide syndrome is an autosomal recessive condition associated with complete or partial absence of the fibula; and defects of the upper limbs that may include partial absence of the radius or ulna as well as hypoplasia of the thumb and fingers. The familial incidence and the high rate of consanguinity in the parents are compatible with autosomal recessive inheritance (69,88,142,196,229).

Aplasia of the fibula in Larsen syndrome has been reported in several cases. There is evidence for autosomal recessive inheritance in some families with Larsen syndrome and for dominant inheritance in others.

Congenital Longitudinal Deficiency of the Tibia (Tibial Hemimelia)

Paraxial tibial hemimelia (tibial meromelia) has an incidence of one per million live births and most occur sporadically (4,31,38,56,217). There are reports of familiar transmission and several syndromes include absence of the tibia as a component (142). These syndromes may include tibial hemimelia with polydactyly and triphalangeal thumb (Worner syndrome), tibial hemimelia; diaplopodia (split hand-foot syndrome), and tibial hemimelia with micromelia (Trico brachycephaly syndrome) (171,207). Congenital dislocation of the hip has been associated with tibial hemimelia in as many as 20% of cases. It occurs bilaterally in about 30% of cases (121).

Lobster Claw Malformation

This condition has a dominant pattern of transmission in some families but many examples of fresh mutations have been reported. The Volkmann syndrome (autosomal dominant subtotal fibular defects with genu valgum) has been described in several families with an autosomal dominant inheritance (196,243).

Congenital Longitudinal Deficiency of the Fibula (Fibular Hemimelia)

Absence of the fibula associated with a short limb and a malformed foot usually due to absent lateral rays represents one of the more common anomalies leading to amputation of the foot in childhood (23,41,62,98,99,116). A classification of fibular hemimelia based on the eventual limb length inequality at skeletal maturity as well as the type of foot abnormality is practical because treatment centers on these two factors (Table 21-1). Generally the affected extremity of children with fibular hemimelia will be significantly shortened and amputation of the foot and fitting with a prosthesis is the most appropriate method of treatment (236,245,246). Early amputation is recommended between 6–18 months of age when it is apparent that the expected limb length inequality will exceed 10 cm (Table 21-2). Ablation of the foot may also be indicated when the projected limb length inequality will be less than 10 cm, but the foot malformation will result in poor function. Kruger (132,133) and others (188,230,231,251,253) have demonstrated that multiple operations to preserve the foot and limb length have not been in the child's best interest. The classification in Table 21-1 allows the development of realistic treatment goals recommended in Table 21-2.

Type A group of patients with fibular hemimelia are the least common. Excision of the fibular anlage is reasonable when the entire fibula is absent and the fibrous band that is invariably present causes tibial tethering with the development of tibial kyphosis or valgus deformity

TABLE 21-1

Classification of Fibular Hemimelia

Type A	-Unilateral, less than 6 em shortening -Minimal foot deformity -Minimal femoral shortening
Type B	-Unilateral, 6–10 em shortening -Minimal foot deformity -Minimal femoral shortening.
Type C	-Unilateral, more than 10 em shortening -Major foot deformity and. -/or major femoral shortening
Type D	-Bilateral

TABLE 21-2

Treatment Protocol

Recommend	**Type A** -Fibular anlage excision -Shoe lifts
Recommend	**Type B** -Fibular anlage excision -Shoe lifts -Limb equalizing procedures
Recommend	**Type C** -Fibular anlage excision -Foot amputation/prosthesis
Recommend	**Type D** -Fibular anlage excision -Bilateral foot amputation/prosthesis

(Figure 21-3). Excision of this band will assist the tibia to grow to its maximum potential (11,23,41). Consideration should be given to a Boyd (21,27,59,134,170) or modified Chopart (145) amputation when a severe foot malformation is coupled with a predicted limb length inequality under 6 cm. The Gruca procedure with tibial splitting to stabilize the foot, thus acting as a foot-sparing technique might also be entertained (230) (Figure 21-4C). This group should also be considered for the Ilizarov type limb-lengthening procedures (109–111).

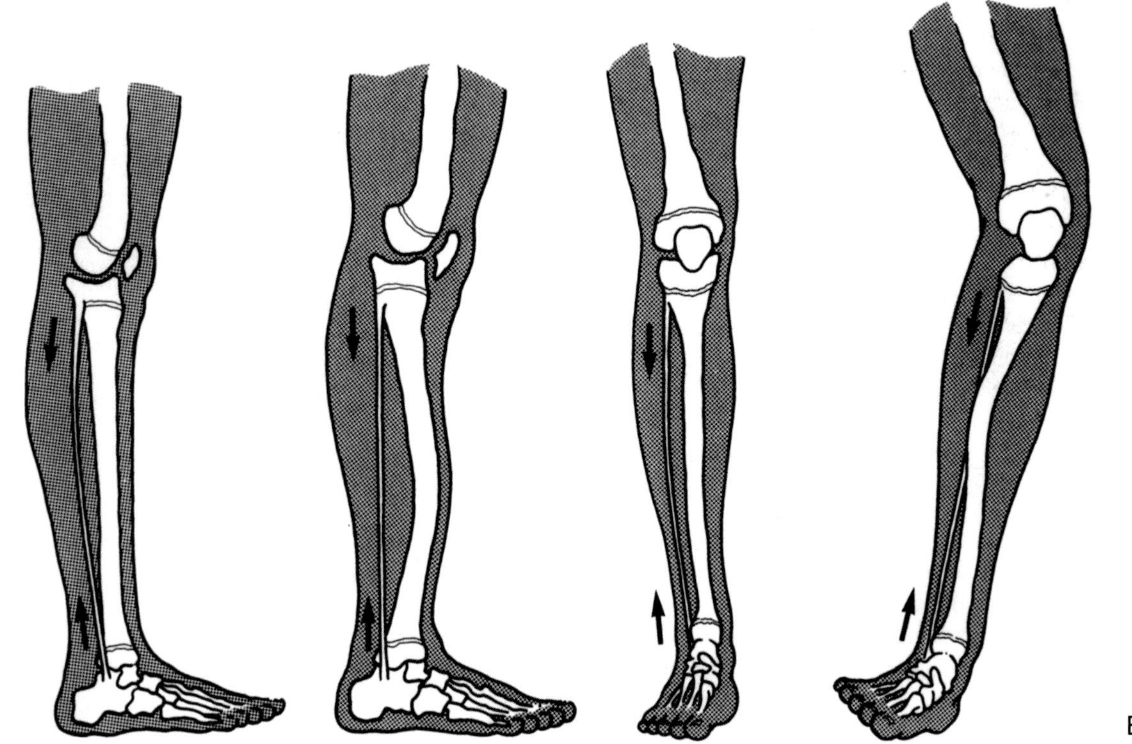

FIGURE 21-3 Tethering effect of fibular analogue producing anterior angulation of tibia (**A**) and valgus deformity of the tibia (**B**).

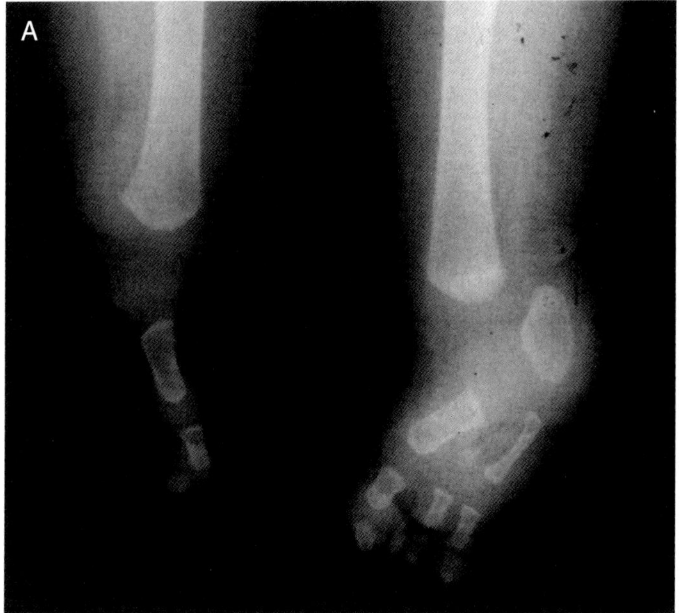

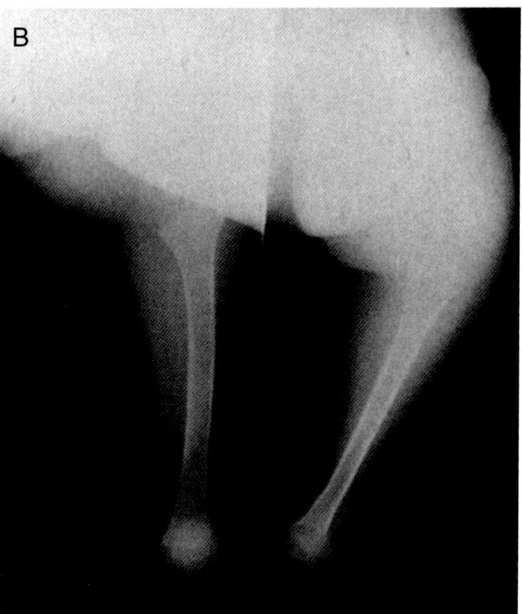

FIGURE 21-4 **A.** Fibular hemimelia with misshapen feet in an 8-month-old child and limb length inequality. **B.** Bilateral Syme amputation was performed with early prosthetic fitting. **C.** The Gruca procedure designed to provide ankle stability in fibular hemimelia. (Modified from Thomas IH, Williams PF. The Gruca operation for congenital absence of the fibula. *J Bone Joint Surg [Br]* 1987;69:587.)

Type B group of fibular hemimelia have predicted shortening of 6–10 cm and amputation of the foot should be considered especially when the foot is malformed. The goal should be a good weight-bearing stump as this will permit the patient to ambulate around the house without a prosthesis (26,37,52). Newer limb-lengthening techniques may result in the need for only a small raise being required.

Type C fibular hemimelia is the most common form. Limb length inequality will be significant and there is usually an associated major foot deformity. Ablation of the foot at an early age combined with a Boyd (27), Syme (86), or modified Chopart amputation is recommended for these children. Children with bilateral fibular hemimelia (type D) usually have very significant predicted limb shortening and will require bilateral amputations of the feet (1,2,6,8). Care should be given to provide good weight-bearing stumps as this will allow them to function around the home without a prosthesis (see Figure 21-4A,B). Although weight bearing is possible with a Syme amputation, the size of the stump is smaller and the gait without the prosthesis is not as functional as that achieved with the Boyd procedure. This Syme amputation does however have the added advantage of easier prosthetic fitting (97,105,113,130,138,145,154,169,174,190).

Parental Refusal of Amputation

Reluctance by parents to agree to amputation of their child's foot at an early age is often encountered when the foot is near normal or the initial limb length inequality does not appear to be excessive (Table 21-3). It is sometimes difficult for parents to appreciate that as the child grows the limb will become progressively shorter and eventually that a prosthesis will be necessary. This is often combined with an unrealistic expectation concerning the technical advances in prosthetics and surgery. The treatment recommendations for the young child with bilateral fibular hemimelia often creates further family concern. These children frequently are capable of functioning independently with minimal orthotic or prosthetic management. As they mature, however, the disproportion between the upper and lower segments of the leg gives them an unusual appearance and their short stature demands prosthetic intervention.

It is most helpful to have families whose child has been advised to have a reconstructive amputation to meet with other families who have had a similar successful experience with their own child. This is a major advantage to the juvenile amputee clinic where such family interaction is facilitated. If the parents still cannot bring themselves to consent to foot amputation despite sound advice from the amputee clinic, a second or even a third opinion from other juvenile amputee teams may be helpful. The clinic team must be patient, respect the parents' dilemma and allow time to assist in choosing the appropriate course. Some children will adapt to modern innovative prosthetic management and function very well (Figure 21-5). A greater number will opt for later amputation when it becomes obvious that this indeed is in their child's best interest. For most families, however, it is best to arrive at a reasoned and informed decision for foot ablation at a very early age (between 6 and 18 months).

TABLE 21-3

Reasons for Parental Refusal

1. Deny natural history
2. Foot near normal
3. Gait functional at present
4. Wish child to participate in decision

In summary, not all children with fibular hemimelia may require ablation of the foot and the decision must be made by the treatment team based on the family unit; the child's prosthetic fitting needs; and the function, appearance, and predicated limb-length discrepancy of the extremity.

Congenital Longitudinal Deficiency of the Tibia (Tibial Hemimelia)

Congenital absence of the tibia is much less common than absence of the fibula and the most children born with this anomaly will require amputation of the foot or a more proximal ablation.

Clinical Picture

Congenital longitudinal deficiency of the tibia can be functionally classified dependent on the amount of tibia remaining (Table 21-4) and the classifications of Jones et al. (118) and Kalamchi (121) are recommended. Absence of the tibia may be complete or partial. The leg below the knee is fixed in a varus position and markedly shortened. The foot is usually in significant varus, and the knee is very unstable when the tibia is completely absent and less unstable when there is a proximal tibial remnant. Quadriceps function is usually absent in type I. There may be an associated knee flexion contracture with a popliteal web. Polydactyly as well as absence of one or two of the medial rays of the foot or shortening of the first metatarsal is often present (100,115,118,121,122) (Figure 21-6).

Treatment

Salvage of a limb with a completely absent tibia is difficult because there is usually associated knee instability and major knee flexion contracture. The limb is always short and the foot very difficult to stabilize. In many instances, the most functional approach is a knee disarticulation with subsequent fitting with a knee disarticulation prosthesis (93,132). There may be an associated femoral hypoplasia and limb length inequality that can be effectively managed by prosthetic fitting. In some instances with marked femoral shortening, a fibular femoral arthrodesis with a modified Chopart amputation of the foot to provide a longer stump may be beneficial. Conversion of the modified Chopart to a Boyd amputation can be considered when the

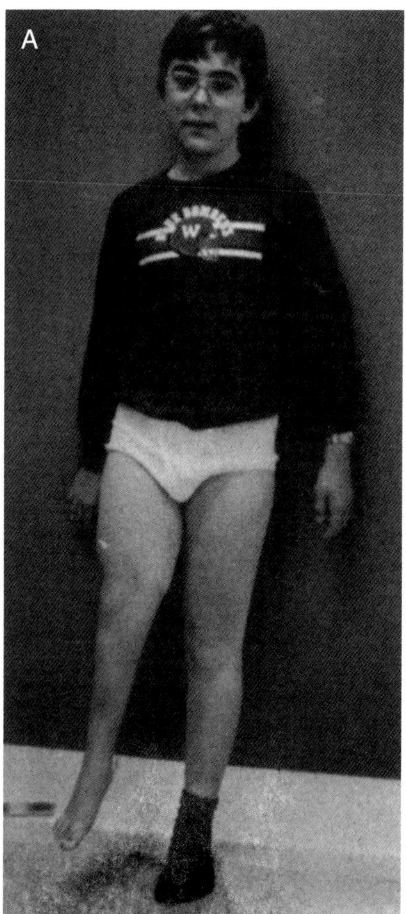

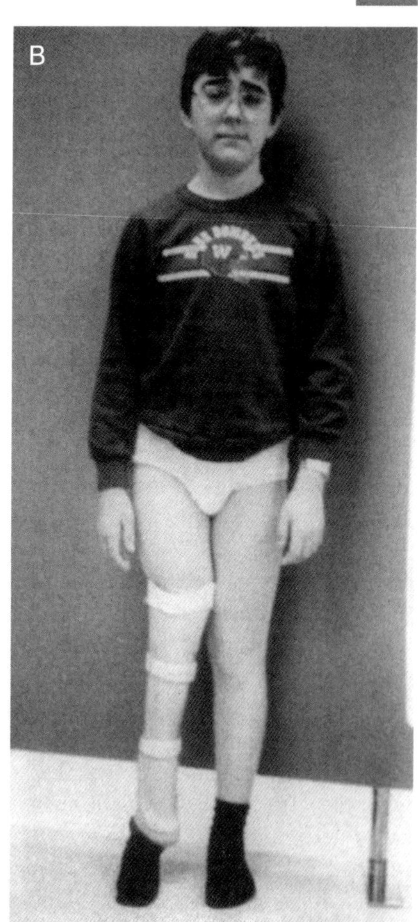

FIGURE 21-5 **A.** This 10-year-old boy's parents refused to allow a Syme amputation with ablation of a normal foot during infancy for fibular hemimelia. **B.** He is currently wearing a modified prosthesis to incorporate his intact foot, and his function is excellent!

TABLE 21-4

Classification of Congenital Longitudinal Deficiency of the Ttibia[1]

TYPE 1a	*TYPE 1b*	*TYPE 2*	*TYPE 3*	*TYPE 4*

[1] Modified after Jones D, Barnes J, Lloyd-Roberts GC. Congenital aplasia and dysplasia of the tibia with intact fibula: Classification and management. *J Bone Joint Surg* 1978; 60B:31.

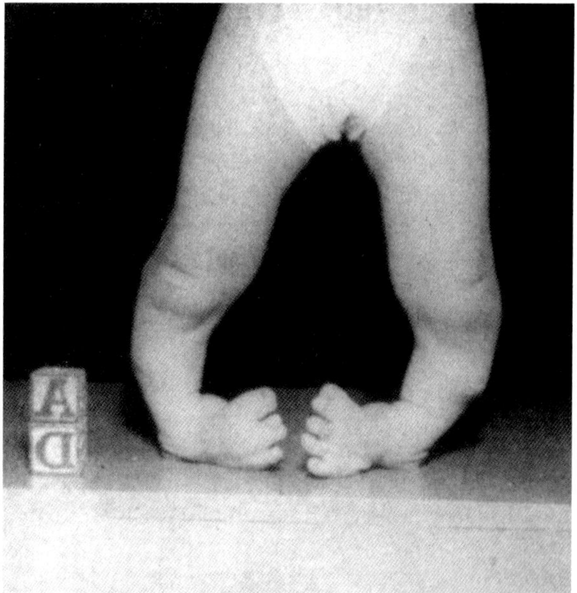

FIGURE 21-6 Tibial hemimelia with marked varus of both feet and knees.

child is older and has mor fibular bone stock to facilitate the calcaneo-fibular arthrodesis if there is varus drift.

Patients with a proximal tibial remnant (types II and IV) whose knees seem to be more stable, may benefit from centralization of the fibula under the femur by fusion to the tibial remnant with removal of the foot (Brown procedure) (31,217). This functions effectively as a below-knee amputation, but the knee will still require prosthetic support to maintain its stability even when the quadriceps are transferred to the transposed fibula when the tibial remnant is very short.

Success has been reported in type IV congenital deficiency of the tibia by ankle reconstruction to create a stable ankle and a plantigrade foot followed by lengthening of the tibia (207,234). By creating a stable ankle through tibial talar arthrodesis and correcting the tibial angulation by osteotomy, a functional stable foot and ankle may be achieved in some type IV children.

Children with type II tibial hemimelia with a long proximal tibial remnant and quadriceps formation will have a more stable knee. In these children, a proximal tibia-fibular synostosis should be created with a Boyd amputation performed as the limb will be short and a below-knee prosthesis will be required.

Children with hypoplastic distal tibia should be considered for a tibio-fibular synostosis to control the diastasis and a Boyd type amputation of the foot. Again, a modified Chopart procedure may buy some time and facilitate prosthetic fitting until a Boyd amputation and fusion is more feasible.

Lengthening of the tibial remnant has not been successful in the past. The Ilizarov method of lengthening may offer more success but its efficacy in this condition remains unproven. Sanctis et al. (207) have reported successful outcomes in three cases of type II tibial agenesis in which they combined correction of the foot shortly after birth by a fibular arthrodesis, followed by fibular transfer to the tibial remnant and alignment of the axis of the leg with the foot coupled with limb lengthening by the Ilizarov technique. Schoenecker et al. (209) have recommended a treatment regimen based on the radiographic classification of Jones, Barnes, and Lloyd-Roberts (118) (see Table 21-4).

Unfortunately, the more severe type I deformity is the most common form. The larger the tibial anlage that is present, the more applicable a Syme, Boyd, or Chopart amputation becomes. Loder and Herring (156) have reported poor results with the Browne fibular centralization procedure due to persistent ligamentous instability at the knee. They also found a very limited range of motion of the knee. The unsatisfactory results in the literature indicate that knee disarticulation provides less mobility, more efficient prosthetic fitting, and rehabilitation as well as reduced costs in the type I congenital longitudinal deficiency of the tibia.

Constriction Band Syndrome

Congenital annular construction bands may result in complete or partial amputations of the foot or lower extremity. This condition is sometimes referred to as "Streeter's syndrome" in recognition of the author who first attributed intrauterine amputation to constriction bands (223). Constriction rings and acrosyndactyly may also be seen in addition to transverse amputations. It is hypothesized that mechanical constriction of the limb occurs when there is entanglement of fetal extremities with amniotic bands following rupture of the amnion (9,12,25,32). Constriction bands may be associated with both the upper and lower extremities, with lower limb involvement being more common (61,119,125,176,187). The toes are often hypoplastic and associated with constriction bands (Figure 21-7). Clubfeet are frequently associated with this syndrome

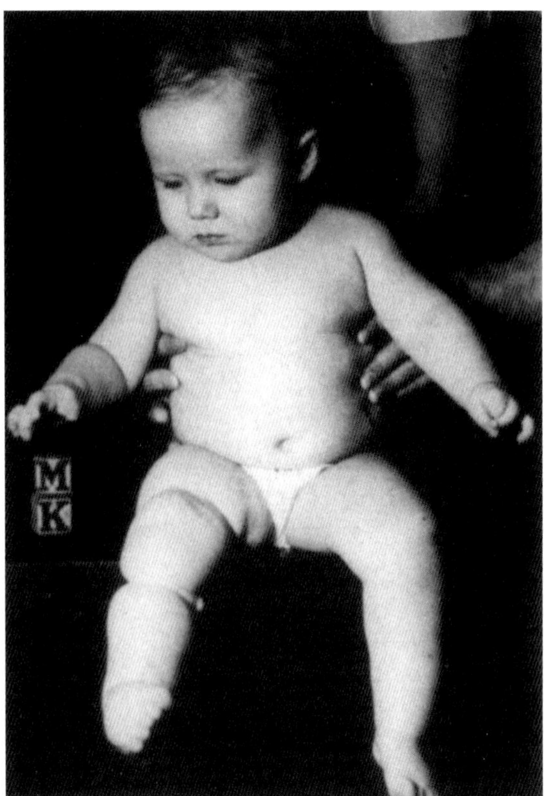

FIGURE 21-7 This eight-month-old child has an obvious above and below knee annular band of the right leg associated with a club foot. The annular bands were released by a staged Z-plasty a short time later together with a club foot release.

(45). Syndactyly affecting the medial two toes is seen in about 20% of patients. Lower limbs affected by constriction bands frequently are associated with a limb-length discrepancy (34,55).

Treatment

Constriction bands with distal edema or neurological impairment require immediate Z-plasty and excision. It is important to emphasize that only one-half of the constriction band should be removed at any one time in order to preserve the vascular integrity to the distal part of the limb. *In utero*, mid-tarsal amputations are often functional and in my experience seldom require revision. The stumps are usually excellent and permit early prosthetic fitting of ankle and mid-foot amputations at the age when the child would normally walk. Release of the syndactyly may be necessary when the toes are bunched up, lending further credence to the concept that they have been bound together by amniotic strands.

The clubfeet may be secondary to the oligohydramnios as a result of amniotic rupture, producing compression and deformity. Another cause of the clubfoot that has been documented as secondary to a proximal constriction, resulting in paralysis of the evertor muscles (228). The clubfoot deformity may be severe but usually responds to surgical release.

Pseudoarthrosis of the tibia has been associated with severe annular constriction bands. The pseudoarthrosis

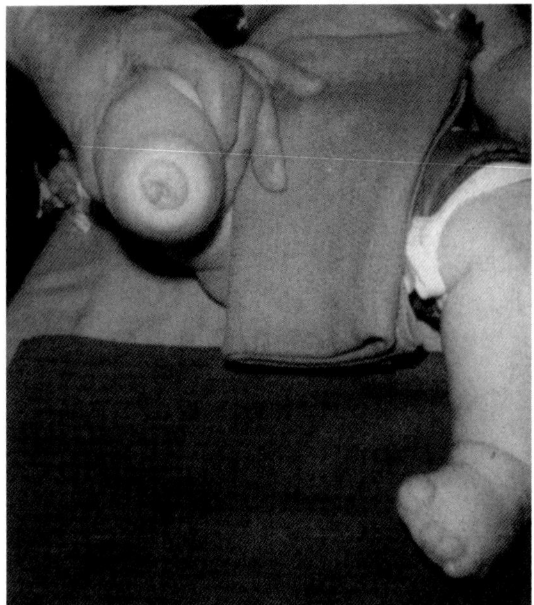

FIGURE 21-8 Amputation at the ankle in an infant with multiple constriction bands. This premature child was born with an open amputation stump which gradually healed over following tibial resection. Note contralateral club foot.

usually heals once the band has been removed. Occasionally, children born with annular constriction bands will have an amputation of the distal tibia or a partial amputation of the foot that results in incomplete skin closure. Local skin care usually results in healing by secondary intention. The exposed avascular bone may occasionally need resection to allow appropriate skin healing (Figure 21-8).

Cleft Feet

Cleft feet are well recognized congenital anomalies with a reported incidence of 1 out of 90,000 live births (55). The anomaly is inherited as an autosomal dominant pattern with varying degrees of penetrance (140,158,184,185). The most frequent presentation is bilateral and usually is associated with cleft hands. The central portion of the foot is absent to a greater or lesser degree. Blauth and Borisch have classified cleft foot deformity into six groups (19) (Figure 21-9). Types I and II are cleft feet with minor deficiencies, both having five metatarsals. The metatarsals are all normal in type I and partially hypoplastic in type II. Type III has four metatarsals, type IV has three metatarsals; which type V has two metatarsals. Type IV represents the monodactylus cleft foot. The type V form is sometimes referred to as "lobster claw foot" and always has a complete deficiency of the second, third, and fourth rays. The type IV and the type V deformities are the most frequently reported although the less dramatic types of cleft foot may not demand treatment and may actually be more common that the literature would indicate (Figure 21-10). The etiology of these central rays defects is speculated to be an insult to apical ectodermal ridge which is responsible for the normal development of the lib buds through the interaction with the underlying myotome (185). A defect in the apical ectodermal ridge may result from a genetic or toxic influence. The former would be plausible because of the strong autosomal dominant pattern of inheritance. The type of defect in the apical ectodermal ridge will determine whether an osseous syndactyly occurs through deficient differentiation; polydactyly by excessive differentiation; or a lack of differentiation resulting in the central defect responsible for formation of cleft feet (247).

Treatment of the more severe deformities (types III, IV, and V) center around approximating the medial and lateral rays to prevent marked splaying of the foot and to provide better weight-bearing support (227,250). This can be accomplished in most feet by syndactylizing the separated medial and lateral rays to prevent marked medial and lateral deviation of the rays and additionally to improve the cosmetic appearance (Figure 21-11).

ACQUIRED AMPUTATIONS

Acquired amputations of the foot and ankle are usually secondary to acute trauma. Malignant tumors seldom involve the foot but occasionally necessitate a foot ablation. Elective amputations of the foot in childhood may be required secondary to vascular malformations, hypertrophic malformations, and a large variety of miscellaneous disorders. The more common traumatic causes of foot loss in childhood result from machinery accidents, motor vehicle trauma, gun shot wounds, and train accidents (Figure 21-12). Although the site and level of amputations is often predicted by the magnitude of the trauma, the surgeon should be knowledgeable about the advantages and disadvantages of the various traditional amputation levels in the foot and ankle (Figure 21-13).

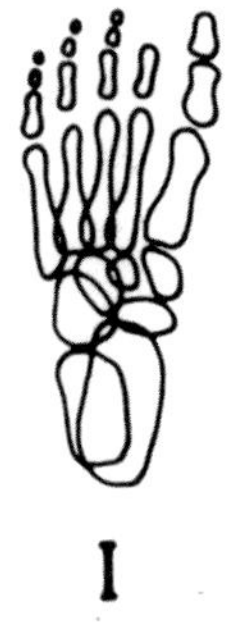

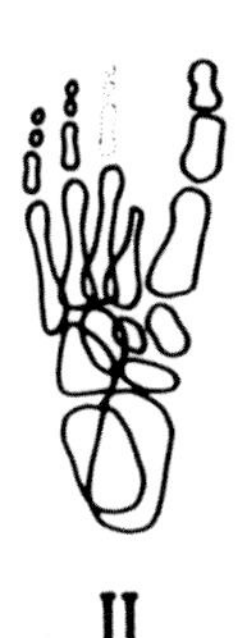

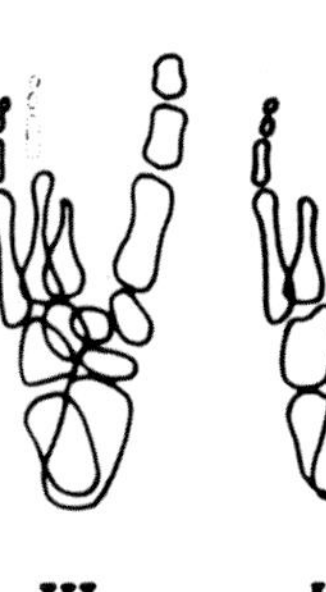

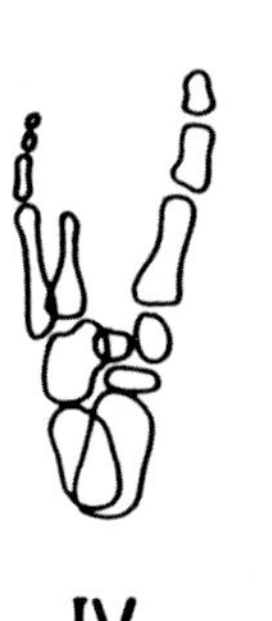

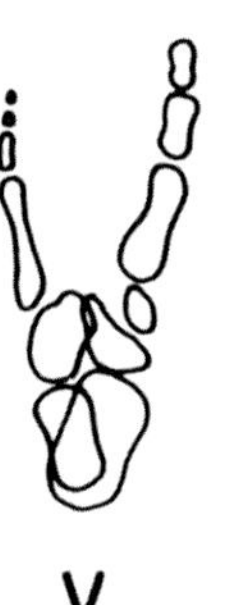

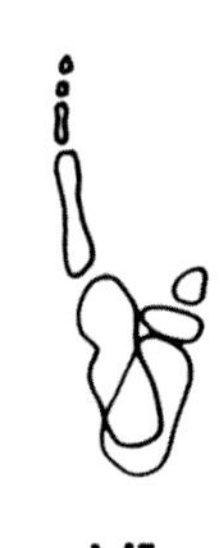

FIGURE 21-9 Classification of cleft foot. (Modified from Blauth W, Borisch NC. Cleft feet. *Clin Orthop* 1990;258:41.)

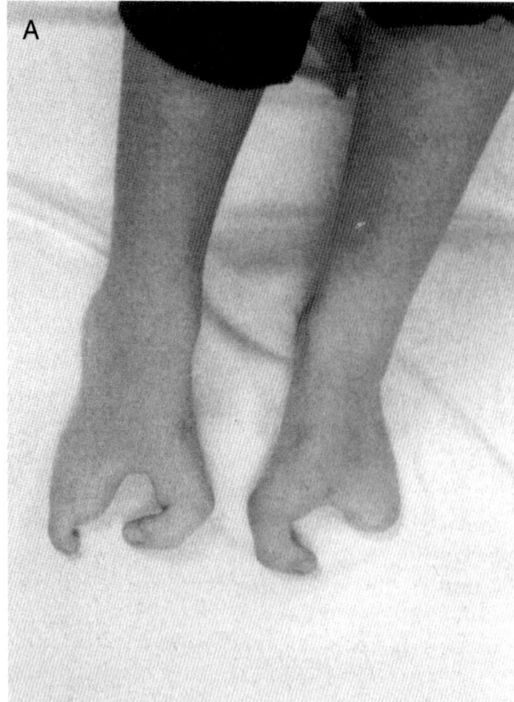

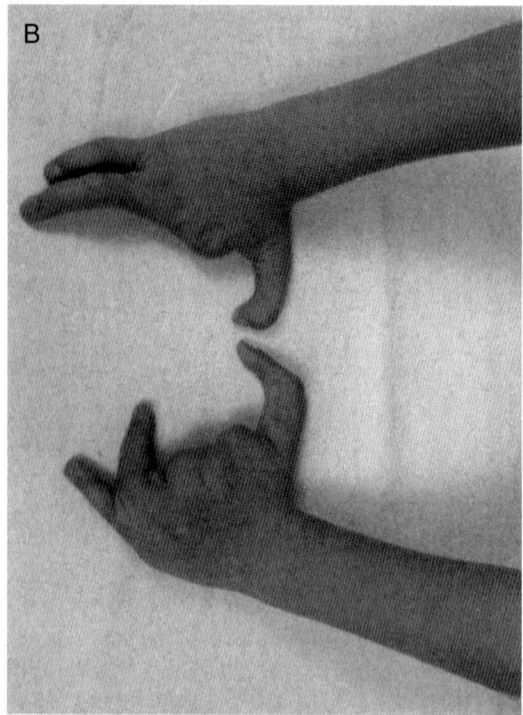

FIGURE 21-10 Lobster claw deformity (central ray amputation) (**A**) in a child with similar deficits in the hands (**B**). (Courtesy of Dr. Jacques D'Astous, Shriner's Hospital, Salt Lake City, Utah.)

Hemangiomatous Hypertrophy and Deformity

Hypertrophy of the foot or portions of the foot or toes is frequently the result of hemangiomatous malformation of the lower extremity (Figure 21-14). The foot enlargement frequently causes the patient the greater disability as it becomes impossible to fit into normal shoe wear. This problem coupled with cosmetics often necessitates partial ablation of the hypertrophied portion, or in severe cases ablation of the entire foot and conversion to a Syme, Boyd, or Lisfranc type of amputation (146,224).

Klippel-Trenaunay syndrome (126,153) and its variants (164) are a common cause of pedal hypertrophy secondary to vascular malformation. This syndrome is a triad of varicose veins, hypertrophy of soft tissue and bone, and port wine cutaneous hemangiomas which are commonly found in the lower extremity (126). Children with this syndrome almost invariably have overgrowth of the extremity, most frequently the foot, secondary to the increased blood supply (Figure 21-15). Multiple arteriovenous fistulae are present but are not localized to any one portion of the extremity. The limb is typically an arm with many dilated superficial veins and cutaneous hemangiomas. Branham's sign of slowing of the pulse with occlusion of the femoral artery frequently is present. Cardiac enlargement and high output cardiac failure is often seen in infancy (44,143).

Radiographs of the extremity demonstrate a course trabecular pattern in the bones indicative of arteriovenous malformations within the bone itself. Arteriography frequently reveals multiple arteriovenous connections and is accompanied by the early venous filling and dilatation of the tortuous proximal segment of the involved arteries (Figure 21-16). Technetium bone scans also show that there is increased bone turnover at the epiphyseal plates of the involved extremity. Excision of the arteriovenous fistulae has been found to be of little value and radiation therapy to obliterate the vessels often results in growth plate damage in addition to the more dire consequence of the later development of osteogenic sarcoma. Limb length

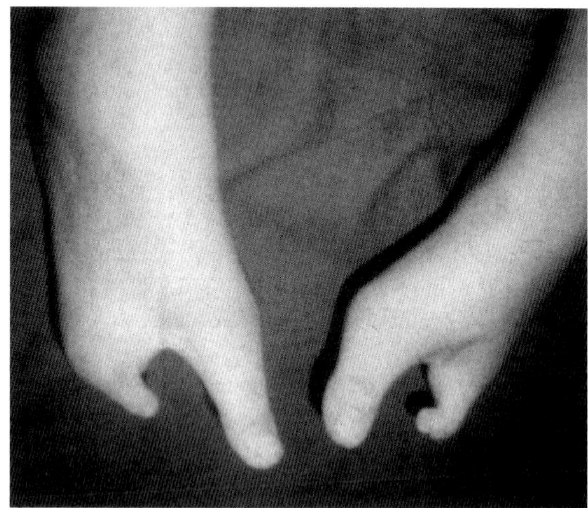

FIGURE 21-11 Surgical syndactyly of a deep central cleft in a child who was able to walk quite normally with ordinary footwear.

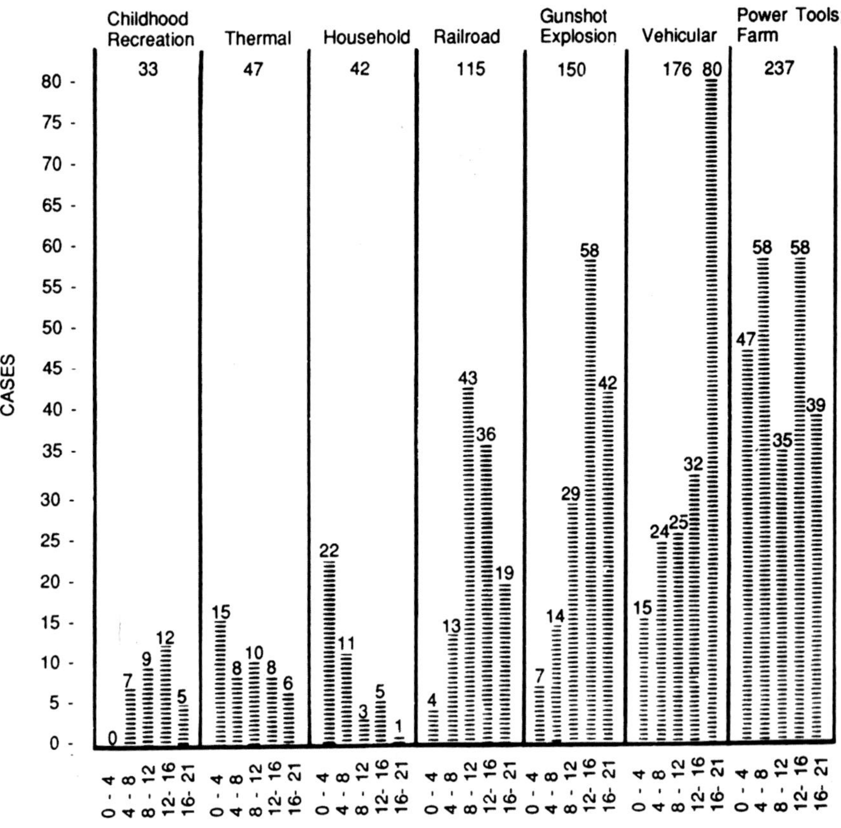

FIGURE 21-12 The etiology of traumatic amputations in 800 juvenile amputees. (From Northwestern University Medical School Juvenile Amputee Course Manual.)

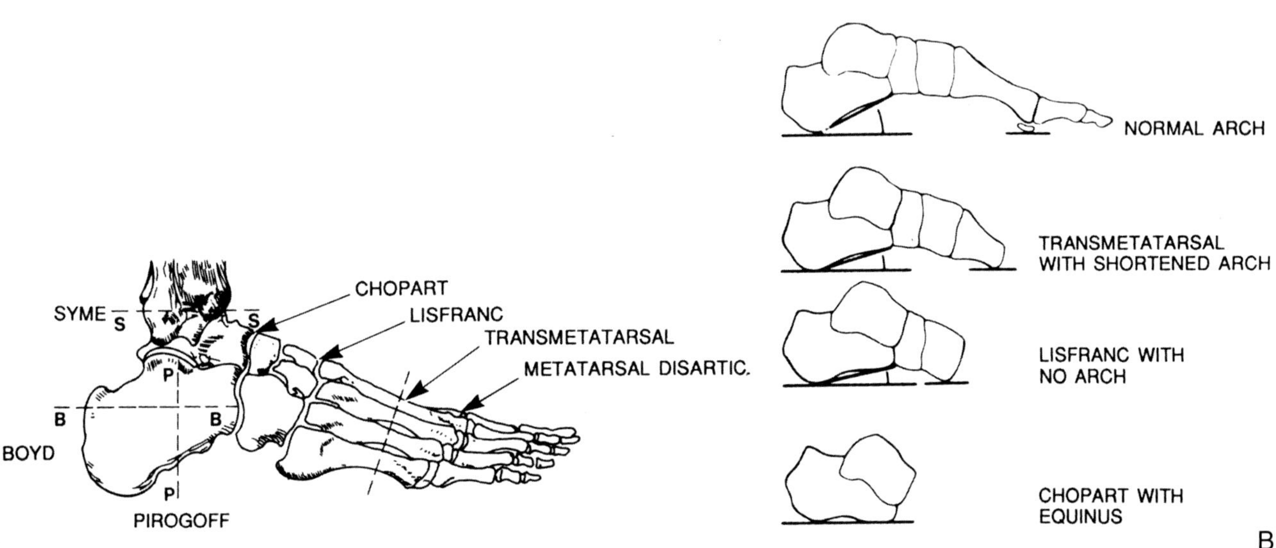

FIGURE 21-13 **A.** Amputation sites in the foot. **B.** The effects of forefoot loss on the maintenance of the longitudinal arch. (Modified from Lange TA, Nasca RJ. Traumatic partial foot amputation. *Clin Orthop* 1984;185:137.)

inequalization and amputation, combined with soft tissue reduction of the foot, are the most practical and appropriate types of procedures for these grossly hypertrophied feet and lower limbs (76,146). Epiphysiodesis of the metatarsals have been helpful in reducing the ultimate length of the foot. This frequently has to be accompanied by soft-tissue reduction and in some instances metatarsal ray excision (Figure 21-17) and even amputation of grossly hypertrophied toes (Figure 21-18). In the very severe cases of total limb hypertrophy, a Syme or a below-knee

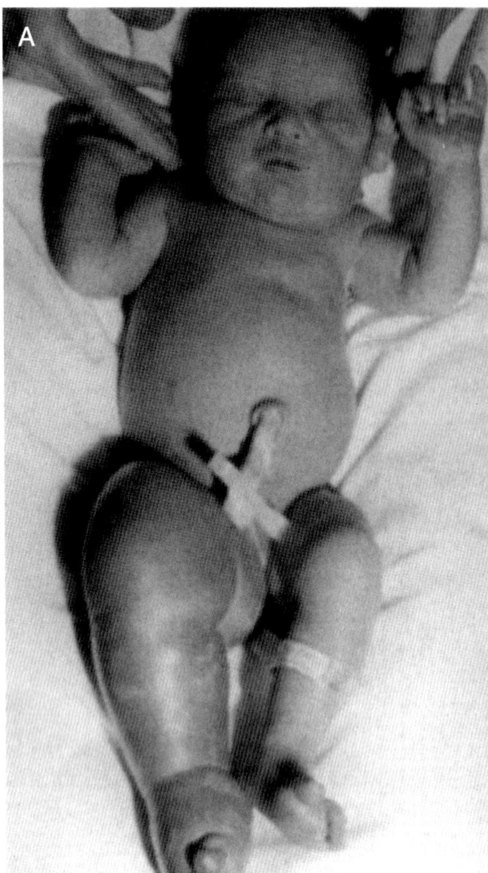

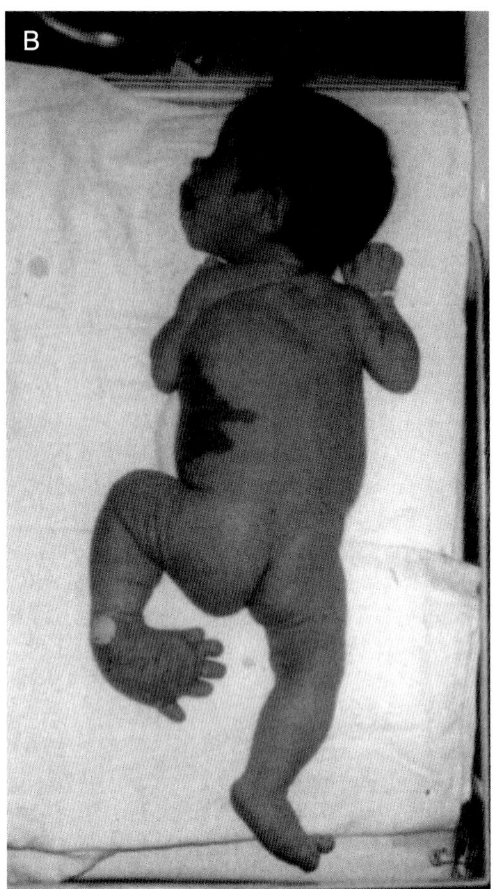

FIGURE 21-14 **A,B.** Two infants with Klippel-Trenaunay syndrome illustrating gross hypertrophy of the affected limb and foot. (From Letts RM. Orthopaedic treatment of hemangiomatous hypertrophy of the lower limb. *J Bone Joint Surg (Am)* 1977;59:777, with permission.)

amputation, or in some rare instances, an above-knee amputation may be required to control the gross deformity (Figure 21-19). An interesting observation has been the marked decrease in size that occurs in the proximal limb following an amputation which includes the majority of the arteriovenous fistulae. This phenomenon often eliminates the anticipated difficulty with prosthetic fitting. Some children with large hemangiomatous malformations have abnormalities in the lymphatic system as well; these areas may be more localized and amenable to soft tissue excision (165,203,224,226).

Surgery on the foot in such children requires meticulous hemostasis, and Hemovac drains should always be used. The sutures should not be removed prematurely and should be retained for a minimum of two to three weeks. When the foot is ablated, prosthetic fitting may initially be difficult. The edema usually subsides within a year or two, and the proximal hypertrophy of the limb decreases to a more normal anatomical size. There are many types of variations of congenital hemangiomatous malformations of the foot and each must be approached in a unique fashion.

Thermal Trauma

Children are frequently the victims of thermal injury resulting from misadventure, accident, or, unfortunately, neglect. The most common type of thermal damage is burn injuries, followed by frostbite and, less commonly, electrical injury. (7).

Burn Amputations

Burns to the feet frequently result in the loss of toes and severe scarring of the dorsal skin of the foot. Fortunately, the plantar skin is very thick and resistant to burn trauma but when lost, maintenance of the viability of the foot is difficult (78). Tissue transfer with microvascular techniques can provide more durable plantar coverage.

Frostbite

The foot of a child is less likely to sustain severe frostbite injury than the hand (7,47,79,193). However, frostbite injuries are seen in Northern cold climates. Amputation should be deferred until there is a clear line of demarcation of the tissue loss (192,200,202) (Figures 21-20 and 21-21). Ablation may require an open or Guillotine technique with subsequent skin grafting (124). Severe frostbite in children may also result in growth plate arrest with the length of the foot ultimately being much shorter, depending on the age of the child at the time of frostbite injury (200) (Figure 21-22).

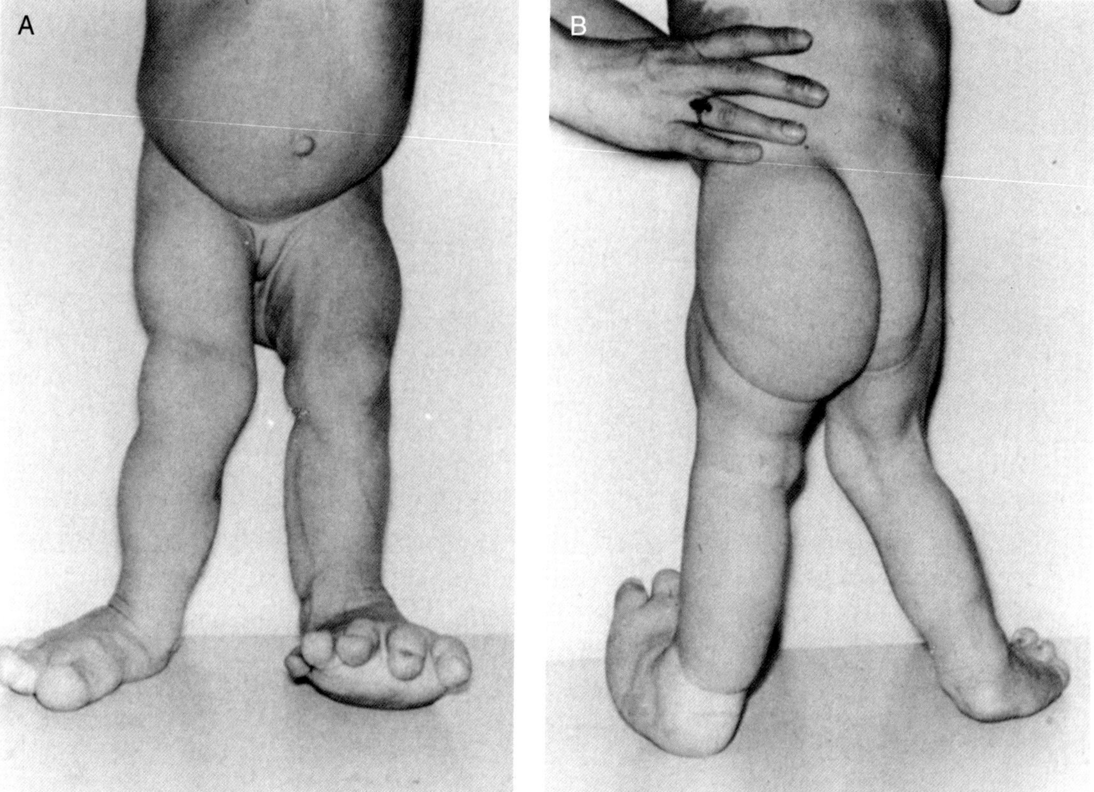

FIGURE 21-15 **A,B.** Marked hypertrophy of both feet secondary to arteriovenous malformation (Klippel-Trenaunay syndrome). These feet were narrowed by ray excision and epiphysiodesis of the metatarsals allowing the child to wear commercially available footwear.

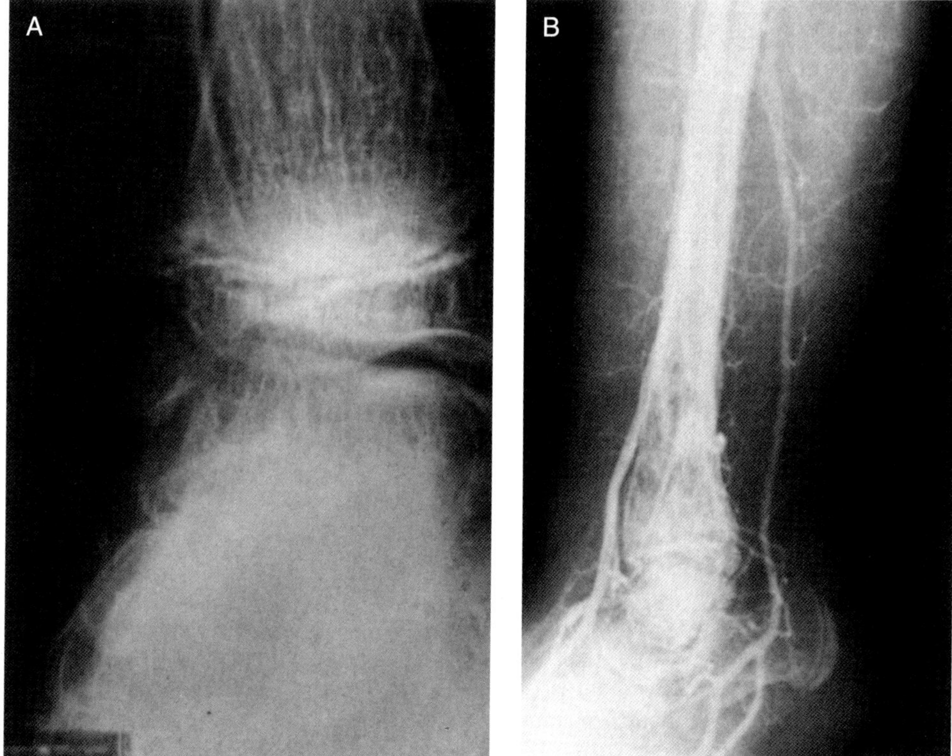

FIGURE 21-16 **A.** Coarse trabeculation of the talus and distal tibia characteristic of arteriovenous malformation. **B.** Hypervascularity of the leg and foot illustrated by a femoral arteriogram.

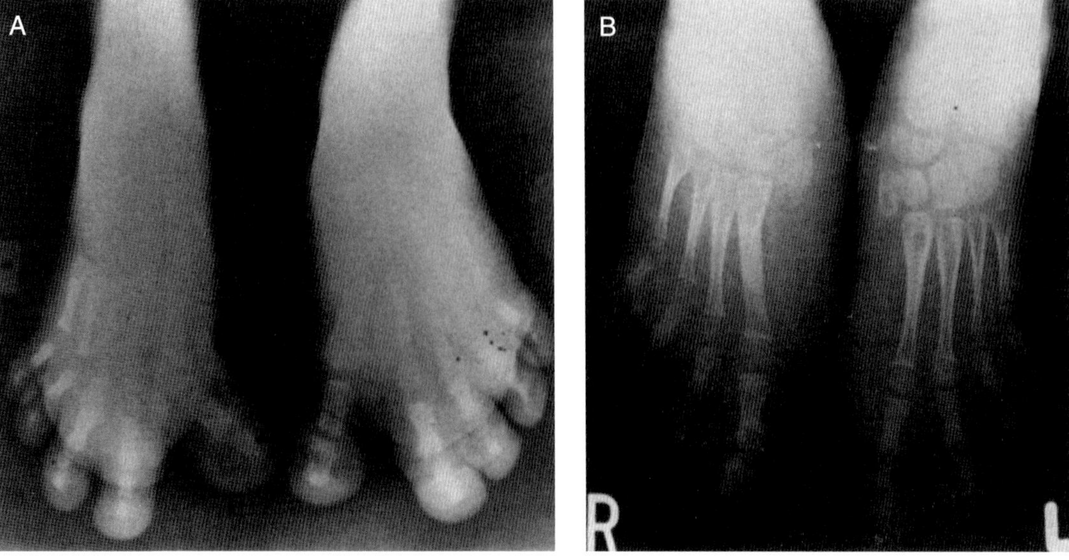

FIGURE 21-17 **A,B.** Excision of grossly hypertrophied and misshapen great toes by bilateral first ray amputations, providing much narrower feet that allowed the child to be fitted with ordinary footwear.

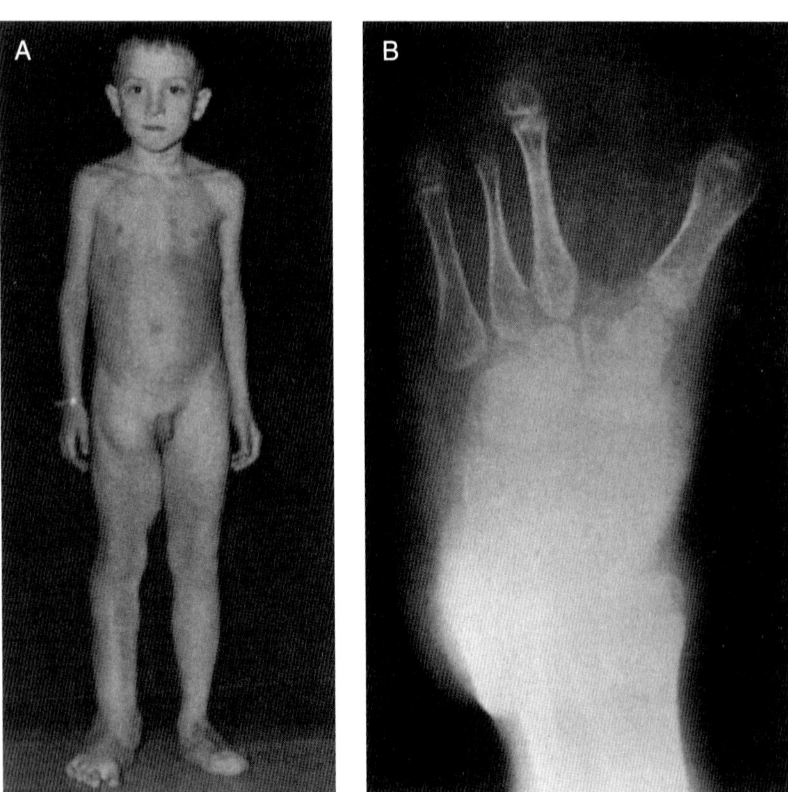

FIGURE 21-18 **A,B.** Amputation of all toes of left foot plus a second ray excision provided a very functional foot that could be fitted with normal shoes.

Electrical Burns

Electrical burns of the feet are much less common than finger burns as the foot seldom comes in contact with an electrical plug or outlet. However, electrical burns are often severe, and the incidence of amputation is much higher than with a thermal burn or frostbite. The level of the amputation is also often more proximal and unfortunately more than the foot may be lost (139).

Machinery Trauma

Children have a particular propensity to entangle their foot into moving parts of machinery, be it a train, an auger, power take-off, or the more ubiquitous lawnmower (see Figure 21-12). Unfortunately, such injuries usually result in complete amputation of the foot or a foot so traumatized that amputation is necessary (127,162). In North America, farm machinery accidents are a common

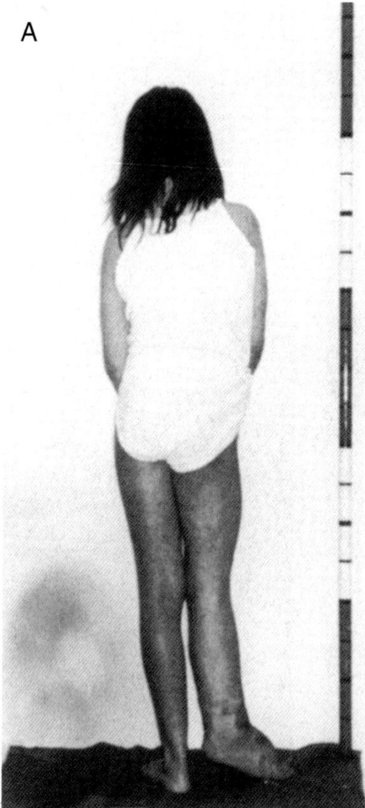

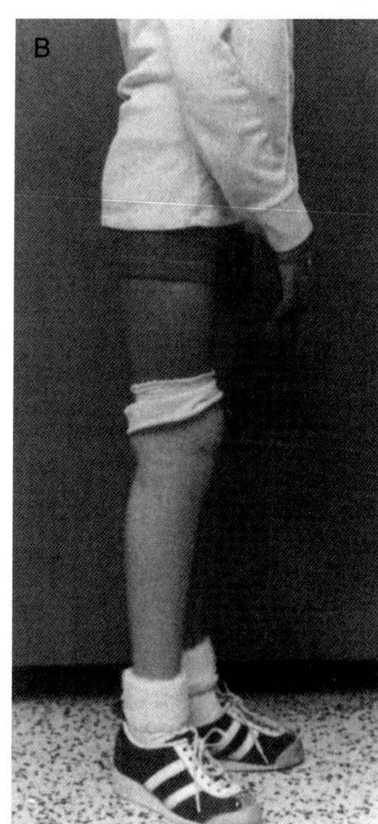

FIGURE 21-19 **A.** Major hypertrophy of the foot which resulted in a significant functional and cosmetic deformity. **B.** Post-amputation of the foot resulting in a much more practical and pleasing limb.

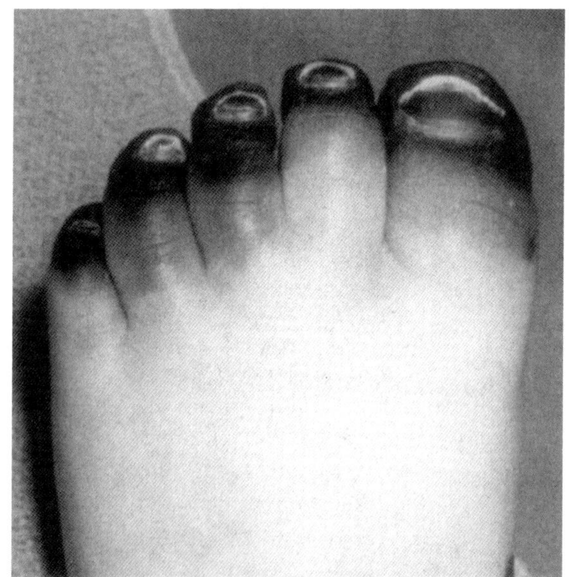

FIGURE 21-20 Frostbite of toes with lines of demarcation forming eight days after injury.

cause of amputation in childhood. These accidents account for 50% of all of the deaths from machinery accidents despite the fact that farms account for only 7% of the population (182,219). A major review of farm accidents in Saskatchewan, revealed that over 50% involved children under 16 years of age and many of these resulted in amputations (107).

The auger is one of the most common pieces of equipment used in the farm environment. Archimedes designed the first auger to deliver water up a hill by encasing a screw device within a cylinder. The principles of today's auger are the same with the exception that the power has increased from that of a singer ox to that of a modern tractor. Portable grain augers, the most common form used by farmers on the prairies, vary in diameter up to s20 cm and have speeds of 500 to 600 revolutions per minute (81,197) (Figure 21-23). Even with protective shields a child's limb can still become caught in this fascinating device (Figure 21-24). Few limbs can be salvaged after becoming entangled in such a piece of equipment and prevention is the most effective treatment for such potential amputations. Often the auger shields are removed during buy harvesting becausw the shields tend to slow the flow of grain by up to 60%. In many areas of the world, safety shielding for power taking-off shafts, cutting blades, and augers are optional accessories and because of cost and the real or imagined decrease in efficiency of the auger, are often not purchased by farmers. There remains a need for additional research in safety engineering and design for these types of farm equipment.

The wounds from such highly powered machinery are absolutely devastating and usually result in amputation on the spot (Figure 21-25), often at a level higher than the foot (Figure 21-26), or result in an extremity that is so severely traumatized that partial or complete surgical amputation will be necessary. The general surgical principles for management of a major contaminated wound are called for: the debris must be completely removed; the wound must be left open; the osseous structures must be

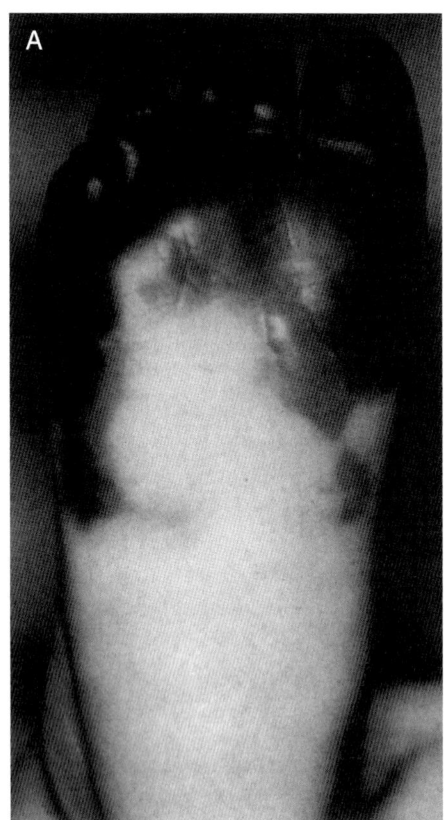

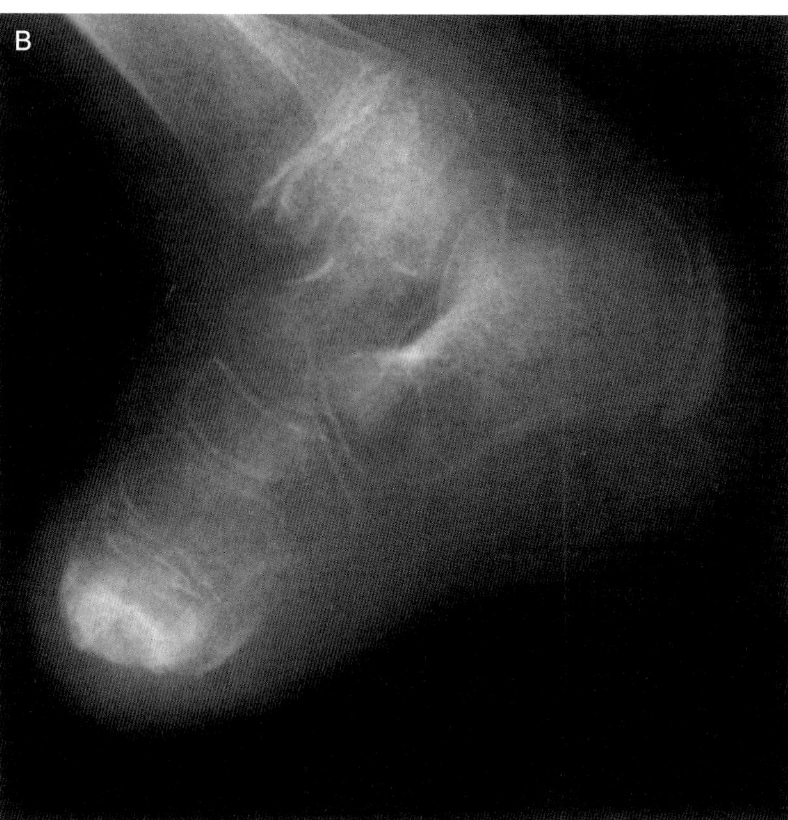

FIGURE 21-21 **A.** Severe frostbite in a child lost in the woods in -10°F temperature. Note the fairly clear demarcation line which allowed a Lisfranc amputation to be performed through the tarsal metatarsal joints **(B)**. The foot has remained very functional with only a shoe filler being required.

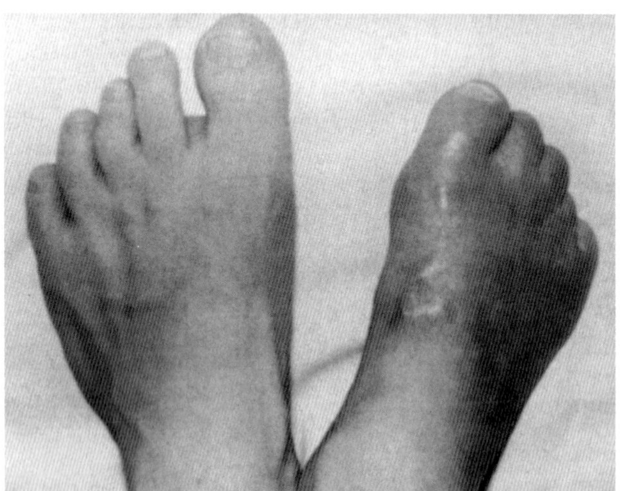

FIGURE 21-22 Eight years post-severe frost bite to the right foot sustained at six years of age, illustrating the continued decreased perfusion rendering the foot susceptible to the cold as well as the decreased size of the foot due to growth plate arrest produced by the freezing.

reduced and immobilized by skeletal traction; and the skin, if degloved, should be replaced as a full-thickness graft (150). The reconstruction of a severely traumatized foot may require free tissue transfer with microsurgical techniques in order to provide a functional extremity with adequate skin cover especially on the weight-bearing plantar surface (49,51,211). Donor tissues potentially available for such transfers are latissimus dorsi muscle (166), scapular skin (238), deltoid muscle, and lateral arm skin (128,212). Success rates as high as 95% have been reported by experienced microvascular surgical teams (168,175).

Another common cause of foot amputation in children occurs when a child falls off a moving box car on which he has hitched a ride. Thompson et al. (231) described these children falling under the wheels of the moving train in such a way that an amputation occurred proximally on one lower limb and through the ankle or foot on the opposite limb as the child falls obliquely under the wheels (Figure 21-27). This results in a bilateral amputee; a devastating way to begin the productive wage-earning years. Many of these children become emotionally compromised and they may require considerable psychiatric support to enable them to cope with their disability (48).

Loss of a major portion of the foot or lower limb in a child demands psychological support and juvenile amputee clinics should have a trained psychologist or psychiatrist who is used to coping with the child's reactions to loss of a limb segment (70,136). The question of salvage versus primary amputation with severely traumatized feet is usually clear cut in children. Waiting for two or three days before deciding on a definitive procedure will often

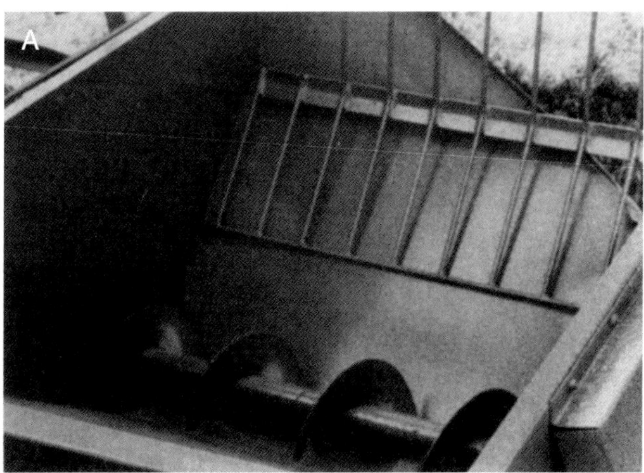

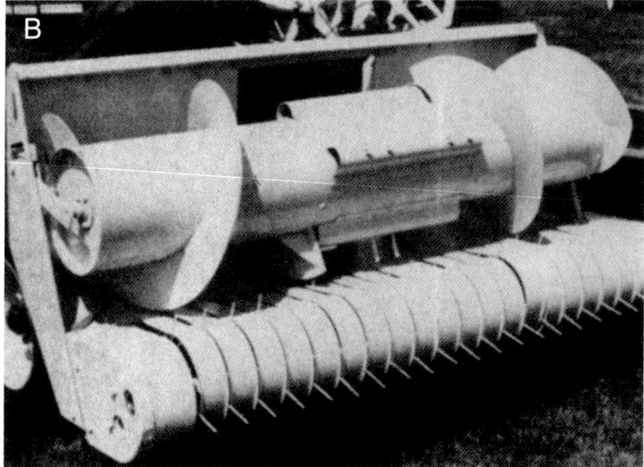

FIGURE 21-23 A. Auger with safety shield removed. B: Combine auger.

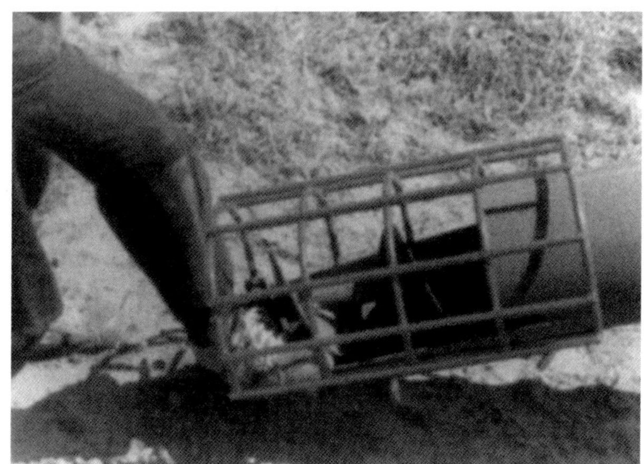

FIGURE 21-24 Safety shields as currently constructed are not completely protective and will allow the intrusion of "inquisitive" limbs.

permit delineation of the viable tissue and assist in decision making (137). Prolonged ischemia of a portion of a foot in children for longer than six to eight hours is still a major criterion for amputation. Absent posterior tibial nerve function is a less absolute indication in a child because of the tremendous growth potential of injured nerves in a child (84,85,90). The results are often much better in a child when it is possible to suture a severed posterior tibial nerve (129). The mangled extremities severity score (MESS) which has been shown to be useful in severe trauma to adult extremities must not be applied as strictly for children, but similar principles apply (90).

Lawnmower Injuries to the Foot in Children

Children's feet are prone to many types of machinery accidents from misadventure or lack of respect for the machine itself (43,155). The power lawnmower is one of the most common causes of foot amputation in children (15). The

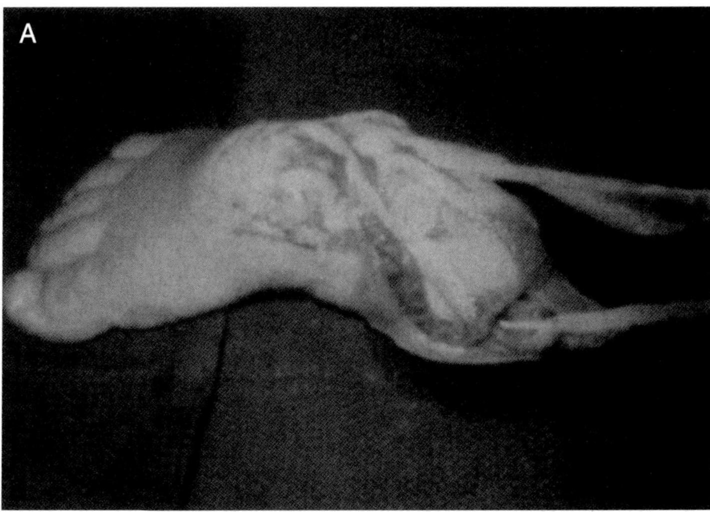

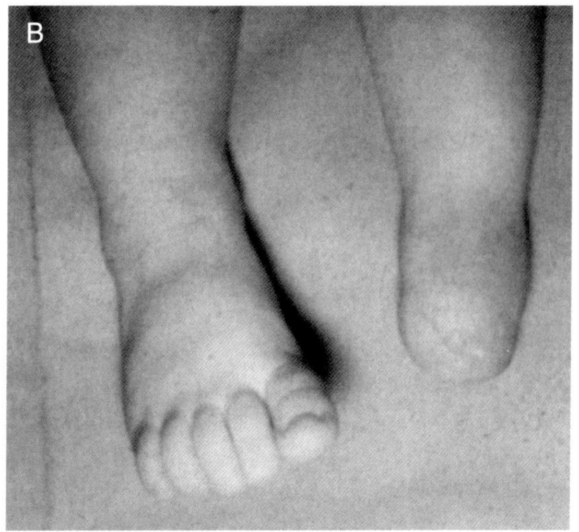

FIGURE 21-25 A. A six-year-old child's foot amputated at the ankle by an auger and brought in with the child in a bag. B. A Syme amputation was performed and the child has an excellent gait with a Syme prosthesis.

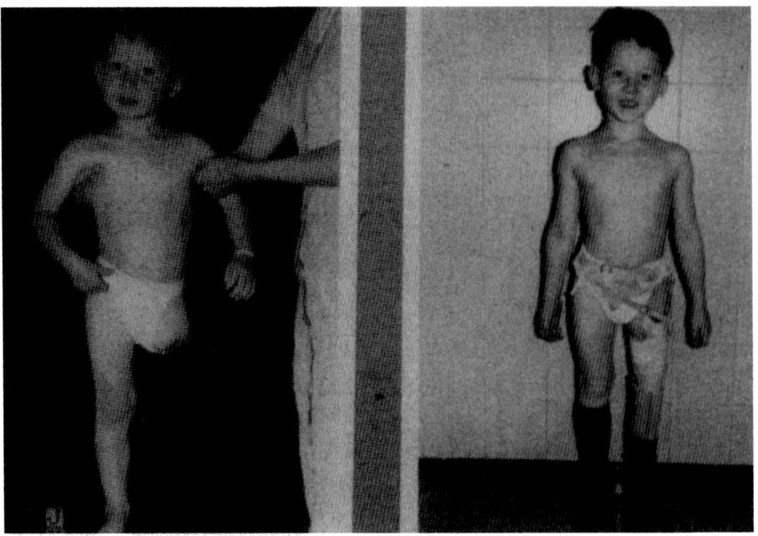

FIGURE 21-26 Auger injuries often "screw" the entire limb into the machine resulting in high level amputations as in this five-year-old boy.

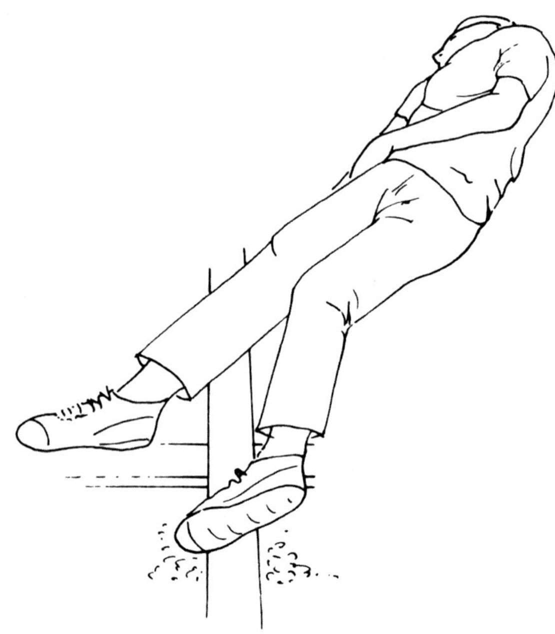

FIGURE 21-27 Oblique positioning of limbs as they slide under a moving train during a fall off a moving boxcar frequently results in bilateral amputations high on one side and involving the foot or ankle on the contralateral side. (From Thompson GH, Balourdas GM, Marcus RE. Rail yard amputations in children. *J Pediatr Orthop* 1983;3:443, with permission.)

injury frequently occurs when a child, sitting with an adult on a tractor lawnmower, falls off and the foot becomes entangled under the blades (117,148,160,189). A Canadian review of lawnmower injuries (148) demonstrated that the most common cause of injury was the child playing near the mower (Table 21-5) and generally results in amputation of the foot or a portion of the foot (Table 21-6).

The wounding capacity of power rotary lawnmowers is immense. An extremity encountered a blade rotating at 3,000 revolutions per minute cannot be extricated before either the limb has been ablated or the blade has had several passes at the limb, causing several areas of major laceration (Figure 21-28). Unfortunately because of the contamination with soil, complications of infection, skin coverage and primary healing in such wounds are frequent (77). Portions of the skin may be degloved by the blade and secondary skin slough is not uncommon. These wounds have to be treated with considerable concern, left open, and the child given a broad spectrum antibiotic and immunizations for tetanus. Fortunately, the wounds inflicted by the lawnmower usually command respect and hence the major wounds are treated very appropriately. The significance of smaller lacerations is sometimes not

TABLE 21-5

Mechanism of Lawnmower Injury of 31 Children

Mechanism	*No: of Children*
Playing near mower	19
Fell off tractor mower	4
Struck by mower	3
Operating mower	3
Missile injury	2

TABLE 21-6

Types of Lawnmower Amputation in 20 Children

Amputation	*No. of Children*
Toes	
Great toe only	3
Multiple	3
Fingers	5
Metatarsal rays	4
Transmetatarsal	2
Below knee	3

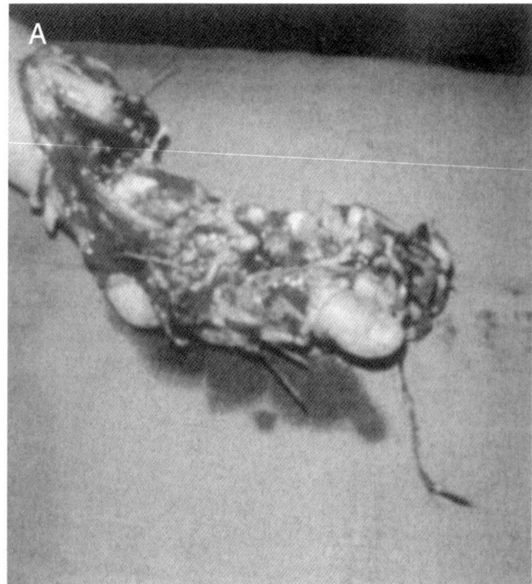

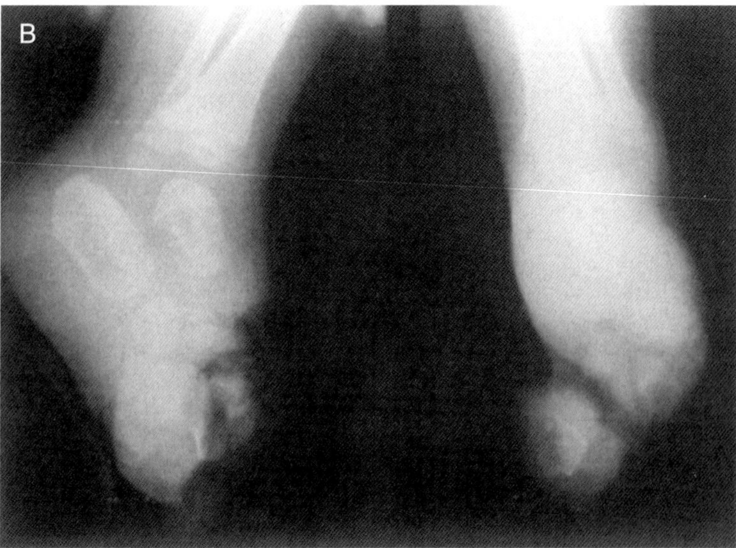

FIGURE 21-28 **A.** Severe trauma sustained when this child's foot was run over by a power lawnmower requiring a Syme amputation. **B.** Loss of the forefoot in a four-year-old child from a lawnmower injury. This was converted to a modified Chopart amputation.

appreciated and it is this type of wound that may result in the most serious clostridial infections. All wounds sustained by the foot resulting from lawnmower injury must be treated aggressively and assumed to be severely contaminated. The use of a vacuum pump for these wounds following debridement often assists the development of granulation tissue facilitating skin grafting (215).

Thorough washing before debridement of these wounds is mandatory. Unfortunately, lawnmower wounds may deceive emergency medical officers who initially do not appreciate the depth and complexity of the wounds because the tissue may fall back together after the blade has passed through. All wounds should be explored thoroughly under general anesthesia. Foreign bodies are frequently found in association with these wounds and radiographs should always be taken to detect unsuspected foreign material (101). Skin that has been degloved, providing it has not been severely traumatized, should be cleaned, defatted, and reapplied as full-thickness grafts. The skin should not simply be reapplied without defatting no matter how healthy it looks as it will inevitably slough if simply sutured back in place. Degloving injuries of the heel are particularly devastating and may result in amputation due to loss of the heel pad unless adequate tissue can be transferred from another site (Figure 21-30).

The wounds should be reinspected and redressed in the operating room at 2–3 days. At 6–8 days, the wound can be closed and skin grafts applied if the tissue is clean and granulating. With the loss of a portion of the foot, a prosthetic "filler" for the shoe may be required to maintain the foot's contour and to provide stability and comfort for the remaining foot mass (Figure 21-31). The filler can be made of polystyrene plastic foam or another plastic material with the opposite foot serving as the mold.

Virtually every lawnmower injury is preventable. A set of guidelines formulated as a result of a review of lawnmower injuries in children in 1977 is still relevant today.

1. Educate children about the dangers of lawnmowers.
2. Prevent children from riding on tractor mowers.
3. Use the grass catcher whenever possible to reduce the number of projectiles.
4. Avoid unnecessary use of powered wheel-driven mowers around children.
5. Have hand controls mounted on the handle so that the mower can be turned off quickly.

Degloving Injuries

Serious degloving injuries are uncommon but currently are being encountered with increasing frequency in children. This form of injury often contributes to amputation of the foot because of loss of soft tissue coverage (144). It is especially devastating when the heel is degloved because split-skin grafting of this area is notoriously unsuccessful. The injury occurs most commonly when a motor vehicle runs over a portion of the foot or when the foot is caught in a piece of moving machinery. The degloved area invariably becomes gangrenous when the skin is simply sutured back in place because of loss of the cutaneous blood supply. The destruction of soft tissue coverage predisposes these foot injuries to infection, contracture, and unsatisfactory cosmesis while the underlying fractured bones are subject to delay or non-union (Figure 21-32).

Degloving occurs when a sudden severe shearing strain is applied to the foot, e.g., by a moving vehicle tire (Figure 21-33). The degloving may be very obvious or it may masquerade as a small break in the skin while there is complete disruption of all attachments between the skin and the underlying fascia, particularly in areas where the skin is densely attached to the underlying fascia as in the palm or the sole of the foot (Figure 21-34). The plane of separation may also occur between fascia and the layers of the tenosynovium or periosteum. This constitutes a more devastating degloving injury which is more difficult to replace without subsequent loss of skin

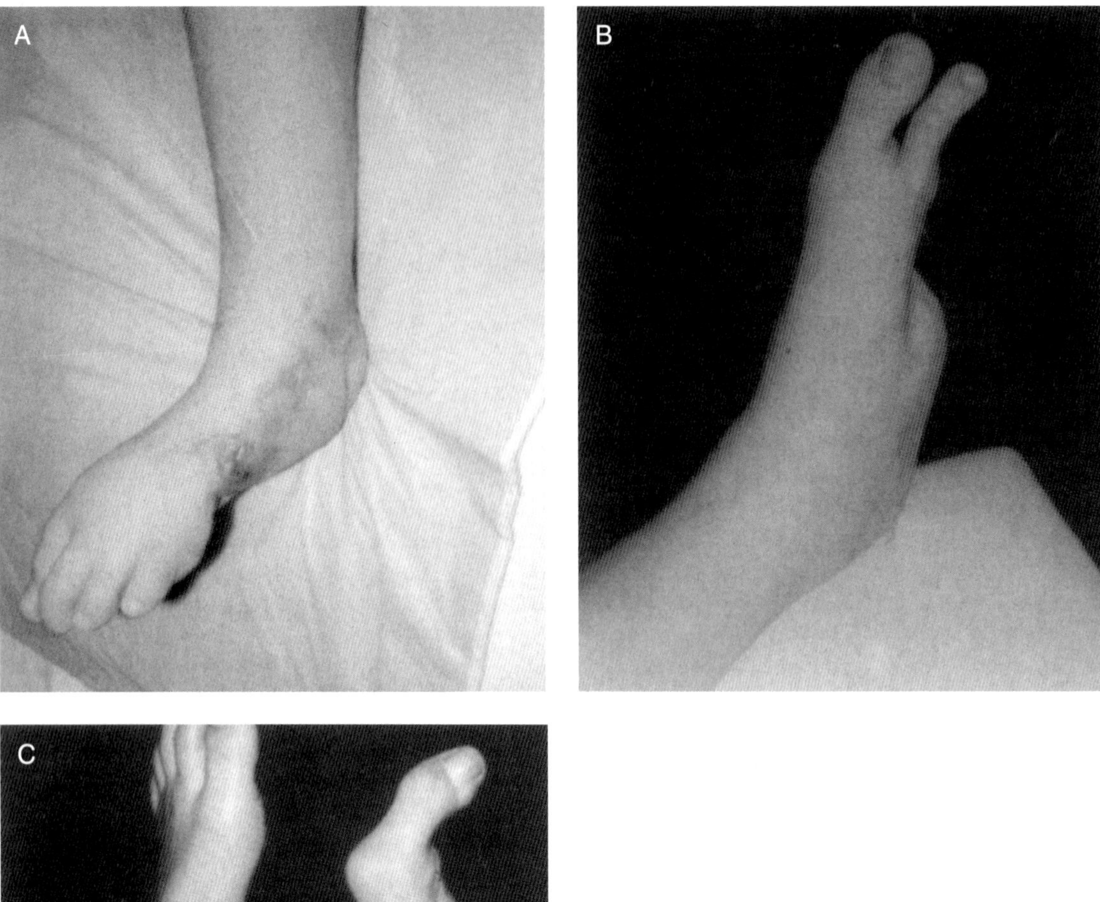

FIGURE 21-29 **A,B,C.** Examples of traumatic amputations of the foot sustained as a result of childhood lawnmower injury. The lateral rays of the foot are most vulnerable.

(159,165,173,196,204,206,208,209,218,239). The foot may undergo degloving and soft tissue causing simultaneously and this makes skin salvage extremely difficult. In these instances, a vascularized tissue graft from another site will frequently be necessary to avoid amputation. Removing the subcutaneous fat from the skin that is degloved and reapplying the skin as a full-thickness graft is often an effective way to salvage and cover the dorsum of the foot. Farmer (62) recorded the first successful replacement of degloved skin as a full-thickness graft in 1943, but many surgeons have not yet appreciated the importance of this concept and as a result keep repeating the error of simply re-suturing the degloved skin and subsequently watching the slough (40,42,49).

The heel and sole are the most difficult sites of degloving. Unfortunately, this area is frequently injured in farm machine accidents and motor cycle trauma. In these instances a microvascular myocutaneous flap may be required for coverage (see Figure 21-30).

Degloving of the foot has in the past necessitated amputations when the underlying pedal structures are relatively intact and neurovascular integrity of the foot is retained. Techniques of microvascular tissue transfers can now salvage many severely traumatized pediatric feet (67,102,112,128,141).

Gun Shot Wounds

An increase in pediatric gun shot wounds is being experienced in many sectors of North America. The increased availability of firearms has resulted in greater access to these weapons by children (106,149,181,186,225,242). The

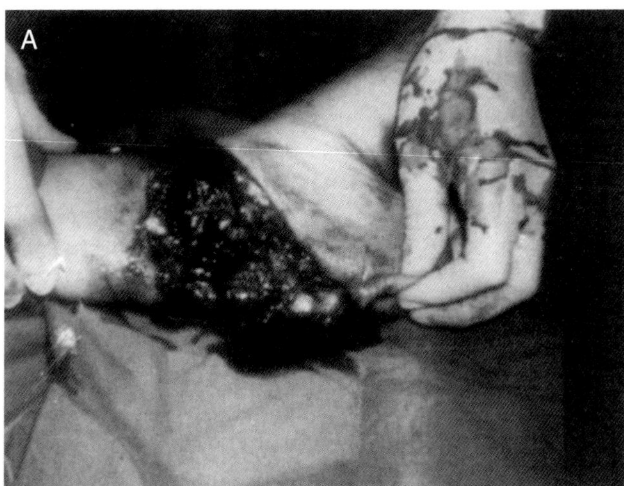

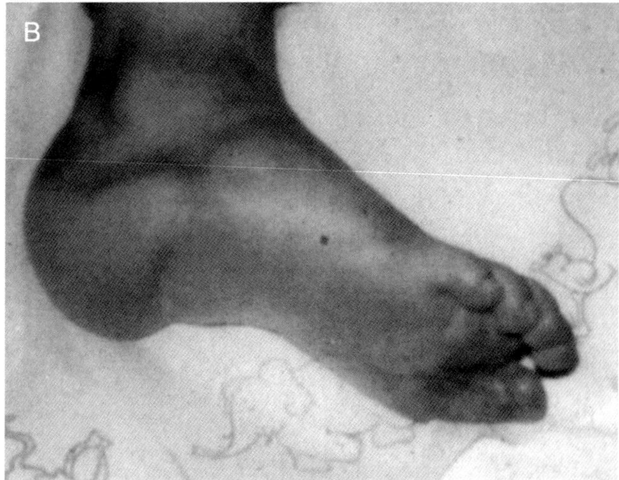

FIGURE 21-30 **A.** Degloved heel. **B.** Heel coverage utilizing a deltoid myocutaneous transplant.

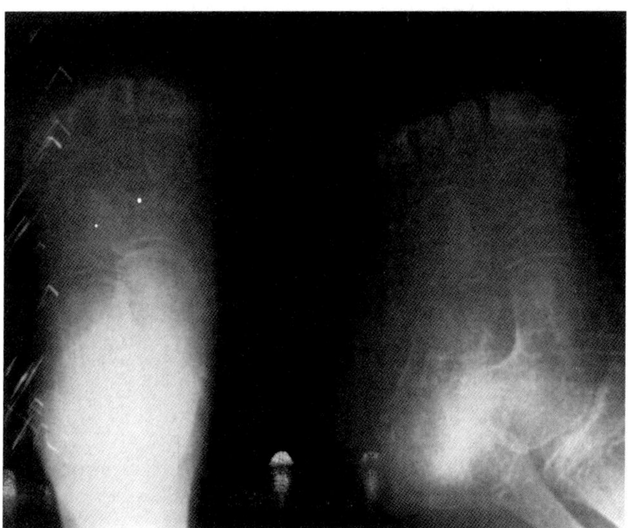

FIGURE 21-31 Amputation of forefoot by a lawnmower. The foot was ultimately functional with a shoe filler.

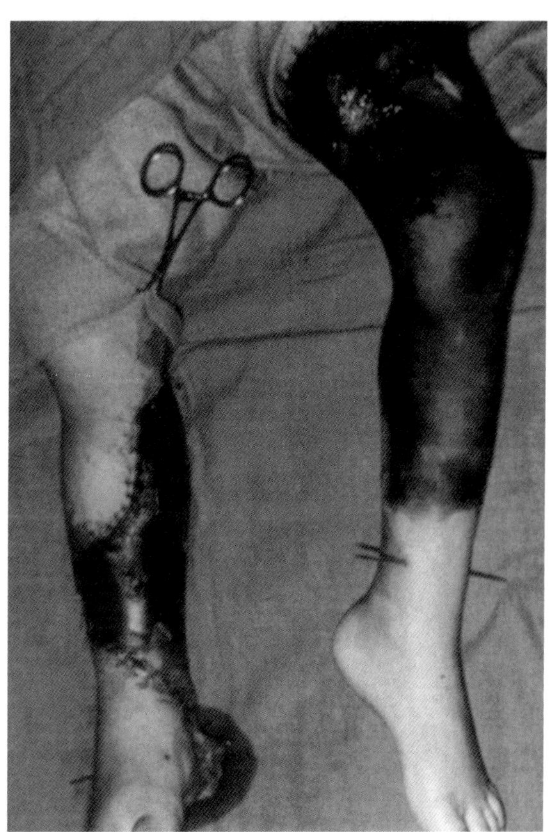

FIGURE 21-32 Complete loss of skin viability including the sole and heel of the right foot, following simple replacement of degloving skin without prior defatting. (From Letts RM. Degloving injuries in children. *J Pediatr Orthop* 1986;6:193, with permission.)

lower extremity is frequently the site of missile injury with the foot being a not-uncommon site of penetration. Gun shot wounds to the foot are inflicted by the child himself in the majority of instances. Because kinetic energy = (mass $\times$ velocity^2) it is the velocity of the missile that is most important in determining the wound character (54). High-velocity missile wounds can result in amputation of portions of the foot. The tremendous energy brought to bear on the surrounding tissues may result in growth plate arrest (149). The small immature tarsal bones have increased vulnerability to this type of trauma and may be completely shattered and destroyed (Figure 21-35). Shotgun injuries devastate the foot and frequently result in major loss of a part of the foot with significant loss of skin and soft tissue (149). High-velocity weapons and shotgun injuries require aggressive treatment because infection and subsequent skin coverage may become major problems. Operative debridement, broad spectrum antibiotic coverage, and secondary grafting are recommended to avoid partial or complete loss of the foot (13,36). This may necessitate free muscle microsurgical flaps where skin coverage is required over weight-bearing portions of the foot (83,89,103). K-wire fixation to realign the metatarsals and phalanges is an effective way to maintain the integrity of the osseous anatomy until soft tissue coverage can be effected (254).

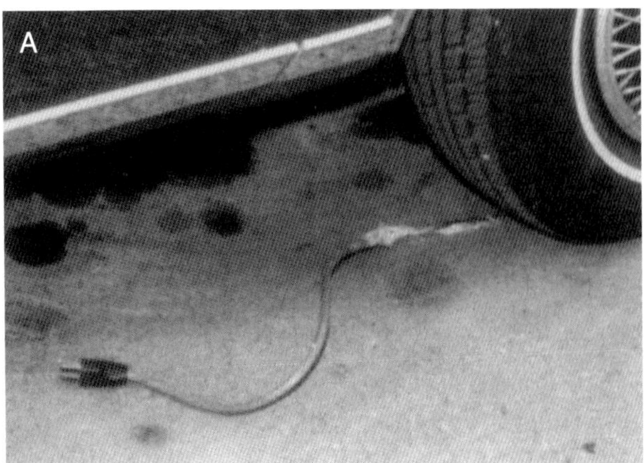

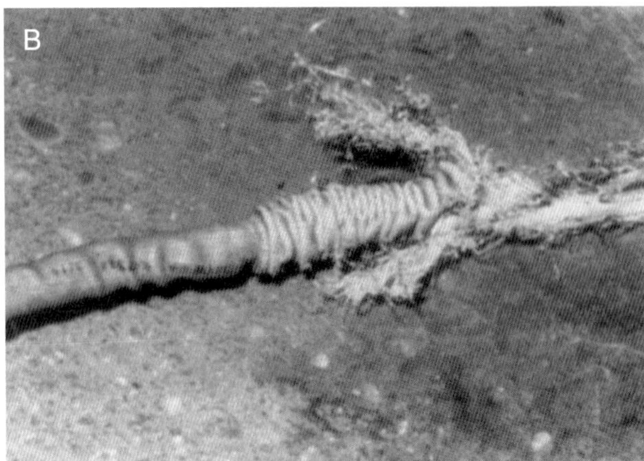

FIGURE 21-33 **A,B.** Degloving of the foot is analogous to an electrical cord being run over by a wheel.

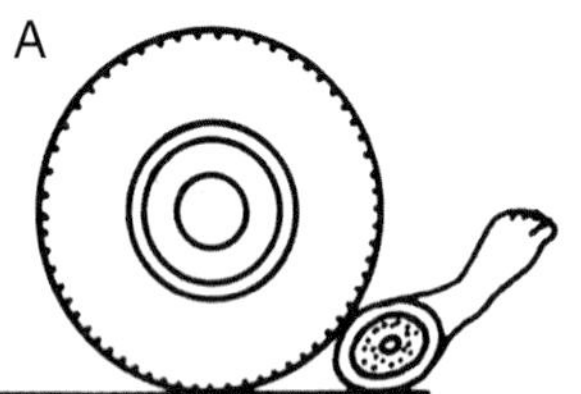

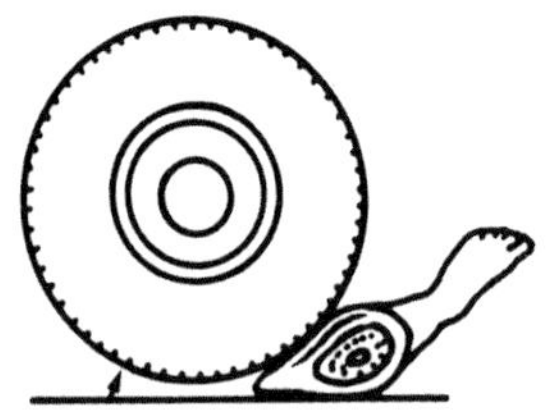

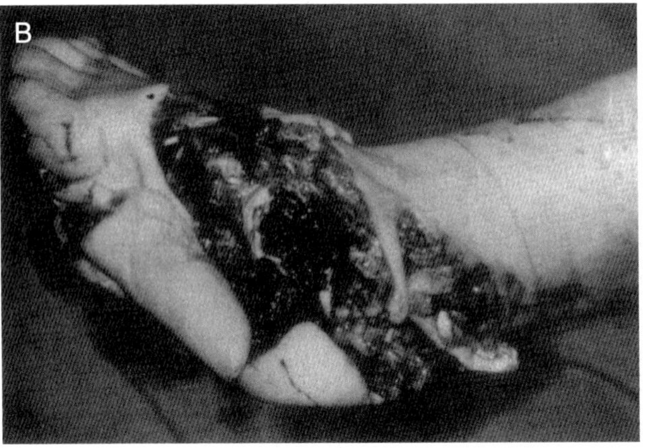

FIGURE 21-34 **A.** Shear force from a tire passing over area of a limb with loose skin attachment may cause a concealed degloving injury. **B.** In the foot where the skin is more adherent the degloving is overt and obvious. (From Letts RM. Degloving injuries in children. *J Pediatr Orthop* 1986;6:193, with permission.)

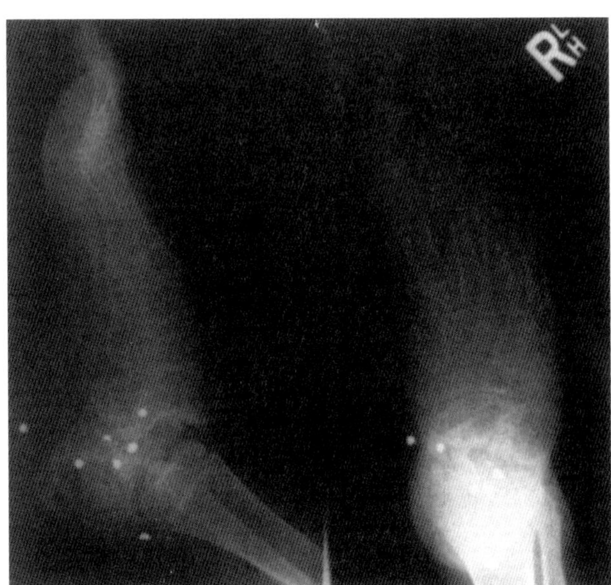

FIGURE 21-35 Gun shot injury to foot which has blown away the talus and a portion of the calcaneus.

Gangrene of the Newborn

Extremity gangrene due to arterial insufficiency is an uncommon cause of amputation in the newborn and was first described by Martini in 1828 (18). Although rare, this type of disastrous event is frequently seen in infants reputing intensive care and the precipitating event can be arterial puncture, indwelling vascular catheters, or other invasive arterial events. Thrombotic or embolic phenomenon may also occur as a complication of the normal obliteration of the ductus arteriosus or the umbilical arteries, as well as the rare occurrence of one twin bleeding into the other *in utero* (Figure 21-36). (10,18,24,28,29,74,91,92,147,163,252).

Treatment

The orthopedist must be aware that arterial insufficiency is a possible cause of peripheral gangrene in the newborn. Early angiography and surgical removal of the obstruction is ideal, but unfortunately not always possible. Supportive care of the limb to avoid trauma and further compromise of the blood supply may result in complete recovery in some instances. The more frequent result however, is progressive ischemia with loss of the distal limb, usually including a portion of the foot or lower extremity. Care must be taken to await appropriate demarcation, avoid sepsis, and remove only the ischemic portion with a good viable skin closure effected.

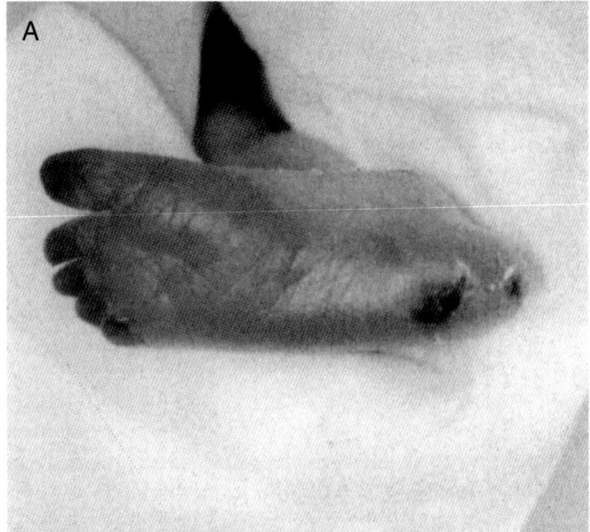

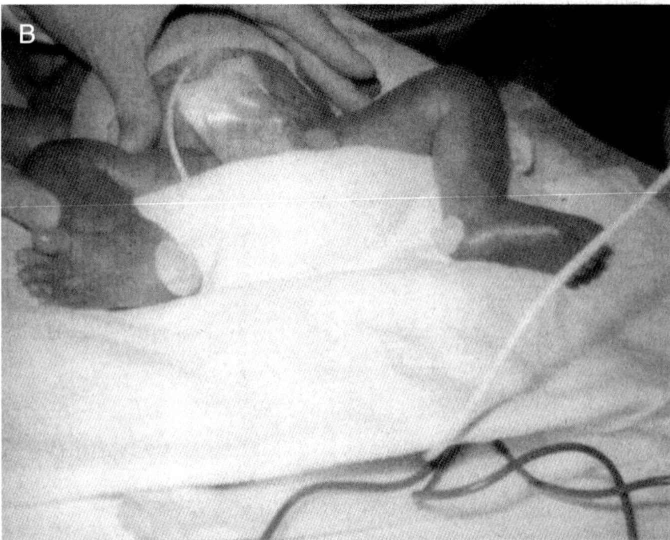

FIGURE 21-36 **A.** Newborn infant who required umbilical catheterization developed vascular insufficiency of both lower extremities resulting in Syme amputation of the feet. **B.** Demarcation of the gangrenous foot developing after several days.

Meningococcemia with Vascular Insufficiency of the Extremities

Meningococcemia is occasionally associated with disseminated intravascular coagulation (DIC) resulting in skin and muscle tissue loss primarily affecting the extremities (16,216,233,238). In some instances, only skin is lost, but in more severe cases, the entire extremity may require amputation (Figure 21-37). Unfortunately, there is little that one can do except to provide supportive treatment for the child and wait the demarcation of the extent of tissue lost (53). A guillotine type amputation of the foot or lower extremity may be the safest approach when infection is a problem. The stump is left open and traction placed on the surrounding skin. Over a period of two to three weeks, the skin will gradually cover the granulation tissue and in most instances an excellent stump will be produced (113). Damage to the growth plates of the remaining extremity may be associated with vascular insufficiency (14,35,58). This may be secondary to thrombosis of the metaphyseal and epiphyseal vessels and may necessitate the early resection of bony bridges and corrective osteotomies to manage the deformities produced by the epiphyseal tethering (248). Families should be provided with psychiatric care to assist them in coping with this devastating disease (213).

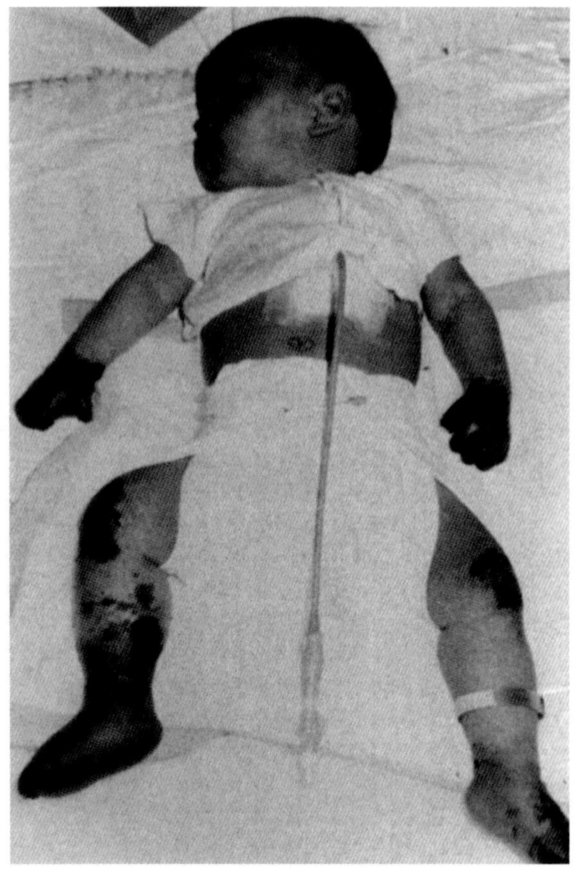

FIGURE 21-37 Meningococcemia resulted in severe vascular insufficiency to the extremities in this six-month-old infant culminating in the loss of both hands, right foot, and a Lisfranc amputation of the left foot.

Compartment Syndrome

Compartment syndrome in the foot is a poorly recognized phenomenon that probably occurs more frequently in the foot than most clinicians appreciate. A high index of suspicion should be entertained when there are clinical signs and symptoms of a compartment syndrome in a foot that has sustained a crushing type of injury. The symptom of pain is difficult to assess in children as a crushed foot will be generally painful in all areas. Pain on passive dorsiflexion of the foot in older children should be viewed with suspicion and evidence of decreased circulation carefully searched for. Increasing pain in the foot and complaints of new numbness or tingling in the toes should be of particular concern. The dorsalis pedis and posterior tibial pulses may be present and should not lull the clinician into a false sense of security

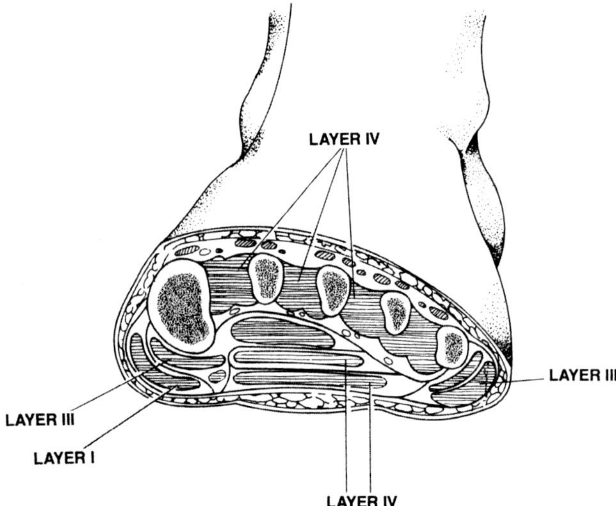

FIGURE 21-38 Muscle layers in the four compartments of the foot which should be decompressed in a severe crush injury to aintain muscle viability. (Modified from Mubarak SJ, Hargens AR. *Compartmental syndrome and its relation to the crush syndrome.* Philadelphia: WB Saunders, 1981.)

that their presence assures that the circulation to all parts of the foot is intact. Associated toe pallor and inability to voluntarily move the toes in an otherwise cooperative child should lend further concern about the possibility of pedal compartment syndrome. Measuring compartment pressures is usually not practical in young children, although in older children this may be helpful.

Early recognition of increased compartment pressures within the fascial spaces of the foot followed by prompt fasciotomy will avoid muscle ischemia and contracture as well as possible amputation of the foot (24,201). The perception of increased compartment pressures can result in the avoidance of amputation or loss of significant interossei muscle function. Compartment syndrome may occur both as a result of burns or direct trauma (214). Gissane (73) described a Lisfranc fracture of the foot that resulted in arterial injury with concomitant bleeding into the foot that ultimately resulted in a below-knee amputation.

The compartments of the foot have been described as four in number by Mubarak and Hergens (177) and are separated by fascia layers which include: (i) medial, (ii) lateral, (iii) central, and (iv) interosseous (Figure 21-38).

Decompression of these compartments can be accomplished by two dorsal incisions or through the medial approach of Henry. The medial approach offers decompression of all four compartments through a single incision and also allows decompression of the medial neurovascular bundle (Figure 21-39) (179,214).

FOOT AMPUTATIONS

The Boyd Amputation

Boyd (27) credited Watson with the first description of this procedure given during a presentation to the Clinical Society of London in 1907.

The Boyd procedure includes foot amputation coupled with a calcaneal tibial fusion. This has the advantage of retaining the heel pad attached to the calcaneal remnant and thus provides a very stable stump which can be used for independent weight bearing without requiring the child to wear a prosthesis (21,170).

The application of this technique in the skeletally immature child necessitates modifications in order to preserve the distal tibial growth plate (59,134).

Surgical Technique

The technique of the pediatric amputation includes modifications described by Kalamchi (21). The midpoint of the calcaneus is marked both medially and laterally, and a fish mouth type of incision is fashioned. The foot is removed through the Chopart joint, and the talus is carefully removed (Figure 21-40). During the dissection, a bone hook to pull the talus forward assists in the removal of the astragalus. The calcaneus is then "squared off" with the anterior portion being removed by an osteotomy which includes the articular surface. The superior surface of the calcaneus is then excised by a second osteotomy which leaves a straight edge to the cancellous surface. The distal tibial cartilage is then resected back to cancellous bone, taking care to preserve the growth plate. This may be done by sharp dissection with a scalpel or an osteotome, depending on the age of the child. When the fibula is present, it too may be trimmed to provide a cancellous surface to fuse to the calcaneus. This procedure is most frequently applicable to patients with congenital fibular hemimelia and the fibular will often be absent.

The calcaneus should then be positioned to sit square under the tibia. The redundant heelcord may require shortening when scar tissue or the tendo-Achillis prevents proper positioning. The tibialis anterior and posterior tendons can be utilized as a sling beneath the calcaneus to assist in holding the bone in proper position. The calcaneus can also be fixed and placed with K-wires. The wound is then closed with the skin edges trimmed appropriately to allow for an anterior closure. A Hemovac drain is inserted and a long leg cast applied (Figure 21-41). The Hemovac drain is removed within 48 hours and the cast changed at three weeks. Sutures are removed at this time and another weight-bearing cast is applied. At six to eight weeks the K-wires can be removed, and fitting for a prosthesis can be started in another two weeks.

Advantages of the Boyd Amputation

This type of amputation results in a good functional end-bearing stump with much less chance of pad migration than the Syme procedure. The preservation of the distal tibial growth plate allows the limb to continue growing even though these limbs are often short and the child usually requires a prosthesis. The procedure is preferred to a below-knee amputation because it allows weight bearing without a prosthesis and thereby permits the child to get up at night to the bathroom and walk around the house without the artificial limb.

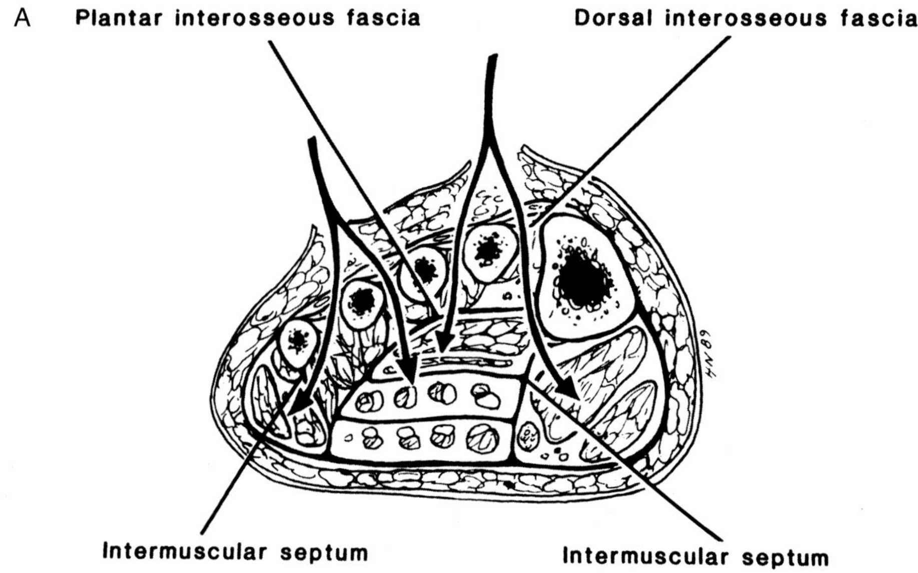

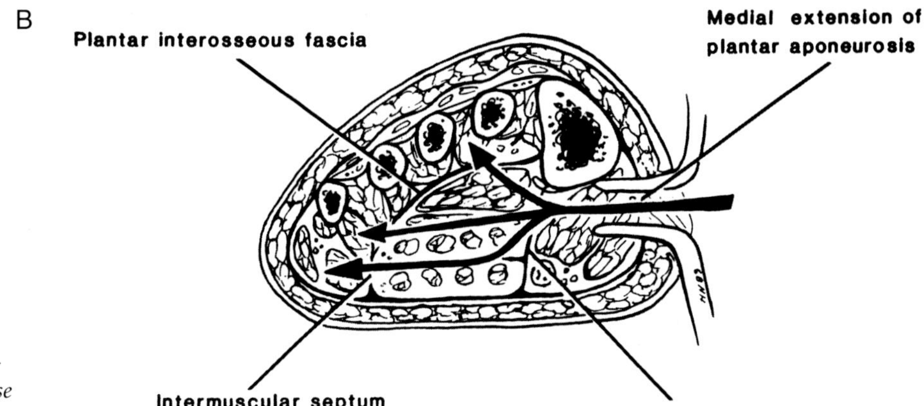

FIGURE 21-39 **A.** Dorsal approach to interosseous compartment decompression. **B.** Medial decompression approach. (From Shereff MJ. Compartment syndromes of the foot. *Inst Course Lect* 1990;39:127, with permission.)

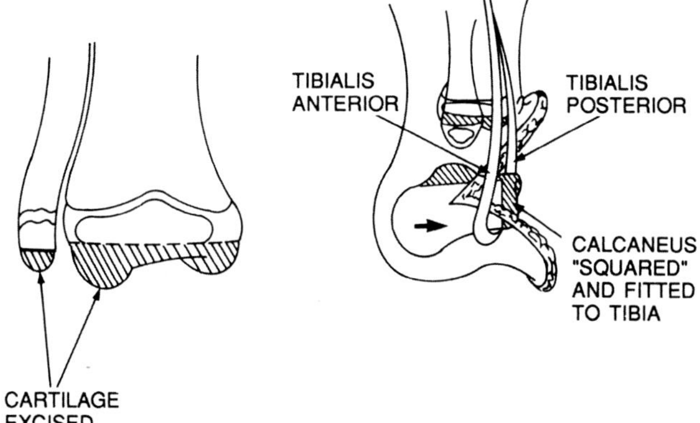

FIGURE 21-40 Modified Boyd amputation with added support from tibialis anterior and posterior sling.

Because the Boyd amputation requires an arthrodesis between the calcaneus and tibia, there is the possibility of a non-union, although I have personally not seen this complication in a child. A corrective osteotomy can be performed at the same time in patients with severe tibial bowing.

The Chopart Amputation

The Chopart amputation, performed at the interface between the talus and calcaneus and the navicular and cuboid, (Figure 21-42), has been associated with a number of complications. Problems include: (i) persistent equinus of the stump, (ii) skin breakdown over the poorly covered anterior talus, and (iii) the very large bulbous stump created prosthetic fitting problems (Figure 21-43). However, the Chopart amputation is a very functional weight-bearing stump when accompanied by muscle balance which prevents the equinus deformity from developing (Figure 21-44).

Children born with congenital Chopart amputations have very functional feet and do not share the complications of increasing equinus seen with the acquired Chopart procedure (17) (see Figures 21-43 and 21-44). This permits the child with the congenital amputation to walk either with or without a prosthesis; indeed, when there is no significant limb-length inequality, a formal prosthesis is often not necessary and a slipper style shoe filler prosthesis similar to one described by Filleauer or Collins may be possible (65).

The Chopart procedure may be appropriate for children who are being considered for elective amputation

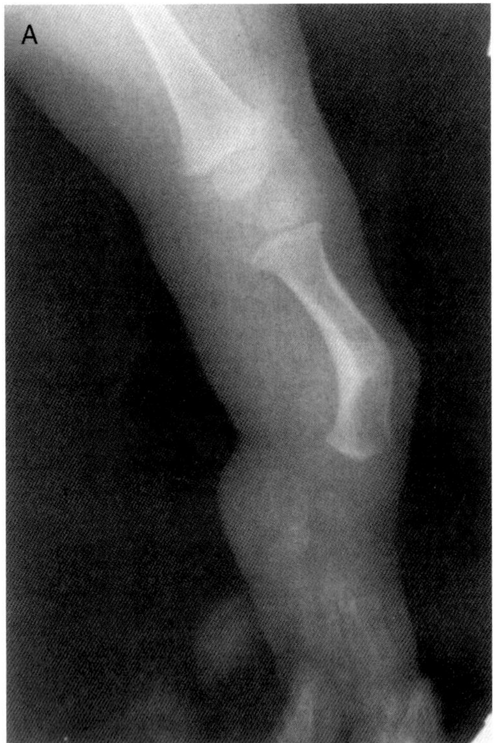

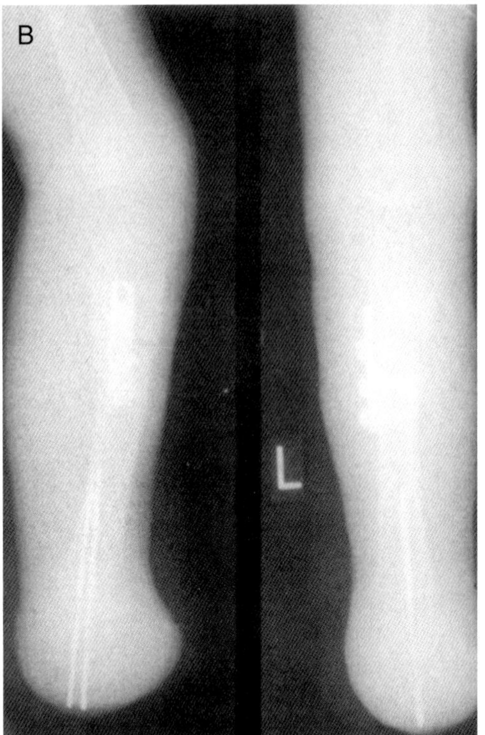

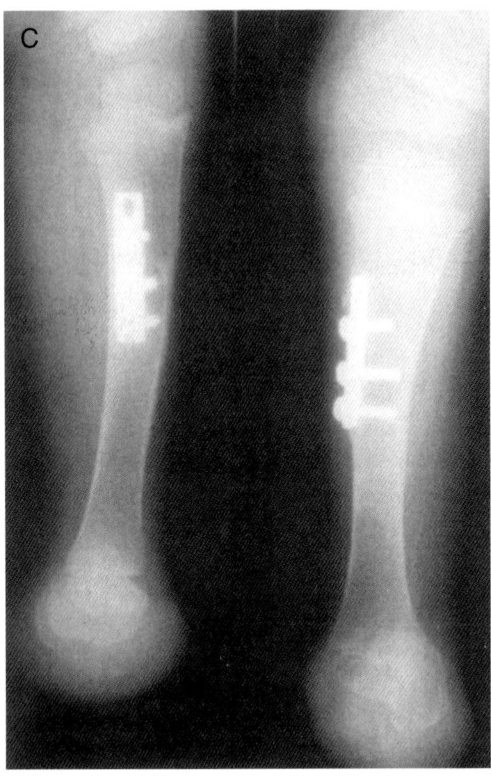

FIGURE 21-41 **A.** This two-year-old child with a unilateral fibular hemimelia and increasing tibial kyphosis underwent a simultaneous corrective osteotomy (**B**) and Boyd amputation. **C.** Fusion between the calcaneous and tibia was complete by two months post-surgery.

because of fibular hemimelia. This group comprises a significant percentage of the children requiring elective foot ablation and the absent fibular eliminates the disadvantage of the bulbous stump.

Syme himself extolled the virtues of the Chopart amputation:

> The operation of Chopart which leaves only the astragalus and calcis is the most valuable of all partial amputations, as it commands the largest portion of the foot requiring removal of disease or injury and at the same time preserves a support for the patient not less useful than that which is afforded by the whole of the tarsus. I performed this operation in 1829, so far as I know, for the first time in Edinburgh and have frequently done so since with the most satisfactory results (191).

Many other types of mid-tarsal amputations have been recommended primarily to preserve the heel pad,

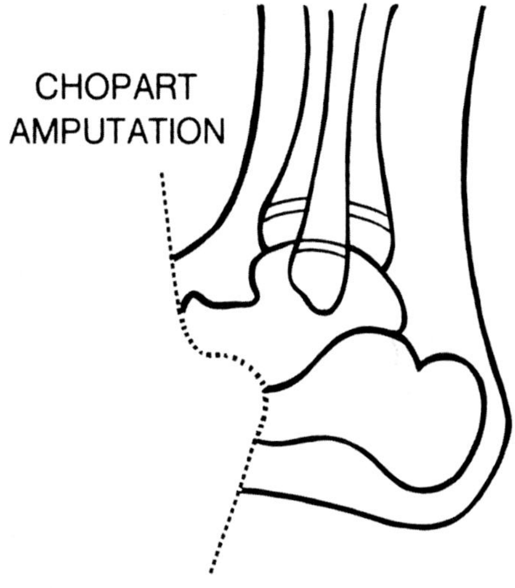

FIGURE 21-42 The traditional Chopart amputation level through the midfoot preserving the calcaneus and talus. (From Letts M, Pyper A. The modified Chopart's amputation. *Clin Orthop* 1990;256:44, with permission.)

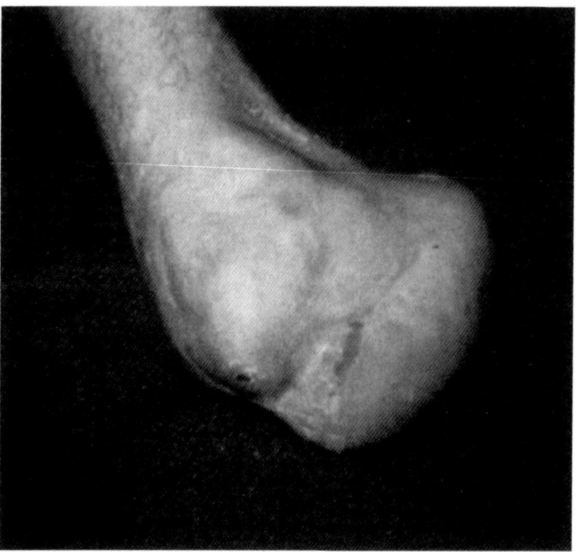

FIGURE 21-43 The "traditional" Chopart amputation is frequently complicated by equinus of the calcaneus and ulceration over the exposed and inadequately covered anterior talus.

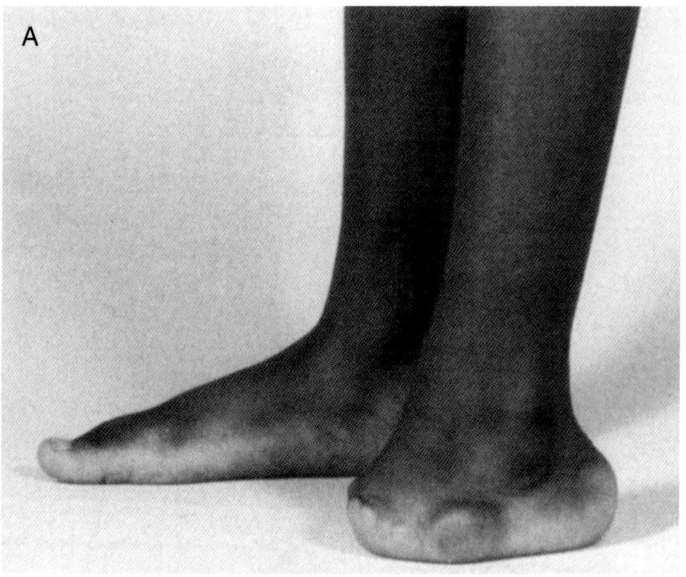

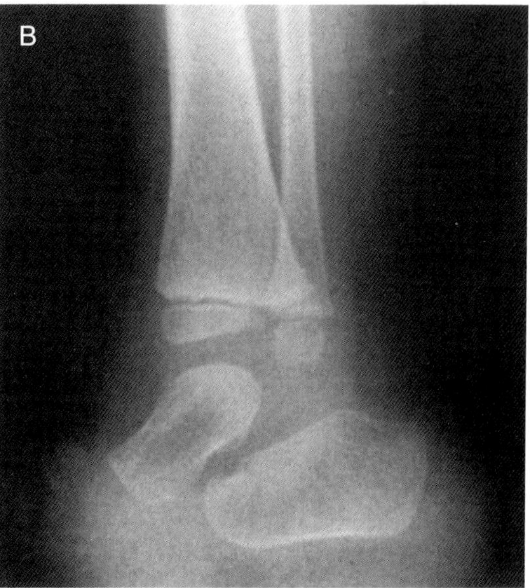

FIGURE 21-44 **A,B.** Congenital Chopart amputation with excellent weight-bearing function. (From Blanco JS, Herring JA. Congenital Chopart amputation: a functional assessment. *Clin Orthop* 1990;256:14, with permission.)

but most have not met with widespread acceptance. The Pirogoff amputation was designed to preserve the posterior surface of the calcaneus. However, the weight-bearing area of the preserved os calcis is not a physiological weight-bearing surface, especially in children who have large cartilaginous calcaneal apophysis (154). Richard modified the Pirogoff amputation by using the normal weight-bearing surface of the calcaneus but failed to fuse the calcaneus to the tibia (130). He sutured the anterior and posterior and plantar tendons together to form a sling to maintain the calcaneal shell and heel pad in a functional position. Kofmann further modified Richards' procedure by transplanting the anterior tendons into the anterior portion of the sustentaculum tali (130). Unfortunately, these procedures did not preserve normal articulations with the resultant development of traumatic arthritis in addition to instability from a weight-bearing joint being maintained primarily by tendon suspension. Boyd (27) corrected many of these deficiencies by fusing the calcaneus to the ankle mortis and provided a relatively successful end-bearing stump but resulted in an extremely shortened limb because of the removal of the talus.

Modified Chopart Amputation

There has been a recent rekindling of interest in the pediatric Chopart amputation primarily because of the good results seen with congenital Chopart amputations as well as the need to provide a functional weight-bearing stump and

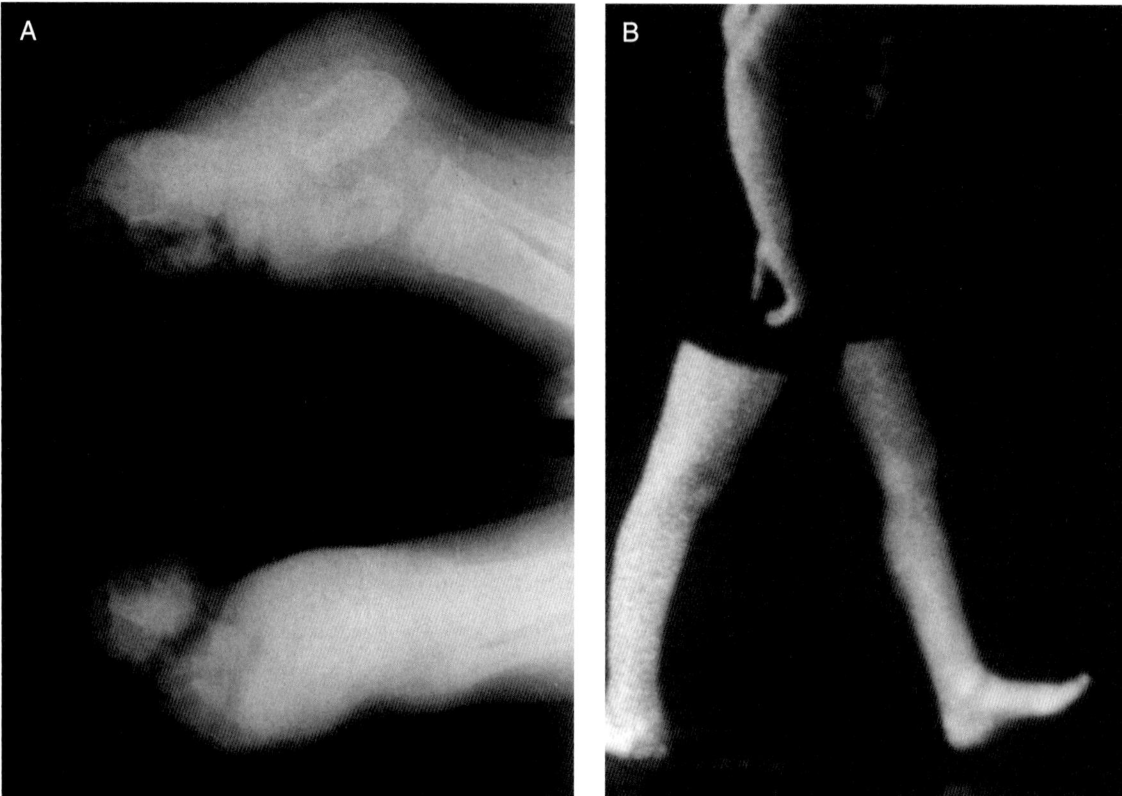

FIGURE 21-45 **A,B.** Traumatic amputation of the foot with the performance of a modified Chopart amputation. The residual hindfoot is very functional and only an AFO with shoe filler was needed with a shoe.

equal limb lengths. When traumatic amputation of a childs foot has occurred in the region of the Chopart joint (Figure 21-45), the option of performing a Syme or Boyd amputation would result in significant shortening of the extremity and require the child to permanently wear a formal prosthesis. Letts and Pyper (145) designed a series of modifications to the pediatric Chopart amputation that have greatly improved the functional results of this procedure.

The basic changes are designed to avoid the problems of equinus and skin breakdown over the anterior stump and include:

1. *Contouring of the anterior talus and inferior calcaneus.* This relieves pressure areas that tend to develop. Excision of these prominent points at the time of amputation minimizes pressure from both shoe wear and weight bearing (Figure 21-46).
2. *Tendon transfer to the neck of talus and sustentaculum tali.* The constant pull of the tendo-Achillis posteriorly is counterbalanced by the transfer of the tibialis anterior, tibialis posterior, extensor communis and extensor hallucis tendons into the talus and/or sustentaculum tali. This also provides moderate dorsi flexion power to the stump (Figure 21-47).
3. *Anterior extension of the plantar skin flap.* The skin flap is designed to extend anteriorly, well over the neck of the talus, to avoid skin breakdown over the anterior aspect of the amputation stump. There is little danger of flap necrosis as the blood supply of this flap is usually excellent. This also counteracts the tendency for the tendo-Achilles to constantly plantar flex the stump by the formation of a plantar skin and fascial sling (Figure 21-48).
4. *Tendo-Achilles lengthening.* Tendo-Achilles lengthening is performed by traditional Z-plasty of the Achilles tendon. This weakens the plantar flexion power of the

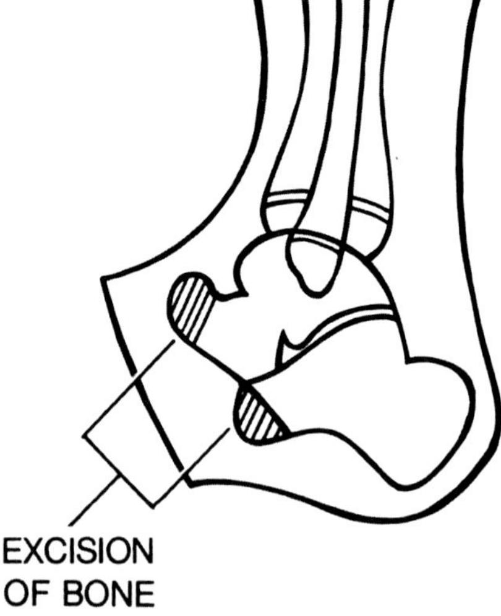

FIGURE 21-46 Excision of bony protuberances of talus and calcaneus to provide a smoothly contoured anterior stump. (From Letts M, Pyper A. The modified Chopart's amputation. *Clin Orthop* 1990;256:44, with permission.)

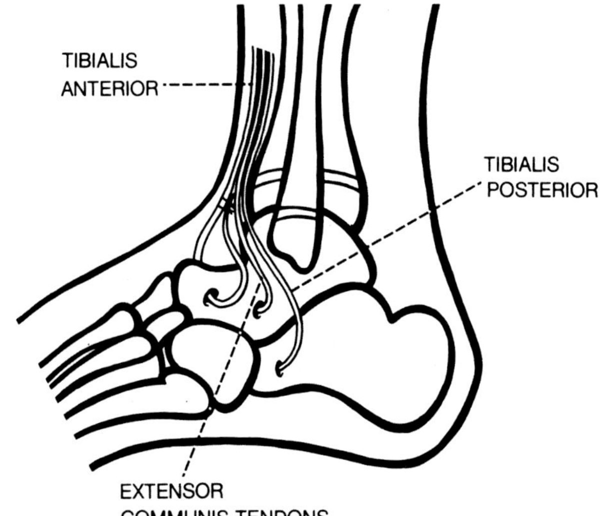

FIGURE 21-47 Transplantation of the tibialis anterior and posterior and extensor tendons into the neck of the talus and sustentaculum tali to provide a dorsiflexion force and avoid the development of equinus. (From Letts M, Pyper A. The modified Chopart's amputation. *Clin Orthop* 1990;256:44, with permission.)

tendo-Achilles and allows the tendons transferred anteriorly to firmly attach to their new osseous beds before dynamic equinus function is regained by the triceps surae (see Figure 21-48).

Advantages If the Modified Chopart Amputation

The Chopart stump provides an extremely functional weight-bearing surface in a child with no limb length inequality, real or anticipated, and allows a near normal gait due to the preservation of the ankle joint and a large heel pad. Prosthetic fitting can be simplified in children with no limb-length inequality by using a polypropylene ankle foot orthosis and a shoe filler or a boot with a shoe filler. When the Chopart amputation has been performed in patients with congenital fibular hemimelia or proximal femoral focal deficiency, the smaller stump resulting from the absence of the fibula permits fitting with the traditional Syme prosthesis (Figure 21-49). Where the stump is too large for this type of prosthesis, a modified Syme prosthesis such as the Tucker-Syme prosthesis provides a more forgiving type of fitting than the traditional Syme prosthesis (Figure 21-50). In children with an absent fibula there is a tendency for the heel to drift into valgus but this can often be avoided by the counter balancing achieved by transferring the tibialis anterior and posterior into the talus and sustentaculum tali to provide a dynamic medial tether. The Chopart amputation allows excellent household ambulation without the prosthesis in both unilateral and bilateral amputees (Figure 21-51). A migrating heel pad or retention of part of the calcaneal apophysis can sometimes complicate the outcome of Syme amputation and can be extremely annoying and present difficult problems for the patient as well as the prosthetics (Figure 21-52). Patients with Syme amputation can bear partial weight but are not comfortable with weight bearing for extended periods of time without their prosthesis. The Boyd procedure is technically difficult to perform in younger patients due to the relatively large amount of cartilage which frequently requires the addition of bone grafting.

The modified Chopart amputation is an attractive alternative amputation site for children who require foot ablations secondary to congenital malformations or severe trauma especially when no significant limb length inequality is anticipated.

The Pirogoff Amputation

The renowned Russian surgeon, Nicolai Ivanovitch Pirogoff (1810–1888) designed his operation in 1854 to solve some of the shortcomings of the Syme amputation which he found technically very difficult to perform (86). This skin incision and the procedure itself are similar to the Syme amputation except that the posterior portion of the calcaneus is retained by dividing it obliquely downward at the junction of the posterior third with the anterior two-thirds of the bone (Figure 21-53). The heel flap therefore does not have to be peeled away from the calcaneus, a part of the Syme amputation that Pirogoff felt to be a

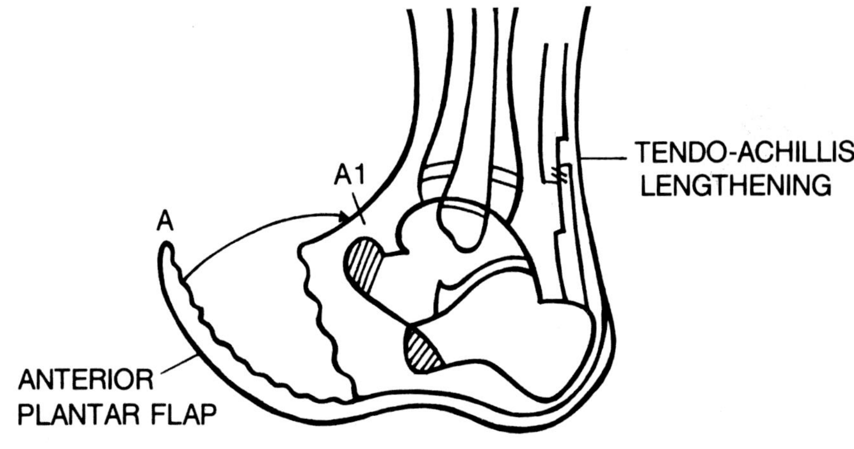

FIGURE 21-48 The "modified Chopart amputation." Illustrating preservation of the plantar skin to cover the anterior stump and tendo-Achilles lengthening to avoid equinus development. (From Letts M, Pyper A. The modified Chopart's amputation. *Clin Orthop* 1990;256:44, with permission.)

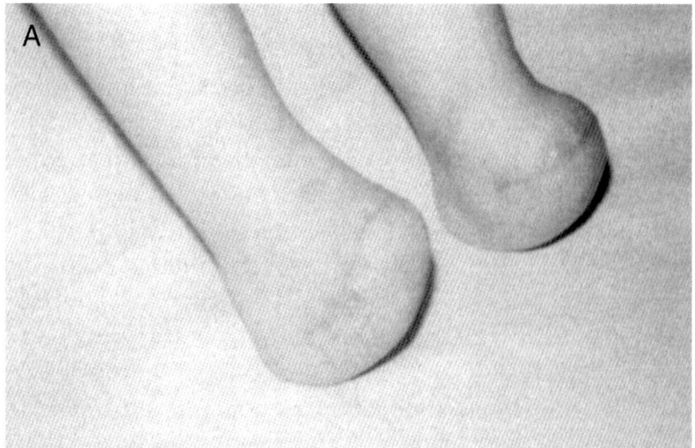

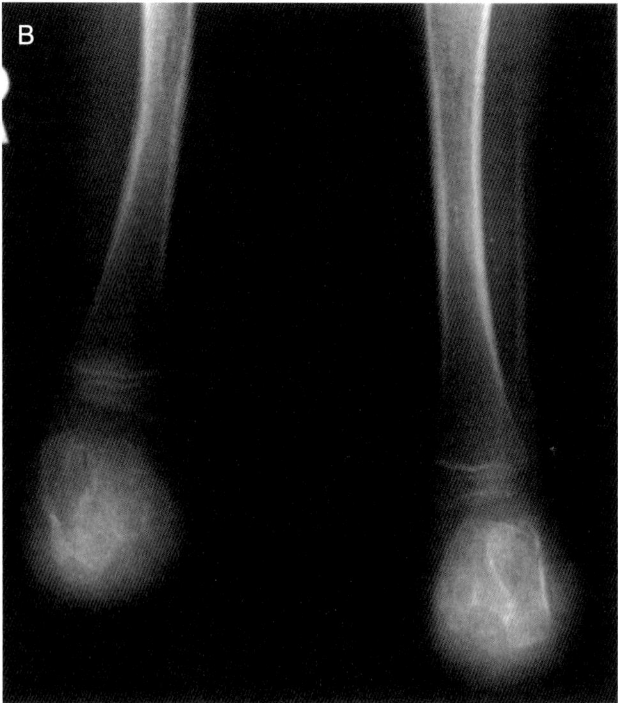

FIGURE 21-49 Modified Chopart amputation in a child with fibular hemimelia. **A.** Note plantar pad brought up well anteriorly over the talar neck. **B.** An excellent weight-bearing platform is afforded by the calcaneus and its heel pad.

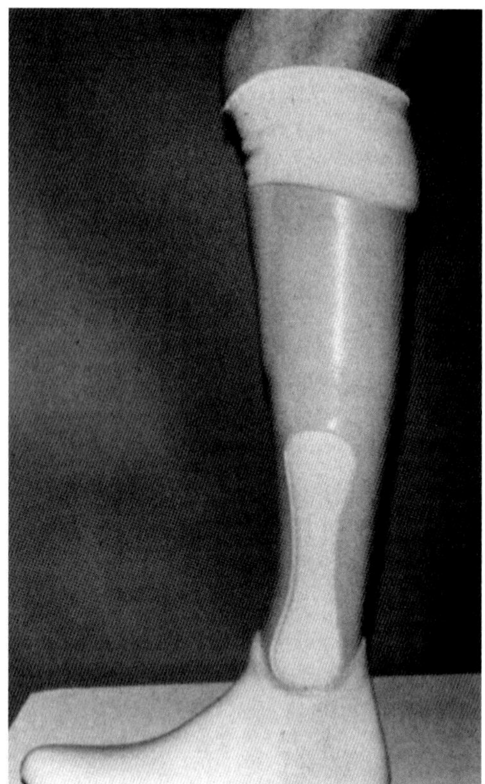

FIGURE 21-50 Prosthetic innovations such as the Tucker-Syme prosthesis facilitate the fitting of the modified Chopart amputation. (From Letts M, Pyper A. The modified Chopart's amputation. *Clin Orthop* 1990;256:44, with permission.)

major shortcoming. The osteotomized surface of the calcaneus is then brought up to the lower end of the tibia and the malleoli divided level with the inferior surface of the tibia. The actual surface of the tibia other than the malleoli is left intact (95).

Pirogoff's operation provides an end-bearing stump which is longer than a Syme stump. The heel flap is always firmly fixed and does not migrate.

The Pirogoff amputation offers children little advantage over the Boyd procedure and is anatomically not physiologic because the child would be weight bearing on the calcaneal apophysis. However, there may be traumatic instances when the Pirogoff type of amputation offers a method of salvaging a more functional weight-bearing extremity, and hence, pediatric orthopedic surgeons should be aware of this technical option (154) (Figure 21-54).

The Syme Amputation

The Syme procedure is the most common form of amputation currently used for both congenital pedal malformation requiring amputation as well as for severe trauma of the foot necessitating ablation of the foot (Figure 21-55). James Syme, an Edinburgh orthopedic surgeon, designed the operation with amputation through the ankle joint because of the high incidence of infection associated with other forms of pedal and tibial amputation at that time. He first published his procedure in 1843 (191). The technique requires meticulous attention to detail especially in the dissection of the heel flap to ensure that damage to the posterior tibial artery is avoided and careful separation of the heel pad from the calcaneus is accomplished by subperiosteal dissection (86). The Syme amputation for children is modified by preserving the distal tibial growth plate (Figure 21-56). The retention of a portion of the calcaneal apophysis is a complication seen in children. This is a cartilaginous structure and will continue to grow and ultimately ossify resulting in a bony protuberance and interference with weight bearing and prosthetic fitting (114,169) (see Figure 21-52). Postoperatively, the heel pad is maintained in the correct position by the use of two-inch tape applied directly to the skin. Alternatively, two K-wires can be inserted through the heel pad and into the tibia to secure the position of the heel pad (Figure 21-57).

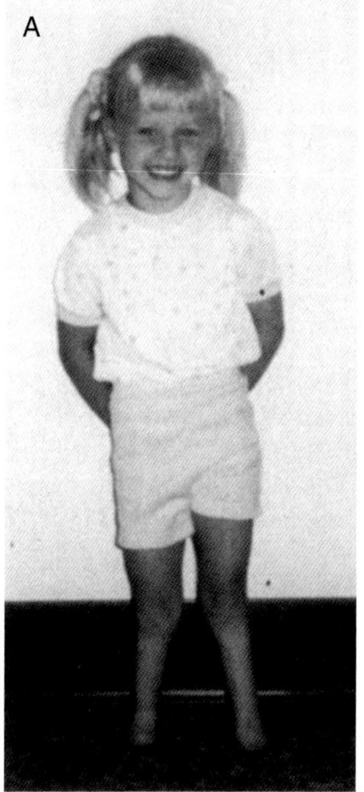

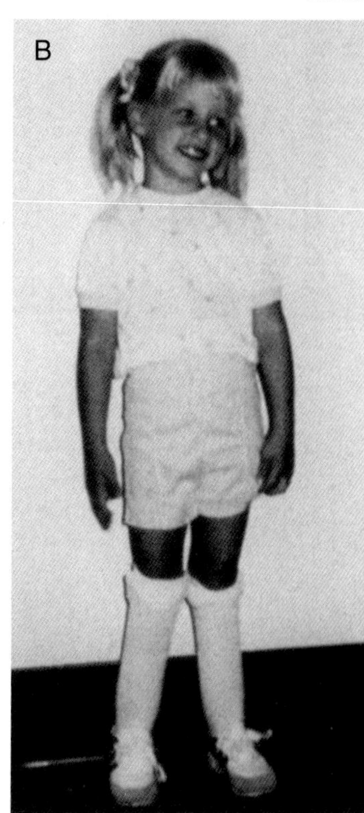

FIGURE 21-51 **A,B.** This four-year-old girl with bilateral fibular hemimelia underwent bilateral modified Chopart amputation. The absent fibula decreases the tendency to a bulbous stump, and full weight bearing is possible with or without her prosthesis.

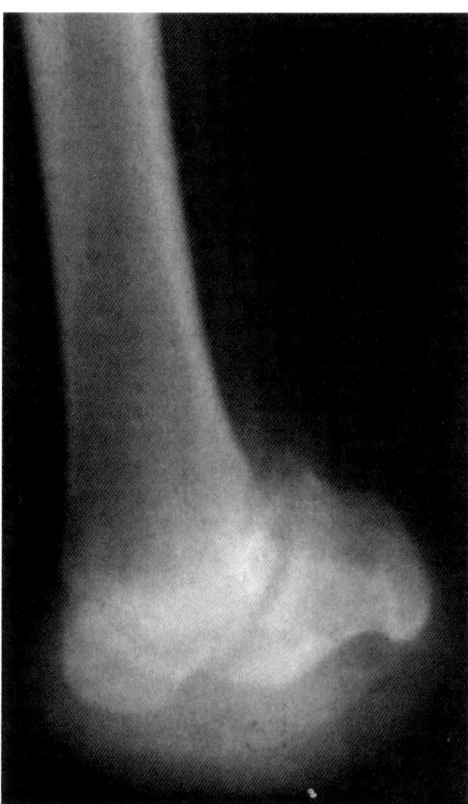

FIGURE 21-52 Retained calcaneal apophysis inadvertently left behind during the performance of a Syme amputation that has continued to grow and ossify.

The Syme amputation is an excellent amputation site for congenital malformations when the limb is already short or will require prosthetic management to equalize

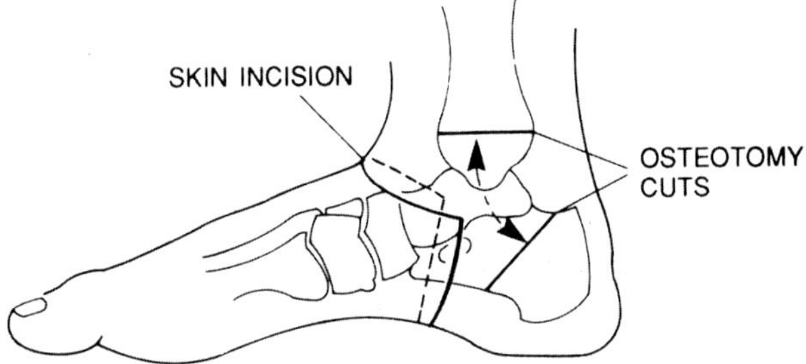

FIGURE 21-53 The Pirogoff amputation designed to preserve the posterior calcaneous with fusion to the tibia, maintaining the heel pad.

the limb length. The Syme procedure may be the only alternative in severe pedal trauma where amputation is necessary. However, it does have the disadvantage of shortening the limb which will necessitate prosthetics for ambulation. When there is an option, the Boyd procedure or even a modified Chopart may be a more practical and functional type of amputation as length is preserved as well as a durable weight-bearing stump.

Applications of the Syme Amputation

Limb Length Inequality with Malformation of the Foot

Common indications for the Syme procedure include patients with malformations of the lower extremities including fibular hemimelia, tibial meromelia, or severe proximal femoral focal deficiency (see Figure 21-13). The amputation allows these children to have a functional stump that can be fitted very effectively with a Syme prosthesis which can be changed with growth to ensure limb

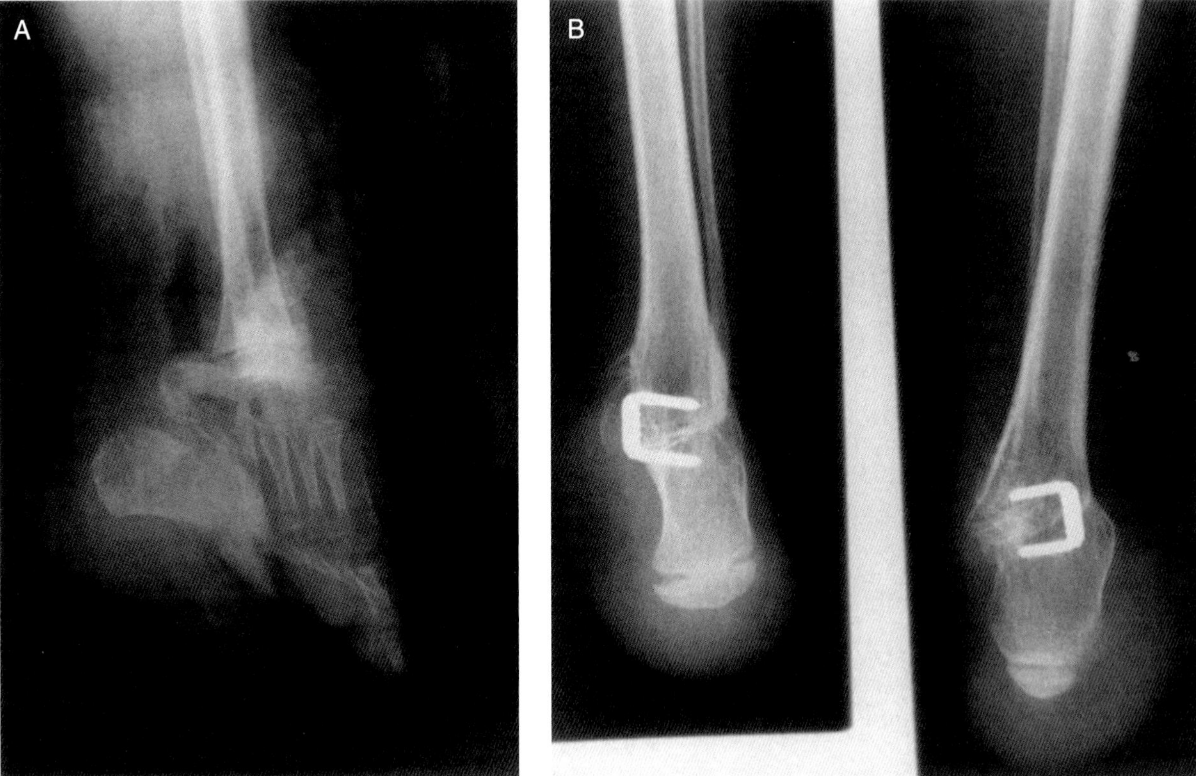

FIGURE 21-54 **A.** Severe foot trauma secondary to a lawnmower injury in which only the distal heel and heel pad were viable. **B.** Pirogoff type of amputation which was successful in providing a functional weight-bearing stump. (Case contributed by Dr. Bill Mcintyre, Children's Hospital of Eastern Ontario, Ottawa, Canada.)

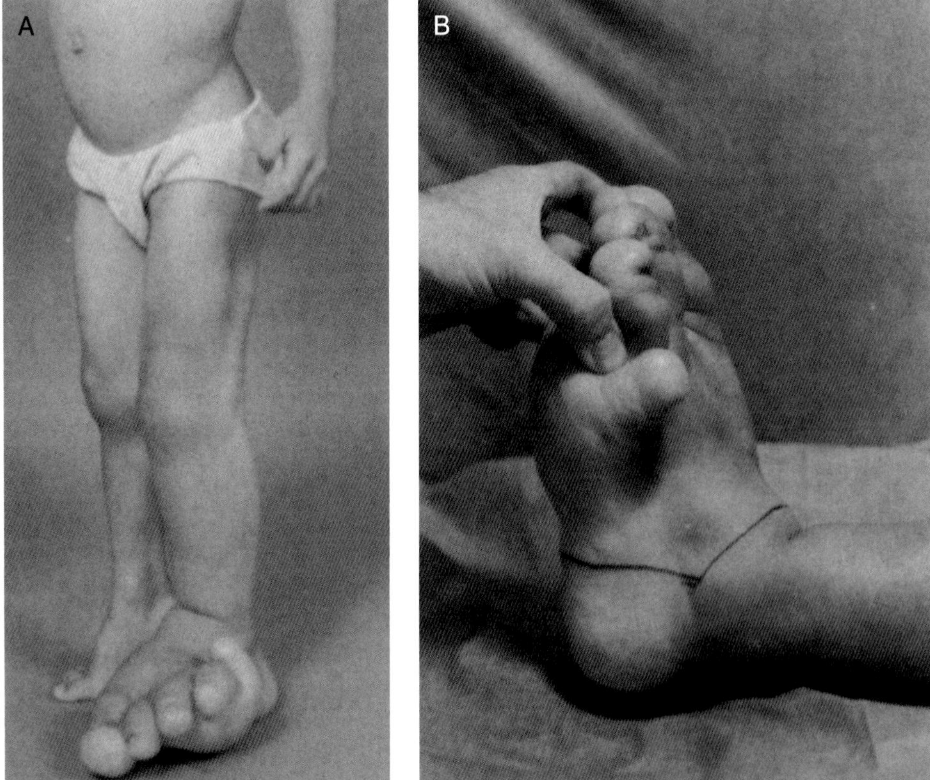

FIGURE 21-55 **A.** Grossly hypertrophied left foot due to congenital arteriovenous malformation. **B.** Skin incision for the Syme amputation. (Courtesy of Dr. Jacques D'Astous, Shriner's Hospital, Salt Lake City, Utah.)

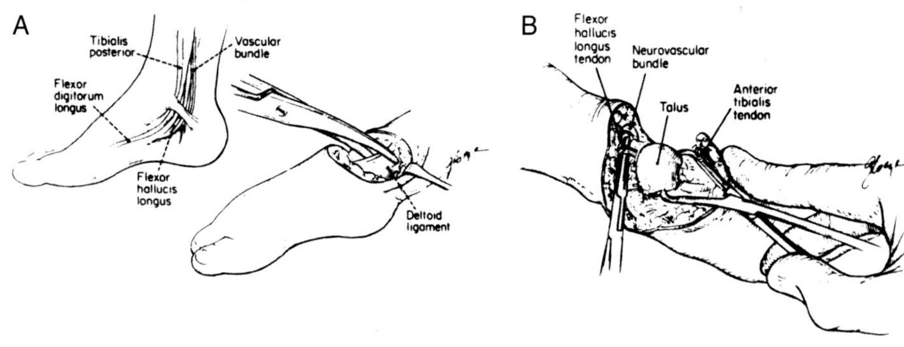

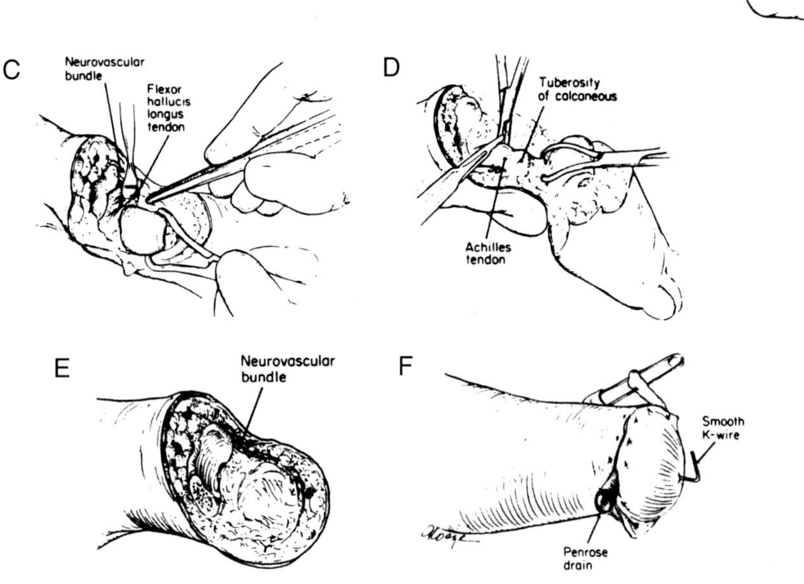

FIGURE 21-56 Technique of Syme amputation in children. **A.** Ligamentous division. **B.** Talus pulled into plantar flexion with bone hook or large towel clip. **C.** Sharp dissection staying close to talus and calcaneus is essential. **D.** Section of tendo-Achillis taking care to remove entire calcaneal apophysis. **E.** Preservation of neurovascular bundle throughout course in the posterior flap. **F.** Closure of the posterior flap anteriorly over a Penrose drain with K-wire holding heel pad in correct position. (Modified from Anderson L, Westin W, Oppenheim WL. Syme amputation in children. *J Pediatr Orthop* 1984;4:550, with permission.)

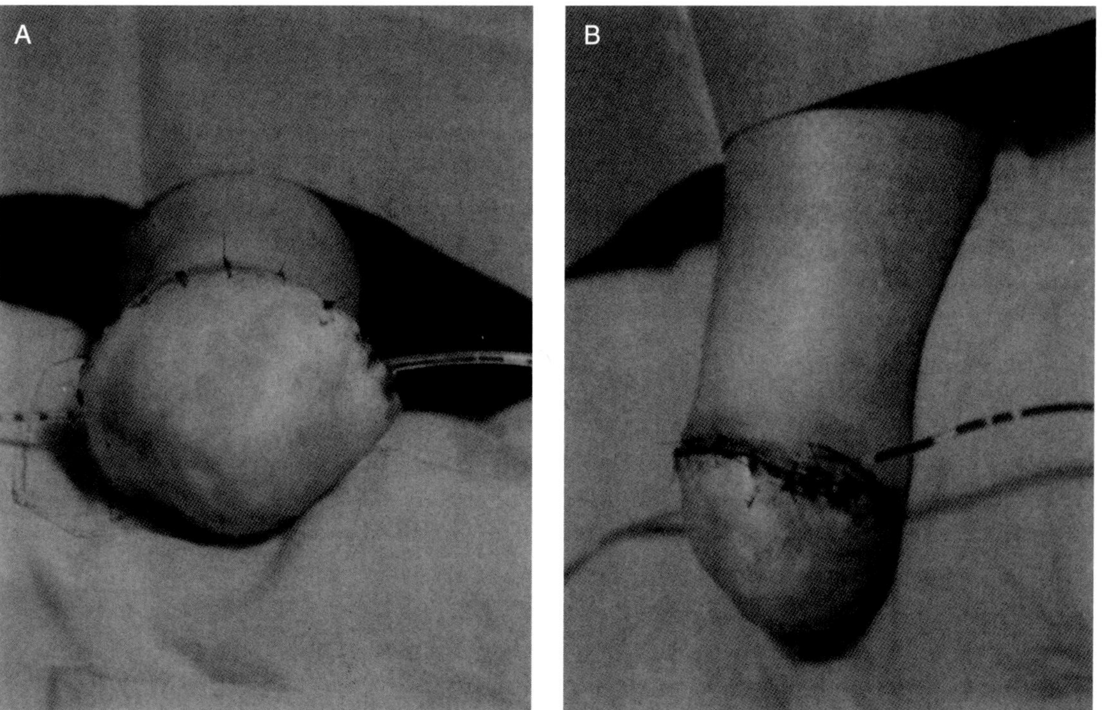

FIGURE 21-57 **A,B.** Syme amputation stump with Hemovac drains and closure of the plantar flap anteriorly.

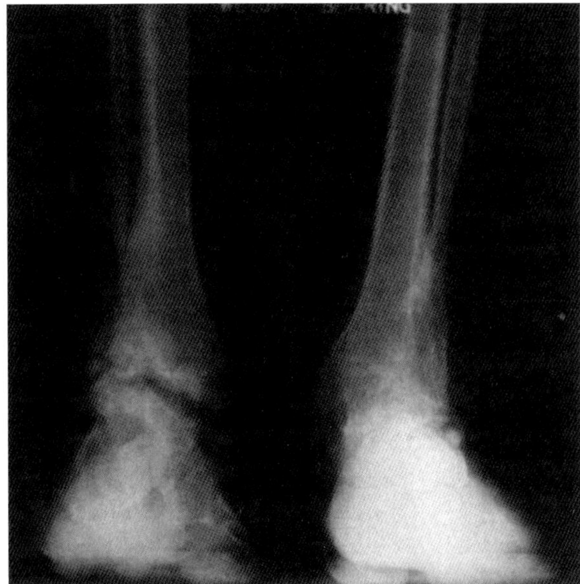

FIGURE 21-58 Severe Charcot ankle and subtalar joint of the right foot with an insensate heel and sole in a child with L-5 myelomeningocele. The associated perforating ulcers on the forefoot necessitated a Syme amputation and in spite of an insensate heel pad, this child functioned well.

length equality (1,2,6,8). Early ablation of the foot in such children is ideal. If possible the procedure should be performed between 6 to 18 months to permit the child to adapt to the prosthesis from the time of initiating ambulation. Problems may arise in convincing parents to have a foot amputation in a child with a near normal foot and whose limb length inequality may not be as obvious when the child is an infant but where the predicted limb length inequality will be 15 cm or more.

Syme Amputation in Congenital Pseudoarthrosis of the Tibia

The Syme amputation may be the most appropriate procedure for children with established congenital Pseudoarthrosis of the tibia particularly when limb-length inequality will contribute to a significant disability. This procedure maintains the distal tibial growth plate and avoids the development of osseous spurs which may develop following diaphyseal amputation (114). The Syme prosthesis controls the pseudoarthrosis adequately and function with the prosthesis is usually excellent.

Severe Congenital or Acquired Malformations of the Foot

Children may develop severe pedal malformations associated with Charcot joint (Figure 21-58), overgrowth of the feet secondary to arteriovenous malformations, lipomas, or gigantism of the foot. In such instances the Syme amputation frequently provides a functional extremity for the child.

Amputation of the Great Toe

The great toe is an important contributor to normal gait. It has been demonstrated by Hicks (96) that the great toe provides stability to the medial aspect of the foot. The plantar

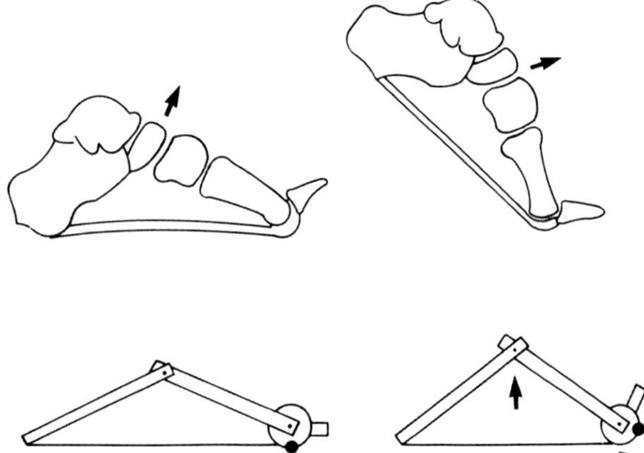

FIGURE 21-59 Windlass action of plantar fascia in maintaining plantar arch as described by Hicks. Amputation of the great toe or forefoot destroys this action contributing to loss of the longitudinal arch.

aponeurosis, which contributes to the maintenance of the medial longitudinal arch, originates from the calcaneal tubercle and passes through the sesamoid to insert into the flexor aspect of the base of the distal phalanx. The proximal phalanx is hyperextended during push-off and this passively tightens the plantar aponeurosis and creates a windlass mechanism which elevates and stabilizes the medial longitudinal arch. This passive mechanism permits the first metatarsal to bear two-fifths of the body weight (Figure 21-59). Amputation of the hallux or first ray results in disruption of the windlass mechanism and body weight is transferred to the second and third metatarsals. There is also a loss of gait cadence and the patient tends to shuffle rather than walk with a normal heel-to-toe gait pattern (82). However, individuals can successfully compensate for loss of the great toe, especially when the remaining toes are intact. There is considerable loss of the spring or bounce in the step when all digits are amputated. Whenever possible, the great toe should be preserved to maintain the windlass action which is important to a normal gait pattern (166,183,222).

Ablation of the great toe may be necessitated by severe malformation of the toe such as gigantism or arteriovenous malformations or secondary to trauma including severe crush injury or amputation from a lawnmower accident (108).

Amputation of Lesser Toes

Amputation of the lesser toes may result from trauma, frost bite, or burns. In general, toes in a child are very resistant to trauma and every effort should be made to salvage the digit. Minor amputations of the tips of the toe should be re-sutured and approached in much the same manner as fingertip injuries in children. Ablation should not be undertaken until it is obvious that the toe is nonviable and a clear demarcation line has been established.

A more common indication for amputation of small toes is polydactyly (20). This condition is often inherited as an autosomy dominant and may be accompanied by accessory fingers. Polydactyly shows racial and geographic variation and is more common in the black race.

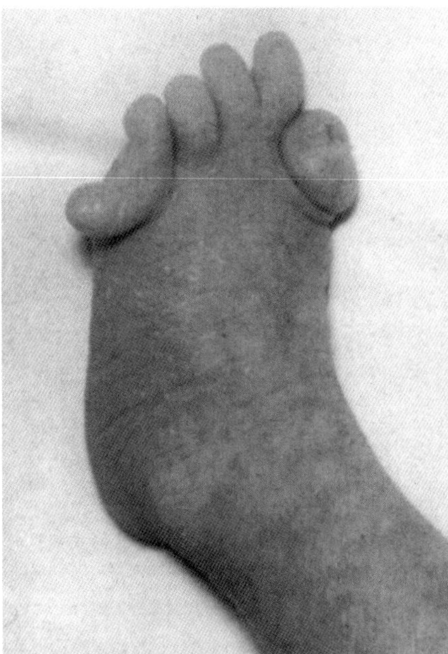

FIGURE 21-60 Accessory or supernumerary little toe with bifid great toe. Amputation of the lateral lying little toe is indicated to facilitate shoe fitting.

Postaxial polydactyly accounts for 80% of the duplication with 15% being preaxial and 6% centrally duplicated (194). Preaxial polydactyly can be induced by the injection of cytotoxic agents into pregnant rates (210). An insult to the ectodermal ridge and a loss of control over the process of digitation results in excessive tissue and subsequent polydactyly. Exposure to radiation has also been shown to induce polydactyly (210).

Many variations of pedal polydactyly can occur and may include duplication of the entire toe or simply the terminal phalanges. Radiographs demonstrate the degree of duplication and have a bearing on treatment. When the entire ray is duplicated, it is necessary to excise the entire ray to ensure that the foot will not be wide and splayed and interfere with shoe fitting. Care must be taken to ensure that the toe with the best tendon function as well as the most cosmetically pleasing digit will be maintained (222). I prefer to remove a supernumerary toe around six months of age prior to the child walking. This reduces the physiological trauma from losing the body part and its effect on body image. It also permits the child to use standard foot wear and learn to walk with a normal foot.

Duplication of the fifth toe is generally best treated by amputation of the most lateral lying toe while duplication of the great toe is commonly treated by amputation of the most medial portion of the toe (Figure 21-60).

PROSTHETIC AND SALVAGE PROCEDURES

Reimplantation of Feet in Children

There are few opportunities for foot re-implantation because injuries to the foot are frequently of a crushing variety. The literature contains few reports of re-implantation of the lower limb (33,120,135,220,237,241,255). In children, clean amputations with no crushing deserves consideration for this procedure. A significant proportion of the re-implantations of fees in the literature have been associated with self amputation in psychiatric patients (135,220). Excellent results are reported because the injuries were clean with no crushing, the feet were properly dealt with by the emergency services, and early weight bearing was protected until bony union and recovery of sensation was obtained.

Clean sharp pedal amputations should be considered for re-implantation. The decision depends on the ability to accomplish the procedure within six hours of the injury, proper care of the amputated portion of the extremity, absence of associated crush injury to the foot, and the availability of a microvascular surgical team. Good clinical judgment is necessary before embarking on this approach with children.

Stump Lengthening Following Amputation of the Foot

The application of the Ilizarov method of limb lengthening in an attempt to provide a more functional foot following metatarsal and mid-tarsal amputation is an exciting development (60,109). Experience as present is meager but Ilizarov has reported very impressive elongation of the foot with his technique (Figure 21-61). He has lengthened the talus, cuboid, and tarsal bones by the technique of corticotomy, stable external fixation, latency, and distraction (110,111). The use of motorized auto distracters for limb lengthening procedures may in the future offer a reliable method of reconstituting major portions of the foot following amputation and may indeed change the emphasis on the type of amputation performed in order to preserve bone stock for future lengthening.

Prosthetic Management of Partial and Complete Foot Amputation in Children

Frequently most children are able to effectively cope with the loss of a foot so that the gait may be virtually normal combined with modern prosthetic fitting. The ground reaction force in children with a below-knee prosthesis is slightly less than in the normal extremity (152). Little difference was found by Lewallen et al. (152) in the joint movement about the ankle in children wearing a below-knee prosthesis when compared to a group of normal children of the same group. They also noted that the walking speed and stride length were only slightly decreased from normal controls.

Partial amputations of the toes and forefoot can usually be managed effectively with an ordinary shoe and prosthetic filler (221). More proximal pedal ablation include the Lisfranc or Chopart amputations which can also be frequently managed with polypropylene AFO and a shoe filler (Figure 21-62), a boot and shoe filler, or a "slipper" prosthesis (Figure 21-63) (17). Amputations of the Syme or Boyd type will require a more formal type of

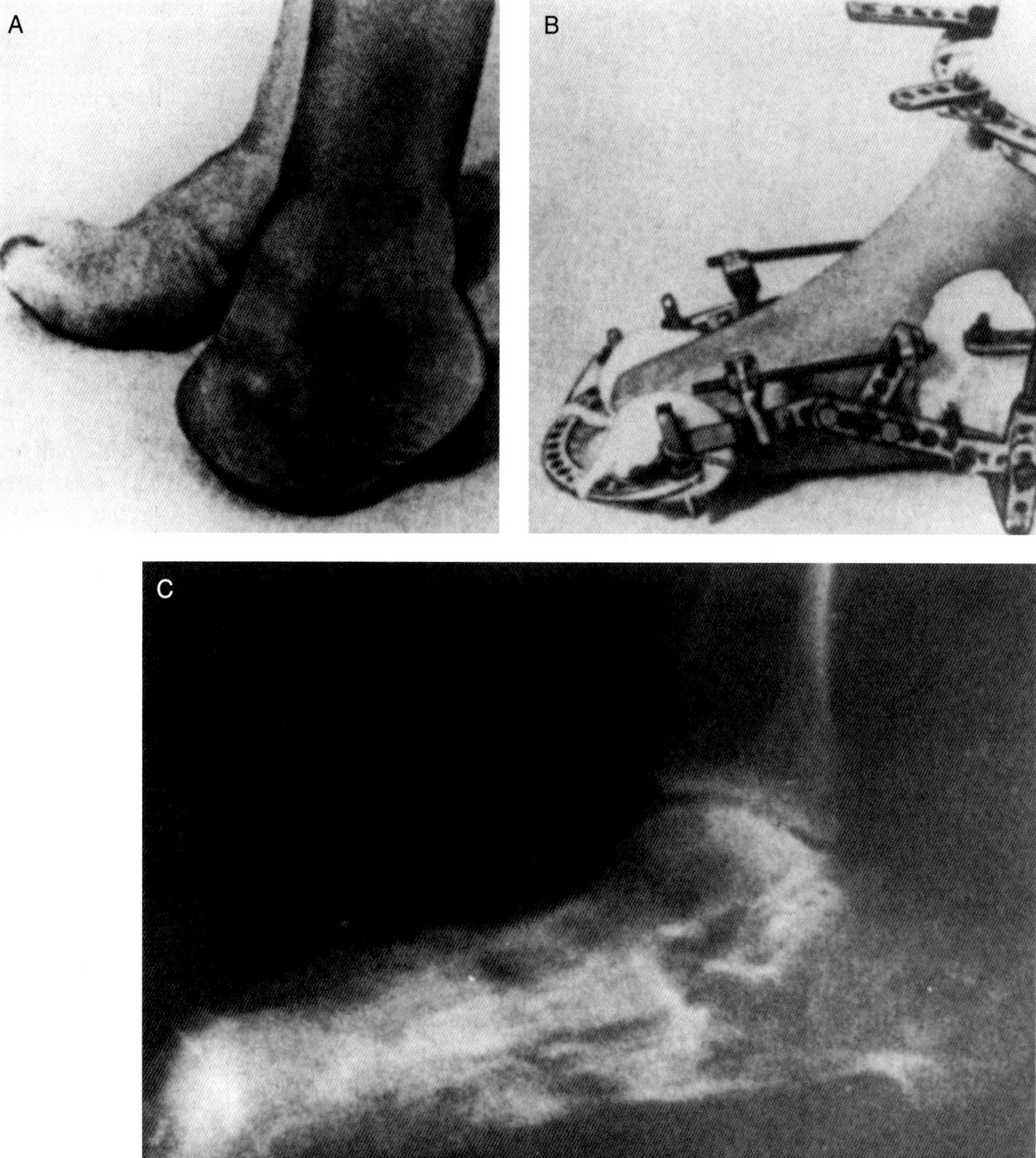

FIGURE 21-61 **A.** Partial amputation of foot. **B.** Lengthening of the foot by the Ilizarov technique. **C.** Radiograph of elongation achieved by this technique. (From Ilizarov GA. Clinical applications of the tension-stress effect for limb lengthening. *Clin Orthop* 1990;250:8, with permission.)

below-knee prosthesis especially modified to incorporate the more bulbous stump (39,205). This may necessitate the removal of a panel on the medial, anterior, and/or lateral portion of the distal prosthesis (22) (Figure 21-64). The most common type of prosthetic foot that is utilized is the solid ankle-cushion heel (SACH foot) (66,75) which is very functional and allows a pseudo-type of plantar and dorsiflexion because of the cushion heel (Figure 21-65). This type of foot prosthesis is cosmetic and can be fitted into most types of childrens' shoes. Other designs provide additional spring for the wearer such as the "flex foot" which enhances push-off at the end of the stance phase (Figure 21-66)(172,173,180,199).

Replacement is frequently required because of rapid growth as well as the child's unforgiving use of the prosthesis. During growth spurts, the prosthesis may have to be changed at 6 to 8 month intervals and usually annually up to the age of 7 to 8 years; then every 18 to 24 months from 8 to 15 years and about every 2 to 3 years to adulthood.

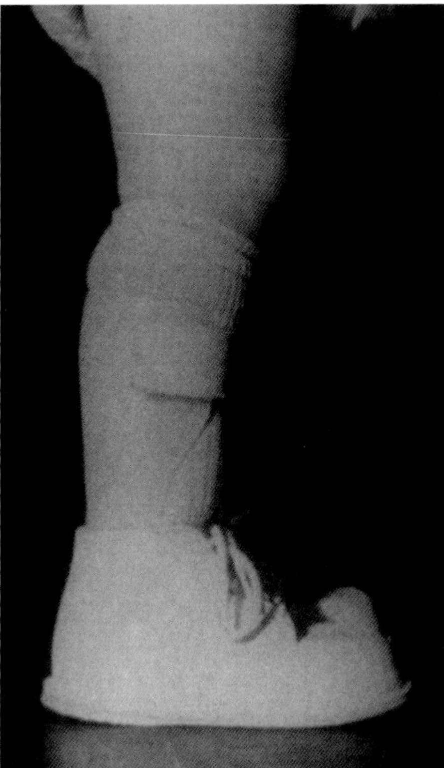

FIGURE 21-62 Children with Chopart or more distal amputations of the foot may be managed with simply an AFO and shoe filler.

Prosthetic Fitting in Children with Congenital Amputation of the Feet

Infants with severe congenital malformations of the feet or with partial amputations secondary to constriction bands will pull to standing and will begin walking at about the same age as other children, i.e., between 8 and 18 months. Even bilateral partial amputees and indeed even those with below knee amputations will also stand and attempt to walk at an average of 12 months. This is the appropriate time for prosthetic assistance and the child should be seen by the juvenile amputee clinic. For partial amputations of the feet, initially only a shoe filler may be required or an AFO to hold the shoe on the partially amputated extremity (65). When the foot is very misshapen a supportive shoe with a filler may be all that is required at this age. Prosthetic fitting can also be instituted for bilateral lesions such as bilateral fibular hemimelia that has undergone Syme amputation. Close observation is necessary to ensure that the infant is comfortable with the prosthesis and careful monitoring of the skin for areas of pressure is necessary. This necessitates close cooperation between the prosthetist, amputee physiotherapist, and the family unit (57). Once the child has mastered balance in the prosthesis or modified orthosis, follow up at three-month intervals is necessary to ensure proper fit and the need for change with growth. This is especially important after the first fitting when there is a rapid change in socket fit due to

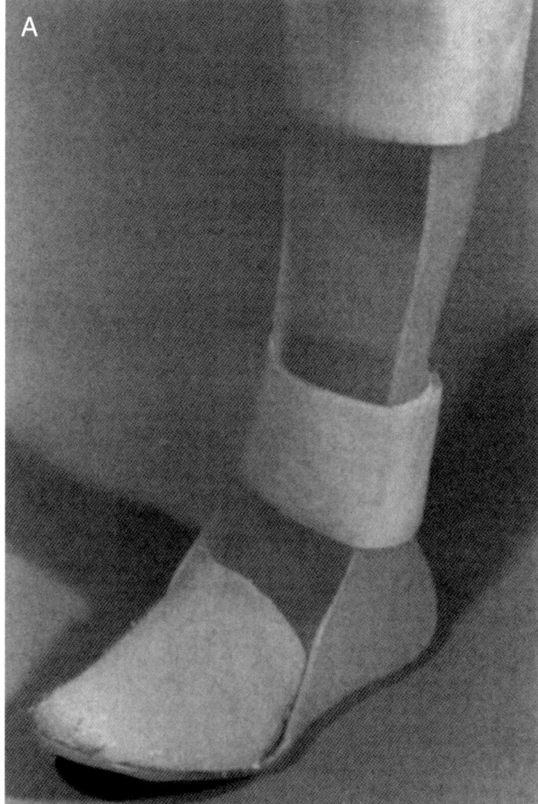

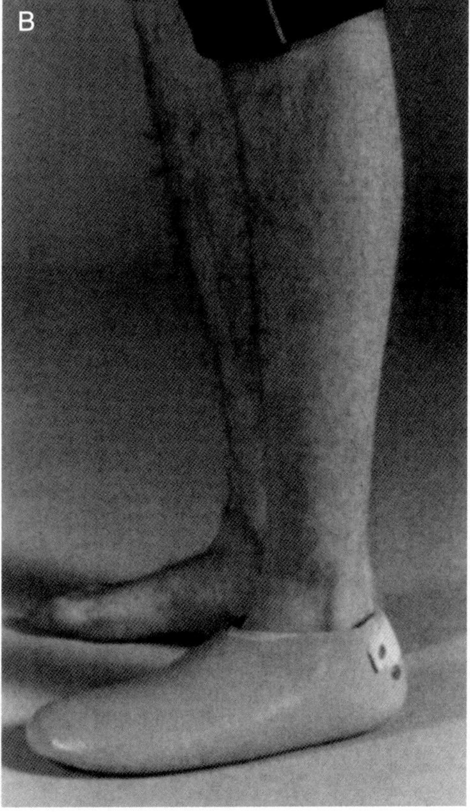

FIGURE 21-63 **A.** Polypropylene AFO with shoe filler. **B.** "Slipper" prosthesis applicable for a Chopart amputation with no limb length inequality. (From Blanco JS, Herring JA. Congenital Chopart amputation: a functional assessment. *Clin Orthop* 1990;256:14, with permission.)

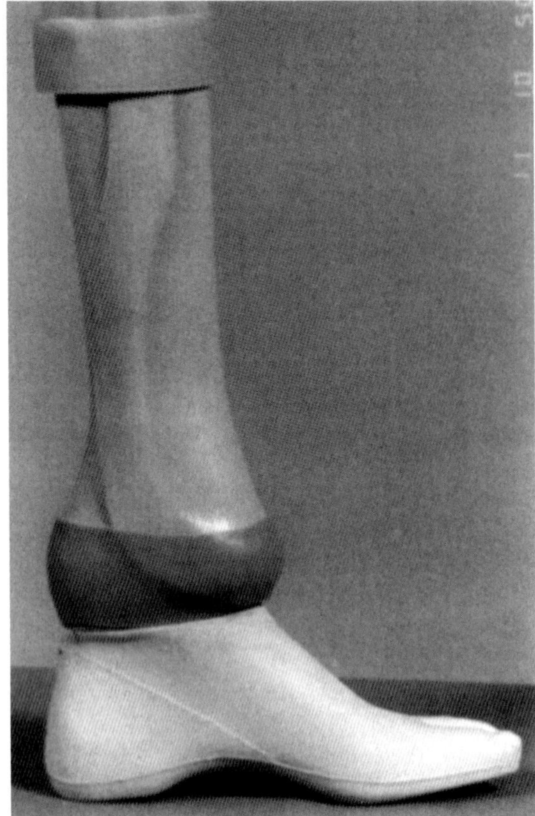

FIGURE 21-64 SACH foot used in conjunction with a below knee prosthesis modified for a Chopart amputation. (From Wiseman NE, Briggs IN, Bolton VS. Neonatal arterial occlusion and ischemic limb gangrene. *J Pediatr Surg* 1977;12:707, with permission)

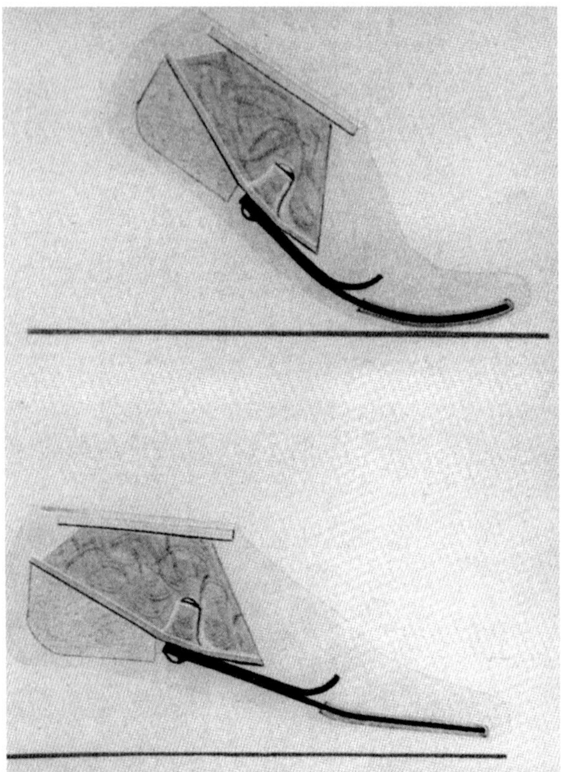

FIGURE 21-66 Prosthetic foot with compressible plastic leaf spring in the forefoot which improves push-off at terminal stance.

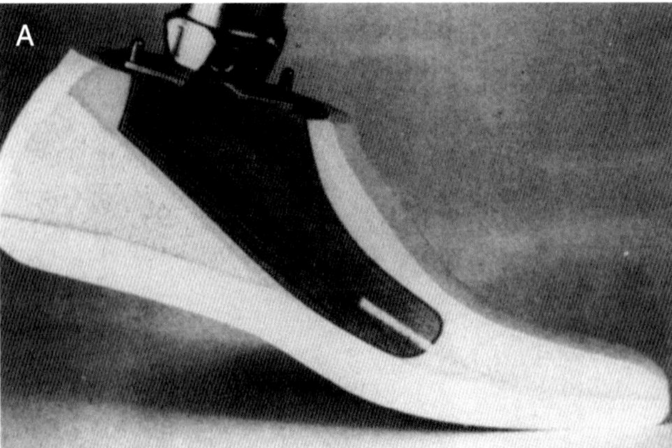

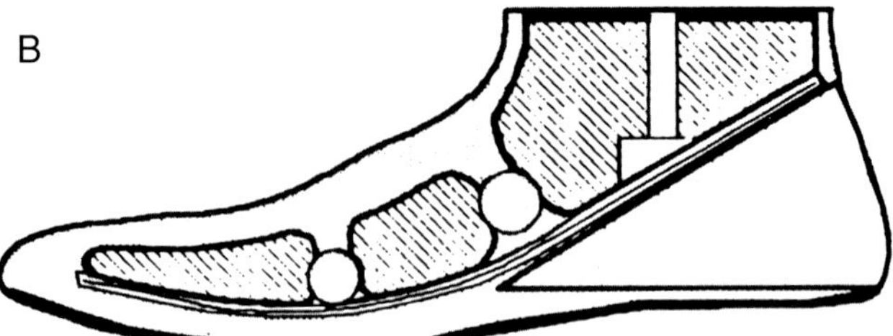

FIGURE 21-65 **A.** Cut-away model of the SACH foot. **B.** Flexible keel type foot provides a smoother roll over than SACH due to round rubber plugs that allow forefoot to bend. (From Michael JW. Overview of prosthetic feet. *Instr Course Lect* 1990;39:367, with permission.)

atrophy of the tissue around the prosthesis. Children with associated upper limb malformations or amputations may be slower in becoming ambulatory but these children should be treated in as normal a manner as possible compared to their physically normal peer group.

In general, the child with a foot or lower limb amputation is best cared for in a specialized child amputee program. Frequent adjustment of the length of the prosthesis may be required in these children who are rapidly growing and who may also require changes in the configuration and socket. An annual new prosthesis is generally necessary up to five years, biannually from five to twelve years; and then every two to three years depending on the child's activities during adolescence.

REFERENCES

1. Achterman C, Kalamchi A. Congenital deficiency of the fibula. *J Bone Joint Surg [Br]* 1979;61:133.
2. Aitken GT. Amputation as a treatment for certain lower extremity congenital abnormalities. *J Bone Joint Surg [Am]* 1959;41:1267.
3. Aitken GT. The child amputee: an overview. *Orthop Clin North Am* 1972;3:447.
4. Aitken GT. Tibial hemimelia in selected lower limb anomalies. In: Aitken GT, ed. *Surgical and prosthetics management.* Washington, DC: National Academy of Sciences, 1971;1–9.
5. American Academy of Orthopaedic Surgeons, ed. *The juvenile amputee atlas of limb prosthesis surgical and prosthetic principles.* St. Louis: CV Mosby, 1981;493.
6. Amstutz HC. Natural history and treatment of congenital absence of the fibula. *J Bone Joint Surg (Am)* 1972;54:1349.

7. Annunziato EJ, Pressman MM, Gorecki GA. Frostbite arthritis of the foot. *J Foot Surg* 1984;23:116.
8. Arnold WD. Congenital absence of the fibula. *Clin Orthop* 1959;14:20.
9. Askins GN, Ger E. Congenital constriction band syndrome. *J Pediatr Orthop* 1988;8:461.
10. Askue WE, Wong R. Gangrene ofthe extremities in the newborn infant. *J Pediatr* 1952;40:58.
11. Badgley CE, O'Connor SJ, Kudner DF. Congenital kyphoscoliotic tibia. *J Bone Joint Surg (Am)* 1952;34:349.
12. Baker CJ, Rudolph AJ. Congenital ring constrictions and intrauterine amputation. *Am J Dis Child* 1971;121:393.
13. Barlow B, Niemirski M, Ghandi RP. Ten years experience with pediatric gun shot wounds. *J Pediatr Surg* 1982;17:927.
14. Barre BS, Thompson GH, Morison SC. Late skeletal deformities: following meningococcal sepsis and disseminated intravascular coagulation. *J Pediatr Orthop* 1985;5:584.
15. Bartholomeusz H. Motor mower ankle trauma. *Aust Fam Physician* 1987;16:977.
16. Belthus MV, Bradish CF, Gibbons PJ. Late orthopaedic sequelae following meningococcal septicemia: a multicenter study. *J Bone Joint Surg (Brit)* 205; 87:236.
17. Blanco JS, Herring JA. Congenital Chopart amputation: a functional assessment. *Clin Orthop* 1990;256:14.
18. Blank JE, Dormans JP, Dowedson RS. Perinatal limb ischemia: orthopaedic implications. *J Pediatr Orthop* 1996; 16:90.
19. Blauth W, Borisch NC. Cleft feet. *Clin Orthop* 1990;258:41.
20. Blauth W, Olason AT. Ossification of the polydactyly of the hands and fat. *Arch Orthop Trauma Surg* 1988;107:334.
21. Blum CE, Kalamchi A. Boyd amputations in children. *Clin Orthop* 1982;165:138.
22. Bochmann D. Prosthesis for the limb-deficient child. In: Kostui KJ, ed. *Amputation surgery and rehabilitation: the Toronto Experience.* Edinburgh: Churchill Livingston, 1981;293.
23. Bohne WHD, Root L. Hypoplasia of the fibula. *Clin Orthop* 1977;125:107.
24. Bonutti PM, Bell GR. Compartment syndrome of the foot: a case report. *J Bone Joint Surg [Am]* 1986;68:1449.
25. Bourne MH, Klassen R. Congenital annular constriction bands; review of the literature and case report. *J Pediatr Orthop* 1987;7:218.
26. Bowker JH. Partial foot and Syme amputations: an overview. *Clin Prosthet Orthot* 1987;12:10.
27. Boyd HB. Amputation of the foot with calcaneal tibial arthrodesis. *J Bone Joint Surg* 1939;21:997.
28. Braly RD. Neonatal arterial thrombosis and embolism. *Surgery* 1965;58:869.
29. Broadbent RS. Recipient twin ischemia with postnatal onset. *J Paediatr* 2007; 150:207.
30. Brooks B, Beal L, Ogg L, Blakeslee B. The child with deformed or missing limbs: his problems and prosthesis. *Am J Nursing* 1962;62:89.
31. Brown FW. Constriction of a knee joint in congenital total absence of the tibia (paraxial hemimelia tibia). A preliminary report. *J Bone Joint Surg [Am]* 1965;47:695.
32. Browne D. The pathology of congenital ring constrictions. *Arch Dis Child* 1957;32:517.
33. Buckely JR, Dunkley P. Successful reimplantation of both feet: brief report. *J Bone Joint Surg (Br)* 1988;70:667.
34. Byrne J, Blanc W A, Baker D. Amniotic band syndrome in early fetal life. *Birth Dejects* 1982; 18:43.
35. Canale ST, Kard S. The orthopaedic implications of purpura fulminans. *J Bone Joint Surg (Am)* 1984;66:765.
36. Carr CR, Stevenson CA. The treatment of missile wounds of the extremities.1st *Course Lect* 1954;11:189.
37. Christie J, Clowes CB, Lamb DW. Amputations through the middle part of the foot. *J Bone Joint Surg (Br)* 1980;62:473.
38. Clark MW. Autosomal dominant inheritance of tibial meromelia. Report of a kindred. *J Bone Joint Surg (Am)* 1975;57:262.
39. Collins IN. A partial foot prosthesis for the transmetatarsal level. *Clin Prosthet Orthot* 1987;12:19–23.
40. Corps BY., Littlewood M. Full thickness skin replacement after traumatic avulsion. *Br J Plast Surg* 1966; 12:229.
41. Cory JM. Fibula hemimelia with tibial angulation: the identification of a problem. *Interclinic Information Bulletin* 1977;17:7.
42. Coryllos E, Dabbert O, Tracey E, Richmond H, David DA. Treatment of an avulsed skin flap involving the circumferences of the entire lower leg. *Ann Surg* 1960; 151:437.
43. Costilla V. Lawnmower injuries in the United States 1996–2004. *Ann Emerg Med* 206; 47:567.
44. Coursley G, Ivans JC, Barker NW. Congenital arteriovenous fistulas in the extremities and an analysis of 69 cases. *Angiology* 1956;7:201.
45. Coventry MD. Congenital absence of the fibula. *J Bone Joint Surg (Am)* 1952;34:911.
46. Cowell HR, Hessinger RN. The relationship of clubfoot to congenital annular bands. In: Bateman JE, ed. *Foot Science.* Philadelphia: WB Saunders, 1976.
47. Crouch C, Smith WI. Long-term sequelae of frostbite. *J Pediatr Radiol* 1990;20:356.
48. Cummings Y, Molnar G. Traumatic amputations in children resulting from "train-electric-bum" injuries: a social-environmental syndrome? *Arch Phys Med Rehab* 1974;55:71.
49. Daniel RK, May JW Jr. Free flaps: an overview. *Clin Orthop* 1978; 133: 122–131.
50. Daniel RK, May JW Jr. Free flaps: an overview. *Clin Orthopedics* 1978;133:122.
51. Daniel RK, Taylor GI. Distant transfer of an island flap by microvascular anastomoses: a clinical technique. *Plast Reconstr Surg* 1983;52: 111.
52. Davidson WH, Bohne WH. The Syme amputation. *J Bone Joint Surg [Am]* 1975;57:905.
53. Davis MS, Nadel S, Habibi P, Levin M, Hunt DM. The orthopaedic management of peripheral ischemia in meningococcal septicemia in children. *J Bone Joint Surg [Brit]* 2000; 82:489.
54. DeMuth W Jr. Bullet velocity and design as determinates of wounding capability. *J Trauma* 1966;6:222.
55. DeMyer W, Baird I. Mortality and skeletal malformations from amniocentesis and oligohydramnios in rats. Cleft palate, clubfoot, macrostomia and adactyly. *Teratology* 1969;2:33.
56. DeSanctis N, Razzano E, Scognamiglio R, Rega AN. Tibial agenesis: a new rational in management of type IIBreport of three cases with a long-term follow-up. *J Pediatr Orthop* 1990; 10: 198.
57. Downie JR. Limb deficiencies and prosthetic devices. *Orthop Clin North Am* 1976;7:465.
58. Duncan JS, Ramsy LE. Widespread bone infarction complicating the meningococcal septicemia and disseminated intravascular coagulation. *Br Med J* 1984;288:111.
59. Eilert RE, Jayakumar SS. Boyd and Syme amputation in children. *J Bone Joint Surg (Am)* 1976;58:1130.
60. Eldridge JC, Armstrong PF, Krajbick JI. Amputation stump lengthening with the Ilizarov technique. *Clin Orthop* 1990;.256:76.
61. Etches PC, Stewart AR, Ives AJ. Familial congenital amputations. *J Pediatr* 1983;101:448.
62. Farmer AW, Laurin CA. Congenital absence of the fibula. *J Bone Joint Surg (Am)* 1960;42:1.
63. Farmer AW. Whole skin removal and replacement. *Surg Clin North Am* 1943;23:1440.
64. Ferguson CM, Morrison JD, Kenwright J. Leg-length inequality in children treated by Syme's amputation. *J Bone Joint Surg [Br]*1987;69:433.
65. Fillauer K. A prosthesis for foot amputation near the tarsal-metatarsal junction. *Orthot Prosthet Int* 30:9–11.
66. Foort J. Prosthetic fitting and components of lower extremity prosthesis. In: Banerjee SN, ed. *Rehabilitation management of amputees,* Baltimore: Williams & Wilkins, 1982;42.

67. Frackleton WH. Surface covering of traumatic lower extremity defects. *Surg Clin North Am* 1958;38:1093.
68. Freie-Maia N. A newly recognized genetic syndrome of tetramelic deficiencies, ectodermal dysplasia, deformed ears and. other abnormalities. *Am J Hum Genet* 1970;22:370.
69. Fried K, Goldberg MD, Mundel G, Rief R. Severe lower limb malformation associated with other deformities and death in infancy in two brothers. *J Med Genet* 1977;14:352.
70. Galaway HR, Hubbard S, Morobrag M. Traumatic amputations in children. In: Kostuik J, ed. *Amputation surgery and rehabilitation: the Toronto experience.* Edinburgh: Churchill Livingston, 1981;137–143.
71. Gibson DA. Child and juvenile amputee. In: Banerjee SN, *ed. Rehabilitation management of amputees.* Baltimore: Williams & Wilkins, 1982.
72. Gillespie R. Congenital limb deformities and amputation surgery. in children. In: Kostuik J, ed. *Amputation surgery and rehabilitation: the Toronto Experience.* Edinburgh: Churchill Livingston, 1981; 105.
73. Gissane W. A dangerous type of fracture of the foot. *J Bone Joint Surg (Br)* 1951; 33:535.
74. Glaun VP, Weinberg EG, Malin AF. Peripheral gangrene in a newborn. *Arch Dis Child* 1971;46:105.
75. Goh JC, Solomonides SF, Spence WD. Biomechanical evaluation of SACH and uniaxial feet. *Prosthet Orthot Int* 1984;8:147.
76. Gomes MMR, Bernatz PE. Anterior venous fistulasBa review of ten year's experience at the Mayo Clinic. *Mayo Clinic Proc* 1973;45:81.
77. Gooperman EM. Anaerobes in clinical practice; frequently for gotten. *Can Med Assoc J* 1976;115:298.
78. Gore D. Comparison of complications during rehabilitation. *J Burn Care Rehab* 1988;9:92.
79. Grace TG. Cold exposure injuries and the Winter athlete. *Clin Orthop* 1987;216:55.
80. Green WB, Cary JM. Partial foot amputations in children. *J Bone Joint Surg (Am)* 1982;64:438.
81. Grogono BJ. Auger injuries. *Injury* 1972;4:247.
82. Grundy M, Tosh T A, Mcleish RG, Smidt L. An investigation of centers of pressure under the foot while walking. *J Bone Joint Surg [Br]* 1975;57:98.
83. Hampton OP Jr. The indication for debridement of gun shot (bullet) wounds of the extremities in civilian practice. *J Trauma* 1961;1:354.
84. Hansen ST. Overview of the severely traumatized lower limb, reconstruction versus amputation. *Clin Orthop* 1989;243:17.
85. Hansen ST. The type III-C tibial fracture: salvage or amputation [Editorial]. *J Bone Joint Surg (Am)* 1987;69:799.
86. Harris RI. Syme's amputation, the technical details essential for success. *J Bone Joint Surg (Br)* 1956;38:614.
87. Harris WR, Silverstein EA. Partial amputations of the foot: a follow-up study. *Can J Surg* 1964;7:6.
88. Heggdekatti RM. Congenital malformation of hands and feet in man. *J Hered* 1939;30:191.
89. Heins M, Khan R, Bjordnat J. Gun shot wounds in children. *Am J Pub Health* 1974;64:326.
90. Helfet DL, Howey T, Johamnon K. Limb salvage vs. amputation: preliminary results of the mangled extremity score (MESS). *Clin Orthop* 1990.
91. Heller G, Alvari G. Gangrene of the extremities in the newborn. *Am J Dis Child* 1941;62.
92. Hensinger RN. Gangrene of the newborn. *J Bone Joint Surg* 1975;57:121.
93. Herring JA, Barnhill B, Gaffney C. Syme amputation: an evaluation of the physical and psychological function in young patients. *J Bone Joint Surg* 1986;68:573.
94. Herring JA. Instructional case-management of tibial dysplasia. *J Pediatr Orthop* 1981;1:339.
95. Herzenberg JE. Congenital limb deficiency and limb length discrepancy. In: Canale B, ed. *Operative pediatric orthopaedics.* St.Louis: Mosby Year Books, 1991;187–215.
96. Hicks JH. The mechanics of the foot. II. The plantar aponeurosis of the arch. *J Anatomy* 1954;88:25.
97. Hodge MJ, Peters TG, Efird WG. Amputations of the distal part of the foot. *South Med J* 1989;82:1138.
98. Hootnick D, Boyd NA, Fixsen JA, Lloyd-Roberts GC. The natural history and management of congenital short tibia with dysplasia or absence of the fibula. A preliminary report. *J Bone Joint Surg [Br]* 1977;59:267.
99. Hootnick DR, Boyd NA, Fixsen A, Lloyd-Roberts GC. Congenital short, tibia with dysplasia or absence of the fibula. A preliminary report. *J Bone Joint Surg [Br]* 1977;59:267.
100. Hootnick DR, Boyd NA, Fixsen A, Lloyd-Roberts GC. Midline metatarsal dysplasia' associated with absent fibula. *Clin Or/hop* 1980;150:203.
101. Horowitz JH, Nichter LS, Kenny JG, Morgan RF. Lawnmower injuries in children: lower extremity reconstruction. *J Trauma* 1985;25: 1138.
102. Houston JW, Gunter GS. Primary cross leg flaps. *Plast Reconstr Surg* 1967;4:58.
103. Howland WC, Ritchey SJ. Gun shot fractures in civilian practice. *J Bone Joint Surg (Am)* 1971;53:47.
104. Hubbard S. Social and psychological problems of the child amputee. In: Kostuik J, ed. *Amputation surgery and rehabilitation.* New York: Churchill Livingston, 1981.
105. Hunter GA. Minor foot amputations. In: Kostiuk JP, ed. *Amputation surgery and rehabilitation: the Toronto Experience.* New York: Churchill Livingston, 1981.
106. Hurst JM, Rybczynski J, Wertheimer SJ. The physis, pathophysiology and management of high velocity gun shot wounds. *J Foot Surg* 1986;25:440.
107. Huston AF, Smith C. Farm accidents in Saskatchewan. *Can Med Assoc J* 1969;100:746.
108. Huurman WW. Congenital foot deformities. In: Mann RA, ed. *Duvries' surgery of the foot.* St. Louis: CV Mosby, 1978.
109. Ilizarov GA. Clinical applications of the tension-stress effect for limb lengthening. *Clin Orthop* 1990;250:8.
110. Ilizarov GA. The tension-stress effect on the genesis and growth of tissue: part I, the influence of stability of fixation and soft tissue preservation. *Clin Orthop* 1989;238:249.
111. Ilizarov GA. The tension-stress effect on the genesis and growth of tissue: part II, the influence of the rate and frequency of distraction. *C/in Orthop* 1989;239:263.
112. Innes CO. Treatment of skin avulsion injuries of the extremities. *Br J Plast Surg* 1967;10:122.
113. Jacobsen ST, Crawford AH, Millar EA, Steel HH. The Syme amputation in patients with congenital pseudoarthrosis of the tibia. *J Bone Joint Surg [Am]* 1983;65:533.
114. Jacobson ST, Crawford AH. Amputation following meningococcemia;. the sequelae to purpura fulminans. *Clin Orthop* 1984;185:214.
115. Jajakumar SS, Eilert RE. Fibular transfer for congenital absence of the tibia. *Clin Orthop* 1979; 139:97.
116. Jansen K, Anderson KS. Congenital absence of the fibula. *Acta Orthop Scand* 1974;45:446.
117. Johnstone BR, Bennett CS. Lawnmower injuries in children. *Aust NZJ Surg* 1989;59:713.
118. Jones D, Barnes J, Lloyd-Roberts GC. Congenital aplasia and dysplasia of the tibia with intact fibula. Ossification and management. *J Bone Joint Surg [Br]* 1978;60:31.
119. Jones KL, Smith EW, Hall BD, et al. A pattern of craniofacial and limb defects secondary to agar tissue bands. *J Pediatr* 1974;84:90.
120. Jupiter JB, Tsai TM, Kleinert HE. Salvage replantation of lower limb amputations. *Plast Reconstr Surg* 1982;69: 1.
121. Kalamchi A, Dave RV. Congenital deficiency of the tibia. *J Bone Joint Surg (Br)* 1985;67:581.
122. Kalamchi A. Congenital deficiency of the tibia. In: Kalamchi A, ed. *Congenital lower limb deficiencies.*, New York: Springer-Verlag, 1989;140.

123. Kamel R, Sakala FB. Anatomical compartments of the sole of the human foot. *NATA Rec* 1961;140:57.
124. Kelly KJ, Glaeser P, Rice TB, Wendelberger KJ. Profound accidental hypothermia and freeze injury of the extremities in a child. *J Crit Care Med* 1990;18:679.
125. Kino Y. Clinical and experimental studies of the congenital constriction band syndrome with an emphasis on its etiology. *J Bone Joint Surg [Am]* 1975;57:636.
126. Klippel M, Trenaunay P. Du noevus variqueux osteoBhypertrophique. *Arch Jen Med (Paris)* 1900;185,3:641.
127. Knapp LW Jr. Occupational and rural accidents. *Arch Environ Health* 1966;13:501.
128. Koman AL, Pennell TC. Salvage of lower extremities following combined orthopaedic and vascular trauma: a predictive salvage index. *Am J Surg* 1987;53:205.
129. Koman AL. Free flaps for coverage of foot and ankle. *Orthopaedics* 1986;9:857.
130. Kritter AE. A technique for salvage of the infected diabetic gangrenous foot. *Orthop Clin North Am* 1973;4:21.
131. Kruger LM, Talbot RD. Amputation and prosthesis as definitive treatment in congenital absence of the fibula. *J Bone Joint Surg [Am]* 1962;43:625.
132. Kruger LM. Congenital lower limb deficiencies. In: American Academy of Orthopaedic Surgery, ed. *Atlas of limb prosthesis surgical and prosthetic principles.* St. Louis: CV Mosby, 1981; 522.
133. Kruger LM. Recent advances in surgery of lower limb deficiencies. *Clin Orthop* 1980;148:97.
134. Kumar SJ. Syme and Boyd amputations in children. In: Kalamchi A, ed. *Congenital Lower Limb Deficiencies.* New York: 2 Springer-Verlag, 1989;163.
135. Kutz JR, Jupiter JB, Tsi TM. Lower limb reimplantation: a report of nine cases. *Foot Ankle* 1983;3:197.
136. Lambert CN, Hamilton RC, Tellicore RI. The juvenile amputation program: its social and economic value: a follow-up study after the age of twenty-one. *J Bone Joint Surg [Am]* 1969;51: 1135.
137. Lange RH. Limb reconstruction versus amputation: decision making in massive lower extremity trauma. *Clin Orthop* 1989;243:92.
138. Lange TA, Nasca RJ. Traumatic partial foot amputation. *Clin Orthop* 1984;185:137.
139. Lazarus HM, Hutto W. Electric burns and frostbite: patterns of vascular injury. *J Trauma* 1982;22:581.
140. Lees DH, Lawler SD, Renwick JH, Thoday 1M. Anonychia with ectrodactyly. Clinical and linkage data. *Ann Hum Genet* 1957;22:69.
141. Lehr HB, Fitts WT. Management of avulsion injuries of soft tissue. *J Trauma* 1969;9:261.
142. Lenz W. Genetics and limb deficiencies. *Clin Orthop* 1980;148:9.
143. Leonard FC, Vassos GA Jr. Congenital arteriovenous fistulation of the lower limb. *N Engl J Med* 1951;245:85.
144. Letts M, Blastorah B, Al-Azzam S. Neonatal gangrene of the extremities. *J Pediatr Orthop* 1997; 17:397.
145. Letts M, Pyper A. The modified Chopart's amputation. *Clin Orthop* 1990;256:44.
146. Letts M, Stevens L, Coleman J, Kettner R. Puppetry and doll play as an adjunct to pediatric orthopaedics. *J Pediatr Orthop* 1983;3:605.
147. Letts RM, Gammon W. Auger injuries in children. *Can Med Assoc J* 1978;118:519.
148. Letts RM, Mardirosian A. Lawnmower injuries in children. *Can Med Assoc J* 1977;116:1151.
149. Letts RM, Miller DD. Gun shot wounds of the extremities in children. *J Trauma* 1976;16:807.
150. Letts RM. Degloving injuries in children. *J Pediatr Orthop* 1986;6:193.
151. Letts RM. Orthopaedic treatment of hemangiomatous hypertrophy of the lower limb. *J Bone Joint Surg (Am)* 1977;59:777.
152. Lewallen R, Dyck G, Quanbury A, Ross K, Letts M. Gait kinematics in below-knee child amputees: a force plate analysis. *J Pediatr Orthop* 1986;6:219.
153. Lindenauer SM. Congenital arteriovenous fistu1a and the Klippel-Tranaunay syndrome. *Ann Surg* 1971;174:248.
154. Lindquist C, Riska EB. Chopart, Pirogott and Syme amputations. *Acta Orthop Scand* 1966;37: 110.
155. Loder RT, Brown K, Zoleske DJ, Jones, E. Extremity lawnmower injuries in children: Report by the Research Committee of the Pediatric Orthopaedic Society of North America. *J Pediatr Orthop* 1997; 17:360.
156. Loder RT, Herring JA. Fibular transfer for congenital absence of the tibia: a reassessment. *J Pediatr Orthop* 1987;7:8.
157. Loeftler RD Jr, Ballard A. Plantar facial spaces of the foot and a proposed surgical approach. *Foot Ankle* 1980;1:11.
158. Louis T, Embleton D. Split hand and split foot deformities, types, origin and transmission. *Biometrics* 1908;6:26.
159. Louton RB, Harley RA, Hagerty RC. A fasciocutaneous transposition flap for coverage of defects of the lower extremity. *J Bone Joint Surg [Am]* 1989;71: 988.
160. Love SM, Grogan DP, Ogden JA. Lawnmower injuries in children. *J Orthop Trauma* 1988;2:94.
161. Lowry RB. Congenital absence of the fibula and carniosynostosis in sibs. *J Med Genet* 1972;9:227.
162. Lucas GL, Wirka HW. Farm accidents occurring in children. *Wis Med J* 1963;62:405.
163. Mackereth M, Lennihan R. Gangrene of the extremity in infants and children. *Angiology* 1972;23:668.
164. MacPherson RI, Letts RM. Skeletal diseases associated with angiomatosis. *J Can Assoc Radiol* 1978;29:90.
165. Malan E, Publionisi A. Congenital angiodyspl~a of the extremities. *J Cardiovascular Surg* 1965;6:255.
166. Mann RA, Poppen NK, Okonski M. Amputation of the great toe. A clinical and biomechanical study. *Clin Orthop* 1988;226:192.
167. Maxwell GP, Manson TN, Hoopes JE. Experience with latissimus dorsi myocutaneous free flaps. *Plast Reconstr Surg.* 1979;64:1.
168. May JW, Gallico GG, Lukash FN. Microvascular transfer of free tissue for closure of bone wounds of the distal lower extremity. *N Engl J Med* 1982;306:256–257.
169. Mazet R. Symes amputation: a follow-up study of fifty-one adults and thirty-two children. *J Bone Joint Surg (Am)* 1968;50:1549.
170. McCollough NC, Matthews JG, Traut A, Caldwell CP. Early opinions concerning the importance of bone fixation of the heel pad of the tibia in the juvenile amputee. *NYU Inter-Clinic Bulletin* 1964;3:1.4
171. McKay M, Clarren SK, Zorn R. Isolated tibial hemimelia in sibs: an autosomal recessive disorder. *Am J Med Genet* 1984;17:603.
172. Michael J. Energy storing feet. A clinical comparison. *Clin Prosthet Orthot* 1987;11:154.
173. Michael JW. Overview of prosthetic feet. *Instr Course Lect* 1990;39:367.
174. Millstein SG, McGowan SA, Hunter GA. Traumatic partial foot amputation in adults. *J Bone Joint Surg (Br)* 1988;70:251.
175. Morrison WA, O'Brien CB, Maclode A. Clinical experiences in free flap transfer. *Clin Orthop* 1986;206:104.
176. Moses JM, Flatt AE, Cooper RR. Annular constricting bands. *J Bone Joint Surg* 1979; 61:565.
177. Mubarak SJ, Hargens AR. *Compartmental syndrome and its relation to the crush syndrome.* Philadelphia: WB Saunders, 1981.
178. Mubarak SJ, Owen CA. Compartmental syndrome and its relation to the crush syndrome. *Clin Orthop* 1975;113:81.
179. Myerson MS. Experimental decompression of the facial compartments of the foot: bases for fasciotomy in acute compartment syndromes. *Foot Ankle* 1988;8:308.
180. Nelson D, Shurr D, Golden J, Meier K. Comparison of energy cost and gait efficiency during ambulation using different prosthetic feet. A preliminary report. *J Prosthet Orthot* 1988;1:24.

181. Nelson KG. The innocent. bystander: the child as unintended victim of domestic violence involving deadly weapons. *Pediatrics* 1984;73:251.
182. Nolan WA. Farm trauma. *Minn Med* 1963;46:337.
183. Oppen NK, Mann RA, O'Konski M, Buncke HJ. Amputation of the great toe. *J Foot Ankle* 1981;1:333.
184. O'Rahilly R, Gardner E, Gray DJ. The ectodermal thickening and ridge in the limbs of staged human embryos. *J Embryol Exp Morphol* 1956;4:254.
185. O'Rahilly R. Morphological patterns in limb deficiencies in duplications. *Am J Anatomy* 1951;89:135.
186. Ordog GJ, Prakash A, Wasserberger J, Balasubramanim S. Pediatric gun shot wounds. *J Trauma* 1987;27:1272.
187. Ossipoff V, Hall BD. Etiologic factors in the amniotic band syndrome: a study of twenty-
188. Pappas AM, Hanawalt BA, Anderson M. Congenital defects of the fibula. *Orthop Clin North Am* 1972;3: 187.
189. Park WH, DennMuth WE Jr. Wounding capacity of rotary lawnmowers. *J Trauma* 1975;15:36.
190. Parziale JR, Hahn KAK. Functional considerations in partial foot amputations, *Orthop Rev* 1988;27:262.
191. Paterson R. *Memorial of the life of James Syme.* Edinburgh: Edmonton and Douglas, 1874.
192. Perdue GF, Lewis SA, Hunt JL. Pyrophosphate scanning in early frostbite injury. *J Am Surg* 1985;49:619.189.
193. Pham,TN. Thermal and electrical injuries. *Surg Clin North Am* 2007; 87:185.
194. Phelps DA, Grogan DP. Polydactylyofthe foot. *J Pediatr Orthop* 1985;5:446.
195. Philipps RS. Congenital split foot (lobster claw) and triphalangeal thumb. *J Bone Joint Surg (Br)* 1971;53:247.
196. Porter EL, Naddelhofter L. A familial lobster claw deformity of the feet and hands in a mother and two children. *J Hered* 1947;38:331.
197. Powers JW. Hazards to health: the hazards off arming. *N Engl J Med* 1964;270:839.
198. Prendiville JB, Louis E. The pneumatic type torsion avulsion injury. *Br J Surg* 1954;42:582.
199. Radcliffe CW, Foort J. The patellar-tendon-bearing below knee prosthesis. Berkeley: University of California.
200. Reed MH. Growth disturbances in the hands following thermal injuries in children. *Can Assoc Radiol J* 1988;39:95.
201. Reis ND, Michaelson M. Crush injury to the lower limbs. *J Bone Joint Surg (Am)* 1986;68:414.
202. Ristkari SK, Vorne M, Mokka RE. Early assessment of amputation level in frost bite by 99M TC-pertechnetate scan. *Acta Chir Scand* 1988;154:403.
203. Robertson DJ. Congenital arteriovenous fistulae of the extremities. *Ann R Coli Surg Engl* 1956;18:73.
204. Robinson DW, Masters FW. The management of complicated avulsion injuries in the extremities. *South Med J* 1967;60:1039.
205. Rubin G. Prosthetic fitting problems of the quasi-Syme. *Clin Orthop* 1981;l60:233.
206. Saact MN. The problems of traumatic skin loss of the lower limbs especially when associated with skeletal injury. *Br J Surg* 1970;57:6601.
207. Sanctis N, Rezzonoano E, Scognaminglio R, Rega AN. Tibulagenesis: a new rational in management of type 2-report of three L cases with long-term follow-up. *J Pediatr Orthop* 1990; 10: 198.
208. Sarant BG, Kagan BM. Prenatal constricting bands and pseudoarthrosis of the lower leg. *Plastic Reconst Surg* 1971;47:547.
209. Schoenecker PL, Capelli AM, Millar EA, et al. Congenital longitudinal deficiency of the tibia. *J Bone Joint Surg (Am)* 1989;71: 278.
210. Scott WJ, Ritter EJ, Wilson JG. Ectodermal and mesodermal cell death patterns in 6-mercaptopurine riboside induced digital deformities. *Teratology* 1980;21: 271.
211. Shapiro J, Akbamia BA, Hanel DP. Free tissue transfer in children. *J Pediatr Orthop* 1989;9:590.
212. Shaw WW. Microvascu1ar free flaps the first decade. Clin *Plast Surg* 1983;10:3.
213. Shears D. Psychiatric adjustment in the year after meningococcal disease in childhood. *J Am Acad Child Adolesc Psychiatry* 2007; 46:76.
214. Shereff MJ. Compartment syndromes of the foot. *Inst Course Lect* 1990;39:127.
215. Shilt JS, Yoder JS, Manuck TA, et al. Role of vacuum-assisted closure in the treatment of pediatric lawnmower injuries. *J Pediatr Orthop* 204;24:482.
216. Silbart S, Oppenheim W. Purpura fulminans medical, surgical rehabilitative considerations. *Clin Orthop* 1985;193:206.
217. Simmons, ED, Ginsberg, GM, Hall, JE. Brown=s procedure for congenital absence of the tibia revisited. *J Pediatr Orthop* 1996; 16:85.
218. Slack CC. Friction injuries following road accidents. *Br Med J* 1952;2:262.
219. Small DD, Dennis CAR. An analysis of grain auger accidents. Regina: Praire Institute of Environmental Health, no. 3.
220. Stewart DE, Lpwery M. Replantation surgery following self inflicted amputation. *Can J Psychol* 1980;25:143.
221. Stills ML. Partial foot prostheses/orthoses. *Clin Prosthet Orthot* 1987;12:14–18.
222. Stokes AP, Hutton WC, Stott JR, Lowe LW. Forces under the "hallux valgus foot before and after surgery. *Clin Orthop* 1979;142:64.
223. Streeter GL. Focal deficiencies in fetal tissues and their relation to interuterine amputation. *Contrib Embryol* 1930;22:1.
224. Stringel G, D'Astous J. Klippel-Trenaunay syndrome and other cases of lower limb hypertrophy: pediatric surgical implications. *J Pediatr Surg* 1987;22:645–650.
225. Stucky W, Loder RT. Extremity gun shot wounds in children. *J Pediatr Orthop* 1991;11:64.
226. Szilagyi DE, Elliot JP, DeRousso FJ, Smith RF. Peripheral congenital arteriovenous fistulae. *Surgery* 1965;57:61.
227. Tachdjian MO. *The Child's Foot.* Philadelphia: WB Saunders,1985;317.
228. Tada K, Yonenobu K., Swanson AB. Congenital constriction band syndrome. *J Pediatr Orthop* 1984;4:726.
229. Tamtamy SA, McKusick VA. The genetics of hand malformations. *Birth Defects* 1978;14:3.
230. Thomas IH, Williams PF. The Gruca operation for congenital absence of the fibula. *J Bone Joint Surg (Br)* 1987;69:587.
231. Thompson GH, Balourdas GM, Marcus RE. Rail yard amputations in children. *J Pediatr Orthop* 1983;3:443.
232. Thompson TC, Straub LR, Arnold WD. Congenital absence of the fibula. *J Bone Joint Surg (Am)* 1957;39:1229.
233. Tochen ML. Bone lesions in the child with meningococcal meningitis and disseminated intravascular coagulation. *J Pediatr* 1977;91:342.
234. Tokmakova, K, Riddler, PA-S, Kumar, SJ. Type IV congenital deficiency of the tibia. *J Pediatr Orthop* 2003; 23:649.
235. Tooms RE. Acquired amputations in children. In: American Academy of Orthopaedic Surgery, ed. *Atlas of limb prosthesis surgical and prosthetic principles.* St. Louis: CV Mosby, 1981; 553.
236. Tooms RE. Amputations of the lower extremity. In: Crenshaw AH, ed. *Campbell's operative orthopaedics,* 6th ed, vol 1. St. Louis: CV Mosby, 1987;607–627.
237. Tsai TM. Successful replantation of a forefoot. *Clin Orthop.* 1979;139:182.
238. Urbaniak JR, Emmial MT, Myer LC. Purpura fulminans. *J Bone Joint Surg (Am)* 1973;55:69.
239. Urbaniak JR, Koman LA, Goldner RD, Armstrong NB, Nunley JA. The vascularized cutaneous scapular flap. *Plast Reconstr Surg* 1982;69:772.
240. Urschel JD. Frostbite: predisposing factors and predictors of poor outcome. *J Trauma* 1990;30:340.
241. Usui M, Minami M, Ishu S. Successful replantation of an amputated leg in a child. *Plast Reconstr Surg* 1979;63:613.
242. Valentine J, Blocker S, Chang JHT. Gun shot injuries in children. *J Trauma* 1984;24:952.

243. Verghe H, Dequeker J, Frins JP, David G. Familial occurrence of severe ulnar aplasia and lobster claw feet: a new syndrome. *Hum Gen* 1978;42:109.
244. Vergsma D, Lenz W. Morphogenesis and malformation of the limb. *Birth Defects* 1977;12:1.
245. Wagner FW. Amputations of the foot and ankle. *Clin Orthop* 1977;122:62–69.
246. Wagner FW. Partial foot amputations. In: American Academy of Orthopaedic Surgeons, ed. *Atlas of limb prosthesis surgical and prosthetic principles.* St. Louis: CV Mosby, 1981.
247. Watson AG, Bonde RK. Congenital malformations of the flipper in three West Indian manatees. *Clin Orthop* 1986;202:294.
248. Watson C, Ashworth A. Growth disturbance and meningococcal septicemia. *J Bone Joint Surg (Am)* 1983;65:1181.
249. Wehbe MA, Weinstein SL, Ponseti IV. Tibial agenesis. *J Pediatr Orthop* 1981;1:395.
250. Weissman SL, Plaschkes Y. Surgical correction of lobster claw-feet: case report. *Plastic Reconstr Surg* 1972;49:89.
251. Westin W, Sakai D, Wood WL. Congenital longitudinal deficiency of the fibula: follow-up of treatment of Syme amputation. *J Bone Joint Surg [Am]* 1976;58:492.
252. Wiseman NE, Briggs IN, Bolton VS. Neonatal arterial occlusion and ischemic limb gangrene. *J Pediatr Surg* 1977;12:707.
253. Wood WL, Ziotsky N, Westin GW. Congenital absence of the fibula: treatment with Syme amputation: indications and techniques. *J Bone Joint Surg [Am]* 1965;47:1159.
254. Wu KK. *Surgery of the foot.* Philadelphia: Lea and Febiger, 1986; Chapter 7.
255. Zhong C, Meyer VE, Kleinart HE, Beasley RW. Present indication and central indications for replantation as reflected by long term functional results. *Orthop Clin North Am* 1981;12:849.

CHAPTER 22

Ankle Fractures in Children

Martin J. Herman and Ashish Ranade

INTRODUCTION

Ankle fractures in children include tibial and fibular fractures that occur at or distal to the metaphyses and frequently involve the physes (growth plates) of these bones. Physeal fractures of the distal tibia and fibula account for as many as 38% of all physeal injuries in children (16,24,29,30). Salter-Harris (SH) type 1 and 2 fractures are more common than other types (Table 22-1). Ankle physeal fractures are the third most commonly injured growth plates, after injuries of the phalanges and distal radius (30). The annual incidence in children is 0.1% (24,29,30). Pediatric ankle fractures occur twice as frequently in boys compared to girls (24). The peak incidence is seen in children between the ages of 8 and 15 years (24,29,30). The fracture patterns vary in a predictable way based on the child's age at the time of injury (36) (Figure 22-1).

Fractures of the ankle in children occur most commonly during sports activities (14). While basketball is the sport with the highest risk of these injuries (8), in-line skating, skateboarding, trampoline jumping, and other recreational activities have also been identified as other causes for these fractures. High-energy mechanisms including falls from heights and motor vehicle trauma are less common causes. Distal tibial and fibular fractures are infrequently the result of child abuse (18) (Figure 22-2).

Children's ligaments are generally stronger than their physes. Compared to adults, torsional forces applied to the immature ankle more frequently result in physeal fractures than in ankle ligament sprains. Management of displaced ankle fractures, particularly those that involve the growth plate, is challenging. As for adults who sustain ankle fractures, restoration of ankle joint stability and anatomic reconstruction of the joint surface are critical to prevent secondary ankle stiffness and premature osteoarthritis after these fractures in children. The surgeon, however, must achieve these goals while minimizing additional injury to a physis already potentially compromised by the initial trauma. Joint surface deformity, angular deviation, and leg-length discrepancy are complications that are unique to children who sustain ankle fractures.

ANATOMY

The ankle is a hinge joint. Ankle stability is achieved by a combination of the osseous restraints of the talus within the distal tibia/fibula mortise configuration and the soft-tissue connections of the ankle ligaments. The syndesmosis between the distal tibia and fibula is sustained by the distal interosseous membrane and the anterior and posterior tibio-fibular ligaments which are dense bands of tissue that connect the distal fibular metaphysis to the lateral distal tibial epiphysis. These strong connections allow only limited physiologic motion between the bones, mostly rotation of the distal fibula with knee flexion and extension. The talus is most constrained by the distal fibula (lateral malleolus) and the distal medial tibia (medial malleolus) in dorsiflexion because the talar dome is wider anteriorly than posteriorly.

The ligaments of the ankle secure the talus in the mortise. The deltoid ligament originates from the distal medial malleolus and supports the ankle medially by providing a check-rein against valgus ankle forces. The superficial deltoid ligament inserts on the talus, calcaneus, and navicular while the deep deltoid ligament inserts on the talus only. The anterior talofibular, calcaneofibular, and posterior talofibular ligaments provide lprimary ankle support against varus and internal torsional forces predominantly. The medial and lateral ankle ligaments originate distal to the physes of the tibia and fibula respectively. The sites of ligament origin and the inherent strength of the ligaments compared to the weaker physes provide an anatomic explanation for the observation that ankle fractures are more common than sprains in children.

The ossification center of the distal tibia appears between 6 and 24 months of age (28). The medial

TABLE 22-1

Distribution of Fracture Types

	Total # of cases	*SH 1/2 (%)*	*SH 3/4 (%)*	*Triplane (%)*	*Tillaux (%)*
Spiegel et al. (36)	237	127(53.6%)	52(21.9%)	15(6.3%)	6(2.5%)
De Sanctis et al. (9)	113	46(40.7%)	21(18.6%)	NA	4(3.5%)
Barmada et al. (1)	92	51(55.4%)	8(8.5%)	19(21%)	14(15.2%)

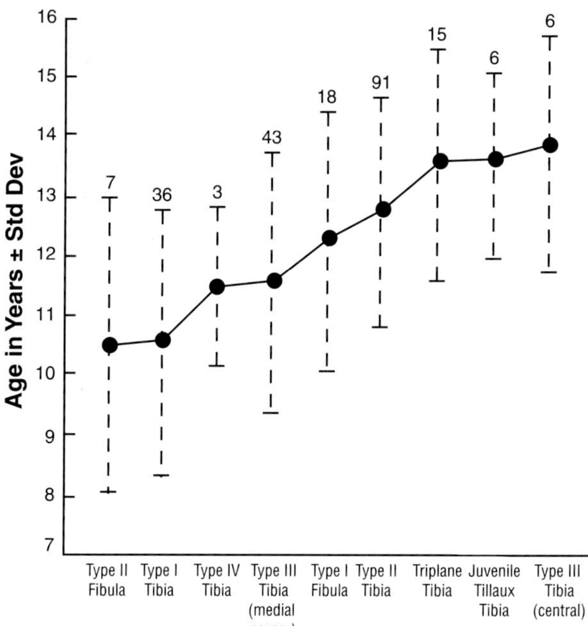

FIGURE 22-1 Graphic depiction of peak age of occurrence for each fracture type. Adapted from Spiegel, PG, et al. Triplane fractures of the distal tibial epiphysis. *Clin Orthop Relat Res* 1984(188): 74–89.

malleolus begins to ossify at about age 7, with most of its growth completed by age 10. Twenty percent of children develop a secondary ossification center (os subtibiale) of the medial malleous between age 6 and 12 years. The physis of the distal tibia accounts for 18% of the overall limb length and 32% of the overall length of the tibia. The distal tibial physis closes at approximately 15 years of age in girls and 17 in boys. Physeal closure begins centrally, extends medially, and then proceeds laterally; the anterolateral quadrant of the physis closes last (Figure 22-3). This gradual and asymmetric closure occurs over 18 month to 2 years and explains the unique fracture patterns of the adolescent transitional fractures of the ankle (juvenile Tillaux and triplane ankle fractures).

The distal fibular ossification center appears at approximately nine months to two years of age. This physis accounts for 45% of the overall length of the fibula. The physis is located at the level of the talar dome. Complete closure of the distal fibular physis occurs approximately two years after closure of the distal tibial physis. Ten percent of children develop a secondary ossification center of the distal fibula (os subfilbulare) between six and twelve years of age.

CLASSIFICATION

Classification systems are useful for communication of fracture patterns in a comprehensive way, to guide treatment, and, ideally, to predict outcomes. The best schemes are easily remembered and can be applied consistently. The two broad categories of classifications that have been applied to children's ankle fractures are mechanism-of-injury and anatomic schemes. To classify adult ankle fractures, the Lauge-Hansen classification (a mechanism-of-injury type) (20) and Weber schemes (anatomic type) are most widely used.(26). Neither of these systems, however, is ideal for the classifying children's fractures. Dias and Tachjdian (11,12) modified the Lauge-Hansen scheme to create a mechanism-of-injury classification for physeal ankle fractures. The initial classification defined four types of injuries in children, describing the foot position (first word) and the direction of force applied (second word). The categories included supination–inversion, pronation–eversion external rotation, supination–plantar flexion, and supination–external rotation (Figure 22-4). The classification was later modified to include fractures unique to children that cannot be described by the original types. These include axial compression distal tibial physeal injuries that result in growth disturbance,juvenile Tillaux fractures, and triplane ankle fractures.

The Salter-Harris (SH) classification (33) (Figure 22-5), an anatomic scheme, is easily applied to physeal ankle fractures (39). Familiarity makes this scheme useful and practical for the orthopedic surgeon. Some difficulties arise, however, when classifying the transitional ankle fractures. The triplane ankle fracture, for example, is a complex fracture of the distal tibia that traverses the physis in anteroposterior, lateral, and axial planes, resulting in multiple fracture fragments. The typical triplane fracture appears to be a type SH 3 or 4 fracture in the AP radiograph and a type SH 2 or 4 fracture in the lateral view (Figure 22-6). Many pediatric orthopedic surgeons, therefore, use the SH classification to describe physeal ankle fractures and apply eponyms (e.g., juvenile Tillaux) and other descriptive terms to identify specific ankle

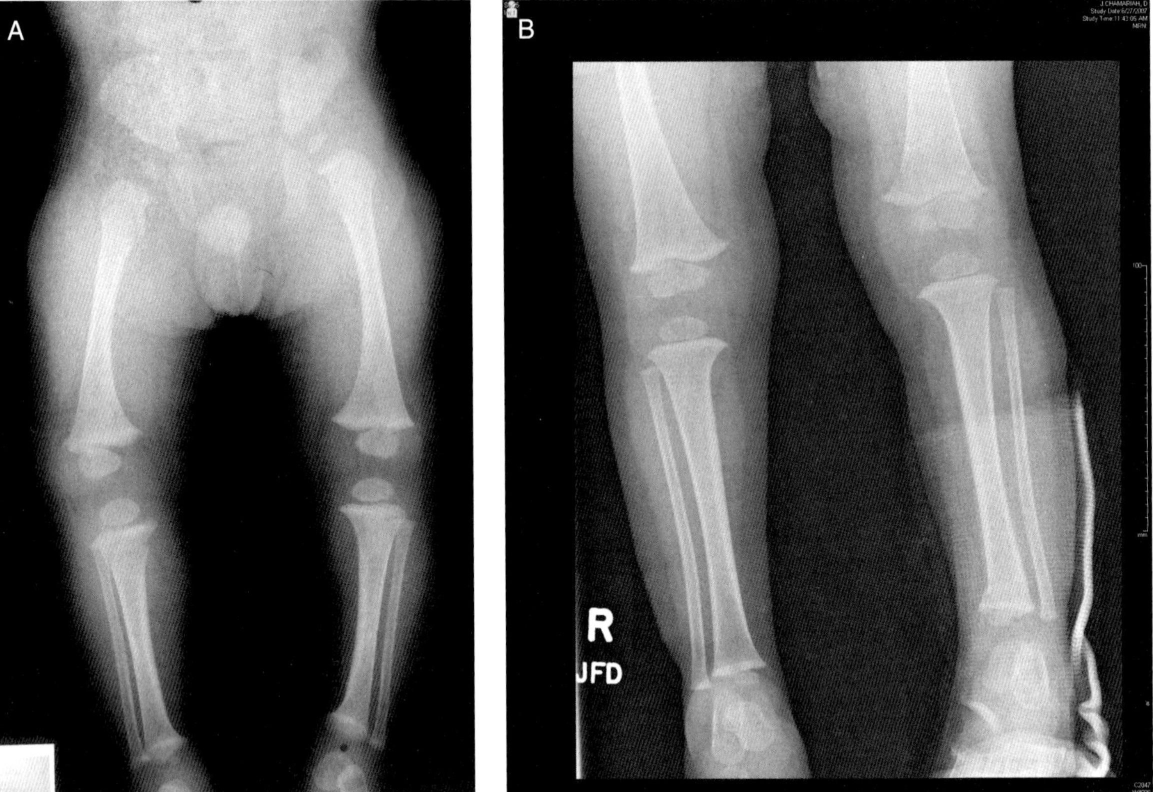

FIGURE 22-2 (**A**) Seven month old admitted with a swollen knee. Radiograph reveals right distal femur and distal tibia metaphyseal corner fractures and a right proximal tibial metaphyseal fracture. The diagnosis of child abuse was confirmed after investigation by social services. (**B**) Twelve-month-old girl presented to her primary care physician with left ankle swelling for three days. The child's mother reported no trauma. After an investigation because of the delay in presentation and incomplete history, the child's older brother admitted that he had stepped on the child when she wouldn't stop crying. Radiograph reveals a left metaphyseal distal tibia fracture.

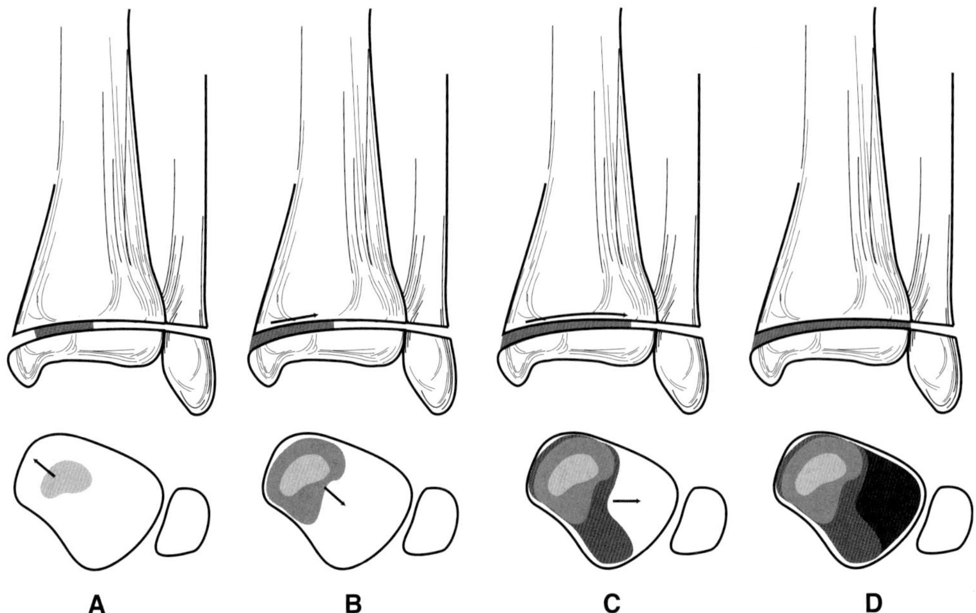

FIGURE 22-3 Closure of the distal tibial physis. The physis of the distal tibia closes gradually over a period of 18 months to 2 years, beginning centrally, progressing medially then posterolaterally. The anterolateral quadrant is the last segment to close. Juvenile Tillaux and triplane ankle fractures occur in adolescents with partial physeal closure. (Adapted from Schnetzler K, Hoernschemeyer D. *J Am Acad Orthop Surg* 2007;15:739.)

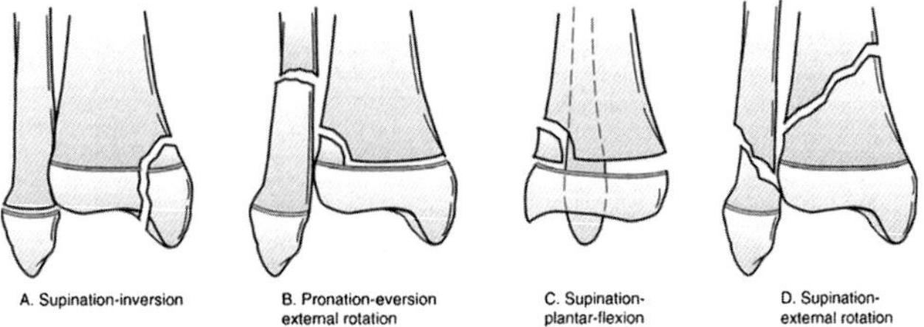

FIGURE 22-4 Dias-Tachjdian classification. The original classification described these 4 fracture patterns and their mechanisms of injury. The classification was later modified to include fractures unique to children that cannot be described by the original types; these include axial compression distal tibial physeal injuries that result in growth disturbance, juvenile Tillaux fractures, and triplane ankle fractures. From Beaty JH, Kasser JR. *Fractures in children.* Rockwood and Wilkins, eds. Philadelphia: Lippincott Williams & Wilkins, 2001.

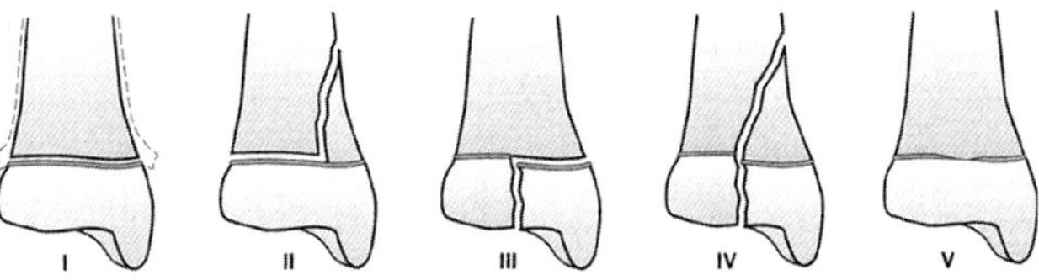

FIGURE 22-5 Salter-Harris classification of distal tibia fractures. From Beaty JH, Kasser JR. *Fractures in children*, Rockwood and Wilkins, eds. Philadelphia: Lippincott Williams & Wilkins, 2001.

injury patterns that are not easily classified by the SH classification (Table 22-2).

Other less common pediatric ankle injuries have been described. The pediatric pilon fracture involves the tibial plafond with both articular and physeal displacement, with or without fibular and talar injuries (21). These fractures are most commonly the result of combined torsional and axial forces resulting in comminuted fracture patterns. The incisural fracture is a linear fracture of the lateral distal tibial metaphysis caused by an avulsion of the distal interosseous membrane from an extreme external rotation force applied to the hindfoot (7). This injury, like the pilon fracture, is best defined by computed tomography (CT).

DIAGNOSTICS

History and Physical Examination

A thorough clinical evaluation begins with a detailed history of the injury mechanism, distinguishing high-energy mechanisms from low-energy ones. Children who sustain ankle injuries from high-energy mechanisms, such as motor vehicle trauma or potential child abuse, must first have a comprehensive multi-system emergency evaluation to diagnose other potentially more serious injuries. Most ankle fractures, however, are isolated injuries, resulting from low-energy trauma such as sports activities. When prompted, the child or parent often is able to remember the circumstances of the injury, including when it occurred, the position of the foot and ankle at the time of injury, and the type of force that caused it. This information may provide important clues to the type of ankle injury sustained. A complete history also includes any history of significant ankle or leg injuries and past medical or surgical conditions.

The physical examination begins with inspection of the ankle for soft-tissue swelling and obvious angular or rotational lower leg deformity. The ankle joint line is palpated for tenderness and evidence of hemarthrosis. Next, the distal tibia and fibula are examined systematically. Based on surface anatomy, the examiner palpates the deltoid ligament, the anterolateral ankle ligaments, and the sydesmosis, starting at the ankle joint line and proceeding proximally. The metaphyses and physes of the distal fibula and tibia and the tips of the malleoli are then individually palpated for point tenderness. Proceeding proximally and distally from the ankle, the shafts of the fibula and tibia, the hindfoot and the base of the metatarsals, especially the fifth metatarsal, are also examined for swelling and tenderness. Neurovascular assessment of the limb, evaluation of skin integrity, and palpation of compartments of the lower leg complete the examination.

IMAGING

Radiographs

High-quality anteroposterior (AP), lateral, and mortise radiographic views of the ankle and AP and lateral views of the entire tibia are necessary to appropriately evaluate the child with a suspected ankle fracture. For children without gross deformity or instability, the radiographs are best taken without a splint or cast so that subtle findings such as non-displaced fractures or physeal widening are not obscured. A complete skeletal survey is prescribed for

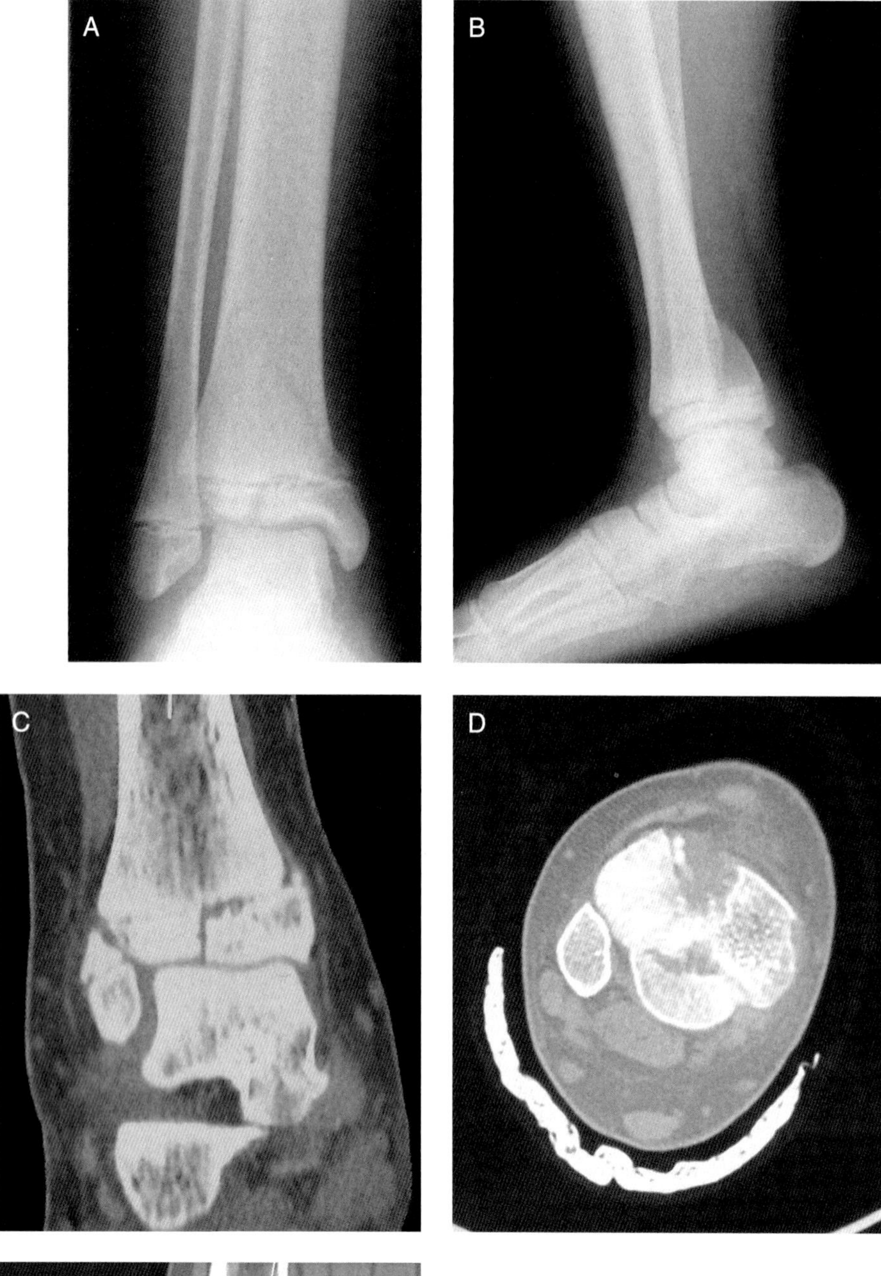

FIGURE 22-6 Triplane fracture. The triplane ankle fracture is a complex injury of the distal tibia that occurs in children approaching skeletal maturity. The fracture line traverses the distal tibia in the transverse, coronal, and axial planes. On radiographs ((**A**) *mortise*, (**B**) *lateral*), the triplane fracture appears as a Salter-Harris 3 or 4 fracture on the AP view and a Salter-Harris 2 or 4 fracture on the lateral view. CT ((**C**) *coronal*, (**D**) *axial*, (**E**) *sagittal images*) best defines the fracture pattern.

TABLE 22-2

Radiographic Classification of Ankle Fractures in Children

1. Describe the distal tibia fracture
   a. Metaphyseal fracture
   b. Physeal fracture (Salter-Harris types 1 through 4)
   c. Transitional type
      i. Juvenile Tillaux fracture
      ii. Triplane ankle fracture
   d. Medial malleolus fracture
   e. Fracture through os subtibiale
2. Describe the distal fibula fracture
   a. Metaphyseal
   b. Physeal fracture (Salter-Harris types 1 through 4)
   c. Fracture through os fibulare
3. Assess ankle ligaments
   a. Deltoid ligament
   b. Anterolateral ankle complex
   c. Syndesmosis ligaments

children whose history and physical examination are suspicious for child abuse.

Computed Tomography (CT)

Thin-cut (2 mm) CT images with multiplanar reconstruction are useful to fully assess intra-articular fracture patterns, such as the juvenile Tillaux and triplane ankle fractures (2). CT is utilized to identify fracture comminution, to measure the amount of articular surface displacement after closed reduction, and to assist the surgeon with planning of operative reduction and fixation. CT is not routinely prescribed because CT images may overestimate the degree of intra-articular displacement of minimally displaced fractures (15).

Magnetic Resonance Imaging (MRI)

MRI has a limited role in the evaluation of acute ankle injuries. This modality is prescribed to identify occult fractures or stress fractures, to assess osteochondral injuries of the distal tibia and talus, and to evaluate the ankle ligaments. MRI may also be a useful tool to identify premature physeal closure after trauma and to map the extent and precise location of a physeal bar. Pathologic fractures of the distal tibia and ankle are rare and seen most commonly in the distal tibial metaphysis. MRI is the best modality for evaluating bony abnormalities and soft tissue masses associated with neoplasms.

TIBIAL FRACTURE TREATMENT

Salter-Harris 1 and 2 Distal Tibial Fractures

Nonoperative Management

Type SH 1 fractures account for approximately 15% of distal tibial physeal fractures, while type SH 2 occur in 40% of these injuries (24,29,30,36). Most type SH 1 and 2 fractures of the distal tibia are managed non-operatively. Non-displaced fractures are immobilized in a long leg cast at the time of diagnosis. For displaced fractures, closed reduction in the emergency room is the best initial treatment. The same basic approach to ankle fracture reduction applies to all displaced fractures. After administration of conscious sedation, the injured limb is suspended over the end of the stretcher, flexing the knee to relax the gastocnemius-soleus muscle complex. The surgeon first applies gentle longitudinal traction to the hindfoot. Next, reduction of the distal fragment is performed by reversing the mechanism of injury based on the history and fragment displacement on the injury radiographs. For those fractures displaced posterolaterally and externally rotated (the most common deformity), the hindfoot is translated anteriomedially and internally rotated while the tibia is pushed posterolaterally. After realignment, the hindfoot is maintained in internal rotation and the ankle is dorsiflexed to 90 degrees. While the foot is held by an assistant, a long-leg cast is applied, usually done by first applying and carefully molding the short-leg portion of the cast, followed by the above-knee portion. After reduction, AP, lateral, and mortise views of the ankle are obtained in the cast.

Acceptable parameters of reduction vary by age because of the potential for remodeling in younger children. For those with more than two years of growth remaining, the surgeon can accept less than or equal to 5 degrees of varus displacement, less than or equal to 10 degrees of valgus and less than or equal to 10 degrees of anterior or posterior displacement. Gapping of the distal tibial physis must also be assessed after reduction. A gap measuring more than 3 mm between the metaphysis and epiphysis on post-reduction radiographs, caused by infolded periosteum preventing reduction, has been correlated with an increased rate of premature physeal closure and is unacceptable in most cases (1) (see Figure 22-6). For children approaching skeletal maturity with less than two years of growth remaining, less deformity is acceptable because little remodeling can be expected: less than or equal to 0 degrees of varus, less than or equal to 5 degrees of valgus, and less than or equal to 10 degrees of AP displacement are satisfactory parameters of reduction.

If the initial reduction is not acceptable, a second manipulation may be attempted in the emergency room if the child remains adequately sedated. More than two attempts at reduction in the emergency room, the use of excessive force, and manipulation with inadequate analgesia are not recommended in order to minimize the risk of an iatrogenic physeal injury.

Operative Management

Surgical management is indicated for those fractures that fail closed reduction under conscious sedation, open fractures, and those rare injuries associated with severe soft-tissue damage or vascular compromise. In the operating room under general anesthesia with muscle relaxation and adequate assistance, an acceptable closed reduction of SH

1 and 2 distal tibia fractures can generally be achieved. After reduction, stable fractures are immobilized in a long-leg cast. Fractures that are unstable after reduction require internal fixation, often placed percutaneously.

Unstable type SH 1 and SH 2 fractures with a very small metaphyseal fragment are best stabilized by crossed smooth wires (0.062 mm or 5/64 in) placed retrograde from the tips of the medial and lateral malleoli across the physis. Type SH 2 fractures with a large metaphyseal (Thurston-Holland) fragment require 4.0 or 4.5 mm cannulated screws. The ideal screw is inserted in the metaphysis parallel and proximal to the physis, achieving fixation through the Thurston-Holland fragment. Transphyseal screws are indicated only for those children with less than two years of growth remaining. For screws placed anteriorly, a 2-cm incision is made just lateral to the midline. The extensor retinaculum is divided longitudinally and the extensor tendons are separated bluntly, taking care to avoid injury to the branches of the superficial peroneal nerve and the neurovascular bundle. Screws may be placed posteriorly, utilizing a small posterolateral incision made just lateral to the Achilles tendon at the level of the metaphysis. While holding the fracture reduced, a guide wire is drilled through a soft tissue protector across the fracture site. Adequacy of reduction and wire location and length are confirmed by fluoroscopy. A self-drilling, self-tapping screw is then inserted under direct vision to prevent entrapment of tendons and neurovascular structures under the screw head. One or two metaphyseal screws provide sufficient fixation. Alternatively, smooth wires may be used for fixation in place of screws.

Open reduction is necessary for irreducible SH type 1 and 2 fractures. The incision is placed at the most likely site of soft-tissue entrapment, usually at the angular apex where physeal widening is apparent. After extrication of muscle, tendon, or periosteum from the fracture site, the fragments are reduced. The surgeon must take care to avoid excessive stripping of additional periosteum or physeal perichondrium while performing the open reduction to avoid iatrogenic physeal injury. Excision of the Thurston-Holland fragment is not recommended. Fixation may then be applied either through the same incision or percutaneously in a fashion similar to that used for closed fractures (Figure 22-7).

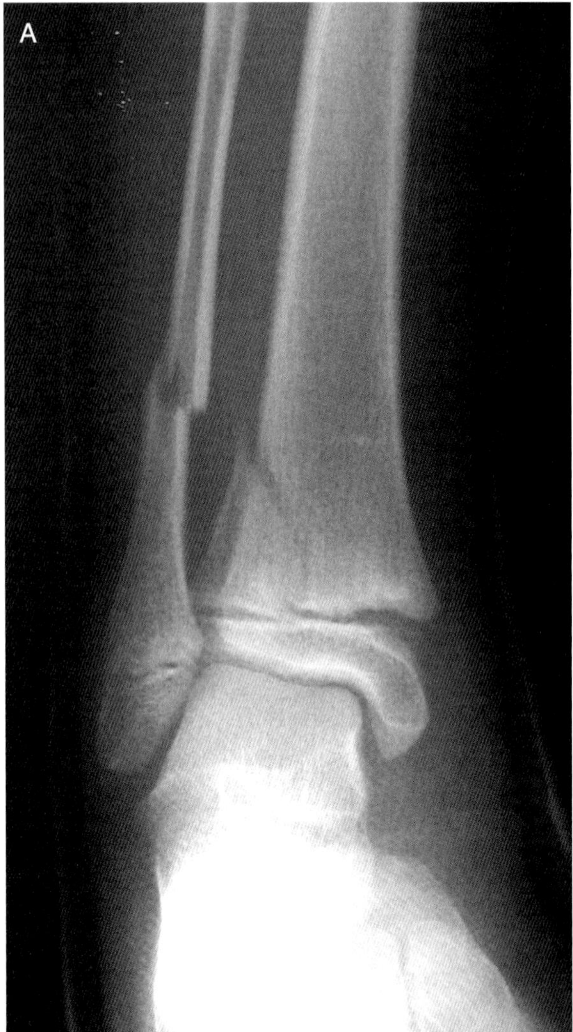

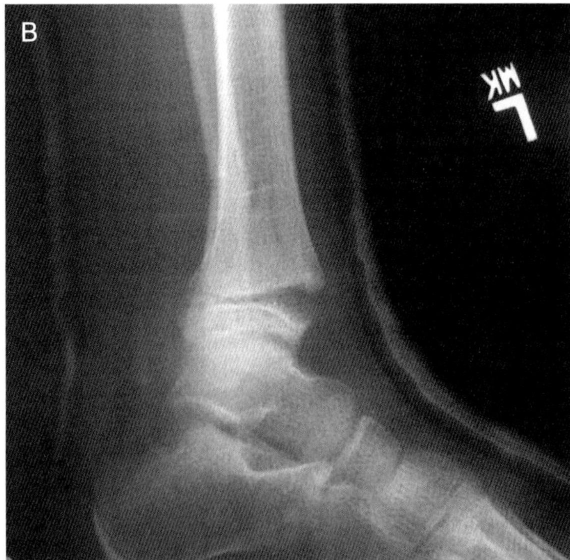

FIGURE 22-7 Eleven-year-old girl who underwent closed reduction of a distal tibia Salter-Harris type 2 fracture. Post-reduction radiographs reveal acceptable AP (**A**) and lateral (**B**) alignment but a physeal gap of 3.5 mm. She underwent open reduction; the gap was caused by infolded periosteum.

Care After Reduction

SH type 1 and 2 fractures are managed without fixation are immobilized for four weeks after injury in a non-weight bearing long-leg cast. Fractures treated with fixation may be immobilized in a non–weight-bearing short leg cast. After cast removal, weight bearing is gradually advanced, protected in a short-leg weight-bearing cast or removable cast-boot for an additional two to four weeks. Radiographs are obtained after removal of these casts to confirm progression of healing. After a short period of rehabilitation, most children return to normal activities within three to four months of injury (Table 22-3). Long-term radiographic follow-up is necessary and is

TABLE 22-3

Care After Closed Reduction of Displaced Ankle Fractures

1. Long-leg non–weight-bearing cast for initial four weeks (may use short-leg non–weight bearing cast with stable fixation).
2. Short-leg weight-bearing cast or removable walking boot for additional two to four weeks.
3. Rehabilitation for 6 to 12 weeks, emphasizing ankle range of motion, strengthening, and proprioceptive training.

done at six-month intervals after initial healing until skeletal maturity, to detect early signs of growth disturbance of the distal tibia.

Late Presentation of Fractures

After two weeks from injury, physeal healing will have progressed to such a degree that simple repeat manipulation will not be effective because of fracture immobility and the potential for iatrogenic physeal. Displaced fractures that present more than two weeks after injury and those that lose reduction but are identified after two weeks from closed reduction are challenging problems. Because of their significant remodeling potential, younger children with unacceptable alignment are immobilized in situ until healing has occurred. Remodeling is then observed for one to two years, after which surgical realignment by hemiepiphyseodesis or osteotomies may be planned. Younger children with severe malalignment of the fracture and older children with less than two years of growth remaining are best treated with open reduction at the time of presentation.

Salter-Harris 3 and 4 Distal Tibia Fractures

Nonoperative Management

Type SH 3 and SH 4 fractures account for approximately 25% of distal tibial physeal fractures, with type SH 3 injuries occurring much more frequently than type SH 4 (24,29,30,36). Non-displaced SH type 3 and 4 fractures are effectively managed with long-leg cast immobilization and careful follow-up with weekly radiographs for two weeks after injury to detect possible displacement. For some displaced fractures, closed reduction under sedation in the emergency room is the best treatment. The same basic approach to closed reduction described for type SH 1 and 2 fractures is utilized. Type SH 3 and 4 fractures most commonly require abduction and external rotation reduction forces to reverse the most mechanism of injury and achieve realignment. The surgeon initially applies gentle longitudinal traction to the hindfoot. Next, reduction of the distal fragment is performed by reversing the mechanism of injury based on the history and fragment displacement on the injury radiographs. Because most type SH 3 and 4 fractures are displaced medially, adducted, and internally rotated, reduction is accomplished by everting the hindfoot and then externally rotating and laterally translating it while the tibia is pushed posteromedially. After realignment, the hindfoot is maintained in slight eversion and external rotation and the ankle is dorsiflexed to 90 degrees. While the foot is held by an assistant, a long-leg cast is applied, usually performed by first applying and carefully molding the short-leg portion of the cast followed by the above-knee portion. After reduction, AP, lateral, and mortise views of the ankle are obtained in the cast.

Acceptable reduction parameters do not vary significantly with the age of the child because these injuries are intra-articular: 2 mm or less of step-off or gapping measured at the joint line and physis is acceptable. High-quality radiographs and CT obtained in the cast after reduction must be critically evaluated to confirm a satisfactory reduction. Follow-up imaging is necessary for nondisplaced fractures to detect possible displacement.

Operative Management

Fixation of most displaced type SH 3 and 4 fractures is recommended because closed reduction may be inadequate or not stable enough to be maintained with cast immobilization alone, and also because non-displaced fractures can displace in a cast. Under general anesthesia with muscle relaxation, closed reduction is first attempted. If an acceptable closed reduction can be achieved easily without forceful or excessive manipulation, the fracture is best stabilized by percutaneous 4.0 or 4.5 mm cannulated screws. While the reduction is maintained by an assistant, a guide wire is placed through a small medial incision crossing the epiphyseal fracture site parallel to the joint line and physis. After confirming adequacy of reduction and wire placement and length with fluoroscopy, a short-thread, self-tapping, self-drilling screw is then inserted, achieving compression across the epiphyseal fracture line. One or two screws are necessary to achieve stable fixation. After screw fixation, the surgeon must critically assess reduction and screw position with fluoroscopy or intra-operative plain radiographs. Screws that violate the joint surface or penetrate the physis must be repositioned.

Open reduction is necessary for irreducible fractures, fractures with comminution and intra-articular fragments, and open fractures. A limited anterior exposure and fracture reduction, combined with percutaneous fixation, is an effective method of treatment of type SH 3 and 4 fractures (22) (Figure 22-8). After marking the site of the epiphyseal fracture line by fluoroscopy on the anterior ankle, a 2–4 cm longitudinal incision is made. The fracture is exposed taking care to identify and retract branches of the superficial peroneal nerve, the neurovascular bundle, and the tendons of the anterior compartment that cross the ankle joint. A small capsular incision is then made and open reduction of the joint line and physis are done under direct vision. A bone reduction clamp facilitates reduction by compressing the fragments. Percutaneous fixation is accomplished as described above (Figure 22-9).

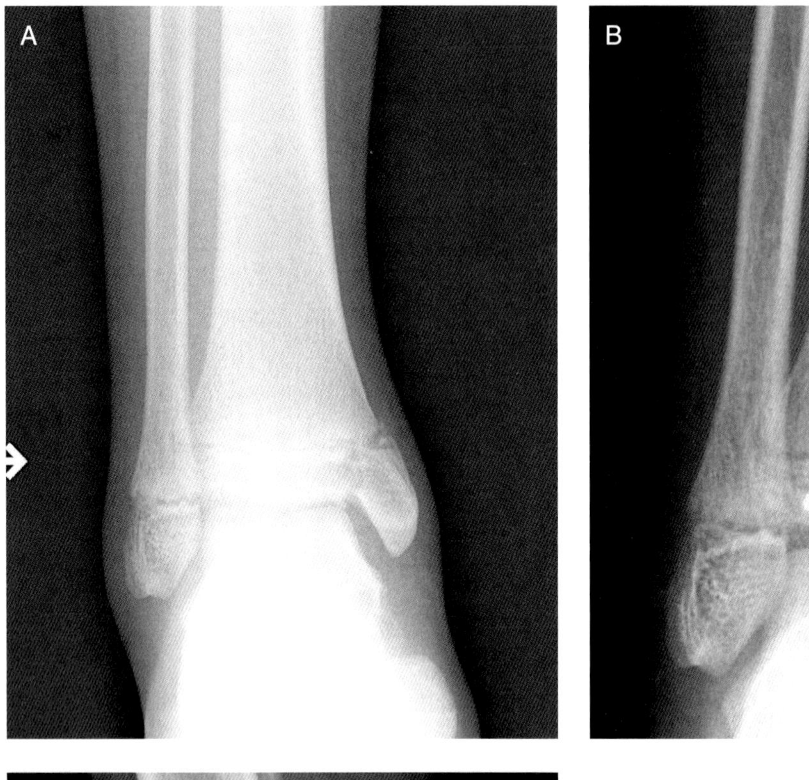

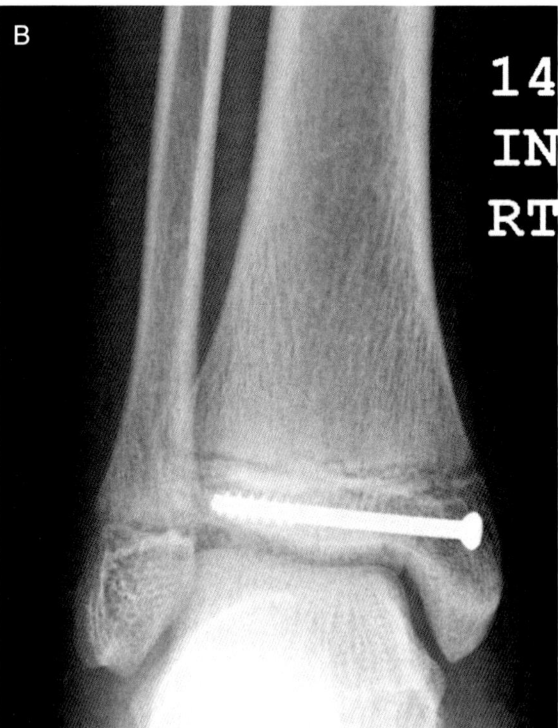

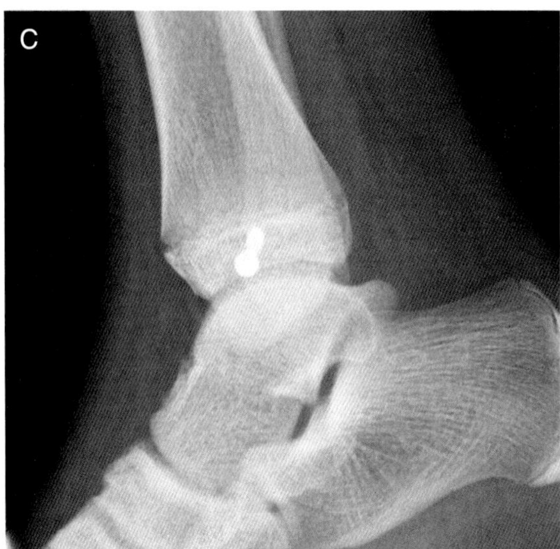

FIGURE 22-10 Salter-Harris 3 fracture. Thirteen-year-old boy who twisted his ankle when tripping over another player during a soccer game. Mortise ankle view (**A**) reveals a displaced Salter-Harris 3 fracture of the medial malleolus. He underwent open reduction and fixation ((**B**) mortise, (**C**) lateral views).

evidence, epiphyseal screws may also alter the distribution of forces across the subchondral bone of the tibial plafond, leading to uneven joint cartilage wear (4).

Salter-Harris Type 5 Distal Tibia Fractures

The true incidence of SH type 5 fractures of the tibia is not known. They result from a crush injury to the physis after high-energy axial loading such as from a fall or motor vehicle trauma. The diagnosis is made retrospectively when a growth disturbance is identified but initial radiographs at the time of injury are interpreted as normal. Treatment of type SH 5 fractures is limited to management of the subsequent growth disturbance.

Transitional Ankle Fractures

Juvenile Tillaux and Triplane Ankle Fractures

The distal tibial physis closes gradually in a predictable fashion during the final 18 months to 2 years of skeletal growth. Closure begins centrally in the physis and progresses to the medial and posterolateral segments. The anterolateral quadrant is the last portion of the growth plate to close. Ankle injuries that occur during this period of transition from an

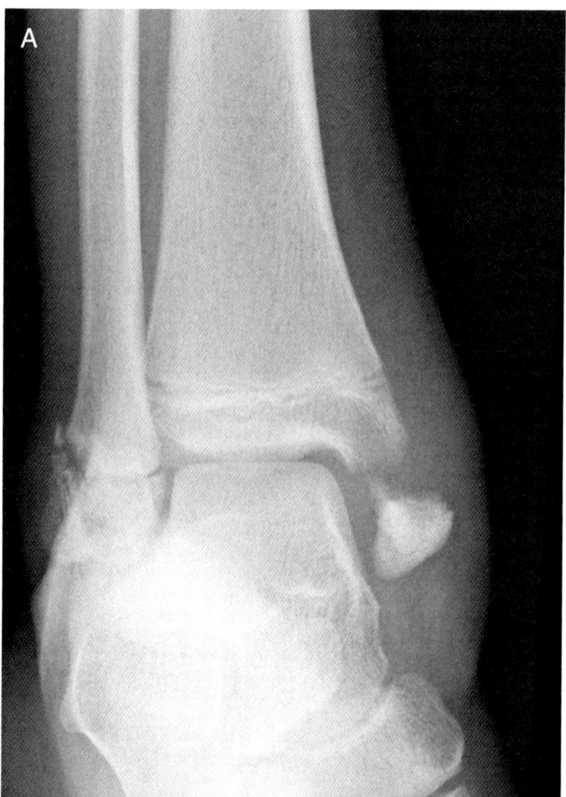

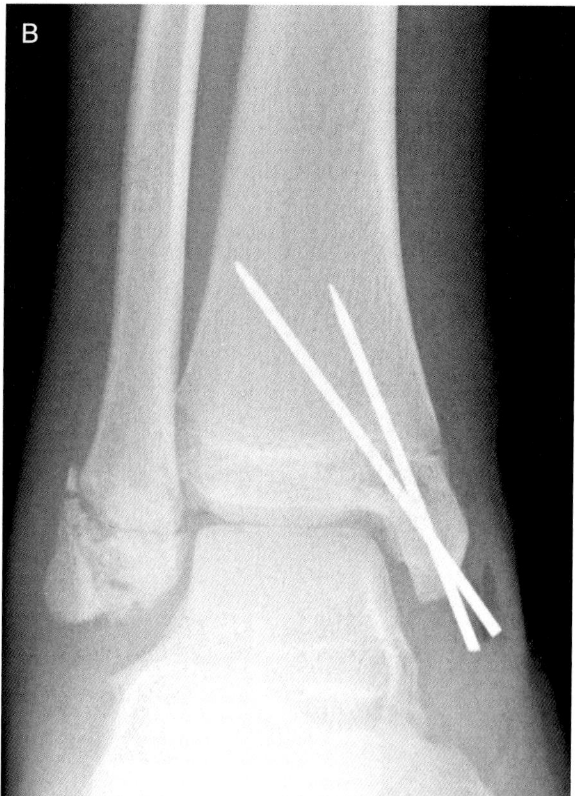

FIGURE 22-11 Medial malleolus fracture. Twn-year-old boy who was hit by a car while on his bicycle. He sustained a Salter-Harris 3 fracture of the fibula and a medial malleolus fracture (**A**). He underwent open reduction of the medial malleolus and fixation with smooth wires to avoid injury to the physis (**B**).

actively growing physis to a closed one are called transitional ankle fractures and result in unique fractures patterns. The juvenile Tillaux fracture and the triplane ankle fracture are the most common transitional ankle fractures.

Juvenile Tillaux

The juvenile Tillaux fracture accounts for 3% of pediatric ankle fractures (24,29,30,36). The result of external rotation forces applied to the distal tibia and foot, the juvenile Tillaux fracture is an avulsion fracture of the anterolateral quadrant of the epiphysis caused by the anterior tibiofibular syndesmosis ligament (Figures 22-11 and 22-12). The diagnosis is often apparent on plain radiographs, appearing as a type SH 3 fracture of the distal tibia. CT imaging is useful for confirming the diagnosis when radiographs are suspicious for the injury as well as defining the degree of joint line displacement.

Nonoperative Management

Fractures with 2 mm or less of joint line displacement are best treated with long-leg cast immobilization. Closed reduction of fractures with greater displacement is sometimes possible. Under conscious sedation in the emergency room per the protocol outline above for type SH 1 and 2 fractures, the surgeon internally rotates the hindfoot, which is positioned in slight equinus, while pushing directly with a posteromedial force on the fragment. The ankle is then dorsifexed to 90 degrees with internal rotation maintained and the foot is held by an assistant while a long-leg cast is applied. High-quality plain radiographs and/or CT images are obtained to assess the reduction. An acceptable reduction is one with 2 mm or less of joint line gapping or step-off.

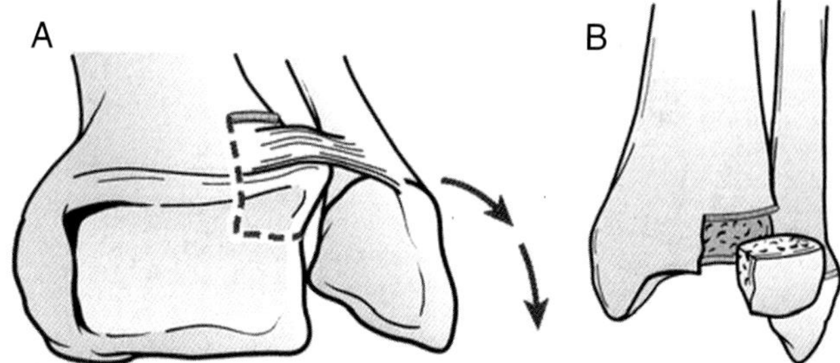

FIGURE 22-12 Juvenile Tillaux fracture: **A.** Forced external rotation of the foot results in an avulsion fracture of the anterolateral quadrant of the epiphysis caused by the pull of the anterior tibiofibular syndesmosis ligament. This injury occurs in children approaching skeletal maturity with incomplete closure of the distal tibial physis. **B.** Fracture reduction can often be done by manipulation of the fragment with a stiff guide wire ("joystick") placed percutaneously into the fragment. A cannulated screw can then be placed over the wire to achieve fracture fixation. (From Rockwood and Wilkins *Fractures in children*, eds. Beaty JH, Kasser JR. Philadelphia: Lippincott Williams & Wilkins, 2001.)

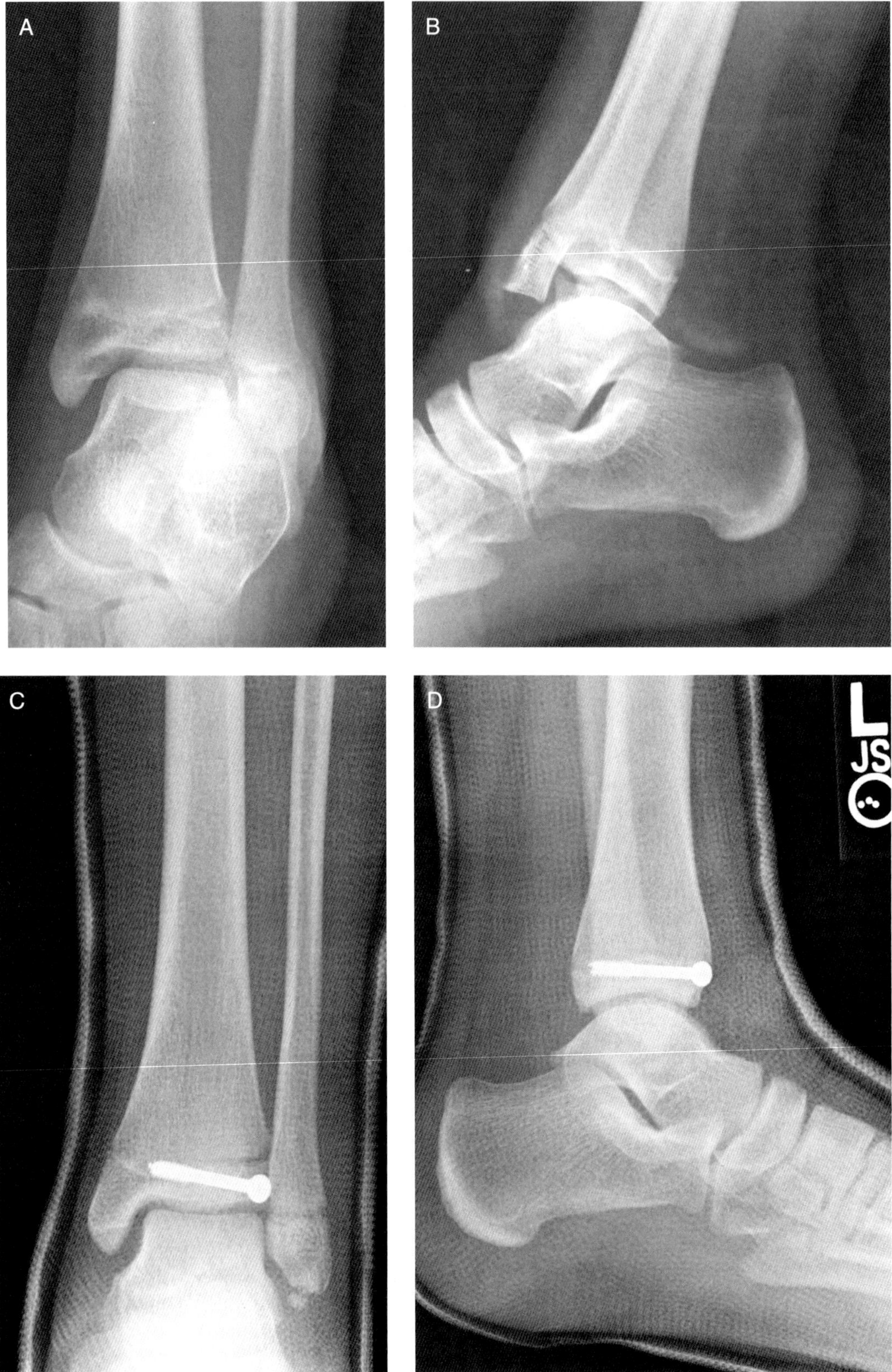

FIGURE 22-13 Juvenile Tillaux fracture. Twelve-year-old girl who tripped off of a curb, catching her foot in a storm grate as she fell. Radiographs reveal a displaced juvenile Tillaux fracture with a physeal fracture of the fibula ((**A**) mortise, and (**B**) lateral views). She underwent open reduction and screw fixation ((**C**) AP and (**D**) lateral views).

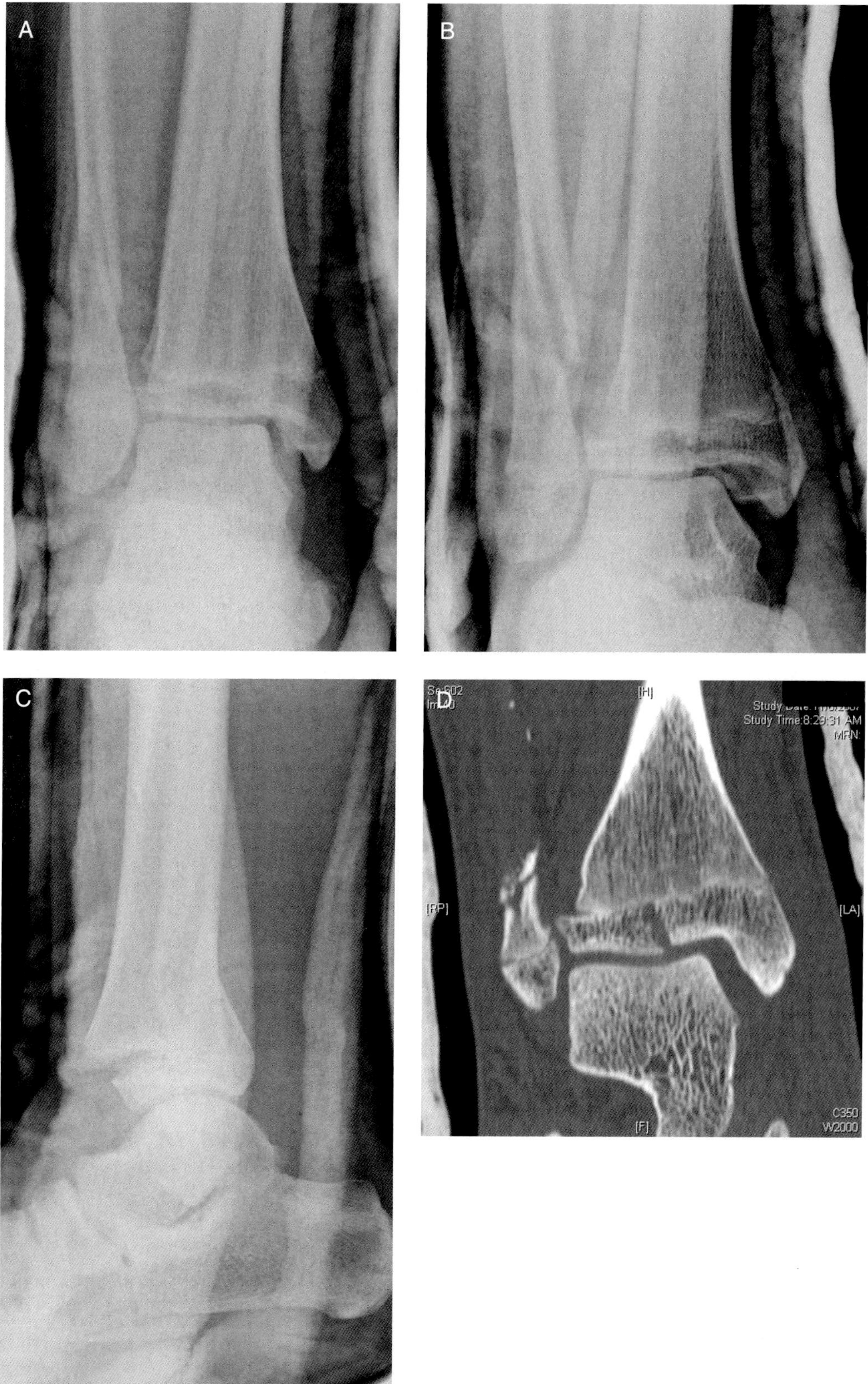

FIGURE 22-14 Two-part triplane fracture. Fourteen-year-old boy who was injured while playing tackle football. AP (**A**) and lateral (**B**) and mortise views (**C**) of the ankle are suggestive of a triplane ankle fracture but the plaster splint obscures the fracture. Coronal (**D**), axial (**E**), and sagittal CT views confirm a 2-part triplane ankle fracture. He underwent closed reduction and internal fixation. Post-operative radiographs (**F, G**) reveal anatomic realignment.

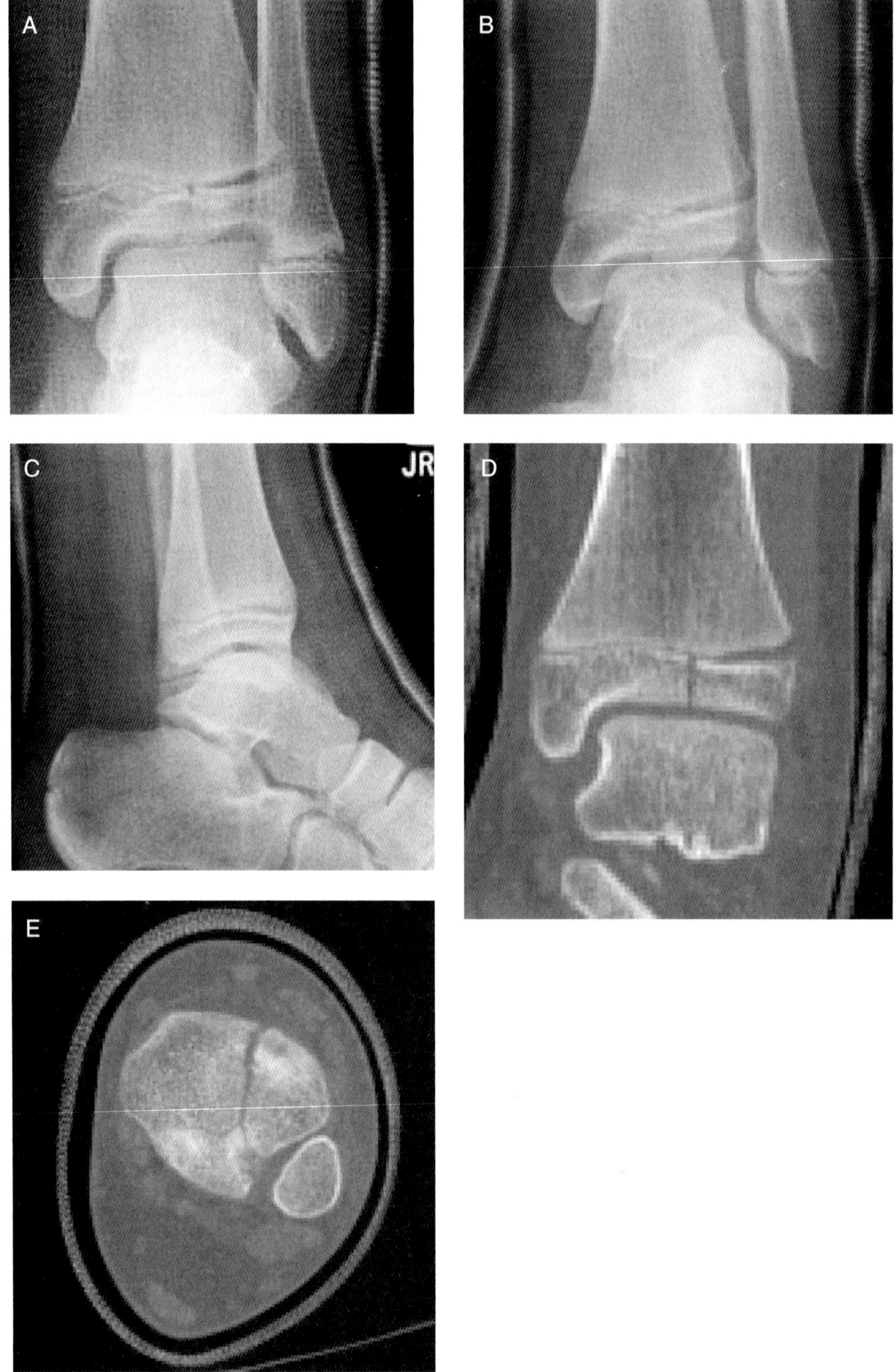

FIGURE 22-15 Three-part triplane fracture. Thirteen-year-old boy who tripped while playing basketball. Radiographs are suggestive of a triplane fracture ((**A**) AP, (**B**) mortise, (**C**) lateral views). ((**D**) CT coronal, (**E**) axial) reveals a minimally displaced three-part triplane fracture. He was treated with long-leg cast immobilization.

Operative Management

Operative reduction is indicated for irreducible fractures. The "joystick" method (34) is a technique of achieving reduction and fixation of juvenile Tillaux fractures percutaneously. Under fluoroscopic guidance, a smooth wire (0.062 mm or 5/64 in) or the guide wire from a cannulated screw system (4.0 or 4.5 mm) is placed into the Tillaux fragment percutaneously in the anterolateral ankle.

The fragment is then reduced by applying a posteromedial force directly to it. After reduction, the smooth wire or guide wire is advanced across the fracture site. The smooth wire may be left as definitive fixation. Improved fixation and fracture site compression, however, are accomplished by placing a cannulated screw over a guide wire. A single wire or screw provides stable fixation. Because most of these fractures occur in nearly skeletally mature children, screw placement across the physis is acceptable.

Open Reduction

Open reduction is performed through a small longitudinal anterolateral incision placed in line with the fracture site, usually approximately 1 cm medial to the medial border of the fibula, and traversing the joint line. After retracting and protecting the small branches of the superficial peroneal nerve and the tendons of the anterior compartment, a longitudinal capsular incision is made, exposing the fracture line and joint surface with limited periosteal stripping. Reduction is then accomplished under direct visualization and fixation is placed through the same incision.

Care After Reduction

The protocol outlined for care after reduction of SH 1 and 2 fractures is utilized for juvenile Tillaux fractures. Radiographic surveillance for growth disturbance is not

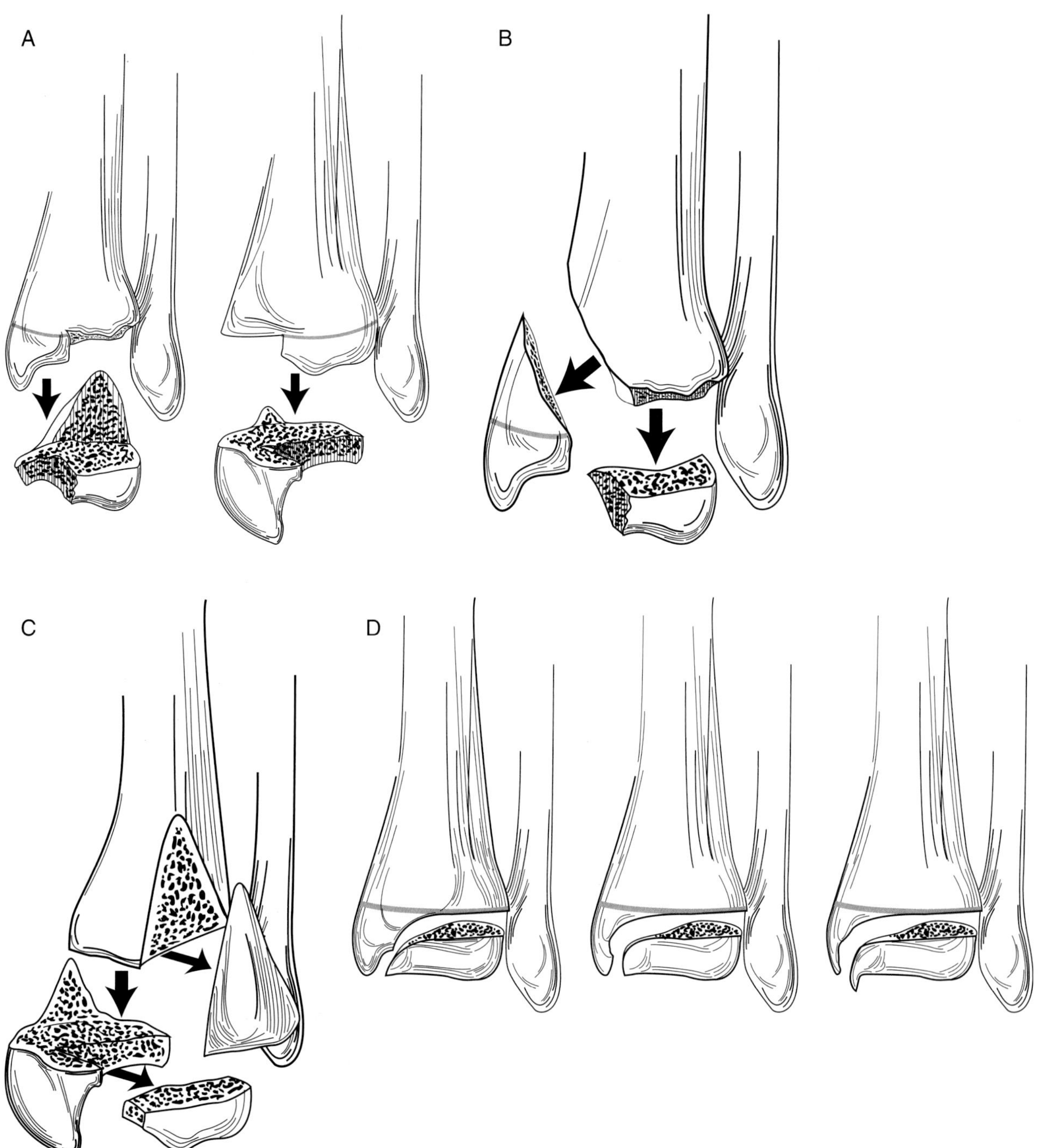

necessary because these injuries occur in children nearing skeletal maturity.

The Triplane Ankle Fracture

The triplane ankle fracture is more common than the juvenile Tillaux fracture and accounts for slightly less than 10% of pediatric ankle fractures. While most of these fractures are transitional, triplane fractures may occur in children with open physes. Torsional and angular forces applied to the foot result in transverse, sagittal, and coronal plane fracture lines through the distal tibia. The two-part variant is the most frequent type (2,5) (Figure 22-13). The epiphyseal fracture line occurs more commonly in the lateral half of the joint line (lateral triplane fracture) because the majority of triplane fractures result from predominantly abduction and external rotation forces, but may also occur in the medial half of the epiphysis (medial triplane fracture) from adduction. Three-part (Figure 22-14), four-part, intra-malleolar, and comminuted types (5,17,37,35) are other reported triplane fracture configurations (Figure 22-15). CT is required in most cases to define the fracture configuration. Application of an axial load to the distal tibia, in addition to rotational and other forces, may result in comminution of the fragments. While similar to triplane fractures, these fractures are best described as pediatric "pilon" fractures (21). Plain radiographs, in combination with CT imaging, are used for defining the specific injury patterns and the degree of comminution.

Nonoperative Management

Minimally displaced fractures are immobilized at the time of diagnosis in a long-leg cast. The majority of triplane fractures are have greater than 2 mm of displacement at presentation, however, and require reduction; many of these fractures can be adequately reduced by closed manipulation (5), especially two-part triplane fractures. The protocol for reduction is similar to that described for reduction of type SH 1 and 2 fractures of the distal tibia. The surgeon first applies gentle longitudinal traction to the hindfoot. Next, reduction of the distal fragment is performed by reversing the mechanism of injury based on the history and fragment displacement on the injury radiographs. For reduction of most lateral two- and three-part triplane fractures, the hindfoot is translated anteromedially and internally rotated while the tibia is pushed posterolaterally; medial triplane fractures, require application of forces in the opposite direction. After realignment, the ankle is dorsiflexed to 90 degrees. While the foot is held by an assistant, a long-leg cast is applied, usually done by first applying and carefully molding the short-leg portion of the cast followed by the above-knee portion. High-quality radiographs and CT are obtained after reduction to assess the reduction. At the joint line, step-off or gapping of 2 mm or less is acceptable. Five degrees or less of varus or valgus displacement and 10 degrees or less of anterior or posterior displacement are acceptable parameters for distal tibial alignment after reduction.

Operative Management

Prior to the scheduled surgery, a CT of the distal tibia is obtained to assist the surgeon in planning the surgical approach and fixation. Closed manipulation under anesthesia often yields an acceptable reduction. Although long-leg cast immobilization is adequate to maintain reduction in some cases, the authors prefer to stabilize

FIGURE 22-16 Triplane ankle fracture patterns. (**A**) Two-part triplane: This pattern consists of one fragment that includes part of the epiphysis attached to the posterior metaphyseal fragment and a second fragment that includes the remaining epiphysis attached to the remaining metaphysis and tibial shaft. In medial triplane fractures, the epiphyseal fracture line occurs in the medial half of the epiphysis, with the metaphyseal fracture line extending proximally in the sagittal plane; the lateral triplane has a more lateral epiphyseal fracture line and its metaphyseal fracture line extends proximally in the coronal plane. (Adapted from Schnetzler K, Hoernschemeyer D., *J Am Acad Orthop Surg* 2007; 15: 741, redrawn from Denton, JR, Fischer, SJ. The medial triplane fracture: Report of an unusual injury. *J Trauam* 1981;21:991.) (**B**) Three-part triplane: The classic pattern is comprised of the anterolateral epiphysis (part 1), the remaining epiphysis attached to a metaphyseal fragment (part 2), and the remaining metaphysis attached to the tibial shaft (part 3). (**C**) Four-part triplane: While variable, this pattern is typically comprised of the anterolateral epiphysis (part 1), a medial malleolus fragment (part 2), the remaining epiphysis attached to a metaphyseal fragment (part 3), and the remaining metaphysis attached to the tibial shaft (part 4). From Rockwood and Wilkins, *Fractures in children*, Beaty, JH, Kasser JR, eds. Philadelphia: Lippincott Williams & Wilkins, 2001.) (**D**) Intra-malleolar triplane. In type 1 fractures (a), the fracture line traverses the epiphysis at the junction of the plafond and medial malleolus. In type 2 injuries, the fracture is intramalleolar, entering the joint medial to the plafond. In type 3 fractures, the fracture line is intramalleolar and extra-articular. (Adapted from Schnetzler K, Hoernschemeyer D. *J Am Acad Orthop Surg* 2007;15:741.)

most triplane fractures with percutaneously placed fixation after reduction in the operating room. For the three-part fracture, the distal tibial metaphysis is fixed first with cannulated screws (see type SH 2 fixation), effectively converting the triplane fracture into a juvenile Tillaux fracture. The Tillaux fragment is then stabilized with an anterolateral cannulated screw. Alternatively, fractures which are partially reducible may be treated with a

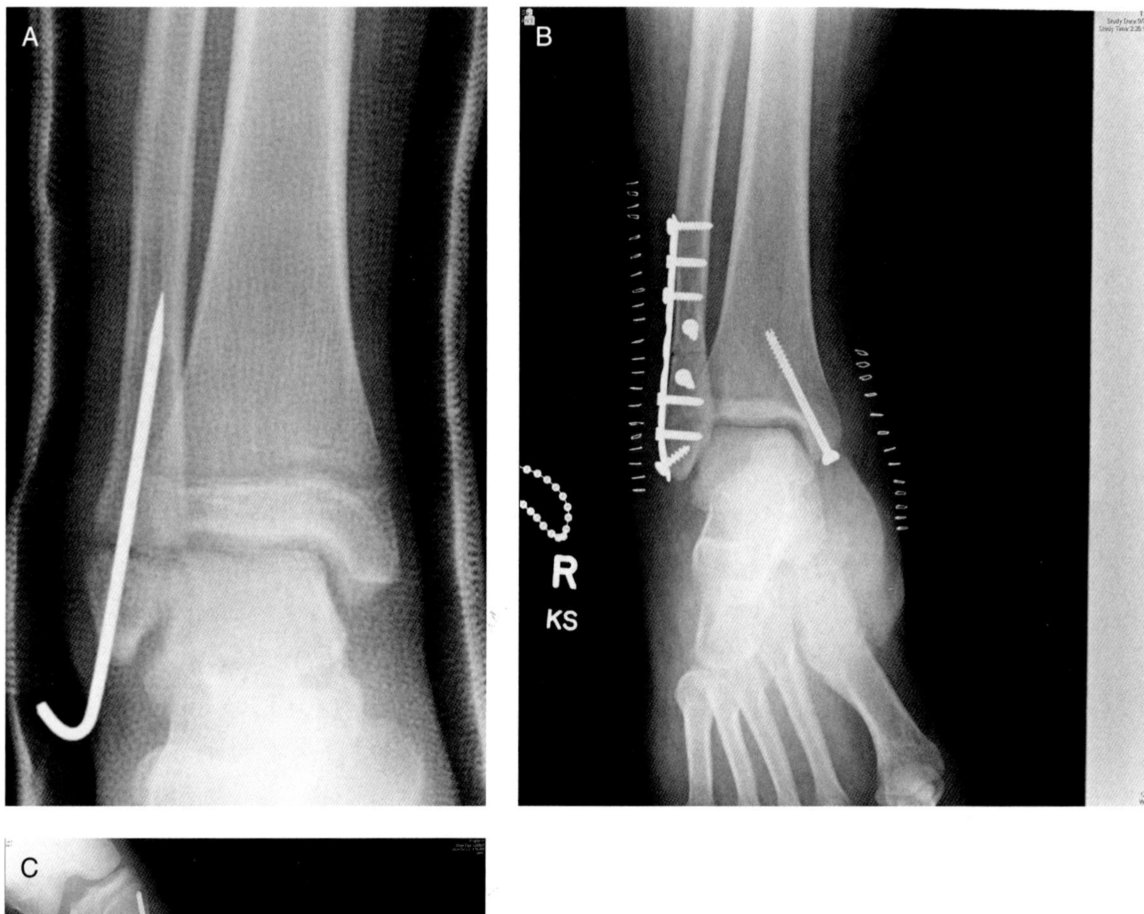

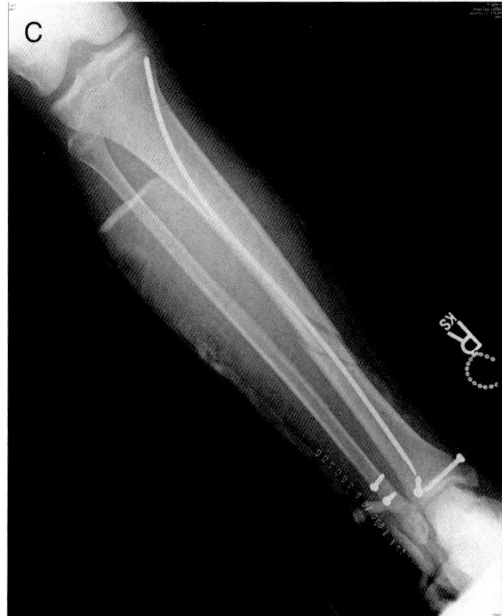

FIGURE 22-17 Fibular fixation. Displaced fractures of the distal fibula frequently occur in association with displaced fractures of the distal tibia. Fibular alignment is frequently restored when the distal tibia fracture is reduced and does not often require fixation. Fixation, when necessary to improve mortise stability or prevent severe fibular deformity, is accomplished by smooth wire(s) (**A**), sideplate-screw constructs (**B**), and lag screws (**C**). The boy in example c. had sustained a spiral tibia fracture and an ipsilateral two-part triplane fracture. Ipsilateral shaft fractures occur in as many as 10% of children with triplane ankle fractures.

TABLE 22-4

Risk of Premature Physeal Closure by Fracture Type

	Total # of cases	*SH 1/2 (%)*	*SH 3/4 (%)*	*Triplane (%)*	*Tillaux (%)*
Spiegel et al. (36)	237	14(11%)	4(7.7%)	4(26.6%)	1(16.7%)
De Sanctis et al. (9)	113	1(2.2%)	6(28.6%)	NA	NA
Barmada et al. (1)	92	17(36%)	3(38%)	4(21%)	0

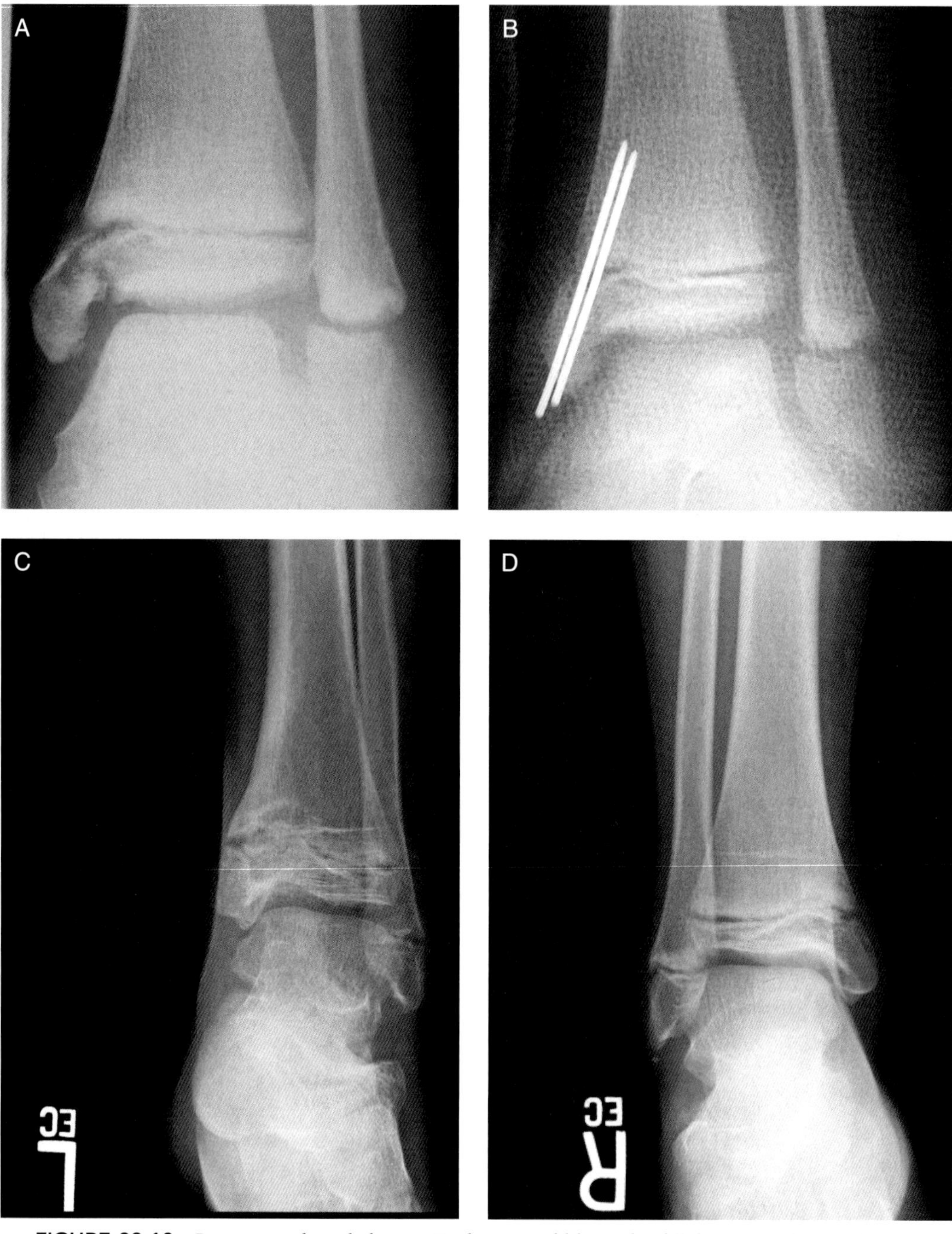

FIGURE 22-18 Premature physeal closure. Twelve-year-old boy who fell from a 10 foot-high wall. He sustained a Salter-Harris 3 tibia fracture with comminution and a Salter-Harris 1 fibula fracture (**A**). He underwent open reduction and smooth wire fixation of the medial malleolus (**B**). He presented 18 months later with a premature physeal closure. On the injured side, the growth line is parallel to the physis in the lateral half but turns obliquely toward the physis and terminates in the medial portion of it, indicative of a medial premature physeal closure. Note the distal tibial varus, joint line deformity and slight overgrowth of the fibula (**C**). The Harris growth lines are parallel to the physis on the opposite normal side (**D**).

limited open reduction and fixation of the joint line (22) combined with closed realignment and percutaneously placed fixation of the metaphysis.

Most four-part triplane fractures, irreducible fractures and those with severe comminution, including pediatric pilon fractures, are best treated with open reduction. Through a 3–5 cm longitudinal curvilinear or J-shaped anteromedial ankle incision, the joint line and medial malleolar fragments are exposed and reduced. Small osteoarticular and cartilage fragments are debrided. While often the metaphyseal fracture line is also reducible by anterior translation of posteriorly displaced fragment(s) through this anterior incision, a second posterolateral incision may be necessary to adequately expose the posterior metaphysis to achieve anatomic reduction. The fracture is then stabilized with cannulated screws or smooth wires. Transphyseal screw fixation may be utilized for most children when necessary similar to the juvenile Tillaux fracture,. For those triplane fractures that occur in children with open physes and more than two years of growth remaining, transphyseal screw fixation should be avoided.

Care After Reduction The protocol outlined for care after reduction of type SH 1 and 2 fractures is utilized for triplane fractures. Radiographic surveillance for growth disturbance is not necessary because these injuries occur in children close to skeletal maturity.

Fibular Fractures

Nonoperative Management Non-displaced or minimally displaced type SH 1 and 2 fractures of the distal fibula result from low-energy inversion ankle injuries and are the most common lower extremity fractures in children. While anterolateral ankle ligament sprains do occur in children, fractures occur more frequently because the ankle ligaments, which originate distal to the physis, are stronger than the physis. While clinically both injuries present with lateral ankle swelling, fibular tenderness 1–2 cm proximal to the tip of the lateral malleolus, as opposed to tenderness directly on the anterolateral ligaments, confirms the diagnosis of fracture, even if radiographs are normal. These injuries are treated with protected weight bearing in a short-leg cast or a removable cast-boot for four weeks.

Displaced fractures of the distal fibular metaphysis and physis are often associated with distal tibia fractures or, less commonly, deltoid ligament injuries (bimalleolar equivalent injuries). While performing reduction of the distal tibial fracture or ankle mortise in children, these fractures tend to reduce indirectly and rarely require fixation. Acceptable reduction parameters are 10 degrees or less of angulation and 1 cm or less of shortening.

Operative Management Indications for stabilization of distal fibular fractures include failure to achieve adequate alignment with closed manipulation, fracture instability (including length instability sometimes seen in comminuted metaphyseal fractures), and fractures in those approaching skeletal maturity. For children with more than two years of growth remaining, metaphyseal and physeal fibular fractures are best stabilized with smooth wires. With the hindfoot held in inversion, a small incision is made at the tip of the lateral malleolus. A smooth wire (0.062 mm or 5/64 inch) is then driven retrograde under fluoroscopic guidance longitudinally across the fracture site and it into the medullary canal of the fibula, stopping 3–4 cm proximal to the fracture site. Alternatively, the wire may be advanced obliquely from the tip of the lateral malleolus, crossing the fracture site and perforating the cortex of the fibula just proximal to the fracture site. One or two wires are adequate to achieve stability. Wires are generally cut outside the skin and removed after four weeks. Lag screw fixation of oblique fractures is also an option (Figure 22-16). For older children and those who are skeletally mature, open reduction and fixation with a one-third tubular plate secured with 3.5 mm screws, crossing the physis if necessary to achieve adequate stability, is the best method of fibular stabilization.

Care After Reduction

Metaphyseal and physeal fibular fractures heal within four to six weeks of injury. Post-operative management, however, is determined by the associated distal tibia fracture type.

Outcomes

Most children who sustain pediatric ankle fractures have satisfactory outcomes (1,9,18,27,36). Anatomic restoration of the joint line and preservation of physeal growth in those children who sustain fractures with more than two years of growth remaining are the most important factors in achieving these outcomes. Poor outcomes occur most frequently in children whose fractures are complicated by premature physeal closure (PCC) and premature osteoarthritis. Some fractures are at particularly high risk for developing these complications (Figure 22-17).

Complications

Malunion

Rotational and angular malunions may occur after ankle fractures in children. Excessive external rotation of the distal tibia is most common after treatment of type SH 1 and 2 fractures (31) and triplane fractures (5). Clinical asymmetry of tibial torsion between the injured and uninjured side after reduction, and a residual physeal gap of more than 2 mm measured on post-reduction radiographs, are suggestive of rotational malreduction (31). Malunions in the frontal and sagittal planes may occur and have a limited potential to remodel in younger children, the true extent of which is unpredictable. Rotational malunions do not remodel. Hemiepiphyseodesis of the distal tibia for small angular deformities in those children with at least two years of growth remaining and osteotomies of the distal tibia and fibula are treatment options.

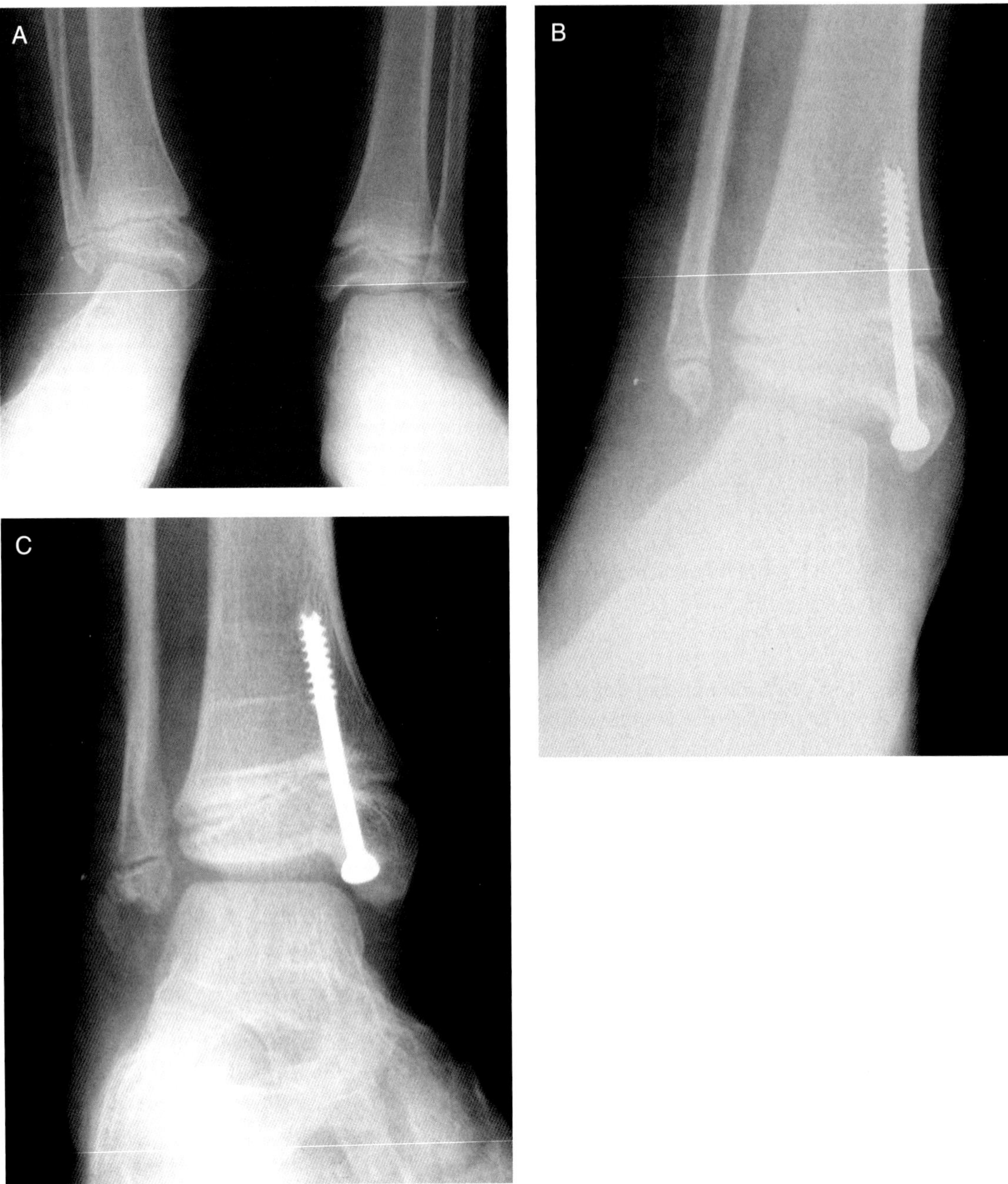

FIGURE 22-19 Valgus deformity secondary to fibula physeal abnormality. Nine-year-old boy who was struck by a truck. He sustained a severe degloving injury of the anterolateral ankle including a partial loss of the distal fibular epiphysis. Two years after injury he has undergrowth of the fibula and a valgus deformity of the distal tibia (**A**). He underwent a medial screw hemi-epiphyseodesis (**B**). Eighteen months later the deformity is improved (**C**) and the screw was removed. He had recurrent varus deformity with growth. A second screw hemiepiphyseodesis was successful in re-correcting the deformity. After the second correction, he had an epiphyseodesis of the entire of the distal tibia.

Premature Physeal Closure (PPC)

The overall rates of PPC reported after distal tibial physeal fractures vary from 7% to 56% of cases. While anatomic open reduction and fixation decreases the occurrence of PPC (19), surgical treatment does not guarantee that PPC will be prevented. SH 3 and 4 fractures are at highest risk for PPC, followed by type SH 1 and 2 fractures, triplane fractures, and juvenile Tillaux injuries (Table 22-4).

PPC may result in leg-length discrepancy (LLD), angular deformities of the ankle and a mismatch of growth between the fibula and tibia. Because the growth potential of the distal tibia is limited, only fractures that occur in younger children are at risk for developing a significant LLD. Distal tibial varus deformity is the most common angular deformity (19,27). This results from a partial growth disturbance secondary to physeal damage

TABLE 22-5

Ankle Fractures at Risk for Poor Outcomes

1. SH 1 and 2 fractures that result from pronation-abduction injuries, especially those with a residual physeal gap greater than 3 mm (20).
2. SH 3 and 4 fractures that result from adduction-supination injuries (29).
3. Fractures with more than 2 mm of residual displacement of the joint line or physis (25,32,36).
4. Fractures that result from high-energy mechanisms, especially axial loading (16,29).

or physeal malalignment, and occurs most frequently after type SH 3 and 4 fractures. Early identification by radiographic surveillance in children with at least two years of growth remaining allows the surgeon to intervene before significant angular and joint line deformity has occurred (Figure 22-18). Physeal bar resection, for those with less than 50% physeal bridging, or epiphyseodesis of the remaining distal tibia and the distal fibula, for those with larger bars, are the best treatment options. Osteotomies of the distal tibia and fibula are indicated for children with severe deformities.

A mismatch of growth of the distal tibia and fibula infrequently results in clinically significant deformity. Continued growth of the fibula after distal tibial arrest is often compensated for by proximal migration of the fibula (17). Epiphyseodesis of the distal fibula after PPC of the tibia is necessary only for those children with two to three years of growth remaining to prevent impingement of the fibula on the lateral calcaneus with hind foot eversion. Fibular growth arrest with normal distal tibial growth may result in valgus deformity in younger children (Figure 22-19). Hemiephyseodesis of the tibia or osteotomies of the tibia and fibula are treatment options.

Post-traumatic Arthritis

Cadaveric studies have shown that more than 2 mm of joint line displacement and 10 degrees of distal tibial malalignment increase ankle joint stresses (32,38), an etiology of premature osteoarthritis. As many as 12% of children who sustained ankle fractures (3) reported ankle pain and had radiographic evidence of osteoarthritis in adulthood. More than 50% of children who sustained triplane ankle fractures followed for more than three years reported symptoms (13). Anatomic restoration of the joint line and anatomic realignment of the distal tibia improves outcomes but does not guarantee a satisfactory result.

Other complications

Delayed union and nonunion are exceedingly rare (6). Inadequate immobilization, premature removal of fixation or inadequate fixation, and infection are potential etiologies. Osteonecrosis of the distal tibial epiphysis after fracture has been reported (10). Extensor retinaculum syndrome (25) may occur after distal tibial physeal fractures in children. This syndrome presents with excessive ankle pain and swelling, anesthesia of the first web space, isolated weakness of the extensor hallucis longus and extensor digitorum communis, and painful passive flexion of the toes. The result of excessive compression beneath the superior retinaculum of the ankle, prompt relief of pain and resolution of symptoms is seen in most cases after fracture stabilization and release of the retinaculum. Reflex sympathetic dystrophy, or complex regional pain syndrome, in children is more common in girls than boys and most frequently involves the lower extremity after minor trauma (40). The surgeon must consider this diagnosis in those children with disproportionately severe pain and findings of autonomic dysfunction after a minor ankle injury. Early recognition of this diagnosis and aggressive treatment improves outcomes.

REFERENCES

1. Barmada A, Gaynor T, Mubarak SJ. Premature physeal closure following distal tibia physeal fractures: A new radiographic predictor. *J Pediatr Orthop* 2003; 23(6): 733–739.
2. Brown SD, et al. Analysis of 51 tibial triplane fractures using CT with multiplanar reconstruction. *AJR Am J Roentgenol* 2004; 183(5): 1489–1495.
3. Caterini R, Farsetti P, Ippolito E. Long-term followup of physeal injury to the ankle. *Foot Ankle* 1991; 11(6): 372–383.
4. Charlton M, et al. Ankle joint biomechanics following transepiphyseal screw fixation of the distal tibia. *J Pediatr Orthop* 2005; 25(5): 635–640.
5. Cooperman DR, Spiegel PG, Laros GS. Tibial fractures involving the ankle in children. The so-called triplane epiphyseal fracture. *J Bone Joint Surg Am* 1978; 60(8): 1040–1046.
6. Cummings RJ. Distal tibial and fibular fractures. In Rockwood and Wilkins' *Fractures in children,* J.H. Beaty and J.R. Kasser, eds. Philadelphia: Lippincott Williams & Wilkins, 2005; 1121.
7. Cummings, RJ, Hahn, Jr. GA. The incisural fracture. *Foot Ankle Int* 2004; 25(3): 132–135.
8. Damore DT, et al. Patterns in childhood sports injury. *Pediatr Emerg Care* 2003; 19(2): 65–67.
9. De Sanctis N, Della Corte S, Pempinello C. Distal tibial and fibular epiphyseal fractures in children: Prognostic criteria and long-term results in 158 patients. *J Pediatr Orthop B* 2000; 9(1): 40–44.
10. Dias L. Fractures of the tibia and fibula. In *Fractures in children.* W.K. Rockwood CA, Kling RE, ed. Philadelphia: JB Lippincott, 1991; 1271–1381.
11. Dias LS, Giegerich CR. Fractures of the distal tibial epiphysis in adolescence. *J Bone Joint Surg Am* 1983; 65(4): 438–444.
12. Dias LS, Tachdjian MO. Physeal injuries of the ankle in children: classification. *Clin Orthop Relat Res* 1978(136): 230–233.
13. Ertl JP, et al. Triplane fracture of the distal tibial epiphysis. Long-term follow-up. *J Bone Joint Surg Am* 1988; 70(7): 967–976.
14. Goldberg VM, Aadalen R. Distal tibial epiphyseal injuries: The role of athletics in 53 cases. *Am J Sports Med* 1978; 6(5): 263–268.
15. Horn BD, et al. Radiologic evaluation of juvenile tillaux fractures of the distal tibia. *J Pediatr Orthop* 2001; 21(2): 162–164.
16. Hynes D, O'Brien T. Growth disturbance lines after injury of the distal tibial physis. Their significance in prognosis. *J Bone Joint Surg Br* 1988; 70(2): 231–233.

17. Karrholm J. The triplane fracture: four years of follow-up of 21 cases and review of the literature. *J Pediatr Orthop Br* 1997; 6(2): 91–102.
18. King J, et al. Analysis of 429 fractures in 189 battered children. *J Pediatr Orthop* 1988; 8(5): 585–589.
19. Kling TF Jr, Bright RW, Hensinger RN. Distal tibial physeal fractures in children that may require open reduction. *J Bone Joint Surg Am* 1984; 66(5): 647–657.
20. Lauge-Hansen N. Fractures of the ankle. II. Combined experimental-surgical and experimental-roentgenologic investigations. *Arch Surg* 1950; 60(5): 957–985.
21. Letts M, Davidson D, McCaffrey M. The adolescent pilon fracture: Management and outcome. *J Pediatr Orthop* 2001; 21(1): 20–26.
22. Lintecum N, Blasier RD. Direct reduction with indirect fixation of distal tibial physeal fractures: A report of a technique. *J Pediatr Orthop* 1996; 16(1): 107–112.
23. Lynn MD. The triplane distal tibial epiphyseal fracture. *Clin Orthop Relat Res* 1972; 86: 187–190.
24. Mizuta T, et al. Statistical analysis of the incidence of physeal injuries. *J Pediatr Orthop* 1987; 7(5): 518–523.
25. Mubarak SJ. Extensor retinaculum syndrome of the ankle after injury to the distal tibial physis. *J Bone Joint Surg Br* 2002; 84(1): 11–14.
26. Muller M, Allgower M, Schneider R, Willenegger H. ed. Manual of internal fixation: Techniques recommended by the AO-group, 2nd ed. New York: Springer-Verlag, 1979.
27. Nenopoulos SP, Papavasiliou VA, Papavasiliou AV. Outcome of physeal and epiphyseal injuries of the distal tibia with intra-articular involvement. *J Pediatr Orthop* 2005; 25(4): 518–522.
28. Ogden JA, Lee J. Accessory ossification patterns and injuries of the malleoli. *J Pediatr Orthop* 1990; 10(3): 306–316.
29. Peterson CA, Peterson HA. Analysis of the incidence of injuries to the epiphyseal growth plate. *J Trauma* 1972; 12(4): 275–281.
30. Peterson HA, et al. Physeal fractures: Part 1. Epidemiology in Olmsted County, Minnesota, 1979–1988. *J Pediatr Orthop* 1994; 14(4): 423–430.
31. Phan VC, Wroten E, Yngve DA. Foot progression angle after distal tibial physeal fractures. *J Pediatr Orthop* 2002; 22(1): 31–35.
32. Ramsey PL, Hamilton W. Changes in tibiotalar area of contact caused by lateral talar shift. *J Bone Joint Surg Am* 1976; 58(3): 356–357.
33. Salter RB. Injuries of the ankle in children. *Orthop Clin North Am* 1974; 5(1): 147–152.
34. Schlesinger I, Wedge JH. Percutaneous reduction and fixation of displaced juvenile Tillaux fractures: a new surgical technique. *J Pediatr Orthop* 1993; 13(3): 389–391.
35. Shin AY, Moran ME, Wenger DR. Intramalleolar triplane fractures of the distal tibial epiphysis. *J Pediatr Orthop* 1997; 17(3): 352–355.
36. Spiegel PG, Cooperman DR, Laros GS. Epiphyseal fractures of the distal ends of the tibia and fibula. A retrospective study of two hundred and thirty-seven cases in children. *J Bone Joint Surg Am* 1978; 60(8): 1046–1050.
37. Spiegel PG, et al. Triplane fractures of the distal tibial epiphysis. *Clin Orthop Relat Res* 1984(188): 74–89.
38. Tarr RR, et al. Changes in tibiotalar joint contact areas following experimentally induced tibial angular deformities. *Clin Orthop Relat Res* 1985(199): 72–80.
39. Vahvanen V, Aalto K. Classification of ankle fractures in children. *Arch Orthop Trauma Surg* 1980; 97(1): 1–5.
40. Wilder RT, et al. Reflex sympathetic dystrophy in children. Clinical characteristics and follow-up of seventy patients. *J Bone Joint Surg Am* 1992; 74(6): 910–919.

CHAPTER 23

Fractures of the Foot in Children and Adolescents

James McCarthy, Theodore J. Ganley, Martin Herman and Hua Ming Siow

INTRODUCTION

Fractures and dislocations about the foot in children are common, accounting for up to 10% of all pediatric fractures (19). Fractures of the metatarsals and phalanges occur most frequently. Most foot injuries in children and adolescents are treated non-surgically and heal without complications. High-energy injuries, including lawnmower injuries, may result in significant damage that requires aggressive operative treatment. Foot injuries sometimes occur in the poly-traumatized child and may be missed because of other distracting injuries or an inability to detect these by exam because of the patient's altered level of consciousness (18,22). Osteochondroses are common in children. While these are discussed in chapter 28, it is important to recognize these disorders, such as Köhler's disorder, and to be able to differentiate them from acute fractures.

Soft-tissue injuries of the foot are difficult to identify and may be more devastating than bony injuries. Direct injuries to the foot are common and sometimes result in massive circumferential swelling of the entire foot that is more dramatic than would be expected from the isolated radiographic findings alone. Lisfranc injuries and compartment syndromes of the foot are uncommon but serious injuries in children that require careful assessment and a high index of suspicion to diagnosis. Recognition and aggressive treatment of these injuries improves outcomes.

Thorough knowledge of the osseous, physeal, and ligamentous anatomy, and its relationship to clinical findings, are critical to making the correct diagnosis of traumatic injuries. A detailed discussion of the anatomy of the foot and ankle is discussed in the first chapter. In particular, accessory ossicles may masquerade as fractures, especially the os vesalianum or os peroneum at the base of the fifth metatarsal, the os fibulare, and the os tibiale. Fracture-specific anatomy will be discussed under the particular injury.

DIAGNOSTICS

Physical Exam

The physical exam is the cornerstone of the diagnostic evaluation for foot injuries and is anatomically based. Assessment of the skin for swelling, ecchymosis, and abrasions or skin loss is the first part of the evaluation. Palpation of bony and ligamentous structures is key to diagnosis for most injuries. The "Ottawa ankle rules" are useful to guide the physical examination when assessing for possible fractures of the ankle or mid-foot. The rules, conceived to aid physicians in deciding which patients need radiographs after an ankle injury, combines the ability to walk four steps (immediately after the injury or in the emergency department) with physical findings of localized tenderness at the posterior edge or tip of either malleolus, the navicular, or the base of the fifth metatarsal, to achieve a score that is correlated with the presence of a fracture. A modified version of these rules has been utilized for assessing children but is not as widely used compared to the adult criteria and may not be useful for children younger than five years of age (31). The Ottawa ankle rules have been shown to be an accurate instrument for excluding fractures of the ankle and mid-foot with a sensitivity of approaching 100% (2). Because other skeletal injures occur in as many as 15% to 20% of patients with foot injuries, the examiner must evaluate the entire lower extremity and other anatomic sites when applicable based on the mechanism of injury to complete the evaluation of the child with a foot injury (11).

While neurovascular injury is uncommon in most fractures, a careful exam, assessing and documenting motor function, sensation, and vascular perfusion, is critical for the severely swollen or traumatized foot. The use of a Doppler to confirm distal pulses may be needed, especially in a small, swollen foot. Compartment pressures may need to be monitored carefully, with frequent reassessment of the injured limb to detect changes consistent with the diagnosis before permanent injury of the soft tissues from increased tissue pressure and decreased perfusion has occurred. Compartment syndrome monitoring must continue for 24–48 hours after a significant traumatic injury. An increase in the need for pain medication to maintain the child's comfort is the most consistent sign of a developing compartment syndrome in children.

A compartment syndrome in the foot can be difficult to diagnosis because changes in sensation and motor function may occur late, and toe movement from the long flexors and extensors may mask intrinsic motor function deficits. The existence of nine foot compartments and frequent presence of complicating injuries necessitate needle catheterization of multiple sites for direct measurement of compartment pressures. Fasciotomy is indicated when compartment pressure exceeds 30 mm Hg, or if compartment pressure is greater than 10–30 mm Hg below diastolic pressure. The surgical approaches (Figure 23-1) for compartment decompression generally include two dorsal incisions for access to forefoot compartments, and one medial incision for decompression of the calcaneal, medial, superficial, and lateral compartments (10). A missed compartment syndrome results in foot stiffness, pain, and an intrinsic minus foot deformity with claw toes.

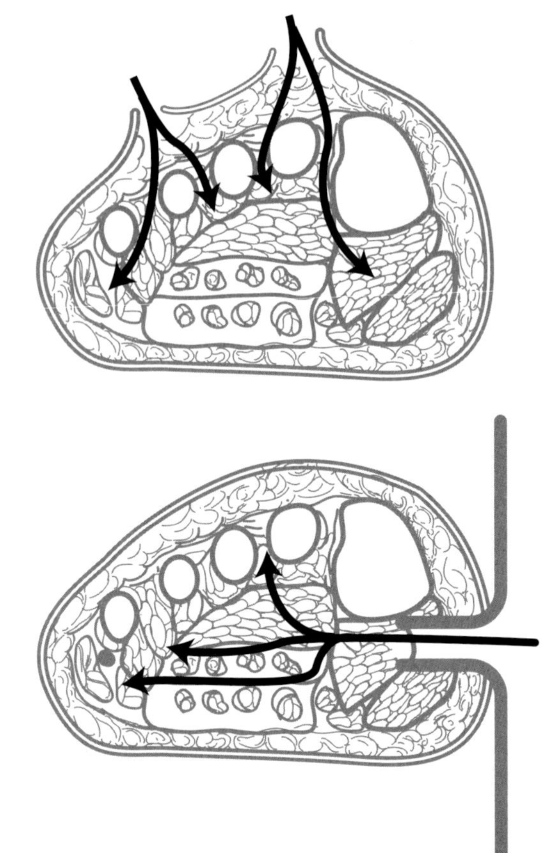

FIGURE 23-1 Surgical technique for release of foot compartments. (Adapted from Silas SI, Herzenberg JE, Myerson MS, Sponseller PD. Compartment syndrome of the foot in children. *J Bone Joint Surg Am.* 1995 Mar;77(3): 356–361.)

Imaging

Initial radiographic examination includes anteroposterior (AP), lateral, and oblique images of the foot. Anteroposterior and lateral radiographs taken with the child weight bearing are useful to diagnose some injuries, such as a Lisfranc fracture-dislocation, which may be missed with non–weight-bearing films. Computed tomography (CT) is best for assessing bone injuries, especially those with intra-articular extension. Magnetic resonance imaging (MRI) is useful for assessment of ligamentous and osteochondral injuries in particular. A bone scan may be indicated to identify occult foot fractures in the child.

TALUS FRACTURES

Fractures of the talus are rare, accounting for about 2% of pediatric foot fractures. These injuries most commonly involve the neck, although the body, medial, lateral, or posterior processes can also be injured. Because young children have a higher cartilage-to-bone ratio than adults, they may better resist bending and be at lower risk for talar fractures (21) compared to adults. Anatomically, the talus is comprised of the head, constricted neck, and body. Most of the blood supply enters through the neck. The artery of the tarsal canal has contributions from the posterior tibial and dorsalis pedis arteries. The artery of the tarsal sinus is formed from branches of the dorsalis pedis and peroneal arteries. In the interosseous canal, an anastomosis is formed between the arteries of the tarsal canal and tarsal sinus. The blood supply to the talus is at risk after displaced fractures of the talar neck, potentially resulting in avascular necrosis.

The majority of talar neck fractures occur from forced dorsiflexion, with the neck impinging against the anterior lip of the fibula. In some cases, there may be an element of supination (12). The child with a talus fracture presents unable to walk, with pain, swelling, and tenderness anterior to the ankle joint. Non-displaced fractures are less symptomatic and may be missed if the diagnosis is not kept in mind (Figure 23-2).

Standard radiographic views are useful for identifying most fractures. For those patients in whom the diagnosis is suspected but the standard views are negative, the "Canale" view, obtained with foot in 15° of pronation and the x-ray tube angulated 75° to the table, may help improve visualization of the fracture. A CT scan is best to assess displacement and articular surface involvement. An MRI and bone scan are useful to assess vascularity at follow-up visits.

Hawkins (12) devised a classification of talar neck fractures in adults, which correlates with the risk of avascular necrosis. Type I fractures are non-displaced fractures of the neck and have a minimal risk of avascular necrosis in adults. In one study by Rammelt (26), the incidence of avascular necrosis in children with non-displaced talar fractures was 16%, higher than the incidence in adults. Eight of eleven cases of avascular necrosis occurred in

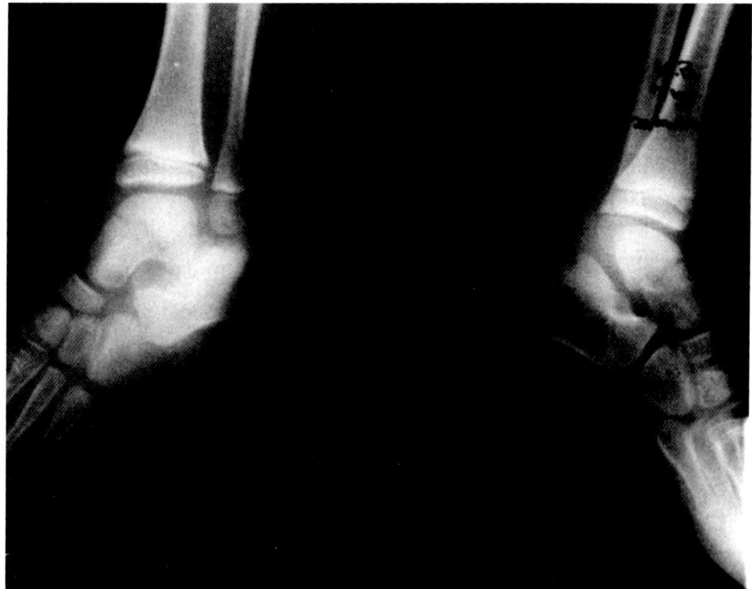

FIGURE 23-2 Seven-year-old boy who fell from a tree. Oblique and lateral x-rays illustrate a non-displaced talar neck fracture. The fracture was satisfactorily aligned and cast immobilization for eight weeks permitted radiographic evidence of healing. Avascular necrosis did not occur. (Courtesy of Dennis Roy, M.D., Cincinnati, Ohio.)

children under five years of age. Half of these fractures were missed initially, which underlines the importance of detecting these injuries. Hawkins type II fractures are displaced fractures of the neck with subluxation or dislocation of the subtalar joint. The risk of avascular necrosis is 41% for patients with this injury. Type III injuries are fractures, combined with subluxation or dislocation of the ankle as well as the subtalar joint, and are associated with a risk of avascular necrosis of 91%. Canale (4) added a type IV talar neck fracture that is associated with subluxation or dislocation of the ankle, subtalar, and talonavicular joints. Patients with this injury have greater than a 90% risk of developing avascular necrosis.

Non-displaced fractures are treated with a non–weight-bearing long-leg cast for six to eight weeks. The talus has good remodeling potential and less than 5° of malalignment on AP radiographs and less than 5 mm of displacement are acceptable. Displaced fractures require closed or open reduction and internal fixation. Fixation may be achieved with wires or screws placed posterior to anterior from the posterior body of the talus toward the distal talar head or from the distal talar head on the non-articular surface across the fracture site and into the body (16).

Avascular necrosis is a serious complication and usually appears between one to six months after injury. The appearance of the Hawkin's sign, a subchondral lucency in the dome of the talus seen on radiographs at follow-up, signifies viability of the talar body. This sign sometimes does not appear in children with non-displaced fractures who are immobilized for a short period; its absence does not always correlate with avascular necrosis in children. Children with an absent Hawkin's sign, however, or established avascular necrosis require close follow-up with serial x-rays, bone scans, or MRI. Non-weight bearing is recommended until revascularization can be identified on follow-up imaging. Because revascularization may take a prolonged time, and the talus has the ability to remodel, Hawkins suggested allowing weight bearing after union has occurred regardless of the presence or absence of the Hawkin's sign.

Other fractures of the talus involving the body and medial, lateral, and posterior processes are rare. Lateral process fractures are associated with skateboarding or snowboarding injuries. Peritalar dislocations are extremely uncommon in children, and are usually the result of high-energy trauma. The surgeon must be careful to assess for associated neurovascular injuries and fractures of the foot. Closed reduction is generally possible if the dislocation is treated in a timely fashion (8). Otherwise, open reduction is necessary, taking care to avoid injury of interposed tendons or neurovascular structures.

CALCANEAL FRACTURES

Calcaneal fractures, like fractures of the talus, are uncommon injuries in children. They usually occur as a result of falls from height or as open injuries from lawnmower accidents. The majority of calcaneal fractures in children are extra-articular, with only 35% associated with intra-articular extension, usually into the subtalar joint (Figure 23-3). Intra-articular fractures are classified into two groups like adult calcaneal fractures, according to Essex-Lopresti (9). Typically with impact after a fall, for example, the inferiorly protruding lateral process of the talus impinges on the superiorly displaced calcaneus. This results in a primary fracture line that extends obliquely from plantar-medial to dorso-lateral and exits into the posterior facet of the subtalar joint and two fracture fragments, an anteromedial sustentacular fragment and a posterolateral tuberosity fragment. Secondary fracture lines then determine which of the two Essex-Lopresti groups the fracture falls into. In the

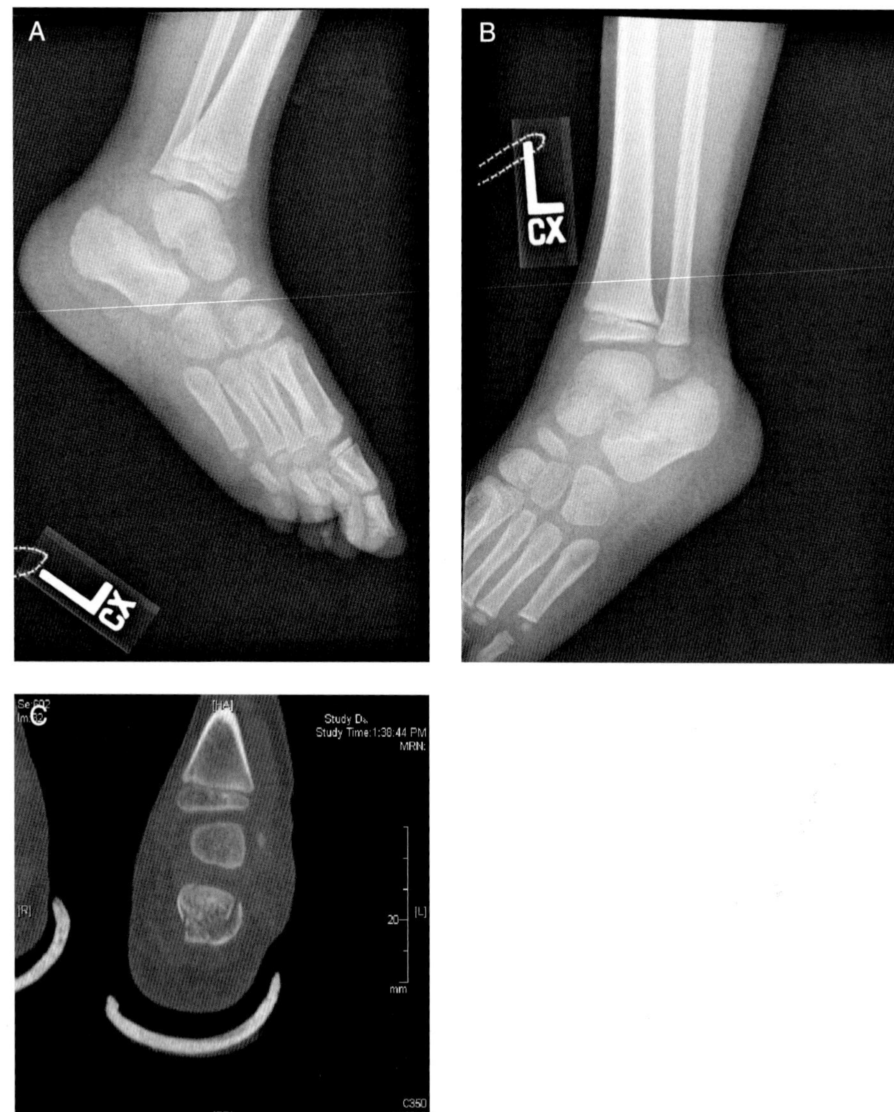

FIGURE 23-3 Six-year-old girl who jumped off a porch, landing on her left foot. Lateral (**A**) and oblique (**B**) x-rays of the foot reveal a calcaneus fracture. Axial CT (**C**) confirms subtalar joint depression without intra-articular step-off. She was treated non-surgically.

tongue-type fracture, the secondary fracture line extends posteriorly through the body, and includes a portion of the posterior facet and dorsal cortex of the tuberosity. In the joint depression fracture, the secondary fracture line deviates dorsally and exits just posterior to the posterior facet. Extra-articular fractures are more common compared to intra-articular fractures and are frequently the result of lower energy mechanisms.

Patients with calcaneus fractures present with a history of a fall from a height or a direct blow to the heel. Typically, the child experiences heel pain on impact associated with an inability to walk, localized swelling, and tenderness. Anteroposterior, lateral, and oblique views of the foot and an axial radiograph of the heel are standard views used to diagnose these fractures. CT is essential for assessing comminuted intra-articular fractures or other complex fracture patterns. Based on the mechanism of injury and physical findings, radiographic assessment of the spine or extremities may also be indicated (29).

Most calcaneal fractures in children are treated non-surgically. Non–weight-bearing immobilization for six weeks is adequate for the majority of fractures and yields good results (3,28). In general, extra-articular fractures have better outcomes compared to intra-articular fractures (15), but even intra-articular fractures with some displacement can remodel with good congruency between the talar and calcaneal surfaces.

Severely displaced fractures in younger children or displaced fractures in children approaching skeletal maturity may warrant open reduction and internal fixation (23,24). One recent study showed good results for displaced fractures treated with open reduction and lateral buttress plating. The average subjective Association of Foot and

Ankle Surgery (AOFAS) hindfoot score for all patients was 64 out of a possible 68 points. One patient who had fixation with a single 3.5-mm cortical screw had the lowest AOFAS hindfoot score, presumably because of loss of articular reduction from inadequate fixation (23).

CUBOID FRACTURES

Cuboid fractures in children and adolescents are also uncommon and may be associated with more severe injuries of the mid-foot such as a Lisfranc injury. Hermel (13) described a nutcracker mechanism of indirect injury whereby the cuboid is compressed between the bases of the third and fourth metatarsals and the anterior process of the calcaneus by forced abduction of a fixed plantar flexed foot. Most cuboid fractures, however, are the result of low-energy injuries and are treated with cast immobilization or symptomatically with good outcomes. Senaran (30) reported a series of 28 preschool children who presented with unwillingness to weight bear on the lateral aspect of the foot who were diagnosed with cuboid fractures. Eight children had no history of injury and the rest sustained minor trauma. Twenty-one children were treated with immobilization for four weeks, and were asymptomatic in an additional four weeks. The remainder was observed without immobilization and was asymptomatic at 7.9 weeks. Ceroni (5) reported four cases in children that resulted from an injury while horseback riding and recommended surgical treatment for displaced injuries to prevent long-term alterations in foot biomechanics and function.

TARSOMETATARSAL (LISFRANC) INJURIES

Lisfranc injuries in children are uncommon. In younger children, fractures of the metatarsals are more common than ligamentous injuries of the Lisfranc joint. This is because the metatarsal bases are attached to each other and to the tarsals with strong ligaments, except for the first and second metatarsals. The second metatarsal base, however, is recessed more proximally, like a keystone in a Roman arch, in relation to the other tarsometatarsal joints and is attached by tough ligaments to all the cuneiforms. This complex is crucial to the strength of the tarsometatarsal joint. When force is applied, failure of the metaphyses at the base of the metatarsals occurs more commonly than injury of the ligaments in immature bone.

Lisfranc injuries can occur directly or indirectly, with the latter mechanism being more common. Direct injuries occur when a falling object hits the foot and disrupts the plantar ligaments, displacing the metatarsals plantarward. Severe soft-tissue swelling is the hallmark of these injuries. Indirect Lisfranc sprains and dislocations occur from violent plantar flexion, abduction, or a combination of these mechanisms. In plantar flexion injuries, the foot is axially loaded with the ankle plantar flexed, resulting in rupture of the dorsal ligaments of the tarsometatarsal joints and occasionally metatarsal shaft or neck fractures. Common scenarios include landing on tiptoes or attempting to brace for a fall from a bicycle. In abduction injuries, the metatarsals are impacted medially, fracturing the base of the second and causing a nutcracker fracture of the cuboid.

The patient with a Lisfranc injury presents with inability to weight bear, pain, severe swelling, and tenderness on the dorsum of the foot overlying the tarsometatarsal joints. Spontaneous reduction often occurs, necessitating a high level of clinical suspicion to avoid missing the diagnosis. Weight-bearing AP and lateral views of the foot are essential if non–weight-bearing studies are normal. Computed tomography, often done with comparison views of the uninjured foot, is useful to detect subtle displacement and associated fractures but is non-weight bearing. Stressing of the mid-foot in the operating room under fluoroscopy is also helpful to diagnose Lisfranc instability if imaging is equivocal and the diagnosis is suspected, based on mechanism and clinical findings.

Immediate treatment includes elevation of the foot and evaluation for compartment syndrome. When swelling has diminished, usually within several days, patients with minimally displaced tarsometatarsal dislocations can be treated in a non–weight-bearing short-leg cast for four to six weeks. Lisfranc ligamentous injuries with greater than 2 mm of displacement can usually be reduced by closed reduction in the operating room, aided by manually applied longitudinal traction or by Chinese finger traps placed on the toes. Percutaneous wires or cannulated screws are then used to stabilize the second metatarsal base, as well as the first and fifth metatarsal bases as dictated by the pattern of injury. Open reduction, when necessary, is accomplished through dorsal incisions. Wiley (34) reported good short-term operative results with 13 out of 18 patients treated with reduction and fixation; only one patient required further treatment.

METATARSAL FRACTURES

Metatarsal fractures are the most common injuries of the pediatric foot. They may occur through direct trauma, resulting in shaft fractures and soft-tissue injury, or indirectly from torsional forces that result most commonly in neck fractures. Fractures at the base of the metatarsals require a proper assessment to exclude associated tarsometatarsal joint injuries. The patient with a metatarsal fracture typically presents limping with localized pain, swelling, and tenderness over the fracture site. Radiographs confirm the diagnosis. While most metatarsal fractures result from low-energy mechanisms, the surgeon must also be aware of the possibility of compartment syndrome when multiple metatarsal fractures are diagnosed or severe soft-tissue swelling is present.

Most metatarsal fractures are minimally displaced and may be treated with cast immobilization for three to six

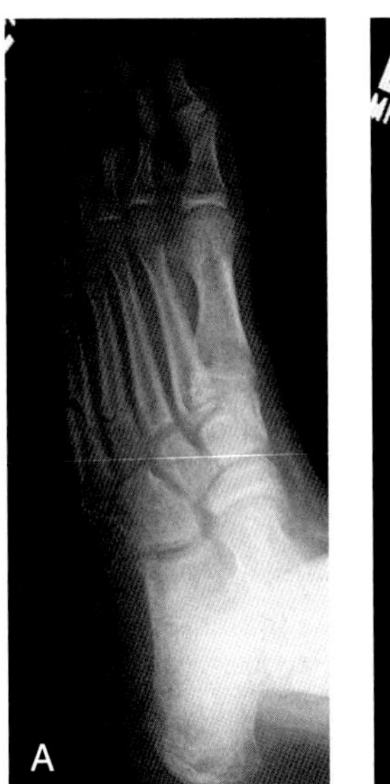

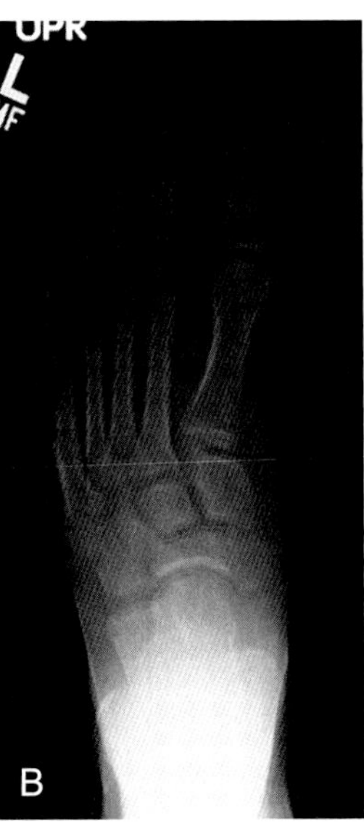

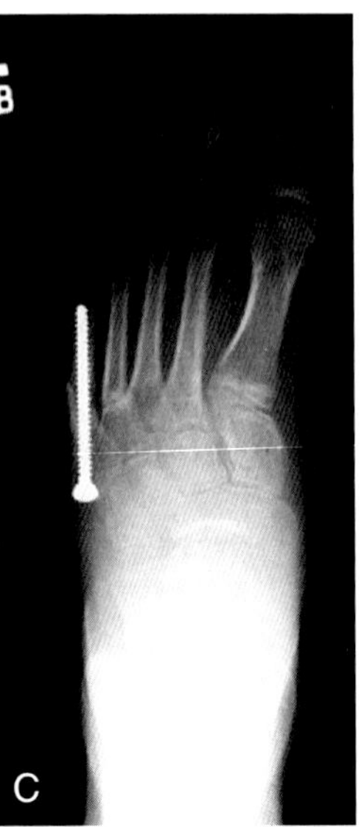

FIGURE 23-4 Fourteen-year-old soccer player presents six weeks after casting for fractures of the fourth and fifth metatarsals. He was tender to palpation over the fifth metatarsal and x-rays showed minimal healing (**A**). He underwent open reduction and screw fixation (**B**).

weeks; weight bearing is permitted based on the patient's level of comfort. Diaphyseal fractures with severe displacement are treated by closed reduction and fixation, usually with a retrograde intramedullary smooth wire placed through the metatarsal head or anterograde from the proximal metaphysis. In the fifth metatarsal diaphysis, an anterograde screw may be utilized for older children (Figure 23-4). Giannestras (11) described the use of Chinese finger traps to aid reduction. Open reduction is rarely required but is best done through a dorsal incision over the fracture site. Displaced intra-articular fractures generally require open reduction and fixation (Figure 23-5). If a concomitant compartment syndrome is suspected, fasciotomies should be performed at the time of reduction and fixation.

Fifth Metatarsal

The fifth metatarsal is the most commonly fractured metatarsal in children, except in those under age five who are more likely to fracture the first metatarsal. Sports activities, such as football or basketball, account for 45% of metatarsal fractures (6). Diaphyseal and neck fractures of the fifth metatarsal heal well and are treated in a similar fashion to the other metatarsals. Fractures in the proximal fifth metatarsal, however, tend to be more complicated in their management. One study examined 103 fractures of the fifth metatarsal in children (14). While most fractures were successfully treated with walking cast immobilization for several weeks, displaced intra-articular fractures and some diaphyseal fractures required more aggressive treatment.

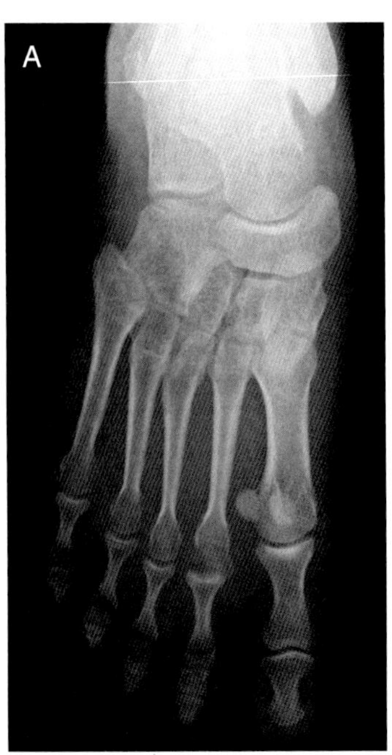

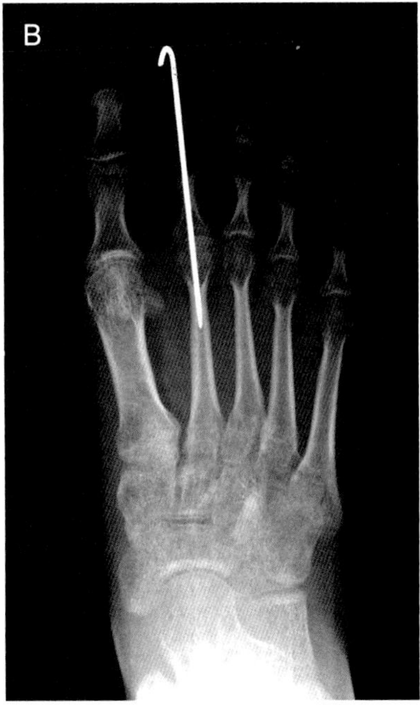

FIGURE 23-5 Thirteen-year-old girl who was stepped on while playing lacrosse. She sustained a displaced intra-articular fracture of the metatarsal head (**A**). She underwent open reduction and fixation (**B**).

Avulsion Fractures

Avulsion fractures of the base of the fifth metatarsal result from an inversion or adduction force (Figure 23-6). The pull of the peroneus brevis is believed to be responsible for this injury but Richli (27) suggested that the tendinous portion of abductor digiti minimi and the tough lateral cord of the plantar aponeurosis may be culpable. The fracture line is typically perpendicular to the long axis of the shaft in the proximal metaphysis and is minimally displaced. Occasionally, there is confusion between this fracture and the incidental finding of an accessory ossicle of the fifth metatarsal such as the os peroneum or os vesalianum (7). An incidental finding of the apophysis typically is not tender to palpation and on radiographs appears parallel to the shaft, not perpendicular as seen with the avulsion fracture. Treatment of avulsion fractures is with a weight-bearing short-leg cast for four to six weeks. Most heal uneventfully.

Intra-articular fractures of the base of the fifth metatarsal also occur (14,20). These avulsion fractures are mostly metaphyseal but extend into the proximal articular surface of the fifth metatarsal. Unlike the typical avulsion fracture, these are best treated with a non–weight-bearing short-leg casts for four to eight weeks based on healing. Widely displaced fractures and those that do not heal after cast immobilization alone require open reduction and fixation with a wire or screw (Figure 23-7).

Jones Fractures

A fracture of the fifth metatarsal at the junction of the proximal metaphysis and diaphysis or just distal to this area is called a Jones fracture. This injury is the result of a vertical or lateral-to-medial force applied to the metatarsophalangeal joint with the ankle in plantar flexion. Healing of this fracture is inconsistent because disruption of the nutrient artery to this anatomic area sometimes occurs, resulting in devascularization and subsequent poor bone healing.

Non-displaced Jones fractures are treated with non-weight bearing in a short-leg cast for six to eight weeks (Figure 23-8). Some studies, however, have shown delayed union rates of 25% to 66%, and nonunion rates of 7% to 28% (17,25,27,32). Refracture is another concern when treating these injuries. Herrera-Soto (14) reported refractures in 3 of 13 children treated with casting while Quill (25) showed that up to one-third of patients sustained a refracture on commencement of sporting activities.

Surgical treatment is indicated for those fractures that do not heal after a minimum of six weeks of cast immobilization. Because refractures are seen almost exclusively in children older than 13 years of age, Herrera-Soto (14) has recommended consideration for surgical treatment for this age group. Competitive athletes who require a faster return to sports and place greater stress on the fracture site may also be surgical candidates at the time of injury. Percutaneous anterograde intramedullary placement of a cannulated screw is the method of choice for immediate treatment of these fractures. Open reduction through a limited lateral exposure, combined with screw fixation and bone grafting, may be necessary to achieve healing of established nonunions. After a short period of non-weight bearing in a cast, weight bearing is initiated gradually as dictated by clinical and radiographic healing. Healing after internal fixation in children takes an average of seven weeks (14).

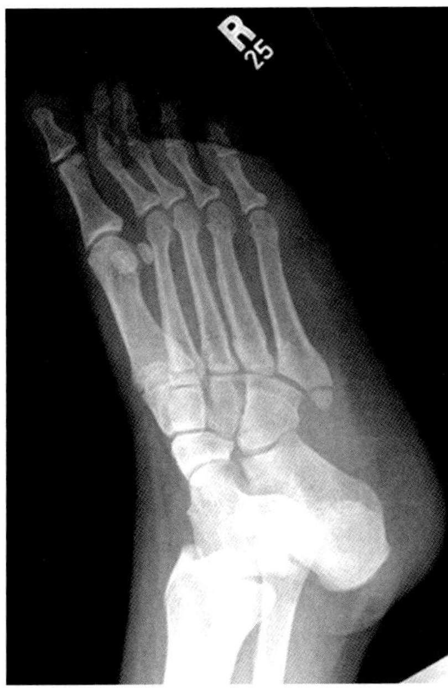

FIGURE 23-6 Fifteen-year-old runner who twisted his foot. He sustained a minimally displaced fifth metatarsal avulsion fracture. He healed after five weeks of casting.

Phalangeal Fractures and Interphalangeal Dislocations

Phalangeal fractures of the foot are common and most frequently result from a falling object or stubbing of the toes. Fractures without severe deformity are best treated with simple "buddy taping" of the injured toe to the adjacent uninjured toe combined with a hard-sole shoe for comfort with weight bearing. For fractures with unacceptable rotation or angulation, closed reduction and buddy taping under digital block is sufficient. Rotational malunion is avoided by assessment of the nailbed angle relative to the adjacent toes. Closed or open reduction and wire fixation is rarely indicated for phalangeal fractures unless gross realignment cannot be achieved and maintained after reduction and buddy taping. Displaced fractures of the proximal phalanx of the great toe require near-anatomic reduction and are more likely to require surgical treatment (Figure 23-9).

Interphalangeal dislocations are less common and typically occur in the lesser toes. Most occur at the proximal interphalangeal joint and are dorsal. These are typically readily reduced under digital block by gentle extension of the joint, followed by longitudinal traction and flexion.

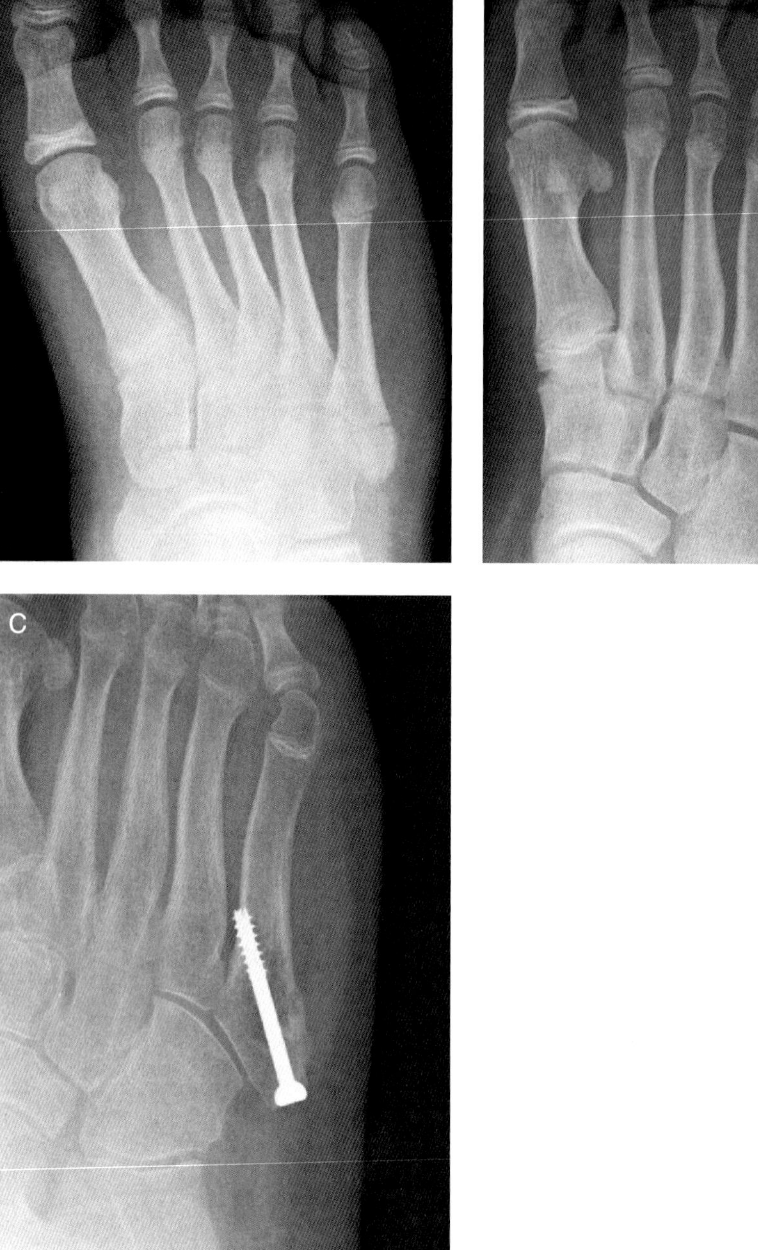

FIGURE 23-7 Thirteen-year-old boy who fell from a tree. He sustained an intra-articular fracture of the base of the fifth metatarsal (**A**). He was treated with cast immobilization for five weeks without clinical and radiographic healing (**B**). He underwent cannulated screw fixation (**C**).

After reduction, buddy taping is applied for a short period of one to two weeks. Open reduction is needed for the rare irreducible dislocation. Through a dorsal incision, the joint is opened and the obstacle to reduction, generally an infolded volar plate or capsule, is removed, allowing joint realignment. While most are stable after open reduction, fixation with a wire may be necessary for unstable fractures or those with associated soft-tissue injury (Figure 23-10).

LAWNMOWER INJURIES

Each year, approximately 9,400 children younger than 18 years require emergency care for lawnmower-related injuries in the United States. In one study, the mean age was 7.6 years and 65% of patients were boys, 40% required hospital admission, and 35% required surgical intervention (33). The injuries sustained included lacerations (30%), fractures (25%), amputations (21%), and burns

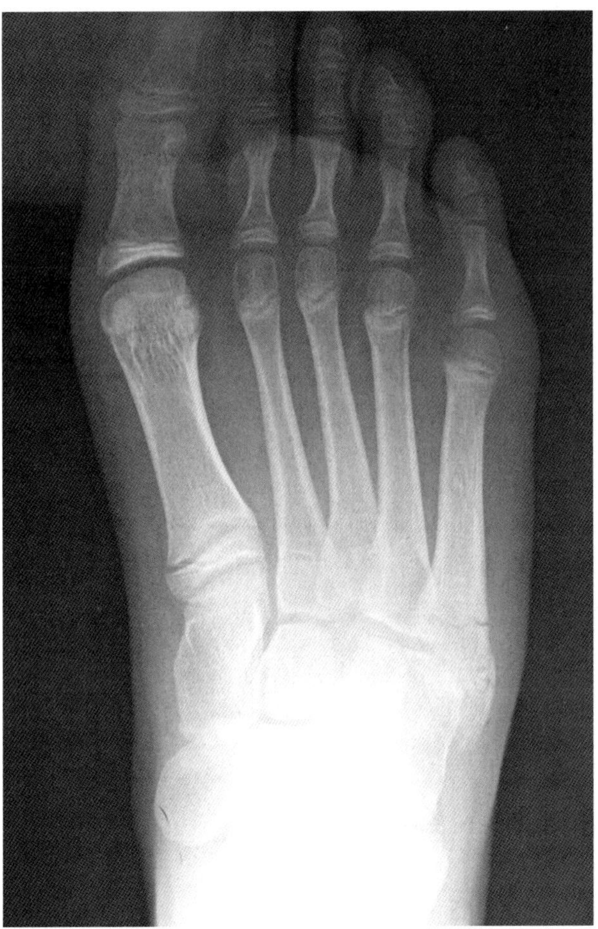

FIGURE 23-8 Eleven-year-old soccer player who was kicked and fell during a game. He sustained a Jones fracture of the fifth metatarsal. He healed after five weeks of non–weight-bearing cast immobilization.

(12%). Lawnmower injuries are particularly destructive to a child's foot and lower extremity, which are the most common sites of injury. Small children are injured while riding on the mower with a parent or are run over when unseen while chasing the mower (33). Older children are injured when using rotary mowers during the process of pulling the mower backward toward their feet. The power blades generate tremendous destructive force that cuts through soft tissue and bone, degloving the skin. The spinning blades blow fragments of grass, dirt, and debris into the wound under pressure. Embedded debris is often incompletely removed by pulse lavage alone and meticulous mechanical debridement must be done to satisfactorily debride the wound. A sterile tooth brush is one effective tool which can help mechanically cleanse the wound.

Treatment of these injuries requires a thorough knowledge of foot anatomy and considerable judgment on the part of the surgeon. Wounds that result from lawnmower injuries are best managed by urgent inspection in the operating room under general anesthesia to fully assess the damage tissue. While the orthopedic surgeon usually has the primary responsibility for care of children with these injuries, assistance from a plastic surgeon is frequently necessary. Thorough debridement should be done gently in order to not compromise the blood supply of marginal tissues. Once cleansed, the tissues are inspected to determine the extent of the injury and the viability of the remaining tissue. Obviously, non-viable tissue must be debrided. Any tissue with questionable viability is preserved and re-evaluated in 24 to 48 hours. Intact but avulsed muscle tendon units are preserved and tacked down out to length to facilitate reattachment later.

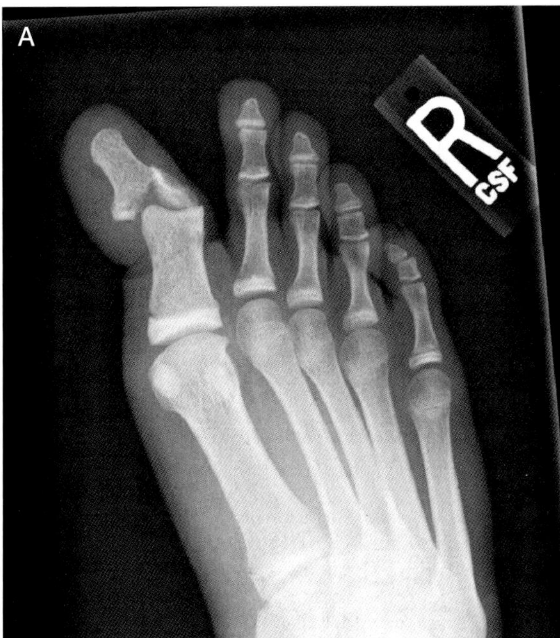

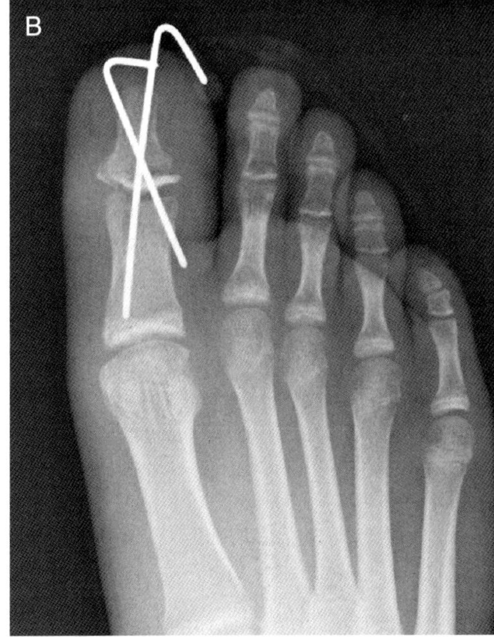

FIGURE 23-9 Fifteen-year-old girl involved in a bicycle accident. She sustained a displaced intra-articular fracture of the distal phalanx of the great toe (**A**). She underwent open reduction and internal fixation (**B**).

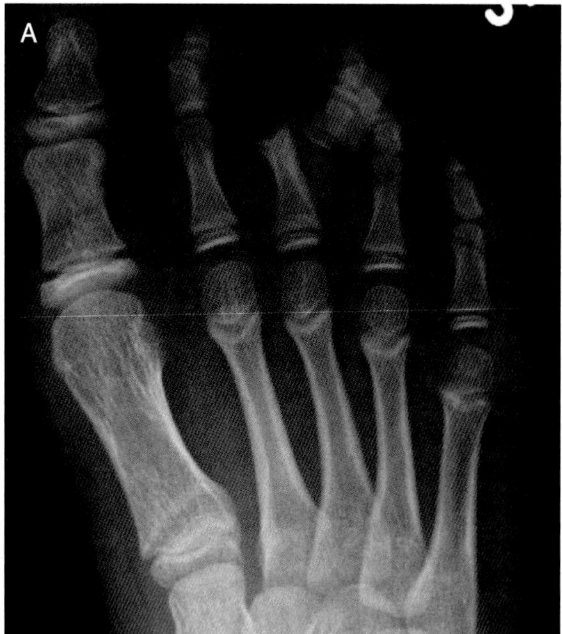

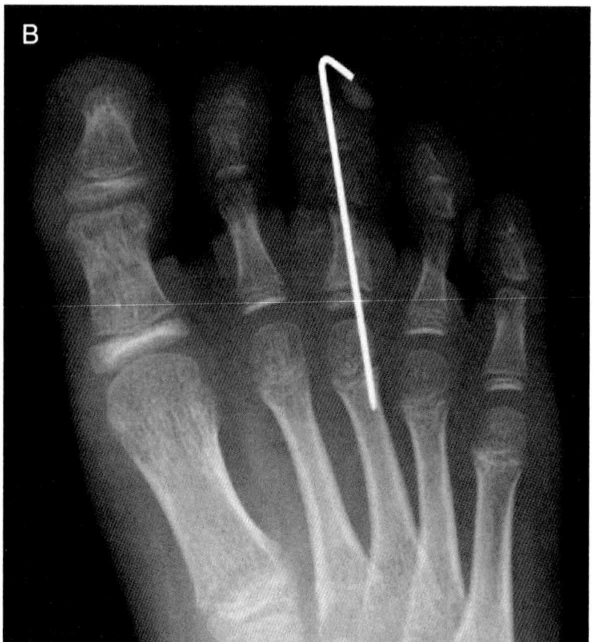

FIGURE 23-10 Eleven-year-old boy who fell off a dirt bike. He sustained an open PIP dislocation of the third toe (**A**). He underwent irrigation, debridement, and ORIF (**B**).

Fracture fixation is best done during the first debridement unless the wound is severely contaminated. Smooth wires and external fixation are most commonly used for stabilization. Following the initial debridement, the foot is protected in a rigid, bulky dressing with the ankle positioned as close as possible to a plantigrade position depending on tissue swelling. The wound may either closed loosely over a drain or covered with a VAC dressing.

Repeat debridements are carried out every 24 to 48 hours until all non-viable tissue and debris have been removed and healthy tissue remains. The ingenuity of the surgeon and knowledge of anatomy and foot biomechanics are used to reconstruct the most functional foot possible using the remaining viable tissues. Muscle tendon units should be reattached to bone in their most functional position. Injured physes generally continue to grow if part of the physeal blood supply remains intact and should be left in place if at all possible. Split thickness skin grafts can be used initially to close small wounds. Healthy-appearing but non-viable skin which is removed during the initial procedure should be preserved for this purpose when possible to avoid the need for a secondary donor site. The use of the VAC system has decreased the need for skin grafting and additional soft-tissue coverage. Those patients with large soft-tissue defects, especially when bone is exposed, may require flap coverage. Long-term follow up is needed to identify and treat late infections and secondary deformities of the foot and ankle, as well as leg-length inequality that may develop in those children with physeal injuries of the long bones of the leg. Because functional recovery is surprisingly good in children despite devastating injuries, the surgeon must make every effort to avoid amputation if possible.

REFERENCES

1. *Acad Emerg Med.* 2009 Apr;16(4):277–287. Epub 2009 Feb 2.
2. Bachmann LM, Kolb E, Koller MT, Steurer J, ter Riet G. Accuracy of Ottawa ankle rules to exclude fractures of the ankle and mid-foot: systematic review. *BMJ.* 2003 Feb 22;326(7386):417.
3. Brunet JA. Calcaneal fractures in children. Long-term results of treatment. *J Bone Joint Surg Br.* Mar 2000;82(2):211–216.
4. Canale ST, Kelly FB, Jr. Fractures of the neck of the talus. Long-term evaluation of seventy-one cases. *J Bone Joint Surg Am.* Mar 1978;60(2):143–156.
5. Ceroni D, De Rosa V, De Coulon G, Kaelin A. Cuboid nutcracker fracture due to horseback riding in children: case series and review of the literature. *J Pediatr Orthop.* Jul–Aug 2007;27(5):557–561.
6. Clapper MF, O'Brien TJ, Lyons PM. Fractures of the fifth metatarsal. Analysis of a fracture registry. *Clin Orthop Relat Res.* Jun 1995(315):238–241.
7. Dameron TB, Jr. Fractures and anatomical variations of the proximal portion of the fifth metatarsal. *J Bone Joint Surg Am.* Sep 1975;57(6):788–792.
8. Dimentberg R, Rosman M: Peritalar dislocations in children. *J Pediatr Orthop* 1993;13:89–93.
9. Essex-Lopresti P. The mechanism, reduction technique, and results in fractures of the os calcis. *Br J Surg.* Mar 1952;39(157):395–419.
10. Fulkerson E, Razi A, Tejwani N. Review: acute compartment syndrome of the foot. *Foot Ankle Int.* 2003 Feb;24(2):180–187.
11. Giannestras N. *Foot disorders.* Vol 558. Philadelphia: Lea & Febiger; 1973.
12. Hawkins LG. Fractures of the neck of the talus. *J Bone Joint Surg Am.* Jul 1970;52(5):991–1002.
13. Hermel M, Gershon-Cohen J. Nutcracker fracture of the cuboid by indirect violence. *Radiology.* 1953;60:850–854.
14. Herrera-Soto JA, Scherb M, Duffy MF, Albright JC. Fractures of the fifth metatarsal bone in children and adolescents. *J Pediatr Orthop.* 2007 Jun;27(4):427–431.
15. Inokuchi S, Usami N, Hiraishi E, Hashimoto T. Calcaneal fractures in children. *J Pediatr Orthop.* Jul–Aug 1998;18(4):469–474.

16. Jensen I, Wester JU, Rasmussen F, Lindequist S, Schantz K. Prognosis of fracture of the talus in children. 21 (7–34)-year follow-up of 14 cases. *Acta Orthop Scand.* Aug 1994;65(4): 398–400.
17. Kavanaugh J, Browser T, Mann R. The Jones fracture revisited. *J Bone Joint Surg Am.* 1978;60A:776–782.
18. Kay RM, Tang CW. Pediatric foot and ankle fractures: evaluation and treatment. *J Am Acad Orthop Surg* 2001;9:303–319.
19. Landin LA. Epidemiology in children's fractures. *J Pediatr Orthop* 1997;6B:79
20. Lawrence SJ, Botte MJ. Jones' fractures and related fractures of the proximal fifth metatarsal. *Foot Ankle.* Jul–Aug 1993;14(6): 358–365.
21. Letts RM, Gibeault D. Fractures of the neck of the talus in children. *Foot Ankle.* Sep 1980;1(2):74–77.
22. Omey ML, Micheli LJ. Foot and ankle problems in the young athlete. *Med Sci Sports Exerc.* Jul 1999;31(7 Suppl):S470–486.
23. Petit CJ, Lee BM, Kasser JR, Kocher MS. Operative treatment f intra-articular fractures of the calcaneus in the pediatric population. *J Pediatr Orthop.* 2007 Dec;27(8):856–862.
24. Pickle A, Benaroch TE, Guy P, Harvey EJ. Clinical outcome of pediatric calcaneal fractures treated with open reduction and internal fixation. *J Pediatr Orthop.* Mar–Apr 2004;24(2): 178–180.
25. Quill GE, Jr. Fractures of the proximal fifth metatarsal. *Orthop Clin North Am.* Apr 1995;26(2):353–361.
26. Rammelt S, Zwipp H, Gavlik JM. Avascular necrosis after minimally displaced talus fracture in a child. *Foot Ankle Int.* Dec 2000;21(12):1030–1036.
27. Richli WR, Rosenthal DI. Avulsion fracture of the fifth metatarsal: experimental study of pathomechanics. *AJR Am J Roentgenol.* Oct 1984;143(4):889–891.
28. Schantz K, Rasmussen F. Good prognosis after calcaneal fracture in childhood. *Acta Orthop Scand.* Oct 1988;59(5):560–563.
29. Schmidt TL, Weiner DS. Calcaneal fractures in children. An evaluation of the nature of the injury in 56 children. *Clin Orthop Relat Res.* Nov–Dec 1982(171):150–155.
30. Senaran H, Mason D, De Pellegrin M. Cuboid fractures in preschool children. *J Pediatr Orthop.* Nov–Dec 2006;26(6): 741–744.
31. Singer G, Cichocki M, Schalamon J, Eberl R, Höllwarth ME. A study of metatarsal fractures in children. *J Bone Joint Surg Am.* 2008 Apr;90(4):772–776.
32. Torg JS, Balduini FC, Zelko RR, Pavlov H, Peff TC, Das M. Fractures of the base of the fifth metatarsal distal to the tuberosity. Classification and guidelines for non-surgical and surgical management. J *Bone Joint Surg Am.* Feb 1984;66(2):209–214.
33. Vollman D, Khosla K, Shields BJ, Beeghly BC, Bonsu B, Smith GA. Lawn mower-related injuries to children. *J Trauma.* 2005 Sep;59(3):724–728.
34. Wiley JJ. Tarso-metatarsal joint injuries in children. *J Pediatr Orthop.* 1981;1(3):255–260.

CHAPTER 24

Foot Infections in Children and Adolescents

Patricia M. de Moraes Barros Fucs, Marco Túlio Costa, Ricardo Cardenuto Ferreira and Karen Myung

INTRODUCTION

Foot infections in children and adolescents are not unusual in the clinical practice of orthopedists. The principles underlying care of infections of the foot are much the same as those underlying infections elsewhere in the body. The foot may be a locus of infection due to wounds, osteomyelitis, septic arthritis, and mycosis. Knowledge of these pathological conditions, along with their differential diagnoses, is necessary in order to prescribe the correct treatment.

DIFFERENTIAL DIAGNOSIS

Other pathological conditions unrelated to bacterial infection may affect the foot in children yet may have similar sets of symptoms. Fractures, neoplasm, synovitis, juvenile rheumatoid arthritis and other types of autoimmune arthritis, and avascular necrosis should be investigated in children with clinical conditions similar to those described above. It is important to remember that there are a number of bone tumors that can simulate subacute and chronic osteomyelitis. The most common scenario is Ewing's sarcoma, but eosinophilic granuloma and leukemia can also present in a similar fashion as osteomyelitis and should be included in the differential diagnosis (10,43). Importantly, 30% of children with leukemia present with bone pain.

Infections can be organized according to tissues involved or by the infecting organism. A convenient outline includes:

1. Bacterial infections
   a. Soft tissue infections of fat; fascia; lymphatics; tendons; and bursae (includes felons, puncture wounds, necrotizing fasciitis, and animal bites)
   b. Bone infections
   c. Joint infections
2. Mycobacterial infections
3. Fungal infections

BACTERIAL INFECTIONS

Soft Tissue Infections

Cellulitis, Lymphangitis and Soft Tissue Abscess

The soft tissue of the foot and ankle may be a locus of infection disseminated hematogenously or by local inoculation of the organism into a wound (24,68). Most soft tissue infections in the uncompromised host are caused by *Staphylococcus aureus* (*S. aureus*) and β-hemolytic streptococci. In puncture wounds, *Pseudomonas aeruginosa* is a frequent offending organism. Generally, *S. aureus* causes cellulitis and abscess formation, and β-hemolytic streptococci typically causes cellulitis and lymphangitis. Some authors hypothesize that these microorganisms are present in the normal bacterial flora of the foot and that they take advantage of a wound or a decrease in host immunity to start the infectious condition (71). According to Giannestras, the frequency of soft-tissue infections has been declining over recent years because of greater foot care (24). Other important factors have been the development of better antibiotics and greater access to medical care. For these reasons, infections are now treated in their initial stages, thus preventing the symptoms of systemic and extensive local involvement.

The clinical presentation resembles soft-tissue infections that occur elsewhere in the body. Fever, pain, erythema, tenderness, and swelling are common symptoms. Weight bearing is generally difficult, and the gait is sometimes impaired. There may or may not be fever or lymphadenopathy. In immunocompromised hosts or after trauma or surgery, the clinical picture may be supplemented with varying degrees of necrosis, foul odor, and bullae. Laboratory tests show leukocytosis and increased erythrocyte sedimentation rate (ESR) and C-reactive protein (CRP) levels.

The treatment of cellulitis and lymphangitis consists of rest and elevation of the affected limb and administration of appropriate antibiotic therapy. Immobilization may help to relieve pain. If the infection is superficial, it can almost always be treated with an antibiotic directed against *S. aureus* and hemolytic streptococci. These agents are dicloxacillin, cephalexin, clindamycin, as well as newer, more broad-spectrum cephalosporins and fluoroquinolones. In cases of more complicated cellulitis, antibiotic therapy should be based on culture data and consultation with infectious disease specialists. Prompt surgical drainage is also indicated if an abscess forms.

Felon

A felon is an infection of the pulp space of the distal portion of a toe near the nailbed. The pulp region is a closed compartment. Obvious or inconspicuous trauma can penetrate the closed pulp space, deposit bacteria, and lead to pus formation. Collection of pus in this area creates pressure, impairing tissue perfusion and causing considerable pain. Generally, the infecting organism is *S. aureus*. However, when lymphangitic streaks are present, hemolytic streptococci should be suspected. In immunocompromised patients, gram-negative organisms may be the offending agents. Failure to decompress a felon may result in contiguous spread to the distal phalanx (local osteomyelitis), distal interphalangeal joint (septic arthritis), or flexor tendon sheath (flexor tenosynovitis). A neglected felon may eventually lead to extrusion or avascular necrosis of the distal phalanx.

Treatment of felons involves surgical debridement. The pulp is widely opened through two lateral incisions or a single incision. If necrotic bone is present, it must be debrided. The wound is often left open to allow for drainage. Delayed primary closure is achieved once swelling and cellulitis subside and the wound appears clean. Partial or complete amputation is indicated when the infection spreads rapidly with extensive soft-tissue or bony involvement, especially in the immunocompromised patient.

Puncture Wounds

Attention must be paid to perforating wounds in the foot. They are common in children and are frequently due to nails, as well as splinters, tacks, glass, thorns, and other objects. Bits of clothing are often carried into the wound. It has been estimated that 8% to 15% of the perforating injuries to feet become infected and require medical attention (22). When infections occur in this type of injury, *Pseudomonas aeruginosa* may be the causal agent. Diabetic patients are apt to have polymicrobial infections (56).

Early complications from puncture wounds include cellulitis and abscess formation. Late complications may include osteomyelitis, osteochondritis, and septic arthritis (26,62). Osteomyelitis occurs in 0.8% to 1.6% of cases and most often affects the metatarsals or calcaneus (60). There are generally few systemic symptoms and laboratory tests present with few abnormalities, which may make early diagnosis more difficult.

Treatment involves careful early attention and vigilance. In such cases of perforating wounds in the foot, the possibility of infection due to *Pseudomonas* should not change the basic principles of wound treatment. Tetanus prophylaxis should always be administered as outlined by the American College of Surgeons. If the patient is seen early, it is important to ensure careful cleansing of the wound, debridement of devitalized tissue, and removal of foreign bodies (63). An iodophor wick and bandage may be used as dressing to allow drainage. According to Tachibana, wound infection after taking these measures would be rare (71). On the other hand, retained foreign material is often found as the nidus of both early and late complications. When a retained foreign body is suspected, radiographs should be obtained with an appropriate soft-tissue technique. If suspicion persists despite negative radiographs, then magnetic resonance imaging (MRI) may be considered.

The exact role of prophylactic antibiotic therapy is controversial. Some surgeons argue that prophylactic antibiotic therapy must not be administered in cases of perforating wounds of the foot (63). Wide-spectrum antibiotics against gram-positive organisms may select the local flora and favor infection by *Pseudomonas*. Others support a judicious use of prophylactic antibiotic therapy (20). If the wound is "clean," as in the case of a needle puncture, no prophylactic therapy is indicated. However, it the wound is more heavily contaminated or if the wound extends to bone, cartilage, or joint, then prophylactic anti-staphylococcal and anti-streptococcal therapy is advised. While it is tempting to administer anti-pseudomonal therapy as well, this treatment has not been fully studied (12). Regardless of initial management, it is important to observe these patients carefully and with early reassessment. When infection has become established, which is generally some days or a few weeks after the injury, careful surgical debridement of the wound is recommended, with removal of all the devitalized tissue and exploration of the wound to search for foreign bodies and obtain cultures. Thereafter, appropriate intravenous antibiotic therapy should be administered which may include initial empiric coverage of gram-positive organisms and *Pseudomonas*, followed by culture-directed therapy. *Staphylococcus* may also cause secondary infection in this type of wound.

Necrotizing Fasciitis

Necrotizing fasciitis is a rapidly progressive soft-tissue infection that may threaten both life and limb. Although uncommon in children, familiarity with this disorder is crucial due to the deceivingly benign presentation of the infection and the devastating consequences of a missed or delayed diagnosis (21). It generally involves the skin and underlying soft tissues, while initially sparing muscle involvement. This condition may rapidly progress toward septic shock and end-organ failure. Multiple etiologies are recognized, including trauma, puncture wounds, and postoperative infection. Group A β-hemolytic *Streptococcus pyogenes* is the organism most commonly found in necrotizing fasciitis, but the infections are also commonly polymicrobial (51). Immunocompromised patients are at increased risk.

Initial physical findings are frequently subtle, and rarely is the diagnosis made at the time of admission.

Early in the course of the disease, necrotizing fasciitis may present as an unremarkable cellulitis which is surprisingly tender. Later, necrotizing fasciitis generally presents as a tense, swollen extremity with erythema and cellulitis that does not respond to antibiotics and elevation. The patient may appear toxic, and bullae and mottled skin discoloration may appear over the affected area. A high index of suspicion must be maintained when evaluating an immunocompromised patient with an acute severe soft tissue infection.

Necrotizing fasciitis is primarily a surgical problem. Emergent and aggressive incision and debridement are critical, along with supportive care by critical care specialists and initial broad-spectrum empiric antibiotic therapy. Antibiotics include penicillin and, for penicillinase-resistant *Staphylococcus,* an aminoglycoside is usually added. Surgery includes thorough debridement of all five plantar fascial spaces through which infection may spread, and is usually accomplished through a single extensile plantar medial incision. Additional incisions may be used to release all of the foot compartments with fasciotomies to prevent compartment syndrome. The wound is initially left open and then closed by secondary intention, grafting, or delayed primary closure when appropriate. After initial debridement, antibiotic therapy may be selected as offending organisms are identified. Multiple surgical debridements may be necessary prior to closure. Amputation may be warranted when limb salvage options have been exhausted or the infection threatens the life of the patient. Even with this aggressive treatment, mortality is as high as 18% in children and can be higher in adults (21).

Animal Bites

Cat and dog bites can introduce *Pasteurella multocida,* an organism that behaves aggressively and can lead to cellulitis, tissue destruction, invasion of tendons and bone, and abscess formation (38,49). Over 1 million dog-bite injuries are treated in the United States each year. More than 50% of the dog bites affect children under the age of 12 years (70). Even more frightening, approximately a dozen people die each year from dog bites and one-third of these deaths are infants less than 12 months of age (70). Similar to the human mouth, the dog oral cavity is full of organisms, including *Staphylococcus aureus, Streptococcus viridans, Pasteurella multocida,* and *Bacteroides* species. The possibility of rabies is also a consideration. Fortunately, rabies is rare after dog bites and surveillance of the dog for 10 days is the simplest monitoring method. In contrast, wild animal bites require prophylactic treatment for rabies, as skunks and raccoons are responsible for the majority of rabid bites. Cat bites are less common than dog bites. However, since cats have needle-sharp canines that drive bacteria deep into tissue, cat bites more commonly result in a deep infection (50% of the time). Typical causative organisms of infection after a cat bite also include *P. multiocida, S. aureus,* and *S. viridans.* Bites by other domestic animals, such as pet rabbits, hamsters, or guinea pigs are treated in the same manner as cat bites.

Treatment principles are similar to human bites with urgent recognition and immediate irrigation and debridement of all nonviable tissue. Prophylactic antibiotic therapy should be administered. Penicillin, ampicillin, or amoxicillin will cover *P. multocida,* as well as mouth flora. Cephalosporins and amoxicillin-clavulanate have the advantage of also covering *Staphylococcus.* Tetanus toxoid should be administered when appropriate. Vigilant follow up is necessary as deep infection may occur despite these measures.

Community-Associated Methicillin-Resistant Staphylococcus Aureus (CA-MRSA) Soft Tissue Infections

Community-associated methicillin-resistant *Staphylococcus aureus* (CA-MRSA) infection in children is an increasing problem (3,58). CA-MRSA infections are caused by different strains than health care-associated MRSA infections and demonstrate different epidemiological patterns and clinical features (3). The CA-MRSA harbor one to two unique staphylococcal chromosome cassettes (SCC) carrying the *mec*A gene. The only virulence factor consistently found in these staphylococci is the extracellular toxin Panton-Valentine leukocidin (PVL) encoded by the *luk*F and *luk*S genes. It has been associated with necrotizing pneumonia and skin infections in otherwise healthy children and young adults, resulting in complications such as subperiosteal abscesses, septic thrombophlebitis, endocarditis, septic pulmonary emboli, and large muscle abscesses (3,58).

Higher-risk groups in the pediatric population include athletes, institutionalized children, and urban children (5). Contact sports, particularly involving skin-to-skin contact, are the primary sources for CA-MRSA outbreaks, namely football, wrestling, and rugby. The typical clinical presentation is an athlete with pain, redness, swelling, and/or an area of drainage on the skin. The onset of symptoms, a history of skin trauma, breaks, or concurrent conditions such as eczema, and any exposure to other symptomatic athletes should be noted. These infections can spread rapidly. Associated systemic symptoms such as fever, malaise, dyspnea, and/or mental status changes should warrant emergent admission and treatment.

Patients without bacteremia or identifiable abscesses are not easily cultured. It is not clear whether it is beneficial to obtain surface cultures of nares, axilla, and groin to help guide diagnosis and therapy, as many CA-MRSA outbreaks have occurred in athletes without detectable nasal colonization (5). Therefore, currently, there are no evidence-based recommendations for routine screening of all athletes.

The gold standard of treatment for CA-MRSA abscesses remains incision and drainage with acquisition of cultures for definitive diagnosis and susceptibility patterns (5) (Figure 24-1). Antimicrobials are used adjunctively with incision and drainage for CA-MRSA infections. First line empiric treatment of suspected CA-MRSA infections is either trimethoprim-sulfamethoxizole for mild infections

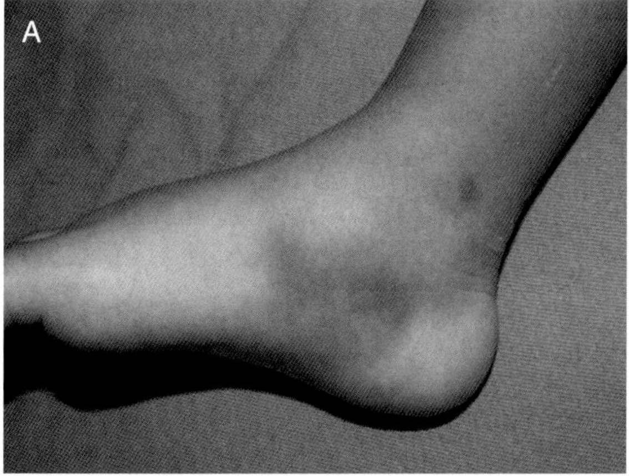

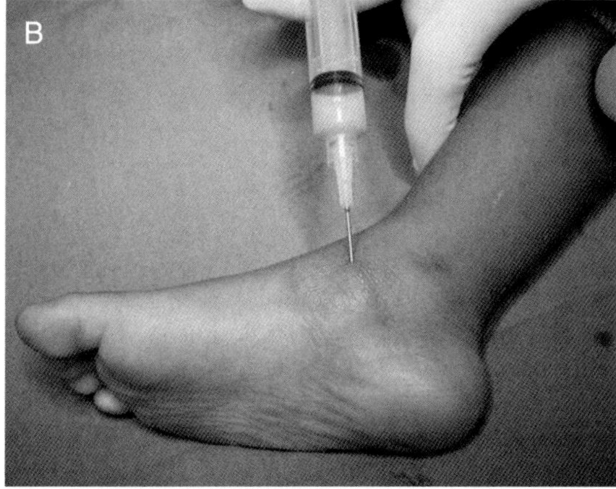

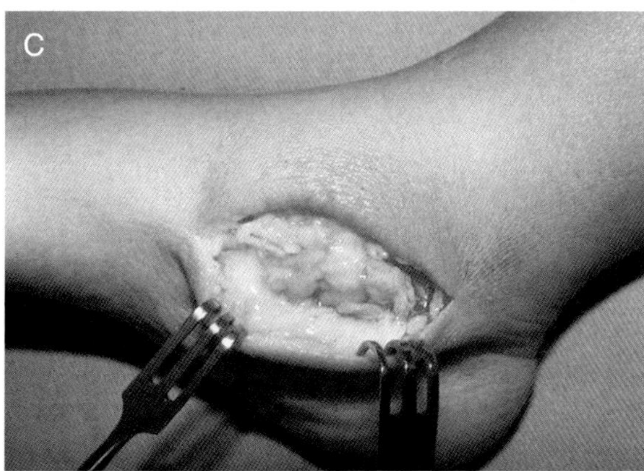

FIGURE 24-1 **A.** Medial aspect of the right foot in a five-year-old patient, history of fever and pain. Clinical signs of erythema, swelling, and increased temperature. **B.** Needle aspiration showing pus. **C.** Intra-operative drainage of the abscess in the midfoot, using medial surgical approach.

and clindamycin or vancomycin for more severe infections (5). Rifampin may be used as a synergistic agent for any one of these antimicrobials, but should never be used alone. Doxycyline is not approved for use under age 12 years. Beta-lactams and first-generation cephalosporins no longer have a role in the treatment of CA-MRSA and should not be used. Close follow up is mandatory. Length of treatment usually continues for at least 14 days and depends on severity and response to treatment (5). Bony involvement requires a longer course. Clindamycin resistance is emerging and varies depending on local resistance patterns (3,5,58). Furthermore, treatment failures on clindamycin have been reported due to an inducible clindamycin resistance during therapy (3,5,58).

According to the guidelines set forth by the National Collegiate Athletic Association, wrestlers with mild to moderate skin infections may return to competition 72 hours after initiation of therapy as long as there is demonstrable clinical improvement, no evidence of new skin lesions for 48 hours, and application of occlusive dressings (74). If the wounds cannot be adequately covered, the athlete should be excluded from play. All breaches in skin should be promptly washed with soap and water and covered. Importantly, proper hygiene in high risk groups should be instructed and enforced.

Bone Infections

Acute Hematogenous Osteomyelitis (AHO)

Acute hematogeneous osteomyelitis (AHO) is an inflammation of bone caused by bacteria that reach bone through a bloodborne route. Sources include adjacent soft tissue and joints or direct inoculation through trauma, even minor, or surgery. AHO is more common in children, usually occurring in the first decade. The presence of the growth plate favors the onset of bacterial infections that are disseminated hematogenously, into the metaphysis of bones. The growth plate is avascular and is maintained by nutrient diffusion. Thus, the circulation is slower in the metaphysis. This provides a niche in which bacteria can become established and multiply. Although the local anatomy favors the onset of acute osteomyelitis, it seems that there is a need for some type of associated local trauma for infection to begin (14,27,63,67). Bacterial infection initially causes an exudate in the metaphysis. When this infection is ineffectively controlled, it develops into pus, thus forming an abscess within the bone. Metaphyseal bone is porous in children and the purulent material extravasates from the metaphysis. Since the periosteum in children is thicker and adheres less strongly to the bone than in adults, the extravasated pus elevates the periosteum to form so-called subperiosteal abscesses. The

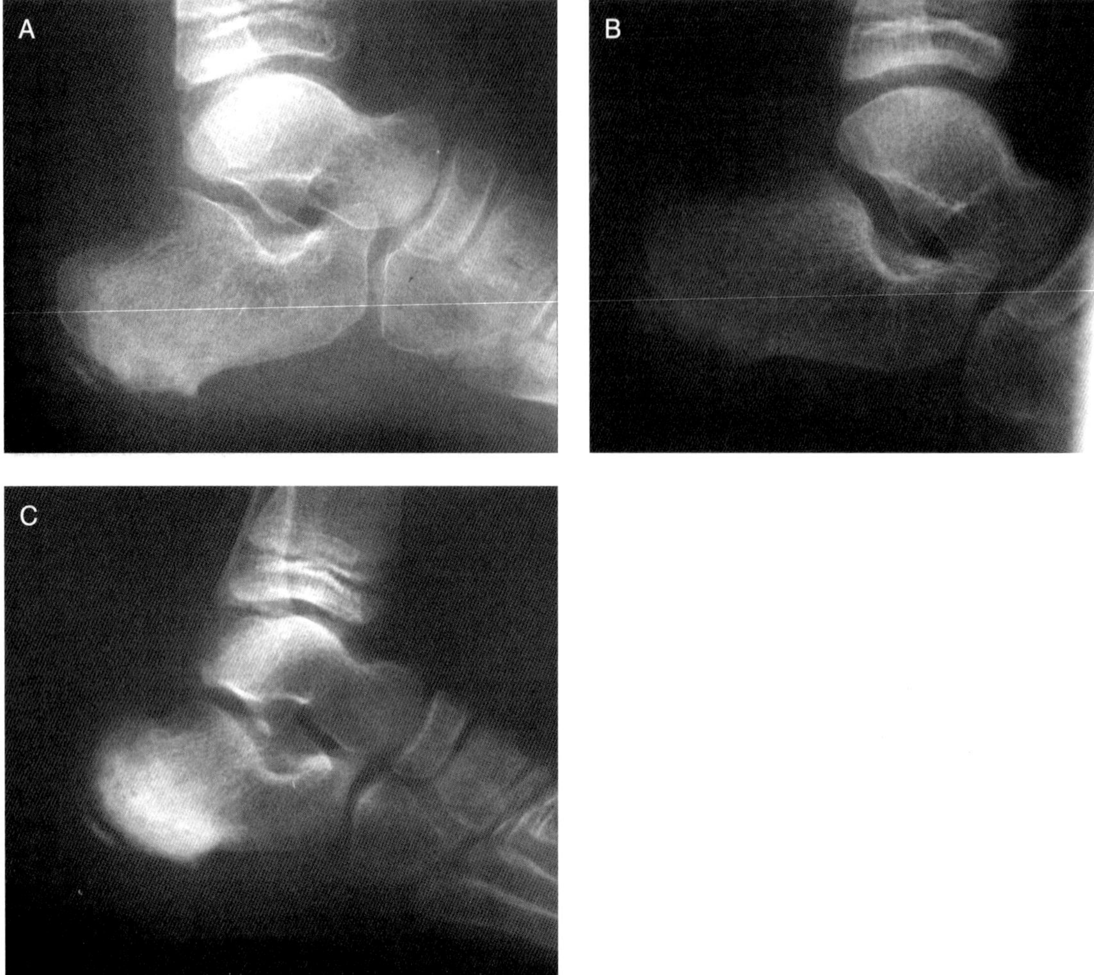

FIGURE 24-2 Radiograph of the right foot, lateral view, of an eight-year-old child. **A.** After a perforating injury by a nail on the plantar surface. **B.** Evolution with a bone lesion in the calcaneus. The clinical abscess required surgical drainage. **C.** Presence of osteomyelitis of the calcaneus.

detached periosteum continues to produce bone and, over time, may form an involucrum. The adjoining cortex can become non-viable and becomes a sequestrum. Septic arthritis, discussed later, may arise when this abscess is in communication with a joint (27,67).

Diagnosis

The diagnosis of pediatric AHO is difficult and is still often delayed. The most important factor in making the diagnosis is the clinical picture, and a high index of suspicion on the part of the clinician is essential. Unexplained bone pain with fever indicates osteomyelitis until proven otherwise.

The onset of pediatric AHO is usually sudden, with a recent or concurrent non-muscular infection in 30% to 50% of patients. Children with AHO often present with refusal to walk. These infants and children may appear systemically ill, with localization of the cardinal signs of infection: swelling, redness, warmth, and pain. The patient may have findings of an adjacent sympathetic joint effusion, with joint irritability and limited range of motion or even pseudoparalysis. Pain and restricted movement are generally the earliest signs. The place where the pain is greatest is usually the infection site (63,67). The diagnosis can often be made by careful physical examination, after the child's trust has been gained. It is recommended to get the child undressed and start the examination in non-painful regions, leaving the affected area until last. Deep soft tissue swelling is the key finding early in the process.

An elevated white blood cell count and erythrocyte sedimentation rate is seen in the majority of these children, but these elevations are not reliable in the neonate. It must be remembered that children with diseases that affect the immunological system may not present with leukocytosis. Blood cultures are positive in 30% to 50% of infants and children, and may identify the causal agent of the infection, thus facilitating the choice of antibiotic (63,67).

For initial assessments, radiographs are generally useful only to rule out fracture or neoplasm, as abnormalities due to the infection are usually only visible seven to ten days after the process starts (14,63,67). At this stage, radiographs may only show osteopenia caused by disuse and increased local circulation. Later, evidence of osteolysis at the infection site, periosteal detachment and, in some cases, even bone sequestration may be present on plain radiographs

(Figure 24-2). MRI, the imaging modality of choice, is especially useful in the axial skeleton and is better able to differentiate abnormal bone marrow involvement than bone scans, CT scans, or radiographs (30,40). However, it lacks the specificity for determining if the abnormal changes are due to osteomyelitis.

Other imaging studies may be helpful, including technetium (Tc 99m) diphosphonate bone scan, a three-phase scan which usually demonstrates increased uptake due to alteration in the physiology of involved bone (53). An abnormal technetium bone scan is non-specific and may show false-positive results associated with trauma or tumors. The presence of several growth plates in the foot makes bone scan difficult to interpret (14). False-negatives (lack of increased uptake with AHO) occur in 4% to 20% and may be seen with avascular necrosis or in very early cases; it takes awhile before there is stimulation of new bone matrix (53). An advantage of bone scan is the possibility of detecting multiple foci of osteomyelitis.

Early studies found that technetium scans were unreliable in infants and neonates, detecting only 50% of foci, but high-resolution techniques have improved the sensitivity in up to 100% in proven sites (4,9,32). Its use in the neonate is particularly helpful, especially when attempting to find multiple sites of infection. Bone scans or other diagnostic imaging should not delay treatment (11). If needed, accuracy of technetium may be increased by repeating the scan in 48 to 72 hours (35).

With osteomyelitis there is an increased uptake almost immediately with 67-gallium citrate leukocyte labeled bone scans (15). These scans are performed less frequently, primarily because they are more expensive and are associated with more radiation exposure as well as increased time to complete (48 to 72 hours). The accuracy of early diagnosis may be increased by following a negative technetium scan with a gallium scan (23). Indium-labeled-leukocyte bone scan requires labeling of leukocytes and thus can be performed only at a highly sophisticated facility (54). Although very accurate, indium-labeled-leukocyte bone scans are limited primarily to difficult diagnostic situations in which other imaging modalities are less ideal, such as chronic osteomyelitis (54).

Local puncture biopsy or open biopsy may play an important role when the infection is refractory to treatment, presents in an atypical fashion, or is advanced on presentation (63, 67). It facilitates bacteriologic diagnosis. The technique of local puncture biopsy involves locating the point of maximum tenderness and swelling (usually metaphyseal) and then using a 16- or 18-gauge (trochared) spinal needle to aspirate. Following careful antisepsis, the needle should be introduced and the deep tissue should first be aspirated, searching for local abscesses. If this is negative, the needle is advanced deeper. When pus comes out after going through the periosteum, the diagnosis of a subperiosteal abscess is confirmed. When subperiosteal puncture is negative, the needle should be introduced into the bone metaphysis to search for intraosseous accumulations. All material should be smeared and cultured and antibiotics begun based on the most likely suspected organism while awaiting definitive cultures. Aspirate is positive in 60% of the cases and bone biopsy in 90% (16,50).

Treatment

The treatment for acute osteomyelitis is based on surgical drainage and intravenous antibiotic therapy (63,67). In most cases, the organism responsible for the infection is *Staphylococcus aureus*, followed by *Streptococcus* species. However, among children under two years of age, organisms like *Haemophilus influenzae* and *Streptococcus pneumoniae* are also frequently seen (14,67). *Salmonella* should always be considered in the differential diagnosis in children with sickle cell disease.

Antibiotic therapy should be guided by the culture results whenever possible, and its duration should be linked to the clinical improvement seen in the patient (31). Two to three weeks of intravenous antibiotic therapy is initially recommended, followed by medication administered orally in selected cases. On rare occasions, if there is a prompt response to IV antibiotics, then oral medication can be initiated earlier, at five to seven days. Ten percent of infants and children do not respond to oral medication and need continued IV antibiotic treatment (50). Prerequisite criteria often described for the switch to oral medications include: identification of the organism; determination of antibiotic sensitivities and susceptibilities; and the confirmation of bactericidal antibiotic levels. Today, the clinical and laboratory (usually CRP) response to treatment is used as the determination for transfer to oral medications. Traditionally, total duration of treatment has been six weeks, but now a shorter duration of antibiotics may be adequate; there is no proven established duration. The length of antibiotic treatment is dependent on the clinical characteristics such as the site, amount of destruction, treatment, and response to treatment. The CRP rises faster and returns to normal more quickly and is the lab indicator of choice for following the treatment of osteomyelitis in infants and children with musculoskeletal infections. In children over the age of one year with duration of symptoms less than 48 hours, most will respond to antibiotic treatment without surgery. If there is no early response to antibiotics (within 36 hours), surgical debridement should be considered.

For cases in which no purulent material is obtained from joint or bone puncture (initial stage of the infection), treatment with antibiotics alone may be possible. For cases in which an intraosseous or subperiosteal abscess has already formed, surgical drainage becomes necessary. The primary role of surgery is to evacuate purulent material. The periosteum can be destroyed if the pus remains accumulated under the periosteum for any length of time. The periosteum may serve as the only source of osteogenic regeneration of the dead bone. If the bone does not regenerate, a permanent defect may result. After draining the subperiosteal abscess, there is debate regarding the need for investigating the bone metaphysis. Some authors have stated that, if there is a subperiosteal abscess, the abscess inside the bone will already have been drained, and investigation inside the bone is unnecessary. According to Green and Edwards, it would be prudent to perforate the metaphysis to verify that there is no intraosseous sequestrated abscess (27). If there is no purulent accumulation in the subperiosteal space, the abscess inside the bone will not have been drained, and both the subperiosteal space and the metaphysis will need to be opened. All purulent material must be drained, with the removal of all the avascular tissue and any devitalized bone fragments. However, whenever possible, damage to the growth plates must be avoided, since this could lead to secondary deformities in the foot (24). Injuries to tendons must also be avoided as these will subsequently trigger muscle imbalance and future deformity. In the case of abscess, prolonged intravenous antibiotic therapy without adequate surgical debridement is ineffective (27). If suction irrigation tubes are used, they should be removed by 48 hours. Placement of long-term IV access under the same anesthetic should be considered.

Special Considerations

Neonatal Osteomyelitis

Acute hematogenous osteomyelitis generally occurs in the metaphyseal region of the bone. However, in children aged up to 12 to 18 months, blood vessels may cross the growth plate to feed the epiphysis (14,63,67). Therefore, infections may be introduced into the epiphysis, thereby destroying the growth plate and causing bone deformity (51). This type of infection is usually found in low-weight neonates that require catheterization of the umbilical vein or other invasive procedures (27,67). The most common clinical signs are edema, erythema, and flexion contracture of the affected joint. Neonatal osteomyelitis tends to be multifocal and involve other joints. Although the causative organism may be *Staphylococcus aureus*, gram-negative organisms, and β-hemolytic *Streptococcus* are also common. Therefore, antibiotics that are efficient against these microorganisms must be administered until culture results have been obtained (27). The treatment should be the same as for acute hematogenous osteomyelitis, described above.

Pseudomonas *Osteomyelitis*

Osteomyelitis caused by *Pseudomonas* may occur in the feet of children and adolescents. These infections occur after puncture wounds to the feet when wearing shoes (22,41,55,67). *Pseudomonas* has already been isolated from the insoles of children's shoes, and deep inoculation by perforating objects is believed to be possible (55). Typical histories involve children who suffered perforating injuries to a foot some days or weeks earlier. Such patients are generally not febrile, but they present pain, elevated temperature, and local erythema that often impede their gait. Systemic symptoms are generally absent (22). Radiographs may already present bone abnormalities because of the time elapsed since the onset of the infection. Abnormalities on plain radiographs, such as bone destruction and periosteal reaction, generally first appear 10 to 14 days after the onset of infection. According to Lau et al., radiography should be the initial examination in these cases (41). However, when no abnormalities are seen on plain radiographs, the examination of choice for confirming the diagnosis of osteomyelitis due to *Pseudomonas* is MRI. The treatment should be the same as for AHO, described above, along with antibiotic therapy directed at *Pseudomonas* as well. The sequelae of osteomyelitis due to *Pseudomonas* that may occur include premature closure of the growth plate, chronic fistulae, joint destruction with loss of movement, and chronic pain (22).

Calcaneal Osteomyelitis

It is believed that in approximately 10% of the children with osteomyelitis, the infection is in the foot. The bone most frequently affected is the calcaneus. Infection of the calcaneus may be caused both hematogenously and by perforating wounds in the foot. Giannestras also highlighted the possibility that osteomyelitis could be secondary to the introduction of Kirschner wires into the foot following orthopedic surgery (24). Loss of the normal trabecular pattern may be the first radiographic sign. Usually, there is very little periosteal bone reaction. Periosteal reaction and signs of bone reabsorption appear later. Lastly, bone sequestration may develop. Most cases responded to antibiotics with or without curettage. At the initial stage, particularly in cases of hematogenous origin, bone puncture biopsy may greatly assist in the diagnosis.

Most early cases respond to antibiotics with or without curettage. Surgical approaches in the plantar region of the foot should be avoided because they may produce painful scars in this support area of the foot. When choosing lateral approaches, attention must be paid to the fibular tendons and sural nerve. When choosing medial incisions, attention must be paid to the posterior tibial neurovascular bundle and the tendons of tibialis posterior and the long flexors of the toes and hallux. Whenever possible, the growth plate of the calcaneus should not be violated, as this could lead to deformity in its growth. After removing all the devitalized tissue and draining the infection, the empty space in the bone can be initially filled with bone cement with antibiotic. After resolving the infectious condition, and with the appearance of granulation tissue on the edges of the bone and surgical wound, the bone cavity can be filled with bone graft and the wound can be closed. It is advisable to follow up such cases until adulthood, in order to monitor any recurrence of infection and to evaluate for any possible bone deformities caused by lesions in the growth plate of the calcaneus.

Subacute Hematogenous Osteomyelitis (SHO)

Subacute hematogenous osteomyelitis (SHO) differs from AHO in that the child is typically less symptomatic, with less pain and often no fever. Usually, no systemic signs are reported, and therefore there is often a delay of several months in the diagnosis. Some children (30% to 40%) have had a trial of antibiotics (50).

Laboratory assessment is more commonly normal (including blood and tissue cultures). Although most commonly located in the metaphysis or diaphysis of the bone, it can occur in the epiphysis. Subacute osteomyelitis of the talus and metatarsals has been reported (2,64,66). There may be no radiographic changes. If present, radiographic changes are slow to develop but may show a lytic lesion.

The organism is usually coagulase-negative *Staphylococcus*. The most important aspect of treating children and adolescents with SHO is to rule out tumors. In addition to cultures of involved tissue, biopsy is needed, and this is the classic situation for which the mantra "Culture all biopsies, and biopsy all cultures" is applied. Treatment thereafter consists of surgical curettage, antibiotics, and rest.

Chronic Recurrent Multifocal Osteomyelitis (CRMO)

Although recognized as a clinical and radiological pathological condition, the etiology and pathogenesis of CRMO is unknown (47). Both infectious and autoimmune etiologies have been proposed. Chronic CRMO differs from AHO in that it has an insidious onset of bone pain and tenderness. It occurs preferentially in Scandinavian children and has associations with dermatological abnormalities like vulgar psoriasis and palmoplantar pustulosis (14,47). SAPHO syndrome (synovitis, acne, pustulosis, hyperostosis, osteitis) is not uncommon in children who present with similar manifestations as CRMO and skin lesions, most commonly palmoplantar pustulosis (6).

It is characterized by involvement of the metaphyses of tubular bones and the clavicle but can also occur in the spine, ischiopubic bone and the sacroiliac joint, sometimes symmetrically. Periods of remission and exacerbation of the clinical condition occur, sometimes with complete remission without sequelae. The symptoms are typical of local infection, with pain, elevated temperature, local rubor, and edema. There may be low-grade fever, while systemic symptoms are rare. Radiographs often demonstrate eccentric metaphyseal sclerotic lucencies.

No organisms are typically isolated with CRMO. Furthermore, CRMO does not typically respond to antibiotic treatment. Corticosteroids or non-steroidal anti-inflammatory drugs, along with symptomatic treatment, may help in some cases, but their efficacy for all cases is unproven (47,67). In one series of patients with CRMO, five of twelve patients had a leg length inequality of greater than 1.5 cm, and other orthopedic deformities may occur (17). The long-term outcome of patients with CRMO is generally good, although a recurrence may manifest months or years later. As many as 26% have active disease at follow-up (mean of 13 years) (36). One of twelve patients had difficulty with school or maintaining a job at maturity; only two had complete resolution of symptoms (17).

Joint Infections

Septic arthritis in children can occur in any joint. Septic arthritis can occur from primary seeding of synovium of the joint or from secondary joint involvement from the adjacent metaphyseal bone or directly from the adjoining epiphysis. Destruction of the articular cartilage begins quickly and is secondary to proteolytic enzymes released from synovial cells.

Diagnosis

The diagnosis of septic arthritis is based on the clinical findings. Typically, this is an acute onset in which the child is irritable, febrile, and anorexic. In the foot, the child will have a limp or will refuse to bear weight. They will have severe pain with attempted passive motion of the joint. The neonate may display only anorexia, irritability, and lethargy, and may not move the affected limb (pseudoparalysis) (57,59).

Laboratory studies include peripheral blood studies which typically demonstrate leukocytosis and an elevated ESR and CRP. Blood cultures are positive in 30% to 50% of patients. The CRP is a very good indicator of disease progression, although non-specific. It is elevated in over 90% of children with musculoskeletal infections at the time of admission and quickly returns to normal after treatment. It may also be helpful in the identification of septic arthritis in children with underlying AHO (72).

Joint aspiration typically reveals a white blood cell (WBC) count greater than 50,000 mm^3, with 75% PMNs. Gram stains from the aspirate are positive in 30% to 50%, and cultures from the aspirate are positive in 50% to 80%. Synovial protein levels of 40 mg/dl and less than the serum protein level is consistent with septic arthritis. Lactate levels are typically elevated in septic arthritis (except in *Gonococcal* infection), and glucose measured in the aspirate is lower than serum level. On direct exam, the aspirate may demonstrate gross pus, and there should be a poor mucin (string) test if infection is present.

Imaging evaluation may assist in the diagnosis. Plain radiography may reveal subtle signs early in the disease process, such as capsular distention, joint space widening, and metaphyseal lucency later in the disease course. Technetium bone scan may show decreased uptake ("cold") early in disease process and increased uptake ("hot") later due to hyperemic response (93% sensitivity). Gallium and indium-labeled-leukocyte scans may be helpful in diagnosis of atypical cases but are difficult to perform and, as mentioned in the previous section, take 48 to 72 hours to perform (37).

Ultrasound is quick, painless, and imparts no ionizing radiation. It can detect effusion in 100% of cases, with a criteria being capsule-to-bone distance greater than two millimeters wider than on the other side. This is not specific for septic arthritis, but the absence of an effusion makes septic arthritis unlikely. Ultrasound is also a useful tool to guide aspiration and confirm needle location.

Treatment

The treatment of septic arthritis is a true emergency that often involves the emergency department as well as radiology and orthopedics. It is therefore important to have an established algorithm for treatment.

Treatment consists of constitutional support, including hydration and antibiotics. The cornerstone of treatment is surgical drainage and irrigation of the joint. A capsular window should be removed to ensure continued drainage and a drain left in place until drainage volume decreases. If rapid reversal of clinical symptoms and vital signs does not occur, re-exploration to foster continued drainage should be considered.

The antibiotic regimen should be started immediately after aspiration and based initially on the suspected organism, and later tailored to the culture results. Intravenous antibiotics should be continued until constitutional signs improve. Switching to oral antibiotics may be considered if no concurrent osteomyelitis is present. There is a trend to decreasing the duration of treatment with parental antibiotics (39,48). In the presence of concurrent osteomyelitis, intravenous antibiotics should be continued as described in the preceding section on osteomyelitis.

The causative organisms vary depending primarily on age. In neonates (0 to 28 days old), Group B *Streptococcus* is most common in healthy neonates, and *Staphylococcus aureus* is most common in high-risk neonates. Gram-negative bacilli must also be considered as a possible organism. Recommended antibiotic treatment includes oxacillin or cefotaxime, with the addition of gentamycin in the high-risk neonate.

In infants to children three years of age, *S. aureus* is the most common organism. *Haemophilus influenza* type B is occurring much less frequently and is virtually nonexistent in children immunized with the *H. influenza* type B vaccine (34). If the child is diagnosed with *H. influenza* type B septic arthritis, 20% to 30% have concomitant meningitis. *Kingella kingae* is becoming more frequently identified, primarily in healthy children less than four years of age, and is often associated with an upper respiratory infection. To identify this organism, the culture must be in a BACTEC bottle and needs to be observed for 14 days. The culture is 87% sensitive for detecting *Kingella kingae.* Recommended antibiotics for patients one to three years of age include cefotaxime or ceftriaxone and penicillin for *Kingella kingae* infection (7,44).

In the older child and adolescent, *S. aureus* infection is still common, but other organisms such as *Neisseria gonorrhea* and *Borrelia bergdorferi* (Lyme disease) must be considered. The recommended antibiotic for *S. aureus* infection is oxacillin.

Special Considerations

Gonococcal Arthritis

Gonococcal arthritis is usually found in sexually active teenagers or in newborns transmitted from their mothers during birth. It is associated with rash, tenosynovitis, and migratory polyarthralgia. The knee is the most common joint affected. Sexual abuse is unfortunately common in children with gonococcal disease (19).

Gonococcal arthritis presents in two ways: In the bacteremic form, there are distinctive skin lesions on the extremities (pustules on a hemorrhagic base), frequently positive blood cultures, and multiple joint involvement but often with sterile effusions (44). The second form is a monoarticular purulent arthritis where the aspirate usually yields the organism. Diagnosis of gonococcal arthritis is confirmed by culture, which needs to be grown under special conditions (warm incubation, with low CO_2 and on either chocolate blood agar or Thayer-Martin culture media).

Treatment is initiated with antibiotics. There is growing resistance to penicillin and, therefore, a third-generation cephalosporin is the initial treatment.

Lyme Disease

Lyme disease is caused by the spirochete *Borrelia burgdorferi,* which is carried by the deer tick. It is typically described to occur in three stages: Stage I is a localized infection (erythema migrans); Stage II is early disseminated (myocarditis and/or Bell's palsy); and Stage III is persistent infection (arthritis). However, the clinical manifestations can be variable, and only 40% of those presenting with Lyme disease have classic Lyme arthritis. It often presents as an episodic synovitis affecting one to four joints with asymptomatic intervals and is considered a great mimicker in that the presentation can be similar to other forms of chronic or even acute arthritis. Heel pain may also occur (65).

The laboratory diagnosis for Lyme disease is made by the use of the ELISA serologic test, which is sensitive but not specific. When negative, no further testing is needed. When positive, a western blot test is needed to further confirm the diagnosis. Synovial fluid findings are generally nonspecific. Other laboratory testing, such as the antinuclear antibody (ANA), may also be positive in 30% of cases.

Treatment consists of antibiotic therapy (penicillin or ceftriaxone), with few long-term problems in treated children (65). Surgical intervention is rarely needed (52).

MYCOBACTERIAL INFECTIONS

Mycobacterial infections of the foot are uncommon in children and adults. Most cases involve infections with *Mycobacterium tuberculosis.* Only 2% of cases of musculoskeletal tuberculosis involve the hands or feet, usually by hematogeneous spread (1, 8). Tuberculosis of the ankle is the most common site of distal extremity presentation. When the foot is involved, the talus, subtalar joint, tarsal bones, talonavicular joint, calcaneus, and first metatarsophalangeal joint are frequent sites. Clinical presentation includes indolent swelling and pain. Atypical mycobacterial infections include *Mycobacterium marinum* in feet exposed to tropical fish or marine life and *Mycobacterium fortuitum* in soil-contaminated wounds (13).

The diagnosis should be suspected in high risk groups. Synovial fluid analysis is generally variable with modest WBC counts, averaging 20,000 cells (25). A biopsy of the synovium or bone is needed to confirm the diagnosis and to characterize the organism. Synovial fluid cultures may yield the organism in 80% of the cases (73). Radiographs eventually demonstrate subchondral osteopenia, bony destruction, periosteal thickening, and periarticular erosion.

Treatment with two or more anti-tubercular drugs for at least nine months is indicated. The specific chemotherapeutic regimen should be catered to the organism's susceptibility profile, as multidrug resistance is emerging. Surgery has a secondary role when joint instability requires fusion. *M. fortuitum* has a tendency to form abscesses, and drainage and debridement may be necessary.

FUNGAL INFECTIONS

Tinea Pedis

Perhaps the most common fungal infection on children's feet and ankles is tinea pedis, also known as "athlete's foot." Children are mostly contaminated by their parents (28). Constant use of footwear seems to favor the appearance of this infection (29). There are three forms of clinical presentation: intertriginous (interdigital), moccasin pattern, and vesicular presentation (29). *Tricophyton rubrum* and *Trichophyton mentagrophytes* are the most commonly encountered organisms.

Intertriginous dermatitis is characterized by scaliness, maceration, and cracks in the spaces between the toes. It may spread to the underside of the toes and the dorsum of the foot. Pruritus is the predominant symptom. The moccasin pattern may start with dry, scaly, or hyperkeratotic stains with erythema, on the plantar or lateral surface of the foot. The symptoms are pain and pruritus, and this form is generally chronic and difficult to treat. The third form of tinea pedis is the vesicular type. It manifests as vesicles or pustules on the sole of the foot and is common in the summer.

The treatment consists of the use of local antifungal agents for three to six weeks (28,29). Parents and other family members need to be evaluated and treated in order to efficiently combat this infection. Adequate hygiene for the feet is essential if recurrence is to be avoided. Keeping the feet dry with the aid of talc, using cotton socks, and alternating between different footwear are measures that help in the treatment (29).

Onychomycosis is rare among children. It is thought that the faster nail growth in children and adolescents may make it difficult for fungal infection to appear. However, it is believed that the prevalence of onychomycosis has been increasing among children (61). Onychomycosis is generally associated with tinea pedis. The following risk factors are related to onychomycosis: trauma, hyperhidrosis of the feet, poor personal hygiene, sports activities, contact with animals, positive family history and immunosuppression (61).

Miscellaneous Fungal Infections

Other fungi can infect deeper tissues in the foot, although this is uncommon. In California and the southwestern United States, *Coccidiodes imitis* is found. *Cryptococcus neoformans* may uncommonly infect the foot and ankle. Mycetoma (Madura foot) is a chronic foot infection mainly found in developing countries. Actinomycetes (such as *Nocardia*) or fungi are thought to be introduced through puncture wounds, forming nodules and then gradually spreading through fascial planes in the foot. Advanced cases are severe and may require amputation (45).

FOOT INFECTION WITH NEUROPATHY

The presence of recurrent ulceration among children with sensory deficits should be diligently managed. Congenital malformations of the central nervous system (myelodysplasia); congenital peripheral neuropathy (congenital insensitivity to pain or hereditary motorsensory neuropathy); or acquired peripheral neuropathy (leprosy, diabetes, or Guillain-Barré disease) constitute the main disorders that may result in loss of pedal sensation in children (18). When sensory deficit is associated with significant motor loss, deformities affecting both the foot and the ankle may develop. These deformities result in areas of abnormal pressure and subsequent ulceration. Continuous presence of skin breakdown functions as a gateway for infections through local contamination (42). Correction of deformity is an essential component of long-term treatment of infection in these cases. Once the infection has been cured and the deformities have been corrected, protection with special footwear and orthoses is needed in order to prevent the appearance of new pressure ulcers and reduce the risk of new infection (42,46).

REFERENCES

1. Alvarez S, McCabe W. Extrapulmonary tuberculosis revisited: a review of the experience at Boston City and other hospitals. *Medicine (Baltimore)* 1984;63:25–55.
2. Antoniou D, Conner AN. Osteomyelitis of the calcaneus and talus. *J Bone Joint Surg Am.* 1974;56:338–345.
3. Arnold SR, Elias D, Buckingham SC, et al. Changing patterns of acute hematogeneous osteomyelitis and septic arthritis: emergence of community-associated methicillin-resistant Staphylococcus aureus. *J Pediatr Orthop.* 2006;26:703–708.
4. Ash J, Gilday D. The futility of bone scanning in neonatal osteomyelitis: concise communication. *J Nucl Med.* 1980;21: 417–420.
5. Benjamin HJ, Nikore V, Takagishi J. Practical management: community-associated methicillin-resistant Staphylococcus aureus (CA-MRSA): the latest sports epidemic. *Clin J Sport Med.* 2007;17:393–397.
6. Beretta-Piccoli BC, Sauvain MJ, Gal I, et al. Synovitis, acne, pustulosis, hyperostosis, osteitis (SAPHO) syndrome in childhood: a report of ten cases and review of the literature. *Eur J Pediatr.* 2000;159:594–601.
7. Birgisson H, Steingrimsson O, Gudnason T. Kingella kingae infections in pediatric patients: 5 cases of septic arthritis, osteomyelitis, and bacteraemia. *Scand J Infect Dis* 1997;29: 495–498.
8. Boulware D, Lopez M, Gum O. Tuberculosis podagra. *J Rheumatol.* 1985;12:1022–1024.
9. Bressler EL, Conway JJ, Weiss SC. Neonatal osteomyelitis examined by bone scintigraphy. *Radiology* 1984;152:685–688.
10. Cabanela ME, Sim FH, Beabout JW, et al. Osteomyelitis appearing as neoplasms. A diagnostic problem. *Arch Surg.* 1974;109: 68–72.

11. Canale S, Harkness R, Thomas P, et al. Does aspiration of bones and joints affect results of later bone scanning? *J Pediatr Orthop.* 1985;5:23–26.
12. Chisholm CD, Schlesser JF. Plantar puncture wounds: controversies and treatment recommendations. *Ann Emerg Med.* 1989;18:1352–1357.
13. Colver G, Chattopadhay B, Francis R, et al. Arthritis of the subtalar joint due to Mycobacterium fortuitum. *B M J.* 1981;283:469–470.
14. Crim JR, Seeger LL. Imaging evaluation of osteomyelitis. *Crit Rev Diagn imaging* 1994;35:201–256.
15. Deysine M, Rafkin H, Russell R, et al. The detection of acute experimental osteomyelitis with 67Ga citrate scannings. *Surg Gynecol Obstet.* 1975;141:40–42.
16. Dich V, Nelson J, Haltalin K. Osteomyelitis in infants and children. A review of 163 cases. *Am J Dis Child.* 1975;129:1273–1278.
17. Duffy CM, Lam PY, Ditchfield M, et al. Chronic recurrent multifocal osteomyelitis: review of orthopaedic complications at maturity. *J Pediatr Orthop.* 2002;22:501–505.
18. Dyck PJ, Thomas P eds. *Peripheral neuropathy,* 4th ed. Philadelphia: Saunders, 2005.
19. Folland DS, Burke RE, Hinman AR, et al. Gonorrhea in preadolescent children: an inquiry into source of infection and mode of transmission. *Pediatr.* 1977;60:153–156.
20. Frierson JG, Hecht PJ. Infections of the foot. In Coughlin MJ, Mann RA, eds. *Surg Foot Ankle.* 7th ed. Amsterdam: Elsevier, 1999:880–893.
21. Fustes-Morales A, GutierrezCastrellon P, Duran-Mckinster C, et al. Necrotizing fasciitis: a report of 39 pediatric cases. *Arch Dermatol.* 2002;138:893–899.
22. Gallo JJ. Pseudomonas osteomyelitis secondary to puncture wound of the foot. *J Fam Pract.* 1988;27:529–532.
23. Ganel A, Horozowski H, Zaltzman S, et al. Sequential use of Tc-MDP and GA imaging in bone infection. *Orthop Rev.* 1981;9:73–77.
24. Giannestras NJ. Infections of the foot. In Giannestras NJ, ed. *Foot disorders, medical and surgical management,* 2nd ed. Philadelphia: Lea and Febiger, 1973:631–641.
25. Goldenberg D, Reed J. Bacterial arthritis. *N Engl J Med.* 1985;312:764–771.
26. Green NE, Bruno J. Pseudomonas infections of the foot after puncture wound. *South Med J.* 1989;73:146.
27. Green NE, Edwards K. Bone and joint infection in children. *Orthop Clin North Am.* 1987;18:555–576.
28. Griffin L. Common sports injuries of the foot and ankle seen in children and adolescents. *Orthop Clin North Am.* 1994;25: 83–93.
29. Guest B. Common pediatric foot dermatoses. *J Pediatr Health Care* 1999;13:68–71.
30. Hald J, Sudmann E. Acute hematogenous osteomyelitis: early diagnosis with computed tomography. *Acta Radiol: Diagnosis* 1982;23:55–58.
31. Hamed K, Tam J, Probwe C. Pharmacokinetic optimization of the treatment of septic arthritis. *Clin Pharmacokinet.* 1996;31:156–163.
32. Herndon W, Alexieva B. Nuclear imaging for musculoskeletal infections in children. *J Pediatr Orthop.* 1985;5:343–347.
33. Holmes K, Counts G, Beaty H. Disseminated gonococcal infection. *Ann Intern Med.* 1971;74.
34. Howard AW, Viskontas D, Sabbagh C. Reduction in osteomyelitis and septic arthritis related to Haemophilus influenzae type B vaccination. *J Pediatr Orthop.* 1999;19:705–709.
35. Howie D, Savage J, Wilson T, et al. The technetium phosphate bone scan in the diagnosis of osteomyelitis in childhood. *J Bone Joint Surg Am.* 1983;65:431–437.
36. Huber AM, Lam PY, Duffy CM, et al. Chronic recurrent multifocal osteomyelitis: clinical outcomes after more than five years of follow-up. *J Pediatr.* 2002;141:198–203.
37. Jaramillo D, Treves ST, Kasser JR, et al. Osteomyelitis and septic arthritis in children: appropriate use of imaging to guide treatment. *Am J Roentgenol.* 1995;165:399–403.
38. Jarvis WR, Banko S, Snyder E, et al. Pasteurella multocida: osteomyelitis following dog bites. *Am J Dis Child.* 1981;135:625–627.
39. Kim HK, Alman B, Cole WG. A shortened course of parenteral antibiotic therapy in the management of acute septic arthritis of the hip. *J Pediatr Orthop.* 2000;20:44–47.
40. Kuhn J, Berger P. Computed tomographic analysis of osteomyelitis. *Radiol.* 1979;130:503–506.
41. Lau L, Bin G, Jaovisidua S, et al. Cost effectiveness of magnetic resonance imaging in diagnosing Pseudomonas aeruginosa infection after puncture wound. *J Foot Ankle Surg.* 1997;36:36–43.
42. Levin M, O'Neal L, eds. *The diabetic foot,* 7th ed. St. Louis: Mosby-Year Book Inc., 2007.
43. Lindenbaum S, Alexander H. Infections simulating bone tumors. A review of subacute osteomyelitis. *Clin Orthop Relat Res.* 1984;184:193–203.
44. Lundy DW, Kehl DK. Increasing prevalence of Kingella kingae in osteoarticular infections in young children. *J Pediatr Orthop.* 1998;18:262–267.
45. Mahgoub E. Mycetoma. *Semin Dermatol.* 1985;4:230–239.
46. Mann RA, Coughlin MJ, Saltzman CL, eds. *Surgery of the foot and ankle,* 8th ed. Philadelphia: Mosby, 2008.
47. Manson D, Wilmot D, King S, et al. Physeal involvement in chronic recurrent multifocal osteomyelitis. *Pediatr Radiol.* 1989;20:76–79.
48. Maraqa NF, Gomez MM, Rathore MH. Outpatient parenteral antimicrobial therapy in osteoarticular infections in children. *J Pediatr Orthop.* 2002;22:506–510.
49. Marcy S. Infections due to dog and cat bites. *Pediatr Infect Dis.* 1982;1:351–6.
50. McCarthy JJ, Dormans JP, Kozin SH, et al. Musculoskeletal infections in children. Basic treatment principles and recent advancements. *J Bone Joint Surg Am.* 2004;86:850–863.
51. McHenry CR, Piotrowski JJ, Petrinic D, et al. Determinants of mortality for necrotizing soft tissue infections. *Ann Surg.* 1995;221:558–565.
52. McLaughlin TP, Zemel L, Fisher RL, et al. Chronic arthritis of the knee in Lyme disease. Review of the literature and report of two cases treated by synovectomy. *J Bone Joint Surg Am.* 1986;68:1057–1061.
53. Merkel K, Fitzgerald RJ, Brown M. Scintigraphic evaluation in musculoskeletal sepsis. *Orthop Clin North Am.* 1984;15:401–416.
54. Merkel KD, Brown ML, Dewanjee MK, et al. Comparison of indium-labeled-leukocyte imaging with sequential technetium-gallium scanning in the diagnosis of low-grade musculoskeletal sepsis. A prospective study. *J Bone Joint Surg Am.* 1985;67:465–476.
55. Miron D, Raz R, Kaufman B, et al. Infections following nail puncture wound of the foot: case reports and review of the literature. *Isr J Med Sci.* 1993;29:194–197.
56. Morrison WB, Schweitzer ME, Wapner KL, et al. Osteomyelitis in feet of diabetics: clinical accuracy, surgical utility and cost effectiveness of MR imaging. *Radiol.* 1995;196:557–564.
57. Obletz BE. Acute suppurative arthritis of the hip in the neonatal period. *Am J Orthop.* 1960;42:23–30.
58. Ochoa TJ, Mohr J, Wanger A, et al. Community-associated methicillin-resistant Staphylococcus aureus in pediatric patients. *Emerg Infect Dis.* 2005;11:966–968.
59. Ogden JA, Lister G. The pathophysiology of neonatal osteomyelitis. *Pediatr.* 1975;55:474–478.
60. Patzakis WJ, Wilkins J, Brien WW, et al. Wound site as a predictor of complications following deep nail punctures to the foot. *West J Med.* 1989;150:545–547.
61. Ploysangum T, Lucky A. Childhood white superficial onychomycosis caused by Trichophyton rubrum: report of seven cases and review of the literature. *J Am Acad Dermatol.* 1997;36:29–32.
62. Riegler HF, Routson G. Complications of deep puncture wounds of the foot. *J Trauma.* 1979;19:18–22.

63. Ritterbusch JF. Infections. In Drennan JC, ed. *The child's foot and ankle.* New York: Raven Press, 1992:377–388.
64. Robb J. Primary acute haematogenous osteomyelitis of an isolated metatarsal in children. *Acta Orthop Scand.* 1984;55: 334–338.
65. Rose CD, Fawcett PT, Eppes SC, et al. Pediatric Lyme arthritis: clinical spectrum and outcome. *J Pediatr Orthop.* 1994;14: 238–241.
66. Skevis X. Primary subacute osteomyelitis of the talus. *J Bone Joint Surg Br.* 1984;66-B:101–103.
67. Staheli LT. Infections. In Staheli LT, ed. *Practice of pediatric orthopedics,* 2nd ed. Philadelphia: Lippincott Williams & Wilkins, 2006:345–364.
68. Stazzone MM, Hubbard AM. The pediatric foot and ankle. *Magn Reson Imaging Clin N Am.* 1998;6:661–675.
69. Steere A, Schoen R, Taylor E. The clinical evolution of Lyme arthritis. *Ann Intern Med.* 1987;107:725–731.
70. Synder CC. Animal bite infections of the hand. *Hand Clin.* 1998;14:691–711.
71. Tachibana DK. Microbiology of the foot. *Annu Rev Microbiol.* 1976;30:351–376.
72. Unkila-Kallio L, Kallio MJ, Peltola H. The usefulness of C-reactive protein levels in the identification of concurrent septic arthritis in children who have acute hematogenous osteomyelitis. A comparison with the usefulness of the erythrocyte sedimentation rate and the white blood-cell count. *J Bone Joint Surg Br.* 1994;76:848–853.
73. Valdazo J, Perez-Ruiz F, Albarracin A, et al. Tuberculous arthritis: report of a case with multiple joint involvement and periarticular tuberculous abscesses. *J Rheumatol.* 1990;17: 399–401.
74. *Wrestling rules and interpretations: Appendix D.* In National Collegiate Athletic Association ed. Indianapolis, 2005.

CHAPTER 25

Foot & Ankle Injuries in Adolescent Athletes

Hua Ming Siow, Danielle B. Cameron and Theodore J. Ganley

INTRODUCTION

Adolescence is a period of rapid growth, development, and maturation, which predisposes adolescent athletes to injury. They tend to incur more severe injuries and these occur more frequently than in young children (39,105). This is contributed to by increased body mass and strength, and alterations in flexibility (70,89). Peak muscle strength occurs at peak height velocity for girls and 6–12 months later for boys (1). Other factors which increase injury rates include an increased participation in year-round sports; less protective equipment available; and inadequate stretching, training, and conditioning drills (40). Over one-half of boys and one-quarter of girls in the United States are involved in competitive sport every year (99). Certain activities have a higher risk for injuries, including basketball, soccer, and football (44%, 27% and 16% of all injuries respectively)(23). Foot and ankle injuries are common and occurred in 12.1% of adolescents attending a sports medicine clinic (110). The physician in charge of adolescent athletes must be aware of their unique characteristics and understand the injuries which they incur. This allows the physician to counsel the patient and their families as to the prognosis, treatment, rehabilitation, and eventual return to activities.

ANATOMY

The ankle is a congruous hinge joint with the talus mortised between the medial and lateral malleoli. The dome of the talus is wider anteriorly than posteriorly, resulting in a higher likelihood of injury from translation and rotation when in ankle plantar flexion. The medial and lateral malleoli are held together by the anterior and posterior inferior tibiofibular ligaments and the distal interosseous membrane, creating a tibiofibular syndesmosis. The anterior tibiofibular ligament is important in the pathomechanism of transitional (Tillaux and triplane) fractures.

Medial and collateral ligaments aid in the stability of the ankle. The thick medial deltoid ligament consists of superficial and deep portions. The superficial portion originates from the medial malleolus and inserts into the talus, calcaneus and navicular. The deep portion has the same origin and inserts into the talus. This ligament resists eversion of the ankle. The lateral ligaments consist of the anterior and posterior talofibular ligaments and the calcaneofibular ligament. These ligaments resist inversion of the ankle. The medial and lateral collateral ligaments originate from the tibial and fibular epiphyses and excessive acute stress transmitted through these ligaments commonly result in physeal injuries. The distal tibial physis closes from central to medial and then lateral over a period of 18 months at around the age of 14 (59). Because fractures commonly propagate through the physis, this progression of closure plays an important role on the development of transitional fractures.

MORPHOLOGY

We see many children brought in by concerned parents for in- or out-toeing. An internal foot progression angle is very common in early childhood and is mainly due to internal tibial torsion or femoral anteversion. This improves or resolves in most patients and does not impact their activities (33). However, persisting variations of foot progression angle from the norm may enhance or detract from their performance. Fuchs (32) found that sprinters had a significantly lower thigh-foot angle and foot progression angle while running, as compared to non-sprinters. An external tibial torsion or foot progression angle can hinder gait. Fabry (27) found that compensatory external tibial torsion develops in children with femoral anteversion, and can be permanent. It creates a "miserable malalignment" which consists of femoral anteversion, increased Q angle, and external tibial torsion, which often leads to patellofemoral problems.

Many patients are also seen for pes planus and the incidence in the population is related to age and sex. In one series it was found that 54% of three-year-olds and 24% of six-year-olds had flat feet. (86) Painful flat feet with diminished subtalar motion should alert one to exclude a tarsal coalition or an accessory navicular ossicle. Stress fractures in military recruits have been shown to occur less frequently in those with pes planus. Studies suggest that flexible pes planus is a common benign condition which rarely causes disability and causes discomfort only when the gastroscoleus was tight (38). Surgery is rarely required to correct hindfoot valgus and forefoot supination (14). Hindfoot varus has been studied for its influence on the development of Sever's apophysitis. McKenzie (74) found that subtalar and forefoot varus was a common finding whereas others (78) found that most children had normal alignment and pronation was the most common deformity found.

Pes cavus is more likely to cause problems than pes planus. Children with pes cavus, especially unilateral pes cavus, should be evaluated for an underlying neurological cause such as Charcot-Marie-Tooth disease, Friedreich's ataxia a tethered cord or other spinal pathology. Griffin (40) recommended orthotics for the treatment of metatarsalgia or clawing of the toes. Sneyers (96) found that patients with pes cavus had a higher rate of lower limb injury due to inadequate shock absorption during locomotion. He noted that the relative load under the forefoot was higher in pes cavus.

Flexibility and strength also seem to play a role in foot and ankle injuries in adolescent athletes. Baumhauer (4) studied predisposing factors to ankle injury in 145 college athletes. General ligamentous laxity, ankle alignment, and ankle ligament stability were not found to be predisposing factors. It was noted that the injured group had a significant strength imbalance with a greater plantar flexion-to-dorsiflexion and eversion-to-inversion strength ratio. Kibler (59) showed that athletes with plantar fasciitis had strength and flexibility deficits in the calf and foot of the affected side. Similar findings have been found in Sever's apophysitis.

PHYSICAL EXAMINATION

The history is often unreliable in the pediatric population, and the entire lower limb should be evaluated, with special attention to the symptomatic areas. Inspection will reveal swelling, deformity, or ecchymosis. Significant swelling or ecchymosis frequently indicates physeal or bony injury. Palpation should assess the distal tibial and fibular physes, the most common areas of injury in the lower limbs of children (22). Tenderness over the deltoid and lateral ligaments may imply instability of the ankle from ligamentous injury. This may be assessed with an anterior "drawer" maneuver. The range of motions of the ankle, subtalar, and knee joints should be assessed, as well as ankle strength and alignment of the lower limb. The proximal fibula should be palpated for swelling or tenderness to exclude Maisonneuve fractures.

It is important to exclude child abuse or pathological fractures if the mechanism of injury does not match the presenting injury. Systemic signs and symptoms or chronic pain should bring suspicion to bear on entities such as juvenile rheumatoid arthritis, seronegative spondyloarthropathy, septic arthritis, osteomyelitis, hemophilia, sickle cell disease, neurological disorders, leukemia, and other tumors.

RADIOGRAPHY

Radiography is used to correlate clinical findings and is not a substitute for a thorough examination of the limbs. If an ankle injury is suspected, anteroposterior (AP), lateral, and mortise views are taken (Figures 25-1 and 25-2). The mortise view is important to detect syndesmotic rupture and may aid visualization of Tillaux fractures or osteochondral lesions. Pain localized to the foot necessitates AP, lateral, and oblique films of the foot. Fractures such as Salter-Harris I fractures may reveal only soft-tissue swelling or slight widening of the physis. In such cases, clinical suspicion of a fracture will have to suffice if the radiographic signs are too subtle. There are also multiple ossification centers in the foot and ankle which may be confused with a fracture. In such cases, a comparison view of the opposite limb may be helpful.

Further investigation by computed tomography (CT) for complex intra-articular fractures, or magnetic resonance imaging (MRI) for intra-articular cartilaginous lesions, may be necessary according to clinical indications.

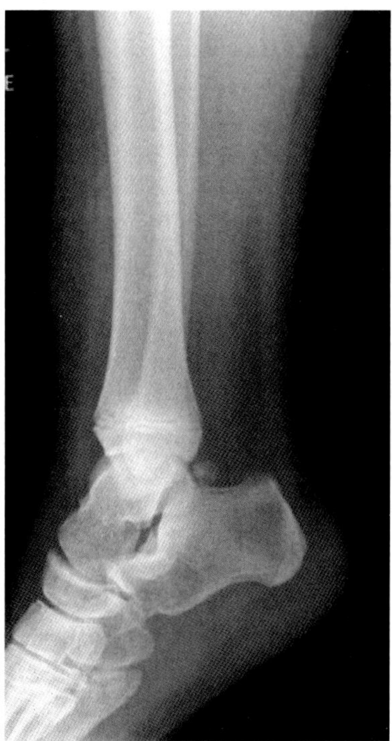

FIGURE 25-1 Os trigonum.

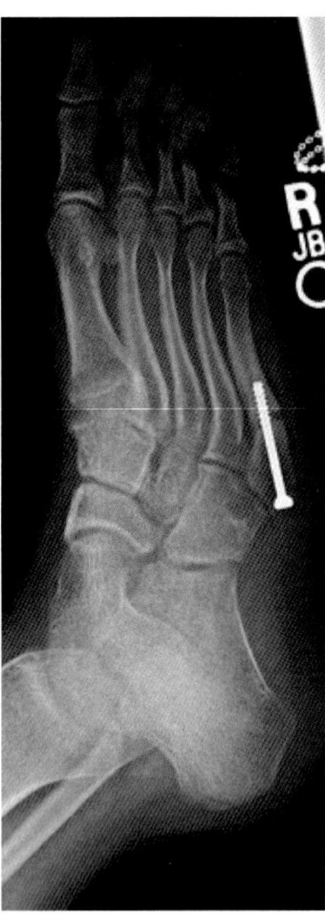

FIGURE 25-2 Jones fracture with half-threaded screw fixation.

CONGENITAL AND DEVELOPMENTAL CONDITIONS

Tarsal Coalition

Tarsal coalition should be suspected in children with recurrent ankle sprains or distal fibular physeal fractures (26,85). These might be due to an increase in stress on the ankle from loss of subtalar motion (6). This is covered in Chapter 11.

Accessory Ossicles

Accessory Navicular

The accessory navicular is the most common accessory bone in the foot and occurs in 4% to 21% of the population, but few become symptomatic (81). It is located at the site of the tibialis posterior tendon insertion into the navicular. Grogan (41) conducted a histological study and concluded that pain was caused by microfractures through the cartilage synchondrosis. Pain may also arise through pressure over the bony prominence or from tibialis posterior tendonitis (15). Adolescent athletes may present with a painful and tender navicular prominence, exacerbated by foot inversion against resistance (104). There may also be erythema or a bursa over a large accessory navicular. The diagnosis is confirmed with an AP or 45° eversion oblique radiograph. Management of symptomatic patients is by shoe wear modification, orthotics, and physical therapy. Excision is reserved for persistently symptomatic patients.

Os Trigonum

An os trigonum occurs in 10% of the population and arises from failure of fusion of an ossification center in the posterior aspect of the talus (9). In some cases, it may occur from nonunion of a fracture caused by acute hyperplantarflexion or plantar inversion (82). It is frequently unilateral and asymptomatic. However it can cause mechanical impingement of the posterior talus and capsule between the posterior tibia and the calcaneus. This occurs in athletes who regularly plantar flex their ankles such as ballet dancers, ice skaters, gymnasts, or soccer players (48). Pain occurs in the posterolateral ankle, and is reproduced on plantar flexion. Associated posteromedial pain may point toward a concurrent flexor hallucis longus tendonitis (44). A lateral radiograph will reveal the os trigonum and plantar flexion views may demonstrate compression (Figure 25-1). Conservative treatment consists of rest, anti-inflammatories, activity modification, casting, and injection (9,48). Resection is usually successful and flexor hallucis longus tenolysis may be required if that tendon is also involved.

Medial Malleolus Ossification Center

Stanitski (98) described 11 cases in children who had pain, swelling, and tenderness over the medial malleolus without a history of acute injury. Radiographs revealed an irregular ossification center at the tip of the medial malleolus, with some having ossicles. They were treated with three weeks of rest, with another three weeks of casting if persistently symptomatic. They rarely require surgical excision.

Bunions

Adolescent bunions have an incidence of up to 35% (37). They have been attributed to metatarsus primus varus (67) and heredity (71). They are more common in girls involved in dancing and gymnastics, sports which place stress on the metatarsophalangeal joint of the hallux (14). Flat feet do not appear to affect its occurrence or recurrence after surgery (21).They differ from adult bunions in that there is typically no arthritic change in the metatarsophalangeal joint or a medial bursa (20). Hallux valgus is more likely in children with an intermetatarsal angle of more than 10° (71). Symptomatic treatment is through selection of broader footwear, orthotics, and activity modification. Surgery is reserved for recalcitrant symptomatic cases, consisting of a combination of a soft-tissue procedure with a proximal or distal osteotomy of the first metatarsal. This is covered in greater detail in Chapter 18.

FRACTURES (SEE CHAPTER 22)

Ankle Fractures

Ankle and foot fractures commonly occur in children and adolescents participating in sports activities. Acute fractures are covered in detail in Chapter 22.

Classification

Stress Fractures

Stress fractures occur following repetitive trauma in athletes and military recruits. DeLee (24) has described them as being spontaneous fractures of normal bones which result from the summation of stresses which would be harmless individually. With sudden increased training intensity, muscle strength increases while osteoclastic resorption of bone occurs for two weeks (42). During the third and fourth week, increased periosteal and endosteal bone formation occurs and the risk of stress fracture decreases henceforth. Decreasing the intensity of training in the third week may decrease the incidence of stress fractures. Other preventative measures include correcting training errors, improving nutrition, addressing medical issues and ensuring the proper use of equipment. Shock-absorbing insoles are also useful in prevention (34,80).

Stress fractures present with localized pain which is aggravated by weight bearing or exercise. There is tenderness of the affected site. Radiographs may show a radiolucent line initially, followed by a periosteal reaction and callus formation after two weeks. Bone scans or CT may be useful if there is any uncertainty in the diagnosis. Treatment mainly consists of abstention from activity until the fracture is shown to be healing well, followed by a gradual increase in the level of training. Particular attention needs to be focused on navicular, proximal second and fifth metatarsal, and sesamoid stress fractures. These fractures are prone to result in chronic pain or poor healing. They are generally treated with six to eight weeks in a short leg cast. Persisting symptoms may necessitate screw fixation (Figure 25-2) and possibly bone grafting for the navicular and metatarsals, or resection for the sesamoids.

Osteochondral Lesions of the Talus

These lesions occur in the talar dome, often after an innocuous ankle sprain, and must be considered in the diagnosis should an ankle sprain not respond to treatment within six to eight weeks (11,24). Berndt and Harty (5) conducted cadaver studies and produced lateral osteochondral injuries with inversion and dorsiflexion, and medial lesions with inversion, plantar flexion, and lateral rotation of the tibia on the talus (Figure 25-3). The atraumatic lesions are believed to result from impaired circulation to the subchondral bone of the talar dome. Canale and Belding (10) noted in their series that all lateral lesions and 64% of medial lesion were caused by trauma, whereas 77% of our patients sustained trauma with no difference between medial and lateral lesions (93).

Patients present with pain and swelling in the ankle associated with occasional catching, popping or locking. Plain radiographs will identify most lesions, with MRI having a high sensitivity for smaller lesions and CT able to aid in staging or preoperative planning. Correlation has not been found between plain radiographic images and findings at arthroscopy (33) (Figure 25-4). Berndt and Harty (5) developed a classification system as follows:

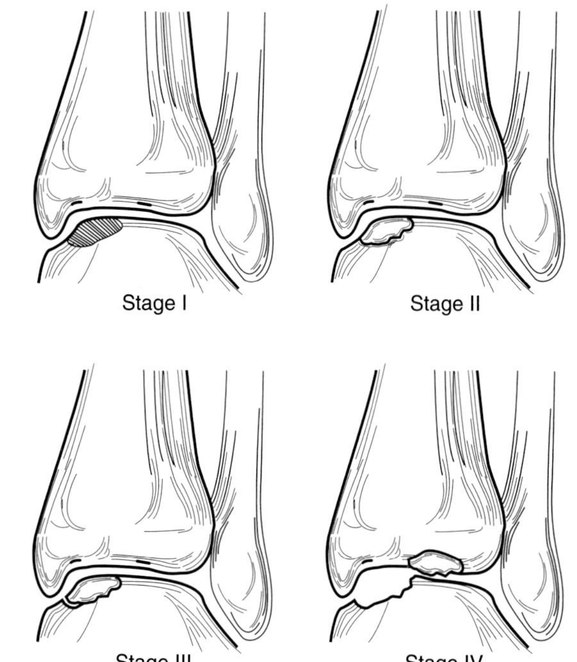

FIGURE 25-3 Berndt and Harty OCD classification.

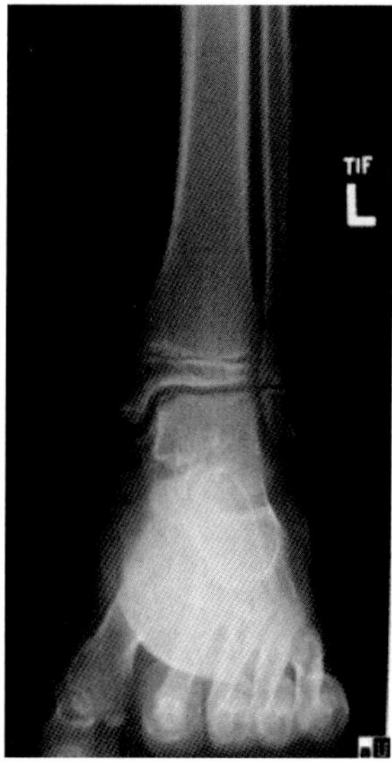

FIGURE 25-4 OCD lesion on medial talar dome.

Stage I had a small area of subchondral compression; Stage II had a partially detached fragment; Stage III had a completely detached fragment in the crater; and Stage IV had a fragment which was loose in the joint (fig 25.3).

Treatment for children with open physes and Stage I and II lesions consists of immobilization and non-weight-bearing for six weeks, with follow up at three months and six months. Patients with symptoms for more than six months or have Stage III and IV lesions are treated arthroscopically. This consists of removal of loose bodies and drilling of the defect, with fixation reserved for large fragments. Debridement and curettage have also been reported with good results (64,88,93).

Osteochondroses

These are a group of conditions of unknown etiology. On radiographs, they are initially sclerotic, followed by fragmentation and gradual reossification over one or two years. This is covered in greater detail in chapter 28.

Kohler's Disease

This is an osteochondrosis of the navicular which usually affects active boys between the ages of four to seven years (84). It is usually unilateral, but may be bilateral in up to one-fourth of all cases (47). It is usually caused by repetitive trauma to the maturing epiphysis (47). Patients present with mid-foot pain which is worse on weight bearing, along with tenderness, swelling, and erythema of the navicular. Radiographs demonstrate increased sclerosis and narrowing of the navicular. However, irregular ossification in this bone can be a normal finding, and this can cause confusion. Patients do well with activity restriction and non-steroidal anti-inflammatory drugs (NSAIDs), or four to six weeks in a short leg cast for the more severe cases.

Freiberg's Infraction

This is an osteonecrosis of the second metatarsal distal epiphysis. It is rarely seen in the third, fourth, or fifth metatarsal heads. The etiology may be due to repetitive trauma in athletics or foot pronation with a hypermobile first metatarsal, with resultant increased pressure under the second metatarsal (76). The average age at presentation is 13 years, and 75% of patients are female. They present with forefoot pain which is worse on weight bearing and activity. Examination reveals tenderness over the affected metatarsal head. Radiographs initially show widening of the metatarsophalangeal joint space, followed by collapse and sclerosis of the articular surface of the metatarsal head (14,47,103). Reossification occurs in two or three years. Treatment consists of avoidance of weight bearing on the affected metatarsal, an orthosis to correct pronation in pes planus, (46) or a short leg cast for six to twelve weeks for more severe cases. Refractory cases are treated by surgical debridement or dorsiflexion osteotomy (12,60).

Apophysitis

The apophyses are the bony insertion sites of tendons which develop as accessory ossification centers and mimic the maturation of an epiphyseal plate. They are placed under constant stress from muscle contraction, which can result in irritation of the physis, known as an apophysitis (13).

Sever's Disease

Sever's disease is a traction apophysitis of the calcaneus which accounts for 8% of all overuse injuries in children (69). It occurs most commonly in athletes between the ages of 8 and 13 (99) and occurs bilaterally in 61% (78). It has been attributed to chronic repetitive shear stress on the vertically oriented apophysis by the triceps surae and the plantar fascia. Aggravating factors include starting a new sport or season, foot pronation, and a tight gastrocnemius-soleus complex secondary to a recent growth spurt (77).

Patients present with heel pain aggravated by activity, especially running and jumping, which is found in sports such as soccer and basketball. Examination reveals localized tenderness of the posterior heel at the insertion of the Achilles tendon, tightness of the Achilles tendons, and weakness of the ankle dorsiflexors (78). Radiographs may reveal fragmentation and sclerosis of the calcaneal apophysitis, but the appearance can be normal as well. In addition, irregularity of the apophysis is a common finding in normal children. It is important to rule out other causes of heel pain such as Achilles tendonitis due to a tight Achilles tendon, infection, tumors, and fractures. Treatment consists of rest, activity modification, NSAIDs, Achilles stretching, ankle dorsiflexion strengthening, and shoe inserts such as heel cups, pads, or lifts.

Iselin's Disease

This is a traction apophysitis of the base of the fifth metatarsal. It appears a small bone fleck on the lateral plantar aspect of the tuberosity, and is located within the insertion of the peroneus brevis tendon. It is best seen on oblique radiographs. The apophysis is located parallel to the shaft of the metatarsal and is differentiated from an avulsion fracture, which is usually transverse (Figure 25-5). The apophysis appears at the age of ten in girls and twelve in boys, fusing about two years later. (12)

The patient is usually a young athlete involved in sports that entail running, cutting, or jumping as these may produce an inversion stress to the area. They present with pain over the lateral aspect of the foot, with tenderness and swelling of the tuberosity. Resisted eversion, extreme

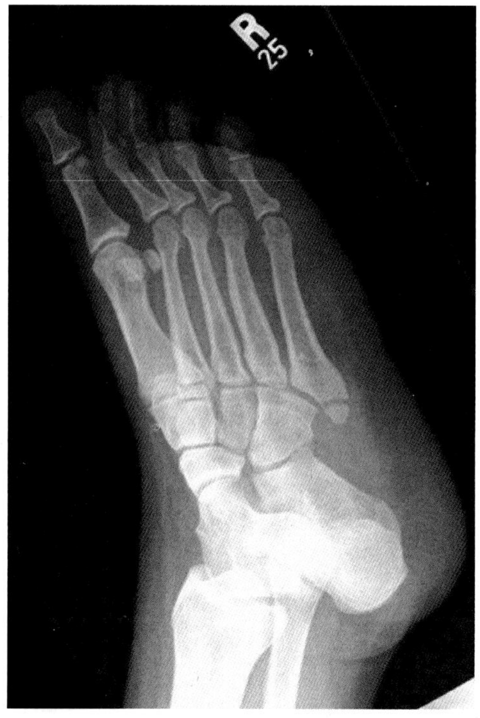

FIGURE 25-5 Fifth metatarsal base avulsion fracture.

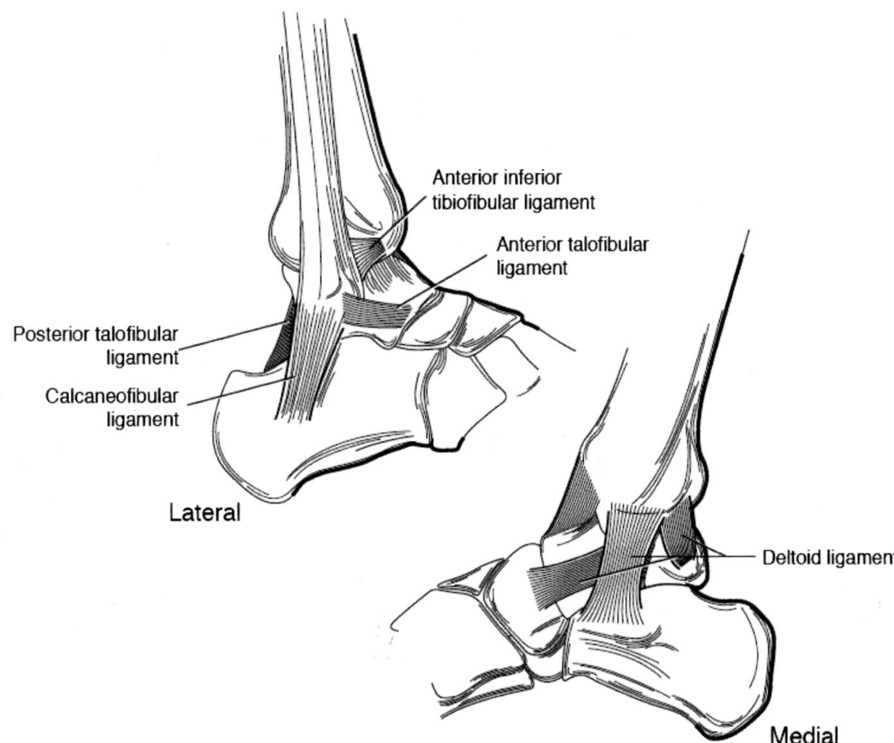

FIGURE 25-6 The medial and lateral ligaments of the ankle.

dorsiflextion, and plantar flexion of the foot exacerbate the pain. A bone scan is usually positive. Treatment consists of immobilization for more severe cases, activity modification, NSAIDs, stretching, and strengthening of the peroneal tendon.

Ankle Sprains

Ankle sprains are the most frequent injury sustained by athletes, estimated to comprise up to 45% of all injuries (35,36,90,109). These usually occur during jumping and cutting sports, such as basketball, football, soccer, and volleyball. Younger children usually injure the distal fibular physis and do not get lateral ankle sprains; however, more mature children and adolescents do. Patients with previous ankle sprains or those who are younger at the time of injury are at risk for recurrent injury (66). Smith (66) found that high school basketball players had an 80% recurrence of ankle sprains and 15% had residual symptoms. Baumhauer (4) has shown that athletes with higher eversion to inversion and lower dorsiflexion to plantar flexion strength ratios had a higher incidence of ankle sprains.

Lateral ankle stability is provided by static and dynamic restraints. The static stabilizers include the anterior talofibular (ATFL) and posterior talofibular ligaments (PTFL) and the calcaneofibular ligament (CFL). They also serve an important proprioceptive role in balance. Dynamic stability is provided by the peroneal muscles, which increase in importance if the lateral ligaments are deficient. The ATFL is the most taut in plantar flexion and is the main stabilizer to ankle inversion in plantarflexion. It is also the weakest lateral ankle ligament. The CFL is most taut in dorsiflexion and also aids in subtalar stability. The PTFL is the strongest ligament and is rarely injured, being taut only in severe dorsiflexion (Figure 25-6).

Lateral ankle sprains most commonly occur during inversion of a plantar flexed ankle, resulting in injury to the ATFL in two-thirds of injuries, and more severe combined ATFL and CFL injuries in one quarter of injuries (36,66,90). Patients usually report hearing a "pop" with acute pain and swelling at the time of injury. The location of swelling and tenderness allows the examiner to distinguish fibular physeal fractures from lateral ankle sprains. Grade 1 sprains consist of a stretched ATFL with no associated instability. These are the most common, with minimal swelling. They usually return to sports in one to two weeks. Grade 2 sprains signify a complete ATFL tear and partial tear of the CFL, with increased swelling and mild joint laxity and instability. They usually take six weeks to return to sports. Grade 3 sprains result from complete rupture of the ATFL and CFL, with gross instability, marked swelling and usually severe pain. Recovery can take three months or more.

Functional rehabilitation is advised for Grade 1 and 2 injuries. This consists of RICE (Rest, Ice, Compression, Elevation) therapy initially. This is followed by protective bracing or taping and early weight bearing. Finally range of motion exercises, strengthening of the dynamic ankle stabilizers, Achilles stretching, proprioceptive and endurance training is carried out. Most Grade 3 injuries respond well to early functional treatment. This provides the fastest recovery of ankle mobility and earliest return to work and physical activity without affecting late mechanical stability, compared to immobilization or

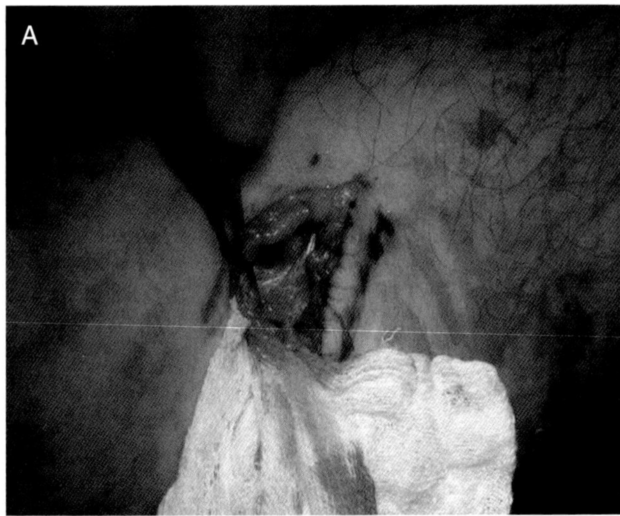

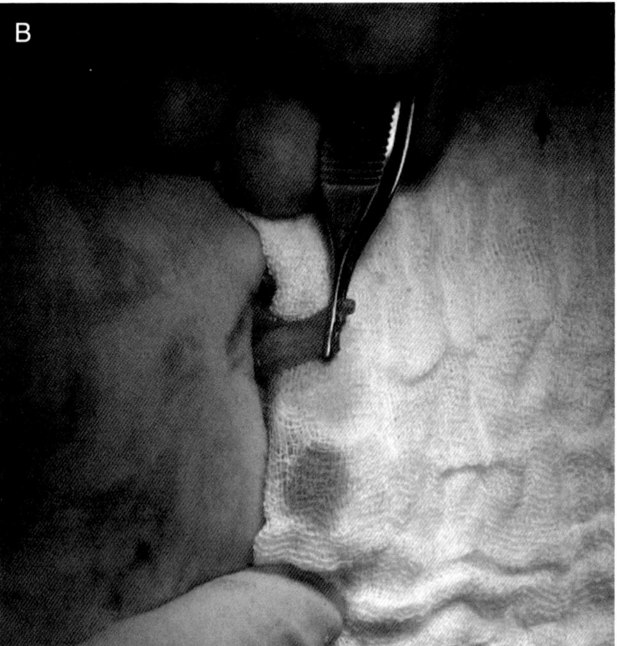

FIGURE 25-7 **A.** Torn ATFL: superior portion. **B.** Inferior portion.

surgery (63,68). Secondary surgical repair, even years after an injury, has results comparable to those of primary repair (Figure 25-7). Thus competitive athletes can initially receive conservative treatment, unless certain circumstances are present which would prevent them from reaching their full potential. These circumstances include severe AP laxity, severe medial and lateral ligamentous injury, associated large avulsion fracture of the fibula, displaced osteochondral lesion of the talus, and a history of recurrent severe ankle sprains (16,89,109). Marsh (72) has described a modified Chrisman-Snook repair on children with a mean age of 14.5 years, with good results in terms of return to sports and high patient satisfaction. However it is important to consider the potential for complications with surgery, including poor wound healing, infection, and nerve injury (87).

Distal syndesmotic or "high" ankle sprains account for 10% to 20% of all ankle sprains, but result in more disability and greater lost playing time compared to lateral ankle sprains (7,50,56,106). The syndesmotic complex is composed of the anteroinferior tibiofibular (AITFL), posteroinferior tibiofibular (PITFL), transverse tibiofibular, and interosseous ligaments. The AITFL provides the majority of the stability to the syndesmosis and is the most frequently injured.

High impact and collision sports cause these injuries by imparting a violent external rotation force to the foot. They usually present with inability to bear weight, although some will only have pain with ankle dorsiflexion or push off. Normally, there is tenderness anteriorly over the AITFL, with mild swelling. The squeeze test may indicate syndesmotic injury if there is distal pain on compressing the fibula to the tibia in the mid-calf (50). Pain may also occur with the external rotation test when the foot is externally rotated with the knee flexed to 90° (7). Radiographs should include a mortise view of the ankle with possible stress external rotation views to reveal an occult diastasis of the ankle.

Stable, isolated syndesmotic sprain is treated with a walking cast for two to six weeks, followed by functional rehabilitation. Recovery may take twice as long as a comparable lateral ankle sprain (113,114). Unstable injuries with diastasis require surgical stabilization, which may consist of repair of the AITFL, debridement of the distal tibiofibular joint space, or fixation of the syndesmosis with a screw (45,92,113). The ankle is immobilized in a short leg cast for four weeks after surgery, followed by progressive weight bearing, removal of any syndesmotic screws at eight to twelve weeks, and the use of an ankle brace for six months.

Medial ankle sprains are less common and are associated with a higher incidence of syndesmotic injury. They are more unstable than lateral ankle sprains and are treated with non–weight-bearing casts for three weeks, followed by rehabilitation (111). Recurrent ankle sprains should bring to mind the possibility of tarsal coalition.

Anterior Ankle Impingement Syndrome

Anterior ankle impingement can be bony or soft tissue related. Bony impingement is seen in ballet dancers and gymnasts who exercise in extreme ankle dorsiflexion, resulting in talar neck periosteal irritation and exostosis formation (77). Soft-tissue impingement can occur due to synovitis or capsulitis from acute or recurrent episodes of inversion ankle sprain, or from repeated forced dorsiflexion on landing in gymnasts (84). Examination reveals tenderness anteriorly, frequently with a tight Achilles tendon. An MRI is useful for diagnosis. Treatment consists of activity modification, icing, NSAIDs, stretching for the Achilles tendon, and dorsiflexion strengthening exercises. Arthroscopic partial synovectomy or osteophyte resection is indicated if conservative treatment fails (108).

Recurrent ankle sprains, especially in soccer players, can cause a "meniscoid lesion." This is a band of white, fibrous, meniscus-like tissue between the fibula and talus which causes anterolateral swelling and pain. Repetitive microtrauma can also result in a hypertrophied ATFL. Patients present with increased pain on ankle dorsiflexion and tenderness over the ATFL. Both the "meniscoid lesion" and hypertrophied ATFL can be treated with arthroscopic debridement.

Posterior Ankle Impingement Syndrome

This is seen most commonly in gymnasts, ballet dancers, divers, and ice skaters. These sports require extreme plantar flexion of the ankle, resulting in compression of the posterior structures of the ankle. There are various causes for pain including os trigonum, flexor hallucis longus (FHL) tendonitis, bursitis, synovitis, or calcified inflammatory tissue (43,51,53). Os trigonum has been covered earlier in the chapter under *Accessory Ossicles.* Patients typically have tenderness over the posterior ankle, which is worsened by forced plantar flexion. Radiographs will help visualize a bony etiology, while MRI is useful for soft-tissue pathology.

Dancers with posteromedial ankle pain may have FHL tendonitis. With chronic inflammation and hypertrophy, the tendon gets compressed in plantar flexion over the posterior talar tubercle (43). With dorsiflexion, the FHL is stretched between the posterior talar tubercle and the sustentaculum tali. Some patients develop a stenosing FHL tenosynovitis with locking of the hallux interphalangeal joint in flexion. These are treated with rest, NSAIDs and physical therapy. Occasionally, the tendon sheath is released if symptoms persist. (62)

Retrocalcaneal bursitis results from inflammation of the bursa anterior to the Achilles tendon. There will be tenderness just superior and anterior to the insertion of the Achilles tendon, (30) which will help distinguish it from Achilles tendonitis. This condition occurs more commonly in ice skaters. Treatment is usually conservative, and bursectomy with partial calcaneal resection is rarely required (55).

Ankle trauma may cause articular chondral damage or bone injury, resulting in chronic impingement of soft tissues. This can cause synovitis, capsulitis, and development of calcified inflammatory tissue. Treatment includes rest and NSAIDs, with arthroscopic resection of the pathological tissue rarely required.

Tarsal Tunnel Syndrome

This is an entrapment neuropathy of the tibial nerve within the tarsal tunnel. Kinoshita (61) noted that this occurred for young athletes mainly involved in repetitive motions such as sprinting, jumping, or performing martial arts. It is covered in more detail in chapter 26. It can be caused by ganglia, bony prominence from tarsal coalition or previous bony injury, accessory muscles or pes planus. Symptoms comprise of pain, paraesthesiae, or numbness of the sole, mainly in the medial aspect. A tendency to walk with the foot in supination is noted in children (2). Tinel's sign and nerve compression test over the tibial nerve posterior to the medial malleolus is positive (2,61). Electrodiagnostic studies help confirm the diagnosis. Conservative treatment consisting of rest, NSAIDs, physical therapy, foot orthoses, and injections can be considered, but athletes frequently fail to return to sport. In such cases, decompression of the tibial nerve is indicated and is usually successful in restoring function.

Haglund Deformity

This is an abnormal bony prominence along the posteriosuperior surface of the calcaneus. It is commonly seen in adolescent females as a result of shoewear (65), and also in ice skaters, skiers, runners and soccer players. Examination reveals a bony prominence more on the lateral aspect with overlying dermal thickening. There may be an associated retrocalcaneal bursitis or Achilles tendonitis as well. Treatment is through padding of the prominence, increasing shoe size or using a heel pad to lift the foot slightly out of the shoe (101). Surgical excision of the bony mass may be required if conservative measures fail (107).

Tendonitis

Overuse injuries of the tendons occur when there is excessive physical activity with insufficient rest, or there are muscle contractures secondary to normal longitudinal growth of the bones. Poor technique, or inadequate footwear or protection are also factors. (73) The Achilles tendon is most commonly affected, but the FHL, anterior and posterior tibialis muscle and peroneal muscle tendons can also be involved (18,19,31). Tendonitis presents with acute onset of sharp and severe pain. Examination reveals tenderness over the path of the involved tendon with weakness and stiffness of the affected tendon. For Achilles tendonitis, there is pain and tenderness at the heel over the tendon, together with a lack of adequate ankle dorsiflexion. Treatment consists of Achilles stretching, strengthening, orthotics, NSAIDs, and the addition of a heel cup or lift. Runners should have shoes with a firm heel and a flexible forefoot, to decrease the lever arm of the gastrocnemius-soleus complex (112).

Peroneal Tendon Subluxation

Children are prone to having peroneal tendon subluxation, most of which are asymptomatic. Some of these are congenital, but most are post-traumatic occurring from snow skiing, ice skating, running, basketball, soccer, or football (8,17). The peroneal tendons are located behind the lateral malleolus in a fibro-osseous tunnel formed by a groove in the fibula and the superior peroneal retinaculum. The peroneal muscles serve as both plantar flexors and evertors of the foot. There may be an anatomic predisposition to peroneal tendon subluxation, such as an absent or shallow fibular groove, possibly combined with pes planus, hindfoot valgus, or a lax or absent peroneal retinaculum. The retinaculum can also rupture from a forced dorsiflexion of the ankle with reflex contraction of the peroneal muscles resulting in dislocation (8,17,25,31,76,91,102).

Athletes may present with an apparent ankle sprain with pain and swelling over the posterolateral aspect of the ankle. They more commonly present weeks or months after the injury with recurrent ankle sprains and lateral ankle instability combined with painful snapping across the ankle (58,97). Subluxation is provoked by forceful ankle dorsiflexion and eversion and there may be acute tenderness behind the posterior malleolus. Radiographs may show a bony avulsion "rim fracture" along the posterior border of the fibula, indicating an avulsion of the superior peroneal retinaculum (83,91).

Acute treatment consists of casting in mild plantar flexion and inversion for six weeks. However, athletes tend to have recurrent symptoms with sports and require operative treatment. Many procedures have been described including retinaculum repair and reconstruction, bony procedures to deepen the groove, bone block procedures, and rerouting of tendons behind the calcaneofibular ligament (17,25,28,52,58,75,79,94,100). If a bony procedure is performed, the patient is required to be skeletally mature to avoid injury to the growth plate.

Turf Toe

Turf toe is a hyperextension injury of the hallux metatarsophalangeal (MTP) joint which results in subluxation and a capsular sprain. Less common mechanism include hyperflexion, valgus and varus strains (54). It is linked to athletes competing on hard artificial surfaces, such as in football, soccer, and basketball, combined with the use of flexible lightweight shoes. Patients present with pain over the medial and plantar aspect of the first MTP joint, associated with swelling and ecchymosis. They have difficulty with push-off due to pain.

Grade I injuries result in pain and mild tenderness, but the athlete is able to continue running with toe taping. Grade II injury results in a loss of motion, moderate pain, and ecchymosis, with inability to play sports for one to two weeks. Grade III injury has severe pain, swelling, and ecchymosis. The athlete is unable to bear weight on the injured toe and requires crutches with casting for a week. The athlete is not allowed to return to sports for four to six weeks. Initial treatment consists of ice, compression, and NSAIDs. Follow-up measures include toe taping, stiffer shoe soles, and activity modification.

Injury Prevention

Hergenroeder (49) has outlined six potential strategies for reducing injuries in youth sports. These include: (i) the pre-season physical examination, (ii) medical coverage at sporting events, (iii) proper coaching, (iv) adequate hydration, (v) proper officiating, and (vi) proper equipment and field/surface playing conditions. Other issues correlated with injury include excessive pressure to perform well in sports, poor psychological coping skills, and lack of social support (29).

It is important to ensure that the above strategies to reduce injury are utilized fully, and any medical or psychosocial issues are addressed before allowing young athletes to compete. This will allow them to avoid injury and benefit from sports to improve their fitness, motor coordination, socialization skills, and self-image.

REFERENCES

1. Adirim TA, Cheng TL. Overview of injuries in the young athlete. *Sports Med* 2003;33(1):75–81.
2. Albrektsson B, Rydholm A, Rydholm U. The tarsal tunnel syndrome in children. *J Bone Joint Surg Br* 1982;64(2):215–217.
3. Bailie DS, Kelikian AS. Tarsal tunnel syndrome: diagnosis, surgical technique, and functional outcome. *Foot Ankle Int* Feb 1998;19(2):65–72.
4. Baumhauer JF, Alosa DM, Renstrom AF, Trevino S, Beynnon B. A prospective study of ankle injury risk factors. *Am J Sports Med* Sep–Oct 1995;23(5):564–570.
5. Berndt AL, Harty M. Transchondral fractures (osteochondritis dissecans) of the talus. *J Bone Joint Surg Am* Sep 1959;41-A:988–1020.
6. Bohne WH. Tarsal coalition. *Curr Opin Pediatr* Feb 2001;13(1):29–35.
7. Boytim MJ, Fischer DA, Neumann L. Syndesmotic ankle sprains. *Am J Sports Med* May–Jun 1991;19(3):294–298.
8. Brage ME, Hansen ST, Jr. Traumatic subluxation/dislocation of the peroneal tendons. *Foot Ankle* Sep 1992;13(7):423–431.
9. Brodsky AE, Khalil MA. Talar compression syndrome. *Foot Ankle* Jun 1987;7(6):338–344.
10. Canale ST, Belding RH. Osteochondral lesions of the talus. *J Bone Joint Surg Am* Jan 1980;62(1):97–102.
11. Canale ST. Fractures of the neck of the talus. *Orthopedics* Oct 1990;13(10):1105–1115.
12. Canale ST. *Osteochondroses and related problems of the foot and ankle.* Vol 2. 2 ed. Philadelphia: Saunders; 2003.
13. Carr K. Musculoskeletal injuries in young athletes. *Clin Fam Pract* 2003;5(2):385–406.
14. Chambers HG. Ankle and foot disorders in skeletally immature athletes. *Orthop Clin North Am* Jul 2003;34(3):445–459.
15. Chen YJ, Shih HN, Huang TJ, Hsu RW. Posterior tibial tendon tear combined with a fracture of the accessory navicular: a new subclassification? *J Trauma* Nov 1995;39(5):993–996.
16. Clanton TO, Porter DA. Primary care of foot and ankle injuries in the athlete. *Clin Sports Med* Jul 1997;16(3):435–466.
17. Clarke HD, Kitaoka HB, Ehman RL. Peroneal tendon injuries. *Foot Ankle Int* May 1998;19(5):280–288.
18. Clement DB, Taunton JE, Smart GW. Achilles tendinitis and peritendinitis: etiology and treatment. *Am J Sports Med* May–Jun 1984;12(3):179–184.
19. Conti SF. Posterior tibial tendon problems in athletes. *Orthop Clin North Am* Jan 1994;25(1):109–121.
20. Coughlin MJ, Mann RA. The pathophysiology of the juvenile bunion. *Instr Course Lect* 1987;36:123–136.
21. Coughlin MJ. Roger A. Mann Award. Juvenile hallux valgus: etiology and treatment. *Foot Ankle Int* Nov 1995;16(11):682–697.
22. Crawford A. *Fractures and dislocations of the foot and ankle.* Philadelphia: Saunders Company; 1998.
23. Damore DT, Metzl JD, Ramundo M, Pan S, Van Amerongen R. Patterns in childhood sports injury. *Pediatr Emerg Care* Apr 2003;19(2):65–67.
24. DeLee JC, Evans JP, Julian J. Stress fracture of the fifth metatarsal. *Am J Sports Med* Sep–Oct 1983;11(5):349–353.
25. Eckert WR, Davis EA, Jr. Acute rupture of the peroneal retinaculum. *J Bone Joint Surg Am* Jul 1976;58(5):670–672.
26. Elkus RA. Tarsal coalition in the young athlete. *Am J Sports Med* Nov–Dec 1986;14(6):477–480.
27. Fabry G, Cheng LX, Molenaers G. Normal and abnormal torsional development in children. *Clin Orthop Relat Res* May 1994(302):22–26.

28. Ferran NA, Oliva F, Maffulli N. Recurrent subluxation of the peroneal tendons. *Sports Med* 2006;36(10):839–846.
29. Fox K, Goudas M, Biddle S, Duda J, Armstrong N. Children's task and ego goal profiles in sport. *Br J Educ Psychol* Jun 1994;64 (Pt 2):253–261.
30. Frey C, Rosenberg Z, Shereff MJ, Kim H. The retrocalcaneal bursa: anatomy and bursography. *Foot Ankle* May 1992;13(4):203–207.
31. Frey CC, Shereff MJ. Tendon injuries about the ankle in athletes. *Clin Sports Med* 1988;7:103–118.
32. Fuchs R, Staheli LT. Sprinting and intoeing. *J Pediatr Orthop* Jul–Aug 1996;16(4):489–491.
33. Ganley T, Flynn J, Gregg J. Sports medicine of the adolescent foot and ankle. *Foot and Ankle Clinics* 1998;3(4):767–785.
34. Gardner LI, Jr., Dziados JE, Jones BH, et al. Prevention of lower extremity stress fractures: a controlled trial of a shock absorbent insole. *Am J Public Health* Dec 1988;78(12):1563–1567.
35. Garrick JG. Epidemiologic perspective. *Clin Sports Med* Mar 1982;1(1):13–18.
36. Garrick JG. The frequency of injury, mechanism of injury, and epidemiology of ankle sprains. *Am J Sports Med* Nov–Dec 1977;5(6):241–242.
37. Geissele AE, Stanton RP. Surgical treatment of adolescent hallux valgus. *J Pediatr Orthop* Sep–Oct 1990;10(5):642–648.
38. Giladi M, Milgrom C, Stein M. The low arch, a protective factor in stress fractures. A prospective study of 295 military recruits. *Orthop Rev* 1985;14:81–84.
39. Goldberg B, Rosenthal PP, Robertson LS, Nicholas JA. Injuries in youth football. *Pediatrics* Feb 1988;81(2):255–261.
40. Griffin LY. Common sports injuries of the foot and ankle seen in children and adolescents. *Orthop Clin North Am* Jan 1994;25(1):83–93.
41. Grogan DP, Gasser SI, Ogden JA. The painful accessory navicular: a clinical and histopathological study. *Foot Ankle* Dec 1989;10(3):164–169.
42. Gross RH. Foot and ankle injuries and disorders. *Adolesc Med* Oct 1998;9(3):599–609, vii.
43. Hamilton WG, Geppert MJ, Thompson FM. Pain in the posterior aspect of the ankle in dancers. Differential diagnosis and operative treatment. *J Bone Joint Surg Am* Oct 1996;78(10):1491–1500.
44. Hamilton WG. Foot and ankle injuries in dancers. *Clin Sports Med* Jan 1988;7(1):143–173.
45. Han SH, Lee JW, Kim S, Suh JS, Choi YR. Chronic tibiofibular syndesmosis injury: the diagnostic efficiency of magnetic resonance imaging and comparative analysis of operative treatment. *Foot Ankle Int* Mar 2007;28(3):336–342.
46. Harris R, Beath T. Hypermobile flat-foot with short tendo achillis. *J Bone Joint Surg Am* 1948;30a:116–140.
47. Harty MP. Imaging of pediatric foot disorders. *Radiol Clin North Am* Jul 2001;39(4):733–748.
48. Hedrick MR, McBryde AM. Posterior ankle impingement. *Foot Ankle Int* Jan 1994;15(1):2–8.
49. Hergenroeder AC. Prevention of sports injuries. *Pediatrics* Jun 1998;101(6):1057–1063.
50. Hopkinson WJ, St. Pierre P, Ryan J, al e. Syndesmosis sprains of the ankle. *Foot Ankle Clin* 1990;10:325–330.
51. Howse AJ. Posterior block of the ankle joint in dancers. *Foot Ankle* Sep–Oct 1982;3(2):81–84.
52. Hui JHP, De SD, Balasubramaniam P. The Singapore operation for recurrent dislocation of peroneal tendons. *J Bone Joint Surg Am* 1998;80(B):325–327.
53. Johnson RP, Collier BD, Carrera GF. The os trigonum syndrome: use of bone scan in the diagnosis. *J Trauma* Aug 1984;24(8):761–764.
54. Jones D, Reiner M. Turf Toe. *Foot Ankle Clin* 1999;4(4):911–917.
55. Jones DC, James SL. Partial calcaneal ostectomy for retrocalcaneal bursitis. *Am J Sports Med* Jan–Feb 1984;12(1):72–73.
56. Kannus P, Renstrom P. Treatment for acute tears of the lateral ligaments of the ankle. Operation, cast, or early controlled mobilization. *J Bone Joint Surg Am* Feb 1991;73(2):305–312.
57. Kay RM, Matthys GA. Pediatric ankle fractures: evaluation and treatment. *J Am Acad Orthop Surg* Jul–Aug 2001;9(4):268–278.
58. Keene JS, Lange RH. Diagnostic dilemmas in foot and ankle injuries. *JAMA* Jul 11 1986;256(2):247–251.
59. Kibler WB, Goldberg C, Chandler TJ. Functional biomechanical deficits in running athletes with plantar fasciitis. *Am J Sports Med* Jan–Feb 1991;19(1):66–71.
60. Kinnard P, Lirette R. Dorsiflexion osteotomy in Freiberg's disease. *Foot Ankle* Apr 1989;9(5):226–231.
61. Kinoshita M, Okuda R, Yasuda T, Abe M. Tarsal tunnel syndrome in athletes. *Am J Sports Med* Aug 2006;34(8):1307–1312.
62. Koleitis GJ, Micheli LJ, Klein KD. Release of the flexor hallucis longus tendon in ballet dancers. *J Bone Joint Surg Am* 1996;78A:1386–1390.
63. Konradsen L, Holmer P, Sondergaard L. Early mobilizing treatment for grade III ankle ligament injuries. *Foot Ankle* Oct 1991;12(2):69–73.
64. Kumai T, Takakura Y, Kitada C, Tanaka Y, Hayashi K. Fixation of osteochondral lesions of the talus using cortical bone pegs. *J Bone Joint Surg Br* Apr 2002;84(3):369–374.
65. Leach RE, DiIorio E, Harney RA. Pathologic hindfoot conditions in the athlete. *Clin Orthop Relat Res* Jul–Aug 1983(177):116–121.
66. Liu SH, Jason WJ. Lateral ankle sprains and instability problems. *Clin Sports Med* Oct 1994;13(4):793–809.
67. Lovell W, Price C, Meehan P. *The foot*. 2 ed. Philadelphia: JB Lippincott; 1986.
68. Lynch SA, Renstrom PA. Treatment of acute lateral ankle ligament rupture in the athlete. Conservative versus surgical treatment. *Sports Med* Jan 1999;27(1):61–71.
69. Maffulli N, Wong J, Almekinders LC. Types and epidemiology of tendinopathy. *Clin Sports Med* Oct 2003;22(4):675–692.
70. Maffulli N. Intensive training in young athletes. The orthopaedic surgeon's viewpoint. *Sports Med* Apr 1990;9(4):229–243.
71. Magee D. *Lower leg, ankle, and foot*. Philadelphia: WB Saunders; 1992.
72. Marsh JS, Daigneault JP, Polzhofer GK. Treatment of ankle instability in children and adolescents with a modified Chrisman-Snook repair: a clinical and patient-based outcome study. *J Pediatr Orthop* Jan–Feb 2006;26(1):94–99.
73. Marsh JS, Daigneault JP. Ankle injuries in the pediatric population. *Curr Opin Pediatr* Feb 2000;12(1):52–60.
74. McKenzie DC, Taunton JE, Clement DB, Smart GW, McNicol KL. Calcaneal epiphysitis in adolescent athletes. *Can J Appl Sport Sci* Sep 1981;6(3):123–125.
75. McLennan JG. Treatment of acute and chronic luxations of the peroneal tendons. *Am J Sports Med* 1980;8:432–446.
76. McManama GB, Jr. Ankle injuries in the young athlete. *Clin Sports Med* Jul 1988;7(3):547–562.
77. Meeusen R, Borms J. Gymnastic injuries. *Sports Med* May 1992;13(5):337–356.
78. Micheli LJ, Ireland L. Prevention and management of calcaneal apophysitis in children:An overuse syndrome. *J Pediatr Orthop* 1987;7:34–38.
79. Micheli LJ, Waters PM, Sanders DP. Sliding fibular graft repair for chronic dislocation of the peroneal tendons. *Am J Sports Med* Jan–Feb 1989;17(1):68–71.
80. Milgrom C, Giladi M, Kashtan H, et al. A prospective study of the effect of a shock-absorbing orthotic device on the incidence of stress fractures in military recruits. *Foot Ankle* Oct 1985;6(2):101–104.
81. Miller TT. Painful accessory bones of the foot. *Semin Musculoskelet Radiol* Jun 2002;6(2):153–161.
82. Niek van Dijk C. Anterior and posterior ankle impingement. *Foot Ankle Clin* 2006;11(3):663–683.

83. Niemi WJ, Savidakis J, Jr., DeJesus JM. Peroneal subluxation: a comprehensive review of the literature with case presentations. *J Foot Ankle Surg* Mar–Apr 1997;36(2):141–145.
84. Omey ML, Micheli LJ. Foot and ankle problems in the young athlete. *Med Sci Sports Exerc* Jul 1999;31(7 Suppl):S470–486.
85. O'Neill DB, Micheli LJ. Tarsal coalition. A followup of adolescent athletes. *Am J Sports Med* Jul–Aug 1989;17(4):544–549.
86. Pfeiffer M, Kotz R, Ledl T, Hauser G, Sluga M. Prevalence of flat foot in preschool-aged children. *Pediatrics* Aug 2006; 118(2):634–639.
87. Pijnenburg AC, Van Dijk CN, Bossuyt PM, Marti RK. Treatment of ruptures of the lateral ankle ligaments: a meta-analysis. *J Bone Joint Surg Am* Jun 2000;82(6):761–773.
88. Pritsch M, Horoshovski H, Farine I. Arthroscopic treatment of osteochondral lesions of the talus. *J Bone Joint Surg Am* Jul 1986;68(6):862–865.
89. Rowland T. *Exercise and Children's health.* Champaign, IL; 1990.
90. Safran MR, Benedetti RS, Bartolozzi AR, 3rd, Mandelbaum BR. Lateral ankle sprains: a comprehensive review: part 1: etiology, pathoanatomy, histopathogenesis, and diagnosis. *Med Sci Sports Exerc* Jul 1999;31(7 Suppl):S429–437.
91. Sammarco GJ. Peroneal tendon injuries. *Orthop Clin North Am* Jan 1994;25(1):135–145.
92. Seitz WH, Jr., Bachner EJ, Abram LJ, et al. Repair of the tibiofibular syndesmosis with a flexible implant. *J Orthop Trauma* 1991;5(1):78–82.
93. Siow H, Tay D, Mitra A. Arthroscopic Treatment of Osteochondritis Dissecans of the Talus. *Foot and Ankle Surgery* 2004;10(4): 181–186.
94. Slatis P, Santavirta S, Sandelin J. Surgical treatment of chronic dislocation of the peroneal tendons. *Br J Sports Med* Mar 1988;22(1):16–18.
95. Smith RW, Reischl SF. Treatment of ankle sprains in young athletes. *Am J Sports Med* Nov–Dec 1986;14(6):465–471.
96. Sneyers CJ, Lysens R, Feys H, Andries R. Influence of malalignment of feet on the plantar pressure pattern in running. *Foot Ankle Int* Oct 1995;16(10):624–632.
97. Sobel M, Geppert MJ, Warren RF. Chronic ankle instability as a cause of peroneal tendon injury. *Clin Orthop Relat Res* Nov 1993(296):187–191.
98. Stanitski CL, Micheli LJ. Observations on symptomatic medial malleolar ossification centers. *J Pediatr Orthop* Mar–Apr 1993; 13(2):164–168.
99. Stanitski CL. Management of sports injuries in children and adolescents. *Orthop Clin North Am* Oct 1988;19(4):689–698.
100. Steinbock G, Pinsger M. Treatment of peroneal tendon dislocation by transposition under the calcaneofibular ligament. *Foot Ankle Int* Mar 1994;15(3):107–111.
101. Stephens MM. Haglund's deformity and retrocalcaneal bursitis. *Orthop Clin North Am* Jan 1994;25(1):41–46.
102. Stover CN, Bryan DR. Traumatic dislocation of the peroneal tendons. *Am J Surg* Feb 1962;103:180–186.
103. Sullivan J. *Ligament injuries of the foot/ankle in the pediatric athlete.* Vol 2. 2nd ed. Philadelphia: Saunders; 2003.
104. Sullivan J. *The child's foot.* 4 ed. Philadelphia: Lippincott; 1996.
105. Sullivan JA, Gross RH, Grana WA, Garcia-Moral CA. Evaluation of injuries in youth soccer. *Am J Sports Med* Sep–Oct 1980;8(5):325–327.
106. Taylor D, Engelhardt D, Bassett IF. Syndesmosis sprains of the ankle: the influence of heterotopic ossification. *Am J Sports Med* 1992;20:146–150.
107. Taylor GJ. Prominence of the calcaneus: is operation justified? *J Bone Joint Surg Br* May 1986;68(3):467–470.
108. Thein R, Eichenblat M. Arthroscopic treatment of sports-related synovitis of the ankle. *Am J Sports Med* Sep–Oct 1992;20(5):496–498.
109. Trevino SG, Davis P, Hecht PJ. Management of acute and chronic lateral ligament injuries of the ankle. *Orthop Clin North Am* Jan 1994;25(1):1–16.
110. Trott AW. Foot and ankle problems in adolescents: sports aspects. *AAOS Symposium on Foot and Ankle.* St. Louis, MO; 1979.
111. Tucker AM. Common soccer injuries. Diagnosis, treatment and rehabilitation. *Sports Med* Jan 1997;23(1):21–32.
112. Wojtys EM. Sports injuries in the immature athlete. *Orthop Clin North Am* Oct 1987;18(4):689–708.
113. Wuest TK. Injuries to the Distal Lower Extremity Syndesmosis. *J Am Acad Orthop Surg* May 1997;5(3):172–181.
114. Xenos JS, Hopkinson WJ, Mulligan ME, Olson EJ, Popovic NA. The tibiofibular syndesmosis. Evaluation of the ligamentous structures, methods of fixation, and radiographic assessment. *J Bone Joint Surg Am* Jun 1995;77(6):847–856.

CHAPTER 26

Nerve Compression Syndromes

In Ho Choi and Won Joon Yoo

INTRODUCTION

Nerve compression syndromes of the foot and ankle are uncommon in children and is often overlooked or underdiagnosed. They are caused by partial or complete compression of peripheral nerves by either external or internal forces. Some clinically important nerve compression syndromes are caused by internal compression from space-occupying lesions such as tumors or hematomas secondary to trauma, or changes in anatomic structure secondary to fracture or dislocation. However, many are primary compression syndromes with unknown causes. Nerve entrapment syndrome or entrapment neuropathy can be used to describe nerve compression syndrome caused by internal pathology. External compression, typically caused by direct trauma or tight footwear, can cause nerve compression syndrome, but more frequently they only initiate or aggravate symptoms in the presence of concomitant internal pathology. The most frequently, encountered entrapment syndromes in athletes involve, in decreasing order, the interdigital nerves; first branch of the lateral plantar nerve; isolated medial or lateral plantar nerves; posterior tibial nerve; deep peroneal nerve; superficial peroneal nerve; sural nerve; and saphenous nerve (58).

Elevated extraneural pressure can cause pathologic changes in vessel-nerve barriers, reduce axonal flow, and cause edema of endoneurium or perineurium, and later, intraneural fibrosis. In animal experiments, it has been shown that external pressures as low as 20–30 mm Hg can impair venous flow in the epineurium (21). Moreover, venous congestion caused by a lower venous pressure (10 mm Hg or less) than external pressure, may diminish the oxygen needed for intracellular axonal transport and cause edema of the endoneurium and perineurium. Compression exacerbated by edema may then aggravate venous congestion to create a vicious cycle. Endoneural edema, demyelination, inflammation, distal axonal degeneration, fibrosis, growth of new axons, remyelination, and thickening of the perineurium and endoneurium may occur as a cascade of biological responses to compression (53).

Damage and later functional recovery of a compressed nerve may depend on the magnitude and duration of compression. Although neural function can usually be recovered progressively by eliminating the causes of compression, irreversible fibrotic changes may occur after severe prolonged compression. Moreover, because the degree of nerve damage cannot be precisely assessed before or during surgery, the prognosis of decompressive surgery is often unpredictable. Sometimes it requires one or two years of follow up to determine the outcome of the operation.

Clinical nerve entrapment is divided into three stages: in stage I, patients feel pain at rest and intermittent paresthesias which are worse at night; in stage II, continued nerve compression leads to paresthesias and numbness that occasionally does not disappear during the day; and in stage III, patients describe constant pain, muscle atrophy, and permanent loss (25). It is evident that the outcome of surgical intervention is much better when a clear dermatomal pain distribution is present or when focal weakness and/or sensory symptoms appropriate for the suspected nerve are present. In many situations, however, nonspecific foot and ankle pain or vague non-localizing sensory symptoms are reported. Standard neurologic test findings may be normal when nerves are compressed only during activity. A variety of neurological conditions, such as radicular pain from lumbosacral nerve roots, referred pain, polyneuropathies, myopathies, and various chronic regional pain syndromes may obfuscate the correct diagnosis (44). Therefore, careful history taking is as important as static and dynamic physical examinations. In addition, a thorough understanding of specific nerve anatomy and its variations are essential for the diagnosis and treatment of nerve compression syndrome, as well as familiarity with proper imaging, e.g., muscle magnetic resonance imaging (MRI), MR neurography (19), and electrodiagnostic tools.

This chapter discusses tarsal tunnel syndrome, deep and superficial peroneal nerve entrapment, and sural nerve entrapment of the foot and ankle.

TARSAL TUNNEL SYNDROME

Anatomy

Tarsal tunnel syndrome is caused by compression of the tibial nerve or of its branches in the distal quarter of the leg, medial ankle, or medial heel (57). The tarsal tunnel is a fibro-osseous structure bridged by the flexor retinaculum over the bony wall formed by the medial malleolus, talus, and calcaneus (4). The flexor retinaculum is continuous with the superficial and deep aponeurosis of the distal leg proximally, and its distal border corresponds to the superior border of the abductor hallucis muscle (56).

The tibial nerve is deep to the soleus and gastrocnemius in the proximal lower leg. In the distal third or quarter of the calf, the nerve becomes superficial and is covered only by skin and fascia as it runs distally just medial to the Achilles tendon. In most individuals, the tibial nerve divides into the medial plantar nerve and the lateral plantar nerve within the tarsal tunnel at a point 0–2 cm proximal to an imaginary line drawn from the tip of the medial malleolus to the calcaneal tuberosity (6). However, in 4% to 7% of patients, the bifurcation site is proximal to the flexor retinaculum (35). The first branch of the lateral plantar nerve (nerve to abductor digiti minimi) originates from the lateral plantar nerve just after it splits from the tibial nerve. The medial calcaneal branches are the most posterior branches of the tibial nerve, and they often branch higher in the tarsal tunnel. The medial calcaneal branch is usually a single nerve arising from the tibial nerve, but there can be two to four branches, and in 10% to 30% of patients, the medial calcaneal branch arises from the lateral plantar nerve (24).

The medial plantar nerve, lateral plantar nerve, and the first branch of the lateral plantar nerve run in separate tunnels deep to the fascia of the abductor hallucis muscle (57) (Figure 26-1).

Etiology

The tibial nerve is compressed under the flexor retinaculum in classic tarsal tunnel syndrome, but it can also be compressed distally after division of the nerve (distal tarsal tunnel syndrome) or posterior to the knee or in the proximal calf (high tarsal tunnel syndrome) (4). Tumors and aberrant muscles around the knee have also been known to cause high tarsal tunnel syndrome (16). In the calf proximal to the distal quarter, compression of the tibial nerve has been reported to be caused by hypertrophied or normal soleus and plantaris muscles in athletic patients (65).

Specific etiologies can be found in 60% to 80% of patients (35); the remaining etiologies are attributed to idiopathic primary nerve compression syndrome. Trauma has been identified as the most common cause of tarsal tunnel syndrome (10). Benign bone tumors, including ganglion cysts, or malunited fracture fragments may act as space-occupying lesions. Other causes of tarsal tunnel syndrome include tenosynovitis of long toe flexors, early collagen vascular disease, varicosities, talocalcaneal coalition, and anomalous muscles, e.g., flexor digitorum accessorius longus (15,41,58).

Distal tarsal tunnel syndrome involves one or several branches of the tibial nerve and may occur concomitantly with proximal nerve compression (57). Isolated medial plantar nerve entrapment is known as "jogger's foot," for obvious reasons (4). At the second muscle layer of the foot, the medial plantar nerve runs along the flexor digitorum longus tendon and passes through the fascial sling (the master knot of Henry), and the plantar calcaneonavicular ligament beneath the talus and navicula (Figure 26-2). Runners' feet with excessive heel valgus or forefoot pronation are at risk of medial nerve entrapment in the region of the master knot of Henry (4).

The lateral plantar nerve can be compressed in the abductor hallucis muscle after excessive plantar fascial

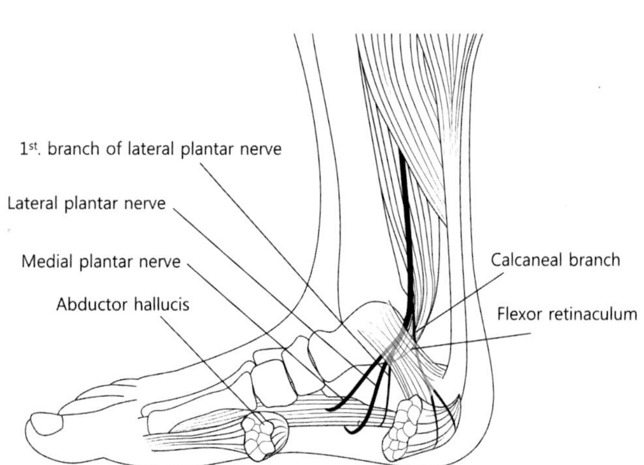

FIGURE 26-1 Tibial nerve and its branches at the medial aspect of foot and ankle.

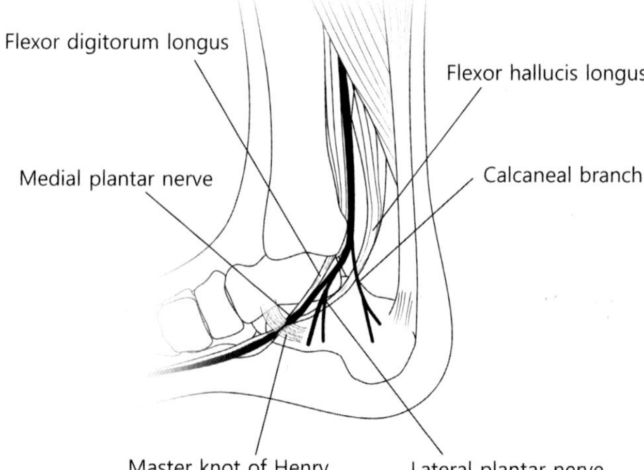

FIGURE 26-2 Entrapment of the medial plantar nerve in "jogger's foot." The nerve may be compressed at the master knot of Henry and the plantar calcaneonavicular ligament beneath the talus and navicula.

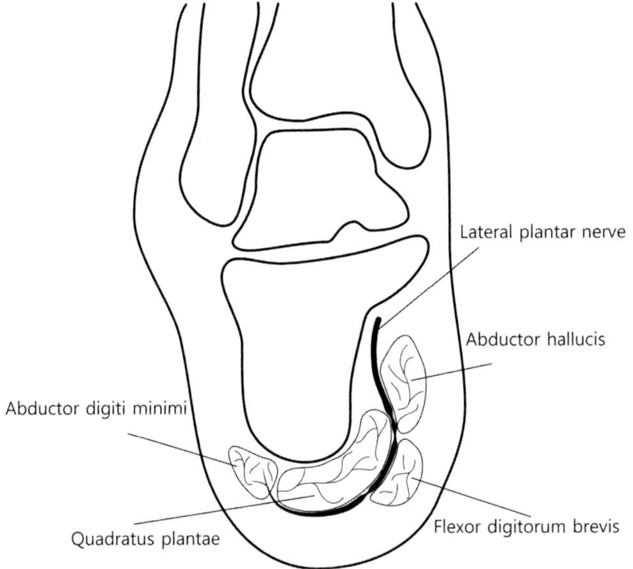

FIGURE 26-3 Entrapment of the first branch of the lateral plantar nerve. The nerve runs between the deep fascia of the abductor hallucis and medial border of the quadratus plantae, where it may be compressed.

release, because the muscle is stretched distally after surgery. The first branch of the lateral plantar nerve runs between the deep fascia of the abductor hallucis and medial border of the quadratus plantae, and hypertrophy of these muscles has been reported to be associated with nerve compression (4,5), which usually occurs at the superior edge of the abductor hallucis and inferior to the muscle where the muscle joins the plantar fascia (Figure 26-3).

Diagnosis

Clinical

The symptoms of tarsal tunnel syndrome are often vague, and the onset may be insidious without a definite history of trauma. Many patients complain of a burning pain or tingling sensation aggravated by activity, but some may experience severe night pain that is relieved by walking (15,30,33,46). There may also be a radiating pain toward the toes or proximally into the calf, with the latter symptom observed in one-third of all patients (35). Sometimes pain and paresthesia are confined to a specific nerve territory. Moreover, in chronic cases, atrophy of the abductor hallucis or abductor digiti minimi may also be observed.

Digital compression of the tarsal tunnel for 30 to 45 seconds yields a radiating pain in many patients, and percussion over the nerve may also yield a radiating pain or paresthesia of the foot. Kinoshita et al. (29) described a provocative maneuver that applies both tensile and compressive force to the tibial nerve: maximal passive dorsiflexion and ankle joint eversion with dorsiflexion of all toes for 5 to 10 seconds. Abnormal bony protrusion and range of motion of the ankle and subtalar joints should be checked to exclude a malunited fracture or a tarsal coalition.

Patients with medial plantar nerve entrapment may typically have a radiating pain from the medial longitudinal arch toward the first and second toes. Moreover, because the long toe flexor tendons are located near the entrapment site, tenosynovitis must be distinguished from medial plantar nerve entrapment. Entrapment of the first branch of the lateral plantar nerve may have a typical tender point at the plantar medial aspect of heel. In cases of distal tarsal tunnel syndrome, local injection of anesthetics into the entrapment site is recommended to confirm the diagnosis and to differentiate it from a concomitant proximal nerve pathology.

Imaging and Electrodiagnostic Testing

Plain radiography may reveal bony lesions including osteochondroma, a displaced fracture fragment, or hypertrophied sustentaculum tali (talocalcaneal coalition). These abnormalities can be delineated more accurately by computed tomography (CT). MRI may be useful in selected cases with soft-tissue lesions, such as, tenosynovitis, varicosities, ganglion cyst, and scar tissue (35). An MRI study (45) showed increased signal intensity in denervated foot muscles using the STIR (short T1 recovery) technique, and this was found to correspond with abnormal spontaneous electromyelogram (EMG) activity. Electrodiagnostic testing may also aid the diagnosis, but results should be interpreted as complimentary to the patient history and physical findings. Decreased conduction velocities in sensory nerves and mixed sensory and motor nerves are known to be highly sensitive and specific for tarsal tunnel syndrome (35). However, difficulty may be experienced performing and interpreting nerve conduction studies in the foot because small amplitudes are produced and nerve conduction may be decreased or absent, even in normal individuals (9). Quantitative sensory testing using the Pressure-Specified Sensory Device (PSSD) can be helpful for the diagnosis of tarsal tunnel syndrome (54,63,64). The device allows cutaneous pressure thresholds to be evaluated painlessly. The PSSD appears to be the most sensitive in identifying the presence of a large-fiber peripheral nerve problem in patients with pain or paresthesias in the foot related to the tibial nerve (52).

Treatment

When the cause of tarsal tunnel syndrome is unclear and symptoms are mild, conservative management should be considered before surgical intervention. Medial arch supports can be tried for patients with a hypermobile valgus heel, and flexor tenosynovitis is managed with a short leg cast or brace. Oral medication with anti-inflammatory drugs or steroid injections help to reduce localized edema caused by tenosynovitis, and depending on the case, tricyclic antidepressants, anticonvulsants, or gabapentin may be useful. When the first branch of the lateral plantar nerve is entrapped, conservative treatment includes shoe modification with heel cups or pads, stretching of the

Achilles tendon and plantar fascia, and medication with anti-inflammatory drugs and steroid injections.

Space-occupying lesions should be removed surgically. The skin incision can be minimal when the location of the lesion is confirmed preoperatively. However, when the cause of compression is uncertain, surgical release should be extensive and include the flexor retinaculum, deep fascia proximal to the flexor retinaculum, and deep fascia of the abductor hallucis. During surgical decompression, perineural fat tissue should be left intact to prevent the formation of adhesions and recurrence of the nerve entrapment. Veins and arteries should not be stripped from the nerve. Usually, the tibial nerve is located posterior to the vena commitans and posterior tibial artery. The medial plantar nerve, lateral plantar nerve, and the first branch of the lateral plantar nerve should be traced distally to the abductor hallucis muscle and tight fascia should be released.

Postoperatively, a short-time splint is helpful for pain control and hemostasis. After two to three days of rest, the splint is removed and early range-of-motion exercise is encouraged. Partial weight bearing can be started at two weeks as tolerated.

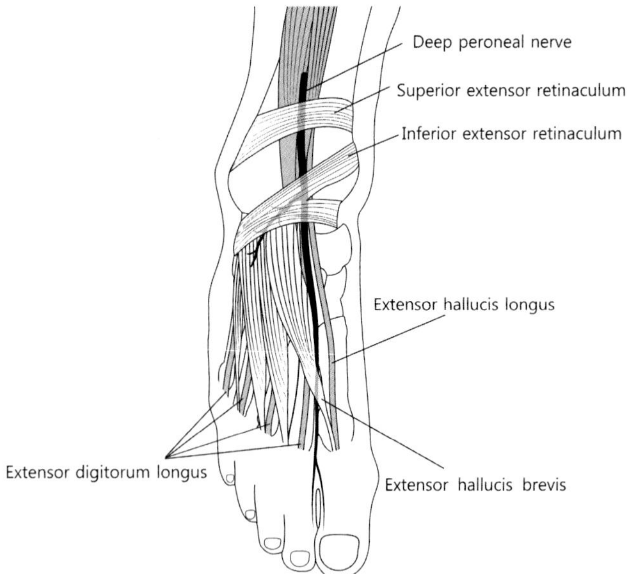

FIGURE 26-4 Anatomic location of the deep peroneal nerve on the dorsum of foot.

DEEP PERONEAL NERVE ENTRAPMENT

Anatomy

The deep peroneal nerve runs between the extensor digitorum longus and the tibialis anterior in the proximal third of the calf, and between the tibialis anterior and the extensor hallucis longus, located superficial to the anterior tibial artery, in the middle and distal third of the leg. The nerve then traverses under the extensor hallucis longus, and then courses between the extensor hallucis longus and extensor digitorum longus proximal to the ankle joint (57). The nerve divides into the lateral and medial branches about 1cm proximal to the ankle joint (1). The lateral terminal branch is a mixed nerve of motor and sensory fibers, whereas the medial terminal branch is a sensory nerve. The lateral terminal branch penetrates the deep surface of the extensor digitorum brevis to provide motor innervation and sensation to the second, third, and fourth metatarsophalangeal joints (1,36,56). The lateral terminal branch arborizes into five main branches, of which two areas are sites of anatomic compression (28). The main medial terminal branch runs lateral to the dorsalis pedis artery and then traverses the artery beneath the oblique inferomedial band of the inferior extensor retinaculum. It may be compressed in this region between the extensor retinaculum and the bony ridges of the talonavicular joint. The nerve then continues distally, passing over the talonavicular joint capsule, between the extensor hallucis brevis and the extensor hallucis longus tendon, and then passes under the extensor hallucis brevis tendon. Finally, it pierces the deep fascia at the first web space to provide sensation to the first toe interspace and the adjacent sides of the first and second toes (Figure 26-4).

Etiology

The deep peroneal nerve lies superficial on the dorsum of foot, and therefore it is vulnerable to compression in several locations along its course. The most commonly described entrapment is anterior tarsal tunnel syndrome, whereby the deep peroneal nerve is compressed in the area formed superiorly by the inferior edge of the inferomedial band of the extensor retinaculum and inferiorly by the talonavicular joint capsule.

Many intrinsic and extrinsic causes produce compression neuropathy of the deep peroneal nerve. The intrinsic mechanism includes compression by dorsal osteophytes of the talonavicular joint; os intermetatarseum, exostoses of the metatarsocueniform joint, fracture fragments; hypertrophied muscles (e.g., extensor digitorum brevis, extensor hallucis brevis, and extensor hallucis longus); ganglia; and nerve stretches resulting from recurrent ankle sprains (4,8,13,25,42,48,50). Os intermetatarseum is an accessory bone found between the base of the first and second metatarsal bones, and it may cause nerve compression especially in athletes (48). The deep peroneal nerve is stretched maximally in a position of ankle plantar flexion with extended toes (8), which may support the clinical history that the syndrome occurs frequently in women wearing high heels, and also the symptoms are aggravated at night when the ankle is plantar flexed during sleep (1,25).

Anterior tarsal tunnel syndrome caused by extrinsic compression was reported to be caused by direct contusion over the dorsum of foot either by single or repeated traumas (31,42) or by increased pressure due to tight-fitting shoes. Sports-related nerve compression may occur in skiers with tight boots (37), ballet dancers in the *pointe* position (57), and in soccer players who have received repetitive blows to the dorsum of the foot (57). Other occasional causes include localized compression by keys in shoe lacings in runners and by a metal bar when the feet are hooked underneath during sit-ups (4).

Diagnosis

Clinical

As with other nerve compression syndromes, symptoms often are non-specific. Patients typically complain of pain on the dorsum of the foot with occasional radiation into the first web space. Pain usually worsens with physical activity and then subsides with rest (4,14), and has been described as burning, aching, dull, or sharp. Patients frequently have a history of recurrent sprains or previous trauma. History taking should also include details of types of footwear worn, aggravating foot positions, sports activities, and the presence of night pain.

The pain may be brought on by forced plantar flexion and inversion of the foot (22), in contrast to the dorsiflexion-eversion test in tarsal tunnel syndrome. Hypoesthesia or paresthesia may be noted in the first web space. If compression occurs before the bifurcation of the nerve, there may be atrophy or weakness of the extensor digitorum brevis. Tinel's sign may be elicited by percussion along the course of the nerve. Osteophytes on the talus or navicular and rarely a small accessory bone between the bases of the first and second metatarsals may compress the deep peroneal nerve.

Differential diagnosis includes lumbosacral nerve root impingement, peripheral neuropathy, tarsal tunnel syndrome, Morton's neuroma, superficial peroneal nerve entrapment, gout, peripheral vascular disease, bony ankle impingement, and ankle sprain or fracture (25).

Imaging and Electrodiagnostic Testing

Plain radiography of the foot may reveal osteophytes or exostoses on the dorsal aspect of talus, navicular, or first metatarsal base.

Electrodiagnostic testing can be useful for diagnosis, when the results correlate with clinical findings. The following techniques are useful in anterior tarsal tunnel syndrome; motor nerve conduction studies of the deep peroneal nerve (recorded at the extensor digitorum brevis muscle), sensory studies of the nerve (recorded at the interspace between the first and second toes), and needle electromyography of the extensor digitorum brevis (9). A delay in nerve conduction of more than 5 ms has been reported to be correlated with compression neuropathy of the deep peroneal nerve (22). Nerve conduction studies are also useful for differentiating more proximal nerve involvement, such as, lumbosacral nerve root compression and common peroneal nerve entrapment, but caution should be exercised when interpreting electrodiagnostic tests, because denervation of extensor digitorum brevis occurs with other peripheral nerve diseases and in some normal subjects (14). In addition, an accessory peroneal nerve, which emanates from the superficial peroneal nerve supplies the extensor digitorum brevis in 28% of individuals, and may confuse the electrodiagnostic test results (34).

Treatment

Conservative management includes convenient shoe wearing, orthotics or accommodative shoes, intermittent bracing or a short leg cast, medication with anti-inflammatory drugs, and steroid injection. Local anesthetics can be used before surgical decompression to localize entrapment sites. When conservative management fails to relieve pain, nerve decompression should be considered. The skin incision extends from proximal to the ankle joint to the base of the first and second metatarsals, and may be straight or lazy S-shaped. Superomedial and inferomedial limbs of the extensor retinaculum are divided, and osteophytes, mass lesions, or scar adhesions should be explored. Extensor hallucis brevis that crosses over the deep peroneal nerve should be resected when the nerve is compressed under a hypertrophied muscle belly or distally by the tendon. Results of surgical decompression depend on the precision of the diagnosis and the duration of nerve compression. Postoperatively, early range-of-motion exercises are encouraged. Weight bearing usually begins two weeks after surgery.

SUPERFICIAL PERONEAL NERVE ENTRAPMENT

Anatomy

The superficial peroneal nerve is a branch of the common peroneal nerve. It branches off at the fibular neck and is usually located in the lateral compartment between the peroneus longus and peroneus brevis muscles. It then passes through a fibrous tunnel (the peroneal tunnel), which varies in length from 3 cm to 11 cm in adults (25) between the anterior intermuscular septum and the fascia of the lateral compartment. The nerve then travels distally in the peroneal tunnel to pierce the deep crural fascia at the junction of the middle and distal third of the lower leg, approximately 10–14 cm above the lateral malleolus in adults (44,57), and subsequently becomes subcutaneous. Approximately 6.5 cm above the lateral malleolus, it divides into two major branches: a smaller more laterally located intermediate dorsal cutaneous nerve and a large medial dorsal cutaneous nerve. The intermediate dorsal cutaneous nerve lies medial to the lateral malleolus and usually provides sensation to the lateral dorsal aspect of the ankle, and fourth and fifth toes, whereas the medial dorsal cutaneous nerve provides sensation to the dorsal medial aspect of the ankle, the medial aspect of the hallux, and to the second and third toes (Figure 26-5).

It should be noted that anatomic variations occur in up to 30% of specimens. For example, the superficial peroneal nerve may exit from the anterior compartment instead of the lateral compartment and the medial and intermediate dorsal cutaneous nerves may pierce the deep

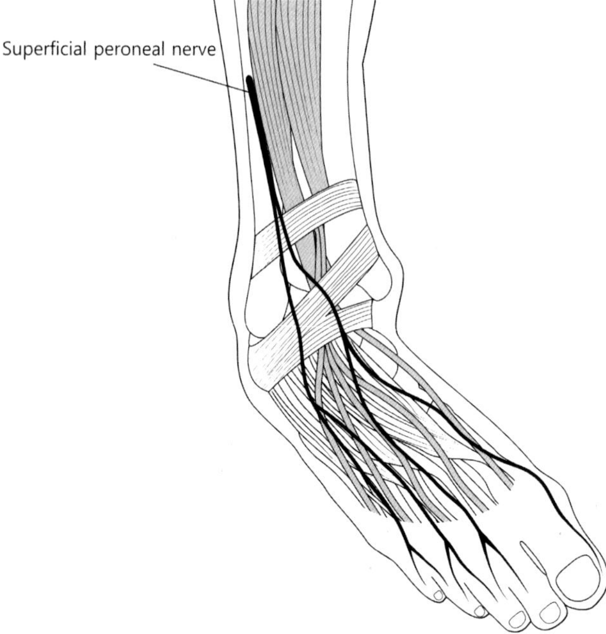

FIGURE 26-5 Anatomic location of the superficial peroneal nerve on the dorsum of foot.

crural fascia independently (2,25). The intermediate dorsal cutaneous nerve may penetrate the crural fascia posterior to the fibula and course medially to cross the lateral aspect of the distal fibula, or the nerve may penetrate the crural fascia anterior to the fibula and continues in close proximity to the anterior fibular border. Both variants are at risk for iatrogenic injury during surgical procedures (7). The accessory deep peroneal nerve may arise from the superficial peroneal nerve and descend in the lateral compartment of the leg, deep to peroneus longus along the posterior border of peroneus brevis. Approaching the ankle joint, this nerve passes through the peroneal tunnel, winds around the lateral malleolus, and it then crosses beneath the peroneus brevis tendon anteriorly to reach the dorsum of the foot. It gives off muscular branches to the peroneus brevis, occasionally to peroneus longus and extensor digitorum brevis, and sensory branches to the lateral region of the ankle (32).

Etiology

The peroneal tunnel usually acts as an impinging structure for the superficial peroneal nerve (38,62). The tunnel is fibrotic and the nerve is often impinged on the edges of the tunnel when local compartment pressure increases. The most common site of entrapment is the point where the nerve pierces the deep fascia. While most entrapments in the peroneal tunnel are caused by compression neuropathy, both compression and tension neuropathies may occur at the exit point from the deep fascia. Overstretching the nerve may be caused by recurrent ankle sprains, or by fascial shift after fasciotomy for compartment syndrome. Muscle herniation through a fascial defect (20,59), fat (43), or a lipoma (3) may also cause impingement. When an anatomic variation is present and the intermediate and medial dorsal cutaneous nerves pierce the deep fascia more distally, tension neuropathy following ankle sprain or iatrogenic nerve damage during fasciotomy may occur more easily. An accessory superficial peroneal nerve which enters the foot by rostro-caudally traversing the lateral malleolus laterally can be entrapped by a fascial band resulting in pain over the lateral malleolus and dorsum of the foot (55).

Diagnosis

Clinical

Many patients have a history of ankle sprains or trauma to the calf, and the majority of patients complain of pain in the middle and distal one-third of the leg with or without local swelling. Pain can radiate onto the dorsum of foot and it is typically elicited or aggravated by physical activities, such as walking, running, or squatting. Pain is usually relieved by rest and night pain is uncommon. Pain relief by conservative treatment is infrequent, unlike that associated with deep peroneal nerve entrapment (2,25,59,60). Sensory changes, such as hypesthesia and paresthesia, may occur along the nerve distribution without specific motor weakness.

Focal mass lesions, such as a lipoma or a herniated muscle may be palpable. Point tenderness is usually elicited where the nerve exits from the deep fascia. When the diagnosis is uncertain, local anesthetic injection can be used to localize the pathology. Styf (60) described three provocative tests to suggest a diagnosis. The first test involves palpating the nerve in the impingement area while the patient exerts active dorsiflexion and eversion against resistance. The second involves stretching the nerve by forced passive plantar flexion and inversion of the ankle joint, and the third test involves percussing the nerve over its course while a physician performs the second test. Pain or paresthesia caused by any of these tests is considered to suggest compression of the superficial peroneal nerve.

Differential diagnosis includes chronic ankle sprains, tumors (e.g., nerve sheath tumor or lipoma), pseudoradicular pain syndrome (38,60), chronic or exertional lateral compartment syndrome, or lumbar radiculopathy.

Imaging and Electrodiagnostic Testing

In typical cases, electrodiagnostic tests may show a reduced nerve conduction velocity with normal peroneal muscle EMG findings. Styf (60) reported that the nerve conduction velocity decreased to less than 44 m/sec in 15 of 21 cases preoperatively, and increased after surgical release, although this increase was not significant. However, electrodiagnostic tests can be normal, as occurs in other nerve entrapment syndromes, and results should be considered complementary during diagnosis and follow up. A lack of intermediate dorsal cutaneous nerve response has also been reported in 2% to 9% of normal individuals (9).

Plain radiographs are used to rule out stress fracture, bone tumors, and other causes of chronic pain. MRI has been used in some studies, but its diagnostic indications have not been defined (12,18,27).

Treatment

Conservative management should be exhausted before surgical treatment, but it rarely provides symptomatic relief.

The skin incision is started 2–3 cm distal to the exit of the superficial peroneal nerve through the deep crural fascia and extended proximally. With careful subcutaneous dissection, the nerve is identified and traced up to the fascial opening, which is usually in the lateral compartment, though sometimes the nerve in the lateral compartment traverses the anterior intermuscular septum, enters the anterior compartment, and then pierces the fascia of the anterior compartment (2,25). The nerve is released by local fasciectomy of the nerve opening. The nerve should then be further traced through the fibrous peroneal tunnel, which is typically located between the anterior intermuscular septum and the fascia of the lateral compartment. The peroneal tunnel should be released sufficiently to allow the nerve to move freely.

Lateral compartment fasciotomy may be effective in symptomatic chronic exertional compartment syndrome, if surgical indications are carefully chosen (11,61).

SURAL NERVE ENTRAPMENT

Anatomy

The sural nerve is formed from contributions from the tibial nerve (medial sural cutaneous nerve) and the common peroneal nerve (lateral sural cutaneous nerve) in 80% of cases and solely from the tibial nerve in the remaining 20% (49). The medial sural cutaneous nerve runs between the two heads of the gastrocnemius muscle and joins the ramus communicans of the lateral sural cutaneous nerve to form the sural nerve at the level of musculotendinous junction of the gastrocnemius. The sural nerve runs distally in the calf and pierces the deep fascia between the middle and distal thirds of the calf. The nerve crosses the Achilles tendon about 10 cm proximal to the calcaneal tuberosity and then runs distally next to the lesser saphenous vein on the lateral border of the Achilles tendon and passes posterior and inferior to the peroneal tendon sheath. It supplies lateral calcaneal branches to the lateral aspect of calcaneus and distally subdivides to a medial and a lateral branch at the level of the tuberosity of the fifth toe. The lateral branch forms the lateral dorsal cutaneous branch of the sural nerve, which provides sensation to the lateral border of the foot and the fifth toe. The medial branch supplies the intermediate dorsal cutaneous nerve from the superficial peroneal nerve, and supplies sensory innervations to the lateral aspect of the fourth toe (25). There is wide variation in the cutaneous innervation patterns of the sural nerve on the dorsum of the foot (39).

Etiology

Sural nerve compression syndrome may occur following fracture of the fibula, talus, calcaneus, cuboid, or fifth metatarsal base (23,51,57). A bony fragment, hematoma, or edema may cause nerve compression during the acute phase, and later, the nerve can become entrapped in a fibrous scar or fracture callus. Repetitive direct contusion to the calf, which usually occurs in soccer players, may lead to fibrous adhesion of the nerve. Chronic repetitive ankle sprain with plantar flexion and inversion injuries may elicit traction neuropathy and later fibrous adhesion at its exit point from the deep crural fascia. In athletes, a thick and unyielding fibrous arch of deep fascia may compromise the sural nerve due to local scar formation or increased muscle mass (17).

Occasionally sural nerve can be entrapped in scar tissue iatrogenically following lateral ankle reconstruction with peroneus brevis tendon (57). Iatrogenic nerve injury and perineural fibrosis also may occur after surgical correction of a peroneal tendon dislocation (posterolateral approach) or a calcaneal fracture (extensive lateral approach). Moreover, percutaneous repair of the Achilles tendon may also lead to sural nerve entrapment (26,40).

Space-occupying lesions, such as an osteochondroma of the talus (47), ganglia and other tumors of the peroneal tendon sheath may cause compression neuropathy (51). Moreover, Achilles peritendinitis (4) and fibroaponeurotic bands from the Achilles tendon (58) can irritate the sural nerve next to the tendon.

Diagnosis

Clinical

Patients may complain of a shooting pain with numbness or paresthesia on the lateral aspect of the foot and ankle. The pain may radiate proximally to the knee. Motor strength and deep tendon reflexes are normal. Careful palpation should be performed along the course of the nerve. In typical cases, local tenderness is positive, and Tinel's sign may be positive in some patients. Stretching of the sural nerve by plantar flexion and inversion of the ankle may elicit radiating pain. In athletes, a dynamic examination may reveal characteristic clinical findings in patients with an unremarkable static physical examination (17).

Imaging and Electrodiagnostic Testing

Plain radiography may reveal a prominent bony fragment or bone tumor, e.g., osteochondroma, at a suspected entrapment site. Ultrasonography and MRI are useful for differentiating soft tissue lesions that compress the sural nerve. Electrodiagnostic tests may show reduced nerve conduction velocity with a reduction in sensory potential amplitude in cases of long-standing entrapment (17).

Treatment

Nonoperative measures should be attempted to reduce external compression or to relieve pain and edema. These include shoe modifications, anti-inflammatory drugs, and steroid injections with or without local anesthetics. Surgery is indicated when symptoms do not respond to conservative management. Displaced or malunited fracture fragments that stretch the nerve should be reduced or resected. Tumors and other space-occupying lesions that compress or stretch the nerve should also be resected. When the sural nerve is entrapped in a fibrous scar, careful decompression of the nerve with neurolysis is necessary, and a tight fascial opening should be released to allow the nerve to move freely.

SUMMARY

Nerve compression syndromes of the foot and ankle are uncommon in pediatric patients and have numerous causes. Diagnosis is not straightforward and is frequently delayed. Detailed history taking often provides a key to the correct diagnosis, especially when nerve compression occurs dynamically only during or after exercise. Types of footwear, an acute or chronic symptom onset, and time-relation with trauma should be obtained by history taking.

Physical examinations along nerve courses should be performed based on a thorough knowledge of the anatomy of the peripheral nerve and its variations. Specific nerve involvement can be suspected by checking the territory affected by numbness or paresthesia. In many cases, tenderness is a typical finding at the entrapment site, and radiating pain may be elicited either by percussion or by stretching maneuvers.

Plain radiography is essential to rule out the presence of a bony lesion, and sometimes specific nerve compression can be suspected for specific types of fracture or dislocation. Although MRI is the modality of choice for differentiating soft-tissue lesions, its diagnostic value in nerve compression syndrome has not been fully established. However, when properly implemented, MR neurography is capable of providing high-quality information about nerve compression and inflammation. Muscle MRI can identify denervation on a precise anatomic basis. In the future, diagnosis of entrapment and compression neuropathy may become easier with advancement of MRI technology. Electrodiagnostic tests, such as nerve conduction studies and needle electromyography, are valuable tools for diagnosing nerve compression syndrome. They provide objective evidence of nerve injury and can differentiate the compression level. However, false-positive or false-negative results are not rare, and anatomic variations of the peripheral nerve may further confuse electrodiagnostic test findings.

Generally, conservative measures including local injections of steroid with or without local anesthetics, and the use of heel cups and/or orthoses are effective at treating nerve compression syndrome. Surgery may be indicated when a patient does not respond to conservative treatment and the site of nerve compression is well documented.

The results of surgical decompression are often unpredictable because functional recovery of a decompressed nerve can be influenced by the severity and duration of compression as well as by the completeness of the decompression. In most cases, it is difficult to correctly assess the degree of nerve damage before or during surgery, and therefore, at least one or two years of follow up is likely to be required to assess the outcome of surgical decompression.

REFERENCES

1. Adelman KA, Wilson G, Wolf JA. Anterior tarsal tunnel syndrome. *J Foot Surg* 27:299–302, 1988.
2. Adkison DP, Bosse MJ, Gaccione DR, et al. Anatomical variations in the course of the superficial peroneal nerve. *J Bone Joint Surg Am* 73:112–114, 1991.
3. Banerjee T, Koons DD. Superficial peroneal nerve entrapment: Report of two cases. *J Neurosurg* 55:991–992, 1981.
4. Baxter DE. Functional nerve disorders in the athlete's foot, ankle, and leg. *Instr Course Lect* 42:185–194, 1993.
5. Baxter DE, Thigpen CM. Heel pain-operative results. *Foot Ankle* 5:16–25, 1984.
6. Baxter DE. *The foot and ankle in sport.* St. Louis: Mosby, 1995.
7. Blair JM, Botte MJ. Surgical anatomy of the superficial peroneal nerve in the foot and ankle. *Clin Orthop Relat Res* 305:229–238, 1994.
8. Borges LF, Hallett M, Selkoe DJ, et al. The anterior tarsal tunnel syndrome: Report of two cases. *J Neurosurg* 54:89–92, 1981.
9. Buxton WG., Dominick JE. Electromyography and nerve conduction studies of the lower extremity: uses and limitations. *Clin Podiatr Med Surg* 23:531–543, 2006.
10. Cimino WR. Tarsal tunnel syndrome: review of the literature. *Foot Ankle* 11:47–52, 1990.
11. Clanton TO, Solcher BW. Chronic leg pain in the athlete. *Clin Sports Med* 13:743–759, 1994.
12. Daghino W, Pasquali M, Faletti C. Superficial peroneal nerve entrapment in a young athlete: the diagnostic contribution of magnetic resonance imaging. *J Foot Ankle Surg* 36:170–172, 1997.
13. Dellon AL. Deep peroneal nerve entrapment on the dorsum of the foot. *Foot Ankle* 11:73–80, 1990.
14. DiDomenico LA, Masternick EB. Anterior tarsal tunnel syndrome. *Clin Podiatr Med* Surg 23:611–620, 2006.
15. Edwards WG., Lincoln CR, Bassett FH, et al. The tarsal tunnel syndrome: Diagnosis and treatment. *JAMA* 207:716–720, 1969.
16. Ekelund AL. Bilateral nerve entrapment in the popliteal space. *Am J Sports Med* 18:108, 1990.
17. Fabre T, Montero C, Gaujard E, et al. Chronic calf pain in athletes due to sural nerve entrapment: A report of 18 cases. *Am J Sports Med* 28:679–682, 2000.
18. Ferkel RD, Karzel RP, Del Pizzo W, et al. Arthroscopic treatment of anterolateral impingement of the ankle. *Am J Sports Med* 19:440–446, 1991.
19. Filler AG., Kliot M, Howe FA, et al. Application of magnetic resonance neurography in the evaluation of patients with peripheral nerve pathology. *J Neurosurg* 85:299–309, 1996.
20. Garfin S, Mubarak SJ, Owen CA. Exertional anterolateral-compartment syndrome: Case report with fascial defect, muscle herniation, and superficial peroneal-nerve entrapment. *J Bone Joint Surg Am* 59:404–405, 1977.
21. Gelberman RH, Eaton RG., Urbaniak JR. Peripheral nerve compression. *Instr Course Lect* 43:31–53, 1994.
22. Gessini L, Jandolo B, Pietrangeli A. The anterior tarsal syndrome: Report of four cases. *J Bone Joint Surg Am* 66:786–787, 1984.
23. Gould N, Trevino S. Sural nerve entrapment by avulsion fracture of the base of the fifth metatarsal bone. *Foot Ankle* 2:153–155, 1981.

24. Havel PE, Ebraheim NA, Clark SE, et al. Tibial nerve branching in the tarsal tunnel. *Foot Ankle* 9:117–119, 1988.
25. Hirose CB, McGarvey WC. Peripheral nerve entrapments. *Foot Ankle* Clin 9:255–269, 2004.
26. Hockenbury RT, Johns JC. A biomechanical in vitro comparison of open versus percutaneous repair of tendon Achilles. *Foot Ankle* 11: 67–72, 1990.
27. Johnston EC, Howell SJ. Tension neuropathy of the superficial peroneal nerve: associated conditions and results of release. *Foot Ankle Int* 20:576–582, 1999.
28. Kennedy JG., Brunner JB, Bohne WH, et al. Clinical importance of the lateral branch of the deep peroneal nerve. *Clin Orthop Relat Res* 459:222–228, 2007.
29. Kinoshita M, Okuda R, Morikawa J, et al. The dorsiflexion-eversion test for diagnosis of tarsal tunnel syndrome. *J Bone Joint Surg Am* 83:1835–1839, 2001.
30. Kopell HP, Thompson WA. Peripheral entrapment neuropathies of the lower extremity. *N Engl J Med* 262:56–60, 1960.
31. Krause KH, Witt T, Ross A. The anterior tarsal tunnel syndrome. *J Neurol* 217:67–74, 1977.
32. Kudoh H, Sakai T, Horiguchi M. The consistent presence of the human accessory deep peroneal nerve. *J Anat* 194:101–108, 1999.
33. Lam SJ. Tarsal tunnel syndrome. *J Bone Joint Surg Br* 49:87–92, 1967.
34. Lambert EH. The accessory deep peroneal nerve: A common variation in innervation of extensor digitorum brevis. *Neurology* 19:1169–1176, 1969.
35. Lau JT, Daniels TR. Tarsal tunnel syndrome: a review of the literature. *Foot Ankle Int* 20:201–209, 1999.
36. Lawrence SJ, Botte MJ. The deep peroneal nerve in the foot and ankle: an anatomic study. *Foot Ankle Int* 16:724–728, 1995.
37. Lindenbaum BL. Ski boot compression syndrome. *Clin Orthop Relat Res* 140:109–110, 1979.
38. Lowdon IM. Superficial peroneal nerve entrapment: A case report. *J Bone Joint Surg Br* 67:58–59, 1985.
39. Madhavi C, Issac B, Antoniswamy B, et al. Anatomic variations of the cutaneous innervation patterns of the sural nerve on the dorsum of the foot. *Clin Anat* 18:206–209, 2005.
40. Maes R, Copin G., Averous C. Is percutaneous repair of the Achilles tendon a safe technique?: A study of 124 cases. *Acta Orthop Belg* 72:179–183, 2006.
41. Mann RA. Tarsal tunnel syndrome. *Orthop Clin North Am* 5:109–115, 1974.
42. Marinacci AA. Neurological syndromes of the tarsal tunnels. *Bull Los Angeles Neurol Soc* 33:90–100, 1968.
43. McAuliffe TB, Fiddian NJ, Browett JP. Entrapment neuropathy of the superficial peroneal nerve: A bilateral case. *J Bone Joint Surg Br* 67: 62–63, 1985.
44. McCrory P, Bell S, Bradshaw C. Nerve entrapments of the lower leg, ankle and foot in sport. *Sports Med* 32:371–391, 2002.
45. McDonald CM, Carter GT, Fritz RC,et al. Magnetic resonance imaging of denervated muscle: comparison to electromyography. *Muscle Nerve* 23:1431–1434, 2000.
46. Menon J, Dorfman HD, Renbaum J, et al. Tarsal tunnel syndrome secondary to neurilemoma of the medial plantar nerve. *J Bone Joint Surg Am* 62:301–303, 1980.
47. Montgomery PQ, Goddard NJ, Kemp HB. Solitary osteochondroma causing sural nerve entrapment neuropathy. *J R Soc Med* 82: 761, 1989.
48. Nakasa T, Fukuhara K, Adachi N, Ochi M. Painful os intermetatarseum in athletes: report of four cases and review of the literature. *Arch Orthop Trauma Surg* 127:261–264, 2007.
49. Ortiguela ME, Wood MB, Cahill DR. Anatomy of the sural nerve complex. *J Hand Surg Am* 12:1119–1123, 1987.
50. Parker RG. Dorsal foot pain due to compression of the deep peroneal nerve by exostosis of the metatarsocuneiform joint. *J Am Podiatr Med Assoc* 95:455–458, 2005.
51. Pringle RM, Protheroe K, Mukherjee S K. Entrapment neuropathy of the sural nerve. *J Bone Joint Surg Br* 56:465–468, 1974.
52. Radoiu H, Rosson GD, Andonian E, et al. Comparison of measures of large-fiber nerve function in patients with chronic nerve compression and neuropathy. *J Am Podiatr Med Assoc* 95: 438–445, 2005.
53. Rempel D, Dahlin L, Lundborg G.. Pathophysiology of nerve compression syndromes: response of peripheral nerves to loading. *J Bone Joint Surg Am* 81:1600–1610, 1999.
54. Rose JD, Malay DS, Sorrento DL. Neurosensory testing of the medial calcaneal and medial plantar nerves in patients with plantar heel pain. *Foot Ankle Surg* 42:173–177, 2003.
55. Rubin M, Menche D, Pitman M. Entrapment of an accessory superficial peroneal sensory nerve. *Can J Neurol Sci* 18:342–343, 1991.
56. Sarrafian S. *Anatomy of the foot and ankle: descriptive, topographical, functional*, 2nd ed. Philadelphia: JB Lippincott, 1993.
57. Schon LC. Nerve entrapment, neuropathy, and nerve dysfunction in athletes. *Orthop Clin North Am* 25:47–59, 1994.
58. Schon LC, Baxter DE. Neuropathies of the foot and ankle in athletes. *Clin Sports Med* 9:489–509, 1990.
59. Styf J. Chronic exercise-induced pain in the anterior aspect of the lower leg: An overview of diagnosis. *Sports Med* 7:331–339, 1989.
60. Sty, J. Entrapment of the superficial peroneal nerve: Diagnosis and results of decompression. *J Bone Joint Surg Br* 71:131–135, 1989.
61. Styf J, Korner LM. Chronic anterior-compartment syndrome of the leg: Results of treatment by fasciotomy. *J Bone Joint Surg Am* 68:1338–1347, 1986.
62. Styf J, Morberg P. The superficial peroneal tunnel syndrome: Results of treatment by decompression. *J Bone Joint Surg Br* 79:801–803, 1997.
63. Tassler PL, Dellon AL. Correlation of measurements of pressure perception using the pressure-specified sensory device with electrodiagnostic testing. *J Occup Environ Med* 37:862–826, 1995.
64. Tassler PL, Dellon AL. Pressure perception in the normal lower extremity and in the tarsal tunnel syndrome. *Muscle Nerve* 19:285–289, 1996.
65. Turnipseed WD, Pozniak M. Popliteal entrapment as a result of neurovascular compression by the soleus and plantaris muscles. *J Vasc Surg* 15:285–293, 1992.

CHAPTER 27

Tumors

Alexandre Arkader and John P. Dormans

INTRODUCTION

Benign and malignant tumors of the foot are rare, especially among children (8, 32,43,57,68). Generally, tumors found in the foot and ankle region are seen more frequently in other parts of the musculoskeletal system and therefore applying the knowledge from other areas to foot tumors may be appropriate. However, one must consider the unique intrinsic anatomy of the foot when planning treatment. The complex anatomic structures include several compartments that are inter-connected, and thus, surgical resection of foot tumors may be very challenging (8). The most common soft-tissue and bone tumors that involve the foot and ankle in children are discussed in further detail in this chapter.

APPROACH

Children with a tumor in the foot and/or ankle often present with a painless growth. Pain, decrease in range of motion, difficulty in wearing shoes, and gait changes also are common presentations. A history of trauma should always be sought, as reactive bone formation may mimic tumorous appearance. Infection must be included in the differential diagnosis. Social history is important, e.g., stress-related injuries such as stress fractures may have radiographic characteristics similar to a tumor.

Due to the complex anatomy, careful physical examination is essential. It is important to determine the exact extent of bony and soft-tissue (joints, vessels, and nerves) involvement. Examination of the skin will rule-out cutaneous forms of sarcomas or vascular abnormalities as well as previous scars or color changes. Elevated skin temperature may indicate inflammatory or infectious conditions (Figure 27-1).

Diagnostic Studies

Radiographs

Plain radiographs should be included in the initial evaluation and consist of at least three views (anterior-posterior, lateral, and oblique). Several benign bone tumors may be diagnosed with plain films (e.g., osteochondroma). Worrisome signs of malignant bone tumors include aggressive, destructive lesions with poorly defined borders. Soft-tissue lesions may also be identified by plain films, because they often contain calcification, or evidence of bone erosion (Figure 27-2).

Ultrasound

Ultrasound is a useful technique that does not involve radiation, and is also inexpensive. It may show fluid collection, such as joint effusion or ganglion cysts. It better defines tumor location, particularly of soft-tissue tumors.

Computerized Tomography (CT)

Computerized tomography (CT) is a good tool for evaluation of the bony architecture, and it helps understanding of the plain films findings (due to the complex foot anatomy). It is especially useful for identification of the nidus in osteoid osteoma and for planning tumor resection.

Magnetic Resonance Imaging (MRI)

Magnetic resonance imaging (MRI) is the best imaging method for evaluation of soft-tissue lesions. It is also very helpful in detecting the extent of soft-tissue invasion associated with bone lesions (see Figure 27-2) as well as assisting in the differential diagnosis (e.g., infection) (Figure 27-3). MRI is essential for the preoperative planning of limb-sparing procedures.

Biopsy

Biopsy is usually necessary for tissue diagnostic confirmation. Exceptions include ganglion cyst, lipoma, and hemangioma that can be diagnosed by physical examination and imaging, especially MRI. All current concepts of biopsy, that are utilized elsewhere, should be applied to foot tumors. Especially important is planning the definitive resection preoperatively and performing the biopsy in line with the definitive surgical approach, avoiding creating flaps and "burning bridges." For most suspicious

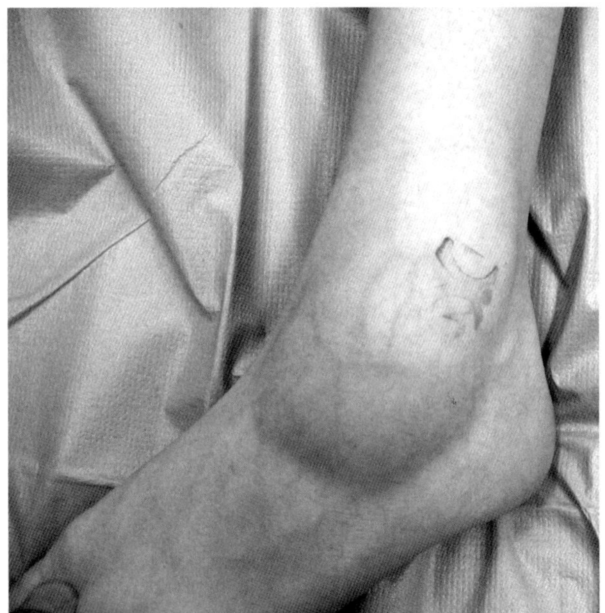

FIGURE 27-1 Inspection; anteroposterior aspect of the left ankle of a 15 year-old girl complaining of a painless mass. Note the prominent vasculature in the area of the mass and the bulging of the skin. (Figures reproduced with permission from The Childrens Orthopaedic Center, Los Angeles, CA)

lesions, we recommend that the biopsy be done by the treating surgeon and referred to a tertiary cancer center. For bony lesions associated with a soft-tissue mass, sampling of the associated mass is usually appropriate and avoids weakening the underlying bone. For purely soft-tissue masses, the biopsy site usually is chosen based on the relationship between the tumor and the underlying surrounding structures, favoring the most superficial area of the tumor.

Staging

This is an essential part of the work-up. Besides being a prognosticator tool, staging helps plan the definitive treatment. Staging is done based on all available imaging studies and the biopsy results. The two most-used staging systems for bone and soft-tissue sarcomas are the criteria devised by the Musculoskeletal Tumor Society (MSTS) – surgical staging (Table 27-1) and by the American Joint Commission of Cancer (AJCC) (6) (Table 27-2). The present AJCC system for sarcomas is based on tumor grade (high vs. low), size (8 cm for bone and 5 cm for soft-tissues), depth (relative to deep fascia), and the presence and location of metastases.

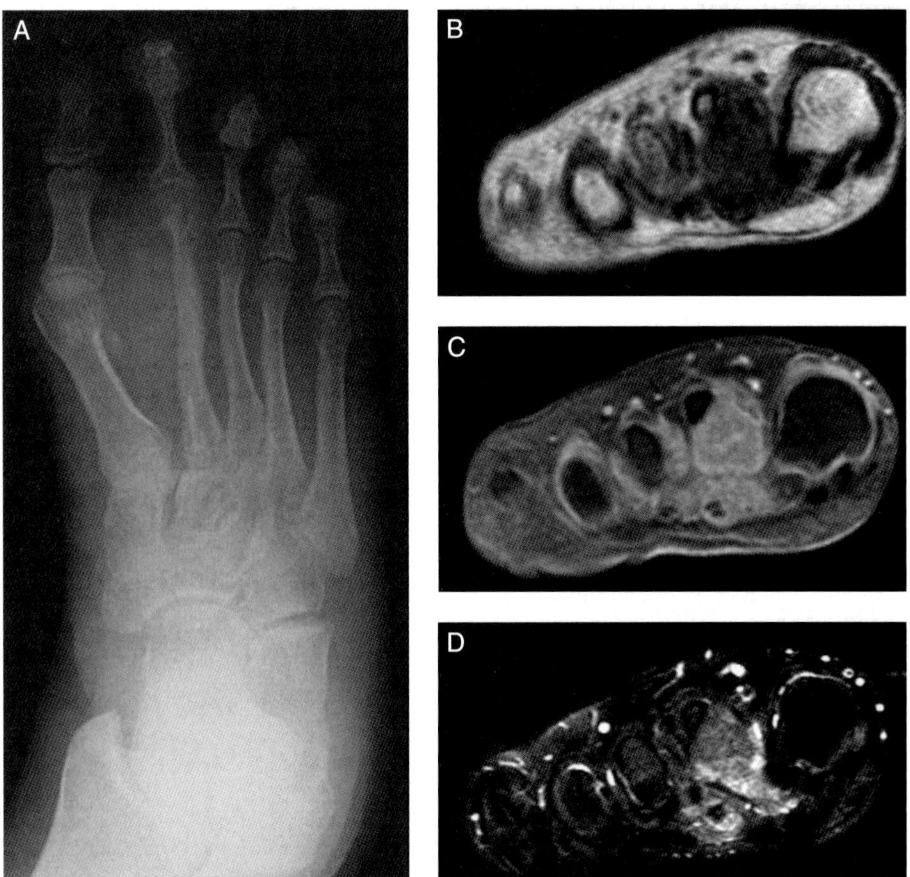

FIGURE 27-2 Anteroposterior radiograph (**A**) shows a poorly visualized soft tissue mass in the first web-space, with a small area of calcification and secondary changes of the second metatarsal with narrowing, hypertrophy and overgrowth. Axial MRI (**B, C** and **D**) better defines this heterogeneous, infiltrative mass, which involves the plantar aspect first web-space and apparently fixed to the 3rd metatarsal but with no invasion or destruction of the bone. This lesion was consistent with benign chondrometaplasia of the foot. (Figures reproduced with permission from The Childrens Orthopaedic Center, Los Angeles, CA)

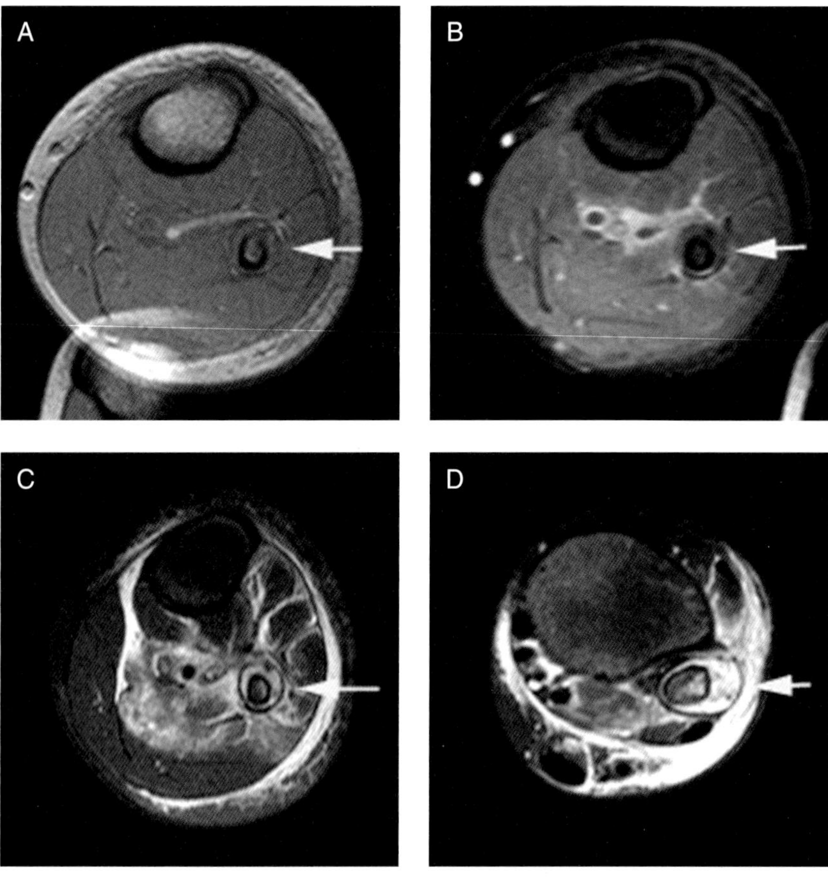

FIGURE 27-3 T1- (**A** and **D**) and T2-weighted (**B** and **C**) MR axial images of the left ankle of a 12 year-old boy, demonstrating subperiosteal abscess (arrow) with surrounding edema caused by acute osteomylelitis of the distal fibula. (Figures reproduced with permission from The Childrens Orthopaedic Center, Los Angeles, CA)

Treatment Methods

The chosen treatment should reflect the expected tumor behavior. Benign tumors should be treated by anatomy-sparing procedures. Benign lesions may be classified as latent (the lesion has been active at some point but now shows no evidence of growth); active (the lesion has been present for some time and continues to grow at a very slow rate, sometimes causing pathologic fracture or angular deformity); or aggressive (the lesion causes bone destruction and grows at a faster pace than active lesions, sometimes is associated with soft-tissue involvement and less frequently distant metastasis). For benign latent and active tumors, intralesional resection or marginal resection is usually appropriate. For benign but locally aggressive lesions, intralesional resection is usually supplemented by an adjuvant (phenol, cryosurgery, etc.). Malignant tumors should be resected with wide margins. Due to the complex bony and soft-tissue anatomy, ray resection and/or amputations are often necessary. Preoperative consultation with a plastic surgeon for anticipated soft-tissue coverage problems is recommended (20).

SOFT-TISSUE TUMORS

Benign Soft-Tissue Tumors

Giant Cell Tumor of the Tendon-Sheath (GCTTS)

GCTTS arises from the synovium, bursa and/or tendon sheaths, and can be classified by its relationship to the joint and growth pattern. The most common form is the localized type. The tumor presents as a circumscribed proliferation of synovial-like cells, foam cells, siderophages

TABLE 27-1

Musculoskeletal Tumor Society (MSTS)

Stage IA	Low grade, intra-low grade
Stage IB	Extra-compartmental high grade
Stage IIA	Intra-compartmental high grade
Stage IIB	Extra-compartmental compartmental
Stage III	Metastatic

TABLE 27-2

American Joint Committee on Cancer (AJCC) (3)

Stage I	Low grade (A or B depending on the size)
Stage II	High grade (A or B depending on the size)
Stage III	Presence of skip metastasis
Stage IV	Distant metastasis (A: lung; B: non-pulmonary metastasis)

and inflammatory cells and is most often in the digits. Approximately 85% of these lesions occur in the fingers and toes.

Any age group may be affected but the tumors are more frequent before the third decade, with a 2:1 female predominance (25). GCTTS usually present as a painless mass or swelling. History of trauma may be obtained. Although GCTTS is a benign active lesion, there is a tendency for recurrence as high as 30% (25). Surgical excision is recommended and ideally the entire synovium involved should be resected (marginal/wide excision) (25,64). These lesions seem to behave similarly in children and adults and meticulous excision has been shown to improve recurrence-free survival (25).

Pigmented Villonodular Synovitis (PVNS)

Pigmented villonodular synovitis (PVNS) is the diffuse form of GCTTS. It is a condition of the synovial membrane and is characterized by the presence of inflammation and hemosiderin deposition. The etiology is unknown. It is typically monoarticular and usually involves the large joints. The knee is the most common site, but hip, ankle, shoulder, and elbow are also common locations (44). The tumor tends to affect the young-adult age group. The lesions can be purely intra-articular (knees and hips represent 90%) or juxta-articular. The clinical symptoms include pain, tenderness, swelling, and limited range of motion (59).

Characteristically PVNS has low signal in both T1- and T2-weighted MRI due to its hemosiderin-laden content. MRI is also helpful differentiating diffuse from localized disease, as well as determining the presence of extra-articular involvement. Erosions of subchondral bone are frequently seen on imaging (64).

Although different treatment modalities have been described, including radiation, injection of radioactive substances and chemotherapy, surgery remains the mainstay of treatment. Resection has the goal of removing all abnormal synovial tissue both to improve the pain management and reduce the risk of secondary joint destruction. Surgical treatment can be performed by an open procedure or by arthroscopy. Joint debridement can be achieved by either method; however the reported results are better with a formal open excision. Most foot lesions are not prone to arthroscopic resection due to the intrinsic anatomy. Recurrence rates as high as 50% have been reported (44,59,61).

Ganglion Cyst

Ganglion cysts present as a fibrous-walled cyst filled with clear mucinous fluid and lacking a differentiated cell lining. They are commonly seen in the soft tissues adjacent to tendons, particularly extensor tendons of feet and hands. Ganglion cysts usually present as a herniation of the synovium and sometimes arise following trauma. Communication between the cyst and the joint may occur but is unusual.

The natural history is one of fluctuation in size and the vast majority are painless. A surgical excision is indicated for symptomatic lesions or when the lesion interferes with shoe wear. Aspiration of the cyst is ineffective and has a very high recurrence rate. Marginal excision is appropriate but should include the capsule.

Plantar Fibromatosis

Plantar fibromatosis is one of the most common forms of fibromatosis. Sometimes referred as superficial fibromatosis or Ledderhose's disease, it typically presents as a solitary, lobular or multilobular mass that averages 0.5 to 2.5 cm in size (21). Histologically, the tumors involve the aponeurosis, forming nodular masses composed of spindle cells with intervening collagen. Some cases are part of an autosomal dominant inheritance pattern. Among adults, there is classic association with alcoholism and diabetes mellitus (4,9).

Clinically, plantar fibromatosis usually presents after age five as a painless nodular mass. There is a slight female predilection (21). Progression to a fibrotic stage associated with joint contractures is not common among children (13). Plantar fibromatosis will often be associated with other symptoms or sites of involvement (knuckle pads, palmar fibromatosis, seizure)(21,62). MRI shows low-intensity (lower than muscle) images in both T1- and T2-weighted images (64). The aggressive forms show displacement and entrapment of adjacent structures.

Although non-surgical treatment has been recommended, the results are fair (i.e., painful extremity and functional compromise) (27,30). Surgery is usually reserved for early stages of contractures. Resection of the nodular lesions has very high recurrence rate.

Lipoma and Lipoblastoma

Lipoma is a benign fat tumor composed of mature white adipocytes. Although it may occur at any age, it is more frequent after the fourth decade. Lipomas are rare in children. They can be superficial (within the subcutaneous tissue) or deep (within deep soft tissues, such as muscle). They usually present as a painless mass. Exceptions are tumors located near a peripheral nerve. Intramuscular lipomas also may be painful and tend to have a higher recurrence rate following surgical resection (6). MRI is a very reliable test for the diagnosis of lipomas (same characteristics as subcutaneous fat), and often precludes the need for a biopsy (Figure 27-4)(64,65).

Lipoblastomas, unlike lipomas, are mainly a childhood condition. A lipoblastoma is a fat tumor that resembles fetal adipose tissue. It can be localized (lipoblastoma) or diffuse (lipoblastomatosis). The tumor occurs more frequently in the first three years and there is a slight male predominance. Clinically, lipoblastoma, presents as a slow growing, often multiple, lobulated, small size masses (approximately 2.5 cm) confined to the subcutaneous tissue (lipoblastoma) or infiltrating the deep muscles (lipoblastomatosis). The imaging differentiation between lipoblastoma/lipoblastomatosis and lipoma or liposarcoma is sometimes difficult (Figure 27-5). Although this is a benign lesion, local recurrences often occur and can be difficult to manage (12,13,39).

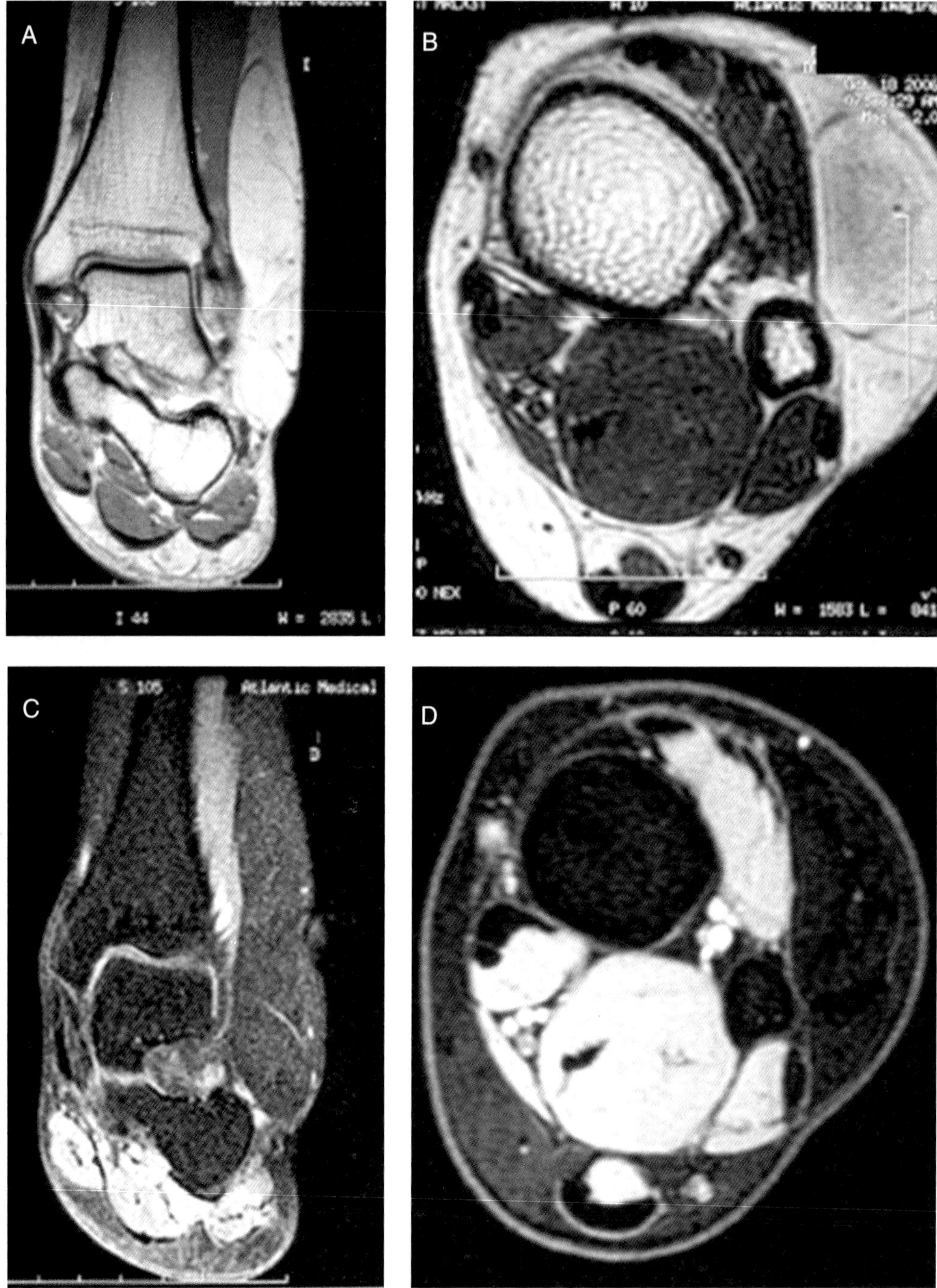

FIGURE 27-4 Coronal (**A** and **C**) and axial (**B** and **D**) T1-weighted (**A** and **B**) and T2-weighted (**C** and **D**) MRI of the left ankle demonstrates a large subcutaneous lesion in the antero-lateral aspect of the ankle. The lesion is homogeneous and has the same signal intensity as the remainder of the subcutaneous fat. This was consistent with lipoma. (Figures reproduced with permission from The Childrens Orthopaedic Center, Los Angeles, CA)

Schwannoma and Neurofibroma

Schwannoma (also known as neurilemoma, neurinoma) is an encapsulated benign nerve sheath tumor that consists of two components: highly ordered cellular component (Antoni A) and a loose myxoid area (Antoni B). They have a predilection for flexion surfaces, especially of feet and hands. Schwannomas are usually solitary, well-encapsulated, and painless lesions that present with a long history of slow growth. Resection is generally easy and because the lesion is superficial, permanent damage to the underlying nerve is uncommon.

Neurofibromas are also a benign tumor of nerve origin. Unlike schwannomas, neurofibromas are not encapsulated. Neurofibromas can present as a solitary (majority) or multiple lesions. The latter is associated with to neurofibromatosis type 1 or von Recklinghausen's disease. Clinically, they present as a painless, superficial mass. Because the neurofibroma is located centrally in the

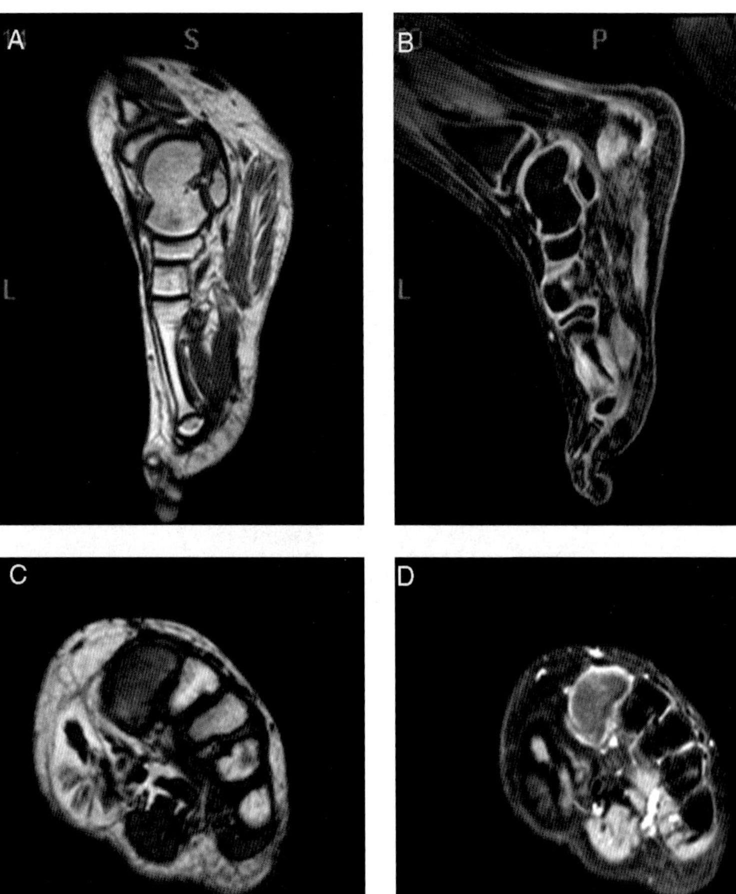

FIGURE 27-5 T1- (**A** and **C**) and T2-weighted (**B** and **D**) MRI of the right foot and ankle of a 9 year-old boy demonstrates an infiltrative, heterogeneous mass of the plantar surface, subcutaneous tissue and hallucis abductor muscle. The patient underwent an open incisional biopsy that was consistent with lipoblastomatosis. (Figures reproduced with permission from The Childrens Orthopaedic Center, Los Angeles, CA)

nerve, function may be permanently impaired prior or following surgical excision. Although extremely rare in children, malignant degeneration may occur, particularly when associated to neurofibromatosis type 1.

Malignant Soft-Tissue Tumors

Synovial Sarcoma

Synovial sarcoma does not originate in the synovium but rather from a mesenchymal spindle cell that resembles epithelial differentiation. The etiology is unknown; however, synovial sarcomas are known to carry a characteristic chromosomal translocation t(X;18) (p11.2;q11.2). Histologically, they can be monophasic composed mainly of spindle cell, or biphasic also presenting with an epithelial (glandular) component.

Synovial sarcoma accounts for 5% to 10% (33) of all soft-tissue sarcomas and occur mainly in young adults between ages 15 and 35. It is the most common malignant tumor of the foot (26,68).

Over 80% of synovial sarcomas arise in deep soft tissue, particularly around the knee, frequently adjacent to the joint or tendon sheaths. Most tumors are slow growing and the size varies especially around the foot and ankle (40,56). There is usually a long delay before diagnosis, averaging up to 20 months in some series (56).

Wide excision is the treatment of choice but depending on the tumor size and location, recurrence rates can be high (40,56). It is still uncertain whether there is a definitive role for chemotherapy, although selected cases may benefit (1). Radiation has been used for improving local control, but it is unclear whether it has any impact on survival (55,67). Pulmonary metastases are frequent (~20%) and impact negatively on the survival rate (56).

Melanoma

Also known as clear cell sarcoma of soft tissue or malignant melanoma of soft parts, melanoma is a rare tumor that involves young adults. The extremities are involved in approximately 80% to 90% of the cases, and foot tumors account for almost 40% (23). Rarely seen in children, melanoma presents as a slow growing, often painful (~50%) mass, that is deep seated and attached to the tendons or aponeurosis (14,29). Almost 50% of these lesions arise from a junctional nevus that present as a flat, tan and non-hairy lesion, often in the plantar aspect of the foot. Indicative signs of malignant degeneration include increase in size (> 5 mm) or skin raising, dark black coloring, or halo pigmentation and ulceration (34).

The overall survival is approximately 50% to 65% at 5 years and 35% at 10 years (15,29). Tumor size and the presence of metastasis impact survival (14,29).

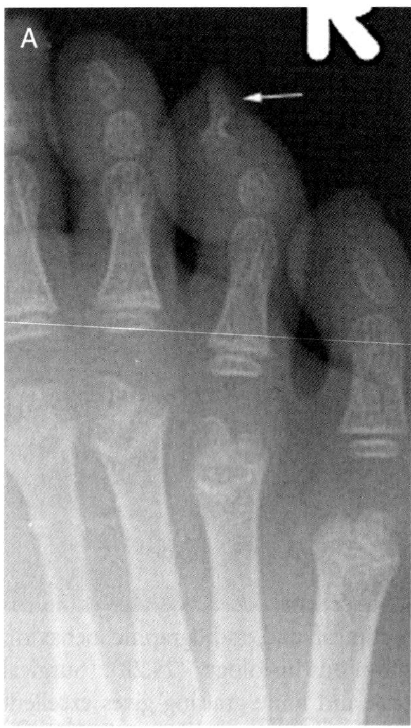

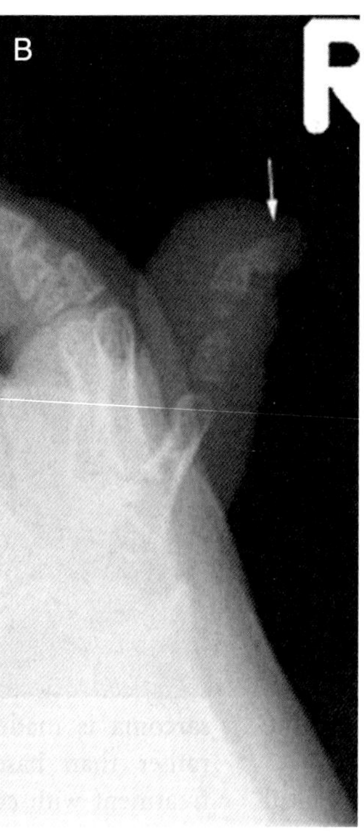

FIGURE 27-8 Anteroposterior (**A**) and lateral (**B**) radiographs of the right 4th toe of a 3 year-old boy demonstrates a pedunculated osteochondroma arising from the distal tip of the distal phalanx. (Figures reproduced with permission from The Childrens Orthopaedic Center, Los Angeles, CA)

to this aggressiveness and tendency for recurrence, surgical treatment includes extended intralesional curettage and the use of adjuvant therapy. Cryosurgery reports with the best long-term results (recurrence free interval) (37,38).

Osteoblastoma and Osteoid Osteoma

Both osteoblastomas and osteoid osteomas are benign bone-forming tumors that are very similar histologically. The differentiation is made based on the size of the lesion and the clinical presentation. Tumors larger than 2 cm are considered osteoblastomas; tumors smaller than 1.5 cm are osteoid osteomas and the remaining are in a "gray zone." Osteoid osteoma presents with the classic history of night pain that responds to NSAIDs or aspirin. Osteoblastoma generate pain that is less characteristic and often unresponsive to those drugs (31,62,66). Osteoid osteoma most commonly involves the long bones, while osteoblastoma also has a tendency to involve the spine. Foot lesions are rare although there are several reports of osteoid osteoma located in the calcaneous, talus, and phalanx (31,42,66). In the author's series, osteoblastoma was not found in the foot (unpublished data).

Malignant Bone Lesions

Ewing Sarcoma (ES)/ Primitive neuro-ectodermal tumor (PNET)

Bone sarcomas rarely occur in the foot and ankle region (62). Ewing sarcoma (ES) is the second most common bony tumor after osteogenic sarcoma but is the most common sarcoma found in the foot and ankle (synovial sarcoma) (2,35). It seems that distal extremity sarcomas have a better overall survival rate than those arising proximal to the knee (68). Ewing sarcoma is characterized by small round blue cells with varying degree of neuroectodermal differentiation. They are often PAS+ and carry a typical immunophenotype CD99. The ES/ PNET family is also characterized by a recurrent t(11;22)(q24;q12) chromosomal translocation (23,62).

There is a slight male predilection and 80% of the patients are younger than 20 years. The presentation is rather nonspecific which may lead to a delay in diagnosis and treatment (2). Ewing sarcoma of the foot will usually present as a painful bony lesion associated with large soft-tissue mass (2,35). Fever, leukocytosis, and elevated sedimentation rate may be present.

Tumors of the hindfoot take a longer time to be diagnosed (average 22 months), and this may contribute to the rate of metastatic disease at presentation and therefore negatively impact the survival (2).

The advances in the chemotherapy regimens have significantly improved the overall survival at five years to approximately 70% (45). The standard of care is neo-adjuvant and adjuvant chemotherapy with wide surgical resection. Radiation therapy (RT) has also been shown to improve the local recurrence and disease-free interval (19,36,55).

Osteogenic Sarcoma (OGS)

Osteogenic sarcoma (OGS) is the most common primary bone tumor. It is most frequently seen around the knee and in other long bones. OGS distal to the ankles is excedingly rare (41).

OGS is a highly anaplastic and pleomorphic spindle cell tumor, characterized by the presence of osteoid produced by the malignant cells (23). It usually has a very aggressive presentation with enlarging painful mass and soft tissue involvement. The vast majority occurs in the first three decades (62). There is a slight higher incidence of OGS of the foot among older patients. The calcaneous seems to be the bone most commonly involved (11).

The treatment is similar to ES and OGS of other locations. Neo-adjuvant chemotherapy is followed by wide surgical resection and adjuvant chemotherapy (11). Unlike ES, OGS does not respond as well to RT, and in case of positive margins or local recurrence, amputation may be necessary.

Chondrosarcoma

Chondrosarcoma is the third most common bone malignancy, and is seen less frequently in young children (28). The average age for chondrosaroma of the foot is in the fifth decade (49). Chondrosarcoma is more prevalent in children with underlying conditions such as Ollier's disease, osteochondromatosis, and Maffucci's syndrome (28,49).

Chondrosarcoma is a malignant tumor with hyaline cartilage differentiation. It encompasses a group of lesions that have similar histology and distinct clinical behavior (23). Differential diagnosis with enchondroma is sometimes difficult since enchondromas of the foot can have a malignant-like histology (28).

Chondrosarcoma can involve any bone of the foot, with the calcaneus most commonly involved (49). Surgery is the mainstay of treatment since chondrosarcomas do not respond to chemotherapy as well as other bone sarcomas. Low-grade lesions may be treated with intralesional resection and cryosurgery. High-grade tumors require wide excision (28).

REFERENCES

1. Adjuvant chemotherapy for localised resectable soft-tissue sarcoma of adults: meta-analysis of individual data. Sarcoma Meta–analysis Collaboration. *Lancet*, 1997. 350(9092): p. 1647–1654.
2. Adkins CD, Kitaoka HB, Seidl RK, et al. Ewing's sarcoma of the foot. *Clin Orthop Relat Res*, 1997(343): p. 173–182.
3. American Joint Commission of Cancer, AJCC Cancer Staging Manual. 6th ed, *A.J.C.o. Cancer*: Springer.
4. Arkkila PE, Kantola IM, Viikari JS, et al. Dupuytren's disease in type 1 diabetic patients: a five-year prospective study. *Clin Exp Rheumatol*, 1996. 14(1): 59–65.
5. Biscaglia R, Bacchini P, Bertoni F. Giant cell tumor of the bones of the hand and foot. *Cancer*, 2000. 88(9): p. 2022–2032.
6. Bjerregaard P, Hagen K, Daugaard S, et al. Intramuscular lipoma of the lower limb. Long-term follow–up after local resection. *J Bone Joint Surg Br*, 1989. 71(5): p. 812–815.
7. Bollini G, Jouve JL, Cottalorda J, et al. Aneurysmal bone cyst in children: analysis of twenty-seven patients. *J Pediatr Orthop B*, 1998. 7(4): p. 274–285.
8. Bos GD, Esther RJ, and Woll TS. Foot tumors: diagnosis and treatment. *J Am Acad Orthop Surg*, 2002. 10(4): p. 259–270.
9. Burge P, Hoy G, Regan P, et al. Smoking, alcohol and the risk of Dupuytren's contracture. *J Bone Joint Surg (Br)*, 1997. 79(2): p. 206–210.
10. Chang CH, Stanton RP, Glutting J. Unicameral bone cysts treated by injection of bone marrow or methylprednisolone. *J Bone Joint Surg Br*, 2002. 84(3): p. 407–412.
11. Choong PF, Qureshi AA, Sim FH, et al. Osteosarcoma of the foot: a review of 52 patients at the Mayo Clinic. *Acta Orthop Scand*, 1999. 70(4): p. 361–364.
12. Chung EB, Enzinger FM. Benign lipoblastomatosis. An analysis of 35 cases. *Cancer*, 1973. 32(2): p. 482–492.
13. Collins MH, Chatten J. Lipoblastoma/lipoblastomatosis: a clinicopathologic study of 25 tumors. *Am J Surg Pathol*, 1997. 21(10): p. 1131–1137.
14. Davila JA, Amrami KK, Sundaram M, et al. Chondroblastoma of the hands and feet. *Skeletal Radiol*, 2004. 33(10): p. 582–587.
15. Deenik W, Mooi WJ, Rutgers EJ, et al. Clear cell sarcoma (malignant melanoma) of soft parts: A clinicopathologic study of 30 cases. *Cancer*, 1999. 86(6): p. 969–975.
16. Dormans JP, Dormans NJ. Use of percutaneous intramedullary decompression and medical-grade calcium sulfate pellets for treatment of unicameral bone cysts of the calcaneus in children. *Orthopedics*, 2004. 27(1 Suppl): p. s137–139.
17. Dormans JP, Hanna BG, Johnston DR, et al. Surgical treatment and recurrence rate of aneurysmal bone cysts in children. *Clin Orthop Relat Res*, 2004(421): p. 205–211.
18. Dubois J, Chigot V, Grimard G, et al. Sclerotherapy in aneurysmal bone cysts in children: a review of 17 cases. *Pediatr Radiol*, 2003. 33(6): p. 365–372.
19. Eralp Y, Bavbek S, Basaran M, et al. Prognostic factors and survival in late adolescent and adult patients with small round cell tumors. *Am J Clin Oncol*, 2002. 25(4): p. 418–424.
20. Ferguson PC. Surgical considerations for management of distal extremity soft tissue sarcomas. *Curr Opin Oncol*, 2005. 17(4): p. 366–369.
21. Fetsch JF, Laskin WB, Miettinen M. Palmar-plantar fibromatosis in children and preadolescents: a clinicopathologic study of 56 cases with newly recognized demographics and extended follow-up information. *Am J Surg Pathol*, 2005. 29(8): p. 1095–1105.
22. Fink BR, Temple HT, Chiricosta FM, et al. Chondroblastoma of the foot. *Foot Ankle Int*, 1997. 18(4): p. 236–242.
23. Fletcher CDM, Unni KK, Mertens F. Pathology & Genetics of Tumours of Soft-Tissue and Bone. World Health Organization Classification of Tumours, ed. P. Kleihues and L.H. Sobin. Lyon: IABC Press, 2002.
24. Gajewski DA, Burnette JB, Murphey MD, et al. Differentiating clinical and radiographic features of enchondroma and secondary chondrosarcoma in the foot. *Foot Ankle Int*, 2006. 27(4): p. 240–244.
25. Gholve PA, Hosalkar HS, Kreiger PA, et al. Giant cell tumor of tendon sheath: largest single series in children. *J Pediatr Orthop*, 2007. 27(1): p. 67–74.
26. Gross E, Rao BN, Bowman L, et al. Outcome of treatment for pediatric sarcoma of the foot: a retrospective review over a 20-year period. *J Pediatr Surg*, 1997. 32(8): p. 1181–1184.
27. Hurst LC, Badalamente MA. Nonoperative treatment of Dupuytren's disease. *Hand Clin*, 1999. 15(1): p. 97–107, vii.
28. Huvos AG, Marcove RC. Chondrosarcoma in the young. A clinicopathologic analysis of 79 patients younger than 21 years of age. *Am J Surg Pathol*, 1987. 11(12): p. 930–942.
29. Kawai A, Hosono A, Nakayama R, et al. Clear cell sarcoma of tendons and aponeuroses: a study of 75 patients. *Cancer*, 2007. 109(1): p. 109–116.
30. Ketchum LD, Donahue TK. The injection of nodules of Dupuytren's disease with triamcinolone acetonide. *J Hand Surg [Am]*, 2000. 25(6): p. 1157–1162.
31. Kilgore WB, Parrish WM. Calcaneal tumors and tumor-like conditions. *Foot Ankle Clin*, 2005. 10(3): p. 541–565, vii.
32. Kirby EJ, Shereff MJ, Lewis MM. Soft-tissue tumors and tumor-like lesions of the foot. An analysis of eighty-three cases. *J Bone Joint Surg Am*, 1989. 71(4): p. 621–626.
33. Kransdorf MJ. Malignant soft-tissue tumors in a large referral population: distribution of diagnoses by age, sex, and location. *AJR Am J Roentgenol*, 1995. 164(1): p. 129–134.

34. Kukita A, Ishihara K. Clinical features and distribution of malignant melanoma and pigmented nevi on the soles of the feet in Japan. *J Invest Dermatol*, 1989. 92(5 Suppl): 210S–213S.
35. Leeson MC, Smith MJ. Ewing's sarcoma of the foot. *Foot Ankle*, 1989. 10(3): p. 147–151.
36. Lin PP, Guzel VB, Pisters PW, et al. Surgical management of soft tissue sarcomas of the hand and foot. *Cancer*, 2002. 95(4): p. 852–861.
37. Malawer MM, Bickels J, Meller I, et al. Cryosurgery in the treatment of giant cell tumor. A long-term followup study. *Clin Orthop Relat Res*, 1999(359): p. 176–188.
38. Marcove RC, Weis LD, Vaghaiwalla MR, et al. Cryosurgery in the treatment of giant cell tumors of bone: a report of 52 consecutive cases. *Clin Orthop Relat Res*, 1978(134): p. 275–289.
39. Mentzel T, Calonje E, Fletcher CD. Lipoblastoma and lipoblastomatosis: a clinicopathological study of 14 cases. *Histopathology*, 1993. 23(6): p. 527–533.
40. Michal M, Fanburg-Smith JC, Lasota J, et al. Minute synovial sarcomas of the hands and feet: a clinicopathologic study of 21 tumors less than 1 cm. *Am J Surg Pathol*, 2006. 30(6): p. 721–726.
41. Mirra JM, Kameda N, Rosen G, et al. Primary osteosarcoma of toe phalanx: first documented case. Review of osteosarcoma of short tubular bones. *Am J Surg Pathol*, 1988. 12(4): p. 300–307.
42. Morris GB, Goldman FD. Osteoid osteoma causing subtalar joint arthralgia: a case report. *J Foot Ankle Surg*, 2003. 42(2): p. 90–94.
43. Murari TM, Callaghan JJ, Berrey Jr. BH, et al. Primary benign and malignant osseous neoplasms of the foot. *Foot Ankle*, 1989. 10(2): 68–80.
44. Myers BW, Masi AT. Pigmented villonodular synovitis and tenosynovitis: a clinical epidemiologic study of 166 cases and literature review. *Medicine (Baltimore)*, 1980. 59(3): p. 223–238.
45. Nesbit ME, Jr., Gehan EA, Burgert, Jr. EO, et al. Multimodal therapy for the management of primary, nonmetastatic Ewing's sarcoma of bone: a long–term follow–up of the First Intergroup study. *J Clin Oncol*, 1990. 8(10): p. 1664–1674.
46. Neville HL, Andrassy RJ, Lobe TE, et al. Preoperative staging, prognostic factors, and outcome for extremity rhabdomyosarcoma: a preliminary report from the Intergroup Rhabdomyosarcoma Study IV (1991–1997). *J Pediatr Surg*, 2000. 35(2): p. 317–321.
47. Newton Jr. WA, Webber B, Hamoudi AB, et al. Early history of pathology studies by the Intergroup Rhabdomyosarcoma Study Group. *Pediatr Dev Pathol*, 1999. 2(3): p. 275–285.
48. Newton Jr. WA, Gehan EA, Webber BL, et al. Classification of rhabdomyosarcomas and related sarcomas. Pathologic aspects and proposal for a new classification—an Intergroup Rhabdomyosarcoma Study. *Cancer*, 1995. 76(6): p. 1073–1085.
49. Ogose A, Unni KK, Swee RG, et al. Chondrosarcoma of small bones of the hands and feet. *Cancer*, 1997. 80(1): p. 50–59.
50. Peltier LF, Jones RH. Treatment of unicameral bone cysts by curettage and packing with plaster-of-Paris pellets. *J Bone Joint Surg Am*, 1978. 60(6): p. 820–822.
51. Punyko JA, Mertens AC, Baker KS, et al. Long-term survival probabilities for childhood rhabdomyosarcoma. A population-based evaluation. *Cancer*, 2005. 103(7): p. 1475–1483.
52. Ramirez AR, Stanton RP. Aneurysmal bone cyst in 29 children. *J Pediatr Orthop*, 2002. 22(4): p. 533–539.
53. Saraph V, Zwick EB, Maizen C, et al. Treatment of unicameral calcaneal bone cysts in children: review of literature and results using a cannulated screw for continuous decompression of the cyst. *J Pediatr Orthop*, 2004. 24(5): p. 568–573.
54. Scaglietti O, Marchetti PG, Bartolozzi P. Final results obtained in the treatment of bone cysts with methylprednisolone acetate (depo–medrol) and a discussion of results achieved in other bone lesions. *Clin Orthop Relat Res*, 1982(165): 33–42.
55. Schoenfeld GS, Morris CG, Scarborough MT, et al. Adjuvant radiotherapy in the management of soft tissue sarcoma involving the distal extremities. *Am J Clin Oncol*, 2006. 29(1): p. 62–65.
56. Scully SP, Temple HT, Harrelson JM. Synovial sarcoma of the foot and ankle. *Clin Orthop Relat Res*, 1999(364): p. 220–226.
57. Seale KS, Lange TA, Monson D, et al. Soft tissue tumors of the foot and ankle. *Foot Ankle*, 1988. 9(1): 19–27.
58. Sessions W, Siegel HJ, Thomas J, et al. Chondroblastoma with associated aneurysmal bone cyst of the cuboid. *J Foot Ankle Surg*, 2005. 44(1): p. 64–67.
59. Sharma H, Jane MJ, Reid R. Pigmented villonodular synovitis of the foot and ankle: Forty years of experience from the Scottish bone tumor registry. *J Foot Ankle Surg*, 2006. 45(5): p. 329–336.
60. Stieber JR, Dormans JP. Manifestations of hereditary multiple exostoses. *J Am Acad Orthop Surg*, 2005. 13(2): p. 110–120.
61. Tyler WK, Vidal AF, Williams RJ, et al. Pigmented villonodular synovitis. *J Am Acad Orthop Surg*, 2006. 14(6): p. 376–385.
62. Unni KK. *Dahlin's Bone Tumors: General aspects and data on 11087 cases*. 5th ed. Philadelphia: Lippincott-Raven, 1996.
63. Vazquez-Flores H, Dominguez-Cherit J, Vega-Memije ME, et al. Subungual osteochondroma: clinical and radiologic features and treatment. *Dermatol Surg*, 2004. 30(7): p. 1031–1034.
64. Waldt S, Rechl H, Rummeny EJ, et al. Imaging of benign and malignant soft tissue masses of the foot. *Eur Radiol*, 2003. 13(5): p. 1125–1136.
65. Woertler K. Soft tissue masses in the foot and ankle: characteristics on MR Imaging. *Semin Musculoskelet Radiol*, 2005. 9(3): p. 227–242.
66. Wu KK. Osteoid osteoma of the foot. *J Foot Surg*, 1991. 30(2): p. 190–194.
67. Yang JC, Chang AE, Baker AR, et al. Randomized prospective study of the benefit of adjuvant radiation therapy in the treatment of soft tissue sarcomas of the extremity. *J Clin Oncol*, 1998. 16(1): 197–203.
68. Zeytoonjian T, Mankin HJ, Gebhardt MC, et al. Distal lower extremity sarcomas: frequency of occurrence and patient survival rate. *Foot Ankle Int*, 2004. 25(5): p. 325–330.

CHAPTER 28

Osteochondoses and Apophysitis

Craig P. Eberson and Jonathan R. Schiller

INTRODUCTION

Osteochondroses and apophysitides are common afflictions of often occur in the pediatric foot. While most are self-limiting, long-term symptoms occasionally result. Apophysitis occurs as an overuse injury and can affect several of the apophyseal plates in the foot, e.g., Sever's disease of the calcaneus. Inflammation of synchondroses between accessory ossicles and the tarsal bones, such as the os trigonum syndrome and symptomatic accessory navicular, are also sources of disability. Finally, the osteochondroses of the child's foot, most notably Kohler's and Freiberg's diseases, are thought to result from a disruption of the normal blood supply to the tarsal navicular and second metatarsal, respectively. These conditions will be reviewed in detail.

APOPHYSITIDES

Apophysitis represents an inflammation of an apophyseal growth plate, usually resulting from chronic traction. Sever's disease, which represents an apophysitis of the calcaneus, is the most commonly seen. These syndromes usually respond to conservative treatments directed toward decreasing inflammation and protecting the involved growth plate from further injury.

Sever's Disease

Heel pain in immature athletes is a common complaint. Frequently, inflammation of the calcaneal apophysis is responsible. The ossification of this secondary nucleus begins typically at seven years of age and usually fuses with the primary calcaneus by age 15 (59). Patients present with complaints of pain after athletic activity. The pain often is located on the plantar or plantar-medial aspect of the foot and is worse after prolonged activity. Pain or stiffness on awakening is also common, similar to patients with plantar faciitis. The average age of onset is 8–13 years old, and 60% of patients have bilateral involvement (40). The condition is often more common in males, with one study demonstrating a rate of almost 4 to 1 (61).

The cause of Sever's disease is debated in the literature. The apophysis serves as the attachment for the Achilles tendon superiorly and the short toe flexors inferiorly. Constant traction from repetitive stress (running, soccer, etc.) often results in inflammation and pain. Ogden (42) felt it represents trabecular microtrauma, rather than a true apophysitis, based on magnetic resonance imaging (MRI) findings. While the condition may represent both apophysitis as well as microtrabecular injury, the treatment is the same regardless of the etiology.

Evaluation of patients with heel pain begins with a thorough history and physical examination. Pain is usually described as activity related. Patients will often be comfortable immediately after sports but will have pain on walking after they "cool down." Symptoms are common after initiating a new sport or at the beginning of the season. Physical exam reveals tenderness of the plantar or medial aspect of the calcaneus in the region of the apophysis, often with pain with palpation of the apophysis. A tight Achilles tendon is almost universally found, although it unclear whether this represents cause or effect. Differential diagnosis of this condition includes stress fracture; infection; inflammatory arthropathy; and calcaneal tumor (unicameral bone cyst, osteoid osteoma). Patients who have atypical pain or symptoms that do not respond to simple measures should have radiographs, particularly for unilateral symptoms (Figure 28-1). While increased density of the apophysis has been reported to be a finding in these patients, Volpon noted this is a normal radiographic finding in children (59). He described an increased degree of fragmentation of the apophysis, although the significance of this is unclear. Radiographs of the contralateral hindfoot often have similar findings. The role of radiographs is primarily to exclude other pathology, and they are usually not indicated for routine cases.

Treatment involves activity modification, and Achilles tendon stretching. Some patients benefit from gel heel

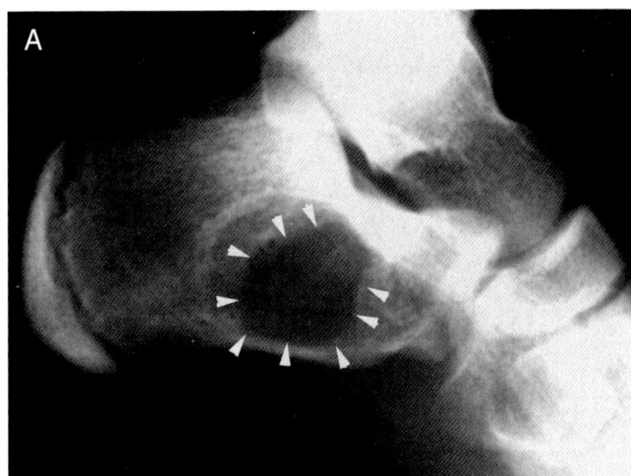

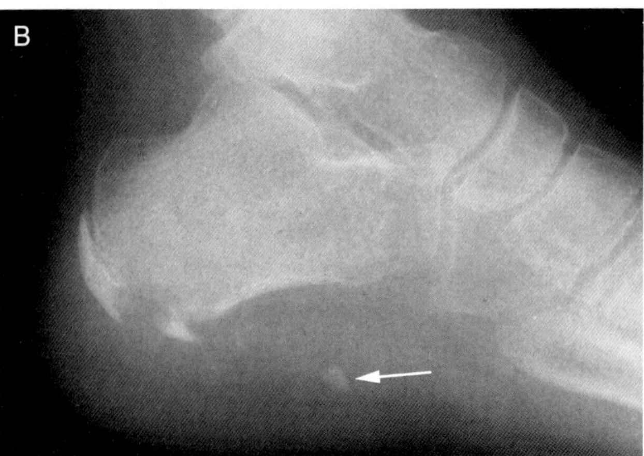

FIGURE 28-1 Differential diagnosis of heel pain. Both of these patients presented with chronic heel pain. **A.** Unicameral bone cyst **B.** Chronic osteomyelitis. Note fragmentation of the apophysis which has "floated" into the forefoot via a large abscess. Interestingly, the patient had no fever and normal laboratory studies. Staph aureus infection diagnosed by intraoperative culture at the time of debridement.

cups to decrease impact trauma to the plantar portion of the apophysis. Usually, casting or complete cessation of sports is not necessary except for extreme cases, although some patients may need to limit their participation in the short term. Patients who limp for more than 12 hours after activity often benefit from a temporary hiatus from activities until symptoms subside.

Other Apophysitides

Children who participate in sports requiring sharp cutting techniques may experience inflammation of the fifth metatarsal apophysis, Iselin's disease (7,46,48). The apophysis is located at the insertion site of the peroneus brevis tendon on the plantar-lateral metatarsal and may become painful in the older child or adolescent. Radiographs may show fragmentation of the apophysis, and bone scans are typically positive; x-ray the contralateral sife for comparison (Figure 28-2). Treatment involves immobilization for acute pain, stretching, and gradual return to activity. While this condition is usually self-limiting, there are reported cases of persistent pain and nonunion (7,46,48). Differential diagnosis includes acute avulsion fracture, as well as peroneal tendonitis. A fracture is usually perpendicular to the axis of the metatarsal (a transverse fracture). The normal apophysis is parallel to the bone, making it possible to differentiate between the two.

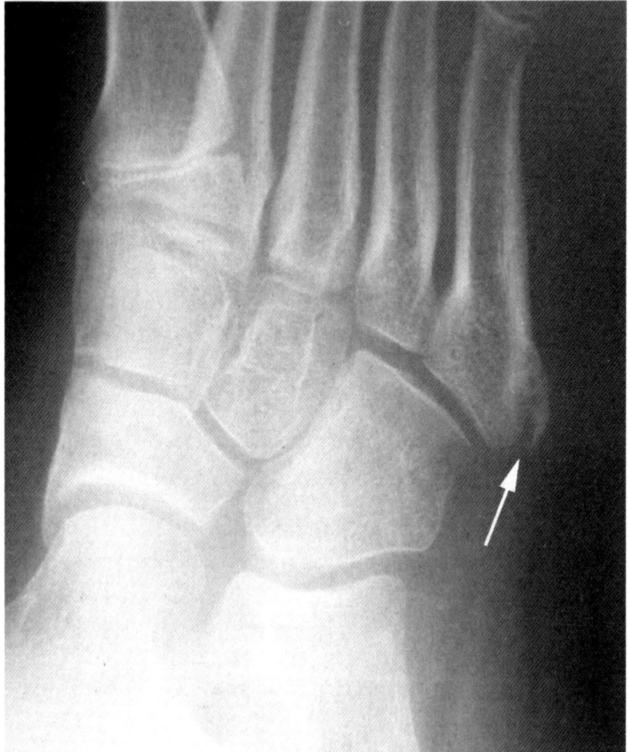

FIGURE 28-2 Radiograph of a 13-year-old female athlete with recurrent "sprains" of her foot. There is fragmentation and sclerosis of the fifth metatarsal apophysis, consistent with a diagnosis of Iselin's disease.

Traction apophysitis of the medial malleolus has also been described (43). Ishii described three patients with pain over the anterior aspect of the medial malleolus (24). Accessory ossification centers were noted on radiographs, and MRI demonstrated injury at the cartilaginous junction between the ossicle and the malleolus proper. Patients presented with a triad of medial swelling, tenderness over the medial malleolus, and pain with valgus stress of the foot. They examined 134 high school basketball players and noted that 25% had tenderness in this region. They concluded that this condition may be more common than reported. Patients generally respond to conservative treatment. Orthotics to control pronation, as well as ankle supportive braces, may be helpful in relieving stress in this region.

Os Trigonum Syndrome /Posterior Ankle Impingement Syndrome (PAIS)

The os trigonum is an accessory bone located at the posterolateral aspect of the talus. It normally appears on radiographs in children between the ages of eight and eleven as a secondary center of ossification and usually fuses to the talus within one year (39). In 1.7% to 7.7% of patients, it remains unfused as an accessory ossicle, known as an os trigonum. Controversy exists as to whether this unfused ossicle is in fact an un-united fracture (16). In either case, the os trigonum may become symptomatic when it is compressed between the calcaneus and the posterior aspect of the tibia. Frequently, there is an associated inflammatory hypertrophy of the ankle capsule (44). The flexor hallucis longus (FHL) tendon runs in a groove on the posteromedial aspect of the talus through a thick tendon sheath. Often inflammation of this tendon may contribute to posterior ankle pain associated with an os trigonum (12,20).

Posterior ankle impingement syndrome (PAIS) is seen in athletic children who participate in activities which require extreme ankle plantar flexion. This includes dancers, divers, martial artists, downhill runners, and others. It can occasionally be seen in older adolescents who wear high heel shoes for extended periods of time (36). Athletes who grip the floor with their toes (gymnasts, martial artists) are also predisposed (12).

Posterior ankle impingement syndrome should be considered in children presenting with posterior ankle pain of a chronic nature. The symptomatic os trigonum presents with pain in the posterior aspect of the ankle, posterior to the peroneal tendons, and is reproduced with extreme plantar flexion. Associated medial pain should raise the question of an associated FHL tendonitis (9,12,20,36,44). The FHL can be palpated in its sheath behind the medial malleolus, and often crepitus can be felt with movement of the great toe. Pain with great toe passive dorsiflexion is another clue to this disorder (12).

Radiologic investigation of PAIS begins with plain radiographs and may also entail computed tomography (CT), MRI, or bone scintigraphy (6,36). On radiographs, the bony os trigonum is identified; sclerotic borders signify chronicity, as opposed to the sharp demarcation seen in an acute fracture (Figure 28-3). Other causes of foot pain (tarsal coalition, calcaneal apophysitis, fracture) are investigated. CT scanning may be helpful in identify a small fragment but is unable to differentiate between acute and chronic processes, bone scintigraphy may be required. A negative study excludes the diagnosis of PAIS although a positive scintigraphic scan is not necessarily confirmatory (26). In a study of 100 soldiers, 14 feet had increased uptake in the os trigonum, while only 10 of these feet had symptoms of PAIS (52).

MRI is the study of choice for PAIS. In addition to identifying edema within the synchondrosis between the os trigonum and the talus, other pathologic processes can be identified, such as osteochondral injury, tendinopathy, subtalar or ankle effusion, and stress fracture (Figure 28-4) (5,6,26,36,60).

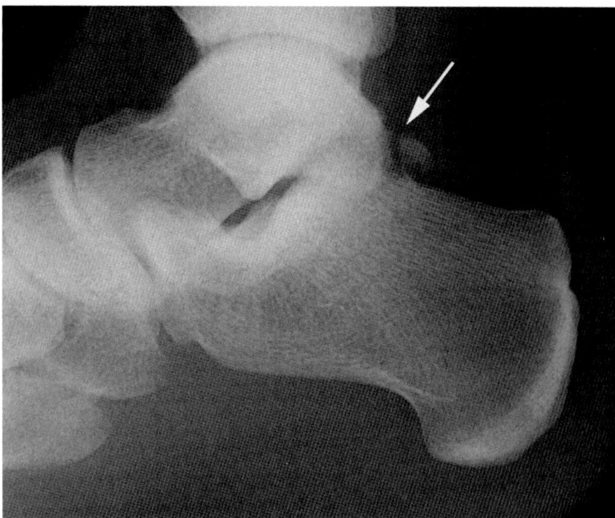

FIGURE 28-3 Os trigonum, seen posterior to the talus. The patient presented with chronic ankle pain during sports.

Differential Diagnosis

A careful history and physical exam is required to rule out other potential causes of posterior ankle pain (Table 28-1).

Treatment

Most patients with PAIS respond to conservative treatment, such as rest and anti-inflammatory medication. Occasionally, a trial of casting is useful. For symptomatic os trigonum, an injection of corticosteroids mixed with a local anesthetic can be helpful as a diagnostic and therapeutic tool; the immediate relief from the anesthetic confirms the diagnosis when the injection is performed under fluoroscopic guidance to confirm location. The corticosteroid may relieve the inflammation, but this may be temporary (9,12,36,44). Steroid injection into the FHL is contraindicated due to concern of tendon rupture, technical difficulty entering the sheath, and the proximity of the tibial nerve (20). Protective dorsiflexion taping will aid some patients after return to sports. The success rate of conservative treatment has been reported to be 60% (22). Some authors feel that some recurrence of symptoms from an os trigonum is certain in a competitive athlete, and resection is recommended (13,44).

For patients who fail conservative treatment, surgery is indicated (1,12,20,36). It is crucial to differentiate among patients who have symptoms from the os trigonum, the FHL, or from both problems. A medial hindfoot approach is utilized for FHL exposure, while a lateral approach is chosen for the os trigonum. A medial approach is used, when there is combined pathology as the FHL cannot be safely released from the lateral exposure. Occasionally, both incisions are needed (20). The specific techniques are described below.

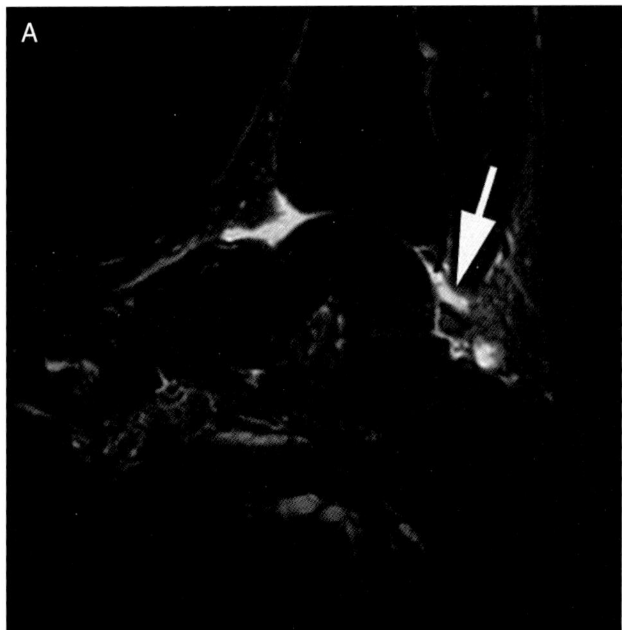

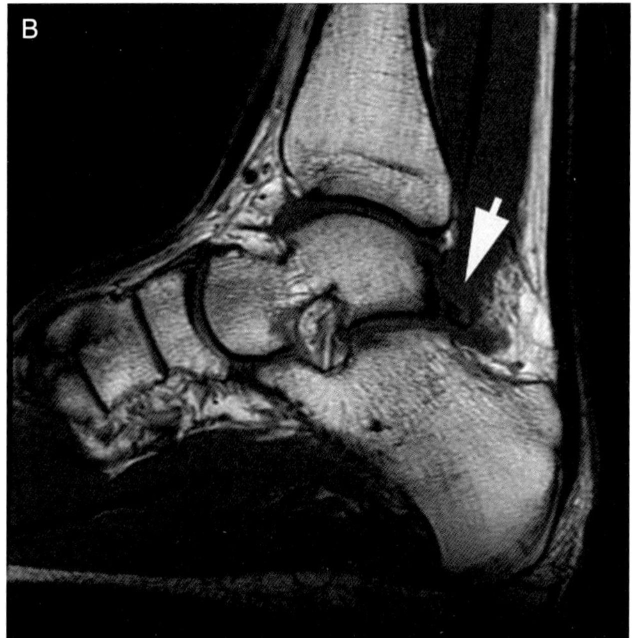

FIGURE 28-4 Magnetic resonance imaging of os trigonum. **A.** edema is noted surrounding the unfused ossicle (*arrow*). **B.** marrow replacement of ossicle due to edema (*arrow*).

Excision of Symptomatic Os Trigonum

The patient is positioned in the lateral or prone position, and a tourniquet is utilized. The incision begins 4 cm proximal to the lateral malleolus and extends 1 cm distal to it. The exposure is slightly proximal to and just posteromedial to the peroneal tendon sheath. After identifying and protecting the sural nerve, the dissection is exposed to the os trigonum by opening the deep posterior compartment fascia, dissecting through the retrocalcaneal fat, and palpating the os trigonum with the foot in dorsiflexion. There is an interval between the FHL medially and the peroneal tendons laterally. The posterior tibiofibular ligament, as well as the posterior ankle capsule, is incised, and the fragment identified just lateral to the FHL. The fragment may have four attachments: superiorly (posterior ankle capsule), inferiorly (posterior talocalcaneal ligament), medially (the FHL sheath), and laterally (the origin of the posterior talofibular ligament). These are released, and the fragment excised. After inspecting the region for additional loose bodies or other pathology, the foot is brought into maximal plantar flexion to ensure that no further impingement occurs.Any residual bony prominence is addressed prior to wound closure. The patient is immobilized in a non–weight bearing short leg cast for one to two weeks, followed by a supervised therapy program (1,20). Abramowitz reported better results in patients who were symptomatic for less than two years, and noted that 8 of 41 patients had postoperative sural nerve sensory loss, 50% of which were permanent. This complication needs to be reviewed with patients prior to surgery (1). Marumoto and Ferkel have described arthroscopic excision of the os trigonum (38). We have no experience with this technique.

TABLE 28-1

Differential Diagnosis of Posterior Ankle Impingement Syndrome

Os trigonum syndrome
Flexor hallucis longus tendosynovitis
Osteochondral injury of the talus
Achilles/peroneal tendonitis
Subtalar inflammatory arthritis
Calcaneal stress fracture/apophysitis
Occult fracture
Posterior tibiotalar ligament injury

Treatment of FHL Tenosynovitis

For patients with isolated FHL pathology, or combined pathology, the patient is placed in the supine position with the leg externally rotated. A curvilinear incision is made over the neurovascular bundle directly behind the medial malleolus. As the branches of the tibial nerve run posteriorly, the safe plane for dissection lies between the bundle and the malleolus. Small vascular branches are ligated, and the bundle is retracted posteriorly. The FHL is identified by moving the great toe and the sheath opened to the level of the sustentaculum tali, where the tendon often impinges as it passes beneath in a fibro-osseous tunnel. The tendon is inspected for nodules, which are debrided, or tears which are repaired. The gliding of the tendon is then observed, and further release of the sheath is done beneath the sustentaculum as needed. Care should be taken to avoid unnecessary release, which could result in tendon subluxation. The tendon is retracted with the neurovascular bundle, and the subtalar joint identified.

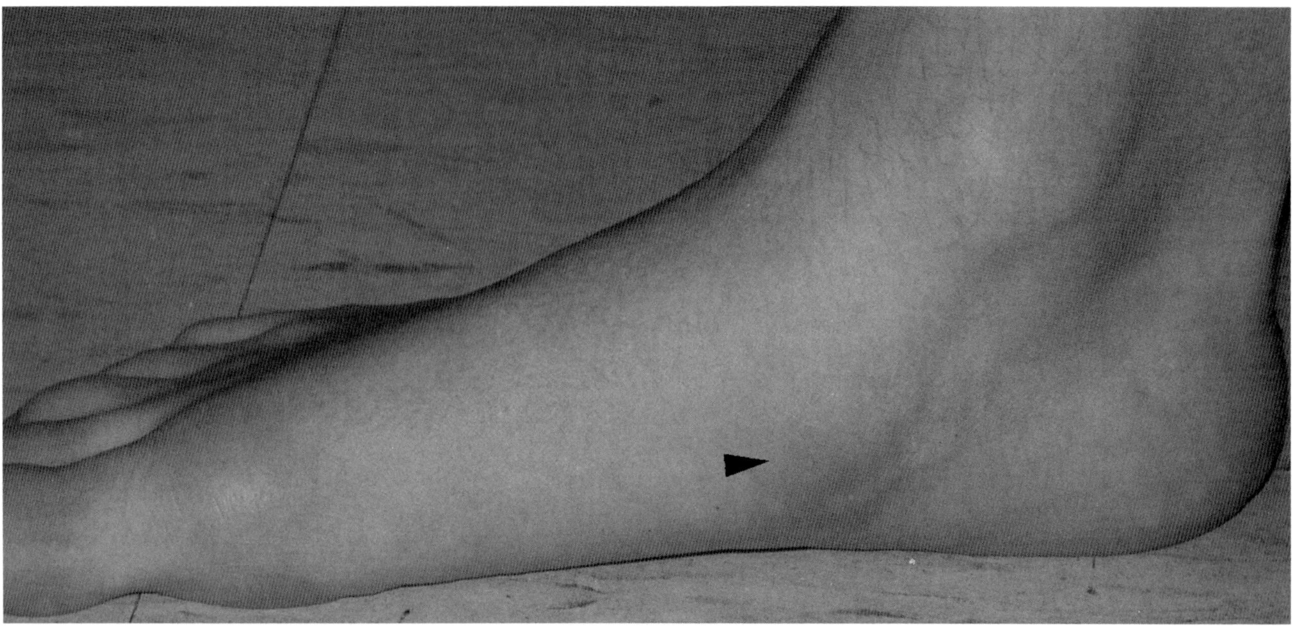

FIGURE 28-5 Flatfoot associated with an accessory navicular. The arch is flat, and there is erythema, callous formation, and tenderness over the navicular (*arrowhead*).

The os trigonum is identified and excised, as described above. The patient is splinted for one week. Formal physical therapy and gradual return to activities is then allowed after sufficient soft-tissue healing (12,20,32,56).

Accessory Navicular

Located on the medial side of the midfoot, an accessory navicular is an accessory ossicle, proximal to the navicular and in continuity with the tibialis posterior tendon (15). It is considered to be a normal anatomic and radiographic variant, present in up to 15% of the population. The accessory navicular is one of the most symptomatic accessory bones in the foot (14,19,34,58). The condition has been observed in multiple family members, and an autosomal dominant pattern with incomplete penetrance has been reported (14,30).

Typically, patients are active adolescents who have a flexible flatfoot, though controversy exists whether the accessory navicular is responsible for loss of the medial arch (3,55). The patient may describe pain and swelling over the medial side of the midfoot and may even have a palpable prominence (Figure 28-5). Shoe wear may become difficult, and pain is often aggravated by tight shoes. Associated erythema directly over the prominence may occur with or without callus formation. There may be tenderness over the prominence of the navicular and resisted inversion may elicit pain, as the tibialis posterior tendon has been shown to insert on the accessory navicular (31). The differential is extensive for medial mid-foot pain and includes: Kohler's disease, tibialis posterior tendon rupture, enthesiopathy of the tibialis anterior tendon, and navicular stress fracture.

Ray and Goldberg classified three types of accessory navicular based on the anatomy of the fragment: type 1, containment of the ossicle within the tibialis posterior tendon, anatomically separate from the navicular; type 2, cartilaginous bridge between ossicle and navicular; and type 3, where the accessory ossicle fuses to the navicular (46). Radiographs are helpful when the navicular and accessory ossicle have ossified and aid in classification and treatment. Standard weight-bearing anteroposterior and lateral foot films, as well as an external oblique view demonstrate the accessory ossicle (Figure 28-6). While the diagnosis is typically based on plain radiographs, occasionally additional imaging may be needed. A bone scan may be useful in the patient when it is unclear what entity is responsible for medial foot pain. MRI has also been utilized in establishing the diagnosis (11,25,29). Histology reveals areas of microfracture at the cartilage bridge (synchondrosis) in type 2 accessory naviculars, with evidence of acute and chronic inflammation and destruction of the cartilage cap; persistent edema suggestive of osteonecrosis, and cellular proliferation suggestive of a reparative process (11,19).

Treatment for asymptomatic pes planus with an accessory navicular is not required. However, a painful prominence or difficulty with shoe wear can be alleviated with a doughnut-shaped piece of mole skin and comfortable wide-based shoes. A molded longitudinal arch support may help relieve pressure over the medial arch and resist pronation of the foot. Cast immobilization for six weeks may be warranted for severe pain. UCLB with medial outflare in the area of prominence controls both pes planus and relieves pressure.

When conservative measures fail, operative intervention is recommended to relieve the symptomatic accessory navicular (3). Traditionally, the Kidner procedure, which excises the accessory ossicle and advances the tibialis posterior tendon plantarly, has been the treatment of choice with adequate success relieving pain (3,49). Ray and Goldberg found good to excellent results with an average of 4.5 years

efficacy has not been demonstrated in the literature thus far. Steroid injections in to the MTP joint have been advocated to alleviate pain. However, the injection can make the arthritis worse and can lead to tendon or ligament rupture if the foot is not immobilized (27). We prefer to avoid these in children. Conservative measures have been helpful in the early stages of the disease process, and most patients respond to nonoperative treatment without long-term consequences (13).

Surgical treatment is rare and is indicated for failure of conservative treatment. Several options exist: debridement and loose body removal, osteotomy, elevation of the loose fragment and bone grafting, core decompression to stimulate revascularization, metatarsal head excision; metatarsal shortening; excision of the proximal phalangeal base; and joint arthroplasty. Unfortunately, there is little agreement as to which procedure is the most beneficial. Early stage Freiberg's managed with joint debridement and synovectomy has been reported to improve joint range of motion, avoid major arthritic changes, and give long-term relief (53). Open-core decompression and osteochondral transplantation have had similar results for early stage Freiberg's (10,17). If there is significant involvement of the metatarsal head with a preserved plantar surface, then a closing-wedge dorsiflexion osteotomy through the metatarsal head and neck is recommended. Initially described by Gauthier and Elbaz in 1979, this procedure moves the healthy cartilage on the plantar surface of the metatarsal head to articulate with the proximal phalanx with reported good outcomes, though potential risk to the remaining blood supply exists, as well as the development of transfer lesions (10,18). MRI may be helpful in deciding the correction angle for dorsal-wedge osteotomy and post-operative confirmation the necrotic focus was decompressed and moved from the proximal phalanx articulation in the rare patient who requires surgery (2,10). Arthroscopy has also been utilized for debridement and core decompression in the treatment of Freiberg's with good results (21,37). Carro et al. performed an arthroscopic Keller excision with debridement and removal of the free body with excellent results at two years follow up (8). Joint arthroplasty using a silastic flexible hinged implant, tendon interposition, and titanium implants have all been attempted with reported good results, though there is a paucity of cases and all require further study to validate their efficacy (16,35,50). The large variety of surgical options emphasizes the lack of a "gold standard" for surgical treatment of this condition, and most surgical approaches to this condition are directed toward treatment in the older, adult patient. It is paramount to remember that the vast majority of children with this condition respond to conservative treatment.

Kohler's Disease

Kohler's disease is an uncommon, self limiting, idiopathic avascular necrosis of the tarsal navicular. Usually unilateral, it affects children between the ages of two and nine, boys more commonly than girls. The prognosis is excellent, with the navicular regaining its normal architecture before the foot completes growth and normal ossification is completed in two years (62). This differs from the adult version, called Müller-Weiss disease, which is often debilitating and leads to surgery for clinical improvement (2).

Although unproven, several theories exist as to the etiology of Kohler's disease. The navicular is subjected to repetitive compressive forces during weight bearing which may lead to avascular necrosis (23,62). Because the navicular is the last bone to ossify, the delay makes the navicular more vulnerable to compressive forces and occlusion of the tenuous vascular supply (47).

The primary complaint is midfoot pain, with children often walking on the lateral border of the foot in an effort to relieve pressure along the medial longitudinal arch. Tenderness and swelling along the navicular may exist, and contraction of the posterior tibialis tendon may elicit pain. Radiographs of the navicular demonstrate areas of sclerosis and flattening, with a loss of the normal trabecular pattern (Figure 28-8). There may be a uniform increase in density with minimal fragmentation, or possibly total collapse.

The mainstay of treatment in the pediatric population is conservative management, with soft longitudinal arch supports, a medial heel wedge, and activity modification leading to excellent results in the majority of cases that require symptomatic treatment (23,62). If pain is severe and persists, a short leg walking cast may be used for four to eight weeks, followed by shoe modifications. Short leg cast immobilization has been shown to decrease the duration of symptoms and morbidity (4,62). Operative treatment is not necessary as patients can be expected to have a normal foot in adulthood.

PEARLS AND KEY POINTS

Most apophyseal and osteochondritic conditions in children respond to conservative treatment. Ruling out other conditions (stress fracture, tumor, infection) is the most important step in the evaluation process. A gradual return to sports activity and avoidance of overtraining will avoid a prolonged debilitating injury.

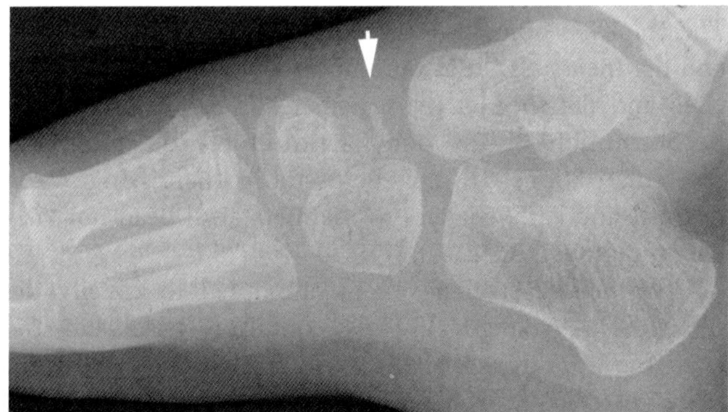

FIGURE 28-8 Radiograph of a 5-year-old patient presenting with medial arch pain. Arrow denotes small, sclerotic navicular seen in Kohler's disease. Symptomatic treatment resulted in reconstitution of normal navicular morphology.

SUMMARY

The growing foot is subject to several disorders related to growth. Accessory bones, such as the accessory navicular can often become symptomatic. Chronic traction to apophyses may result in pain as well. Finally, ill-defined conditions such Kohler's disease, may be related to the cartilaginous nature of developing bone. While most patients do well with nonoperative treatment, indications for surgical intervention should be understood in order to ensure optimal management.

REFERENCES

1. Abramowitz Y, Wollstein R, Barzilay Y, London E, Matan Y, Shabat S, et al. Outcome of resection of a symptomatic os trigonum. *J Bone Joint Surg Am,* 85–A(6): 1051–1057, 2003.
2. Ahmad J, Raikin SM. Osteonecrosis of the second metatarsal head, navicular and talus. *Curr Opin Orthop,* 17: 103–110, 2006.
3. Bennett GL, Weiner DS, Leighley B. Surgical treatment of symptomatic accessory tarsal navicular. *J Pediatr Orthop,* 10(4): 445–449, 1990.
4. Borges JL, Guille JT, Bowen JR. Kohler's bone disease of the tarsal navicular. *J Pediatr Orthop,* 15(5): 596–598, 1995.
5. Bureau NJ, Cardinal E, Hobden R, Aubin B. Posterior ankle impingement syndrome: MR imaging findings in seven patients. *Radiology,* 215(2): 497–503, 2000.
6. Campbell SE. MRI of sports injuries of the ankle. *Clin Sports Med,* 25(4): 727–762, 2006.
7. Canale ST, Williams KD. Iselin's disease. *J Pediatr Orthop,* 12(1): 90–93, 1992.
8. Carro LP, Golano P, Farinas O, Cerezal L, Abad J. Arthroscopic Keller technique for Freiberg disease. *Arthroscopy,* 20 Suppl 2: 60–63, 2004.
9. Chambers HG. Ankle and foot disorders in skeletally immature athletes. *Orthop Clin North Am,* 34(3): 445–459, 2003.
10. Chao KH, Lee CH, Lin LC. Surgery for symptomatic Freiberg's disease: extraarticular dorsal closing-wedge osteotomy in 13 patients followed for 2–4 years. *Acta Orthop Scand,* 70(5): 483–486, 1999.
11. Choi YS, Lee KT, Kang HS, Kim EK. MR imaging findings of painful type II accessory navicular bone: correlation with surgical and pathologic studies. *Korean J Radiol,* 5(4): 274–279, 2004.
12. DeAsla RJ, O'Malley M, Hamilton WG Flexor hallucis tendonitis and posterior ankle impingement in the athlete. *Techniques in foot and ankle surgery* 1(2): 123–130, 2002.
13. DiGiovanni CW, Patel A, Calfee R, Nickisch F. Osteonecrosis in the foot. *J Am Acad Orthop Surg,* 15(4): 208–217, 2007.
14. Dobbs MB, Walton T. Autosomal dominant transmission of accessory navicular. *Iowa Orthop J,* 24: 84–85, 2004.
15. Eberson CP, Schiller J. Common pediatric foot and ankle conditions. In: CW Digiovanni, GJ, ed. *Foot and Ankle. Core Knowledge in Orthopaedics,* pp. 147–170. Elsevier Mosby, 2007; 147–170.
16. el-Tayeby HM. Freiberg's infraction: a new surgical procedure. *J Foot Ankle Surg,* 37(1): 23–27; discussion 79, 1998.
17. Freiberg AA, Freiberg RA. Core decompression as a novel treatment for early Freiberg's infraction of the second metatarsal head. *Orthopedics,* 18(12): 1177–1178, 1995.
18. Gauthier G, Elbaz R. Freiberg's infraction: a subchondral bone fatigue fracture. A new surgical treatment. *Clin Orthop Relat Res,* (142): 93–95, 1979.
19. Grogan DP, Gasser SI, Ogden JA. The painful accessory navicular: a clinical and histopathological study. *Foot Ankle,* 10(3): 164–169, 1989.
20. Hamilton WG, Geppert MJ, Thompson FM. Pain in the posterior aspect of the ankle in dancers. Differential diagnosis and operative treatment. *J Bone Joint Surg Am,* 78(10): 1491–1500, 1996.
21. Hayashi K, Ochi M, Uchio Y, Takao M, Kawasaki K, Yamagami N. A new surgical technique for treating bilateral Freiberg disease. *Arthroscopy,* 18(6): 660–664, 2002.
22. Hedrick MR, McBryde AM. Posterior ankle impingement. *Foot Ankle Int,* 15(1): 2–8, 1994.
23. Ippolito E, Ricciardi Pollini PT, Falez F. Kohler's disease of the tarsal navicular: long-term follow-up of 12 cases. *J Pediatr Orthop,* 4(4): 416–417, 1984.
24. Ishii T, Miyagawa S, Hayashi K. Traction apophysitis of the medial malleolus. *J Bone Joint Surg Br,* 76(5): 802–806, 1994.
25. Issever AS, Minden K, Eshed I, Hermann KG. Accessory navicular bone: when ankle pain does not originate from the ankle. *Clin Rheumatol,* 2007.
26. Karasick D, Schweitzer ME. The os trigonum syndrome: imaging features. *AJR Am J Roentgenol,* 166(1): 125–129, 1996.
27. Katcherian DA. The treatment of Freiberg's disease. In: EG Richardson M, ed. *Foot and Ankle Clinics: Lesser Toe Deformities,* Philadelphia: Saunders, 1998; 323–344.
28. Katcherian DA. Treatment of Freiberg's disease. *Orthop Clin North Am,* 25(1): 69–81, 1994.
29. Kiter E, Erdag N, Karatosun V, Gunal I. Tibialis posterior tendon abnormalities in feet with accessory navicular bone and flatfoot. *Acta Orthop Scand,* 70(6): 618–621, 1999.
30. Kiter E, Erduran M, Gunal I. Inheritance of the accessory navicular bone. *Arch Orthop Trauma Surg,* 120(10): 582–583, 2000.
31. Kiter E, Gunal I, Karatosun V, Korman E. The relationship between the tibialis posterior tendon and the accessory navicular. *Ann Anat,* 182(1): 65–68, 2000.
32. Kolettis GJ, Micheli LJ, Klein JD. Release of the flexor hallucis longus tendon in ballet dancers. *J Bone Joint Surg Am,* 78(9): 1386–1390, 1996.
33. Kopp FJ, Marcus RE. Clinical outcome of surgical treatment of the symptomatic accessory navicular. *Foot Ankle Int,* 25(1): 27–30, 2004.
34. Lawson JP, Ogden JA, Sella E, Barwick KW. The painful accessory navicular. *Skeletal Radiol,* 12(4): 250–262, 1984.
35. Lui TH. Arthroscopic interpositional arthroplasty for Freiberg's disease. *Knee Surg Sports Traumatol Arthrosc,* 15(5): 555–559, 2007.
36. Maquirriain J. Posterior ankle impingement syndrome. *J Am Acad Orthop Surg,* 13(6): 365–371, 2005.
37. Maresca G, Adriani E, Falez F, Mariani PP. Arthroscopic treatment of bilateral Freiberg's infraction. *Arthroscopy,* 12(1): 103–108, 1996.
38. Marumoto JM, Ferkel RD. Arthroscopic excision of the os trigonum: a new technique with preliminary clinical results. *Foot Ankle Int,* 18(12): 777–784, 1997.
39. Mc DA. The os trigonum. *J Bone Joint Surg Br,* 37–B(2): 257–265, 1955.
40. Micheli LJ, Ireland ML. Prevention and management of calcaneal apophysitis in children: an overuse syndrome. *J Pediatr Orthop,* 7(1): 34–38, 1987.
41. Nakayama S, Sugimoto K, Takakura Y, Tanaka Y, Kasanami R. Percutaneous drilling of symptomatic accessory navicular in young athletes. *Am J Sports Med,* 33(4): 531–535, 2005.
42. Ogden JA, Ganey TM, Hill JD, Jaakkola JI. Sever's injury: a stress fracture of the immature calcaneal metaphysis. *J Pediatr Orthop,* 24(5): 488–492, 2004.
43. Ogden JA, Lee J. Accessory ossification patterns and injuries of the malleoli. *J Pediatr Orthop,* 10(3): 306–316, 1990.
44. Omey ML, Micheli LJ. Foot and ankle problems in the young athlete. *Med Sci Sports Exerc,* 31(7 Suppl): S470–86, 1999.
45. Prichasuk S, Sinphurmsukskul O. Kidner procedure for symptomatic accessory navicular and its relation to pes planus. *Foot Ankle Int,* 16(8): 500–503, 1995.
46. Ray S, Goldberg VM. Surgical treatment of the accessory navicular. *Clin Orthop Relat Res,* (177): 61–66, 1983.

47. Sangeorzan BJ, Benirschke SK, Mosca V, Mayo KA, Hansen ST, Jr. Displaced intra-articular fractures of the tarsal navicular. *J Bone Joint Surg Am,* 71(10): 1504–1510, 1989.
48. Schwartz B, Jay RM, Schoenhaus HD. Apophysitis of the fifth metatarsal base. Iselin's disease. *J Am Podiatr Med Assoc,* 81(3): 128–130, 1991.
49. Sella EJ, Lawson JP, Ogden JA. The accessory navicular synchondrosis. *Clin Orthop Relat Res,* (209): 280–285, 1986.
50. Shih AT, Quint RE, Armstrong DG, Nixon BP. Treatment of Freiberg's infraction with the titanium hemi-implant. *J Am Podiatr Med Assoc,* 94(6): 590–593, 2004.
51. Smillie IS. Treatment of Freiberg's infraction. *Proc R Soc Med,* 60(1): 29–31, 1967.
52. Sopov V, Liberson A, Groshar D. Bone scintigraphic findings of os trigonum: a prospective study of 100 soldiers on active duty. *Foot Ankle Int,* 21(10): 822–824, 2000.
53. Sproul J, Klaaren H, Mannarino F. Surgical treatment of Freiberg's infraction in athletes. *Am J Sports Med,* 21(3): 381–384, 1993.
54. Stanley D, Betts RP, Rowley DI, Smith TW. Assessment of etiologic factors in the development of Freiberg's disease. *J Foot Surg,* 29(5): 444–447, 1990.
55. Sullivan JA, Miller WA. The relationship of the accessory navicular to the development of the flat foot. *Clin Orthop Relat Res,* (144): 233–237, 1979.
56. Theodore GH, Kolettis GJ, Micheli LJ. Tenosynovitis of the flexor hallucis longus in a long-distance runner. *Med Sci Sports Exerc,* 28(3): 277–279, 1996.
57. Thompson FM, Hamilton WG. Problems of the second metatarsophalangeal joint. *Orthopedics,* 10(1): 83–89, 1987.
58. Ugolini PA, Raikin SM. The accessory navicular. *Foot Ankle Clin,* 9(1): 165–80, 2004.
59. Volpon JB, de Carvalho Filho G. Calcaneal apophysitis: a quantitative radiographic evaluation of the secondary ossification center. *Arch Orthop Trauma Surg,* 122(6): 338–341, 2002.
60. Wakeley CJ, Johnson DP, Watt I. The value of MR imaging in the diagnosis of the os trigonum syndrome. *Skeletal Radiol,* 25(2): 133–136, 1996.
61. Weiner DS, Morscher M, Dicintio MS. Calcaneal apophysitis: simple diagnosis, simpler treatment. *J Fam Pract,* 56(5): 352–355, 2007.
62. Williams GA, Cowell HR. Kohler's disease of the tarsal navicular. *Clin Orthop Relat Res,* (158): 53–58, 1981.

CHAPTER 29

Macrodactyly

Durga N. Kowtharapu, Dinesh Thawrani and S. Jay Kumar

Macrodactyly is an uncommon congenital malformation characterized by enlargement of both the soft tissue and the osseous elements of the foot or digit. The term "macrodactyly" is derived from two Greek words: *macros* (large) and *dactylos* (digit). The condition differs from macrodactyly of the hand in terms of less neuronal involvement (10). Megalodactyly, dactylomegaly, macrodystrophia lipomatosa, lipofibromatous hamartoma, club toes, digital gigantism, and local gigantism are synonyms for macrodactyly (2,8).

All enlarged digits do not fall into the category of macrodactyly. Enlargement of the fingers may be due to a hemangioma, lymphangioma, lipoma, or tumor mass. In these conditions, only the skin and soft tissues are involved, and roentgenograms show no increase in the size of the phalanges. Barsky published the first large series (64 cases) of this anomaly and preferred to reserve the term "macrodactyly" for digits that shows enlargement of all structures (2). However, enlargement of blood vessels and tendons is not always seen, and the enlargement of nerves is more confined to the hand, and not commonly seen in the foot (7,8,10). In contrast, pseudogigantism is a three-dimensional enlargement of a limb and is associated with a specific disease such as hemangioma, arteriovenous aneurysm, congenital lymphedema, lymphangiectasis, Ollier's disease, Maffucci's syndrome, and Klippel-Trenaunay syndrome (17). Macrodactyly must be differentiated from other conditions that are associated with foot gigantism as a general manifestation or localized manifestation of a systemic disease. This includes conditions such as congenital lipofibromatosis (9), nerve territory-oriented macrodactyly (11), neurofibromatosis (27), proteus syndrome (28), and idiopathic gigantism (1). These conditions are predominantly associated with hypertrophy of fibro-fatty tissue, nerve, bone, or nails.

EPIDEMIOLOGY

Macrodactyly is a rare condition and has an incidence of 1 in 18,000 people (10). Many studies report a larger number of patients with hand involvement, but a few report that foot involvement is more common than the hand (13,21). Macrodactyly, while uncommon in whites, appears to be even less common in blacks. When it does occur in blacks, it involves the toes rather than the fingers, whereas in Caucasians, the fingers are predominantly affected (21). Unilateral involvement is more common (12) with a slight predominance in the male population (4,10,15). Fifty percent of the cases are associated with multiple digit involvement, and 8% of the cases are associated with local malformations like syndactyly or clinodactyly. In cases where multiple digits are involved, the adjacent digits are always affected (10,18).

ETIOLOGY

The exact etiology is unclear. A variety of factors may be involved, and the overgrowth cannot be explained by a single factor. Hemangioma, lymphangioma, lymphangiectasis, and neurofibromatosis have a definite clinical and pathological abnormality that is related to the overgrowth. However, it is hard to explain the phenomena of overgrowth of all the structures like skin, subcutaneous fat, nerves, and bone of the involved part, without overgrowth of the other organs of the body.

Streeter hypothesized that if the germ plasm had an extreme vitality or growth stimulus for some unknown cause, then overgrowth would occur. The cause of these changes in germ plasm growth may be mechanical, drug related, or a result of a deficiency in blood supply or oxygen deprivation (23). Barsky, postulated that macrodactyly is the result of the interaction of two or more extrinsic agents, each unlikely to produce a teratological effect by itself. He further explained his findings as resulting from a disturbance in the growth-limiting factor that allowed the overgrowth to proceed (2). Kelikian believed that the most common variety of macrodactyly should be called nerve territory-oriented macrodactyly. This allowed the association of overgrowth and nerve anomalies without specifying cause and effect and will include both idiopathic gigantism and neurofibromatosis (11). Turra et al., on the basis of anatomic and pathological findings, hypothesized neuroinduction as a cause for foot gigantism (27). Minguella and Cusi studied 16 patients with macrodactyly of the hands and feet and reported that three out of sixteen had a positive family history of macrodactyly (18). However, other studies state that there is no familial history in their study population (2,4,10,15).

PATHOLOGY

Fibro-fatty proliferation leads to enlargement of all the tissues in the digits. This overabundant fibro-fatty tissue resembles adult subcutaneous fat rather than children's fat. Dissection of this fibro-fatty tissue showed large fat globules, which were difficult to extrude with pressure. Dissected specimens showed fibrous bands that radiated between the periosteum and surrounded nerve fibers, blood vessels, and sweat glands (2,19). Moore's microscopic studies on nerve fibers of the patients with macrodactyly revealed an abundant fibro-fatty tissue in the fasciculi of the involved nerve (20). Fibro-fatty tissue is almost always the predominant tissue and concentrates on the plantar and lateral sides of the digits, giving a hyperextended appearance to the digits. A proliferation of the fibroblastic tissue between the cortex and periosteum was the outstanding pathological finding, which probably leads to the phalangeal overgrowth (3).

CLASSIFICATION

Barsky classified macrodactyly into two types, based on the size and progressive growth of the digits (2). Initially, this classification was applied mainly for macrodactyly of the upper extremities, and later it was also adapted to the lower extremities. The two types are:

Static type (macrodactyly simplex congenital): The enlargement is present at birth, and the increased size does not increase disproportionately with growth.

Progressive type (lipomatous macrodystrophy): There is disproportionate growth of the involved digit or digits and the involved digit increases in size at a faster rate than can be attributed to the normal growth pattern.

Chang et al. (4) classified macrodactyly of the foot into two types based on involvement of the great toe. This classification helps in planning treatment.

Group A: Normal great toe and macrodactyly of the lesser toes

Group B: Macrodactyly of the great toe with or without involvement of the lesser toes

CLINICAL FEATURES

Most cases of macrodactyly are evident soon after birth. Occasionally the progressive type may not become apparent until later in infancy, when relentless enlargement occurs.

The second ray is commonly affected followed by the third, first, fourth, and fifth rays of the foot (10,18,24). Syndactyly or brachydactyly may coexist (Figure 29-1).

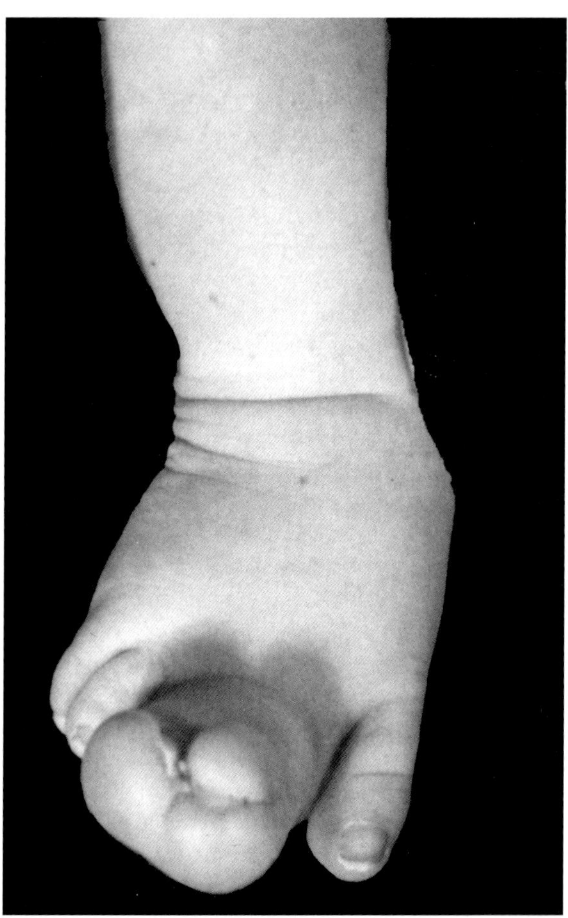

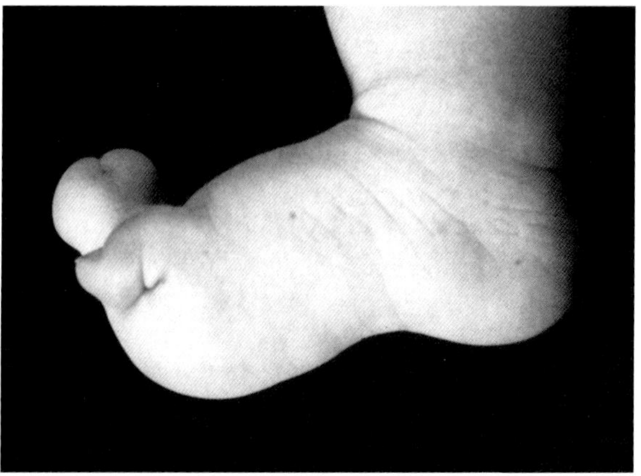

FIGURE 29-1 Clinical pictures showing macrodactyly and syndactyly of the second and third toes with hyperextension deformity of the toes and abundant fibro-fatty tissue on the sole of the foot.

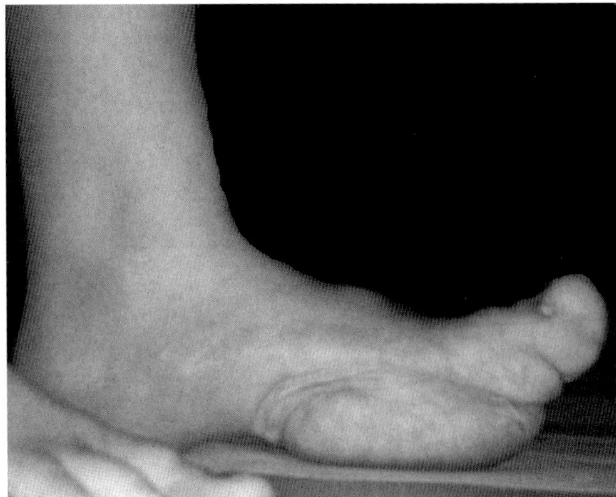

FIGURE 29-2 Clinical picture showing macrodactyly of the foot with hyperextension deformity of the great toe and abundant fibro-fatty tissue on the sole of the foot.

Eighteen percent to seventy-eight percent of cases are associated with different patterns of involvement of the metatarsals (4,5,9,10,18). The plantar surface is more hypertrophied than the dorsal side of the foot. This leads to hyperextension of the toe and restricts joint movements from a distal to proximal level (Figure 29-2) (18). In static macrodactyly, the involved digits are about one and half times the normal length and width, but a more striking enlargement is seen in the progressive type. The bone age is advanced in the involved phalanges in both types. The enlargement of the metatarsals leads to increased size of the foot, and at the same time, the width of the ipsilateral leg, thigh, forearm, and arm may also increase substantially. In patients, where multiple digits are involved, the adjacent digit is likely to be involved and they both grow in a divergent manner. Thus, the problem of local gigantism is compounded by malalignment of the digit and will need further procedures for correction.

Cosmetic concerns or problems with shoe fitting are often the presenting complaints in macrodactyly. If macrodactyly involves the big toe, large, fleshy nail folds become uncontrollable and an ingrown toenail may result (Figure 29-3). Problems with ambulation or pain as a presenting symptom are quite rare. Large creases are not uncommon in the skin, which leads to maceration and these patients need intensive foot care and hygiene.

In summary, overgrowth of all the mesenchymal elements is seen in true macrodactyly, whereas overgrowth of the single element (blood vessels lymphatics, soft tissue, tendon, or bone) is common in hemangioma, lymphangioma, neurofibromatosis, giant cell tumor of the tendon sheath (22), and Ollier's disease.

INVESTIGATIONS

Standing anteroposterior and lateral radiographs of the foot are needed to evaluate the deformity. Increase in the length and width of the phalanges with or without involvement of the metatarsals is an integral feature of macrodactyly. In a standing anteroposterior radiograph Chang et al. (4) recommend measuring the metatarsal spread angle, which is formed by the medial border of the first metatarsal and the lateral border of the fifth metatarsal (Figure 29-4). This angle helps to assess the severity and progression of the deformity. This is useful in patients with unilateral involvement because it can be compared with the measurement of the normal foot. In their study of seventeen patients, the mean metatarsal spread angle of the normal feet was around 19 degrees and that of affected side was around 29 degrees. In the absence of specific clinical features, magnetic resonance imaging (MRI) evaluation of the tissues involved in macrodactyly can be helpful in establishing a diagnosis and also aids in determining the extent of soft-tissue involvement.

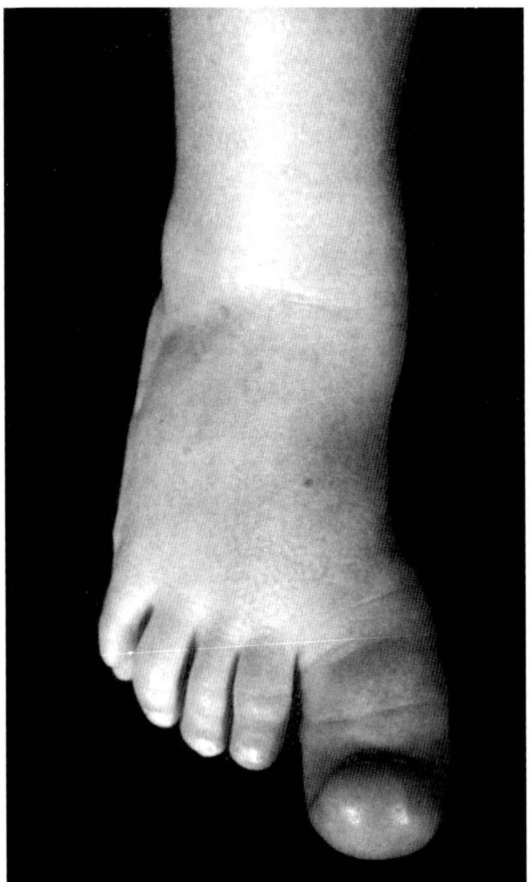

FIGURE 29-3 Clinical picture showing macrodactyly of the great toe with hyperextension of the terminal phalanx, nail bed involvement, and curling of the distal part of the toe.

TREATMENT

The problem associated with macrodactyly of the foot results from an increase in the length, width, and height of the forefoot and toes. The goal of treatment is to

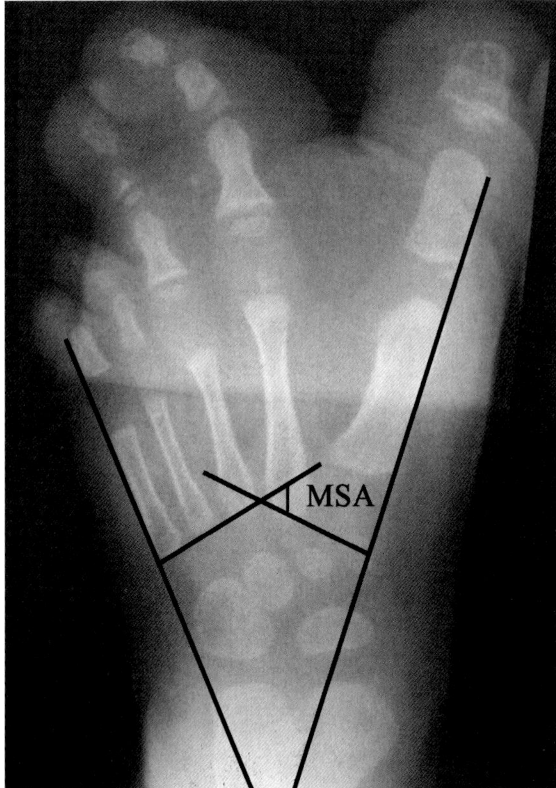

FIGURE 29-4 Radiograph showing the metatarsal spread angle (MSA), which is angle formed between the medial border of the first metatarsal and lateral border of the fifth metatarsals of the foot.

reduce the size of the foot to allow fitting of regular shoes, and, if possible, to achieve an acceptable appearance with a minimum number of procedures (4).

Due to the progressive nature of the deformity, subsequent surgical procedures are often required even after the primary satisfactory management. Dedrick and Kling reported an average of four {range two to six} additional procedures in his series of thirteen patients (6).

Various options are available to treat this rare condition. These are soft-tissue debulking, epiphysiodesis, bony reduction, ray resection, and amputation. The indication for each procedure is different, and a successful outcome after surgery depends on the location, type, and severity of the macrodactyly. Meticulous preoperative assessment and planning are needed.

Soft-Tissue Debulking

This procedure is indicated in children with mild to moderate hypertrophy of the digits. The skin, subcutaneous tissue, and underlying hypertrophic fat are excised by a longitudinal elliptical incision on either side of the involved digit. Usually, it is performed in two stages at an interval of three to six months to preserve circulation. Ligation of the vessels is not recommended. The plantar and digital nerves need to be preserved, but local cutaneous nerves can be sacrificed along with the soft tissue. Debulking surgery alone is not effective in moderate and severe cases and a review of the literature showed a high rate of recurrence (4,6).

Our indication for this procedure is mainly in skeletally immature patients with minimal osseous involvement. However, in moderate and severe cases, it should be considered as a supplemental procedure following osseous correction.

Epiphyseal Arrest

Epiphyseal arrest is advocated at the base of each phalanx when the involved digit approaches the size of the digit of the patient's same-sex parent. This is often successful in limiting longitudinal growth, but it does not alter the circumferential bone growth. Topoleski et al. claim to have halted the longitudinal growth of macrodactyly in their series by proximal phalangeal epiphysiodesis (25). We recommend epiphyseal arrest for the treatment of only great toe macrodactyly, as an alternative to amputation (4).

Bony Reduction

A number of techniques are available to reduce the bone size but almost all procedures have to be combined with soft-tissue reduction. The most popular techniques were described by Barksy (2), Tsuge and Ikuta (26), and Kotwal and Farooque (14). In the Barsky technique, the distal portion of the middle phalanx is excised and arthrodesis of the distal interphalangeal joint is performed. In the Tsuge technique, except for a thin rim of bone, the whole distal phalanx is excised. In the Kotwal procedure, the middle phalanx is excised and the extensor tendons are shortened. These techniques will create a smaller digit at the expense of sacrificing joint movement. However, this is an acceptable compromise because many of the digits showed decreased joint movement prior to surgery. These procedures are frequently associated with recurrence of the deformity. Osteotomies and bone shortening may be necessary when digital gigantism is associated with lateral or medial deviation of the enlarged digit. Diaphyseal shortening of the metatarsal is indicated in macrodactyly of the great toe. Shortening of the metatarsal helps in achieving good correction of the length, but the width of the foot is unchanged (4).

Phalangeal Amputation

Amputation of the phalanges of the big toe may be performed to facilitate shoe wear. Amputation of the lesser toes does not reduce the width of the foot, and it leaves a wide gap, so it is not a preferred procedure. In these instances, ray resection is the best option (Figure 29-5).

Ray Resection

Ray resection and soft-tissue debulking is indicated when there is severe enlargement, patient has had multiple previous failed procedures, and an insensate toe. Complete ray resection, including ample soft-tissue debulking, is the most useful procedure to reduce the width and height of the foot (Figure 29-6). This helps in improving cosmesis and aids in shoe wear. This procedure reduces the need of

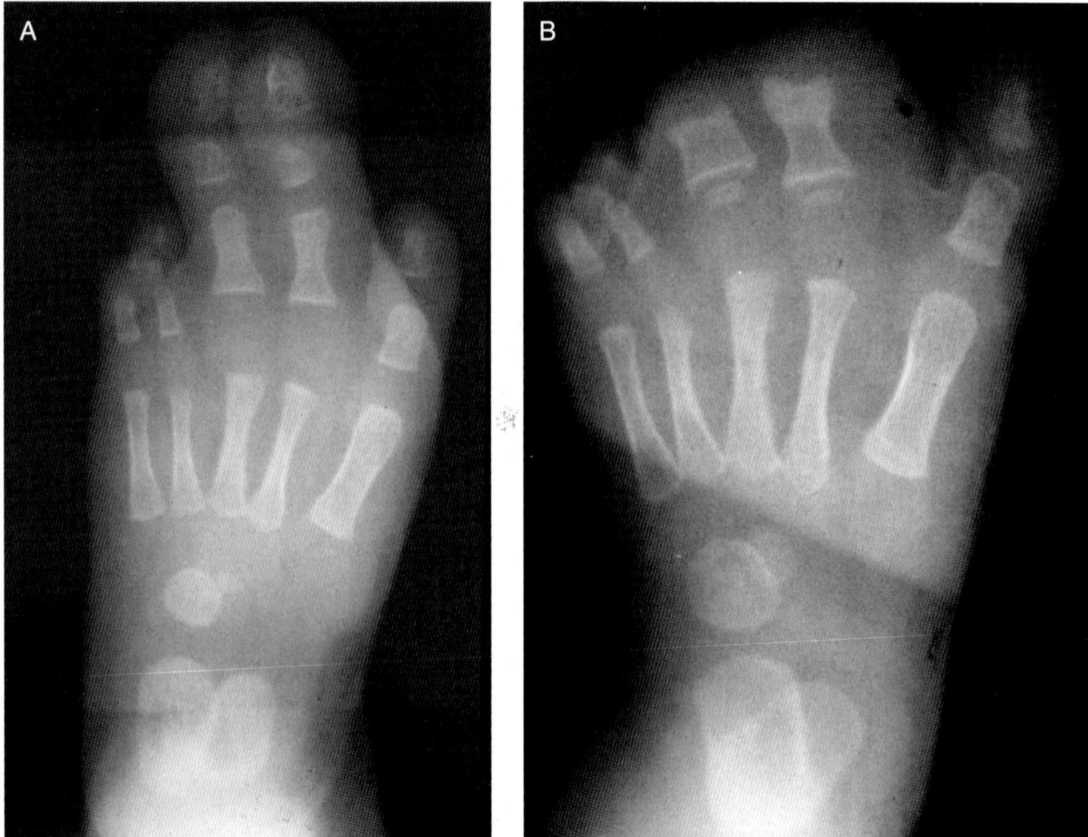

FIGURE 29-5 **A.** Radiograph illustrating macrodactyly and syndactyly of the second and third toes with thickening of the phalanges of the toes and increased width of the foot. **B.** Radiograph of the same patient after amputation of the terminal phalanx of the second and third toes showing persistent widening of the foot.

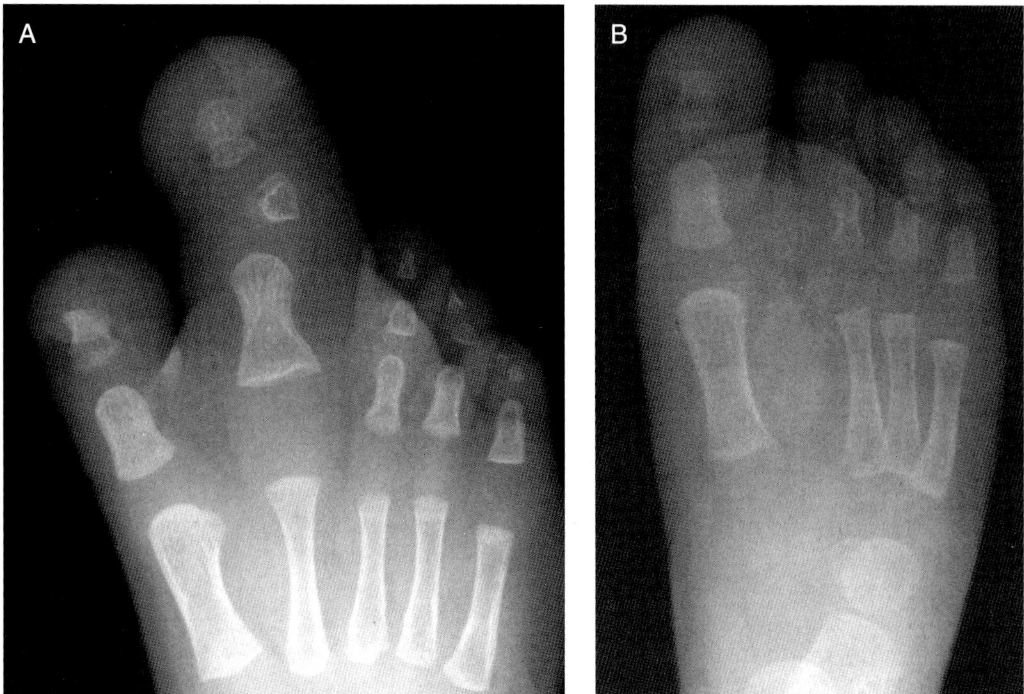

FIGURE 29-6 **A.** Radiograph illustrating macrodactyly of the second toe. There is thickening of the phalanges of the toe and an increase in the width of the foot. **B.** Radiograph of the same patient after second ray resection showing good correction and reduction of the width of the foot.

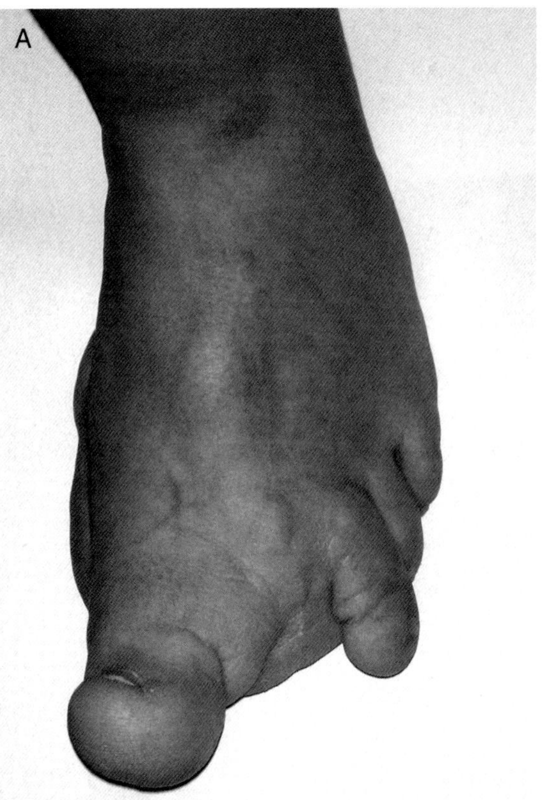

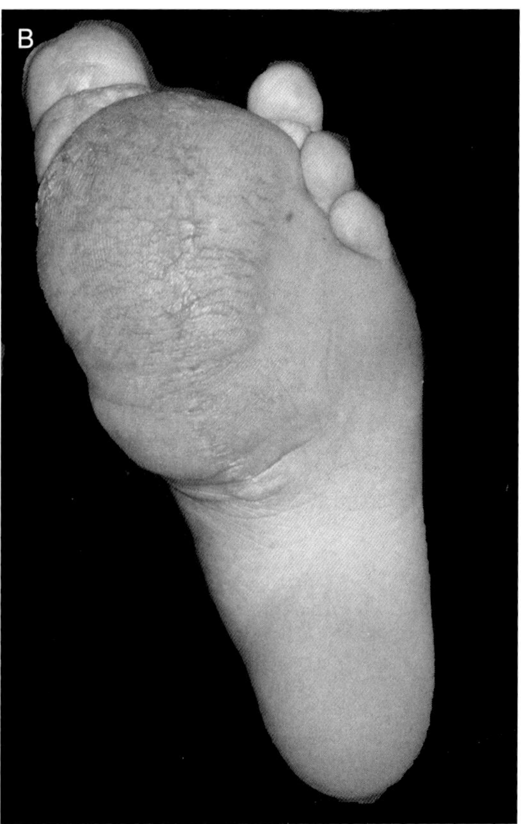

FIGURE 29-7 **A.** Clinical picture showing recurrence of the macrodactyly after second ray resection and soft-tissue debulking. The progressive fibro-fatty infiltration has increased the space between the first and third toe. **B.** There is fibro-fatty infiltration at the distal sole with sparing of the heel of the foot. This patient would be best served with a Syme amputation.

further surgeries and it should be done at an early age when the foot is two standard deviations wider than the foot of a child of the same age (6). The metatarsal spread angle can be reduced by about 10 degrees following resection of one ray. To make the width of the foot as equal as possible to the normal side, ray resection is indicated when the metatarsal spread angle exceeds that on the normal side by more than 10 degrees. For mild cases, where the metatarsal spread angle difference is less than 10 degrees, repeated diaphyseal shortening of the metatarsal and soft tissue debulking may be performed. Except the first ray, the remaining rays can be safely removed either as a single ray or in combination with other rays of the foot. In ray resection, the phalanges, metatarsals, and soft tissues are totally excised and to improve correction and avoid recurrence, a wedge of the adjacent tarsal bones should be resected.

The great toe and first metatarsal contribute significantly in weight bearing and normal gait, so resection is not a viable option (16). In cases with unilateral macrodactyly of the great toe, the length of the phalanges and metatarsal may be reduced by shortening at the diaphyseal level. Because this procedure is usually done in younger patients, they might need a secondary shortening procedure at maturity. Although epiphysiodesis is another option, early epiphysiodesis leads to significant shortening of the metatarsal and it should not be performed until the first metatarsal reaches adult length (4).

Amputation

Amputation of the foot is an excellent option if the deformity is so severe that debulking or resection is not likely to correct the deformity of the foot. If the heel is not involved and the skin of the sole is viable, a Syme or Boyd's amputation is preferred (Figure 29-7). If the skin is scarred and infiltrated to a significant extent, a below knee amputation will enable the patient to become functional very quickly. Amputation does not control the overgrowth of adipose tissue proximal to the site of ablation, and these patients may need secondary procedures.

The overall treatment should be tailored to the functional needs of the patient, taking into account the progressive nature of the disease process, the proximal extent of bony involvement, and the presence of concomitant neural changes.

Timing of the Surgery

The timing of operative intervention depends on the severity of the macrodactyly. When it is mild with only slight enlargement of the toe or toes, the patient may not regard it as a problem until shoe wear becomes difficult or the toe becomes cosmetically unappealing. In severe cases with unsightly enlargement of the toes and forefoot, operative intervention can be deferred until at least six months of the age in order to assess the extent and rate of growth of the lesion. This will help the surgeons to determine the optimal operative procedures.

Turra et al. suggested waiting until the age of three to four years before surgical intervention. He believed that by then the growth potential of the hypertrophic tissue would have manifested itself (27). In our opinion, six months of age is probably the appropriate time to assess the disease. A longer period of observation does not offer any advantage, and reduction of the width of the foot by ray resection may become more difficult after this age because of maturation and stiffness of the tarsometatarsal joint.

SUMMARY

Macrodactyly of the foot is a rare congenital anomaly. The pattern of involvement and the severity of the deformities differ widely. The goal of treatment is to reduce the size of the foot with a minimum number of procedures, so that the individual can wear normal footwear and the foot has an acceptable cosmetic appearance. Ray resection of the lesser toes should be performed, when there is metatarsal involvement and the metatarsal spread angle is greater than 10 degrees compared to that on the normal side, or when toe amputation is likely to create a wide, cosmetically unappealing interphalangeal space. As amputation of the great toe is contraindicated, multiple surgical interventions may be needed to correct macrodactyly of the great toe. These include diaphyseal shortening of the metatarsal and phalanges in addition to soft-tissue debulking. If the terminal phalanx is deformed and the nail is curled in the skin fold, amputation of the terminal phalanx is indicated.

REFERENCES

1. Ackland MK, Uhthoff HK. Idiopathic localized gigantism: a 26-year follow-up. *J Pediatr Ortho,* 6(5): 618–621, 1986.
2. Barsky AJ. Macrodactyly. *J Bone Joint Surg Am* 49(7): 1255–1266, 1967.
3. Ben-Bassat M, Casper J, Kaplan I, Laron Z. Congenital macrodactyly. A case report with a three-year follow-up. *J Bone Joint Surg Br* 48(2): 359–364, 1966.
4. Chang CH, Kumar SJ, Riddle EC, Glutting J. Macrodactyly of the foot. *J Bone Joint Surg Am* 84–A(7): 1189–1194, 2002.
5. Chen SH, Huang SC, Wang JH, Wu CT. Macrodactyly of the feet and hands. *J Formos Med Assoc* 96(11): 901–907, 1997.
6. Dedrick D, Kling TF. Ray resection in the treatment of macrodactyly of the foot in children. *Orthop Trans* 9: 145, 1985.
7. Dell PC. Macrodactyly. *Hand Clin* 1(3): 511–524, 1985.
8. Dennyson WG, Bear JN, Bhoola KD. Macrodactyly in the foot. *J Bone Joint Surg Br* 59(3): 355–359, 1977.
9. Grogan DP, Bernstein RM, Habal MB, Ogden JA. Congenital lipofibromatosis associated with macrodactyly of the foot. *Foot Ankle* 12(1): 40–46, 1991.
10. Kalen V, Burwell DS, Omer GE. Macrodactyly of the hands and feet. *J Pediatr Orthop* 8(3): 311–315, 1988.
11. Kelikian H. *Congenital deformities of the hand and forearm.* Philadelphia: WB Saunders, 1974.
12. Keret D, Ger E, Marks H. Macrodactyly involving both hands and both feet. *J Hand Surg (Am)* 12(4): 610–614, 1987.
13. Khanna N, Gupta S, Khanna S, Tripathi F. Macrodactyly. *Hand* 7(3): 215–222, 1975.
14. Kotwal PP, Farooque M. Macrodactyly. *J Bone Joint Surg Br* 80 B(4): 651–653, 1998.
15. Kumar K, Kumar D, Gadegone WM, Kapahtia NK. Macrodactyly of the hand and foot. *Int Orthop* 9(4): 259–264, 1985.
16. Mackenzie WG, Gabos P. Localized disorder of bone and soft tissue. In: Morrissey RT, Weinstein SL, eds. *Lovell and Winters pediatric orthopedics,* Philadelphia: Lippincott Williams & Wilkins, 350–352, 2001.
17. McGrory BJ, Amadio PC, Dobyns JH, Stickler GB, Unni KK. Anomalies of the fingers and toes associated with Klippel-Trenaunay syndrome. *J Bone Joint Surg Am* 73(10): 1537–1546, 1991.
18. Minguella J, Cusi V. Macrodactyly of the hands and feet. *Int Orthop* 16(3): 245–249, 1992.
19. Minkowitz S, Minkowitz F. A morphological study of macrodactylism: A case report. *J Pathol Bacteriol* 90(1): 323–328, 1965.
20. Moore B. Macrodactyly and associated peripheral nerve changes. *J Bone Joint Surg Am* 24: 617–631, 1942.
21. Ofodile FA. Macrodactyly in blacks. *J Hand Surg (Am)* 7(6): 566–568, 1982.
22. Skaliczki G, Mady F. Giant cell tumor of the tendon sheath of the toe imitating macrodactyly: case report. *Foot Ankle Int* 24(11): 868–870, 2003.
23. Streeter G. Focal deficiencies in foetal tissues and the relation to intrauterine amputation. *Embryo* 22(1), 1930.
24. Temtamy SA, Rogers JG. Macrodactyly, hemihypertrophy, and connective tissue nevi: report of a new syndrome and review of the literature. *J Pediatr* 89(6): 924–927, 1976.
25. Topoleski TA, Ganel A, Grogan DP. Effect of proximal phalangeal epiphysiodesis in the treatment of macrodactyly. *Foot Ankle Int* 18(8): 500–503, 1997.
26. Tsuge K, Ikuta Y. Macrodactyly and fibro-fatty proliferation of the median nerve. *Hiroshima J Med Sci* 22(1): 83–101, 1973.
27. Turra S, Santini S, Cagnoni G, Jacopetti T. Gigantism of the foot: our experience in seven cases. *J Pediatr Orthop* 18(3): 337–345, 1998.
28. Wiedemann HR, Burgio GR, Aldenhoff P, Kunze J, Kaufmann HJ, Schirg E. The proteus syndrome. Partial gigantism of the hands and/or feet, nevi, hemihypertrophy, subcutaneous tumors, macrocephaly or other skull anomalies and possible accelerated growth and visceral affections. *Eur J Pediatr* 140(1): 5–12, 1983.

CHAPTER 30

Rheumatic Diseases of Childhood

Walter B. Greene

INTRODUCTION

Rheumatic diseases in children are multisystem disorders that cause chronic inflammation of joints as well as other tissues and organs. As such, theses disorders may be perplexing at onset and a broad knowledge of their clinical manifestations is required for both timely diagnosis and effective treatment (8,14). For the child whose synovitis does not "go away," the end result can be a painful and disabling arthritis that may affect several joints.

Orthopedic surgeons frequently are the initial physician evaluating a child with an inflammatory arthropathy and their understanding of pediatric rheumatic disorders can be critical in making a timely diagnosis and initiation of medical treatment. Furthermore, using a variety of non-operative and operative modalities, the orthopedic surgeon can make a significant impact on the function of these patients. This is particularly true at the foot and ankle because a well-aligned and plantigrade foot can provide surprisingly good walking function despite marked loss of ankle and hindfoot motion (Figure 30-1).

JUVENILE RHEUMATOID ARTHRITIS

Juvenile rheumatoid arthritis (JRA) is the most common cause of chronic arthritis in children. The incidence is 10 to 20 cases per 100,000 children, but may be decreasing (17,23). The etiology of JRA is uncertain but studies indicate that the disease probably results from a complex choreography initiated by different external events such as bacterial or viral infection or hormonal changes that trigger abnormal, genetically influenced interactions between T cells and antigen-presenting cells (8,14,31,36). A hereditary component is supported by human leukocyte antigen (HLA) associations in the different types of JRA. The primary pathologic event in JRA occurs in the synovium, suggesting that the offending agent is carried to the joint via the bloodstream. The subsequent activation of cytokines, neutrophiles, monocytes, T cells, B cells, and plasma cells secrete catabolic enzymes that not only disrupt proteoglycan and collagen but also intensify and perpetuate synovial hypertrophy and inflammation. Additional stress is caused by the associated joint effusion, which stretches the capsule and causes instability and malalignment.

No laboratory test is definitive in JRA; therefore, JRA is a diagnosis of exclusion. The four criteria for diagnosing JRA include: (i) chronic synovial inflammation of unknown cause, (ii) onset at or before 16 years, (iii) objective evidence of arthritis in one or more joints for six consecutive weeks, and (iv) exclusion of other diseases. In contrast to rheumatoid arthritis (RA) that develops in adults, JRA is more likely to begin in the knees and ankles.

Classification of JRA facilitates recognition of complications and prognosis. *Oligoarticular JRA* has less than four joints affected at six months after disease onset. If a child with oligoarticular JRA subsequently progresses to have more than four affected joints, his or her disease is then reclassified as *oligoarticular extended JRA*. *Polyarticular JRA* has five or more involved joints at six months and most patients eventually have 10 to 20 affected joints. Polyarticular patients are further classified as rheumatoid factor (RF) positive or RF negative. *Systemic JRA* is characterized by systemic symptoms at onset including high, spiking fever, and a characteristic rash. The number of involved joints in systemic JRA is variable.

Oligoarticular Juvenile Rheumatoid Arthritis

Sixty percent of children have oligoarticular involvement (1,8). Females predominate at a 5:1 ratio. The onset of symptoms is usually between one to three years of age and the disease begins in a single joint in approximately half of these children. The knee is most frequently involved, but the ankle is also a common site. The hip is rarely involved at disease onset. The disease may remain confined to a single joint or synovitis may develop in other joints.

At onset, the pain in oligoarticular JRA is typically mild. Common symptoms include morning stiffness, gelling after inactivity, and discomfort with extended play or walking

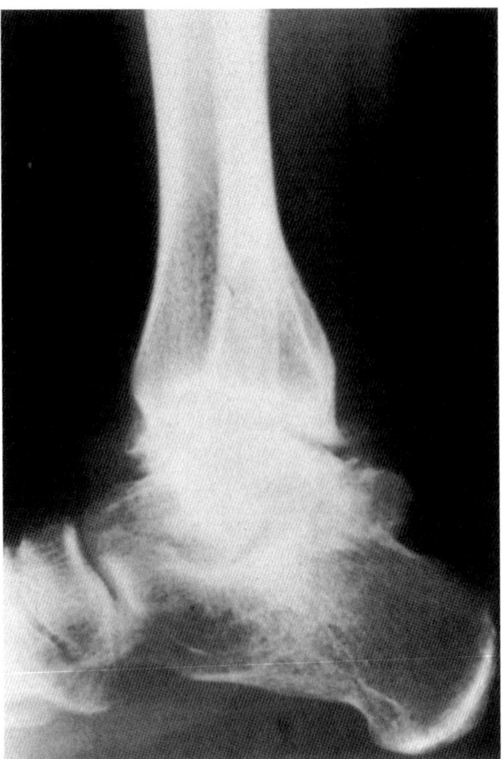

FIGURE 30-1 Lateral radiograph ankle in a 32-year-old male with severe hemophilia. During his first decade, agents that provided effective transfusion therapy were not available; however, he had consistent non-operative treatment for numerous ankle and calf bleeds that included compression dressings, plaster splints, casting, and braces to maintain his foot in a well balanced position. Despite marked joint narrowing and limited motion (arc of ankle motion limited to 6 degrees on the right and 12 degrees on the left as well as virtually no inversion or eversion), the plantigrade posture of his feet permitted regular shoe wear and allowed the patient to work at a job that required frequent standing and walking.

activities. Typical findings include mild swelling of the joint, periarticular warmth, and discomfort at the extremes of motion but relatively mild limitation of motion.

Laboratory tests are often normal including the nonspecific inflammatory studies, i.e., white blood cell count (WBC), erythrocyte sedimentation rate (ESR), and C-reactive protein (CRP). If a patient with oligoarticular JRA is rheumatoid factor (RF) positive, that patient is typically older and will progress to polyarticular JRA. Anti-nuclear antibodies (ANA) testing may be positive at a low titer ($\leq$1:256) in JRA patients, but is most prevalent (approximately 75%) in girls with oligoarticular JRA who develop chronic anterior uveitis, a condition that does not cause prodromal symptoms and may lead to blindness unless recognized at an early stage.

Oligoarticular JRA has the best prognosis for remission of joint disease. Oligoarticular extended children, however, are more likely to have persistent synovitis. In a long term follow-up study ($\geq$10 years after disease onset), 41% of oligoarticular patients still had active joint disease (35). Of note, this study was done before methotrexate was routinely used in an expeditious manner and before biologic agents were available. It is anticipated that future long-term studies will demonstrate improved outcomes.

Polyarticular Juvenile Rheumatoid Arthritis

Polyarticular JRA accounts for 30% of JRA cases. With multiple affected joints, the child with polyarticular JRA is less of a diagnostic dilemma. Symmetric involvement of the knees, wrists, and ankles is most common, but many patients also have involvement of the fingers and toes. Pain and swelling in the ankle joint may mask subtalar synovitis, but subsequent erosion and deformity of the hindfoot demonstrates that the disease also affected these joints. Fatigue, low-grade fever, and obvious joint symptoms are common at onset of disease. These patients are more likely to develop unremitting synovitis as well as anorexia, growth retardation, and psychological regression.

Age at onset and the presence of RF identifies two subgroups of polyarticular JRA. Females predominate in both groups at an approximately 3:1 ratio. Polyarticular JRA in young children has many similarities to oligoarticular JRA including typical onset between ages one to three years, similar HLA patterns, seronegative RF, and uveitis more common in females who are ANA seropositive.

Adolescent onset polyarticular JRA is similar to adult rheumatoid arthritis (RA). These patients are often RF seropositive, have an increased frequency of HLA antigens associated with adult RA, and are more likely to develop rheumatoid nodules, joint erosions, and Felty syndrome (RF positive RA or JRA, splenomegaly, and neutropenia secondary to splenic sequestration and subsequent granulocyte destruction). Remission rates are also lower in RF positive patients.

Systemic Onset Juvenile Rheumatoid Arthritis

Ten percent of children have systemic symptoms at onset that may precede development of joint swelling by weeks to months. The age at onset is variable but is usually less than five years. The sex ratio is equal and there is no HLA association. By definition, the fever is > 39.3° C (103° F). Typically, the fever occurs in the late afternoon or evening and is often accompanied by a rash, intense aching, and malaise. The temperature is normal or subnormal in the morning and the child acts and plays surprisingly well except when the fever is present.

The classic rash is an evanescent, salmon-pink macular or maculopapular reaction noted when the fever is peaking and most commonly seen on the trunk, axilla, and proximal extremities. Central clearing may be present. Hepatosplenomegaly and generalized lymphadenopathy occur in most children. Other visceral problems found in systemic JRA include pericarditis, vasculitis, anemia, growth retardation, and the rare but serious macrophage activation syndrome (acute onset hepatic failure with encephalopathy, purpura, bruising, and mucosal bleeding).

About half of the children with systemic JRA go into remission. This result is more likely in those with oligoarticular disease. Other predictors of an earlier time to remission include absence of active arthritis, an ESR of < 26 mm/hour, and no requirement for corticosteroid therapy at three and six months (28). Compared to other types of JRA, systemic patients with persistent arthritis have a poorer response to second and third line medical therapy and are more likely to progress to end stage arthritis by the adolescent years.

LONG-TERM PROBLEMS

With persistent disease, several long-term conditions may develop (Table 30-1). Ankylosis may develop and compared to both adult RA and other pediatric arthridities, this complication is much more common in JRA. Common sites include the cervical spine and feet (Figure 30-2). Inflammatory synovitis may accelerate growth in adjacent epiphysis, but progression of the resultant limb length discrepancy is usually limited and uncommonly requires epiphysiodesis (27).

Growth retardation may be localized, causing problems such as micrognathia, or generalized with short stature. Generalized growth retardation as well as osteopenia is exacerbated by steroid therapy and is more common in systemic JRA (8,11). Growth hormone may improve the short stature. Calcium, vitamin D, and bisphosphonate therapy can decrease fragility fractures and improve but not normalize the low bone mineral density (19,34). Chronic cardiopulmonary or vascular disorders are uncommon in JRA but are occasionally noted in systemic JRA.

Chronic anterior uveitis may occur in JRA as well as the seronegative spondyloarthropathies (7,8). Although uveitis may precede arthritis, it usually develops five to seven years after onset of arthritis. In a study of 1,081 children, the incidence of uveitis was 21% in oligoarticular JRA, 14% in RF negative polyarticular JRA, 10% in psoriatic arthropathy, 8% in juvenile ankylosing spondylitis, and < 1% in systemic JRA and RF positive JRA (24). Because uveitis may not cause prodromal symptoms and may progress to blindness if not treated early, slit lamp examination is indicated at diagnosis of JRA or a spondyloarthropathy. The frequency of subsequent ocular examination is based on the likelihood of developing uveitis (7). Young females with oligoarticular JRA who are ANA positive are at greatest risk and should have a slit lamp exam every three months for two to four years. Initial treatment of chronic anterior uveitis is glucocococorticoid eye drops and should be directed by an ophthalmologist knowledgeable in the treatment of this disorder.

TABLE 30-1

Potential Long-Term Conditions Associated with JRA

Joint
- Cartilage destruction
- Erosive arthritis
- Ankylosis
- Subluxation

Bone
- Ostoepenia
- Low impact fractures
  - Vertebral compression
  - Metaphyseal or epiphyseal

Growth Abnormalities
- Long bones: retarded or accelerated
- Leg length discrepancy
- Early closure of the physis
- Micrognathia
- Brachydactyly

Growth Retardation
- Short stature
- Weight-for-height below 80th percentile
- Low serum albumin

Spondylitis
- Cervical ankylosis
- Atlantioaxial instability

Tenosynovitis
- Muscle weakness and contractures
- Chronic uveitis
- Vasculitis
- Pericarditis
- Pericardial effusion
- Myocarditis
- Pleuropulmonary disease

MEDICAL TREATMENT OF JUVENILE RHEUMATOID ARTHRITIS

Control of inflammation is the primary goal of medical management of JRA as well as other chronic aseptic inflammatory arthridities. Non-steroidal anti-inflammatory drugs (NSAIDs) are the first line of therapy. Naproxen, tolmetin, and ibuprofen inhibit the activity of cyclo-oxygenase enzymes, COX-1, and COX-2 in the metabolism of arachidonic acid to prostaglandins, thromboxanes, and prostacyclins and are approved for use in children. Naproxen is usually well tolerated in children and its twice-a-day administration and oral suspension (125 mg/5 ml) improves compliance for both school-age children and for younger children whose parents both work. A typical dosage in JRA is 15 to 20 mg/kg/day. Ibuprofen is usually well tolerated in children but has the disadvantage of more frequent dosage requirements. Tablets are prescribed at 30–40 mg/kg/day in four divided doses. The oral suspension (100 mg/5 ml) contains both the S and the R enatiomers; therefore, it is not absorbed as well and should be given at a dose of 40–50 mg/kg/day. Tolmetin is not available in oral suspension and may be more likely to cause gastric irritation in children. Its dosage is 25–30 mg/kg/day in three divided doses. Pseudoporphyria is an uncommon side effect of NSAIDs, is

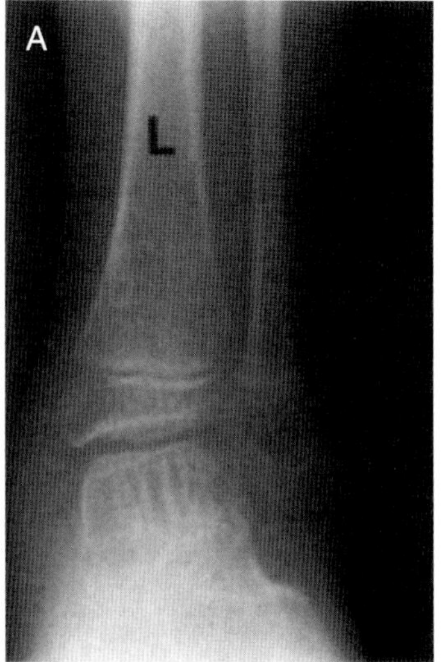

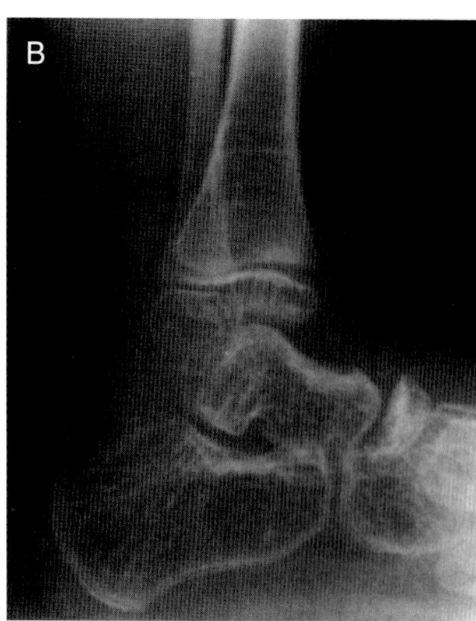

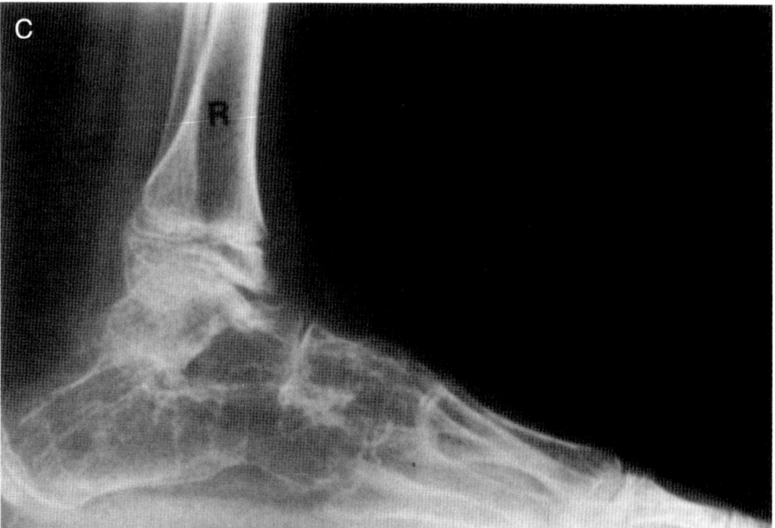

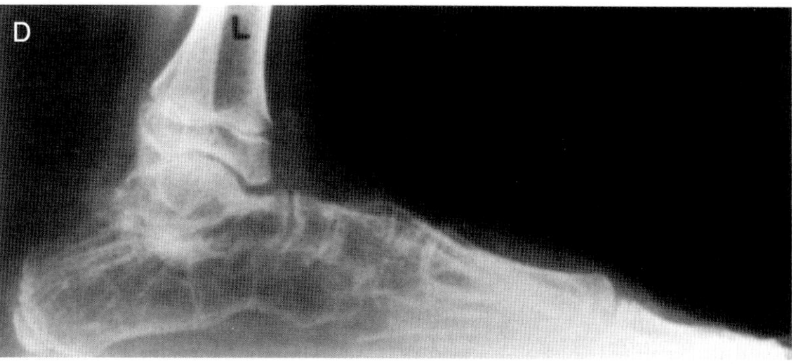

FIGURE 30-2 **A.** AP radiograph left ankle at age six years. **B.** Lateral radiograph left ankle at age 6 years. **C.** Lateral radiograph right foot at age ten years. **D.** Lateral radiograph left foot at age 10 years. AP and lateral radiograph of a six-year-old female who developed systemic JRA at two years of age. Striking osteopenia and early erosions noted in ankle and hindfoot joints. Lateral radiographs of feet at age ten show ankylosis of talocalcaneal, talonavicular, and calcaneocuboid joints as well as erosions in the ankle joint. However, plantigrade posture of the feet and functional ambulation had been maintained by continuous use of night splints and AFOs.

more frequent with naproxen, and although other manifestations of this photodermatis resolve with discontinuation of the NSAID, residual scarring remains.

Other NSAIDs have been used in JRA. Indomethacin is useful in treating the fever and pericarditis of systemic onset JRA. Celecoxib, a COX-2 inhibitor, may be useful for the child that develops gastric irritation. Piroxicam is given only once a day and may be helpful in an older child.

Response to a particular NSAIDs is variable. An adequate trial is 8 to 12 weeks. In a well-documented study, 57% showed significant improvement during a three-month interval with one-half of the responders demonstrating improvement by two weeks, two-thirds by one month, 79% by two months, and the remainder by three months (18). However, analysis of randomized, controlled trials indicate that the long-term control of synovitis in JRA by NSAIDs is mostly limited to those with oligoarthritis (15).

Prior to beginning NSAID long-term therapy, lab studies should include liver function tests (principally serum glutamic transaminase); renal function tests (BUN, creatinine, and urinalysis); and a complete blood count (CBC). The liver function studies should be repeated seven to ten days later. Serum renal and hepatic tests and a CBC should be checked on a three- to six-month interval. These measures are acceptable screening for the hepatitis, proteinuria, hematuria, anemia, and thrombocytopenia that occasionally occur with these medications. If a child responds and then progresses to clinical remission, gradual withdrawal of NSAIDs can be tried 6 months after remission has been maintained.

With the exception of the child with pericarditis, systemic glucocorticoids should be avoided if at all possible in JRA. On the other hand, periodic injection of intra-articular injections can be quite helpful, particularly when there are only a few joints without significant erosions that remain boggy and inflamed despite therapeutic NSAIDs. Triamcinolone hexacetonide may cause skin atrophy and hypopigmentation, but due to its long-lasting effect, is particularly effective for large joints. Due to a shorter half life, triamcinolone acetonide has minimal risk of skin complications and may be a better option for smaller, superficial joints; however, a comparative study of these two agents in oligoarticular JRA demonstrated better short- and long-term results with triamcinolone hexacetonide (38).

Methotrexate is the initial second-line drug typically used in JRA. Multiple studies have demonstrated its efficacy at relatively low doses, ease of administration, low rate of acute adverse reactions, and absence of apparent long-term oncogenic or reproductive consequences. At the lower doses used in JRA, the anti-inflammatory effectiveness of methotrexate is secondary to the increased release of adenosine, a potent inhibitor of neutrophil adherence, and the inhibition of tumor necrosis factor α (31,36).

Methotrexate is classified as one of the disease-modifying antirheumatic drugs (DMARD) and is now prescribed after three to six months of inadequate response to NSAIDs. Other drugs such as hydroxychloroquine, D-penicillamine, and aurnofin were previously considered DMARDs but have failed to demonstrate significant response in better-designed studies (8,36). Gold is now rarely used due to its poorer efficacy and higher rate of complications. Sulfasalazine may be effective in JRA but its use is limited by a relatively high rate of severe toxicity. Compared to methotrexate, leflunomide has similar side effects, but does not have as high a rate of effectiveness (26).

Starting doses of methotrexate are 0.3 mg/kg/week which can be increased to a maximum of 1 mg/kg/week (maximum dose 25 mg/wk orally or 15/m2 subcutaneously to maximum of 50). Supplemental folic acid decreases the most common side effects of gastrointestinal toxicity and oral mucosal ulcerations. Other side effects including hepatotoxicity, immunosuppression, pulmonary disease, pancytopenia, and lymphoproliferative diseases are uncommon in children receiving the doses prescribed for JRA. Methotrexate should be continued longer after remission than NSAIDs because early withdrawal may result in recurrence of synovitis. Gradual decrease should not begin until one year of remission has been sustained.

With a better understanding of the pathogenic mechanisms involved in JRA and other chronic inflammatory disorders, biologic agents have been developed that directly interfere with one or more steps in the immune response. Elevated levels of tumor necrosis factor α (TNFα) and TNFβ are found in JRA and affect the acute-phase inflammatory response and release of destructive proteases in multiple ways. Etanercept, a TNF inhibitor, was the first widely used biologic agent and has been particularly effective in oligoarticular extended and polyarticular patients who had not responded to or were intolerant of methotrexate (15,20). Etanercept is given subcutaneously twice weekly (0.4 mg/kg, maximum 25 mg). This dosage is well tolerated in children. The most common side effects include injection site reactions (39%) and upper respiratory infections (35%). Varicella-susceptible children should be immunized three months prior to initiation of etanercept.

Other newer biologic agents include infliximab and adalimumab (TNFα inhibitors); anakinra (interleukin -1 inhibitor); and rituximab (β-cell depleter). Early studies have demonstrated that they are effective in decreasing inflammation and progressive arthritis in JRA as well as the seronegative arthopathies (6,15,36). Subsequent studies as well as the development of other biologic drugs will undoubtedly advance treatment of chronic inflammation.

In summary, NSAIDs are primarily effective in oligoarticular JRA. Methotrexate is often effective for polyarticular and extended oligoarticular JRA but is less successful in systemic JRA. When methotrexate is inadequate, antitumor necrosis factor medications are usually effective in polyarticular JRA but are less successful in systemic JRA.

ACTIVITIES, BRACING, AND PHYSICAL THERAPY

If joint erosions have not developed and if medical therapy adequately controls the synovitis, then pain and disability are minor and questions concerning activity level, bracing, and physical therapy are relatively moot. These modalities, however, are extremely important with more severe disease. The basic principle is for the child to be as active as possible without exacerbating pain and swelling while maintaining joint motion and alignment.

Play and sports should be directed toward activities that do not accentuate forces across involved joints. Biking and swimming should be encouraged. These activities not only put the joints through a range of motion, but

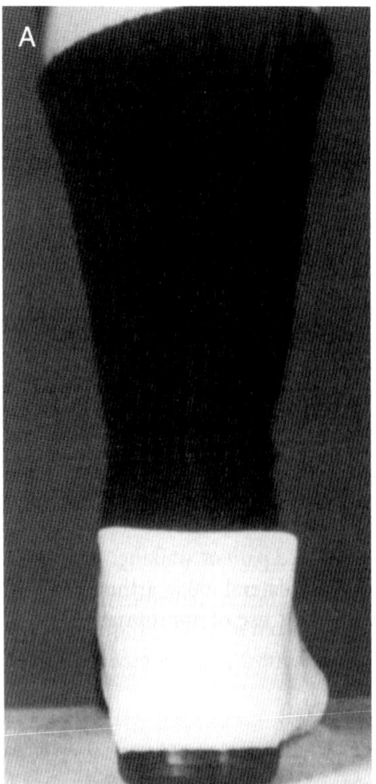

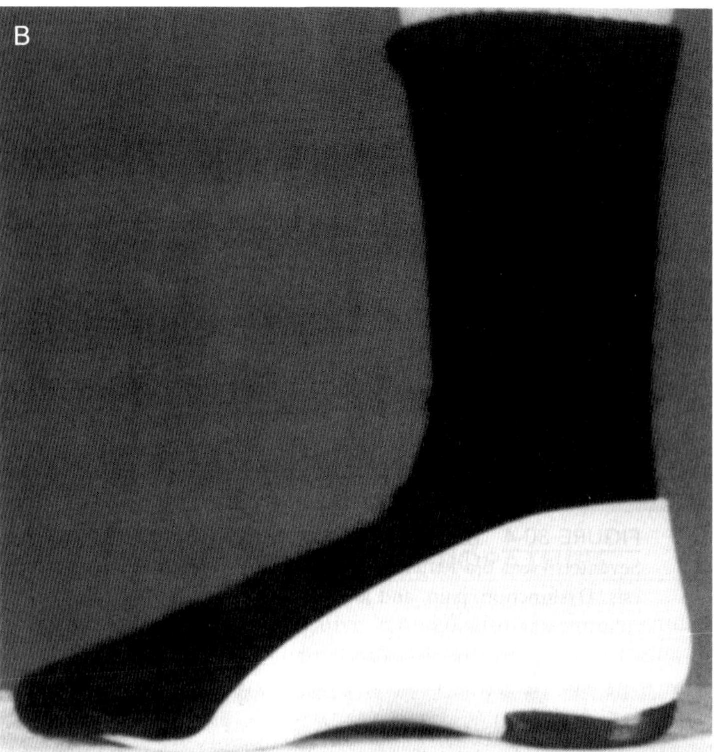

FIGURE 30-3 Two views of UCBL orthotic molded to correct excessive heel valgus and alleviate pressure area beneath the talonavicular joint and metatarsal heads.

they also strengthen muscles about the hip and knee. Other sports can be participated in as tolerated.

Orthoses can be particularly helpful in supporting foot and ankle joints while minimizing progression of deformity. Night-time splinting to prevent equinus contractures and maintain foot alignment should be considered for any child with chronic synovitis of the foot and ankle. With more severe disease, shoe inserts or custom-made orthotics are necessary to alleviate pain. Hindfoot valgus and midtarsal involvement is best managed by a semi-rigid or rigid orthotic fabricated from a plaster mold of the correctly positioned foot. Lining the orthotic with a thermoplastic material will provide pain relief and shock absorption in selected areas, especially the talonavicular joint region (Figure 30-3). Metatarsophalangeal (MTP) joint pain and synovitis can be alleviated by incorporating a metatarsal pad positioned proximal to the MTP joints and grinding out the orthotic underneath the MTP joints. In the older child with severe toe deformities, extra-depth shoes allow greater leeway in orthotic padding and support.

With ankle involvement, a short leg or ankle-foot-orthosis is necessary. A hinged orthosis that will allow some ankle motion is preferred when heel alignment is relatively normal. With severe valgus or varus of the hindfoot and ankle, a solid ankle-foot-orthosis with an appropriate supramalleolar flange or T-strap provides better control of alignment and better alleviation of pain. Although children with severe involvement may progress to ankylosis of their tarsal joints, consistent and effective orthotics can maintain good alignment. With plantigrade posture of the foot, it is striking how well a person can function even with virtually no ankle or foot motion (Figure 30-4).

The goals of physical therapy are (i) to maintain activity; (ii) to maintain and, when possible, improve joint mobility; and (iii) to restore diminished muscle strength associated with inactivity imposed by the synovitis. Obviously, these goals are easier and more effectively achieved when medical therapy can relieve joint swelling and pain.

SURGICAL THERAPY

Ankylosis of the cervical vertebrae without significant prodromal symptoms characteristically occurs in patients with JRA (32). Therefore, preoperative assessment of these patients should include AP, odontoid, and flexion-extension lateral radiographs of the cervical spine (Figure 30-5). Temporomandibular (TM) joint arthritis is also more frequent in JRA and may limit opening of the mouth. The anesthesiologist should have the knowledge and equipment to handle cervical ankylosis and TM arthritis.

Synovectomy has a limited place in JRA (32). Although some reports indicate good results after synovectomy, most show that the procedure does not alter the natural course of a disease that often spontaneously resolves or remits with medical therapy (8,21). Ovregard et al. (21) noted that an early result after synovectomy that was initially rated good was often changed to a poor response when follow up was less than three years; however, this study was done before methotrexate and biologic agents were available and, perhaps more importantly, the

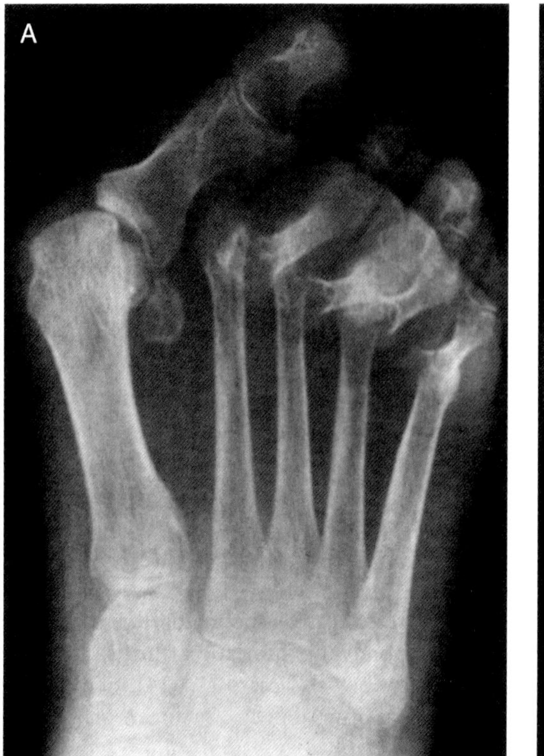

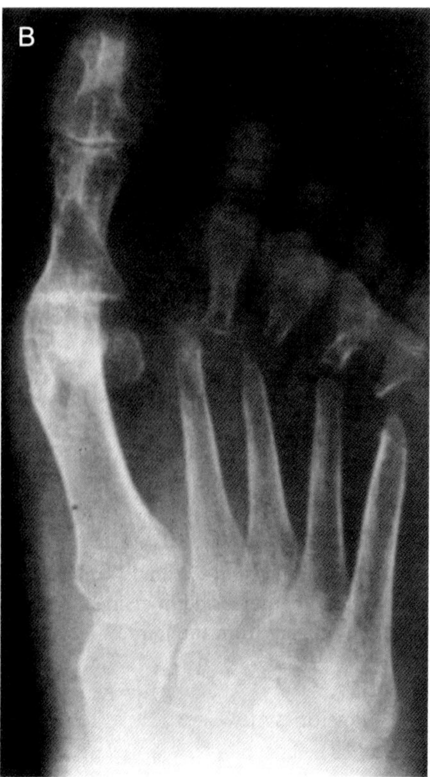

FIGURE 30-7 **A.** AP radiograph of the right foot pre-op. **B.** AP radiograph of the right foot 6 months after operation. Fifty five-year-old-female with onset of polyarticular JRA at age 11 years. Shoe modifications had been satisfactory for many years but pain and deformity had progressed. Preoperative radiograph show severe hallux valgus, dislocation of the 2-5 MTP, and claw toe deformities of the lessor toes. Postoperative radiographs after arthrodesis of the great toe MTP joint and resection arthroplasties of the 2-5 MTP joints. Patient's walking and pain were much improved.

and hip. Typical sites of enthesitis in JAS include the patellar and Achilles tendons and the plantar fascia. The presence of HLA-B27 antigen supports the diagnosis of JAS.

Symptoms of back or sacroiliac pain may be absent in JAS, but limited lumbar motion may be demonstrated by the skin distraction test. With the patient standing, measure a 15-cm span from the posterior iliac spine (dimples of Venus) to the upper lumbar region. Then, ask the child to flex forward as much as possible. Normally, the distance between the two points should increase by 5–7 cm, but in patient with spondylitis, the expected skin distraction is markedly decreased. In JAS, radiographic changes usually develop in the sacroiliac and lumbar spine by late adolescence but may not be present until later adult years. Uveitis and aortitis with aortic regurgitation and conduction defects also occur in JAS, but their frequency seems to be less than that observed in AS.

Treatment begins with NSAIDs, activity modification, and foot orthotics. With continued pain, the TNFα inhibitor drugs have demonstrated good results in AS and it is hoped that early intervention with these agents may prevent severe ankylosis and associated deformities of the spine (5,6,31).

Psoriatic Arthritis

Psoriasis affects 1% to 2% of the general U.S. population (8,14). The disorder is more common in adults, but approximately 20% to 30% have the onset of psoriasis before the age of 16 years. In adults who develop psoriatic arthritis (PsA), the discrete, scaly, erythematous skin lesions typically precede musculoskeletal symptoms; however, approximately 15% of adults develop arthritis or dactylitis before skin manifestations occur. The pattern of joint involvement varies but approximately 70% have an *asymmetric oligoarticular peripheral joint arthritis.* Spinal involvement occurs in approximately 25% of adults with PsA and these patients are more likely to be HLA-B27 positive.

Involvement of the hand and foot is relatively common in PsA (22,25). *Dactylitis* is secondary to inflammation of the tenosynovium, periosteum, and joints. The result is a markedly swollen, "sausage" digit with periarticular erosions and thickening of the phalanges. Some patients develop a characteristic, "pencil point-in-cup" arthropathy of the distal interphalangeal (DIP) joints secondary to resorptive, whittling erosions on the proximal side of the joint. Pitting, ridging, or onycholysis of the nails occurs in 80% of adults with PsA but in only 20%

without joint involvement. Dystrophic nail changes and DIP arthritis are not as common in children as in adults. Chronic uveitis and conjunctivitis is less common in juvenile PsA.

In children, arthritis and dactylitis are more likely to antedate the skin lesions with approximately half of the children with PsA developing joint inflammation first. A positive family history of psoriasis is a helpful clue when joint symptoms occur first. The age of onset of PsA in children is bimodal with the first peak occurring mainly in girls before five years of age and a second peak with more equivalent gender ratio during mid to late childhood (8,30). Compared with children older than five years, younger PsA patients are more likely to be female, exhibit dactylitis and small joint involvement, and be ANA positive. Older children are more likely to have enthesitis, axial joint disease, and persistent oligoarthritis. Both pediatric and adult PsA have a much weaker HLA-B27 association than that observed in AS or arthritis of inflammatory bowel disease.

The lower limbs are more commonly affected in children with PsA. Monoarticular involvement of the knee is the most common presentation, but additional joints are subsequently affected in an asymmetric fashion. During the course of the disease, Shore and Ansell (25) reported knee involvement in 77%, ankle in 66%, hindfoot in 38%, metatarsophalangeal involvement in 33%, and toe involvement in 33%. Non-traumatic swelling of a single, small joint, especially in a toe, suggests PsA because other forms of chronic arthritis rarely cause isolated small joint disease. As in adults, nail pits in children may precede the onset of skin lesions and the severity of nail pits often correlates with the severity of the arthritis (22).

Treatment of PsA is initiated with NSAIDs. Intra-articular glucocorticoids can be effective in oligoarticular PsA. Second line agents include methotrexate, sulfasalazine, and TNF-α inhibitors. Several recent studies have documented increased efficacy of various TNFα inhibitors including etanercept, infliximab, adalimumab, and alefacept in both joint and skin manifestations in adults with PsA (6,16).

Arthritis of Inflammatory Bowel Disease

Peripheral arthritis or sacroilitis occurs in approximately 10% to 20% of patients with inflammatory bowel disease (IBD) secondary to ulcerative colitis or Crohn disease. Arthralgia without joint effusion is more common than arthritis with synovitis. Peripheral arthritis is typically oligoarticular, asymmetric, in the lower extremities, and parallels the course of the bowel disease. The arthritis of IBD is typically of short duration and responds to NSAIDs. Sacroilitis and spondylitis in IBD is associated with presence of HLA-B27 antigen, does not always follow the course of the bowel disease, and is more likely to persist and require second line drug therapy. Inflammatory bowel disease arthritis is unlikely to cause persistent symptoms or require DMARDs; however, biologic agents can be effective in relieving abdominal symptoms.

Systemic Lupus Erythematosus

Systemic lupus erythematosus (SLE) is an autoimmune disease with widespread inflammation of connective tissues and blood vessels (3,8,14). Intermittent symptoms such as malaise, arthritis, dermatitis, nephritis, and pleurisy may precede the diagnosis for several months. Antinuclear antibody (ANA) titers, particularly antibodies to native (double-stranded) DNA are high in symptomatic patients and confirm the diagnosis.

Approximately 15% of all SLE patients have the onset of disease in childhood. The incidence is uncommon in the first decade, but almost as frequent in adolescence as in subsequent age groups. The incidence is higher in female at approximately a 5:1 ratio and more frequent in nonwhite children.

The clinical manifestations in SLE are numerous and multisystem. The classic malar "butterfly" rash is an erythematous, either flat or raised rash that typically spares the nasolabial fold. It is noted in one-third to one-half of children at onset and eventually is observed in three-fourths. Photosensitivity and discoid rash are also common.

Arthralgia and arthritis occur in most children. The joint pain is characteristically of short, 24- to 48-hour duration, is often severe but with minimal objective findings, and it may be migratory. Common sites include the fingers, wrists, elbows, shoulders, knees, and ankles. Tenosynovitis of the extensor tendons often accompanies arthritis of the small joints of the hands. Some patients have swelling and loss of motion that is more persistent; however, joint erosions are uncommon as is chronic arthritis.

Myalgia is common during an acute phase. Steroid myopathy may be noted with chronic disease. Osteonecrosis is a significant complication noted most often in those requiring prolonged steroid medication. Other frequent clinical problems include lupus nephritis, photosensitivity, vasculitis, Raynaud phenomenon, painless ulcer on the hard palate, depression, psychosis, headaches, seizures, pericarditis, decreased pulmonary function without symptoms, pleural effusions, pleuritis, hepatomegaly, and splenomegaly.

Glucocorticoids are the mainstay of medical therapy for SLE. Surgical intervention for musculoskeletal conditions is primarily for various conditions associated with osteonecrosis.

Juvenile Dermatomyositis

Juvenile dermatomyositis (JDM) is a multisystem disorder of uncertain etiology characterized by a vasculopathy and mononuclear inflammatory infiltrates surrounding vessels of striated muscle, skin, and the gastrointestinal tract. An immune-complex vasculitis with perivascular infiltrates of mononuclear cells is noted early in the disease process.

Approximately 15% to 20% of all patients with dermatomyositis have onset during childhood. JDM is more common in girls and the onset is more frequent in four- to ten-year-old children. Compared to adults, in JDM vasculitis is more frequent and often severe, calcinosis is more common, polymyositis is uncommon, and malignancy is very rare.

Juvenile dermatomyositis in most patients evolves through four clinical phases. First is a prodromal period of several weeks with non-specific symptoms that evolves to progressive muscle weakness and dermatitis that lasts days to weeks. The third phase is a plateau period of persistent myositis and dermatitis of one to two years' duration. The recovery phase often has residual muscle atrophy and contractures and sometimes calcinosis.

Typical symptoms at onset include malaise, fatigue, anorexia, and weight loss accompanied by fever, proximal muscle weakness, and rash. The muscle weakness is symmetric and predominantly affects proximal muscles initially in the lower limbs followed by the shoulder girdle and proximal arm. Involved muscles may be tender and occasionally edematous and indurated. *Gower sign* is often present. The child may be unable to climb stairs, dress, or even walk. Weakness of the neck flexors and back muscles may result in the inability to sit unaided or even hold the head upright. In severely affected children, weakness of pharyngeal muscles causes difficulty swallowing and possible aspiration. Distal muscle weakness may be noted with a rapid, severe onset or later in the disease. Although muscle weakness may be severe, deep tendon reflexes are preserved.

Cutaneous abnormalities usually appear a few weeks after onset of weakness. The classic rash occurs in approximately 75% and a less distinctive dermatitis is present in the remainder. The diagnostic cutaneous signs include a heliotrope facial rash, symmetrical papules over the extensor surfaces of joints, and periungual erythema with capillary loop abnormalities. The *heliotrope rash* is a violaceous suffusion of the upper eyelids often accompanied by an erythematous, scaly malar rash that is similar to but less well demarcated than the malar rash in SLE. Edema of the eyelids and face is often present. *Gottron papules* typically are shiny, pink-red, atrophic, scaly plaques that may initially be pale ("collodion patch"). These lesions develop central hypopigmentation. Gottron papules are especially common over the proximal interphalangeal joints of the hands, less common over the metacarpophalangeal and distal interphalangeal joints, and rarely observed over the toes. The knees, elbows, and malleoli may be affected. The periungual skin is strikingly erythematous and telangiectases is noted in the nailfold.

Indurative edema of the skin is often observed in the early phase of JDM. Thinning of the skin, loss of hair, telangiectases, and cutaneous ulcers at the corners of the eye, in the axilla, and in stretch marks may complicate latter phases of JDM.

Calcinosis occurs in approximately 40% of patients. The dystrophic calcification may be subcutaneous nodules, large tumerous deposits typically in proximal muscles (*calcinosis circumscripta*); fascial plane deposition (*calcinosis universalis*); severe exoskeleton-like deposits in the subcutaneous tissue, or mixed forms. Complications of the dystrophic calcification include superficial ulceration and limited joint motion. Limited calcium deposits may resorb with time.

Laboratory abnormalities include elevation of non-specific inflammatory markers and muscle enzymes, particularly aspartate aminotransferase, creatine kinase, aldolase, and lactic dehydrogenase. Electromyography may be helpful in confirming the diagnosis of JDM. Typical findings are consistent with myopathy (decreased amplitude and duration of action potentials) and denervation (increased insertional activity, fibrillations, and positive sharp waves). Muscle biopsy may be needed to confirm the diagnosis of an equivocal case. The biopsy should be performed on an involved but not atrophic muscle. Typical findings are the perivascular infiltrates and patchy areas of muscle degeneration.

The course of the JDM is greatly altered by early diagnosis and initiation of prednisone with an initial dose of 2 mg/kg/day. Serum levels of muscle enzymes are followed to monitor response to therapy. Supportive modalities are helpful. Initial physical therapy focuses on maintaining joint motion. Muscle strengthening should not begin until acute inflammation has decreased.

The duration of active disease is approximately 18–24 months in 60% with one to two episodes of exacerbation and full recovery. The other 40% have longer duration of disease, repeated flares of inflammation, and long term sequelae that ranges from mild atrophy and contractures to severe disability. Immunosuppresive agents can be helpful for disease that does not respond to steroids. Treatment of calcinosis with various medications as well as surgery has produced mixed and limited results. Excision of calcific masses in areas of ulceration or pressure is the surgical procedure that has the best success.

Systemic Sclerodermas

The etiology of the systemic as well as the localized sclerodermas is unknown. Systemic sclerodermas are classified as diffuse, limited, or an overlap syndrome such as mixed connective tissue disease. Diffuse cutaneous systemic scleroderma (DCSS) is a rare disease that is more common in girls (3:1 ratio). Predisposing conditions include diabetes, phenylketonuria, and progeria. Perivascular infiltrates are found in the skin, gastrointestinal tract, lungs, heart, and kidneys.

The onset of DCSS is often insidious and diagnostic delay may be years. Common clinical manifestations include the following: Raynaud phenomenon; atrophy and tightening of the skin of the hands and feet; telangiectases of the face, trunk, and hands; joint contractures; resorption of the tuft of distal phalanges; abnormal esophageal motility, decreased vital capacity, and cardiac arrhythmias.

Limited cutaneous systemic scleroderma (LCSS) is the syndrome previously called CREST syndrome (calcinosis, Raynaud phenomenon, esophageal dysmotility, sclerodactyly, and telangiectases). Sclerosis in LCSS is limited to the distal digits. In LCSS, calcinosis is often severe and Raynaud phenomenon is more likely to cause digital ulceration.

Death may occur in DCSS and LCSS and is usually secondary to cardiac or gastrointestinal complications. Therapy for these disorders often provides limited relief. Raynaud condition is typically managed with calcium channel blockers and appropriate skin protection. Physical therapy can be helpful in minimizing joint contracture progression and maximizing function.

Localized Sclerodermas

The localized sclerodermas are primarily linear scleroderma and morphea. These conditions are more common than systemic sclerodermas and linear scleroderma is twice as frequent as morphea. Fibrosis of connective tissue in localized sclerodermas is limited to dermis, subcutaneous tissue, and superficial striated muscle. Low-titer elevation of ANA titers occurs in approximately 50% of children. Otherwise laboratory studies are normal.

Linear scleroderma has one or more areas of bands of abnormal tissue that most often involves the lower extremities, followed by the upper extremities, trunk, and face. The lesions often affect only one side of the body. Linear scleroderma often spans joints with resultant severe and rigid contractures and associated muscle atrophy and shortening of the limb. At onset the skin is brawny and edematous. Later, the skin is atrophic, indurated, and an ivory or yellow color.

Morphea scleroderma (patches) is classified by the following types: (i) plaque (single or multiple), (ii) generalized (smaller lesions in a more widespread distribution), (iii) bullous, (iv) linear, and (v) deep. These lesions occur on the extremities or trunk and may coalesce or enlarge.

Localized scleroderma may spontaneously resolve, but more severe disease has exacerbations and remissions that may occur over many years. D-penicillamine may be helpful, particularly if used early in the more generalized type of morphea. Bottoni et al. (4) reported surgical results in seven children including release of contractures (4), femoral osteotomy (1), ulnar nerve decompression (1), and tendon transfer (1). Full correction of the deformity was difficult and wound complications necessitated an amputation in one child.

Reactive Arthritis (Reiter Syndrome)

Reactive arthritis (ReA), formerly called Reiter syndrome, is an aseptic inflammatory arthritis that follows enteric or genitourinary bacterial infections in genetically susceptible individuals (2). ReA is highly associated with the presence of HLA-B27, 65% to 85% of affected children being positive. Those who are HLA-B27 negative are frequently positive for cross-reacting antigens. The role of HLA-B27 is uncertain but is probably secondary to similarity of some peptides in some gram negative organisms to peptides in the binding site of the B27 molecule.

ReA secondary to enteritis is primarily associated with *Salmonella enteritidis, Salmonella typimurium, Shigella flexneri, Shigella dysenteriae Yersinia enterocolitica*, and *Campylobacter jejuni*. ReA secondary to urethritis is associated with *Chlamydia trachomatis*. Other gram-negative bacteria can cause ReA but are uncommon. Arthritic symptoms are noted one to four weeks after the triggering infection. Proceeding diarrhea can usually be recalled, but urethritis, found mostly in the adolescent years, may cause an asymptomatic urethral or vaginal mucopurulent discharge or hemorrhagic cystitis.

Acute arthritis with an effusion is most commonly observed, but some ReA children present with or subsequently develop arthralgia, enthesitis, and/or dactylitis. The arthritis is typically asymmetric, oligoarticular, and most commonly in the knees or ankles. Large effusions are common but the joint swelling may be minimal. Common sites of enthesitis are the Achilles tendon, plantar fascia, and patellar tendon. Dactylitis is observed in the toes. Sacroiliitis and back pain may develop but is usually mild and likely to remit in children with ReA.

Conjunctivitis occurs in about two-thirds of children with ReA, but is frequently mild, transient, and may be missed. Acute iritis may occur with persistent disease. Painless ulcers of the oral mucosa are common. Characteristic skin lesions that may occur are keratoderma blennorrhagica (scaly lesions similar to psoriasis), and circinate balanitis (shallow ulcers on the glans penis).

Low-grade anemia and elevated acute phase reactants are common. The joint fluid is sterile and has white blood cell count of 15,000 to 30,000 cells per mm^3. Asymptomatic urethritis may cause a sterile pyuria. If there is no history of preceding infection, elevated antibody titers of associated bacteria may be helpful.

After onset of ReA, the arthritis is usually active for several months, and then enters a remission which may be sustained or the child may develop recurrent episodes of arthritis that persists. Initial treatment of ReA includes NSAIDs and activity modifications. If the ReA is secondary to urethritis, three months of tetracycline probably shortens the duration of the disease; however, the use of antibiotics following enteric infections is less clear. For persistent arthritis and enthesitis, sulfasalazine is recommended. The role of methotrexate and biologic agents is less clear in ReA.

Acute Rheumatic Fever and Poststreptococcal Reactive Arthritis

Acute rheumatic fever (ARF) is an immune disorder characterized by diffuse vasculitis of small vessels. ARF follows a group A β-hemolytic *Streptococcus pyogenes* pharyngitis in genetically predisposed people. The latency period is typically two to three weeks. The five major manifestations of ARF are arthritis, carditis, chorea, erythema marginatum, and subcutaneous nodules (ACCES). The minor manifestations include fever, arthralgia, elevated acute phase reactants (erythrocyte sedimentation rate or C-reactive protein), and prolonged P-R electrocardiac interval. The presence of two major manifestations or one major and two minor signs indicates a high probability of ARF if supported by evidence of preceding group A streptococcal infection (positive throat culture or elevated or rising streptococcal antibody titers).

Arthritis occurs in 70% and is transient and migratory with pain and swelling of a joint sometimes lasting only for hours. Joints primarily affected include the elbow, wrist, knee, and ankle. Pain may be severe and is typically very responsive to aspirin (50–75 mg/kg/day in four divided doses) or NSAIDs. A lack of subsidence of arthritis within five days of therapy warrants consideration of other diagnoses. Persistent arthropathy does not occur in children with ARF.

Poststreptococcal reactive arthritis (PSRA) also follows group A streptococcal pharyngitis. Compared to ARF, the latency period is shorter (< 10 days) in PRA and for that reason the incidence of positive throat cultures or rapid antigen tests is higher. The arthritis is nonmigratory and most commonly affects the knees and ankles. About half of the patients have upper extremity involvement. Axial arthritis is noted in one-fourth. Cardiac disease occurs in 6% and is only noted several months after onset of arthritis.

Treatment includes NSAIDs and antibiotic prophylaxis for one year. Duration of arthritis is protracted in poststreptococcal reactive arthritis, lasting on average two months. The absence of association with HLA-B27 in both ARF or PRA indicates that these disorders have a different pathogenesis than the RA that follows enteric or genitourinary infections.

Lyme Disease

Lyme disease (LD) is a multisystem disease and the most common tickborne infection in North America and Europe. In the United States, LD is caused by infection from the spirochete *B. burgdorferi* which is transmitted by the bite of *Ixodes scapularis* (deer tick) in southern New England, the mid-Atlantic states (to Maryland and Virginia), and the upper Midwest (Wisconsin and Minnesota), and by *Ixodes pacificus* in northern California. Sporadic cases occurring elsewhere are almost always acquired during visits to these endemic areas.

During its two-year life cycle (egg-larva-nymph-adult), the *I. scapularis* larva and nymph require a blood meal, which is usually acquired from a white-footed field mouse. An infected mouse can transmit *B. burgdorferi* to the ticks. An infected nymph may transmit *B. burgdorferi* to an unaffected mouse. Both nymph and adult ticks may transmit the spirochete to humans.

LD can be separated into three stages. Early localized disease occurs one day to a month (mean seven to ten days) after the tick bite. This stage is characterized by the pathognomonic skin lesion *erythema migrans* (EM) which occurs in about 90% of patients. EM is an expanding erythematous papule or macule. Central clearing may occur but a "bull's eye pattern" is only noted in 30%. Common sites include the groin, axilla, thorax, abdomen, and popliteal space. EM is often painless but may be pruritic. Multiple EM lesions occur in 10% of patients. Even without treatment, EM resolves by four weeks. Other symptoms during the early localized phase are nonspecific fatigue, headache, myalgia, and arthralgia.

Early disseminated LD occurs days to ten months after the tick bite. Approximately 50% of untreated patients develop arthritis and/or arthralgia. Intermittent episodes of an oligoarticular, migratory arthritis of large joints is common. Involvement of small joints is uncommon and should suggest another disorder. Stiffness, rather than pain, is the primary complaint. Large effusions are common. The synovial fluid white count is 10,000–25,000 white blood cells/mm^3.

Other possible manifestations of early disseminated LD include carditis in 10% and neurologic conditions in 12% of untreated patients. Atrioventricular heart block is the classic LD cardiac lesion but mild pericarditis can also occur. Neurologic manifestations of early disseminated LD include cranial neuritis (most often facial palsy), lymphocytic meningitis, and peripheral neuropathy. Other conditions found during this stage are less specific and include conjunctivitis, iritis, lymphadenopathy, lymphadenosis benigna cutis, hepatitis, and proteinuria.

Late LD occurs months to years after the tick bite and similar to the early disseminated stage may occur without prior manifestations of LD. Migratory polyarthritis occurs in about 50% and chronic monoarthritis, usually of the knee, occurs in 10% of untreated patients. Neurologic manifestations include a chronic, often subtle, encephalopathy and/or peripheral neuropathy.

Documented EM is diagnostic of LD. Other clinical manifestations, however, require laboratory studies to confirm the diagnosis. Blood, joint fluid, and spinal fluid should be sent for culture and serologic tests. Elevated levels of IgM antibodies to *B. burgdorferi* may not be detectable for four weeks and IgG levels may not be measurable for eight weeks. Early, even insufficient, antibiotic therapy may negate elevated antibody levels and some patients remain seronegative despite continued active disease. Polymerase chain reaction (PCR) studies can identify *B. burgdorferi* in skin, synovial fluid, synovial tissue, serum, and spinal fluid. PCR is more sensitive than culture, more specific than serologic studies, and may detect organisms before antibody titers develop; however, these tests are not routinely done due to expense and the rate of false-positive and false-negative results.

Antibiotic therapy can hasten resolution of LD and also prevent progression to later conditions of the disease. The evidence-based guidelines for type and duration of antibiotic therapy developed by a consensus panel of the Infectious Diseases Society of America varies depending on the stage of the disease, the type of manifestation, and the age of the patient (37). Lyme arthritis initially can be treated with a four-week course of oral antibiotic therapy. If persistent but improved arthritis occurs, a second course of oral antibiotics is recommended. If the arthritis has not changed or worsened, a four-week course of intravenous ceftriaxone can be given. A better understanding of LD has virtually eliminated the need for surgical intervention and long-term disability.

Arthritis Secondary to Hemophilia

Although any of the 14 coagulation factors may be deficient or absent, musculoskeletal problems are primarily limited to deficits in either factor VIII or Factor IX. Factor VIII hemophilia accounts for about 75% of all inherited clotting disorders and Factor IX deficiency constitutes approximately 12% of the total. The other inherited coagulation disorders mostly have mucosal hemorrhages such as epistaxis and menorrhagia, and uncommonly have joint bleeds except after major trauma.

Both Factor VIII and Factor IX hemophilia are sex-linked disorders. Clinical suspicion of these disorders is triggered by bleeding at the time of circumcision, atypical bruising with immunization or play, or excessive bleeding from lip lacerations in toddlers learning to walk. Joint and muscle bleeds become the dominating clinical problem as the child becomes more active. With severe hemophilia (< one unit/dL clotting factor, commonly noted as <1%), a hemarthrosis may occur with trivial trauma during routine play.

Knee bleeds are most frequent in older children but the ankle is the most common site of hemarthrosis in the child less than ten years old. Ankle bleeds are particularly common in the preschool child, probably related to their jumping propensity. Parents note limping and a reluctance to bear weight on the affected limb. An older child frequently notes an aura of pain that precedes any obvious swelling. With deficient clotting, joint bleeds are severe even after a trivial incident and are associated marked swelling and pain.

Muscle bleeds in the calf are also frequent in children with hemophilia. The most common site is the gastrocnemius. Therefore, these patients also hold their foot in equinus, but there is no swelling of the ankle joint and ankle dorsiflexion is increased when the knee is flexed.

Hemophilic arthropathy begins with a major hemarthrosis and is more likely to progress if two or three occur in a joint within a short period. As blood inside the joint is catabolized, the iron from the hemoglobin is absorbed by the synovium. Synovial cells can absorb only a limited amount of iron; when that quantity is exceeded, the cell disintegrates and releases lysozymes that not only destroy articular cartilage but also inflame the synovial tissue. The result is a hypertrophic and hypervascular synovium that, in a person with a clotting deficiency, is fragile and tends to bleed spontaneously. Thus, begins a vicious cycle of recurrent bleeds in the joint followed by more synovitis and joint destruction.

Chondrocytes take up iron as well, and with an excessive amount, the chondrocytes also disintegrate and release lysozymes that also destroy the cartilage matrix. Furthermore, the the chondrocyte may undergo necrosis. This combination of synovitis and primary cartilage erosion explains the rapid and severe arthropathy in hemophilic children who do not have access to adequate replacement therapy.

Radiographic changes in the early stages of hemophilic arthropathy are similar to those observed in other inflammatory arthritidies. Erosions at the joint margin, subchondral cysts, and subchondral irregularity are characteristic. With end-stage arthropathy, narrowing of articular cartilage is obvious, but the subchondral bone is more sclerotic in hemophiliacs.

Transfusion to replace the missing clotting factor is most critical in the management of any hemarthrosis or muscle bleed. Aspiration of the joint can remove the bulk of blood and may reduce the amount or iron that must be absorbed. Major joint bleeding should be followed by a period of prophylactic transfusion therapy that prevents recurrent joint bleeds and allows the synovitis that occurs after single hemarthrosis chance to resolve. If hypertrophic synovitis and recurrent joint bleeds develop, the child may be treated with radiation synovectomy, arthroscopic synovectomy, or open synovectomy.

Equinus contracture may develop after repeated calf bleeds. Early on, these contractures may be corrected by serial casting (Figure 30-8). Patients without access to replacement therapy or those that develop an inhibitor to the clotting factor must be taught to seek medical attention early so that nonoperative modalities such as compression dressings and serial casting can be used minimize arthropathy and contractures.

Sickle Cell Anemia

Approximately 1 of every 300 African Americans has sickle cell disease. The three common genotypes are: (i) SS disease – homozygous for hemoglobin S, (ii) SC disease – heterozygous for hemoglobin S and hemoglobin C, (iii) Sβ disease – heterozygous for hemoglobin S and hemoglobin β-thalassemia. Musculoskeletal problems in these patients include dactylitis, sickle cell crises,

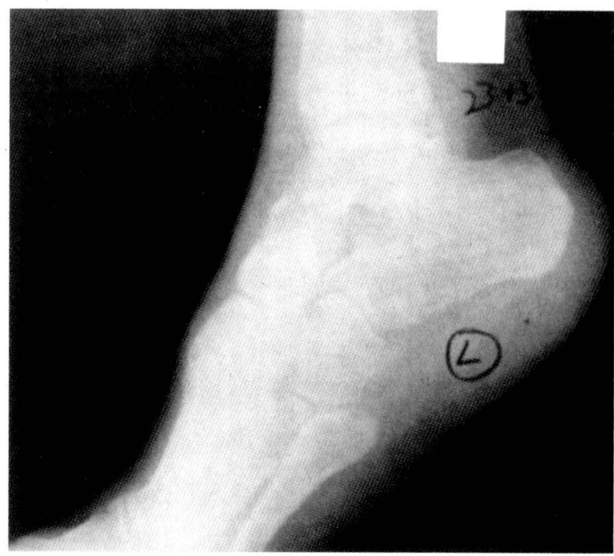

FIGURE 30-8 Lateral radiograph of left foot demonstrate severe equinus contracture in a 22-year-old male with severe equinus contracture but absence of significant ankle arthropathy. Contracture developed secondary to gastrocsoleus hemorrhages during childhood.

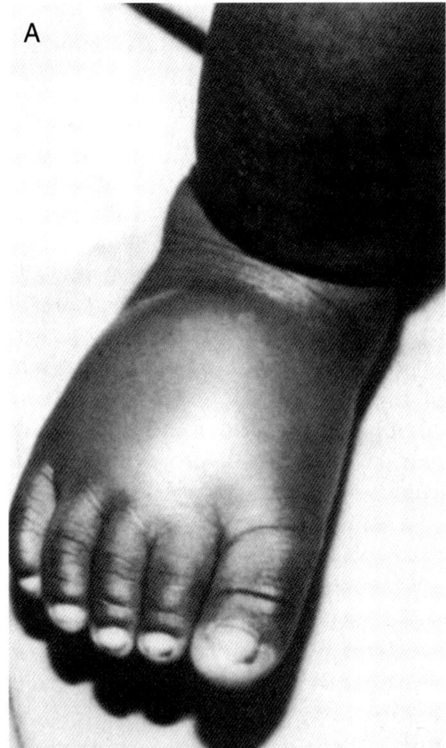

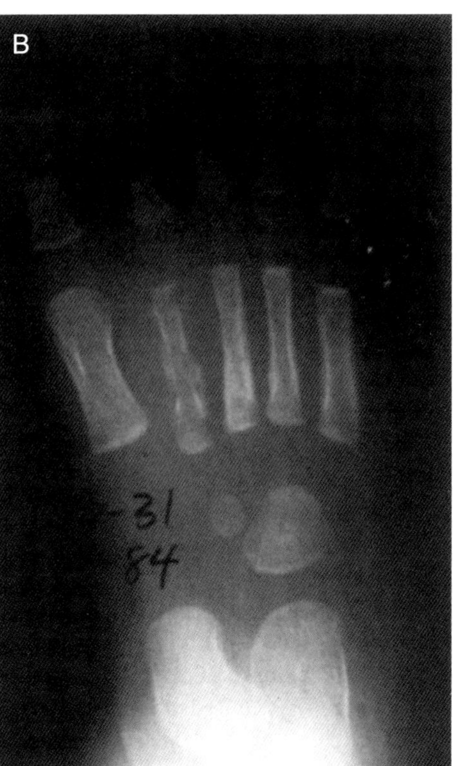

FIGURE 30-9 **A.** Clinical appearance of the right foot 48 hours after hospitalization of this seven-month-old male with sickle cell disease. Marked swelling of the left ring finger was also noted on admission. Diagnosis on admission was hand-foot syndrome and patient was treated with hydration and pain management. When swelling and fever persisted, aspiration of the foot and hand was performed. Purulent material was obtained and then drainage and irrigation of the hand and foot was done in the operating room. Culture from hand and foot grew *Salmonella*. **B.** AP radiograph of the right foot on the 15th hospital day shows bony destruction and periosteal reaction in the second metatarsal. This patient had osteomyelitis but radiographs are consistent with either resolving osteomyelitis or dactylitis.

osteonecrosis, osteomyelitis, septic arthritis, reactive arthritis, and leg ulcers (9).

Dactylitis or hand-foot syndrome is caused by infarction of bone marrow in the hand or foot (29). It occurs after hemoglobin F has been replaced by hemoglobin S and is often the first clinical manifestation of sickle cell disease. Affected children present with a swollen hand or foot or swelling limited to a digit. Cessation of this problem coincides with the disappearance of hematopoietic marrow in the hands and feet. Therefore, no series has reported dactylitis in patients older than six years.

A sickle cell crisis results from a localized area of infarction. Extremity pain from a crisis is secondary to bone marrow infarction. Proximal migration of the hematopoietic marrow explains the infrequent occurrence of sickle cell crisis in the distal tibia.

The incidence of osteomyelitis is increased in SCD. Because the signs and symptoms are similar, it may be difficult to distinguish both dactylitis and sickle cell crises from osteomyelitis (13). Furthermore, osteomyelitis may begin as an infarction that evolves into osteomyelitis. Elevated temperature, white blood cell count, and findings on radiographs, bone scans and MRI frequently overlap in these conditions, but sequential radionuclide bone marrow and bone scans may be helpful in differentiating osteomyelitis from bone infarction.

If clinical signs and laboratory results suggest osteomyelitis, a biopsy should be performed to confirm the diagnosis and to obtain cultures. *Staphylococcus aureus* and salmonellae are common causes of osteomyelitis in SCD and initial antibiotic therapy should cover both organisms.

Compared to osteomyelitis, septic arthritis is relatively uncommon in SCD. Most cases are caused by organisms other than salmonella unless the joint infection was secondary to direct penetration from an adjacent osteomyelitis.

Reactive arthritis is more common in patients with SCD probably secondary to the increased frequency of salmonella dysentery following abdominal infarction. The knees and elbows are most frequently involved, but symptoms may also occur in the ankles and joints of the feet. Polyarticular symptoms are more common. Arthralgia will last for a few days to two months. Joint effusions will typically last one to two weeks.

Leukemia

Leukemia, a myeloproliferative malignancy, is the most common cancer in childhood. Peak incidence is one to five years of age. Musculoskeletal symptoms are present at onset in approximately fifty percent. In many children the symptoms are mild but a significant number have musculoskeletal pain as the primary complaint (33). Back pain with a collapsed vertebra easily directs one to a diagnostic evaluation, but a high index of suspicion is required when evaluating a child with leukemia who has extremity pain as their presenting complaint.

In most cases, the pain is not well localized but diffusely spread over a region. Tenderness is most often in the metaphyseal region of bone. The distal femur area is the most common site, but other areas such as the hands, elbows, and ankle may be painful. Joint effusions also may occur. Infiltration of the bone marrow is the obvious cause of the bone pain but the pathogenesis of the arthritis is uncertain. Multiple joints may be involved. Asymmetric involvement of the large joints is characteristic. The joint pain may be migratory.

Low-grade fever is common in leukemia. Therefore, the differential diagnosis includes JRA, reactive arthritis, osteomyelitis, and septic arthritis. Pain in leukemia is often worse at night (as opposed to the morning stiffness in JRA), is usually disproportionate to the objective findings, and is more severe than the pain observed in JRA. In a child who presents with unexplained back or limb pain, inquiries about lethargy, headache, vomiting, night pain, and easy bruising may be helpful. Marked elevation of ESR and CRP is noted in leukemia and can help exclude JRA. The CBC, white blood cell differential, and platelet count may be normal at onset of symptoms, but dissociation of the acute-phase indices (elevated ESR and CRP with normal or low platelet count) coupled with low WBC suggest the need for bone marrow aspiration. Further indication of leukemia includes blast cells in peripheral smears and elevation of lactic dehydrogenase or urate. Helpful radiographic signs include osteopenia and metaphyseal radiolucent bands.

REFERENCES

1. Allen RC, Ansell BM. Juvenile chronic arthritis: clinical subgroups with particular relationship to adult patterns of disease. *Postgrad Med J* 62: 821–826, 1986.
2. Barth WF, Segal K. Reactive Arthritis (Reiter's Syndrome). *Am Fam Physician.* 60: 499–503, 507, 1999.
3. Benseler SM, Silverman ED. Systemic Lupus Erythematosus. *Pediatr Clin N Am.* 52: 443–467, 2005.
4. Bottoni, CR, Reinker KA, Gardner RD, et al. Scleroderma in childhood: A 35-year history of cases and review of the literature. *J Pediatr Orthop* 20: 442–449, 2000.
5. Brandt J, Listing J, Haibel H, et al. Long-term efficacy and safety of etanercept after readministration in patients with active ankylosing spondylitis. *Rheumatology (Oxford)* 44: 342–348, 2005.
6. Braun J, Sieper J. Biological therapies in the spondyloarthritides – the current state. *Rheumatology* 43: 1072–1084, 2004.
7. Cassidy J, Kivulin J, Lindsley C, et al. Ophthalmologic examinations in children with juvenile rheumatoid arthritis. *Pediatrics* 117: 1843–1845, 2006.
8. Cassidy, JT, Petty RE, eds. *Textbook of Pediatric Rheumatology,* 5th ed. Philadelphia: Saunders, 2005.
9. Diggs LW. Bone and joint lesions in sickle-cell disease. *Clin Orthop* 52: 119–143, 1967.
10. Dunn, AL, Busch MT, Wyly JB, et al. Arthroscopic Synovectomy for Hemophilic Joint Disease in a Pediatric Population. *J Ped Orthop* 21: 414–426, 2004.
11. Felin EM, Prahalad S, Askew EW, et al. Musculoskeletal abnormalities of the tibia in juvenile rheumatoid arthritis. *Arthrits Rheum* 56: 984–994, 2007.
12. Greene WB. Synovectomy of the ankle for hemophilic arthropathy. *J Bone Joint Surg* 76-A: 812–819, 1994.
13. Greene WB, McMillan CW: Salmonella osteomyelitis and hand-foot syndrome in a child with sickle cell anemia. *J Ped Orthop* 7: 716–718, 1987.
14. Harris Jr. ED, Budd RC, Firestein GS, Genovese MC, Sargent JS, Ruddy S, Sledge, CB, ed. *Kelley's Textbook of Rheumatology,* 7th ed. Philadelphia: Saunders, 2005.
15. Hashkes PJ, Laxer RM. Medical treatment of juvenile idiopathic arthritis. *JAMA* 294: 1671–1684, 2005.
16. Krueger G, Callis K. Potential of tumor necrosis factor inhibitors in psoriasis and psoriatic arthritis. *Arch Dermatol* 140: 218–225, 2004.
17. Lawrence RC, Helmick CG, Arnett FC, et al. Estimates of the prevalence of arthritis and selected musculoskeletal disorders in the United States. *Arthritis Rheum* 41: 778–799, 1998.
18. Lovell DJ, Giannini EH, Brewer EJ: Time course of response to nonsteroidal anti-inflammatory drugs in juvenile rheumatoid arthritis. *Arthritis Rheum* 27: 1433–1437, 1984.
19. Lovell DJ, Glass D, Ranz J, et al. A randomized controlled trial of calcium supplementation to increase bone mineral density in children with juvenile rheumatoid arthritis. *Arthritis Rheum* 54: 2235–2242, 2006.
20. Lovell DJ, Reiff A, Jones OY, et al. Long-term safety and efficacy of etanercept in children with polyarticular-course juvenile rheumatoid arthritis. *Arthritis Rheum* 54: 1987–1994, 2006.
21. Ovregard T, Hoyeraal HM, Pahle JA, et al. A three-year retrospective study of synovectomies in children. *Clin Orthop* 259: 76–82, 1990.
22. Perlman SG. Psoriatic arthritis in children. *Pediatr Dermatol* 1: 283–287, 1984.
23. Peterson LS, Mason T, Nelson AM, et al. Juvenile rheumatoid arthritis in Rochester, Minnesota 1960–1993: is the epidemiology changing? *Arthritis Rheum* 39: 1385–1390, 1996.
24. Saurenmann RK, Levin AV, Feldman BM, et al. Prevalence, risk factors, and outcome of uveitis in juvenile idiopathic arthritis: a long-term followup study. *Arthritis Rheum* 56: 647–657, 2007.
25. Shore A, Ansell BM. Juvenile psoriatic arthritis: an analysis of 60 cases. *J Pediatr* 100: 529–535, 1982.
26. Silverman E, Mouy R, Spiegel L, et al. Lefunomide or methotrexate for juvenile rheumatoid arthritis. *N Engl J Med* 352: 1655–1666, 2005.
27. Simon S, Whiffen J, Shapiro F. Leg-length discrepancies in monoarticular and pauciarticular juvenile rheumatoid arthritis. *J Bone Joint Surg* 63-A: 209–215, 1981.
28. Singh-Grewal D, Schneider R, Bayer N, et al. Predictors of disease course and remission in systemic juvenile idiopathic arthritis: significance of early clinical and laboratory features. *Arthritis Rheum* 54: 1595–1601, 2006.
29. Stevens MCG, Padwick M, Serjeant GR. Observations on the natural history of dactylitis in homozygous sickle cell disease. *Clin Pedatr[Phila]*: 20: 311–317, 1981.
30. Stoll ML, Zurakowski D, Nigrovic LE, et al. Patients with juvenile psoriatic arthritis comprise two distinct populations. *Arthritis Rheum* 54: 3564–3572, 2006.

31. Sullivan KE. Inflammation in juvenile idiopathic arthritis. *Pediatr Clin N Am* 52: 335–357, 2005.
32. Swann M. The surgery of juvenile chronic arthritis. An overview. *Clin Orthop* 259: 70–75, 1990.
33. Tuten H, Robert MD, Gabos PG, et al. The limping child: a manifestation of acute leukemia. *J Pediatr Orthop* 18: 625–629, 1998.
34. Thornton J, Ashcroft DM, Mughal MZ, et al. Systematic review of effectiveness of bisphosphonates in treatment of low bone mineral density and fragility fractures in juvenile idiopathic arthritis. *Arch Dis Child* 91: 753–761, 2006.
35. Wallace CA, Levinson JE. Juvenile rheumatoid arthritis: outcome and treatment for the 1990s. *Rheum Dis Clin North Am* 17: 891–905, 1991.
36. Weiss JE, Ilowite NT. Juvenile idiopathic arthritis. *Pediatr Clin North Am* 52: 413–442, 2005.
37. Wormser GP, Dattwyler RJ, Shapiro ED, et al. The clinical assessment, treatment, and prevention of Lyme disease, human granulocytic anaplasmosis and babesiosis: clinical practice guidelines by the Infectious Diseases Society of America. *Clin Inf Diseases* 43: 1089–1134, 2006.
38. Zulian F, Martini G, Gobber D, et al. Triamcinolone acetonide and hexacetonide intra-articular treatment of symmetrical joints in juvenile idiopathic arthritis: a double-blind trial. *Rheumatology (Oxford)* 43: 1288–1291, 2004.

CHAPTER 31

Osteochondrodysplasias

Dennis P. Grogan

INTRODUCTION

The osteochondrodysplasias are a heterogeneous collection of constitutional diseases that are due to primary abnormalities of the growth and development of cartilage or bone. Many have extraskeletal abnormalities as well. Confusing terminology, especially regarding the classification of these disorders, has impeded our understanding of skeletal dysplasias in the past. Rubin's "dynamic classification of bone dysplasias" was one of the first to organize and attempt to establish some logic to our study of this area (68,79). As further cases have been studied and our clinical acumen has developed, the natural refinement of our ability to diagnose and to more accurately define each of these varied disorders has followed. The previous "lumping" of many separate diseases into groups, "achondroplasia" for example, has been followed by the more accurate "splitting" of these diseases into like groups based on more careful clinical assessment. The exact histopathologic mechanism of each disorder is still only partially understood, if at all (82). As knowledge of their basic biochemical defect has become available, a more complete understanding and physiologic classification will be possible. The basic error of genetic or cellular metabolism or chemical malfunction for an increasing number of osteochondrodysplasias is being exposed each year (6).

The large number of different skeletal dysplasias and the relative rarity of each of them make the task of differential diagnosis a demanding one. A multidisciplinary approach to these children, combining the genetic, radiologic, pediatric, and orthopedic aspects of each child's presentation will enable the physician to make an accurate diagnosis in most cases. Establishing an accurate diagnosis will then allow the physician to provide appropriate genetic counseling to the family and a realistic prognosis based on the natural history of the dysplasia, as well as timely and goal-oriented treatment of the patient's present and future problems. Two reports involving four children point out the possibility of skeletal dysplasia presenting as a neuromuscular disorder and reinforce the need to carefully evaluate these children (13,83).

Evaluation of a patient with a known or suspected skeletal dysplasia must carefully consider all of the possible clinical features associated with the dysplasia, and the general medical as well as the orthopaedic implications of each finding on the patient's overall condition. One of the most important orthopaedic considerations for patients with skeletal dysplasias is the increased incidence of atlantoaxial instability. At the time of their initial evaluation, and certainly preoperatively, these children should undergo a thorough evaluation of their cervical spine with flexion-extension lateral radiographs, and a baseline neurological evaluation so that any future changes will be apparent. Flexion-extension magnetic resonance imaging (MRI) has provided more information in some cases regarding the actual pathologic changes, i.e., compression or impingement of the upper spinal cord.

The more common osteochondrodysplasias will be considered in this chapter. Their presenting clinical and radiographic findings will be addressed, with emphasis on the orthopaedic features and treatment. Information regarding the foot and ankle will be provided in detail in those dysplasias with characteristic findings, but many skeletal dysplasias will have no specific changes involving this area.

MULTIPLE HEREDITARY OSTEOCHONDROMATOSES

The disorder of multiple hereditary osteochondromatosis (MHO) is one of the most common of the skeletal dysplasias. It is equally well known as multiple hereditary exostoses, multiple cartilaginous exostoses, or diaphyseal aclasis. This is often one of the most frequently encountered congenital anomalies of skeletal development in the orthopaedist's practice. It is transmitted as an autosomal dominant condition, with males and females equally affected, and often there will be a strong family history present. It is caused by a mutation in one of two EXT genes (EXT 1 or EXT 2) leading to defective heparin

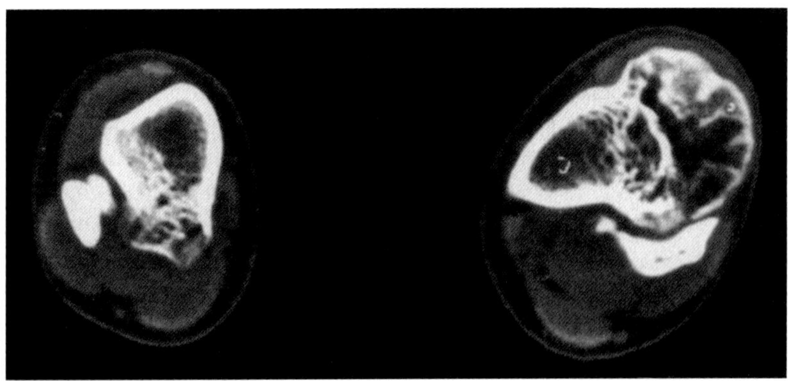

FIGURE 31-3 CT scan through the distal tibia in a boy with multiple hereditary osteochondromatosis. The large anterolateral exostosis on the right is as large as the distal tibia at this level and has displaced the fibula.

the previously expressed belief that the growth retardation of a bone is directly related to the size and number of the exostoses was inaccurate.

Of interest is the fact that although elbow problems related to subluxation of the proximal radius are common secondary to the distal radio-ulnar growth asymmetry and deformity at the wrist, no comparable problems have been reported at the knee subsequent to the deformity at the ankle. Prominence of the proximal fibula secondary to the growth of the osteochondromata is common, however, and may require excision to relieve peroneal nerve symptoms.

Treatment should be directed at minimizing the progression of the deformity once it is noted. Surgical options would include procedures directed toward immediate correction of the current deformity, or those procedures that would allow future correction with growth of the extremity. Jahss and Olives (33) reported 13 ankles with symptomatic osteochondromata that were treated with simple excision. Snearly and Peterson (74) described nine patients who underwent a variety of surgical procedures. Their results allowed them to suggest guidelines for the treatment of these patients. Isolated excision of osteochondromata is best for those patients of any age with symptoms referable to the osteochondromata, and for young patients with early angular deformity or relative length discrepancy between the tibia and fibula. They found that severe angular deformities and length discrepancies were less likely to develop later in young patients whose osteochondromata were excised at an early age. Hemi-epiphyseodesis of the medial distal tibial epiphysis is best for patients who have tibiotalar valgus greater than 15 degrees and with minor fibular relative shortening (defined as the fibular physis at or distal to the level of the tibial physis). Fibular lengthening is performed when the relative fibular shortening is more severe, with the distal fibular physis proximal to the distal tibial epiphysis. A combination of hemi-epiphyseodesis and fibular lengthening can be done in those patients with both deformities. Osteochondromata in the operative field should be excised during any of these procedures (74). We have utilized a similar treatment protocol for these children, operating at an earlier age and with lesser degrees of deformity to prevent severe deformities from developing, and have been pleased with our results. Hemi-epiphyseodesis can easily be achieved utilizing a screw or an 8-plate (Orthofix) across the medial distal tibial epiphysis (Figure 31-5). Osteotomy of the distal tibia and fibula is now required less often, reserved for the older child with significant deformity, and does not specifically address the problem of the fibular shortening. Chin et al. (16) studied the natural history of the osteochondroma of the distal tibia and fibula and formulated treatment recommendations similar to those above. Beals and Shea (8) have recently reported using the bone age to predict correction when using the medial distal tibial surface epiphyseodesis. However, Loder et al. (47) also reported a study involving 40 children with chondrodysplasias and found a 0.6-year delay in bone age compared to chronologic age in this population (children with MHO and enchondromatosis).

Although tibiofibular synostosis has previously been reported in up to 25% of these patients (75), Snearly and Peterson (74) found a much lower incidence of this deformity. Only one of their nine patients was suspected of having a congenital synostosis preoperatively. At the time of operative exploration, an interdigitation of adjacent tibial and fibular osteochondromata was found, separated by a layer of fibrous tissue. They postulated that these exostoses may have gone on to synostosis by skeletal maturity, with further growth and confluence. We have substantiated this anatomic finding in several patients, and suspect that it is a result of observing these children more closely and operating on them at an earlier age than was done in the past when osteotomy of the distal tibia at skeletal maturity was often the treatment of choice. A transfibular approach for resection of distal tibial osteochondromata has recently been reported by Gupte et al. (27).

Deformity of the foot can be produced by the effect of the osteochondromata on the growth of the long bones of the foot, most commonly the metatarsals but including the phalanges (Figure 31-6). Length discrepancies can develop between the metatarsals which then produce secondary toe deformities. Angular deformities of the metatarsals and toes may also result from the progressive deviation. Calluses are not commonly seen under the

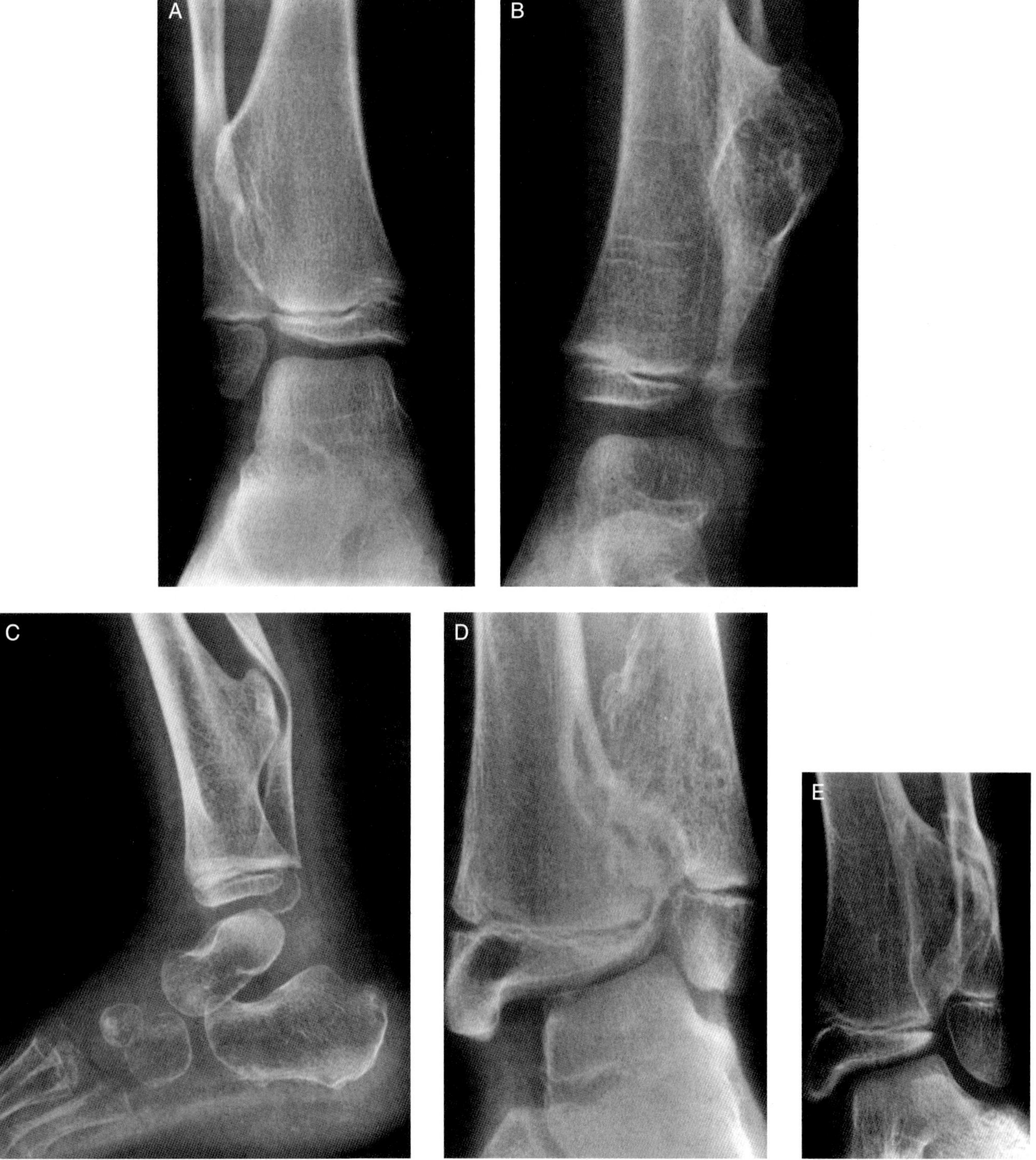

FIGURE 31-4 **A-E.** The range of ankle deformities in patients with multiple hereditary osteochondromatosis. The exostosis may be of any size, originate from either the tibia or the fibula, and have a variable degree of fibular shortening and ankle valgus.

heads of the longer metatarsals (33). Pressure effects may appear on adjacent metatarsals with scalloping of the bone. Loss of subtalar motion has also been reported, related to the growth of exostoses about the medial facet of the subtalar joint (33). Treatment of any of these deformities is based on the specific cause and the degree of deformity or symptomatology.

Two more cautions should be expressed when treating children with HMO. Darilek et al. (20) have recently reported on the increased incidence of pain in this population and recommended treatment directed toward its alleviation, and Hosalkar et al. found an increased incidence of keloid formation following surgical excision of osteochondromas in these children (32).

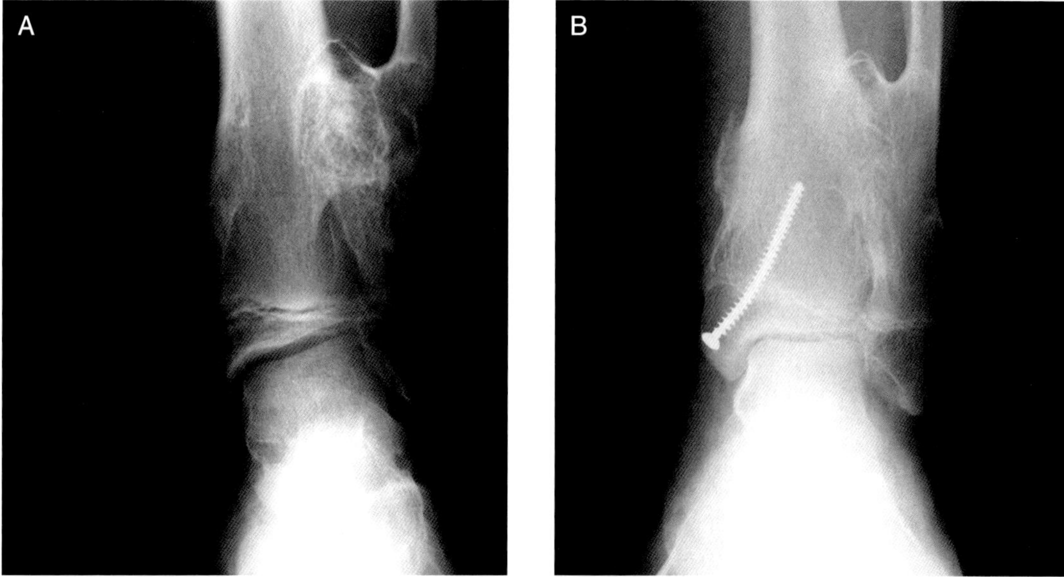

FIGURE 31-5 **A.** Standing AP left ankle of a 12-year-old young man with multiple hereditary osteochondromatosis. Note the significant ankle valgus. **B.** Three years following screw hemi-epiphyseodesis of the medial distal tibia. Note the excellent correction of the ankle deformity.

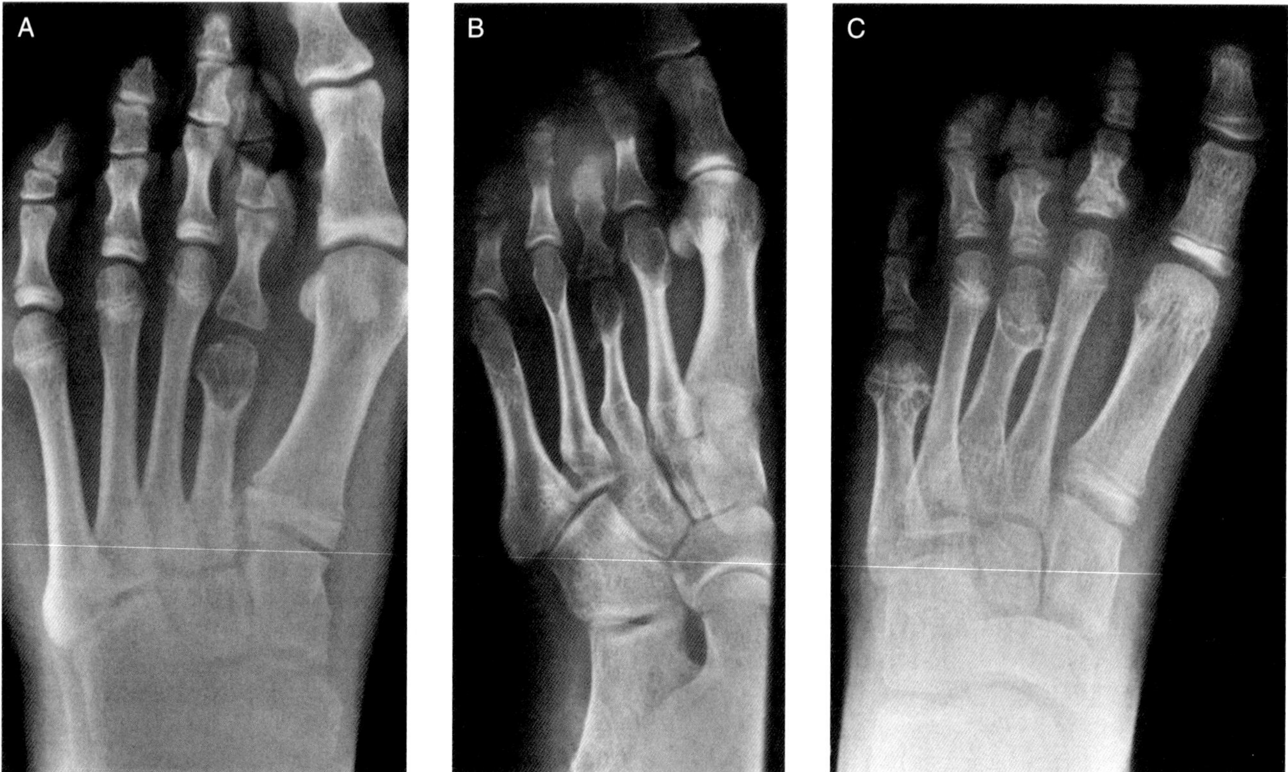

FIGURE 31-6 **A-C.** Multiple hereditary osteochondromatoses in the feet are usually small but can have a significant effect on the growth of the tubular bones and subsequent deformities of the toes.

ENCHONDROMATOSIS

Enchondromatosis, or Ollier disease, is a disorder of normal endochondral ossification in which multiple cartilaginous lesions develop mainly within the metaphyseal regions of the tubular bones, but flat bones and the spine may be involved. The onset is usually noted between the second and tenth year of life. No hereditary factor has been demonstrated, each case appearing to be sporadic.

The multiple enchondromata are indistinguishable from solitary enchondromata, both radiographically and histologically. They appear as oval, pyramidal, or linear

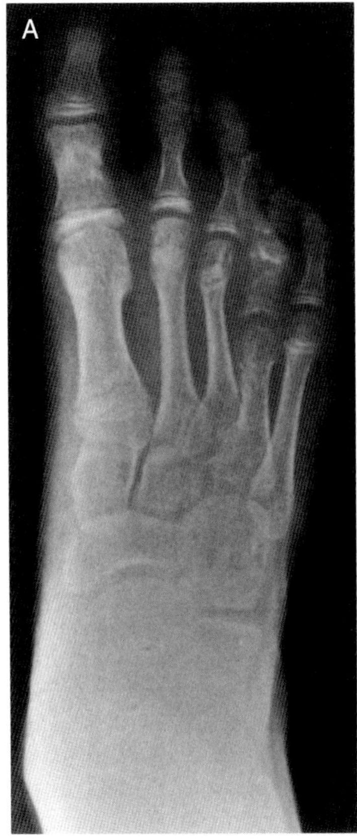

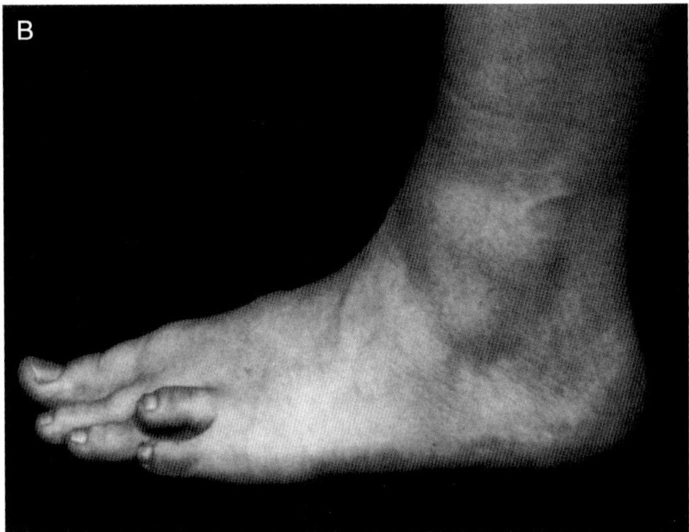

FIGURE 31-7 **A,B.** AP radiograph and lateral photograph of the right foot of a 15-year-old young lady with multiple enchondromatosis. The multiple cartilaginous lesions are visible clinically as "lumps" on the bones. The toe deformity has resulted from enchondromata producing a growth disturbance of the fourth ray. Her other foot was amputated at another institution 3 years previously due to a severe recurrent deformity.

radiolucencies, often causing expansion and cortical thinning, and are usually asymmetric. They are usually seen in the region of the physis, and most likely represent a cellular defect within the growth plate. The enchondromata arise and enlarge in a sporadic manner until puberty. Growth of the lesions after skeletal maturity is evidence of malignant degeneration until proven otherwise (71), although patients with enchondromatosis associated with soft-tissue hemangiomas (Maffucci syndrome) are at higher risk of developing chondrosarcoma from these lesions than are patients with Ollier disease (77). The cartilaginous lesions often appear to remodel as they are replaced by mature bone at maturity (17,49). Involvement may be unilateral or bilateral, but is more commonly bilateral (49).

Patients usually present with the growth of palpable masses from the skeleton (Figure 31-7). Limb length discrepancy and angular deformity may develop from the influence of these cartilaginous lesions on the affected growth plate. The tubular bones of the hands and feet are most commonly involved, but the long bones of the upper and lower extremities are at risk. Significant alteration in the normal contours of the individual bones may develop which may lead to clinical deformity and loss of joint function. Varus and valgus deformities are common in the lower extremity. We have treated one patient who developed progressive scoliosis and required posterior fusion and instrumentation, and another patient who underwent a below knee amputation at another institution for significant and recurrent deformity of the tibia and ankle.

The treatment principles are similar to those of multiple hereditary osteochondromatosis. The lesions are curetted and grafted when their size produces symptoms or dysfunction, particularly in the hands or feet. Angular deformities and limb length discrepancies are treated as in other conditions. Our experience as well as that of others is that the healing of osteotomies, pathological fractures, and spinal fusions is complete (77). The recent study by Loder et al. (47) documented a 0.6-year delay in the bone age compared to chronologic age in children with chondrodysplasias, including children with MHO and Ollier's enchondromatosis.

METACHONDROMATOSIS

Metachondromatosis was first described in 1971 by Maroteaux as a skeletal dysplasia with features of both multiple hereditary osteochondromatosis and multiple enchondromatosis (52). It is transmitted as an autosomal dominant trait, and has been reported in only a small number of patients.

Despite the presence of both osteochondromata and enchondromata, this disorder represents a variant with significant differences from either of the other two conditions. The multiple exostoses characteristically occur in the digits of the hands and feet and in the long bones. They are pedunculated and point toward the adjacent joint, compared to the growth away from the joint characteristic of the solitary or multiple hereditary osteochondromatoses. The histology of the exostoses from both conditions is indistinguishable, however. The biochemical function of the involved chondrocytes does differ from those in MHO, however. The EXT gene mutations involved in MHO are not seen in patients with metachondromatosis (14). Another way in which these dysplasias differ is that spontaneous regression of the exostoses is frequently seen in metachondromatosis. A range of four to ten years has been documented between initial enlargement and regression in these lesions, but during that same time period, new lesions had developed and others had increased in size. Predicting the fate of any individual exostosis in this condition is, therefore, not possible. Periarticular calcifications and ossifications have also been reported in these patients (7,10).

The enchondromata seen in metachondromatosis are found in the iliac crests and in the metaphyseal regions of the long bones of the lower extremities, the proximal humerus, and the distal radius. The absence of enchondromata from the hands or feet differentiates this condition from multiple enchondromatosis, or Ollier disease.

Patients usually present with complaints referable to the enlarging masses. Just as with multiple hereditary osteochondromatosis, treatment is indicated only for those lesions that are causing symptoms (i.e., pain, joint limitation, compression of adjacent structures), especially given the chance for regression of the exostoses in this condition. Necrosis of the skin has been documented in some of these patients with rapidly growing lesions (7). These exostoses do not appear to have the same effect on the growth of the long bones as do the multiple cartilaginous exostoses. Short stature is not a reported feature of metachondromatosis. Mild angular deformities have been noted in the digits of the hands and feet, but not in the long bones. No significant bowing, shortening, joint deformity, or subluxation have been seen. Peroneal nerve palsies have resolved completely after excision of the exostosis from the proximal fibula. No instances of malignant degeneration have been observed (7,10).

DYSPLASIA EPIPHYSEALIS HEMIMELICA

Dysplasia epiphysealis hemimelica (DEH) or Trevor's disease is an uncommon skeletal dysplasia with isolated, rather than systemic findings in involved patients. It is characterized by an osteocartilaginous mass arising from an epiphysis. Trevor (84) originally named this disorder tarso-epiphyseal aclasis, to differentiate it from diaphyseal aclasis (or multiple hereditary osteochondromatosis, MHO), which it resembled except for the site of origin of the osteochondromatous overgrowths. Fairbank (24) formulated the current terminology, accurately describing the process as a true dysplasia rather than a failure of remodeling, or aclasis.

DEH effects the growth of either the medial or lateral half of the epiphysis of a long bone, or a carpal or tarsal bone. The distal femur, distal tibia, and the talus are the most commonly involved bones, with a predilection for medial involvement. It is considered a sporadic occurrence, with more males than females reported (up to 3 males: 1 female), and no evidence for a genetic mode of transmission exists.

Patients are usually seen within the first years of life, with an asymmetric enlargement of a joint (typically the knee or ankle), limitation of motion, or pain. The ossification centers of affected bones will usually appear prematurely and remain larger than those of the opposite bone for several years. Radiographs show an irregular enlargement or protrusion from the epiphysis (Figure 31-8). Multiple ossification centers with areas of radiodensity are usually apparent, which will eventually coalesce. In young children these secondary centers often appear widely separated from their parent epiphysis, but with time and growth will fuse with each other and then with the main body of the epiphysis (24). This radiographic appearance is the result of variable enchondral ossification within the lesion. The histology of these areas demonstrates normal appearing bone covered with normal hyaline cartilage, indistinguishable from that of an osteochondroma. The biochemical function of the involved chondrocytes, however, does differ from those in MHO. The EXT gene mutations involved in MHO are not seen in patients with DEH (14). There is minimal metaphyseal abnormality. Angular deformity or limb length discrepancy may develop because of the effect of this bony overgrowth on the adjacent physis, with either growth stimulation or retardation. One or more bones may be involved in one extremity, but involvement of more than one extremity is rarely seen (24,38). Merzoug (60) recently reported two cases of bilateral DEH and added that only two other cases had ever been reported in the literature. Very few cases of DEH of the upper extremity have been documented.

Treatment is dependent on symptoms related to the bony mass, taking the natural history of these lesions into consideration. If the dysplasia interferes with function, produces significant deformity, or causes pain, then treatment may be indicated. At skeletal maturity, the area of overgrowth will become incorporated into the normal bone, with enlargement of the area of previous involvement, but with an otherwise normal bony appearance. Attempted excision of the entire mass would often be difficult and carries with it a chance of regrowth of the

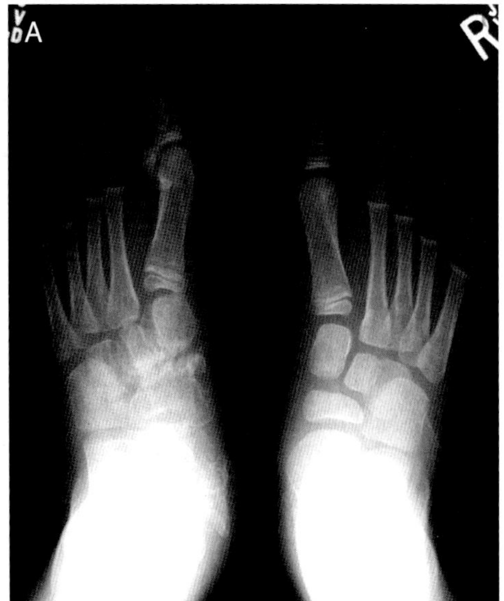

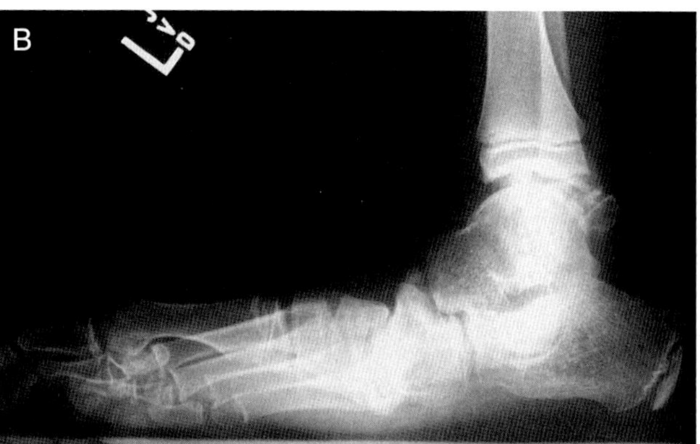

FIGURE 31-8 **A,B.** AP and lateral radiographs of an eight-year-old young man with dysplasia epiphysealis hemimelica. Note the exostoses and deformities involving the ankle, subtalar, and midfoot joints.

lesion. A significant portion of normal articular surface may also have to be removed to excise the abnormal area, and is obviously not indicated to deal with this benign lesion. For these reasons, excision should be limited to the prominent portion of overgrowth that may be causing pain or other symptoms due to its mass effect or from pressure on adjacent structures (44). The parents should be counseled regarding the natural history of this process, so that they too will understand the treatment goals. Treatment of any limb length discrepancy or angular deformity can be handled in a standard fashion, with epiphysiodesis or osteotomy, respectively. Although skeletal maturity has signaled the end of growth of the lesion in most cases, Kettelcamp et al. (38) reported several cases of cartilage proliferation into adult life, and recommended continued observation.

Involvement of the ankle usually consists of changes within the talus and/or the distal tibia, most frequently on the medial aspect. The head of the talus is involved less often than the body. The other medial bones of the midfoot, the navicular, and the medial cuneiform, are commonly included in the dysplastic process, but only rarely are other bones in the foot involved. Treatment of this condition about the foot and ankle should follow the guidelines above. Those masses that are causing significant pain, deformity, or limitation of joint function should be considered for excision. If partial or complete removal can be carried out without damage to the normal architecture of the foot, it should be performed and satisfactory relief of symptoms can be anticipated. There is a chance that further reconstructive surgery (i.e., arthrodesis of the ankle or subtalar joints) may be required in the future if there is severe enlargement or deformity of the talus.

DIASTROPHIC DYSPLASIA

Diastrophic dysplasia, previously referred to as diastrophic dwarfism, is a rare form of skeletal dysplasia characterized by extreme short-limb disproportionate dwarfism. It is transmitted as an autosomal recessive condition, and the sexes are thus affected equally. The incidence is not known, but the disorder is less common than classical achondroplasia (31,89). The clinical presentation is rather unique, with specific hand, ear, and foot abnormalities, a high incidence of severe and progressive kyphoscoliosis, and significant multiple joint flexion contractures. Diastrophic dysplasia has been shown to be caused by mutations in the solute carrier family 26 (sulfate transporter), member 2 gene (SLC26A2) and is thereby related to several other osteochondrodysplasias (achondrogenesis 1B, atelosteogenesis type II and autosomal recessive multiple epiphyseal dysplasia). A genotype-phenotype correlation has been postulated between the exact genetic mutation and the clinical presentation (48).

The hand is characterized by the "hitchhiker thumb," which is proximally set, abducted, and hypermobile, with a disproportionately shortened first metacarpal. Symphalangism of the proximal interphalangeal joint is common. Cystic masses develop in the external ear early in life (during the first three months) in over three-fourths of these patients. The swelling then becomes hard and thickened, deforming the cartilage, and eventually calcifying and ossifying, thus giving rise to the "cauliflower ear." There is considerable infant mortality secondary to respiratory problems, but if patients survive this period, life expectancy appears to be normal (89).

The rhizomelic shortening of the extremities is characterized by moderate to severe flexion contractures, most

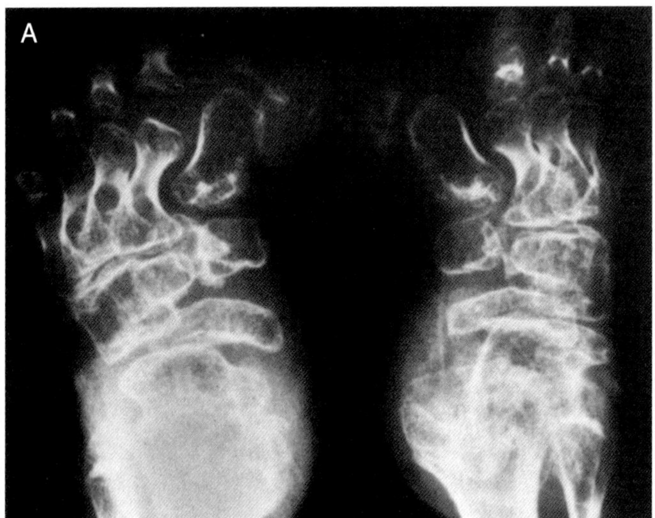

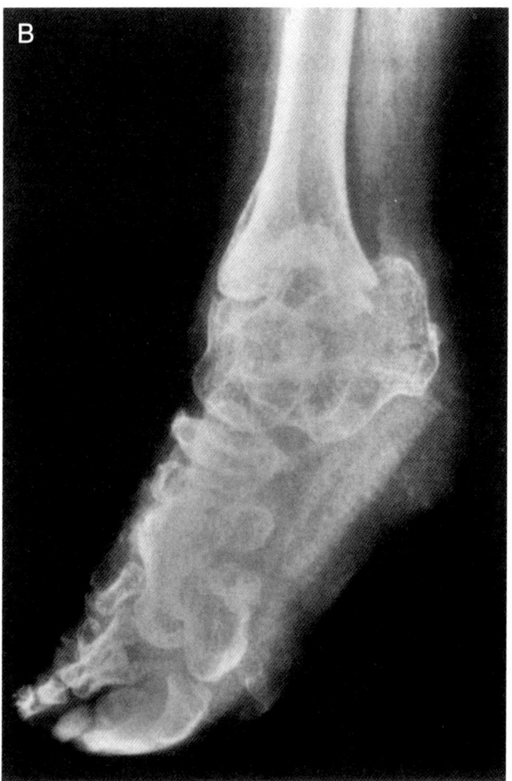

FIGURE 31-9 **A,B.** AP and lateral radiographs of bilateral rigid equinovarus deformities in a child with diastrophic dysplasia. The bones are short and broad. The first metatarsal is particularly affected with medial deviation of the first ray and a large space between the first and second toes.

commonly involving the elbows, hips, and knees. Cervical kyphosis and thoracolumbar kyphoscoliosis are frequently encountered problems.

The feet are classically short and broad with severe equinovarus deformities (Figure 31-9). Each of the components of the clubfoot deformity is extremely rigid. Metatarsus varus with medial twisting of the metatarsals, and particular shortening of the first metatarsal is typical. There is often an increased space between the first and second toes. The tarsal centers of ossification appear early but are irregular in appearance, with dense borders and osteopenic centers. The tubular bones of the feet may have irregular deformities with shortening and metaphyseal flaring, and flattening of the epiphyses. Both metaphyses and epiphyses are affected and premature development of osteoarthritis is a feature (89). Many patients with diastrophic dysplasia have walking difficulties that are often of a multifactorial nature including flexion contractures of the knees, early and rapid osteoarthrosis, equinus or equinovarus foot deformities and obesity, but only rarely spinal stenosis (64).

Treatment for the clubfoot deformities should begin with early serial manipulation and casting. Walker et al. (85) reported that 26 of 51 patients did not adequately correct with casting alone and required surgical correction. The percentages of successful non-operative treatment may increase now that most pediatric orthopaedic surgeons are using the Ponseti technique for treating clubfeet but more experience will be necessary before its effectiveness in these rigid clubfeet will be known. Our experience would indicate that a high percentage of these patients will still require surgical intervention. Posteromedial release is often the primary surgical procedure but treatment should be tailored to the remaining deformities in each individual foot. Because of the size, shape, and rigidity of these feet, attempts at surgical correction are often difficult. Further reconstructive procedures may be indicated for incomplete or persistent deformity at a later age. Talectomy may prove helpful as a secondary procedure for a persistently deformed and rigid foot, as it has for the foot deformity associated with amyoplasia congenita (arthrogryposis).

ACHONDROPLASIA

Achondroplasia is the most common form of dwarfism and is considered the prototype for short trunk dwarfism. It is inherited as an autosomal dominant condition, yet nearly 80% of new cases are the result of spontaneous genetic mutation. In the past, many of the other, rarer forms of dwarfism were inaccurately diagnosed as achondroplasia. A single gene mutation mapped to the short arm of the fourth chromosome is responsible for achondroplasia (band 4p16.3). This has been shown to cause a mutation in fibroblast growth factor receptor 3 (*FGFR3)* and is responsible for achondroplasia, hypochondroplasia,

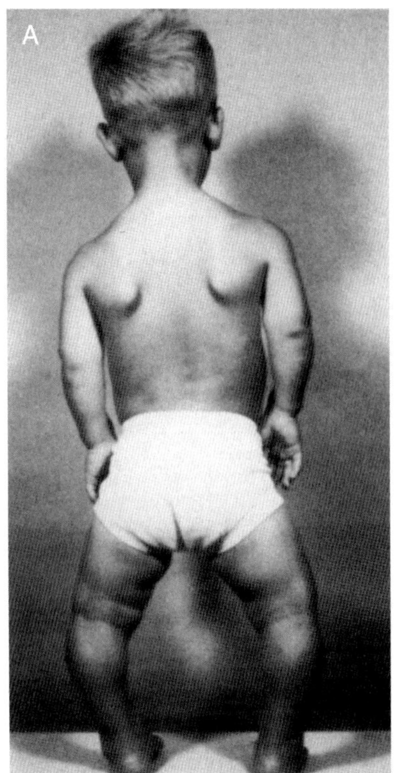

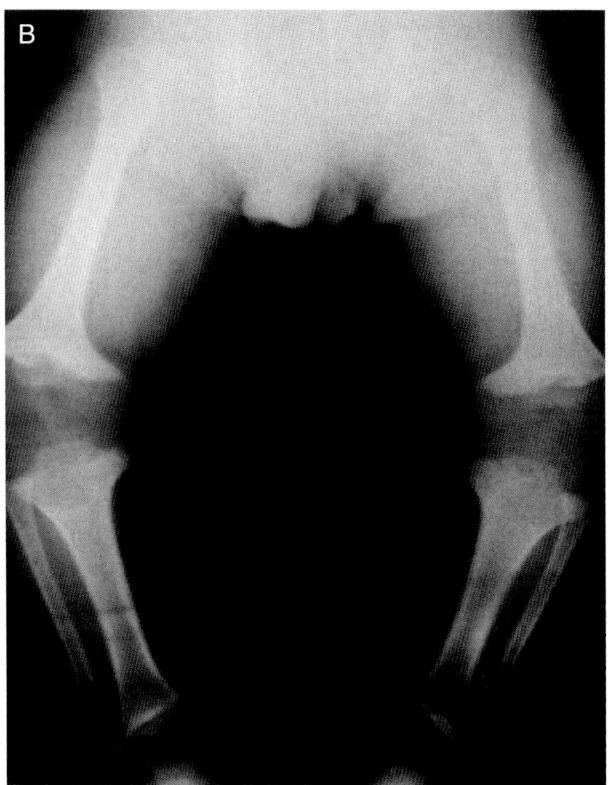

FIGURE 31-10 **A,B.** Standing PA photograph and radiograph of the lower extremities of a six-year-old boy with achondroplasia. The knee and ankle varus with short, broad tubular bones, relative fibular lengthening, and metaphyseal flaring are evident.

and thanatophoric dysplasia. The primary function of *FGFR3* is to limit osteogenesis (87). Mutation in this receptor causes enhancement in its function of limiting endochondral ossification. In achondroplasia the mutation in *FGFR3* is due to transition of a guanine to adenine (G to A) at nucleotide 1138 of complimentary DNA.

Patients with achondroplasia have a disproportionate type of short-limb dwarfism with the proximal segments of the upper extremity relatively shorter than the middle or distal segments (rhizomelic micromelia) (Figure 31-10). The head is disproportionately large in relation to the height, and characteristic facies include a depressed nasal bridge, a prominent forehead, midface hypoplasia, and a prominent mandible. Developmental milestones are typically delayed, in part due to the generalized ligamentous laxity and the muscular hypotonia. Increased lumbar lordosis and narrowing of the lumbar interpedicular distance may cause problems with spinal stenosis. Thoracolumbar kyphosis is common in infancy, most often regressing after the patient begins independent ambulation. Congenital abnormalities at the cranial or cervical level may have serious neurological implications, including hydrocephalus and spinal cord compression. In the absence of these complications, the prognosis for life span and function is good.

The pelvis is short and broad with a horizontal acetabulum. The tubular bones are short and broad due to the disproportion between normal periosteal latitudinal growth and decreased longitudinal growth from the physis. The femoral neck is short and bony muscular attachments are prominent. The metaphyses are broad and may be irregular. Epiphyseal ossification is typically normal except in the distal femur where it may be quite irregular and delayed, with an inverted V-shaped physis in childhood (45,55).

The most frequent finding in the lower extremities is genu varum, possibly related to the disproportionate growth between the tibia and the fibula (63). The fibula is relatively longer and appears to tether the growing leg into progressive varus. A resultant varus deformity at the ankle often accompanies the genu varum (Figure 31-11). One recent study concluded that the fibular overgrowth did not correlate with the severity of genu varum (1). The long-term prognosis of these radiographic abnormalities is not well delineated, but no increased incidence of osteoarthritis has been documented, making the need for treatment unclear (5,41,45). Realignment osteotomy of the proximal tibia and fibula has been the standard of treatment for those children with significant genu varum deformity (greater than 15 degrees of varus), usually for cosmetic and biomechanical alignment reasons. Some authors recommend waiting until skeletal maturity, while others feel it should be done when it is clinically indicated. There is general agreement that bracing for varus deformity in achondroplasia is not indicated because of the inability of braces to effect correction, mainly due to the significant associated ligamentous laxity (5). Supramalleolar osteotomy is rarely indicated, but is effective in

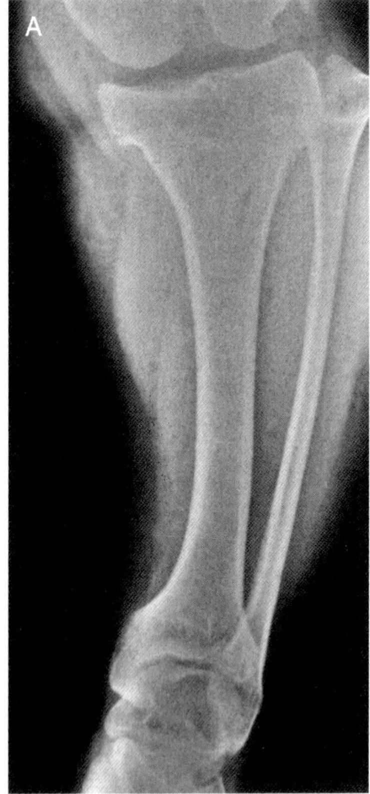

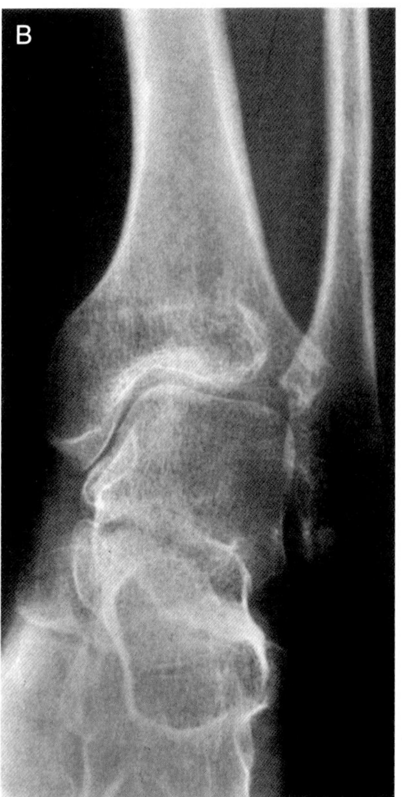

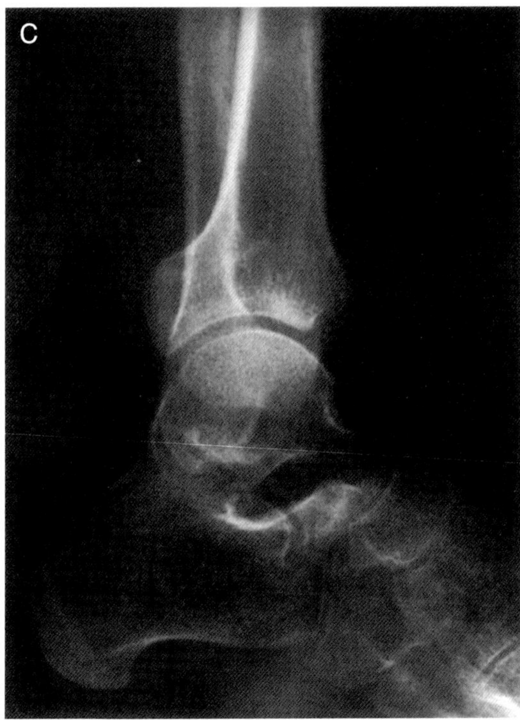

FIGURE 31-11 **A-C.** Thirteen-year-old female with achondroplasia. AP radiograph of the lower leg demonstrates the fibular lengthening relative to the tibia with prominence of both the proximal and distal ends. AP and lateral views of the ankle illustrate the varus deformity at the ankle (related to the length of the fibula), the position of the distal fibula relative to the lateral talus, and the flaring of the distal tibia.

those children with clinically significant varus deformity of the distal tibia and ankle (41). A more physiologic approach to the genu varus deformity is an epiphysiodesis of the proximal and distal fibula done at ages eight to ten (63). This allows a gradual correction of the deformity with further growth. Those older patients with prominence of the fibular head and knee pain at this site may require resection of the fibular head with or without proximal tibial osteotomy.

Specific deformities of the foot are not typical of achondroplasia (Figure 31-12). Mild pes planus may be present related to the ligamentous laxity. The increased length of the fibula may produce a varus position of the heel and hindfoot. Although the varus ankle can be

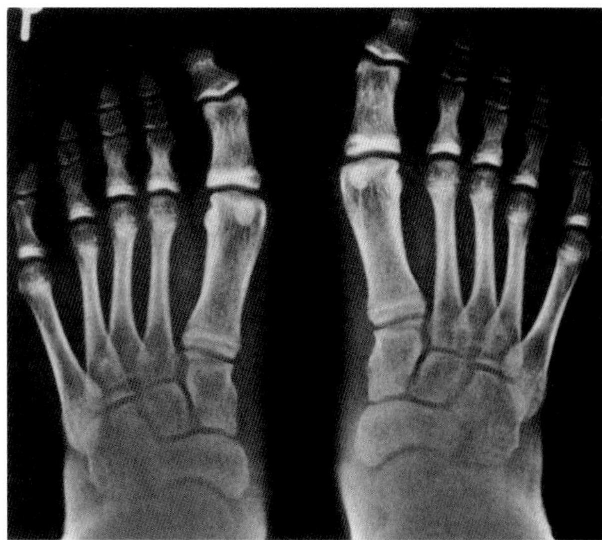

FIGURE 31-12 AP radiograph of the foot of a 15-year-old boy with achondroplasia. The first MTP joints are relatively squared off, as are the cuneiform-metatarsal joints. The middle and distal phalanges of the fifth toes are fused.

radiographically significant, it is most commonly asymptomatic. Complaints referable to lateral weight bearing on the heel, excessive lateral shoe wear and pain from impingement of the lateral malleolus on the calcaneus have been reported, however (5). Leg or foot pain, dysesthesias, paresthesias, or diminished walking tolerance should be seen as signs of spinal rather than foot pathology. Radiculopathy from nerve root compression or cauda equina syndrome occurs in up to 50% of achondroplastic patients (36). Limb lengthening for short stature continues to be controversial but practiced in a number of centers (2).

SPONDYLOEPIPHYSEAL DYSPLASIA CONGENITA

Spondyloepiphyseal dysplasia (SED) congenita is a short-trunk, disproportionate type of dwarfism transmitted as an autosomal dominant trait, although most cases arise from a new mutation. There are two subtypes identified, based on the degree of involvement (78). The more involved subtype is recognizable at birth, with severe spine changes and coxa vara. The milder form has less spine and hip deformity, will not be clinically apparent until three to four years of age, and will have a slightly taller adult height. Both subtypes have a flat face with wide-set eyes. Myopia and/or retinal detachment can be seen in 50% of these patients. Infants with SED congenita are hypotonic, with delayed motor development, and normal mental development. The ligamentous laxity and hypoplasia of the odontoid predispose these children to atlantoaxial instability, which must be considered and evaluated periodically and preoperatively. As with any child with cord compression due to C1-2 instability, the early signs can be as subtle as increased fatigability. Os odontoideum can also be seen associated with cervical instability (Figure 31-13).

A defect in type II collagen with the gene located on chromosome 1293 has been observed to cause an alteration in the length of the alpha 1 chain (30,61).

Radiographic findings include the delayed ossification of the secondary centers. In particular, the proximal femur, knee, talus, and calcaneus are not seen to be ossified at birth. The delay in ossification of the distal femur and proximal tibia leads to flattening and irregularity. The spine shows platyspondyly with flattening and dorsal wedging of the vertebral bodies. Anterior ossification defects of the vertebral bodies are characteristic. Varying degrees of epiphyseal and metaphyseal abnormalities of the long tubular bones are seen, with shortening consistent with the degree of epiphyseal involvement. The hips are usually severely involved with coxa vara and have the appearance of "bilateral Perthes disease" because of the changes and irregularities within the femoral ossification centers. The development of early osteoarthritis is typical, often leading to hip replacement as a young adult. Genu valgum is more common than genu varum. Realignment osteotomy (often of the distal femur) is appropriate for the severe deformity or to relieve symptoms (Figure 31-14).

The hands and feet are typically minimally involved (Figure 31-15). The tubular bones are not shortened or broadened to the extent seen in other dysplasias. The ossification of the carpal and tarsal centers are delayed, however. The most common significant deformity of the foot is a clubfoot deformity. This should be treated with early serial manipulation and casting, and may require surgical soft tissue release. As with clubfeet associated with other conditions, as our experience grows in the use of the Ponseti technique of treatment, we may increase our ability to treat these feet with this minimally invasive technique. These feet are not like the rigid clubfeet seen in diastrophic dysplasia, and usually respond well to appropriate treatment (Figure 31-16).

PSEUDOACHONDROPLASTIC DYSPLASIA

Pseudoachondroplasia is a type of rhizomelic short-limb dwarfism with a normal appearing head and face. It has been referred to as the pseudoachondroplastic type of spondyloepiphyseal dysplasia but is actually distinct both clinically and genetically (28). A mutation in the cartilage oligomeric matrix protein (COMP) has been observed, the same protein that shows abnormalities in multiple epiphyseal dysplasia (MED). COMP is a protein found in the extracellular matrix of cartilage, tendon, and ligament (21). Transmission is by both autosomal dominant and autosomal recessive inheritance, with considerable variability of expression.

Development usually appears normal during the first one to two years. Age at walking may be delayed, with a waddling gait developing. By two to three years of age the

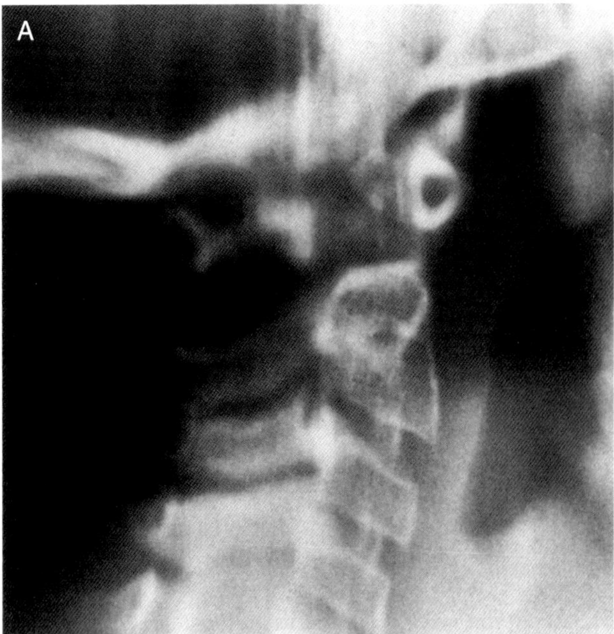

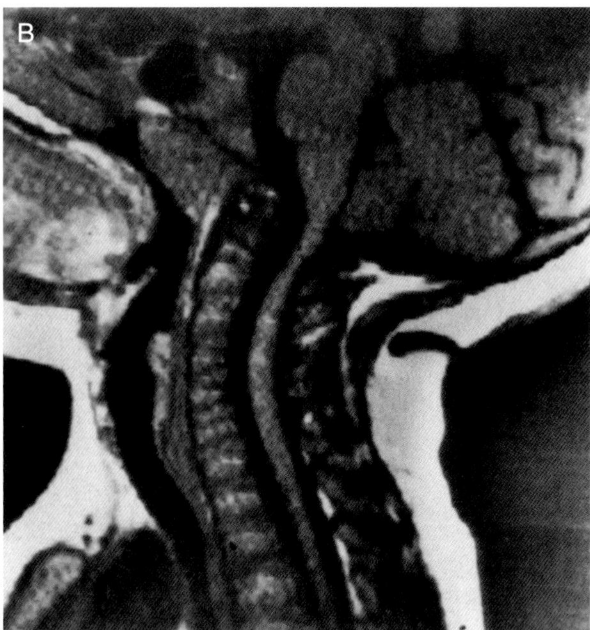

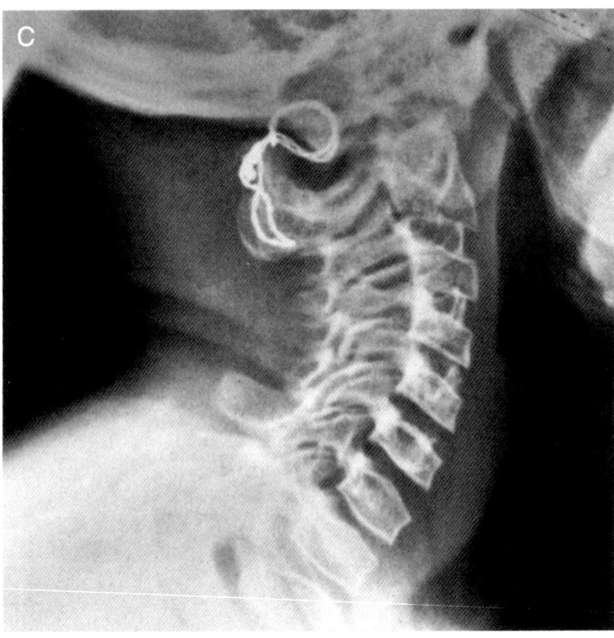

FIGURE 31-13 **A.** Lateral tomogram of the cervical spine demonstrating an os odontoideum in an asymptomatic 15-year-old girl with spondyloepiphyseal dysplasia. **B.** Lateral flexion-extension magnetic resonance images revealed canal compromise and cord narrowing, necessitating C1-2 fusion (**C**).

growth retardation and shortness of stature become apparent. The disproportionately long trunk, shortened extremities, and increased lumbar lordosis resemble those findings in achondroplasia, but these patients have a normal head and facial appearance. Lower limb deformities of progressive severity develop later. Marked ligamentous laxity contributes to the degree of deformity. Both genu varum and genu valgum are common, and asymmetric "windswept" deformities have been reported (40). Evaluation of the upper cervical spine is important in patients with pseudoachondroplasia because of the tendency for atlantoaxial instability and chronic compressive myelopathy to develop secondary to the ligamentous laxity and odontoid hypoplasia. Life expectancy and intellectual development are otherwise normal.

Radiographic findings include epiphyseal and metaphyseal changes (26). The epiphyses are small and deformed with expanded, irregular metaphyses. The long bones are short and thick. The platyspondyly is mild, with irregular flattening and anterior protrusion of the vertebral bodies. By adolescence the shape of the vertebrae tend to normalize. Scoliosis of a mild to moderate degree is seen in some patients. Premature osteoarthritis of the hips and knees often results in disability. The dysplastic

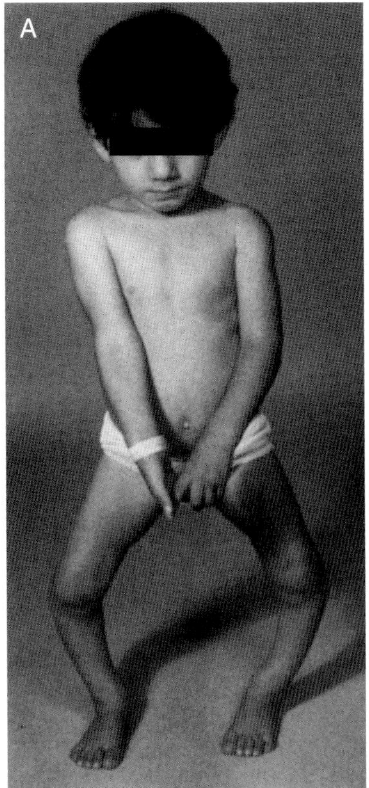

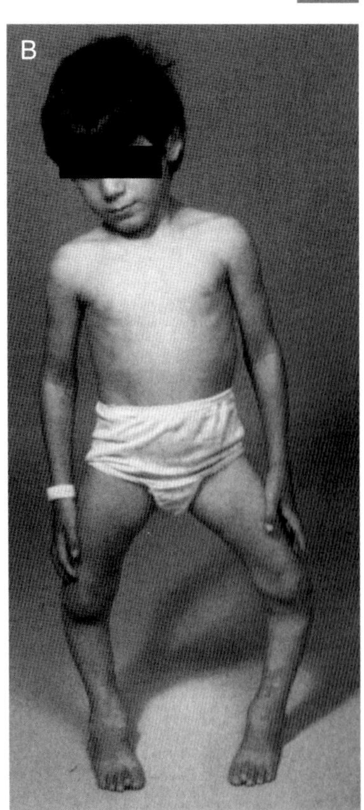

FIGURE 31-14 **A,B.** Photographs of sisters with spondyloepiphyseal dysplasia congenita with marked genu varum bilaterally requiring distal femoral and proximal tibial osteotomies.

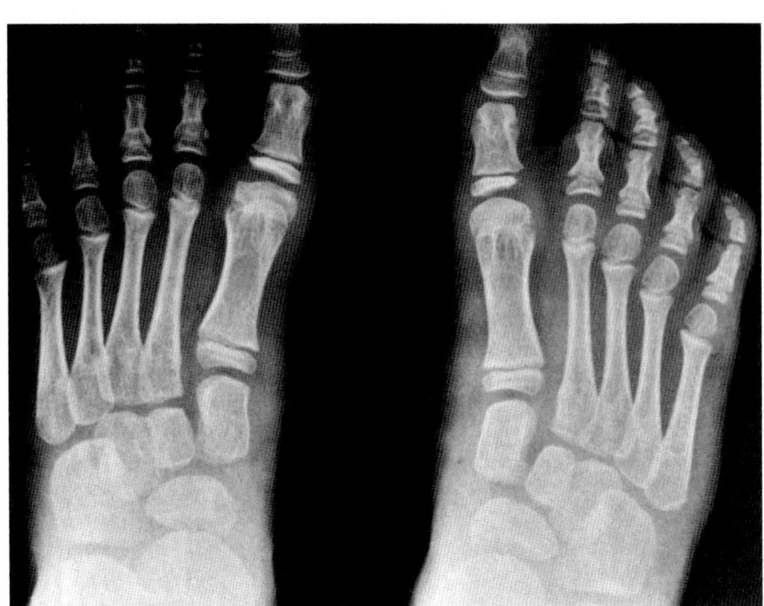

FIGURE 31-15 AP radiograph of the foot of a girl with spondyloepiphyseal dysplasia. The phalangeal epiphyses are cone-shaped.

capital femoral epiphyses and the articular surfaces of the distal femurs become progressively deformed and incongruent, leading to the marked degenerative changes seen in the adult.

The hands and feet are involved to a greater extent than seen in either achondroplasia or spondyloepiphyseal dysplasia. The carpal and tarsal bones have delayed maturation. The metacarpals, metatarsals, and phalanges are short and broad with irregular epiphyses and broadened metaphyses. The fingers and toes have a resulting loss of the normal proximal to distal tapering and a short, stubby appearance (77). Pes planus is common, related to the generalized ligamentous laxity.

In those patients with significant angular deformity, corrective osteotomy is indicated to realign the mechanical axis of the hip, knee, and ankle and, thus, to minimize the tendency for the development of arthrosis (40). This most commonly involves osteotomy of the proximal tibia and fibula, preferably at or toward the end of growth so that the chance of recurrence is lessened. Arthroplasty of the hip and knee may be necessary in adulthood when symptomatic degenerative changes present.

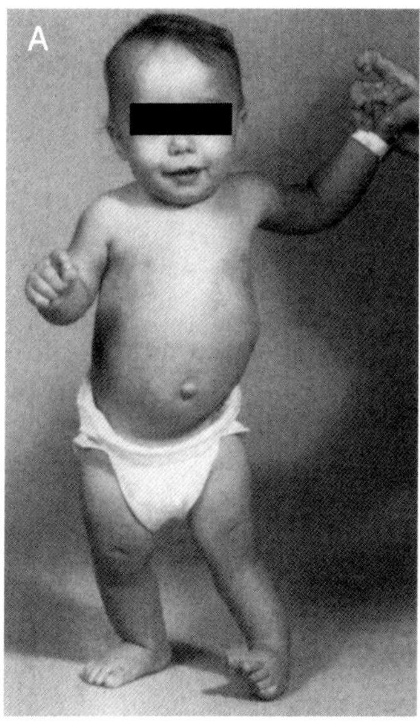

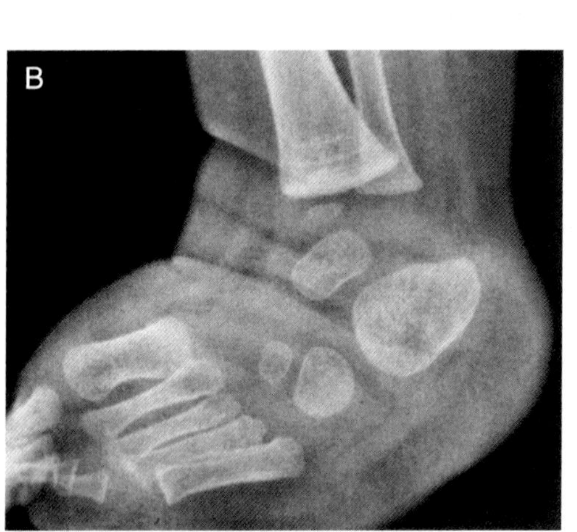

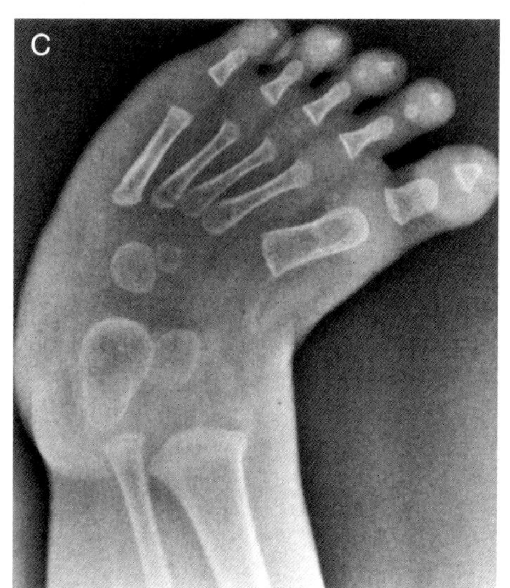

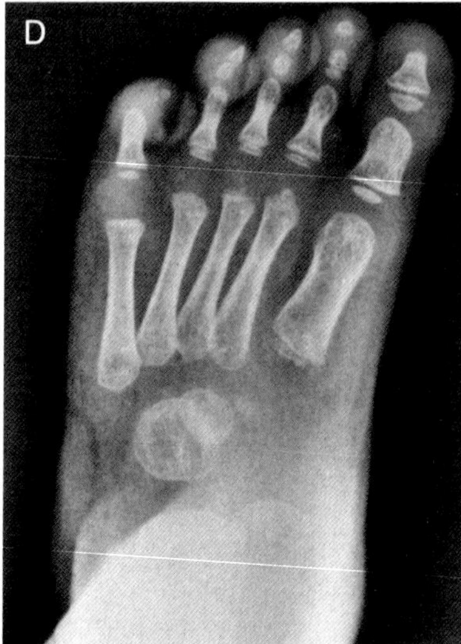

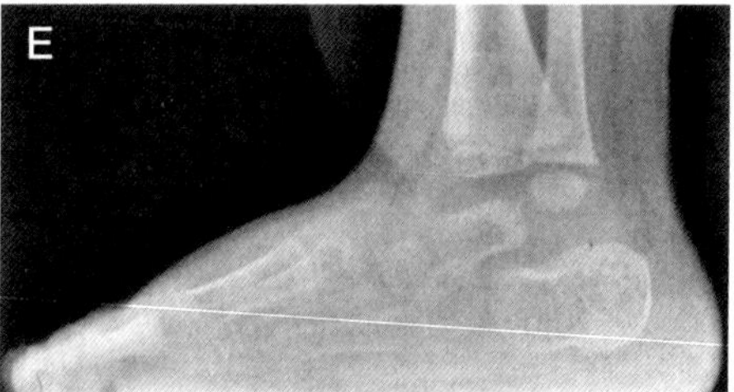

FIGURE 31-16 **A-C.** Photograph and, unilateral clubfoot deformity in a one-year-old child with spondyloepiphyseal dysplasia congenita. His mother also has SED but did not have a clubfoot. She has recently required bilateral total hip arthroplasties for degenerative hip disease at age 28. **D,E.** At age two years and nine months, two years following posteromedial release. The foot is well corrected. Delayed ossification is seen.

HYPOCHONDROPLASIA

Hypochondroplasia is one of the many conditions that in the not too distant past was included within those diagnoses lumped together as "achondroplasia." It is now well recognized as having a consistent presentation that resembles, but is clinically, radiographically, and genetically distinct from achondroplasia. Hypochondroplasia is suitably named because it does appear to be "mild" achondroplasia, but it has been demonstrated that matings between achondroplastic and normal individuals do not result in offspring with the findings of hypochondroplasia (59). It is transmitted by an autosomal dominant gene, but with a high rate of spontaneous mutation. Its incidence has been estimated to be one twelfth that of achondroplasia (35). The mutation is not as specific as that in achondroplasia, but most often occurs in the gene for FGFR-3 on the short arm of the fourth chromosome and appears to result in an increase in the activation of factors that slow cell growth (18).

The most important features of hypochondroplasia that distinguish it from achondroplasia include a later age of diagnosis (due to milder clinical findings), taller stature, near normal appearance of the craniofacies and of the hands, lack of neurological problems (i.e., hydrocephalus or cauda equina compression), and less lumbar lordosis with less narrowing of the interpedicular distances. The tubular bones are short with a metaphyseal flare, but the extremities are not predominantly rhizomelic, mesomelic, or acromelic in appearance (35). There are more affected females reported and mental deficiencies are more common than in achondroplasia (9,35,76).

Genu varum is common but usually mild, and often corrects spontaneously with growth. The fibula is often relatively longer than the tibia and is one of the earliest radiographic signs of hypochondroplasia. A varus tilt to the ankle results, but not usually to a degree requiring treatment. The body of the talus appears flattened and the talar neck slightly foreshortened (9), possibly secondary to the ankle deformity (Figure 31-17). The proximal medial epiphysis of the tibia is squared off. Postaxial polydactyly of the foot can be seen.

MULTIPLE EPIPHYSEAL DYSPLASIA

Multiple epiphyseal dysplasia (MED) is characterized by a primary disturbance of the normal ossification process of many epiphyses. Its genetic transmission is considered autosomal dominant in the majority of cases, but with variable expressivity. Findings similar to but milder than those in pseudoachondroplasia are seen. It is felt to be a heterogeneous disorder with several different mutations (locus heterogeneity) having been reported in the gene encoding cartilage oligomeric matrix protein (COMP) as well as in COL9A2 (21).

The diagnosis is usually made during the first few years of life, but may not be recognized until adolescence or early adulthood in the milder cases. The child is typically of normal to moderately short stature, with normal body proportions. Most problems relate to the lower extremities with prominent, frequently painful joints. Limited motion or gait disturbances are common. The hips, knees, and ankles are primarily involved. Delayed ossification of the secondary centers, with eventual irregularity and fragmentation of the epiphyses leads to flattening and deformation of the articular surfaces. The involvement of bilateral proximal femoral epiphyses may resemble bilateral Perthes disease, but is typically symmetric and synchronous with early acetabular involvement. Early and progressive degenerative arthritis with pain and limitation of motion results, often necessitating treatment. Total hip arthroplasty is frequently required for the patient with severe hip disease. Genu valgum, or less commonly genu varum, may follow the involvement and flattening of the distal femoral condyles. Corrective osteotomy is probably best deferred until skeletal maturity unless the deformity is severe or progressive and symptomatic before then. If the joint involvement in the lower extremities is severe and untreated, the patient may be so incapacitated as to become unable to stand and walk by the fifth to sixth decade (79). Life expectancy is normal.

Deformity at the ankle is typically into valgus. The articular surfaces of both the talus and the distal tibia are predictably irregular. Specific clinical problems with the foot are uncommon.

METAPHYSEAL CHONDRODYSPLASIA

Metaphyseal chondrodysplasia is a heterogeneous condition with rather distinct subtypes, each with its own clinical and genetic characteristics, but with similar skeletal radiographic findings. The dysplastic changes are localized to the metaphyses of the tubular bones, with normal epiphyses. The abnormal maturation of the cartilage cells within the growth plate appears to be the source of these radiographic changes (56).

The most frequent of the metaphyseal chondrodysplasias is the Schmid type (66,70). It is transmitted as an autosomal dominant trait. The genetic defect is in the alpha 1 chain of type X collagen (86). There is mild to moderate shortness of stature with bowed legs usually evident in the second year (Figure 31-18). Although uncommon in other dysplasias, leg pain is common during childhood, with gradual spontaneous improvement. A waddling gait may develop and varus deformities of both the knees and the ankles are often present. The metaphyseal changes are present in all of the short and long tubular bones, including those of the hands and feet. There is variable irregularity with widening and scalloping, and radiolucent metaphyseal cysts may be present (Figure 31-19). The metaphyses may demonstrate splaying and cupping reminiscent of the changes seen in vitamin D resistant (hypophosphatemic) rickets, and should be differentiated by the lack of biochemical abnormalities (3). The proximal

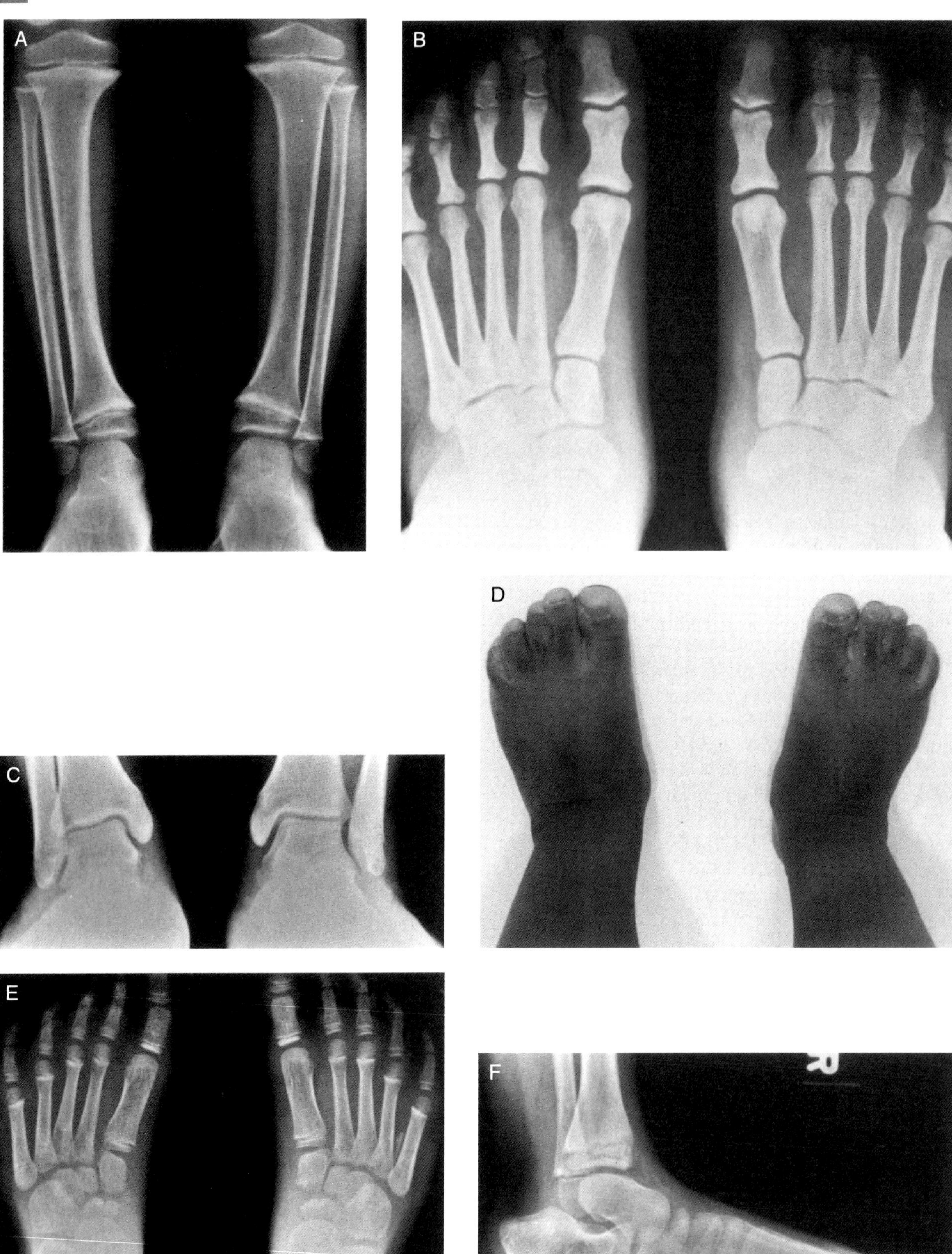

FIGURE 31-17 Three children with hypochondroplasia: **A.** AP of the legs and ankles of a seven-year-old girl. The distal fibulae are long and there is mild varus of the tibiae and ankles. **B-D.** AP radiographs of both feet and ankles and AP photograph of both feet of a 13-year-old girl. Varus tilt of the ankle and relatively longer fibulae are present. The feet are short and broad with mild planovalgus. **E,F.** AP and lateral radiographs of a seven-year-old boy. There is pes planovalgus, the tubular bones are short, and the feet are broad. Ossification irregularities of the navicular and the first cuneiform are present.

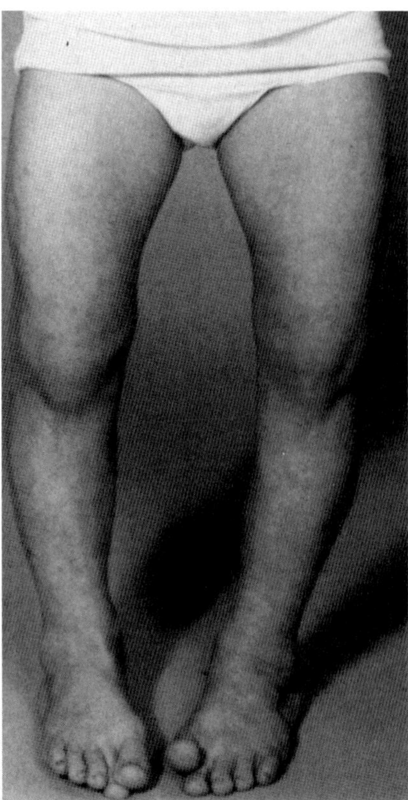

FIGURE 31-18 Genu varum in a girl with metaphyseal chondrodysplasia, Schmid type.

femoral metaphyses are more involved than the distal, and coxa vara is common. The varus deformity of the lower extremity is due to bowing of both the femur and tibia. Progressive improvement in the degree of deformity is not uncommon with growth. Osteotomy of the tibia and fibula is indicated if significant progression is documented, to realign the plane of the knee and ankle. Valgus osteotomy of the hip is often helpful to improve the coxa vara. Other than the varus deformity of the ankle, there are no specific deformities of the foot and ankle. The cervical spine should be evaluated for any evidence of atlantoaxial instability. The normal appearance and shape of the epiphyses and, thus, the articular surfaces, seem to protect these patients from degenerative arthroses later in life.

The McKusick type of metaphyseal chondrodysplasia, also referred to as cartilage-hair hypoplasia, is less common and is transmitted as an autosomal recessive condition (58). The metaphyseal changes are similar, but involvement of the distal femur is more severe than in the proximal femur, and coxa vara is less common and less severe when present. There is greater shortening of the long bones, and a disproportionate growth between the tibia and the fibula is common. This fibular overgrowth results in a significant varus deformity at the ankle that may require corrective osteotomy. Many of these individuals have associated immunological defects, and should have a thorough pediatric evaluation.

Other more rare types of metaphyseal chondrodysplasias include the Jansen type, with severe short stature, severe metaphyseal changes, and flexion deformities of the joints; metaphyseal chondrodysplasia associated with pancreatic insufficiency (malabsorption) and neutropenia; and metaphyseal chondrodysplasia associated with thymolymphopenia (agammaglobulinemia) (35,79).

SPONDYLOMETAPHYSEAL DYSPLASIA (KOZLOWSKI TYPE)

This disorder was established in 1967 by Kozlowski who described several children with dysplastic changes involving both the spine and the metaphyses. It must be differentiated from the metaphyseal chondrodysplasias (43) and metatropic dwarfism (79). The Kozlowski type is the best known and the most common. It is inherited as an autosomal dominant condition, with most cases representing new mutations (35).

The effected children have a moderate growth deficiency, especially of the trunk, with platyspondyly and odontoid hypoplasia. The most characteristic radiographic finding is the irregular metaphyseal ossification in the tubular bones, most marked in the proximal femur. A waddling gait with joint limitation and early degenerative changes and pain may result (Figures 31-20 and 31-21).

SPONDYLOEPIMETAPHYSEAL DYSPLASIA

This rare skeletal dysplasia was only recently appreciated as a unique type of dwarfism, and continues to be differentiated from others with similar characteristics (11,42,67,81). The abnormalities associated with spondyloepimetaphyseal dysplasia (SEMD) have been linked to the collagen type 2 or type 11 molecule or the COMP gene (29) without a definite proven relationship. At least two types have been described with variable clinical findings, the Strudwick and Hall types (4,67).

These children have dwarfism with severe kyphoscoliosis, joint laxity, and generalized epiphyseal and metaphyseal dysplasia, and typical facies. Multiple joint dislocations may be present. It may be inherited in an autosomal dominant or recessive pattern. The author's two patients have shortening of the fibulae with ankle valgus (Figure 31-22) and significant recurvatum deformity at the knee. Radiographs demonstrate the diffuse epiphyseal and metaphyseal changes with irregularities, sclerosis, and flaring, with multiple joint deformities. The feet have not been ascribed any particular problems in SEMD.

CHONDRODYSPLASIA PUNCTATA

As with many other skeletal dysplasias, chondrodysplasia punctata has become recognized as a group of similar disorders rather than as a single condition. This group of osteochondrodysplasias is characterized by small focal

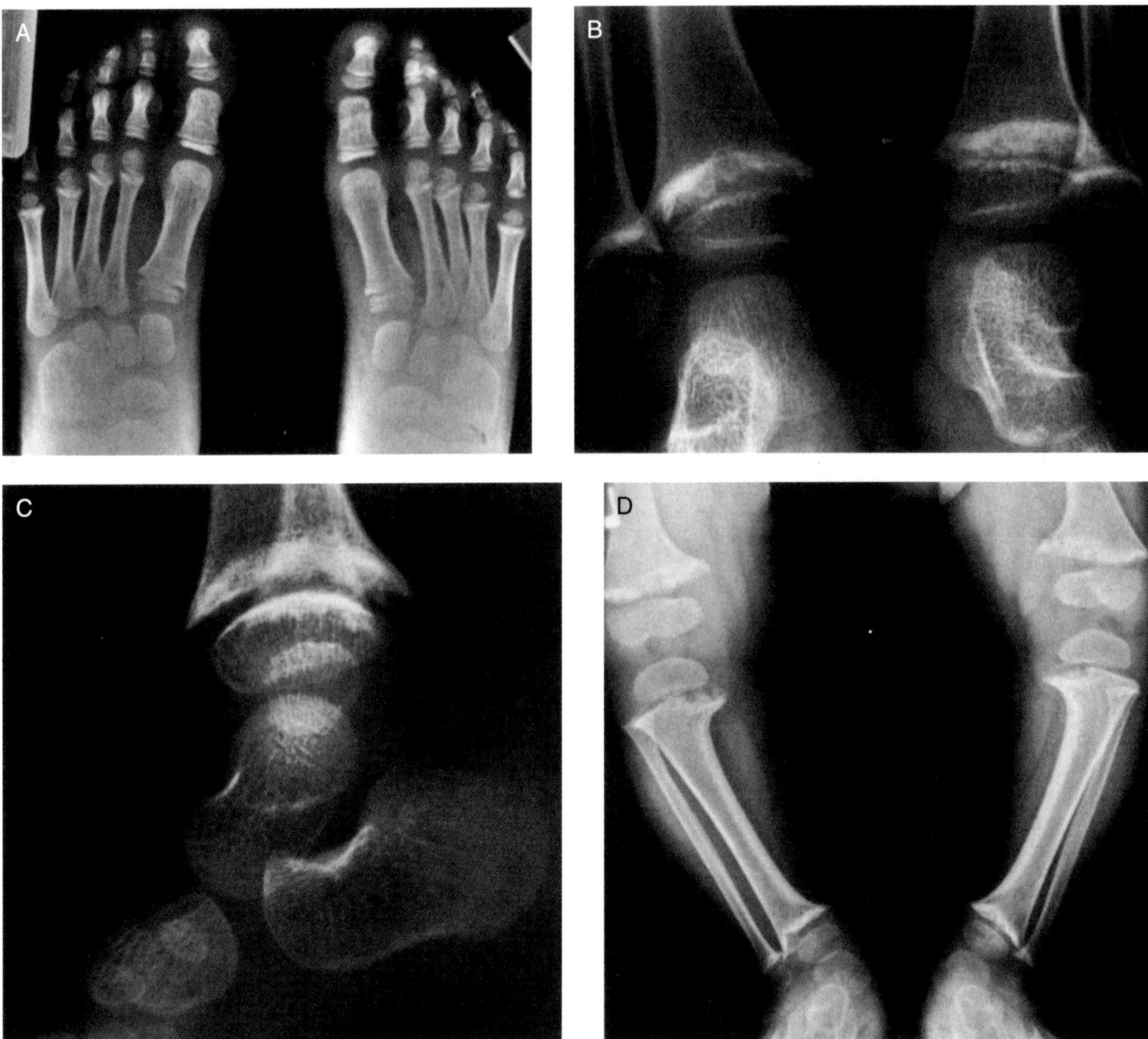

FIGURE 31-19 **A-D.** AP and lateral views of the feet and ankles and AP view of the lower extremities in a boy with metaphyseal chondrodysplasia, Schmid type. The metaphyseal changes include widening, irregularity, scalloping, sclerosis, and early cystic changes. Both the ankles and knees have a significant varus deformity that required a proximal tibial osteotomy for correction.

calcifications in articular, epiphyseal, and other types of cartilage in infancy, with the subsequent development of epiphyseal dysplasia and associated anomalies of the facies, eyes, and skin (80). The most frequent form, Conradi-Hünermann syndrome, is an autosomal dominant disorder with considerable variability in expression and a high incidence of spontaneous mutation (73). A more severe rhizomelic form exists that is transmitted as an autosomal recessive condition, in which death is the rule within the first two years of life, as well as a sex-linked dominant variety (51).

Patients with Conradi-Hünermann syndrome have a mild to moderate growth deficiency, flat facies with a low nasal bridge, and asymmetric shortening of the extremities with areas of punctate calcifications of the epiphyses in infancy. The presence of stippled or punctate calcifications on a radiograph of a newborn is characteristic, but not pathognomonic of this disorder. Similar changes can be seen in a variety of dysplastic conditions. The stippling is typically seen in the cartilaginous portions of the epiphyses of the long bones, the carpal and tarsal bones, and the pelvis, but may be present along the vertebral column or in extraskeletal locations. Congenital cataracts occur in nearly 20% of these patients (80). Scoliosis is the most frequent orthopaedic problem, often developing during the first year of life and related to congenital osseous malformation (i.e., hemivertebrae or unsegmented bars). Patients with progressive congenital scoliosis will require spinal fusion, often during the first two years of life. Bracing has usually not been effective. Cervical instability has

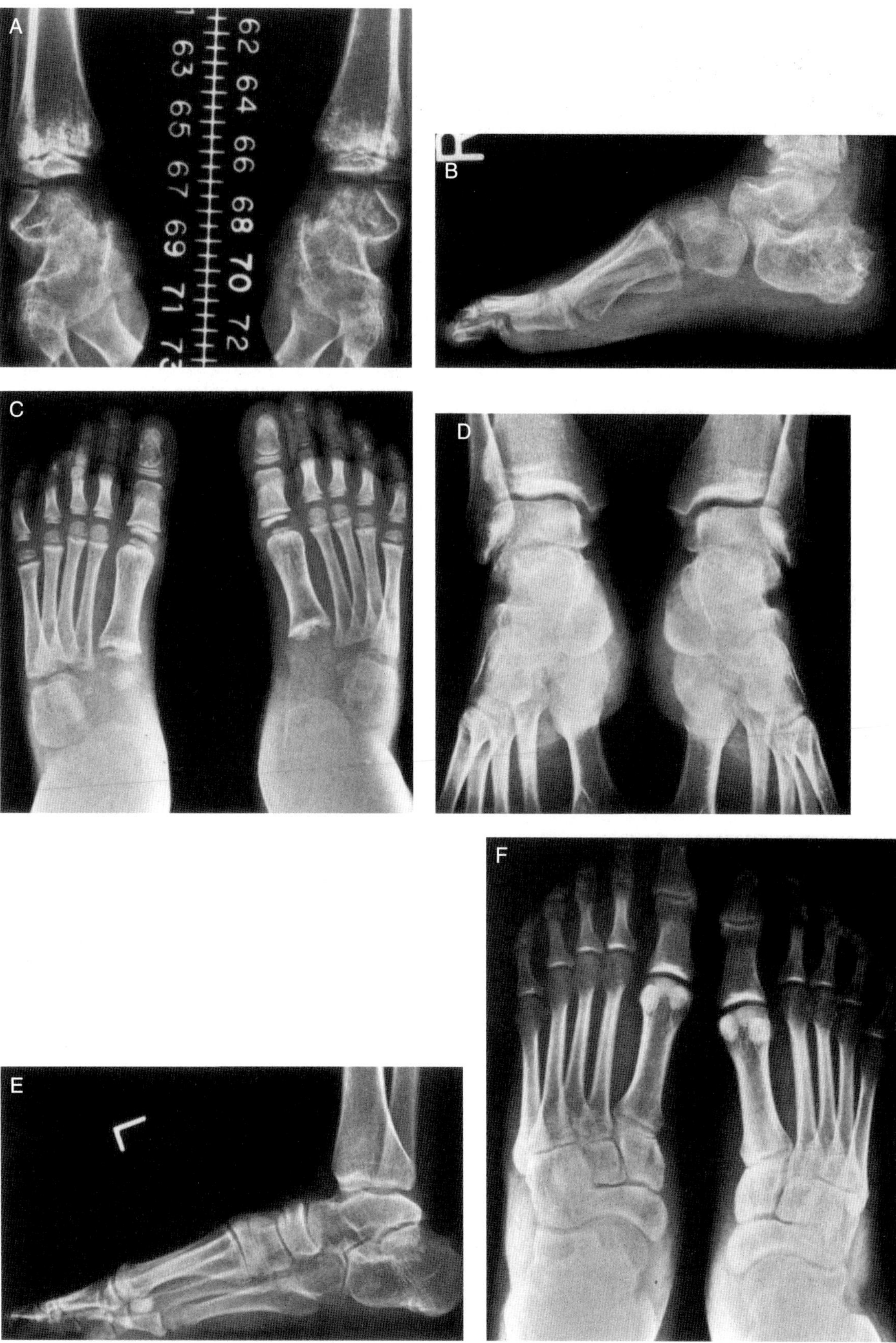

FIGURE 31-20 **A-C.** AP and lateral radiographs of the ankles and feet of a six-year-old boy with spondylometaphyseal dysplasia, Kozlowski type. The metaphyseal areas adjacent to the growth plates are irregular. There is an open growth plate at the distal end of the first metatarsal. **D-F.** AP and lateral views of the ankles and feet of this young man's mother who also has spondylometaphyseal dysplasia but is obviously skeletally mature. She has flattening and irregularity of the talus, with squaring-off of the distal metatarsals, and other areas of mild bony irregularity.

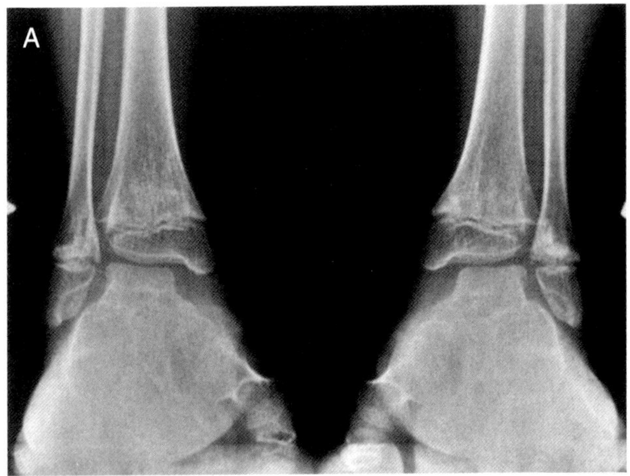

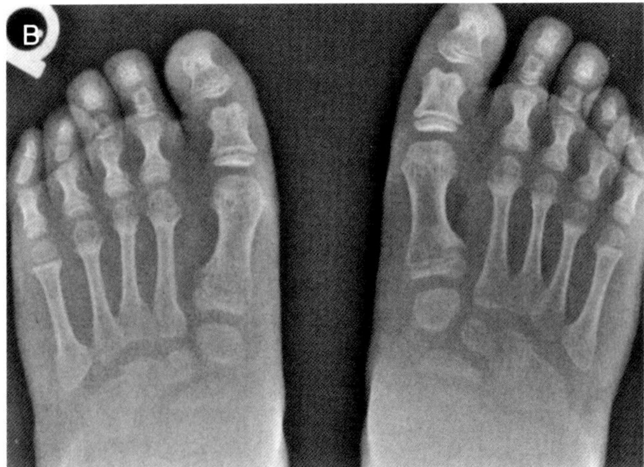

FIGURE 31-21 **A,B.** Standing AP of both ankles and feet of an 11-year-old boy with spondylometaphyseal dysplasia, Kozlowski type.

been reported and should be evaluated (as with most skeletal dysplasias).

Delay in appearance of the secondary centers of ossification is common, especially in the proximal femurs that may contribute to the flattening and subsequent dysplastic changes within the joint. Asymmetric shortening of the long bones related to the areas of punctate mineralization of the epiphyses is common. Limb-length discrepancy is managed by epiphysiodesis or lengthening. Polydactyly has been reported as an occasional finding, in both the Conradi-Hünermann and the sex-linked dominant types of chondrodysplasia punctata (35,51).

CHONDROECTODERMAL DYSPLASIA

Chondroectodermal dysplasia, or Ellis-van Creveld syndrome, represents a unique type of disproportionate short-limb dwarfism with progressive distalward shortening of the extremities. The major clinical findings in this condition include postaxial polydactyly, dysplasia of the fingernails and toenails, congenital heart disease, dental abnormalities, and sparse fine hair (Figure 31-23). It is transmitted as an autosomal recessive trait with a variability of expression, and is typically diagnosed at birth. The genetic defect is in a novel gene called EVC, on the short arm of the fourth chromosome (4p16), which leads to a generalized defect of maturation of endochondral ossification (62). Interestingly, this area on chromosome 4 is just proximal to the FGFR3 receptor, mutations of which result in achondroplasia.

Chondroectodermal dysplasia has an increased frequency in the Old Order Amish community in Lancaster, Pennsylvania, with an incidence of 5 per 1,000 births (57). One-third to one-half of infants with chondroectodermal dysplasia are stillborn or die within the first weeks of life. Death is most often due to congenital heart disease, most frequently associated with an atrial septal defect or a single atrium, or pulmonary insufficiency associated with pulmonary malformations including a small, deformed thoracic cage. Recurrent bronchopulmonary infections may be a problem throughout childhood. The majority of survivors are of normal intelligence.

These children exhibit acromesomelia, in which the distal segments demonstrate progressive shortening compared to the more proximal segments. This phenomenon is seen right out to the phalanges, with the distal and middle phalanges disproportionately shorter than the proximal ones. Postaxial polydactyly is constant in the hands and is commonly seen in the feet (23,57). The fingernails and toenails are typically hypoplastic and syndactyly is frequent. Genu valgum is characteristic, often of a progressive nature and leading to a severe deformity. Both femur and tibia may be externally rotated. Laxity of the medial collateral ligament and superolateral patellar dislocation are frequent (77).

Fusion of the capitate and hamate bones of the wrist, cone-shaped epiphyses of the middle and distal phalanges, and fusion of the metacarpals or phalanges characterize the radiograph of the hand. Pelvic configuration is characteristic, with small iliac crests and a hook-like downward spike of bone from the inner aspect of the acetabulum at the level of the triradiate cartilage. Premature ossification of the capital femoral epiphysis may occur. Hypoplasia of the lateral portion of the proximal tibial epiphysis, and a bony exostosis arising from the proximal medial metaphysis are typical, and relate to the progressive genu valgum that is seen in these patients. The fibulae are also disproportionately short compared to the tibiae, leading to a usually mild degree of ankle valgus.

Once the cardiac status is evaluated, treatment of the postaxial polydactyly of the hands and feet and the syndactyly of the hands is indicated. Excision of the toe that will result in the most normal contour of the foot is the best guideline for treatment. In the majority of cases of postaxial polydactyly, the most lateral toe should be excised, even if that toe has a more normal appearance than the remaining toe. The overall appearance and

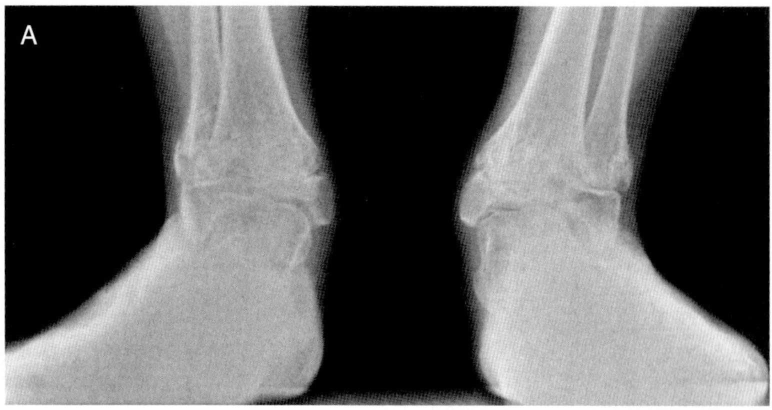

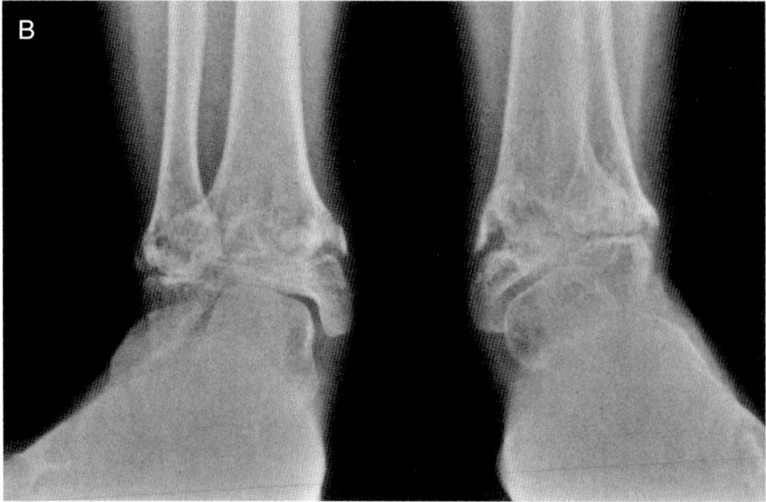

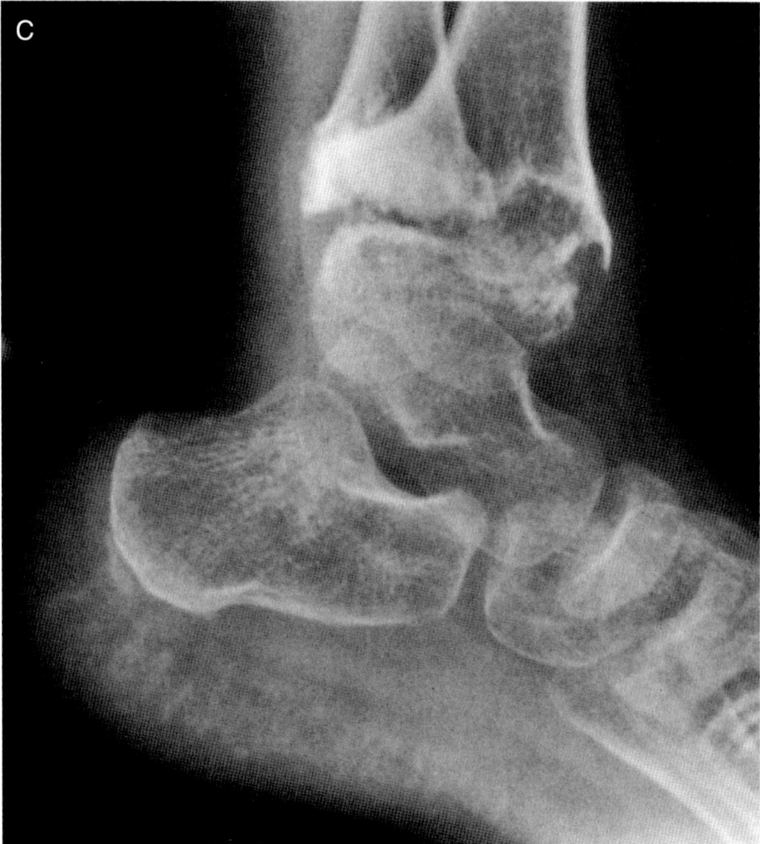

FIGURE 31-22 Spondyloepimetaphyseal dysplasia. **A.** AP radiograph of the ankles of a 12-year-old girl. **B,C.** AP and lateral of her 14-year-old brother demonstrate the fibular shortening and resultant ankle valgus. The epiphyses and metaphyses are irregular, and the metaphyses are widened.

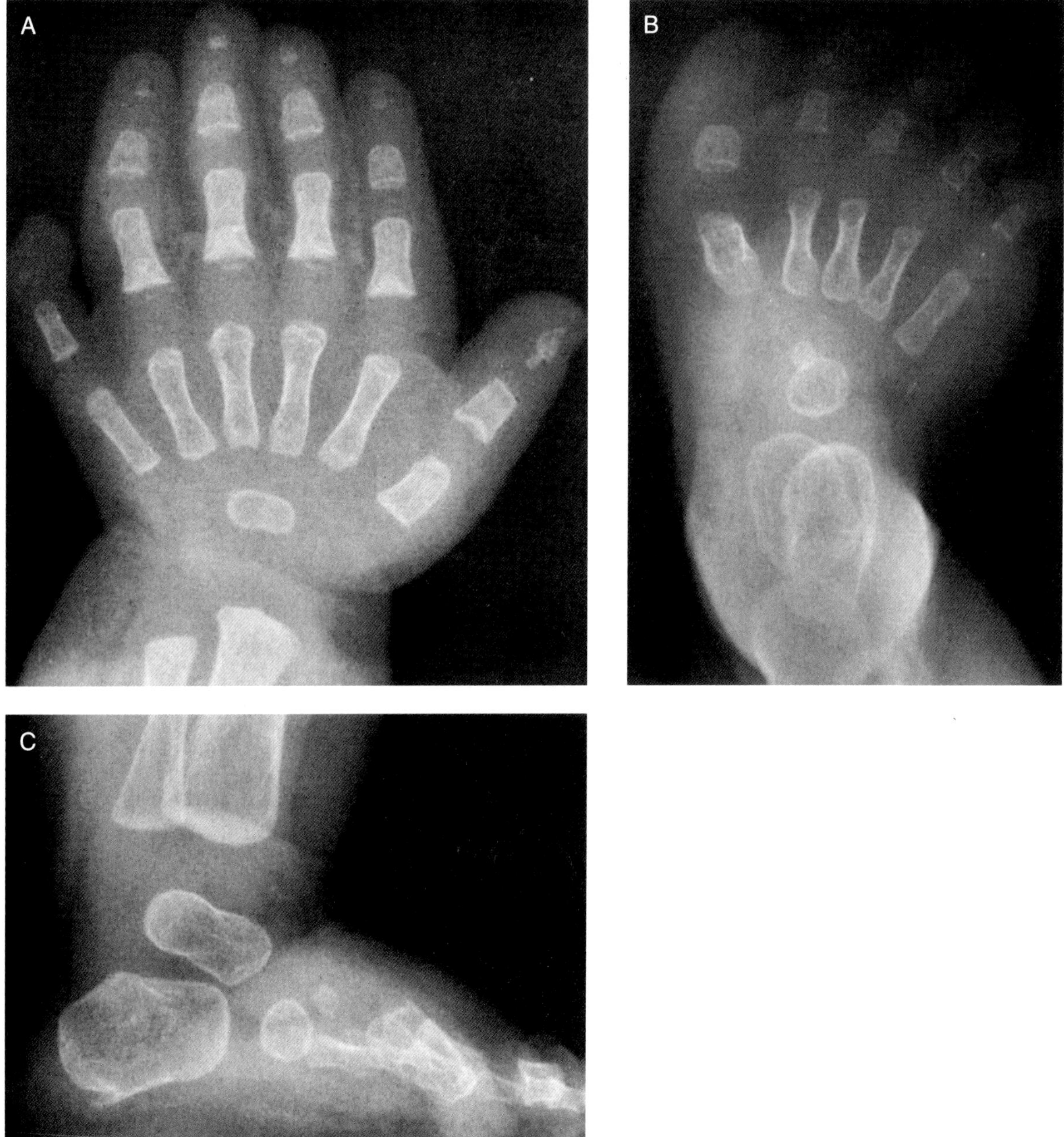

FIGURE 31-23 **A.** AP radiograph of the hand of an eight-month-old girl with chondroectodermal dysplasia. The postaxial polydactyly with fusion of the ossification centers of the wrist, cone-shaped epiphyses of the proximal and middle phalanges, and acromesomelia can be seen. **B,C.** AP and lateral radiographs of the foot. The foot is broad and delayed ossification of the distal tibia, fibula, and phalanges is evident. A small bony spike extends from the plantar aspect of the calcaneus. A similar spicule can be seen in the pelvis at the level of the triradiate cartilage.

weight-bearing ability of the foot are more important than the characteristics of the individual toe.

As with most angular deformities of the lower extremities associated with skeletal dysplasias, bracing does not offer a reasonable treatment option for the valgus deformity of the knee. Corrective proximal tibial osteotomy is indicated for genu valgum deformities greater than 15 to 20 degrees. Because of the primary growth abnormality of the proximal tibia, recurrence of the deformity with growth is a concern until skeletal maturity (77).

MELORHEOSTOSIS

Melorheostosis is a rare skeletal dysplasia characterized by its linear pattern of sclerosis along the long axis of the bone(s), resembling melting wax dripping down one side of a candle, or flowing hyperostosis (15). No hereditary or genetic basis has been established. There are differences between the disease process in children and adults.

Patients present with stiffness, loss of joint motion, deformity, and associated pain. Often the tense, shiny, or erythematous skin changes (overlying the eventual bony findings) will precede the radiographic changes (79). The skin is woody and firm, with tethering of the underlying fascia, particularly of the hand and the foot. Pain is a prominent feature in adults, but is usually not noted in children until late adolescence (90). Growth inhibition and limb length discrepancy frequently occur and will require treatment. The fibrosis and contracture development is usually progressive and may lead to significant disability. Treatment with either soft tissue release or osteotomy is often followed by recurrence of the deformity (15,90). Amputation is sometimes the definitive treatment for the short, rigid, very deformed limb.

Melorheostosis in children is an endosteal hyperostosis, with sclerotic streaking of the long bones and spotting of the small bones. In adults the radiographic pattern is more one of subperiosteal or extracortical hyperostosis (90). The histologic features are nonspecific and similar to the hyperostosis of other conditions. Dense areas of rather normal bone and markedly thickened areas of dense fibrosis in the soft tissues are typical (15,90).

Involvement of the foot and ankle is usually of either the medial or lateral aspect and continuous from the lower leg. Rigid and progressive equinovarus deformity often results from medial involvement (Figures 31-24 and 31-25). The plantar fascia is usually fibrotic and contributes to the deformity as part of the unyielding soft tissues. Shortening procedures such as talectomy and amputations have been recommended for recurrent deformity, rather than submitting the patient to repeat soft tissue release procedures with the high likelihood of future progression and recurrence (90).

ACROMICRIC DYSPLASIA

Acromicric dysplasia is a recently described skeletal dysplasia named for the marked shortening of the hands and feet. Severe growth retardation, mild facial anomalies, and specific radiographic abnormalities of the hands are characteristic. Both sexes are affected and all patients have been isolated cases from normal families, although an autosomal dominant type of transmission has been demonstrated (25,35,53).

The hands and feet in these patients are short and stocky, with short, pudgy fingers and toes with some limitation of flexion. Other joints are normal. The skeletal changes appear localized to the hands and feet, with no changes in the long bones except for shortening. The metacarpals and metatarsals are short and wide with pathognomonic changes. The first metacarpal is short with a round pseudo-epiphysis at its distal end. The other four metacarpals are pointed proximally, with a notch on the proximal radial aspect of the second and on the proximal ulnar aspect of the fifth. Cone-shaped epiphyses are present distally (35,53). The phalanges are short and broad and cone-shaped epiphyses are common. Growth plate biopsy demonstrates disorganization of the growth

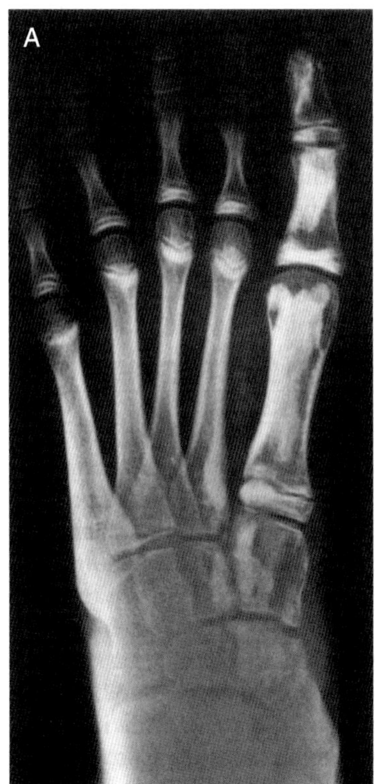

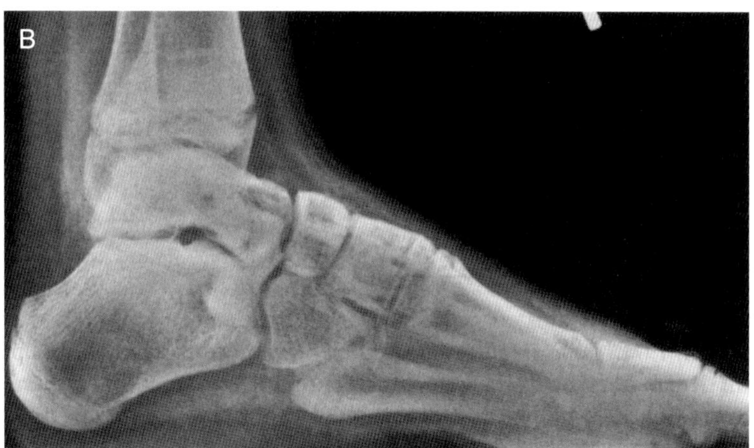

FIGURE 31-24 **A,B.** AP and lateral radiographs of a girl with melorheostosis of the medial aspect of her foot. There are skin changes evident clinically, but no deformity at this time.

Natural history and treatment. *J Bone Joint Surg Am.* 82(9): 1269–1278, 2000.

17. Cleveland M, Fielding JW. Chondrodysplasia (Ollier's disease). Report of a case with a thirty-eight year old follow-up. *J Bone Joint Surg [Am]* 41: 1341–1344, 1959.
18. Cohen MM. Some chondrodysplasias with short limbs: molecular perspectives. *Am J Med Genet* 112:304–313, 2002.
19. Cole WG. Abnormal skeletal growth in Kniest dysplasia caused by type II collagen mutations. *Clin Orthop* 341:162–169, 1997.
20. Darilek S, Wicklund C, Novy D, et al. Hereditary multiple exostosis and pain. J Pediatr Orthop 25(3): 369–376, 2005.
21. Deere M, Sanford T, Francomano CA, et al. Identification of nine novel mutations in cartilage oligomeric matrix protein (COMP) in patients with pseudoachondroplasia and multiple epiphyseal dysplasia. *Am J Med Genet* 85:486–48, 1999.
22. Dias LS. Valgus deformity of the ankle joint: pathogenesis of fibular shortening. *J Pediatr Orthop* 5: 176–180, 1985.
23. Ellis RWB, van Creveld S. Syndrome characterized by ectodermal dysplasia, polydactyly, chondrodysplasia and congenital morbus cordis: report of 3 cases. *Arch Dis Child* 15: 65–84, 1940.
24. Fairbank TJ. Dysplasia epiphysialis hemimelia (tarso-epiphysial aclasis). *J Bone Joint Surg [Br]* 38: 237–257, 1956.
25. Faivre L, Le Merrer M, Baumann C, et al. Acromicric dysplasia: long term outcome and evidence of autosomal dominant inheritance. *J Med Genet* 38(11):745–749, 2001.
26. Ford N, Silverman FN, Kozlowski K. Spondylo-epiphyseal dysplasia (pseudoachondroplastic type). *Am J Roentgenol* 86: 462–472, 1961.
27. Gupte CM, Dasgupta R, Beverly MC. The transfibular approach for distal tibial osteochondroma: an alternative technique for excision. *J Foot Ankle Surg* 42(2): 95–98, 2003.
28. Hall JG. Pseudoachondroplasia. *Birth Defects* 1(6): 187–202, 1975.
29. Hameetman L, David G, Yavas A, et al. Decreased EXT expression and intracellular accumulation of heparan sulphate proteoglycan in osteochondromas and peripheral chondrosarcomas. *J Pathol.* 211(4): 399–409, 2007.
30. Harrod MJ, Friedman JM, Currarino G, et al. Genetic heterogeneity in spondyloepiphyseal dysplasia congenita. *Am J Med Genet* 18:311–320, 1984.
31. Hollister DW, Lachman RS. Diastrophic dwarfism. *Clin Orthop* 114: 61–69, 1976.
32. Hosalkar H, Greenberg J, Gaugler RL, et al. Abnormal scarring with keloid formation after osteochondroma excision in children with multiple hereditary exostoses. *J Pediatr Orthop.* 27(3): 333–337, 2007.
33. Jahss MH, Olives R. The foot and ankle in multiple hereditary exostoses. *Foot Ankle* 1: 128–142, 1980.
34. Jeune M, Beraud C, Carron R. Dystrophie thoracique asphyxiante de caractere familial. *Arch Fr Pediatr* 12: 886–891, 1955.
35. Jones KL. *Smith's Recognizable Patterns of Human Malformation.* Philadelphia: WB Saunders, 1988.
36. Kahanovitz N, Rimoin DL, Sillence DO. The clinical spectrum of lumbar spine disease in achondroplasia. *Spine* 7: 137–140, 1982.
37. Kajantie E, Andersson S, Kaitila I. Familial asphyxiating thoracic dysplasia: clinical variability and impact of improved neonatal intensive care. *J Pediatr* 139(1):130–133, 2001.
38. Kettelcamp DB, Campbell DJ, Bonfiglio M. Dysplasia epiphysialis hemimelica. *J Bone Joint Surg [Am]* 48: 746–766, 1966.
39. Kniest W. Zur abgrenzung der dysostosis enchondralis von der chondrodystrophie. *Z Kinderheilkd* 70: 633–640, 1952.
40. Kopits SE, Lindstrom JA, McKusick VA. Pseudoachondroplastic dysplasia: pathodynamics and management. *Birth Defects* 10: 341–352, 1974.
41. Kopits SE. Orthopaedic complications of dwarfism. *Clin Orthop* 114: 153–179, 1976.
42. Kozlowski K, Beighton P. Radiographic features of spondyloepimetaphyseal dysplasia with joint laxity and progressive kyphoscoliosis. *Fortschr Rontgenstr* 141: 337–341, 1984.
43. Kozlowski K. Metaphyseal and spondylometaphyseal chondrodysplasias. *Clin Orthop* 114: 83–93, 1976.
44. Kuo RS, Bellemore MC, Monsell FP, et al. Dysplasia epiphysealis hemimelica: clinical features and management. *J Pediatr Orthop* 18(4): 543–548, 1998.
45. Langer LO, Baumann PA, Gorlin RJ. Achondroplasia. *Am J Roentgenol* 100: 12–26, 1967.
46. Langer LO, Beals RK, Solomon IL, et al. Acromesomelic dwarfism: manifestations in childhood. *Am J Med Genet* 1: 87–100, 1977.
47. Loder, RT, Sundberg S, Gabriel K, et al. Determination of bone age in children with cartilaginous dysplasia (multiple hereditary osteochondromatosis and Ollier's enchondromatosis). *J Pediatr Orthop* 24: 102–108, 2004.
48. Macias-Gomez NM, Megarbane A, Leal-Ugarte E, et al. Diastrophic dysplasia and atelosteogenesis type II as expression of compound heterozygosis: first report of a Mexican patient and genotype-phenotype correlation. *Am J Med Genet A* 129(2): 190–192, 2004.
49. Mainzer F, Minagi H, Steinbach HL. The variable manifestations of multiple enchondromatosis. *Radiology* 99: 377–388, 1971.
50. Majewski F, Pfeiffer RA, Lenz W, Muller R, Feil G, Seiler R. Polysyndaktylie, verkurzte gliedmassen and genitalfehlbildungen: Kennzeichen eines selbastandigen syndroms? *Z Kinderheilkd* 111: 118–138, 1971.
51. Manzke H, Christophers E, Wiedemann HR. Dominant sex-linked inherited chondrodysplasia punctata: a distinct type of chondrodysplasia punctata. *Clin Genet* 17: 97–107, 1980.
52. Maroteaux P, Spranger J, Opitz JM, et al. Le syndrome camptomelique. *Presse Med* 79: 1157–1162, 1971.
53. Maroteaux P, Stanescu R, Stanescu V, Rappaport R. Acromicric dysplasia. *Am J Med Genet* 24: 447–459, 1986.
54. Maroteaux P. La metachondromatose. *Z Kinderheilkd* 109: 246–261, 1971.
55. Maynard JA, Ippolito EG, Ponseti IV, Mickelson MR. Histochemistry and ultrastructure of the growth plate in achondroplasia. *J Bone Joint Surg [Am]* 63: 969–979, 1981.
56. Maynard JA, Ippolito EG, Ponseti IV, Mickelson MR. Histochemistry and ultrastructure of the growth plate in metaphyseal dysostosis: further observations on the structure of the cartilage matrix. *J Pediatr Orthop* 1: 161–169, 1981.
57. McKusick VA, Egeland JA, Eldridge R, Krusen DE. Dwarfism in the Amish. I. The Ellis-van Creveld syndrome. *Bull Johns Hopkins Hosp* 115: 306–336, 1964.
58. McKusick VA, Eldridge R, Hostetler JA, Ruangwit U, Egeland JA. Dwarfism in the Amish. II. Cartilage-hair hypoplasia. *Bull Johns Hopkins Hosp* 116: 285–326, 1965.
59. McKusick VA, Kelly TE, Dorst JP. Observations suggesting allelism of the achondroplasia and hypochondroplasia genes. *J Med Genet* 10: 11–16, 1973.
60. Merzoug V, Wicard P, Dubousset J, Kalifa G. Bilateral dysplasia epiphysealis hemimelica: report of two cases. *Pediatr Radiol* 32(6): 431–434, 2002.
61. Murray LW, Bautista J, James PL, Rimoin DL. Type II collagen defects in the chondrodysplasias. I. Spondyloepiphyseal dysplasias. *Am J Hum Genet*, 45: 5–15, 1989.
62. Polymeropoulos MH, Ide SE, Wright M, et al. The gene for the Ellis-van Creveld syndrome is located on chromosome 4p16. *Genomics* 35:1–5, 1996.
63. Ponseti IV. Skeletal growth in achondroplasia. *J Bone Joint Surg [Am]* 52: 701–716, 1970.
64. Remes V, Poussa M, Lonnqvist T, et al. Walking ability in patients with diastrophic dysplasia: a clinical, electroneurophysiological, treadmill, and MRI analysis. *J Pediatr Orthop* 24(5): 546–551, 2004.
65. Rimoin DL, Siggers DC, Lachman RS, Silberberg R. Metatropic dwarfism, the Kniest syndrome and the pseudoachondroplastic dysplasias. *Clin Orthop* 114: 70–82, 1976.
66. Rosenbloom AL, Smith DW. The natural history of metaphyseal dysostosis. *J Pediatr* 66: 857–868, 1965.

67. Rossi M, De Brasi D, Hall CM, et al. A new familial case of spondylo-epi-metaphyseal dysplasia with multiple dislocations Hall type (leptodactylic form). *Clin Dysmorphol* 14(1):13–18, 2005.
68. Rubin P. *Dynamic classification of bone dysplasias.* Chicago: Year Book Medical, 1964.
69. Saldino RM, Noonan CD. Severe thoracic dystrophy with striking micromelia, abnormal osseous development, including the spine, and multiple visceral anomalies. *Am J Roentgenol* 114: 257–263, 1972.
70. Schmid F. Beitrag zur dysostosis enchondralis metaphysaria. *Monatsschr Kinderheilkd* 97: 393–397, 1949.
71. Schwartz HS, Zimmerman NB, Simon MA, Wroble RR, Millar EA, Bonfiglio M. The malignant potential of enchondromatosis. *J Bone Joint Surg,* 69–A: 269–274, 1987.
72. Shapiro F, Simon S, Glimcher MJ. Hereditary multiple exostoses: anthropometric, roentgenographic, and clinical aspects. *J Bone Joint Surg* [*Am*] 61: 815–824, 1979.
73. Silengo MC, Luzzatti L, Silverman FN. Clinical and genetic aspects of Conradi-Hunermann disease. A report of three familial cases and review of the literature. *J Pediatr* 97: 911–917, 1980.
74. Snearly WN, Peterson HA. Management of ankle deformities in multiple hereditary osteochondromata. *J Pediatr Orthop* 9: 427–432, 1989.
75. Solomon L. Bone growth in diaphyseal aclasis. *J Bone Joint Surg* [*Br*] 43: 700–716, 1961.
76. Specht EE, Daentl DL. Hypochondroplasia. *Clin Orthop* 110: 249–255, 1975.
77. Sponseller PD, Ain MC. The Skeletal Dysplasias. In: Morrissy R.T., Weinstein S.L. eds.: *Lovell and Winter's Pediatric Orthopaedics,* 6th ed. Philadelphia: Lippincott, Williams, and Wilkins, 2006; 205–250.
78. Spranger JW, Langer LO. Spondyloepiphyseal dysplasia congenita. *Radiology* 94: 313–322, 1970.
79. Spranger JW, Langer LO, Wiedemann HR. *Bone dysplasias. An Atlas of Constitutional Disorders of Skeletal Development.* Philadelphia: WB Saunders, 1974.
80. Spranger JW, Opitz JM, Bidder U. Heterogeneity of chondrodysplasia punctata. *Humangenetik* 11: 190–212, 1971.
81. Spranger JW. The epiphyseal dysplasias. *Clin Orthop* 114: 46–60, 1976.
82. Stanescu V, Stanescu R, Maroteaux P. Pathogenic mechanisms in osteochondrodysplasias. *J Bone Joint Surg* [*Am*] 66: 817–836, 1984.
83. Stenzler S, Grogan DP, Frenchman SM, McClelland S, Ogden JA. Progressive diaphyseal dysplasia presenting as neuromuscular disease. *J Pediatr Orthop* 9: 463–467, 1989.
84. Trevor D. Tarso-epiphysial aclasis. A congenital error of epiphysial development. *J Bone Joint Surg* [*Br*] 32: 204–213, 1950.
85. Walker BA, Scott CI, Hall JG, Murdoch JL, McKusick VA. Diastrophic dwarfism. *Medicine* 51: 41–59, 1972.
86. Wallis GA, Rash B, Sykes B, et al. Mutations within the gene encoding the alpha-1 (X) chain of type X collagen cause metaphyseal chondrodysplasia type Schmid but not several other forms of metaphyseal chondrodysplasia. *J Med Genet* 33:450–457, 1996.
87. Wang Q, Green RP, Zhao G, Ornitz DM. Differential regulation of endochondral bone growth and joint development by FGFR1 and FGFR3 tyrosine kinase domains. *Developmen.* 128(19):3867–76, 2001.
88. Winter RB, Bloom BA. Spine deformity in spondyloepimetaphyseal dysplasia. *J Pediatr Orthop* 10: 535–539, 1990.
89. Wynne-Davies R. Genetics and congenital musculoskeletal disorders. *Obstet Gynecol Annu* 6: 247–260, 1977.
90. Younge D, Drummond D, Herring J, Cruess RL. Melorheostosis in children. *J Bone Joint Surg (Br)* 61: 415–418, 1979.

CHAPTER 32

Genetic Conditions

Kenneth J. Guidera and Gabriela J. Ferski

INTRODUCTION

The child's foot is frequently involved in genetic conditions and syndromes. These disease states vary from Down syndrome with pes planus and toe gaps to caudal regression syndrome and sirenomelia with rigid clubfeet and lower limb fusion. The spectrum ranges from feet with slight variations of normal anatomy, which need no treatment, to those with severe deformity which may preclude ambulation without surgery. There have been many advances in identifying the genetic inheritance patterns of these conditions and these will be referenced here.

Basic Clinical Genetic Principles

These conditions, by definition, must have a genetic basis. Genetic principles include the specificity of individual defects and variation in expression (104). The former relates to the fact that a pattern of disease cannot be made on the basis of a single genetic defect, unless it is a true monogenic condition. This is a single deformity occurring secondary to a mutation of one gene (239). A sequence of anomalies is usually required for a specific diagnosis. In the case of the foot, this may be a minor defect, such as syndactyly, which still plays a significant role in the formation of the diagnosis and the effect on the individual patient. Variance in expression refers to differences in presentation of a genetic condition among individuals with the same disease. This is the usual case with genetic syndromes, and it is rare to find a given anomaly in all patients with the same condition.

Heterogenicity is another genetic principle which implies that similar phenotypes may result from different etiologies. For example, children with Down syndrome and Prader-Willi syndrome have similar morphologic appearances with mental deficiency, obesity, hypotonia, and small feet with minor anomalies. However, the genetics of the two conditions vary significantly with Down syndrome being a trisomy of chromosome 21 and Prader-Willi having a long arm deletion of chromosome 15.

The genetic conditions include chromosomal abnormalities such as trisomies, with extra chromosomal material or deletions. These involve an abnormal phenotype based on an aberration of the genotype. The human genetic pattern consists of 22 pairs of autosomes and 1 pair of sex chromosomes; one of each pair derived from the maternal and paternal parent. Conditions such as Down or Prader-Willi syndrome result from too much or too little chromosome material. Because many genes are carried by a single chromosome, these types of disorders may yield devastating anomalies, affecting multiple organ systems. Risk factors such as increased maternal age account for many of the chromosomal disorders; however, most parents of trisomy patients have normal genotypes with the condition arising *de novo* (239).

Single gene defects are unifactorial disorders that involve the autosomal dominant and autosomal recessive inheritance patterns. The autosomal dominant conditions appear in all generations without skipping, and the affected persons have a 50% chance of transmitting the disorder to their children. Autosomal recessive conditions present when the patient has received the recessive gene from both parents. The condition is seen only in a homozygotic offspring, but not in the heterozygotic parents or siblings. There is no sex relationship, and the recurrence risk of the parents for future offspring is 25%.

Sex-related genetic conditions generally involve X-chromosome linkage of the defect. Most of the conditions are X-linked recessive, with very few being X-linked dominant. These latter conditions have a female predominance (242). In the recessive disease states, the hemizygous male expresses the phenotype of the condition, while the female does not. Therefore, all patients are male, and the father cannot pass the trait on to his son.

A combination of genetic and environmental factors may lead to a multifactorial or polygenic condition. These have a lower risk of penetration than autosomal dominant and recessive conditions, with an increased incidence among relatives. The polygenic load in a particular family can be quantitated and risk factors calculated. For example, clubfoot may be a multifactorial condition in which there is a 1 in 20 risk factor after the first affected offspring, 1 in 7 after the second, and 1 in 2 after the third (239).

The majority of genetic foot deformities will fall into the monogenic, chromosomal, or multifactorial group. Common trends may be seen in each group, and the family history is important in delineating the genetic nature of the condition. The foot disorders discussed here will be presented along the lines of their inheritance patterns. The treatment of these disorders includes observation, orthotics, and surgical intervention. The newer techniques will be referenced here.

THE FOOT IN SPECIFIC GENETIC DISORDERS

Chromosomal Defects

Down Syndrome

Down syndrome or *trisomy 21* is one of the most common genetic disorders. There is an incidence of 1 in 660 newborns (104). Ninety-four percent of the cases are a true trisomy, 2% to 4% are mosaics, and 3% are translocations (135,144). The phenotype consists of hypotonia, a flat face, small ears, slanted palpebral fissures, hypermobility of joints, and mental retardation. The vast majority of affected individuals remain ambulatory. The foot is frequently involved, but usually not to a degree that impairs walking.

The foot disorders consist of first and second toe gaps, dorsiflexed toes, plantar creases, and an open dermal bridge on the plantar surface. The foot is frequently broad, flat, and supple with hindfoot or hallux valgus (Figure 32-1). Merrick et al. described 475 Israeli patients with Down syndrome, noting hallux valgus in 103 and pes planus in 199 (189 bilateral) (139). They recommended early orthotic treatment to avoid shoe fitting problems. Gait studies have shown a decrease in plantar flexion movements and velocity, with increased heel eversion (46,197). The latter was corrected with an orthosis. Foot surgery is rarely indicated in these very functional and active patients unless the bunion or hindfoot becomes severely painful or deformed (38,50).

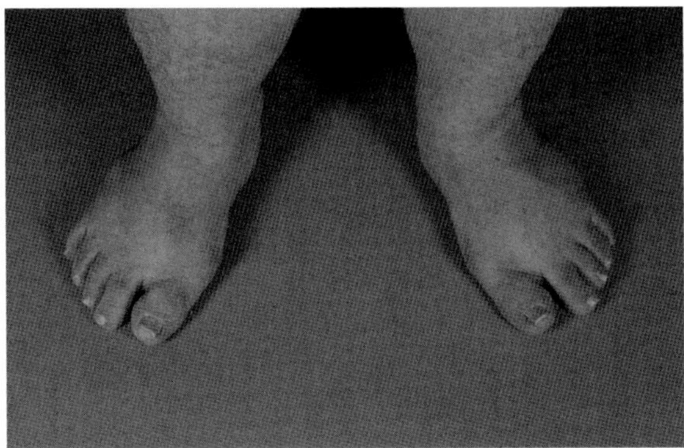

FIGURE 32-1 Down syndrome: Trisomy 21; the typical planovalgus foot in Down syndrome. Hallux valgus is frequently present.

Other Trisomies

Genetic aberrations involving other chromosomes occur at a lesser rate than *trisomy 21* and frequently have lower survival rates. These include *trisomy 18* with an incidence of 0.3 per 1,000 newborns and a 10% survival rate past the first year (104,236). Most die from cardiovascular complications during the first year of life with foot deformity being present in 90% (14). These include a short dorsiflexed hallux, equinovarus, rocker bottom feet, syndactyly, and ectrodactyly (41,126). In *trisomy 18,* arthrogryposis of the wrists and ankles bilaterally has been described as has hexadactyly of the feet (42,44). The presenting characteristics of hand, head, feet, and cardiac anomalies frequently allow ultrasonographic intrauterine diagnosis (91). However, due to the feeble nature of the children, treatment is rarely required. In Arizawa's review (14) all patients died within the first three months of life.

Similarly, children with *trisomy 13,* occurring in 1 of 5,000 newborns, present with equinovarus, first and second toe clefts, and hypoplastic nails. The survival rate for this syndrome is also low, with 18% surviving the first year (104,236).

Other rare trisomies include *trisomy 9* characterized by joint dislocations, contractures, short phalanges, and abnormally positioned digits. Cardiac, brain, and facial anomalies are also presenting features in this trisomy (72). *Trisomy 20 P* involves toe clinodactyly, rocker bottom feet, and prominent heels (196). Interstitial deletion of the long arm of the fourth chromosome results in a phenotype of mental delay, hypotonia, peculiar facies, and small hands or feet (22). *Trisomy 1Q* is a rare condition with facial abnormalities and flexion and valgus deformities of the extremities (169). Foot and ankle deformities are noted in many other trisomies such as rocker bottom feet in *trisomy 4p* (225). These syndromes also have short life expectancies and rarely require intervention (104,196).

Children with *trisomy 10 Q* exhibit mental retardation, growth retardation, facial anomalies, foot positional defects, deep plantar furrows, and toe camptodactyly (248). They are, however, ambulatory and may need soft tissue releases for ankle equinus contractures (Figure 32-2).

Non-Trisomy Chromosomal Anomalies

Prader-Willi syndrome results from a deletion of the long arm of the chromosome 15 (144). The patients are hypotonic, mentally retarded, obese, and small statured with eating disorders. The hands and feet are markedly decreased in size such that some adult patients wear children's shoes. Associated anomalies include scoliosis, hip dysplasia, lower extremity limb inequality, genu valgum, and osteopenia. Foot deformities consisting of pes planus, pes cavus, metatarsus adductus, and hallux valgus are present in approximately half of the patients with this syndrome (119,238,245). Any treatment is complicated by behavioral problems associated with brain abnormalities (244). Gait and developmental motor abnormalities may develop early and also hinder any treatment but ambulation is generally maintained and orthopedic treatment may be minimal (37,104,235).

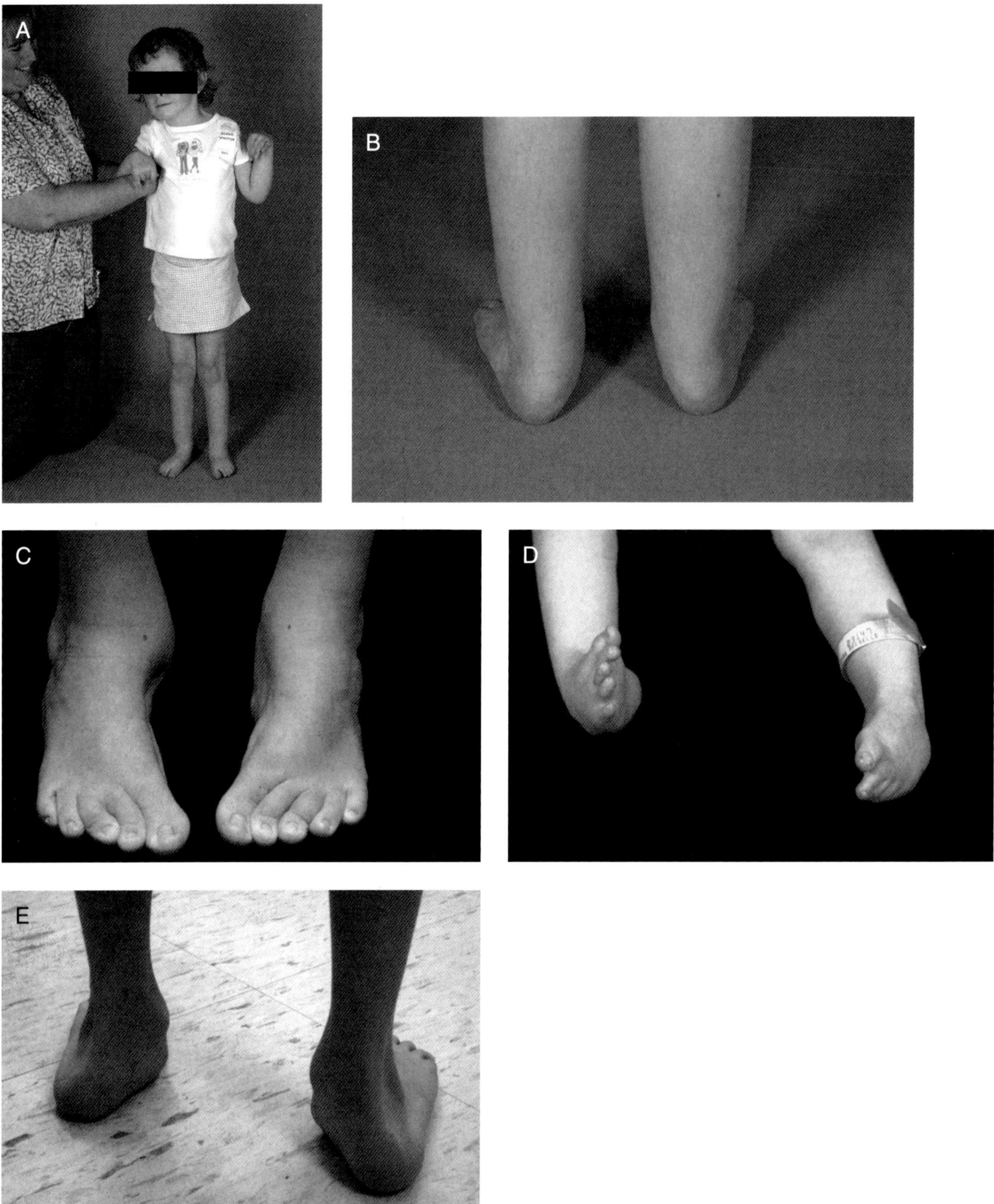

FIGURE 32-2 Other trisomies with foot deformities. **A.** Trisomy 8p. **B.** Trisomy 8p. **C.** Trisomy 12. **D.** Trisomy 6. **E.** Chromosome #5 deletion.

Sex Chromosome Disorders

Abnormalities may also occur in the sex chromosomes. These result in varying phenotypic anomalies, some of which have foot involvement.

The XYY syndrome, with an incidence of 1 per 826 males, is frequently missed due to the subtle nature of its characteristics. The boys are tall and clumsy, with abnormal hand posturing and increased length of the long bones, resulting in feet which are long and narrow (104,233).

In *Kleinfelter's* syndrome (XXY), the affected males were classically described as tall and underweight, with long, slender limbs and feet. The condition may be under diagnosed, and the incidence is reported as high as 1 in 500 males (61). The phenotypic presentation is variable with malignancy, obesity, metabolic syndrome, hypogonadism, and infertility being associated (29,30,61,114, 121). In the XXXY or XXXXY syndromes, the majority of patients present with mental retardation, growth deficiency, and pes planus. Children with *Turner* syndrome (XO) exhibit decreased stature, questionably responsive to androgen therapy, with short fourth metatarsals in 50%. Treatment with testosterone is frequently recommended, but the administration of growth hormone is controversial (8). Associated conditions may include aortic anomalies, cardiac, renal, and auditory problems. Subchondral fractures have also been described. Despite all these phenotypic presentations, there is frequently a delay in diagnosis (63,96,158,182,183,191,210,227). Generally, none of these foot anomalies secondary to sex chromosomal aberrations require treatment (39,104,222,233,236). except for proper shoe wear to avoid a skin breakdown and ingrown toe nails which are frequently present (69). Limb lengthenings for short stature in Turner syndrome were attempted in one series of 10 patients but with poor results (27). Rare sex chromosome anomalies such as 49, XXXXY (71) may exhibit skeletal anomalies involving the feet and lower extremities (Figure 32-3).

Non-Chromosomal Disorders

Autosomal Dominant Conditions

Nail-Patella Syndrome

Autosomal dominant conditions by definition are expressed in 50% of the carriers' offspring. Nail-patella syndrome, hereditary onchyodystrophy, is an example of this. More than 200 cases have been reported (104) with an estimated incidence of 4.5 per million live births in the United States. The incidence currently has been reported as high as 1 in 50,000 births (221). There is an autosomal dominant inheritance pattern related to the ABO blood group locus, with the involved family members having the same blood type (67,128,166,243). This syndrome consists of a tetrad of signs including nail dysplasia, patellar hypoplasia or aplasia, iliac horns, and radial head dislocation. The condition may be associated with other anomalies such as nevi and bony sclerosis (57).

The foot deformity is the chief presenting complaint in this syndrome and frequently requires treatment (Figure 32-4). Twenty-five of 44 patients in this author's review had clubfeet (81). Eighteen underwent corrective

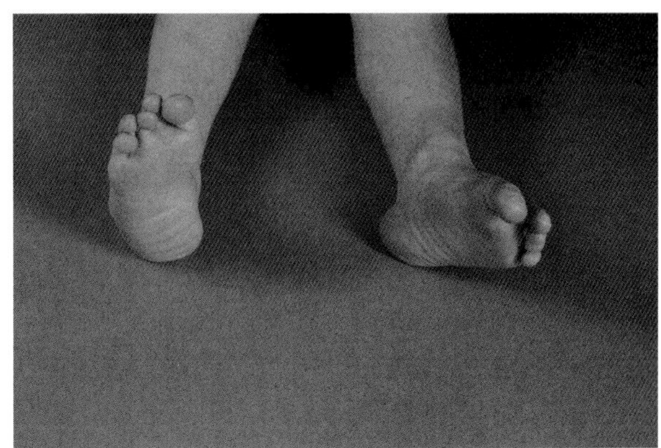

FIGURE 32-3 Sex chromosome disorders: talipes equinovarus seen in XXXXY syndrome.

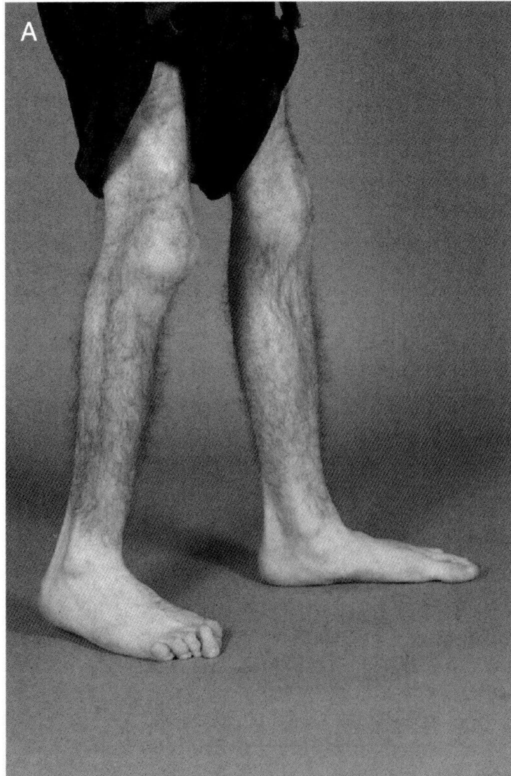

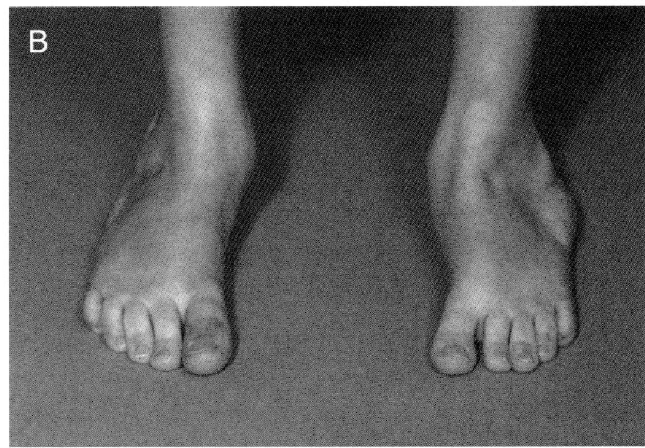

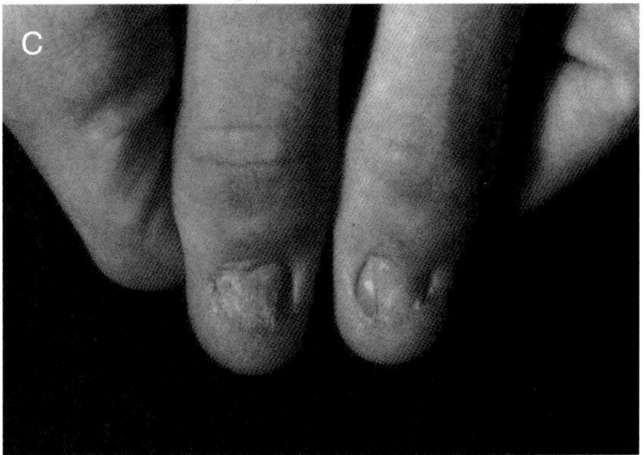

FIGURE 32-4 Nail patella syndrome. **A.** The whole lower extremity is involved, including the knee and foot. **B.** Clubfoot or pes planovalgus may be present. **C.** Finger and toenail abnormalities are part of the diagnostic triad.

surgery consisting of posteromedial releases and/or isolated Achilles tendon lengthenings. Seven patients required later revision surgery for residual deformity consisting of subtalar or triple arthrodeses, and calcaneal osteotomies. Sweeney noted a lower incidence of clubfoot at 19% with 70% being bilateral (221). With ultrasound, this can be diagnosed *in utero* (221).

The clubfoot deformity is frequently rigid in this condition and requires an early posteromedial release to avoid recurrence and repeat surgery. Tendo-Achilles lengthening alone may be inadequate. Calcaneovalgus and congenital convex pes valgus deformities may also be treated successfully with early soft-tissue releases and tendon transfers (81,93). Bracing is recommended after surgery, but prolonged orthotic usage is generally not required. Fieldler (68) described the long-term sequelae consisting of midtarsal joint subluxation with an ankle ball-and-socket deformity and hindfoot valgus in an untreated adult. All patients may remain active and ambulatory with appropriate treatment of the foot and knee deformities.

Rett Syndrome

Rett syndrome is a progressive encephalopathy seen only in females. It was first described by Andreas Rett in 1966 (172). The condition appears during the first 18 months of life and consists of progressive mental deterioration, autistic behavior, and stereotypic hand wringing motions (82,83,84) (Figure 32-5).

The incidence is estimated to be 1 in 15,000 live female births with over 2,000 cases now reported (229). The inheritance pattern is thought to be autosomal dominant with incomplete expression or lethality in males, or possibly related to an inactive X chromosome. Other metabolic and environmental etiologies have been proposed, but at present there is no proven genetic pathway. However, the fact that all patients are female points to the autosomal dominant theory described above (148,152). The responsible gene appears to be dominant mutation on the X q 28 locus (103).

Scoliosis and joint contractures are the prevalent orthopedic problems in this condition. The scoliosis may be rapidly progressive and life threatening (226). Loder and Lee (127) described eight Rett patients with bilateral equinus and equinovarus contractures. Heelcord lengthenings had favorable results but a split posterior tendon transfer failed, requiring a triple arthrodesis as a salvage procedure. Conservative treatment had mixed results. Two of the nine patients in this author's (79) review required tendo-Achilles lengthening for equinus deformity. One had pes planus and was treated orthotically, as were those patients with mild equinus deformities. Early intervention with orthotics appears beneficial to these patients, as do judicious surgical releases if that fails. There are periods of regression and stabilization in this syndrome which can affect any treatment plan (153). The girls are frequently ambulatory until the teenage years; therefore, treating the foot deformity early and appropriately is essential.

Apert Syndrome

Apert syndrome is an autosomal dominant condition also known as acrocephalosyndactyly (104,144). The incidence is reported at 15–16 per 1 million births (132). The majority of cases are new mutations with a 50% risk for offspring of the affected patient. The syndrome affects the head, hands, and feet with an acrocephalic cranial dysplasia and syndactyly of the hands and feet. There is frequently broadening of the thumb and hallux. Generally, the second, third, and fourth toes are syndactylized, and the first and fifth toes are free. The toenails may or may not be continuous. Duplicated first metatarsals were present in

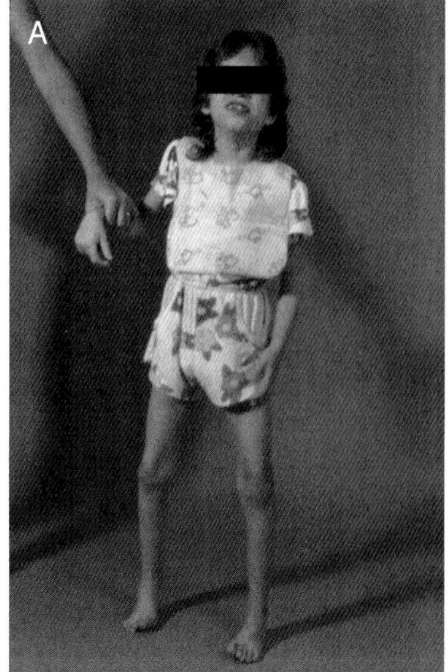

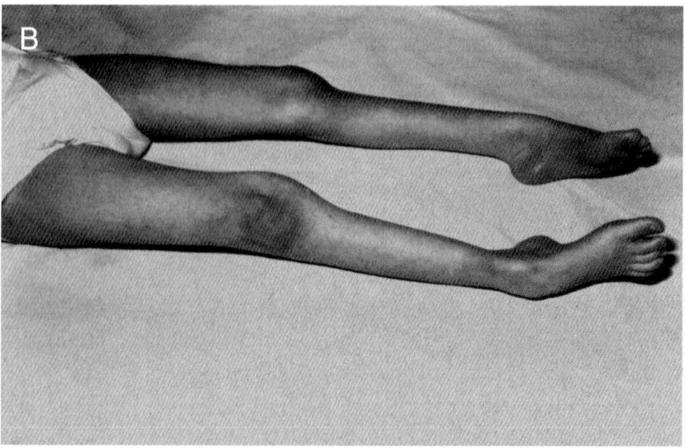

FIGURE 32-5 Rett syndrome. **A.** The patients are initially weight bearing with equinus and equinovarus foot deformities. **B.** The foot deformities become more rigid as the patient matures, and ambulation is frequently lost.

five patients in Blank's series and are not a rare phenomenon, according to Gorlin (28,75). The foot deformities are frequently symmetrical and the toes may be completely absent in severe cases (Figure 32-6). Fearon has described good to excellent results in a series of 43 patients who underwent staged soft-tissue release and later osteotomies for syndactyly of the hands and feet. He stressed the importance of including the feet in this treatment (66).

Conditions similar to Apert syndrome also have foot involvement. *Pfeiffer syndrome*, for example, includes equinus, syndactyly, and broad toes with aberrant positions (104) (Figure 32-7). Martsolf (133) describes short middle phalanges with an oval configuration and trapezoidal shaped proximal phalanges with varus deformities of the first toes. The first and second metatarsals may be broadened with accessory epiphyses and syndactyly of the second, third, and fourth toes. The syndactyly is generally complete and the classic appearance of the foot is a hallmark of Pfeiffer syndrome (184).

Carpenter syndrome is also a related condition consisting of acrocephaly, polydactyly, and partial syndactyly (104). Robinson (177) described preaxial polydactyly, duplication of phalanges, and broadening of the first metatarsal. The first toenail is generally duplicated with mild cutaneous syndactyly between all toes. Surgical intervention was not required for foot disorders in this series.

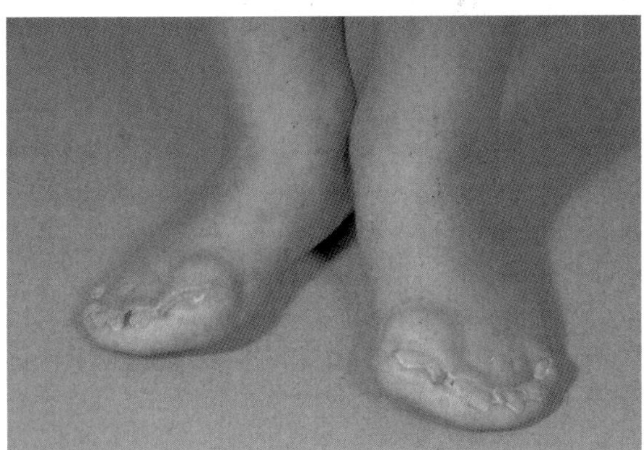

FIGURE 32-6 Apert syndrome: severe bilateral syndactyly seen in Apert syndrome.

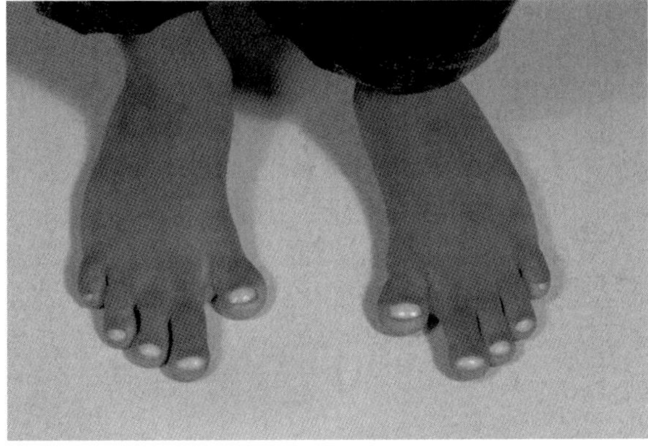

FIGURE 32-7 Pfeiffer syndrome: broad toes with aberrant positions are the hallmark of this syndrome.

Greig syndrome is a similar autosomal dominant cephalosyndactyly. The patients have a peculiar facies with both polydactyly and syndactyly of the toes and fingers. Gollop and Fontes (73) found broad toes with medial deviation, equinovarus deformities, and shortening and fragmentation of the proximal phalanx of the hallux in this syndrome. Surgery may be required to remove extra digits or correct angulation of the existing toes.

Multiple Synostosis Syndrome

Multiple synostosis syndrome is an autosomal dominant dysplasia which results in phalangeal, carpal, and tarsal synostoses (104). The mid-phalangeal joints are frequently fused (symphalangism) with distal digital hypoplasia. The phalanges and toenails may be absent. Da-Silva noted bilateral symmetrical deformities including synostosis of both the hands and midfoot (53). Rigid hindfoot valgus or pes planus are frequently present and may require either subtalar or triple arthrodesis (Figure 32-8).

Jackson-Weiss Syndrome

Jackson-Weiss syndrome is another autosomal dominant condition with foot involvement. This syndrome, similar to Apert and Pfeiffer syndrome, consists of craniosynostosis, mid-facial hypoplasia, and foot anomalies described initially in a large Amish population (100). All patients had foot abnormalities consisting of broad, short first metatarsals and proximal phalanges. The first ray deviates medially with associated changes such as calcaneocuboid or naviculocuneiform coalitions. There may be associated fusions between the first and second metatarsals. Medial deviation of the first toe and hindfoot, or deformities of the midfoot

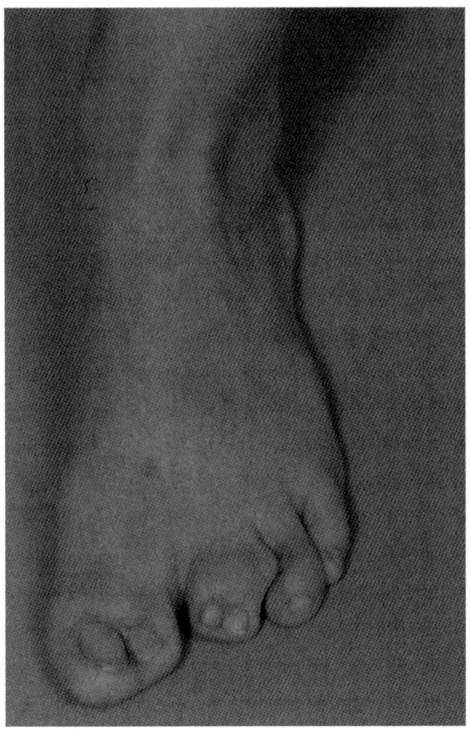

FIGURE 32-8 Multiple synostosis syndrome: this condition has synostosis of the tarsals, carpals, and phalanges with fusion of the mid-phalangeal joints.

occasionally require an osteotomy to maintain a plantigrade foot. The feet have a characteristic radiographic appearance with multiple mid foot metatarsal fusions and short, broad metatarsals (89,130). One patient in Jackson and Weiss' group required toe amputations due to the deformity.

Popliteal Pterygium Syndrome

Popliteal pterygium syndrome or, facio-genito-popliteal syndrome was initially described by Trelat in 1869 (97,104). This autosomal dominant condition consists of popliteal webbing, toenail dysplasia, and toe syndactyly. Facial anomalies may also be present (190). There are fusions of the interphalangeal joints, with valgus deformities of the hindfoot and pyramid-shaped skin over the hallux. The toes are broad, syndactylized, and the hallux may be laterally deviated. Additionally, these patients have cleft lips and lower lip pits, which differentiate them from the autosomal recessive multiple pterygium syndrome. The foot deformities may be treated by standard surgical methods and coordinated with popliteal release surgery and osteotomy (157).

Larsen Syndrome

Multiple joint dislocations, facial anomalies, and clubfoot deformities characterize this condition (175). It is inherited in an autosomal dominant manner, and these individuals have numerous extremity contractures and dislocations. The initial patient described in 1568 may well have had arthrogryposis (9). There is frequently a rigid equinovarus or hindfoot valgus deformity, with a calcaneal ossicle due to delayed ossification as described by Latta (122). Stanley and Seymour (213) illustrated the development of a ball and socket ankle joint, a talocalcaneal coalition, and forefoot varus deformities in their review of eight patients. They found severe progressive foot contractures similar to those in arthrogryposis. The patients generally remain ambulatory, and should be treated with early posteromedial soft-tissue releases of the clubfoot and long-term bracing. Recurrence or late treatment will necessitate a talectomy, osteotomy, or triple arthrodesis. Cervical spine deformities have preoperative radiographic evaluation including lateral flexion and extension views because the instability may be life-threatening (188) (Figure 32-9).

Cornelia de Lange Syndrome

This disorder also referred to as Brachman-de Lange syndrome, exhibits growth retardation, mental deficiency, microbrachiocephaly, and limb malformations including syndactyly and clubfoot. There is a reported incidence of

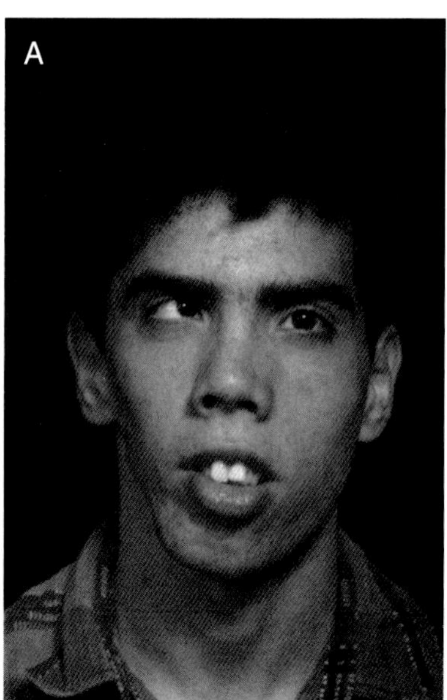

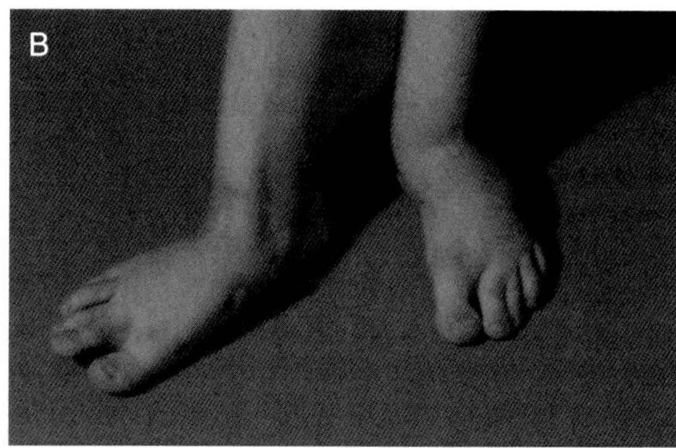

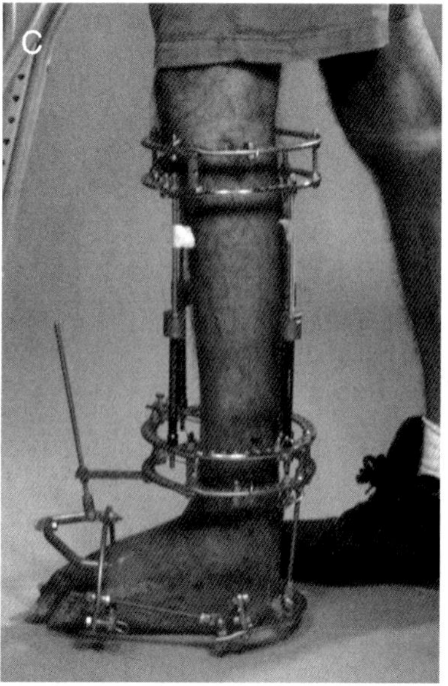

FIGURE 32-9 Larsen syndrome. Consists of facial anomalies (**A**) and equinovarus or valgus deformities (**B**). The rigid foot deformities may require osteotomy or external fixation (**C**).

1 in 10,000 births (113). Robinson (178) has presented evidence suggesting an autosomal dominant inheritance pattern; however, many cases arise sporadically, and Hawley (88) found an increased rate of skeletal and limb malformations in the lower birth weight babies with this syndrome. Smith (104) described micromelia of the feet in 99% and syndactyly of the second and third toes in 81% of those affected with both partial and total syndactyly and bunion formation being reported (113,130).

These patients are mentally deficient, but ambulatory. There are frequent gastrointestinal and cardiac anomalies such as apnea, congestive heart failure, and bowel obstruction, which may affect treatment plans for the patient who needs surgical correction of the equinovarus deformity (25).

Brachiodactyly Type E

The hereditary types of brachydactyly (shortening of digits, metatarsals, and metacarpals) were initially presented by Bell (24) in 1951, and type E was clarified by Riccardi (173). This autosomal dominant condition is more prevalent in females and consists of short metatarsals and phalanges with cone shaped epiphyses (130). The latter may be a result of a localized vascular disturbance at the growth plate. There is a propensity for the shortening to be seen in the fibular-sided rays of the metatarsals and phalanges (142). The feet appear similar to those seen in pseudohypoparathyroidism, but the metabolic and mental deficiencies are lacking, as are the ectopic calcifications and subcutaneous ossifications (77). Surgical treatment for these foot abnormalities has not been necessary unless there is dorsal displacement of the short digit (Figure 32-10).

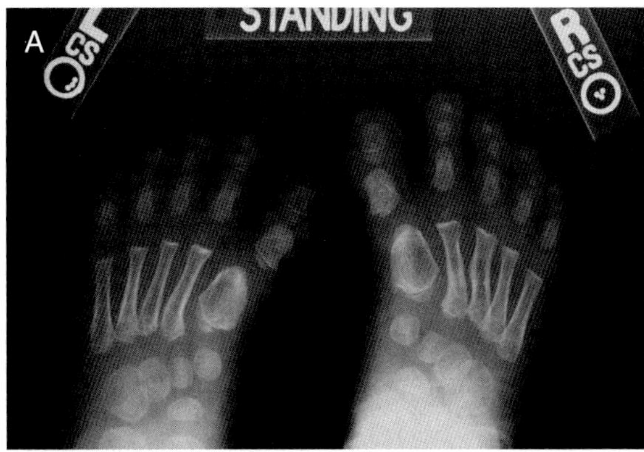

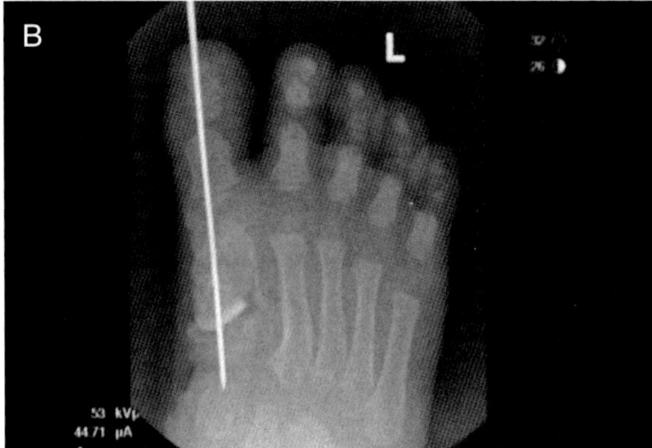

FIGURE 32-10 Brachiodactyly Type E. **A.** Short cone-shaped metatarsals and phalanges of brachiodactyly. **B.** Surgical realignment may be necessary for malaligned toes.

Weaver Syndrome

Patients with accelerated skeletal growth and maturation, camptodactyly, and facial anomalies constitute this syndrome. Large birth weight and hypotonia are also associated (130). Clinodactyly of the toes occurs with associated clubfoot, calcaneovalgus deformity, or metatarsus adductus (104). Cervical instability and neoplasm have also been reported in these patients (111). The bony overgrowth and maturation is dysharmonic and may result from a mesenchymal defect with early mineralization of the ossification centers (13). The patients also exhibit distal splaying or widening of the long bones.

The condition is felt to be autosomal dominant, but males are affected three times more than females, with milder phenotypic expression in girls. The foot deformities are common with 7 of 10 reported cases having pedal malposition (13). The foot anomalies require standard orthopedic treatment consisting of casting, bracing, or posteromedial releases for resistant talipes equinovarus.

Whistling Face Syndrome

This condition also referred to as Freeman-Sheldon syndrome is an autosomal dominant trait having a mask-like face with the mouth in a whistling position. In addition to hand anomalies, the feet exhibit bilaterally symmetrical talipes equinovarus and flexion contractures of the toes (Figure 32-11). Antley reports a high incidence of clubfoot; 21 of 37 cases (11). The patients are ambulatory and require surgical correction of these rigid deformities. Repeat surgery with a lateral cuboid or calcaneal osteotomy may be necessary if there is recurrence after a posteromedial release. Kousseff (117) has described an autosomal recessive variant of this condition in twins with similar clinical features. The syndrome may actually be more of a spectrum of musculoskeletal and neurologic manifestations due to a primary brain anomaly (5,136,249). Scoliosis, respiratory infections and malignant hyperthermia may complicate any treatment (216).

Oculo-Dento-Digital Syndrome

This rare condition reviewed by Gorlin (76) consists of enamel hypoplasia, craniofacial and dental abnormalities, camptodactyly of the fingers, and syndactyly of the toes and fingers. There is broadening of the metatarsals and hypoplasia of the middle phalanges. The toe phalanges may be absent (136). Neurologic changes may occur from abnormal white matter or cervical compression. This genetic disorder generally arises as a new mutation, is inherited in an autosomal dominant manner, and should be considered when evaluating children with poor dentition and syndactyly (99). No treatment is generally required for the feet.

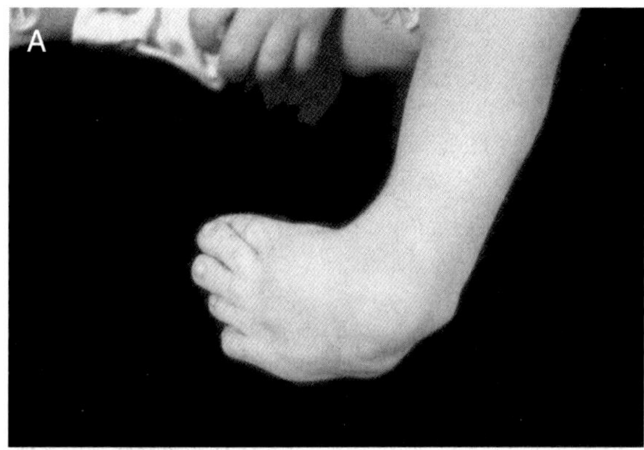

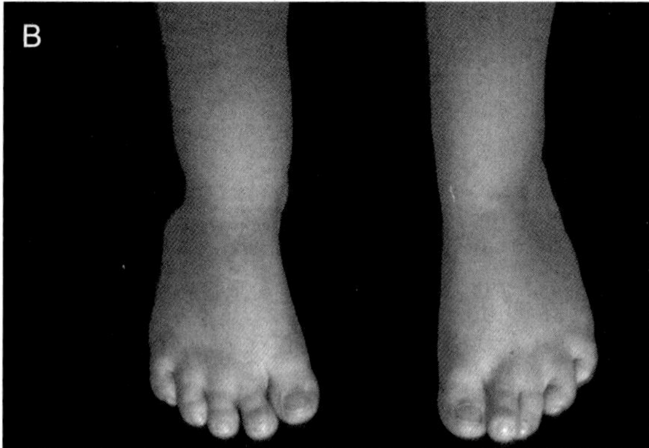

FIGURE 32-11 Freeman-Sheldon syndrome. **A.** The rigid equinovarus of the Freeman-Sheldon syndrome. **B.** Post-operative correction of talipes equinovarus and flexion deformities of the toes.

Adams-Oliver Syndrome

This is also a rare, but interesting, autosomal dominant condition with foot involvement (101). These patients exhibit scalp and hair defects with transverse terminal defects of the feet. The syndrome is also associated with cardiac and vascular anomalies and striking distal limb amputations or defects (7,70,136). The toe anomalies may vary from nail hypoplasia to complete congenital amputation (Figure 32-12). Bonafede (31) described kindred with this condition, one of whose foot defects consisted of ectrodactyly (clawfoot) with rudimentary second and fifth toes. Treatment other than shoe modification for this condition has not been described.

Ectrodactyly

Ectrodactyly itself is an autosomal dominant condition seen in families with the split hand-split foot malformation (23,212). The clinical spectrum is extremely variable. One family member may have both hand and foot involvement, while another may exhibit much less involvement, such as unilateral aplasia of one limb. The feet are usually more affected than the hands. The tarsals may consist of a coalesced mass, while the carpals are normal and the hands bilaterally split or have monodactyly. Corea (51) described this condition in association with congenital absence of the fibula in a patient who required amputation and prosthetic fitting. Robinson (176) presented cases with associated cleft lips, hearing loss, and dental dysplasia. Bhat and co-workers (26) estimate the incidence to be 1 in 90,000. Their minimum criteria for inclusion in this syndrome are the absence of two or more digits. Beck (23) has reported this syndrome in twins with an associated bilateral absence of the ulna, estimating the incidence to be approximately 1 in 35,000–50,000 live births. Zlotogora (251) described a family with this condition which may represent a rare variant with an autosomal recessive inheritance pattern. More cases with an autosomal recessive inheritance pattern have been reported as have associated femoral bifurcations (136). The ectodermal dysplasia group of syndromes, first described by Darwin, comprises over 150 syndromes who present with skin, ear, eye, and oral-facial abnormalities, hearing loss, and ectrodactyly of the upper and lower extremities (199).

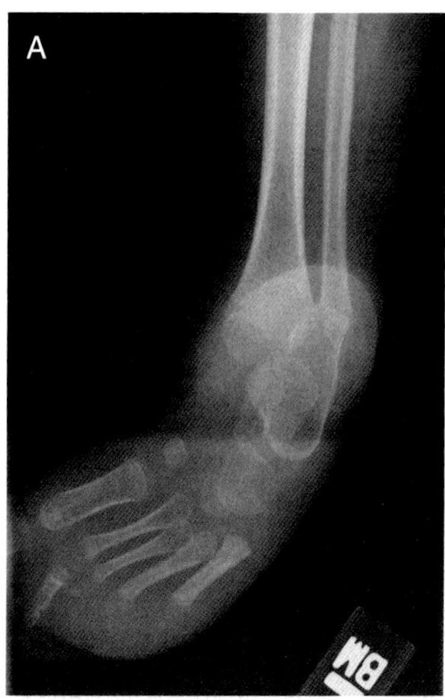

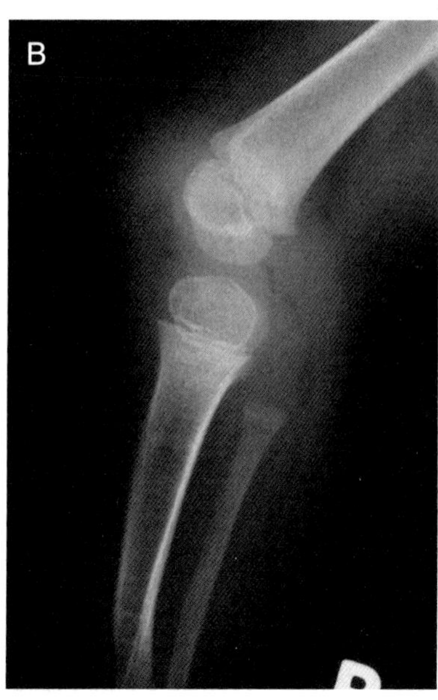

FIGURE 32-12 Adams-Oliver syndrome. **A.** Rigid talipes equinovarus seen in Adams-Oliver syndrome. **B.** Congenital distal limbs amputations are common.

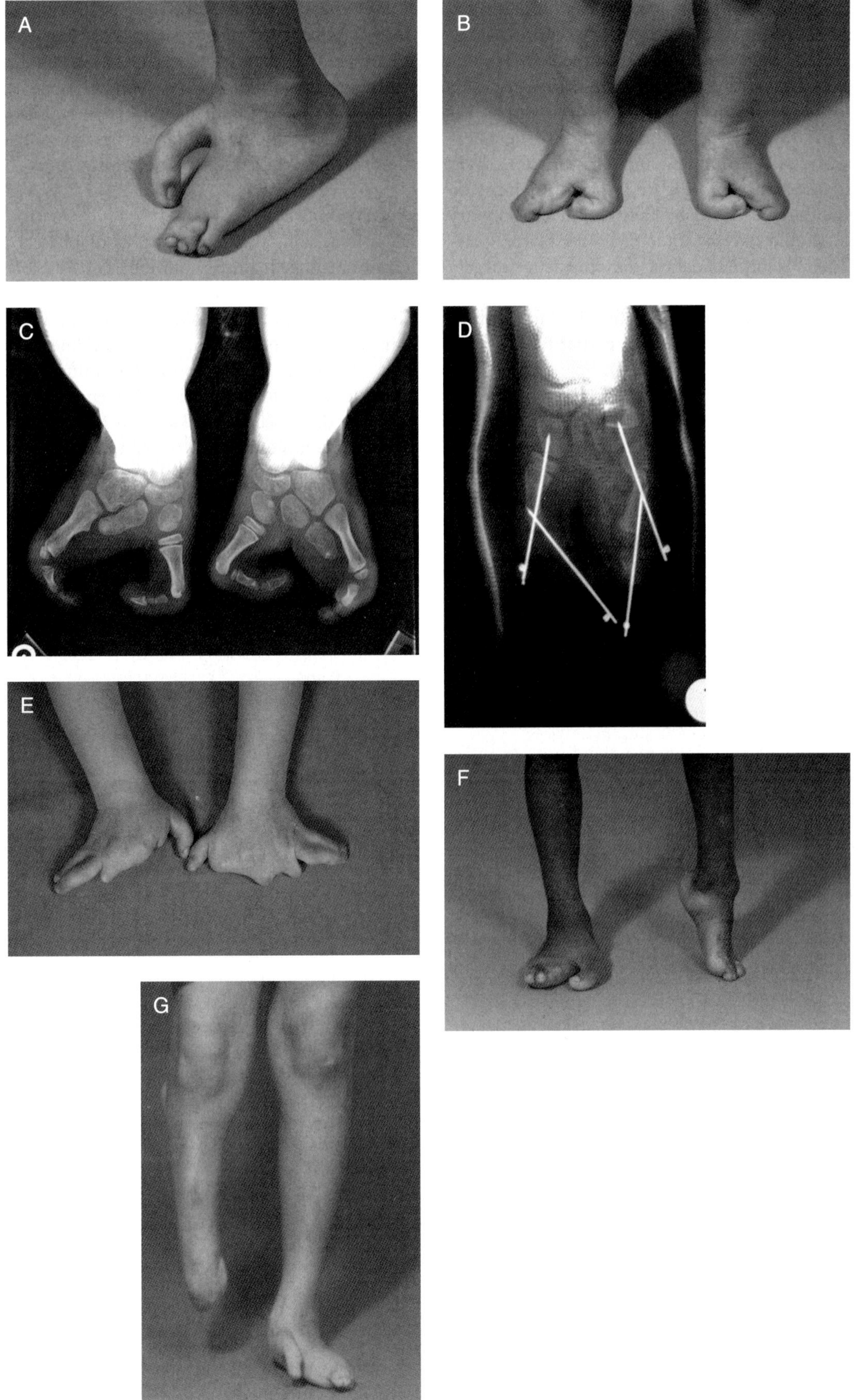

FIGURE 32-13 Ectrodactyly. **A**. Severe split foot seen in ectrodactyly. **B–D**. Symptomatic feet may require osteotomy. **E**. The hands may be also involved. **F–G**. Severe deformities with shortening; may require amputation.

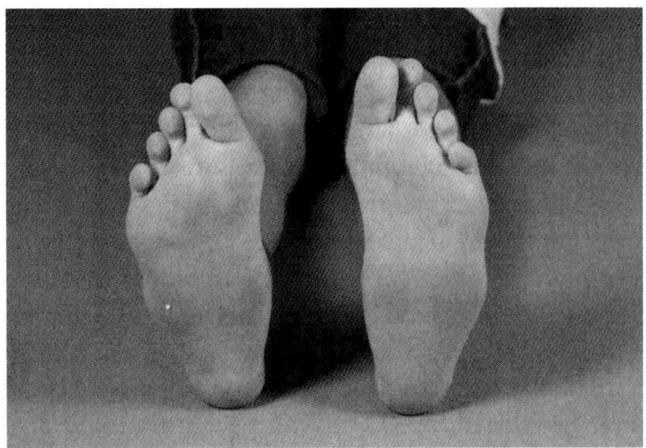

FIGURE 32-16 Ehlers-Danlos syndrome: pes planus and overlapping toes are frequently seen in this condition with ligamentous laxity.

forms (type II). Smith (104) feels that the recessive form may represent a sporadic mutation of the dominant gene. Sillence (201,202) has delineated the phenotypes into 4 types, describing the recessive variety as having more severe involvement, including perinatal demise in type II. The classification is evolving and there are now up to 12 reported types. Its classification as a syndrome may be more appropriate (163).

The orthopedic problems of these patients include fragile bones with multiple fractures and resultant skeletal deformities. There may be flatfeet with joint dislocation, or arachnodactyly (135). Gross ankle deformity secondary to multiple tibial and femoral fractures can result in abnormal positioning of the foot, requiring surgical correction (Figure 32-17). The foot bones themselves are not usually significantly deformed in children. However, adolescents and adults with severe involvement may develop foot degenerative changes secondary to multiple fractures and long-term malposition. The main stay of orthopedic treatment remains intra medullary rodding of the long bones to correct angular deformities although external fixator correction has been proposed (228). Cyclic IV administration of bisphosphonates has been popularized by Fassier and Glorieux with increases in bone density and decreased incidence of bone pain and fracture (250).

Fibrodysplasia Ossificans Progressiva Syndrome

This syndrome also known as myositis ossificans congenita is inherited in an autosomal dominant manner (54). In addition to fibrous dysplasia and ossification of the soft tissues, the most recognizable characteristic is a classic shortening of the first toe with hallux valgus (209). An interesting finding is that the toe is often monophalangic (136). The thumbs may be similarly affected and Rogers (180) found great toe involvement in 40 of 44 patients. Four patients in his report had good results after hallux valgus surgical correction, but the risk of post-operative stiffness is high in any extremity surgery for this population. More than 95% develop restrictive heterotopic ossification which is normal in its histologic appearance, but located in an ectopic site (136). These patients are generally diagnosed early and later develop spine and long bone problems such as humeral-chest wall synostosis and joint subluxation (64,193). The patients may develop classic-appearing cervical spine anomalies such as large posterior elements and narrow vertebral bodies with fusions between C2–C7. These appear morphologically different from the cervical spine anomalies of Klippel-Feil syndrome (195).

McKusick (135) outlined the metatarsal abnormalities leading to hallux valgus. This included shortening of both the metatarsal and phalanges with distortion of their proximal and distal ends. Radiographically, the first metatarsal is shortened and fused with the abnormal epiphysis of the proximal phalanx (87). Surgical correction requires

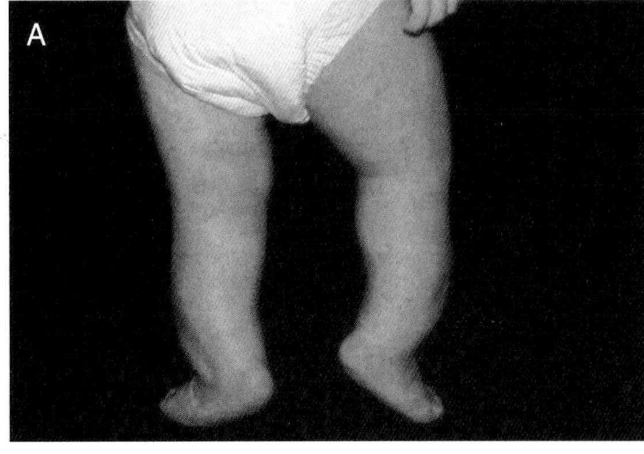

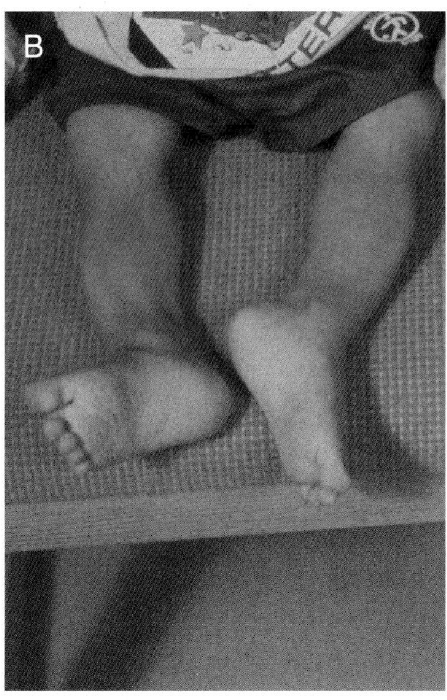

FIGURE 32-17 Osteogenesis imperfecta: the long bone deformities may lead to abnormal foot positions such as equinovarus (**A**) and malrotation (**B**).

not only a soft tissue release medially, but an additional osteotomy of the metatarsal and proximal phalanx.

Soft-tissue trauma and influenza-like viral illness may trigger flare-ups of this condition with new heterotopic ossification production. The incidence of missed diagnosis is very high and surgical or anesthetic procedures can also trigger episodes of this condition. The wrong diagnosis may lead to inappropriate procedures and flare-ups. Acute swelling of the limbs with increased angiogenesis has been noted during flare-ups. The most common erroneous diagnoses are sarcoma and fibromatosis. However, the autosomal dominant inheritance pattern and clinical presentation allow for a more accurate diagnosis (112,143, 194,208,231).

Other auto-dominant conditions arising by mutation affecting the foot and ankle include Saethre-Chotzen syndrome and the Muenke type mutation. These result in tarsal fusions, brachiodactyly, clinidactyly, duplication of the phalanges and epiphyseal deformities (230). The osteolysis syndromes are also autosomal dominant although some are recessive and result in destruction of multiple osseous structures. In the foot, the tarsal bones degenerate and there is synovitis and short metatarsals, commonly the fourth (204).

Autosomal Recessive Conditions

With autosomal recessive conditions the risk of recurrence in a family is 25%. The phenotype is only present clinically in the homozygote, carrying both recessive genes (242). These syndromes are common and frequently have orthopedic and foot involvement.

Storage Diseases

Most mucopolysaccharidoses are autosomal recessive, and for this review may be considered together. These individuals frequently have multiple orthopedic problems resulting from a lysosomal enzyme deficiency. The enzymes are used for glycosaminoglycan degradation and the syndromes result from the accumulation of these mucopolysaccharides in various tissues. There are at least six of these conditions with both similarities and variations (104,135,144). The common entities and their relationship to foot anomalies will be considered. All are autosomal recessive except Hunter syndrome (124,247).

Scheie syndrome results in stiff joints, a broad face with coarse features, corneal opacity, and normal mentation. There is joint limitation with occasional clawhand deformity, secondary to this deficiency of alphaiduronidase. The resulting foot deformity consists of broadening and widening of the feet which is only minimally disabling in these patients who survive into adulthood.

Hurler syndrome (124) also presents with a coarse face and corneal opacity, but has associated mental retardation, hepatosplenomegaly, and elbow contractures. The patients have widened diaphyseal sections of the long bones and metacarpals, but only flatfeet have been described as foot problems. Survival is frequently limited to the first and second decades. Maroteaux-Lamy syndrome has a Hurler phenotype. Foot problems have not been described for this group of patients, but genu valgum has been described which can create an abnormal foot and lower extremity posture. This may be improved with epiphyseal stapling (154).

Hunter syndrome, the most severe of the storage diseases, is X-linked recessive. Facial changes, clouded corneas, and stiff joints are present. There is less flaring of the long bones than in Hurler syndrome, but the contractures can lead to an equinovarus deformity. The more severely affected die in childhood and those with milder types rarely require surgery unless severe contractures impede ambulation.

Sanfilippo syndrome, secondary to heparin sulfatase deficiency, results in mental retardation, behavioral problems and progressive mental deterioration. These patients develop scoliosis and stiff joints. Equinovarus foot deformities may occur due to local contractures (Figure 32-18). Surgery is indicated at an early age prior to development of a rigid clubfoot, subsequent physical deterioration, and loss of ambulation. Progressive foot deformity may be prevented with bracing. Survival may be into the third decade.

Morquio syndrome results from the absence of a sulfatase enzyme with resulting skeletal deformities consisting of genu valgum and kyphoscoliosis. Foot involvement is limited except for short, broad flatfeet with hindfoot valgus reminiscent of Scheie or Hurler syndrome (Figure 32-19). Orthotic control may be warranted to help maintain a normal foot position in these patients who frequently survive into adulthood. Surgery, however, is rarely needed for the foot.

Glycogen storage disease IV is mutation resulting in early liver failure and death with arthrogrypotic-like changes in the lower extremities (136). Myofibrilar myopathy refers to a heterogenesis group of storage diseases affecting skeletal musculature. There is associated cardiac muscle weakness with cardiac arrhythmias and failure. Distal lower extremity weakness results in a flaccid appearance of the foot and ankle (136).

Multiple Pterygium Syndrome

Also known as Escobar syndrome (104), this autosomal recessive condition consists of multiple pterygium about

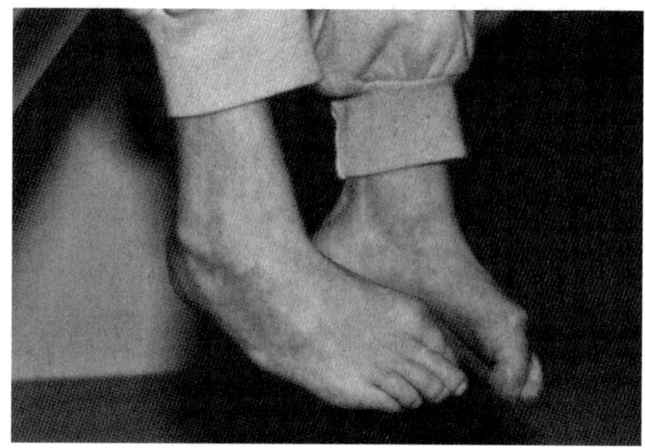

FIGURE 32-18 Storage disease: Sanfilippo syndrome; the rigid equinovarus seen in Sanfilippo syndrome.

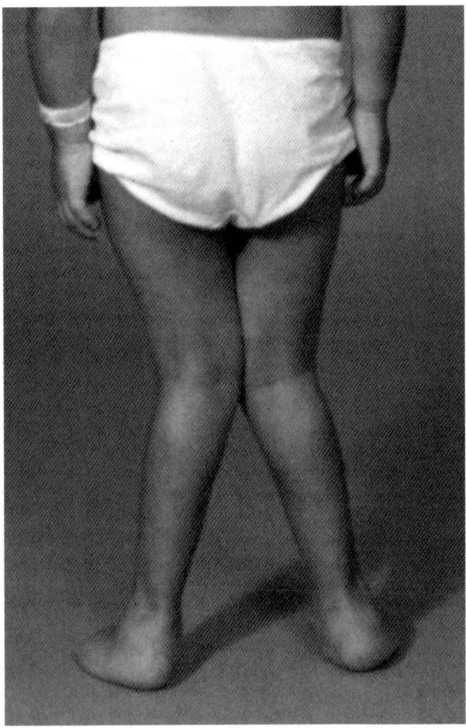

FIGURE 32-19 Storage disease: Morquio syndrome; characteristic broad flat feet and hind foot valgus.

the neck, shoulder, elbow, and knee (62,85), with a characteristic facies and vertebral anomalies. The pterygia may result from fetal akinesia and the condition may arise from a spontaneous mutation (136,156). There may be associated camptodactyly, syndactyly, and contractures leading to a clubfoot or a rocker-bottom foot deformity (Figure 32-20). A lethal form of multiple pterygium syndrome has also been described by Hall. It exhibits multiple contractures and pterygia involving all major joints. Another form presents with complete syndactyly of the hands and feet (16). The presentation of most forms clinically is similar to that of arthrogryposis (156).

The feet are involved with talipes equinovarus, calcanovalgus, and vertical tali. The malposition is extremely rigid due to the underlying soft tissue contractures, requiring extensive soft tissue releases in a young child, or an additional talectomy or lateral osteotomy if older. Similar to arthrogryposis, other joint contractures have to be corrected in order to maintain ambulation.

Cockayne Syndrome

This autosomal recessive condition results in senile-like changes in early infancy with deterioration of vision and hearing, hepatosplenomegaly, arteriosclerosis, and dermatitis of the skin (129). The musculoskeletal changes include kyphosis, joint restriction, and cyanosis of the extremities. Equinus contractures and clubfoot deformities are common (Figure 32-21). The patients require long-term bracing due to frequent recurrence, and ambulation may be lost due to progressive loss of balance. There is a risk of premature demise (average age 12 years) in many patients, but some patients survive into adulthood (149,170). There are defects in DNA nucleotide repair with reduced myelination in the brain (118).

Less Frequent Autosomal Recessive Conditions

Foot involvement may be a minor factor in some of the rare autosomal recessive conditions. This generally does not require treatment, but may aid in the diagnosis. For example, Seckel syndrome (131) exhibits short stature, microcephaly, a beaked nose, mental retardation, and dislocated elbows. There is a characteristic separation between the first and second toes which does not inhibit ambulation. This syndrome exhibits a marked phenotypic

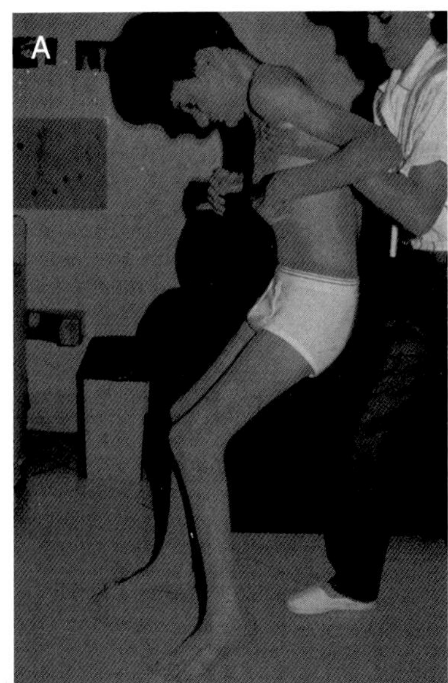

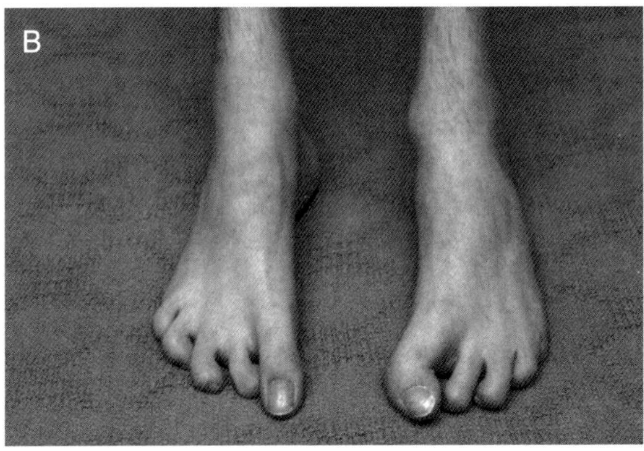

FIGURE 32-20 Multiple pterygium syndrome. **A.** This condition presents with multiple joint contractures. **B.** Toe deformities, clubfoot, or rocker-bottom foot may be present.

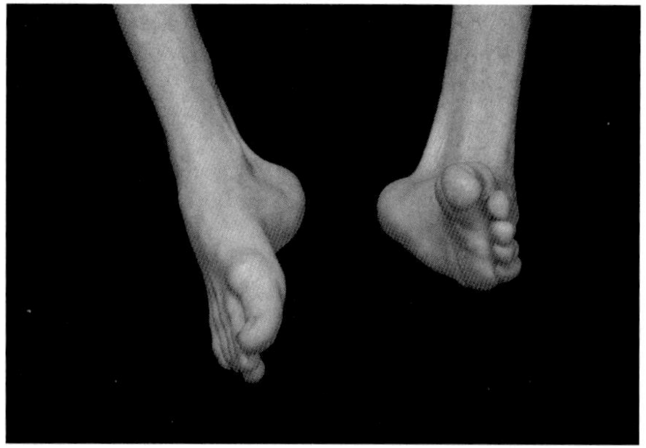

FIGURE 32-21 Cockayne syndrome: senile changes and clubfoot are part of the Cockayne syndrome.

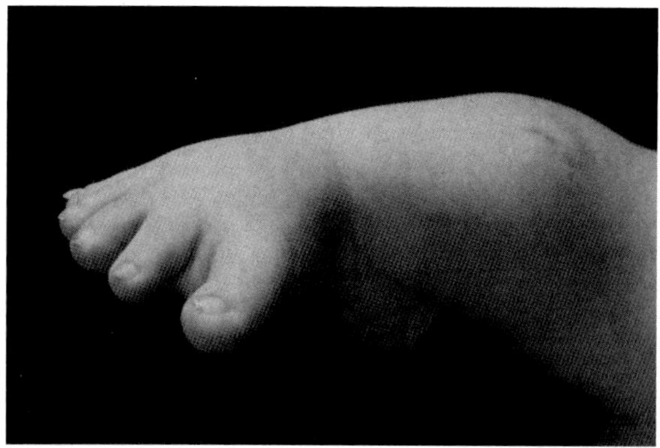

FIGURE 32-22 Camptomelic syndrome: the severe clubfoot seen in Campomelia.

variability which may be related to chromosome fragility during replication (40).

Similarly, patients with *Smith-Lemli-Opitz syndrome* (104,207) present with short stature, microcephaly, mental retardation, and foot disorders consisting of metatarsus adductus, and syndactyly of the second and third toes. Unless grossly affected, these foot anomalies require no correction.

Cerebro-oculo-facioskeletal syndrome is an autosomal recessive condition consisting of microcephaly; hypotonia; eye, nose, and ear defects; and multiple contractures with resultant foot deformities (165,220). These include rocker-bottom feet, vertical tali, and posterior displacement of the second metatarsal. Camptodactyly, scoliosis, and osteoporosis are also frequently present. This condition is possibly related to brain and spinal cord degeneration and may be a variant of neuropathic arthrogryposis. Survival is frequently limited to early childhood due to progressive deterioration and failure to thrive.

The *camptomelic syndrome* is an autosomal recessive (104) skeletal dysplasia with multiple congenital deformities including clubfeet. This syndrome consists of a flat face, macrocephaly, and skeletal changes (95). The cardinal features for this diagnosis are anterior tibial bowing, severe rigid clubfeet, short thin lower extremities, a skin depression over the tibial deformity, and other coexisting anomalies including chest, vertebral, and scapular deformities (Figure 32-22). The deformities may be severe enough to be diagnosed by prenatal ultrasonography (206). Demise is frequently in early childhood, secondary to respiratory compromise, but long-term survival has been reported, and these patients may require surgical intervention for clubfoot and other deformities. The talipes equinovarus is extremely rigid with a proximal tibial defect, making operative correction difficult.

Another rare autosomal recessive condition with clubfeet is *Zellweger syndrome* which consists of hypotonia, facial changes, hepatomegaly, and renal anomalies. There are multiple joint contractures with clubfeet and delayed skeletal maturation, which help distinguish this condition from Down syndrome which has a similar phenotypic appearance of hypotonia and a "mongoloid" appearance (110). Zellweger syndrome also has a metabolic component with disturbances in peroxisome and mitochondrial function. Neuro-imaging, specifically MRI scanning may be helpful in diagnosing this syndrome due to cortical or myelination abnormalities (20,141,218).

A similar condition is *Mohr syndrome,* which has oral and facial changes, and associated toe syndactyly, polydactyly, and bilateral reduplication of the hallux. Silengo (200) described both hand and foot polydactyly and syndactyly in a single patient. Levy (125) presented Mohr patients with broadening of the metatarsals and navicular, and duplication of the cuneiforms. The bifid great toe is the hallmark of this syndrome and the condition resembles oral-facial-digital syndrome but has a lower incidence and different inheritance pattern. There can also be polydactyly and shortening of the upper extremities (94,107).

Polydactyly is also a part of *Grebe syndrome,* an autosomal recessive condition, which has limb shortening and dwarfism. There may be missing digits or polydactyly. The fingers actually resemble toes. Romeo (181) discusses hypoplasia of the metatarsals, tarsal and metatarsal fusion, short phalanges, and hindfoot valgus in this disorder. Fibula hemimelia, digital duplication, and hallux valgus are common associated foot deformities (6,168).

Similarly, the *Bardet-Biedl syndrome* results in a phenotype of obesity, retinal changes, renal disease, virilism, and polydactyly. Haning (86) described a patient with postaxial hexadactyly of the hands and feet who required removal of the extra digits. In a recent study, 17 out of 27 patients had post axial polydactyly and the authors questioned the true existence of epiphyseal dysgenesis which has been described. They felt the changes in the epiphysis were secondary to obesity (167). Bardet-Biedl syndrome may be a complex mutation of three genes (triallelic inheritance), rather than a simple autosomal recessive trait (109). The existence of metatarsal epiphyseal dysgenesis has been supported by the finding of a metatarsal pseudoepiphysis (145). There is an abnormal gait pattern which may be related to the polydactyly and obesity but also to temporal lobe abnormalities noted on MRIs (43).

Radial aplasia-thrombocytopenia syndrome, or TAR, is an autosomal recessive condition with absent radii, ulnar hypoplasia, and multiple limb defects (104). Many of the patients succumb prior to age two, but those who survive have diminishing trouble from the thrombocytopenia. The limb anomalies consist of coxa valga, knee and ankle contractures, femorotibial fusions, hip dislocation, and teratophocomelia, similar to that seen in thalidomide congenital defects (Figure 32-23). Anyane-Yeboa (12) recommends deferring any elective surgery until the platelet count normalizes.

McLaurin et al. noted foot deformities in multiple patients including calcaneovalgus feet, overlapping fifth and second toes, and syndactyly (137). Christensen and Ferguson found lower extremity deformities in all 11 TAR patients in their study, consisting of foot abnormalities such as equinovarus and metatarsal synostosis (45).

Antley-Bixler

This is a rare condition with skeletal cranio-facial and urological abnormalities. This is autosomal recessive and results in lower extremity bowing, clubfoot, syndactyly, and vertebral abnormalities. The toes and feet are elongated and there may be a synostosis between the cuboid and cuneiform. The clubfoot may be present in up to 20% of the cases and there may be prenatal fractures diagnosed by ultrasound (186).

Baller-Gerold Syndrome

Baller-Gerold syndrome is an autorecessive condition with skeletal, cardiac, facial, genitourinary, gastrointestinal and craniosynostosis abnormalities. There are numerous upper extremity anomalies that include club hand, hypoplastic thumbs, and absent metacarpals. In the lower extremities, there is bowing and hip dislocation with hypoplastic first toes and brachiodactyly of the others, along with syndactyly and polydactyly. The extent of treatment depends on the clinical severity (224).

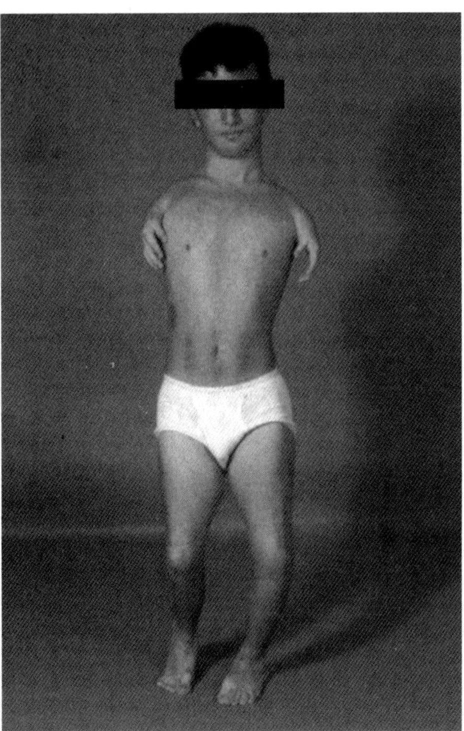

FIGURE 32-23 Radial aplasia-thrombocytopenia syndrome: TAR; phocomelia and lower extremity deformities are part of TAR syndrome.

Sex-Linked Disorders

These types of syndromes are carried on the X or Y chromosome and are related to the sex of the patient. Several such conditions are commonly seen by orthopedists. Hemophilia, Duchenne muscular dystrophy, and hypophosphatemic rickets are examples of this. The above conditions have only rare foot involvement and need not be considered in this discussion, except for Duchenne muscular dystrophy which is presented in another chapter. Other sex-linked conditions are not frequently evaluated by orthopedists, but they do have foot and ankle involvement and may present for treatment.

Oto-palato-digital syndrome, known also as *Taybi syndrome*, has an X-linked semi-dominant etiology with variable expression in females. The phenotype consists of deafness, cleft palate, a characteristic facial appearance, and a generalized skeletal dysplasia (104). Dudding describes short, broad first toes and terminal phalanges, syndactyly, and hypoplasia of the great toenail (58). Toe flexion, equinovarus, or hindfoot valgus deformities may develop with subsequent degeneration of the ankle joint. There is a "distinctive pattern" of radiographic changes in the feet consisting of abnormally shaped first, second and third metatarsals, with midfoot accessory ossification centers, and hypoplasia of the navicular and cuneiforms. The feet may require surgical correction consisting of soft tissue releases, a hindfoot osteotomy, or arthrodesis.

Several authors have described a similar dysplasia, oto-palato-digital syndrome type II, in which patients have more growth retardation, shorter survival, tibial bowing, and absent fibulae (36,215). The feet are also involved with ossification defects, short toes, polydactyly, and syndactyly. This syndrome may be secondary to defective intramembranous ossification (155). Surgery most likely is not being required in this subgroup, which is frequently lethal.

Conditions with Unknown Genetics

Some syndromes are currently without a true definite genetic pathway. However, they appear more frequently in families, and deserve consideration here for their foot and ankle implications.

Rubenstein-Taybi is a syndrome of unknown genetic etiology. It may arise from a genetic mutation that results in a deficiency of histone transferase activity (147,179).

Those affected have a normal chromosomal karyotype. It most likely is a multifactorial trait resulting in a characteristic face, mental retardation, and broad thumbs and toes (185,203). The phalanges of the great toes are prominent, and the toe and thumb broadening is a criterion which may be useful in forming a diagnosis. Foot surgery for this condition has not been reported. Wood and Rubenstein describe "the kissing delta phalanx" in the toes which is a duplicated longitudinal bracked epiphysis (241). This was present in 30 out of 530 patients (241). In those who are symptomatic, they recommend removal of the extra nail and partial resection of the duplicated phalanx (241).

The patello-femoral joint is unstable in this condition in a minority of patients and if symptomatic, Mehlman et al. recommend quadriceplasty or quadricepts lengthening (138). These patients can have severe anesthetic and surgical complications due to airway and cervical spine abnormalities which should be evaluated preoperatively (246).

The overgrowth syndromes result in localized asymmetric growth of the limbs. There is a spectrum of these disease states with foot involvement ranging from congenital gigantism of the toe to Klippel-Trenaunay-Weber syndrome. The genetic pattern of these conditions is uncertain. Pellerin (160) has proposed the term "congenital soft tissue dysplasia" based on the histological appearance of normal differentiated cell overgrowth. He does not feel these are purely vascular disorders. The dysplasia may arise from disturbances of several cell regulation mechanisms secondary to environmental factors or a genetic mutation. The mutation of a growth factor regulatory gene has also been proposed by Kousseff causing the elimination of fine tuning and the dysregulation of growth (115,116). Other overgrowth syndromes may affect the foot size and function. The feet are generally larger and may have toe abnormalities. The inheritance patterns are variable and these syndromes include Beckworth-Weiderman (auto dominant); Sotos (sporadic); Weaver (sporadic); Proteus (sporadic); and Simpson-Golabi-Belmel (X-linked recessive) (174).

Congenital gigantism or *macrodactyly* of the foot falls under this category. In true macrodactyly, there is an increased size of all elements of the toe, not just the soft tissue (19,232). There is a static form present at birth, and as well as a variant with progressive disproportionate growth. The toes may enlarge to a size that affects shoe wear or the position of the adjacent toes. Generally not all toes are affected (171). The medial digits appear more involved, and syndactyly is frequently an associated finding (Figure 32-24). Grogan reviewed ten cases of macrodactyly associated with congenital lipofibromatosis of the foot (78). In this condition, there is fibro-fatty proliferation and an abundance of such tissue on the plantar aspect of the toes and foot.

Treatment ranges from observation to amputation and ray resection depending on the severity of involvement. Debulking procedures and epiphysiodesis of the phalanges may produce acceptable cosmetic results, as will ray resections in severe involvement. Isolated phalangeal resection only corrects part of the problem (78).

Klippel-Trenaunay-Weber syndrome is also part of this spectrum of asymmetric gigantism. In this condition there is variable limb gigantism and hemangiomata which may be capillary or cavernous, with large varicosities (160,214). The skin, brain, and skeletal system may all be involved. The hypertrophy may be so significant as to require amputation or may result in isolated toe enlargement (Figure 32-25). The vascular status of these patients needs to be carefully evaluated prior to any elective procedure. Due to the abnormal vasculature, bleeding problems, poor skin healing, and a high rate of thromboembolism can occur postoperatively (21). These patients can develop cardiopulmonary compromise, spinal cord arterioveneous malformations with cord compromise, rhabdomyosarcoma, debilitating soft-tissue and osseous pain, and genitourinary involvement (3,34,65,98,123).

Similarly, Proteus syndrome produces eccentric limb enlargement with macrodactyly, subcutaneous vascular

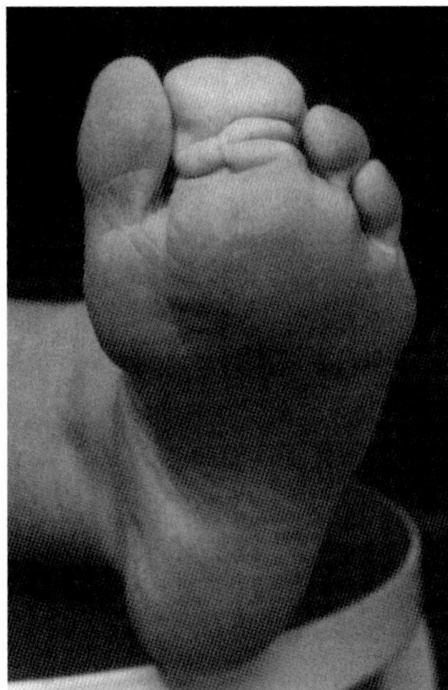

FIGURE 32-24 Macrodactyly: congenital gigantism. In macrodactyly, there may be increased size of all toe components.

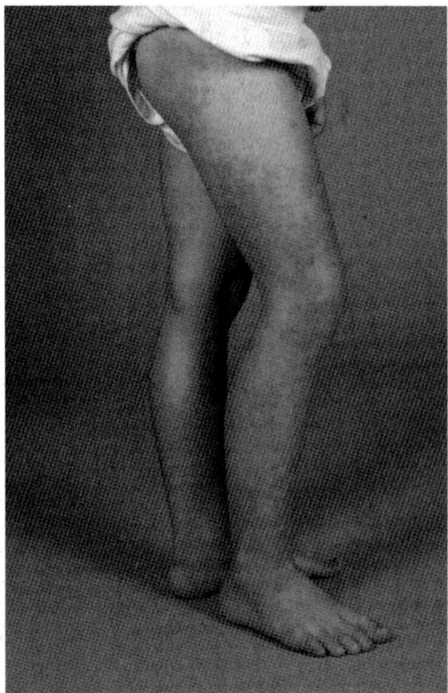

FIGURE 32-25 Klippel-Trenaunay-Weber syndrome. Unilateral hypertrophy seen in Klippel-Trenaunay-Weber syndrome.

tumors, and hyperpigmented nevi or streaks (47). The limbs are frequently normal at birth with progressive enlargement. Additionally, these patients have large fat deposits in the limbs and abdomen. Acetabular dysplasia and focal myositis have also been described as have central nervous system abnormalities and scoliosis (10,55,108,223). The overlap of phenotypes between Klippel-Trenaunay-Weber and Proteus syndromes is significant, and may well be a constellation of similar conditions as proposed by Pellerin (160). Surgical excision of the excess tissue has been proposed, but may be complicated by scars, keloid, recurrence, and further overgrowth after surgery.

Cremin (52) has used MRI scanning to define the mesodermal malformations, and Azouz (17) illustrated radiographic changes including hypertrophy of the first metatarsals and phalanges with aberrant calcification of the navicular and medial cuneiform bones. Jamis-Dow has described the specific radiographic criteria for diagnosing Proteus syndrome, stating the importance of this since specific genetic testing is not available (102). Bone imaging is also helpful with the diagnosis, showing areas of overgrowth (105). Surgery in these complex patients should be approached cautiously.

Intrauterine Environmental Factors

Although not truly genetic in nature, these conditions should be considered in this discussion. They may be idiopathic in origin, but they occur *in utero*, are present at birth, and result in significant skeletal deformities. Having many severe foot anomalies, these conditions should be included in the differential diagnosis, not as truly genetic conditions, but as related disorders.

Congenital constriction band sequence or amniotic band syndrome is one such anomaly. This is also referred to as *Streeter syndrome*. These patients present with congenital amputations, syndactyly, clubfoot, and facial or visceral anomalies (15) (Figure 32-26). The deformities most likely occur secondary to limb compression by the amniotic bands. Jones calls this early amniotic rupture sequence and relates the timing of the rupture to the deformity (104). For example rupture at five weeks' gestation results in limb amputation, polydactyly, and syndactyly, whereas if the insult occurs after seven weeks there is

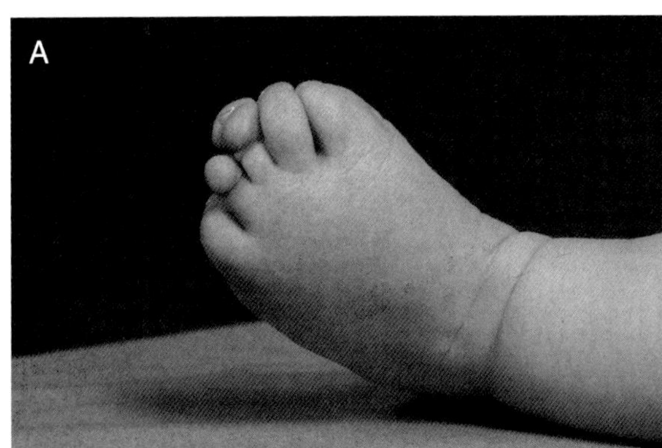

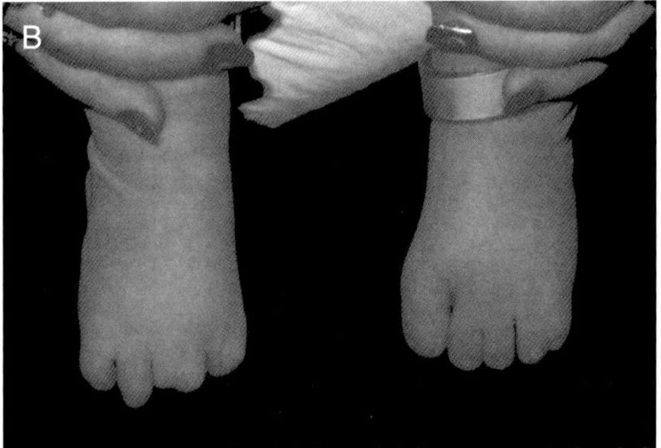

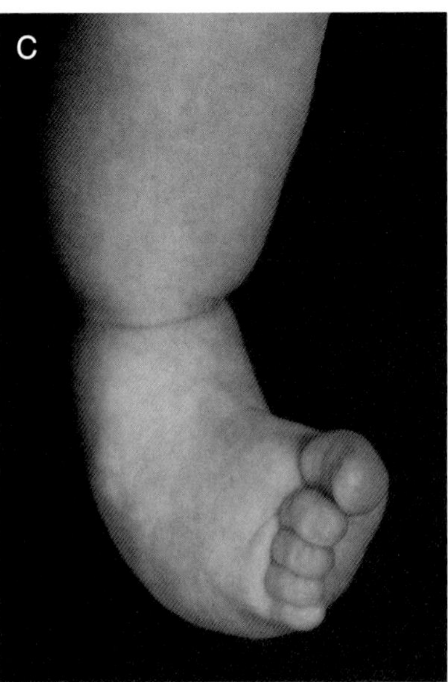

FIGURE 32-26 Streeter syndrome. **A.** Toe abnormalities from amniotic bands. **B.** Toe amputations. **C.** Clubfoot with severe constriction proximally.

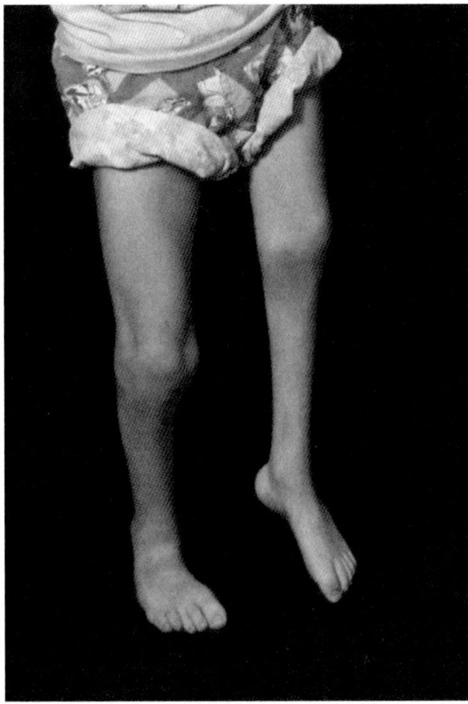

FIGURE 32-27 VATER association. Clubfoot, syndactyly, and polydactyly are all part of the VATER association.

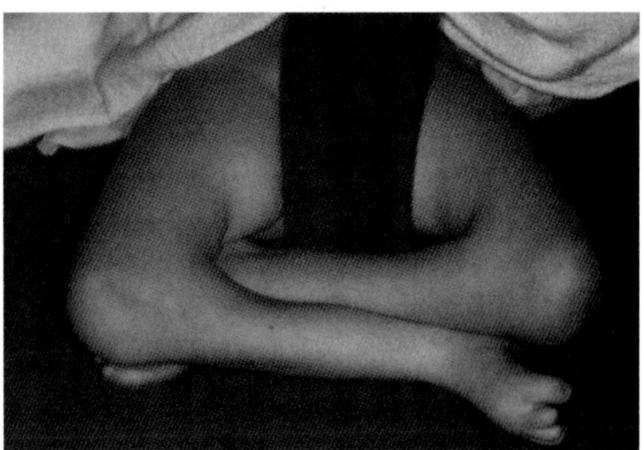

FIGURE 32-28 Caudal regression. **A.** The crossed-leg appearance of caudal regression with rigid lower extremity contractures.

foot deformation such as clubfoot. Others consider this a spectrum of arthrogryposis.

The talipes equinovarus is usually severe and rigid. The constriction bands generally need to be released serially prior to correction of the foot deformity. Forty-two percent of the patients in the Askins study had syndactyly, including both fenestrated (acrosyndactyly) fusion or complex syndactyly in which both the soft tissue and bones are fused (15). The toe syndactyly frequently requires no treatment, but the clubfoot needs to be corrected surgically. Long-term casting and bracing is required to prevent recurrence, but with appropriate treatment, good function and independent mobility can be achieved and maintained (240).

The *VATER* (104) *association* consists of vertebral, anal, tracheal, esophageal, and renal defects. The association is non-random and is seen more frequently in diabetic mothers. There may be subsets of this condition with multiple other anomalies. Up to 78% of VATER association patients have other system defects (32). The condition may be the result of an undefined teratogenic event between the fourth and eighth week of gestation. Skeletal anomalies include scoliosis, clubfoot, polydactyly, syndactyly, and radial aplasia (Figure 32-27). The spine defects include congenital vertebral anomalies, torticollis and scoliosis. These may be diagnosed by intrauterine ultrasound (4,237).

The "lobster claw" foot deformity has also been described, reminiscent of ectrodactyly (60). This may require surgical realignment, as described previously, if the patient thrives and is ambulatory. The syndactyly and polydactyly may need no treatment unless affecting ambulation, but the talipes equinovarus and lower

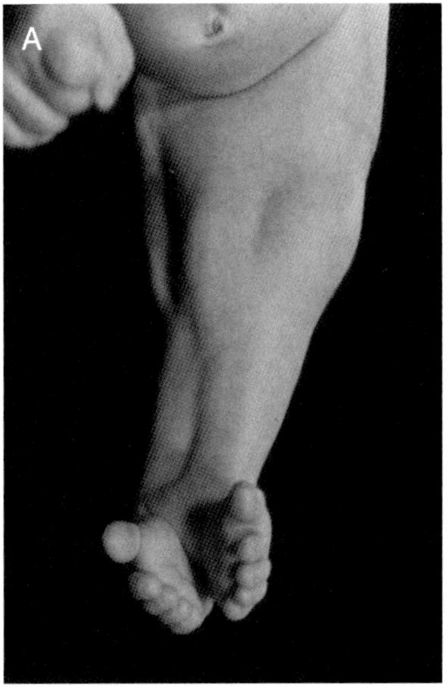

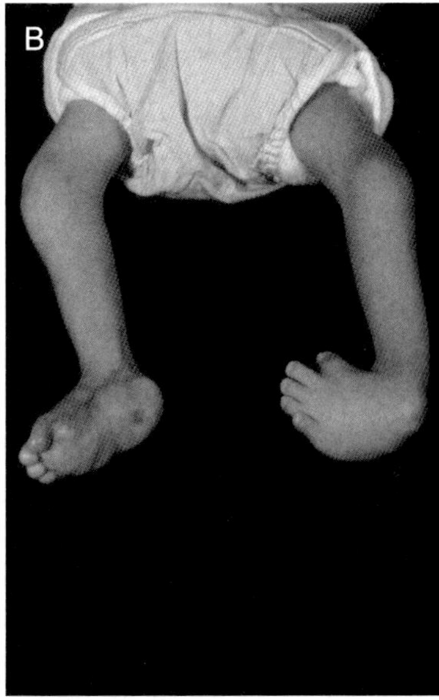

FIGURE 32-29 Sirenomelia. **A.** Complete lower extremity fusion seen in sirenomelia. **B.** Post-separation and prior to final foot reconstruction.

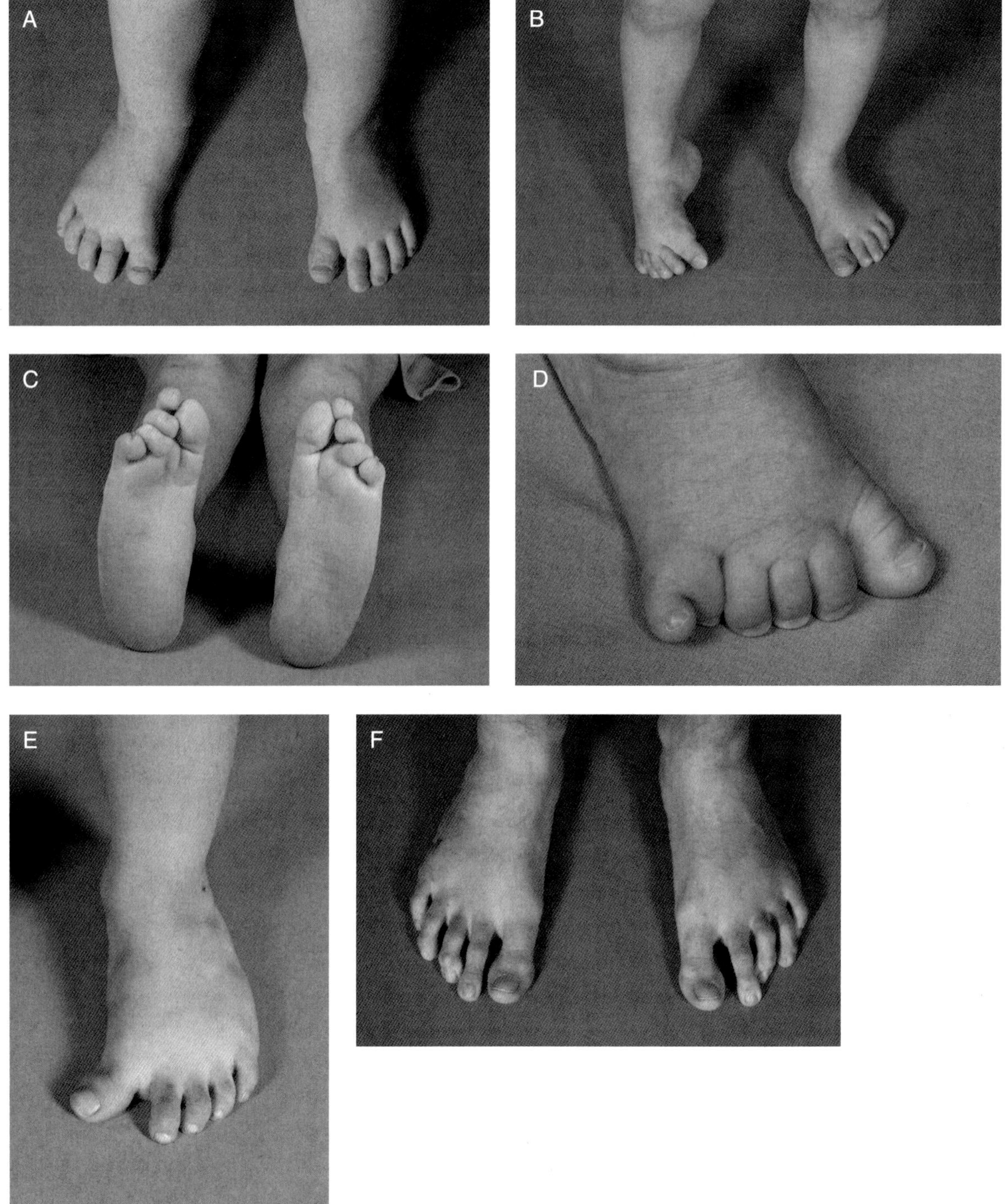

FIGURE 32-30 General manifestations of the foot seen in various genetic conditions. **A.** Brachydactyly. **B.** Cavovarus. **C.** Claw toes. **D.** Duplication. **E.** Hallux varus. **F.** Hammer toes. **G.** Pes planus. **H.** Clubfoot. **I.** Rocker-bottom feet. **J.** Syndactyly.

extremity contractures frequently require surgical intervention. Cardiac, pulmonary, and tracheal abnormalities may complicate any surgical treatment (33).

Caudal regression is also an intrauterine defect seen more commonly in diabetic mothers. Maternal diabetes may also be a factor with 22% of cases having a diabetic mother (219). Vascular insufficiency and teratogens have also been identified as possible etiologies (205). This is a syndrome with sacral agenesis and multiple lower extremity deformities in which maternal drug and alcohol abuse may also play a role (1,80). Spine, bladder, and neural tube anomalies are frequently associated and can be diagnosed *in utero* with scanning (90,106,198). The patients present with severe limb deformities including the "Buddha" crossed-leg appearance (Figure 32-28). The feet have a rigid clubfoot deformity and require both soft tissue releases and osteotomies or talectomy for correction. Many authors have proposed amputation, but with extensive

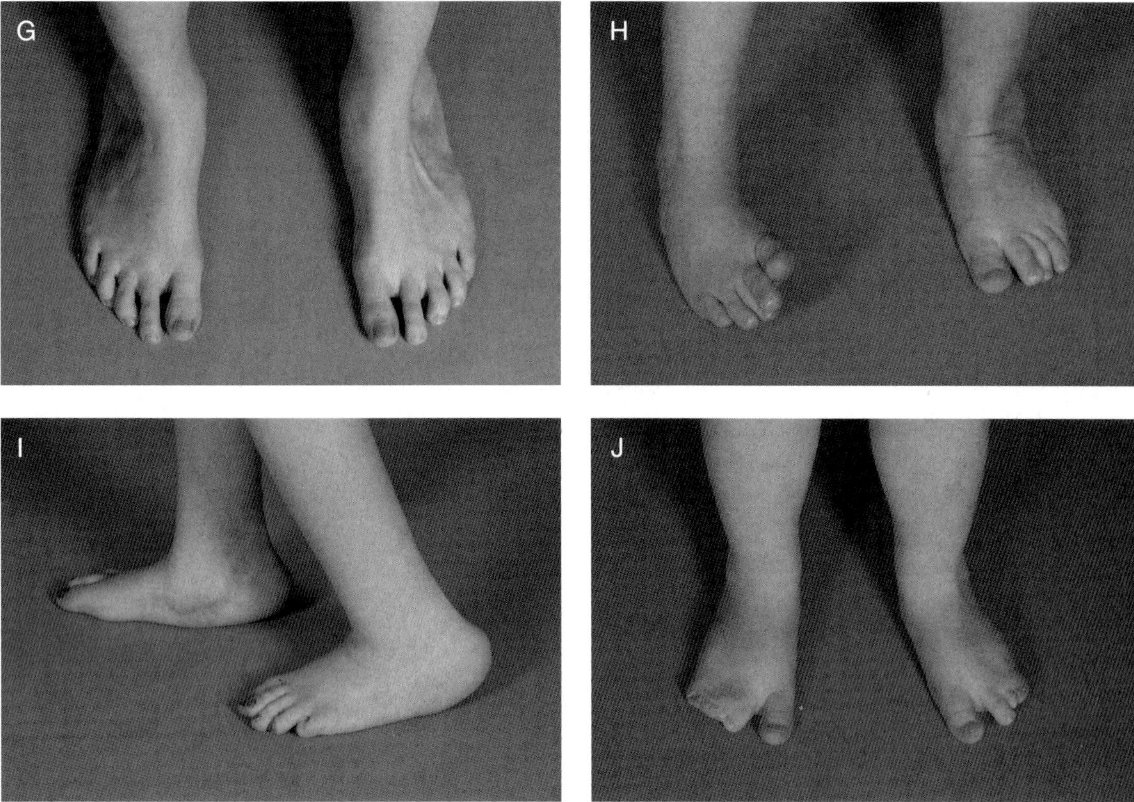

FIGURE 32-30 (*Continued*)

surgery the children may sit and stand with support rather than undergo complete limb ablation (18,80,159,161).

At the far end of the caudal regression spectrum is *sirenomelia* which is a complete fusion of the lower extremities with spine and genitourinary defects (59). Jones feels that this is related to a defect in the caudal blastema and Stevenson states the etiology may be a vascular-steal phenomenon (104,217). This rare condition (1 in 1,000,000 live births) may result from blood being diverted to the placenta from the lower extremities (vascular steal) or a defect in blastogenesis (120). An intrauterine diagnosis can be made with ultrasound or an MRI (150,192,234). The surgical separation of the lower limbs and subsequent reconstruction including the genitourinary and gastrointestinal systems requires a multidisciplinary team approach and numerous staged surgeries (140).

The patient in Figure 32-29 underwent complete limb separation, with skin grafting and clubfoot correction. This required tissue expanders, extensive soft-tissue releases, and a calcaneal osteotomy. This patient, now a teenager, has become independently ambulatory after multiple surgical procedures.

SUMMARY

The genetic basis for disease has many manifestations in the skeletal system, especially in the foot and ankle. These conditions demonstrate great variety from autosomal dominant to sex-linked states. The involvement spans a spectrum from major foot deformity as in nail-patella syndrome with clubfeet, to minor involvement as in Carpenter syndrome with syndactyly and polydactyly (Figure 32-30). In each of these syndromes the foot may be a presenting anomaly, as well as a key to the diagnosis. In treating genetic conditions with foot involvement, one has to evaluate the deformity and decide where it fits into a syndrome. For example syndactyly, polydactyly, and clubfoot are frequent manifestations of genetic diseases, but their involvement varies with each entity, as does the treatment. As always, the surgeon should attempt to preserve and enhance function over appearance and cosmesis. The physician needs to be cognizant of the overall ramifications of each syndrome, prior to attempting correction of the foot deformity. Some patients will have shortened survival, a fragile medical state, or lose ambulation potential early. These factors will greatly affect orthopedic treatment. Knowledge of these conditions and their associated foot involvement hopefully will facilitate diagnosis, treatment, and genetic counseling in these complex patients.

ACKNOWLEDGMENTS

The authors wish to acknowledge the following staff from Shriners Hospitals for Children: Nancy R. Pisciotto, RN,

ONC for her contribution with the chapter figures; Betsy Wehrwein for her work with references; and Kathleen Wielatz, Tim Boehlke, and Donabelle (PT) Hansen for their assistance with media services. The authors also wish to thank the patients and families for their contributions.

REFERENCES

1. Abraham E. Sacral agenesis with associated anomalies (caudal regression syndrome): Autopsy case report. *Clin Orthop* 145:168–171, 1979.
2. Ainsworth SR, Aulicino PL. A survey of patients with Ehlers-Danlos syndrome. *Clin Orthop Relat Res* 286:250–256, 1993.
3. Alexander MJ, Grossi PM, Spetzler RF, et al. Extradural thoracic arteriovenous malformation in a patient with Klippel-Trenaunay-Weber syndrome: Case report. *Neurosurg* 51:1275–1279, 2002.
4. Al Kaissi A, Chehida BF, Safi H, et al. Progressive congenital torticollis in VATER association syndrome. *Spine* 31:e376–e378, 2006.
5. Alves AF, Azevedo ES. Recessive form of Freeman-Sheldon's syndrome or "whistling face." *J Med Genet* 14:139–141, 1997.
6. Al-Yahyaee SA, Al-Kindi MN, Habbal O, et al. Clinical and molecular analysis of Grebe acromesomelic dysplasia in an Omani family. *Am J Med Gen Part A* 121:9–14, 2003.
7. Amor DJ, Leventer RJ, Hayllar S, et al. Polymicrogyria associated with scalp and limb defects: Variant of Adams-Oliver syndrome. *Am J Med Genet* 93:328–334, 2000.
8. Amory JK, Anawalt BD, Paulsen CA, et al. Klinefelter's syndrome. *Lancet* 356:333–335, 2000.
9. Anderson T: Earliest evidence for arthrogryposis multiplex congenita or Larsen syndrome? *Am J Med Gen* 71:127–129, 1997.
10. Andres BM, McCarthy EF, Frassica FJ: A muscular lesion suggestive of focal myositis in a child with Proteus syndrome. *Cl Orthop Rel Res* 404:326–329, 2002.
11. Antley RM, Uga N, Burzynski NJ, et al. Diagnostic criteria for the whistling face syndrome. *Birth Defects* 11:161–168, 1975.
12. Anyane-Yeboa K, Jaramillo S, Nagel C, et al. Brief clinical report: Tetraphocomelia in the syndrome of thrombocytopenia with absent radii (TAR syndrome). *Am J Med Genet* 20:571–576, 1985.
13. Ardinger HH, Hanson JW, Harrod MJ, et al. Further delineation of Weaver syndrome. *J Pediatr* 108:228–235, 1986.
14. Arizawa M, Nakayama M, Suehara N. Clinical spectrum and congenital anomalies in trisomy 18. *Acta Obstet Gynaecol Jpn* 41:1545–1550, 1989.
15. Askins G, Ger E. Congenital constriction band syndrome. *J Pediatr Orthop* 8:461–466, 1988.
16. Aslan Y, Erduran E, Kutlu N. Autosomal recessive multiple pterygium syndrome: A new variant? *Am J Med Genet* 93:194–197, 2000.
17. Azouz EM, Costa T, Fitch N. Radiologic findings in the proteus syndrome. *Pediatr Radiol* 17:481–485, 1987.
18. Banta JV, Nichols O. Sacral agenesis. *J Bone Joint Surg* 51A: 693–703, 1969.
19. Barsky,AJ. Macrodactyly. *J Bone Joint Surg* 49A:1255–1266, 1967.
20. Barth PG, Majoie CB, Gootjes J, et al. Neuroimaging of peroxisome biogenesis disorders (Zellweger spectrum) with prolonged survival. *Neurol* 6:439–444, 2004.
21. Baskerville PA, Ackroyd JS, Thomas ML, et al. The Klippel-Trenaunay syndrome: Clinical, radiological and haemodynamic features and management. *Br J Surg* 72:232–236, 1985.
22. Beal M. H, Falk RE, Ying KL. A patient with an interstitial deletion of the proximal portion of the long arm of chromosome 4. *Am J Med Genet* 31:553–557, 1988.
23. Beck RB, Brudno DS, Rosenbaum KN. Bilateral absence of the ulna in twins as a manifestation of the split hand-split foot deformity. *Am J Perinatol* 6:1–3, 1989.
24. Bell J. On brachydactyly and symphalangism. In: *Treasury of human inheritance.* London: Cambridge University Press, 1–31, 1951.
25. Benson M. Cornelia de Lange syndrome: A case study. *Neonat Net* 21:7–13, 2002.
26. Bhat BV, Ashok BA, Puri RK. Lobster claw hand and foot deformity in a family. *Indian Pediatr* 24:675–677, 1987.
27. Bidwell JP, Bennett GC, Bell MJ, et al. Leg lengthening for short stature in Turner's syndrome. *J Bone Joint Surg* 82 B:1174–1176, 2000.
28. Blank CE. Apert's syndrome (a type of acrocephalosyndactyly)-observations on a British series of thirty-nine cases. *Ann Hum Genet* 24:151–164, 1960.
29. Bojesen A, Juul S, Gravholt C, et al. Prenatal and postnatal prevalence of Klinefelter syndrome: A national registry study. *J Clin Endoc Metab* 88:622–626, 2003.
30. Bojesen A, Kristensen K, Birkebaek NH, et al. The metabolic syndrome is frequent in Klinefelter's syndrome and is associated with abdominal obesity and hypogonadism. *Diabet Care* 29:1591–1598, 2006.
31. Bonafede RP, Beighton P. Autosomal dominant inheritance of scalp defects with ectrodactyly. *Am J Med Genet* 3:35–41, 1979.
32. Botto LD, Khoury MJ, Mastroiacovo P, et al. The spectrum of congenital anomalies of the VATER association: An international study. *Am J Med Genet* 71:8–15, 1997.
33. Braddock SR. A new recessive syndrome with VATER-like defects, pulmonary hypertension, abnormal ears, blue sclera, laryngeal webs, and persistent growth deficiency. *Am J Med Genet* 123A:95–9, 2003.
34. Brandenburg VM, Graf J, Schubert H, et al. Images in cardiovascular medicine. Klippel-Trenaunay-Weber syndrome. *Circ* 111:e23, 2005.
35. Bravo JF, Wolff C. Clinical study of hereditary disorders of connective tissues in a Chilean population. *Arthr Rheumat* 54:515–523, 2006.
36. Brewster TG, Lachman RS, Kushner DC, et al. Oto-palato-digital syndrome, type II-an X-linked skeletal dysplasia. *Am J Med Genet* 20:249–254, 1985.
37. Butler MG, Meaney FJ, Palmer CG. Clinical and cytogenetic survey of 39 individuals with Prader-Labhart-Willi syndrome. *Am J Med Genet* 23:793–809, 1986.
38. Caird MS, Wills BP, Dormans JP. Down syndrome in children: The role of the orthopaedic surgeon. *J Am Acad Orthop Surg* 14:610–619, 2006.
39. Caldwell PD, Smith,DW. The XXY (Klinefelter's) syndrome in childhood: Detection and treatment. *J Pediatr* 80:250–258, 1972.
40. Casper AM, Durkin SG, Arlt MF, et al. Chromosomal instability at common fragile sites in Seckel syndrome. *Am J Hum Genet* 75:654–660, 2004.
41. Castle D, Bernstein R. Trisomy 18 syndrome with cleft foot. *J Med Genet* 25:568–570, 1988.
42. Čekada S, Kilvain S, Brajenović-Milić B, et al: Partial trisomy 13q22→qter and monosomy 18q21→qter as a result of familiar translocation. *Acta Paediatr* 8:675–678, 1999.
43. Chen CL, Chung CY, Cheng PT, et al. Linguistic and gait disturbance in a child with Laurence-Moon-Biedl syndrome. *Am J Phys Med Rehab* 83:69–74, 2004.
44. Chen CP. Arthrogryposis of the wrist and ankle associated with fetal trisomy 18. *Prenat Diag* 25:417–428, 2005.
45. Christensen CP, Ferguson RL. Lower extremity deformities associated with thrombocytopenia and absent radius syndrome. *Cl Orthop Rel Res* 375:202–206, 2000.

46. Cion, M, Cocilovo A, Rossi F, et al. Analysis of ankle kinetics during walking in individuals with Down syndrome. *Am J Assoc Ment Retard* 106:470–476, 2001.
47. Clark RD, Donnai D, Rogers J, et al. Proteus syndrome: An expanded phenotype. *Am J Med Genet* 27:99–117, 1987.
48. Cleveland RH, Holmes LB. Hand-foot-genital syndrome: The importance of hallux varus. *Pediatr Radiol* 20:339–343, 1990.
49. Coleman WB, Aronovitz DC. Surgical management of cleft foot deformity. *J Foot Surg* 27:497–502, 1988.
50. Concolino D, Pasquzzi A, Capalbo G. Early detection of podiatric anomalies in children with Down syndrome. *Acta Paediat* 95:17–20, 2006.
51. Corea JR, Sankaran-Kutty M. Lobster claw leg. *J Bone Joint Surg* 71B:861, 1989.
52. Cremin BJ, Vilgoen DL, Wynchank S, et al. The Proteus syndrome: The magnetic resonance and radiological features. *Pediatr Radiol* 17:486–488, 1987.
53. da-Silva EO, Filho SM, de Albuquerque SC. Multiple synostosis syndrome: Study of a large Brazilian kindred. *Am J Med Genet* 18:237–247, 1984.
54. Delatycki M, Rogers JG. The genetics of fibrodysplasia ossificans progressiva. *Cl Orthop Rel Res* 346:15–18, 1998.
55. Dietrich RB, Glidden DE, Roth GM, et al: The Proteus syndrome: CNS manifestations. *Am J Neuroradiol* 19:987–990, 1998.
56. Do T, Giampietro PF, Burke SW, et al. The incidence of protrusio acetabuli in Marfan's syndrome and its relationship to bone mineral density. J *Pediatr Orthop* 20:718–721, 2000.
57. Drouin CA, Grenon H. The association of Buschke-Ollendorf syndrome and nail-patella syndrome. *J Am Acad Derm* 46:621–625, 2002.
58. Dudding BA, Gorlin RJ, Langer LO. The oto-palato-digital syndrome. A new symptom-complex consisting of deafness, dwarfism, cleft palate, characteristic facies, and a generalized bone dysplasia. *Am J Dis Child* 113:214–221, 1967.
59. Duhamel B. From the mermaid to anal imperforation: The syndrome of caudal regression. *Arch Dis Child* 36:152–155, 1961.
60. Dusmet M, Fete F, Crusi A, et al. VATER association: Report of a case with three unreported malformations. *J Med Genet* 25:57–60, 1988.
61. Eberl MM, Baer MR, Mahoney MC, et al. Unsuspected Klinefelter syndrome diagnosed during oncologic evaluation: A case series. *JABFP* 18:132–139, 2005.
62. Escobar V, Bixle, D, Gleiser S, et al: Multiple pterygium syndrome. *Am J Dis Child* 132:609–611, 1978.
63. Even L, Cohen A, Marbach N, et al: Longitudinal analysis of growth over the first 3 years of life in Turner's syndrome. *J Pediatr* 137:460–464, 2000.
64. Falliner A, Drescher W, Brossmann J. The spine in fibrodysplasia ossificans progressiva: A case report. *Spine* 28:e519–e522, 2003.
65. Fay A, Fynn-Thompson N, Ebb D. Klippel-Trénaunay syndrome and rhabdomyosarcoma in a 3-year old. *Arch Opthalmol* 121:727–729, 2003.
66. Fearon JA: Treatment of the hands and feet in Apert syndrome: An evolution in management. *Plast Reconstr Surg* 112:1–12, 2003.
67. Fidalgo Valdueza A. The nail-patella syndrome. A report of three families. *J Bone Joint Surg* 55B:145–162, 1973.
68. Fiedler BS, De Smet AA, Kling TF, et al: Foot deformity in hereditary onychoosteodysplasia. *J Can Assoc Radiol* 38:305–308, 1987.
69. Findlay CA, Donaldson MD, Watt G. Foot problems in Turner's syndrome. *J Pediatr* 138:775–777, 2001.
70. Fryns JP, Legius E, Demaerel P, et al. Congenital scalp defect, distal limb reduction anomalies, right spastic hemiplegia and hypoplasia of the left arteria cerebri media. *Cl Genet* 50:505–509, 1996.
71. Galasso C, Arpino,C, Fabbri F, et al. Neurologic aspects of 49, XXXXY syndrome. *J Child Neurol* 18:501–504, 2003.
72. Gérard-Blanluet M, Danan C, Sinico M, et al. Mosaic trisomy 9 and lobar holoprosencephaly. *Am J Med Gen* 111:295–300, 2002.
73. Gollop TR, Fontes LR: The Greig cephalopolysyndactyly syndrome: Report of a family and review of the literature. *Am J Med Genet* 22:59–68, 1985.
74. Goodman FR, Bacchelli C, Brady AF, et al. Novel *HOXA 13* mutations and the phenotypic spectrum of hand-foot-genital syndrome. *Am J Hum Genet* 67:197–2002, 2000.
75. Gorlin RJ. Apert syndrome with polysyndactyly of the feet. *Am J Med Genet* 32:557, 1989.
76. Gorlin RJ, Meskin LH St. Geme JW. Oculodentodigital dysplasia. *J Pediatr* 63:69–75, 1963.
77. Graudal N, Galloe A, Christensen H. The pattern of shortened hand and foot bones in D-and E-brachydactyly and pseudohypoparathyroidism/ pseudopseudohypoparathyroidism. *Fortschr Rontgenstr* 148:460–462, 1988.
78. Grogan DP, Bernstein RM, Habal MB, et al. Congenital lipofibromatosis associated with macrodactyly of the foot. *Foot Ankle* 12:46, 1991.
79. Guidera KJ, Borrelli J, Raney E, et al. Orthopaedic manifestations of Rett syndrome. *J Pediatr Orthop* 11:204–208, 1991.
80. Guidera KJ, Raney E, Ogden JA, et al. Caudal regression: A review of seven cases including the mermaid syndrome. *J Pediatr Orthop* 11:743–747, 1991.
81. Guidera KJ, Satterwhite Y, Ogden JA, et al. Nail patella syndrome: A review of 44 orthopaedic patients. *J Pediatr Orthop* 11:737–742, 1991.
82. Hagberg B, Aicardi J, Dias K, et al. A progressive syndrome of autism, dementia, ataxia and loss of purposeful hand use in girls: Rett's syndrome: Report of 35 cases. *Ann Neurol* 14:471–479, 1983.
83. Hagberg B, Goutieres F, Hanefeld F, et al. Rett syndrome: Criteria for inclusion and exclusion. *Brain Dev* 7:372–373, 1983.
84. Hagberg B, Witt-Engerstrom I. Rett syndrome: A suggested staging system for describing impairment profile with increasing age towards adolescence. *Am J Med Genet* 24:183–194, 1986.
85. Hall JG, Reed SD, Rosenbaum KN, et al. Limb pterygium syndromes: A review and report of eleven patients. *Am J Med Genet* 12:377–409, 1982.
86. Haning RV, Carlson IH, Gilbert EF, et al. Virilism as a late manifestation in the Bardet-Biedl syndrome. *Am J Med Genet* 7:279–292, 1980.
87. Harrison RJ, Pitcher JD, Mizel MS, et al. The radiographic morphology of foot deformities in patients with fibrodysplasia ossificans progressiva. *Foot Ankle Internat* 26:937–941, 2005.
88. Hawley PP, Jackson LG, Kurnit DM. Sixty-four patients with Brachmann-de Lange syndrome: A survey. *Am J Med Genet* 20:453–459, 1985.
89. Heike C, Seto M, Hing A, et al. Century of Jackson-Weiss syndrome: Further definition of clinical and radiographic findings in "lost" descendants of the original kindred. *Am J Medic Genet* 100:315–324, 2001.
90. Hentschel J, Stierkorb E, Schneider G, et al. Caudal regression sequence: Vascular origin? *J Perinat* 26:445–447, 2006.
91. Hepper PG, Shahidullah S. Trisomy 18: Behavioral and structural abnormalities. An ultrasonographic case study. *Ultrsound Obstet Gynecol* 2:48–50, 1992.
92. Herzka A, Sponseller PD, Pyeritz RE. Atlantoaxial rotatory subluxation in patients with Marfan syndrome. *Spine* 25:524–526, 2000.
93. Hogh J, Macnicol MF. Foot deformities associated with onycho-osteodysplasia. A familial study and a review of associated features. *Int Orthop* 9:135–138, 1985.
94. Hosalkar HS, Shah H, Gujar P, et al. Mohr syndrome: A rare case and distinction from orofacial digital syndrome 1. *J Postgrad Med* 45:123–124, 1999.

95. Houston CS, Opitz JM, Spranger JW, et al. The campomelic syndrome: Review, report of 17 cases, and follow-up on the currently 17-year-old boy first reported by Maroteaux et al. in 1971. *Am J Med Genet* 15:3–28, 1983.
96. Huang KC, Hsu WH, Lee KF, et al. Subchondral insufficiency fracture with rapid collapse of the femoral head in a patient with Turner's syndrome. *Rheumat* 44:826–827, 2005.
97. Hunter A. The popliteal pterygium syndrome: Report of a new family and review of the literature. *Am J Med Genet* 36:196–208, 1990.
98. Husmann DA, Rathburn SR, Driscoll DJ. Klippel-Trenaunay syndrome: Incidence and treatment of genitourinary sequelae. *J Ur* 177:1244–1249, 2007.
99. Ioan DM, Dagomiz D, Fryns JP. Oculo-dento-digital dysplasia. Full manifestation of the syndrome in a 9.5 year-old girl and type III syndactyly in the father. *Genet Counsel* 13:187–189, 2002.
100. Jackson CE, Weiss L, Reynolds WA, et al. Craniosynostosis, midfacial hypoplasia, and foot abnormalities: An autosomal dominant phenotype in a large Amish kindred. *J Pediatr* 88:963–968, 1976.
101. Jaeggi E, Kind C, Morger R. Congenital scalp and skull defects with terminal transverse limb anomalies (Adams-Oliver syndrome): Report of three additional cases. *Eur J Pediatr* 149:565–566, 1990.
102. Jamis-Dow CA, Turner J, Biesecker LG, et al. Radiologic manifestations of Proteus syndrome. *RG* 24:1051–1068, 2004.
103. Jellinger KA. Rett syndrome-an update. *J Neural Transm* 110:681–701, 2003.
104. Jones KL. *Smith's Recognizable Patterns of Human Malformation*. Philadelphia: WB Saunders, 1988.
105. Joshi U, van der Sluijs JA, Teule GJ, et al. Proteus syndrome: A rare cause of hemihypertrophy and macrodactyly on bone scanning. *Clin Nucl Med* 30:604–605, 2005.
106. Kaciski M, Jaworek M, Skowronek-Bala B. Caudal regression syndrome associated with the white matter lesions and chromosome 18p11.2 deletion. *Br Dev* 29:164–166, 2007.
107. Kahl P, Heukamp LC, Buettner R, et al. Orofaciodigital syndrome type IV (Mohr-Majewski syndrome): Report of a family with two affected siblings. *Ped Dev Path* 10:239–243, 2007.
108. Kalhor M, Parvizi J, Slongo T, et al. Acetabular dysplasia associated with intra-articular lipomatous lesions in Proteus syndrome. *J Bone Joint Surg* 86A: 831–834, 2004.
109. Katsanis N, Ansley SJ, Badano JL, et al. Triallelic inheritance in Bardet-Biedl syndrome, a Mendelian recessive disorder. *Am Ass Adv Scie* 293:2256–2259, 2001.
110. Kelley RI. Review: The cerebrohepatorenal syndrome of Zellweger, morphologic and metabolic aspects. *Am J Med Genet* 16:503–517, 1983.
111. Kelly TE, Alford BA, Abel M. Cervical spine anomalies and tumors in Weaver syndrome. *Am J Med Genet* 95:492–495, 2000.
112. Kitterman JA, Kantanie S, Rocke DM, et al. Iatrogenic harm caused by diagnostic errors in fibrodysplasia ossificans progressiva. *Pediatr* 116:e654–e661, 2005.
113. Kline AD, Krantz ID, Sommer A, et al. Cornelia de Lange syndrome: Clinical review, diagnostic and scoring systems, and anticipatory guidance. *Am J Med Genet Part A* 143:1287–1296, 2007.
114. Komwilaisak R, Komwilaisak P, Ratanasiri T, et al. Three-dimensional ultrasonographic findings of the rare chromosomal abnormality 48, XXY/+18: A case report. *J Med Assoc Thai* 87:198–203, 2004.
115. Kousseff BG. Neurofibromatosis: A prototype of the phakomatoses, paracrine disorders in man? *J Fla Med Assoc* 76:535–538, 1989.
116. Kousseff BG, Madan S. The phakomatoses-an hypothesis: Paracrine growth regulation disorders? *Dysmorph Clin Genet* 2:76–90, 1988.
117. Kousseff BG, McConnachie P, Hadro TA. Autosomal recessive type of whistling face syndrome in twins. *Pediatrics* 69:328–331, 1982.
118. Kraemer KH, Patronas NJ, Schiffmann R, et al. Xeroderma pigmentosum, trichothiodystrophy and Cockayne syndrome: A complex genotype-phenotype relationship. *Neuroscience* 145:1388–1396, 2007.
119. Kroonen LT, Herman M, Pizzutillo PD, et al. Prader-Willi syndrome: Clinical concerns for the orthopaedic surgeon. *J Pediatr Orthop* 26: 673–679, 2006.
120. Kulkarni ML, Abdul Manaf KM, Prasannakumar DG, et al. Sirenomelia with radial dysplasia. *Ind J Pediatr* 71:447–449, 2004.
121. Lanfranco F, Kamischke A, Zitzmann M, et al. Klinefelter's syndrome. *Lancet* 364:273–283, 2004.
122. Latta RJ, Graham CB, Aase J, et al. Larsen's syndrome: A skeletal dysplasia with multiple joint dislocations and unusual facies. *J Pediatr* 78:291–298, 1971.
123. Lee A, Driscoll D, Gloviczki P, et al. Evaluation and management of pain in patients with Klippel-Trenaunay syndrome: A review. *Ped* 115:744–749, 2005.
124. Leroy JG, Crocker AC. Clinical definition of the Hurler-Hunter phenotypes. A review of 50 patients. *Am J Dis Child* 112:518–530, 1966.
125. Levy EP, Fletcher BD, Fraser FC. Mohr syndrome with subclinical expression of the bifid great toe. *Am J Dis Child* 128:531–533, 1974.
126. Lin HY, Lin SP, Chen YJ, et al. Clinical characteristics and survival of trisomy 18 in a medical center in Taipei. *Am J Med Genet* 140 A: 945–951, 2006.
127. Loder RT, Lee CL, Richards BS. Orthopedic aspects of Rett syndrome: A multicenter review. *J Pediatr Orthop* 9:557–562, 1989.
128. Lucas GL, Opitz JM, Wiffler C. The nail-patella syndrome. Clinical and genetic aspects of 5 kindreds with 38 affected family members. *J Pediatr* 68:273–288, 1966.
129. Macdonald WB, Fitch KD, Lewis IC. Cockayne's syndrome. An heredo-familial disorder of growth and development. *Pediatrics* 25:997–1007, 1960.
130. Magalini ST, Magalini SC. *Dictionary of medical syndromes*, 4th ed. Philadelphia: Lippincott-Raven; 1997.
131. Majewski F, Goecke T. Studies of microcephalic primordial dwarfism I: Approach to a delineation of the Seckel syndrome. *Am J Med Genet* 12:7–21, 1982.
132. Mantilla-Capacho JM, Arnaud L, Díaz-Rodrigues M, et al. Apert syndrome with preaxial polydactyly showing the typical mutation Ser252Trp in the FGFR2 gene. *Genet Counsel* 16:403–406, 2005.
133. Martsolf JT, Cracco JB, Carpenter CG, et al. Pfeiffer syndrome. An unusual type of acrocephalosyndactyly with broad thumbs and great toes. *Am J Dis Child* 121:257–262, 1971.
134. McClure SD, Van de Velde S, Fillman R, et al. New finding of protrusio acetabuli in two families with congenital contractural arachnodactyly. *J Bone Joint Surg* 89A:849–854, 2007.
135. McKusick VA. *Heritable disorders of connective tissue*. St. Louis: CV Mosby, 1966.
136. McKusick VA. *Online Mendelian inheritance in man*. OMIM™. John Hopkins University, Baltimore, MD. Available at: http://www.ncbi.nlm.nih.gov/omim. Accessed July 23, 2007.
137. McLaurin TM, Bukrey CD, Lovett RJ, et al. Management of thrombocytopenia-absent radius (TAR) syndrome. *J Pediatr Orthop* 19:289–296, 1999.
138. Mehlman CT, Rubinstein JH, Roy DR. Instability of the patellofemoral joint in Rubinstein-Taybi syndrome. *J Pediatr Orth* 18:508–511, 1998.
139. Merrick J, Ezra E, Josef B, et al. Musculoskeletal problems in Down syndrome- European Paediatric Orthopaedic Society survey: The Israeli sample. *J Pediatr Orthop Part B* 9:185–192, 2000.
140. Messineo A, Innocenti M, Gelli R, et al. Multidisciplinary surgical approach to a surviving infant with sirenomelia. *Pediatr* 118:e220–e223, 2006.

141. Mochel F, Grébille AG, Benachi A, et al. Contribution of fetal MR imaging in the prenatal diagnosis of Zellweger syndrome. *Am J Neuroradiol* 27:333–336, 2006.
142. Morava Ė, Czakó M, Kárteszi J, et al. Ulnar/fibular ray defect and brachydactyly in a family: A possible new autosomal dominant syndrome. *Clin Dysmorphol* 12:161–165, 2003.
143. Moriatis JM, Gannon FH, Shore EM, et al. Limb swelling in patients who have fibrodysplasia ossificans progressiva. *Cl Orthop Rel Res* 336:247–253, 1997.
144. Morrissy RT, ed. *Lovell and Winter's pediatric orthopaedics.* Philadelphia: JB Lippincott, 1990.
145. Moses G, Howard C, Bar-Ziv J, et al. 'Epiphyseal dysgenesis' in Laurence-Moon-Biedl-Bardet syndrome. *J Pediatr Orthop Part B* 7:193–198, 1998.
146. Moumoulidis I, Ramsden R, Moffat D. Unusual otological manifestations in Camurati-Engelmann's disease. *J Larygol Otol* 120:892–895, 2006.
147. Murata T, Kurokawa R, Krones A, et al. Defect of histone acetyltransferase activity of the nuclear transcriptional coactivator CBP in Rubinstein-Taybi syndrome. *Hum Molec Genet* 10:1071–1076, 2001.
148. Naidu S, Chatterjee S, Murphy M, et al. Rett syndrome: New observations. *Brain Dev* 9:525–528, 1987.
149. Nance MA, Berry SA. Cockayne syndrome: Review of 140 cases. *Am J Med Genet* 42:68–84, 1992.
150. Nisenblat V, Leibovitz Z, Paz B, et al. Dizogotic twin pregnancy discordant for sirenomelia. *J Ultrasound Med* 26:97–103, 2007.
151. Nishimura G, Nagai T. Radiographic findings in Shprintzen-Golberg syndrome. *Pediatr Radiol* 26:775–778, 1996.
152. Nomura Y, Honda K, Segawa M. Pathophysiology of Rett syndrome. *Brain Dev* 9:506–513, 1987.
153. Nomura Y, Segawa M. Natural history of Rett syndrome. *J Child Neurol* 20:764–768, 2005.
154. Odunusi E, Peters C, Krivit W, et al. Genu valgum deformity in Hurler syndrome after hematopoietic stem cell transplantation: Correction by surgical intervention. *J Pediatr Orthop* 19:270–274, 1999.
155. Ogata T, Matsuo N, Nishimura G, et al. Oto-palatodigital syndrome, type II: Evidence for defective intramembranous ossification. *Am J Med Genet* 36:226–231, 1990.
156. Parashar SY, Anderson PJ, McLean N, et al. Spectrum of features in pterygium syndrome. *Asian J Surg* 29:104–108, 2006.
157. Parikh SN, Crawford AH, Do TT, et al. Popliteal pterygium syndrome: Implications for orthopaedic management. *J Pediatr Orthop* 13B:197–201, 2004.
158. Parker KL, Wyatt DT, Blethen SL, et al. Screening girls with Turner syndrome: The national cooperative growth study experience. *J Pediatr* 143:133–135, 2003.
159. Passarge E, Lenz W. Syndrome of caudal regression in infants of diabetic mothers: Observations of further cases. *Pediatrics* 37:672–675, 1966.
160. Pellerin D, Martelli H, Latouche X, et al. Congenital soft tissue dysplasia: A new malformation entity and concept. *Prog Pediatr Surg* 22:1–29, 1989.
161. Phillips WA, Cooperman DR, Lindquist TC, et al. Orthopaedic management of lumbosacral agenesis. *J Bone Joint Surg* 64A:1282–1294, 1982.
162. Place HM, Enzenauer RJ. Cervical spine subluxation in Marfan syndrome. *J Bone Joint Surg* 88A:2479–2482, 2006.
163. Plotkin H. Syndromes with congenital brittle bones. *BMC Pediatr* 4, 2004.
164. Pradhan BB, Bhasin M, Otsuka NY. A metatarsal equivalent to the metacarpal index in Marfan syndrome. *Foot Ankle Internat* 26:881–885, 2005.
165. Preus M, Fraser FC. The cerebro-oculo-facioskeletal syndrome. *Clin Genet* 5:294–297, 1974.
166. Raman D, Haslock I. The nail-patella syndrome-a report of two cases and a literature review. *Br J Rheumatol* 22:41–46, 1983.
167. Ramirez N, Marrero L, Carlo S, et al. Orthopaedic manifestations of Bardet-Biedl syndrome. *J Pediatr Orthop* 24:92–96, 2004.
168. Rao N, Joseph B. Grebe syndrome with bilateral fibular hemimelia and thumb duplication. *Skel Radiol* 31:183–187, 2002.
169. Rao VB, Kerketta L, Korgaonkar S, et al. Maternal origin of extra marker chromosome 1Q31.1-qter and 13pter-q12.12 in a child with dysmorphic features. *Genet Counsel* 16:139–143, 2005.
170. Rapin I, Weidenheim K, Lindenbaum Y, et al. Cockayne syndrome in adults: Review with clinical and pathologic study of a new case. *J Child Neurol* 21:991–1006, 2006.
171. Rawat SS. A new operative technique for congenital gigantism of the toes. *Br J Plastic Surg* 43:120–121, 1990.
172. Rett A. On an unusual brain atrophic syndrome with hyperammonemia in childhood. *Wien Med Wochenschr* 116:723–726, 1966.
173. Riccardi VM, Holmes LB. Brachydactyly, type E: Hereditary shortening of digits, metacarpals, metatarsals, and long bones. *J Pediatr* 84:251–254, 1974.
174. Rimoin DL, Connor JM, Pyeritz RE, eds. *Emery and Rimoin's principles and practice of medical genetics,* 3rd ed. London: Churchill Livingstone, 1996.
175. Robertson FW, Kozlowski K, Middleton RW. Larsen's syndrome. Three cases with multiple congenital joint dislocations and distinctive facies. *Clin Pediatr* 14:53–60, 1975.
176. Robinson GC, Wildervanck LS, Chiang TP. Ectrodactyly, ectodermal dysplasia, and cleft lip-palate syndrome. Its association with conductive hearing loss. *J Pediatr* 82:107–109, 1973.
177. Robinson LK, James HE, Mubarek SJ, et al. Carpenter syndrome: Natural history and clinical spectrum. *Am J Med Genet* 20:461–469, 1985.
178. Robinson LK, Wolfsberg E, Jones KL. Brachmann-de Lange syndrome: Evidence for autosomal dominant inheritance. *Am J Med Genet* 22:109–115, 1985.
179. Roelfsema JH, White SJ, Ariyűrek Y, et al. Genetic heterogeneity in Rubinstein-Taybi syndrome: Mutations in both the CBP and EP300 genes cause disease. *Am J Hum Genet* 76:572–580, 2005.
180. Rogers JG, Geho WB. Fibrodysplasia ossificans progressiva. A survey of forty-two cases. *J Bone Joint Surg* 61A:909–914, 1979.
181. Romeo G, Zonana J, Rimoin DL, et al. Heterogeneity of nonlethal severe short-limbed dwarfism. *J Pediatr* 91:918–923, 1977.
182. Rosenfeld RG. Turner's syndrome: A growing concern. *J Pediatr* 137:443–444, 2000.
183. Ross JL, Kowal K, Quigley CA, et al. The phenotype of short stature homeobox gene (SHOX) deficiency in childhood: Contrasting children with Leri-Weill dyschondrosteosis and Turner syndrome. *J Pediatr* 147:499–507, 2005.
184. Rossi M, Jones RL, Norbury G, et al. The appearance of the feet in Pfeiffer syndrome caused by *FGFR1* P252R mutation. *Clin Dysmorphol* 12:269–274, 2003.
185. Rubinstein JH, Taybi H. Broad thumbs and toes and facial abnormalities. *Am J Dis Child* 105:88–108, 1963.
186. Rumball KM, Pang E, Letts RM. Musculoskeletal manifestations of the Antley-Bixler syndrome. *J Pediatr Orthop Part B* 8:139–143, 1999.
187. Sacheti A, Szemere J, Bernstein B, et al. Chronic pain is a manifestation of the Ehlers-Danlos syndrome. *J Pain Sympt Manage* 14:88–93, 1997.
188. Sakaura H, Matsuoka T, Iwasaki M, et al. Surgical treatment of cervical kyphosis in Larsen syndrome. *Spine* 32:e39–e44, 2007.
189. Santini S, Rebeccato A, Schiavon R. Pedal ectrodactyly: A case report with a new surgical management. *J Foot Ankle Surg* 41:320–327, 2002.
190. Sasidharan CK, Ravi KV. Popliteal pterygium syndrome with unusual features. *Indian J Pediatr* 71:269–270, 2004.
191. Sävendabl L, Davenport ML. Delayed diagnoses of Turner's syndrome: Proposed guidelines for change. *J Pediatr* 137: 455–459, 2000.

192. Sawhney S, Jain R, Meka N. Sirenomelia: MRI appearance. *J Post Grad Med 52*: 219–220, 2006.
193. Sawyer JR, Klimkiewicz JJ, Iannotti JP, et al. Mechanism for superior subluxation of the glenohumeral joint in fibrodysplasia ossificans progressiva. *Cl Orthopaed Rel Res* 346:130–133, 1998.
194. Scarlett RF, Rocke DM, Kantanie S, et al. Influenza-like viral illnesses and flare-ups of fibrodysplasia ossificans progressiva. *Clin Orthop Rel Res* 423:275–279, 2004.
195. Schaffer AA, Kaplan FS, Tracy MR, et al. Developmental anomalies of the cervical spine in patients with fibrodysplasia ossificans progressiva are distinctly different from those in patients with Klippel-Feil syndrome. *Spine* 30:1379–1385, 2005.
196. Schinzel A. Trisomy 20pter = to q11 in a malformed boy from a t(13; 20) (p11; q11) translocation-carrier mother. *Hum Genet* 53:169–172, 1980.
197. Selby-Silverstein L, Hillstrom HJ, Palisano RJ. The effect of foot orthoses on standing foot posture and gait of young children with Down syndrome. *Neuro Rehab* 16:183–193, 2001.
198. Shah JR, Sainani N, Patkar DP. Caudal regression syndrome with sacral rib: MRI features. *Acta Radiol* 47: 862–864, 2006.
199. Shin JJ, Hartnick CJ. Otologic manifestations of ectodermal dysplasia. *Arch Otolaryngol Head Neck Surg* 130:1104–1107, 2004.
200. Silengo MC, Bell GL, Bagioli M, et al. Oro-facial-digital syndrome II. Transitional type between the Mohr and the Majewski syndromes: Report of two new cases. *Clin Genet* 31:331–336, 1987.
201. Sillence DO, Barlow KK, Garber AP, et al. Osteogenesis imperfecta type II delineation of the phenotype with reference to genetic heterogeneity. *Am J Med Genet* 17:407–423, 1984.
202. Sillence DO, Senn A, Danks DM. Genetic heterogeneity in osteogenesis imperfecta. *J Med Genet* 16:101–116, 1979.
203. Simpson NE, Brissenden JE. The Rubinstein-Taybi syndrome: familial and dermatoglyphic data. *Am J Med Genet* 25:225–229, 1973.
204. Singh JA, Williams CB, McAlister WH. Talo-patello-scaphoid osteolysis, synovitis, and short fourth metacarpals in sisters: A new syndrome? *Am J Med Genet* 121A:118–125, 2003.
205. Singh SK, Singh RD, Sharma A. Caudal regression syndrome-case report and review of literature. *Pediatr Surg Internat* 21:578–581, 2005.
206. Slater CP, Ross J, Nelson MM, et al. The campomelic syndrome-prenatal ultrasound investigations. A case report. *S African Med J* 67:863–866, 1985.
207. Smith DW, Lemli L, Opitz JM. A newly recognized syndrome of multiple congenital anomalies. *J Pediatr* 64:210–217, 1964.
208. Smith R. Fibrodysplasia (myositis) ossificans progressiva. *Cl Orth Rel Res* 346:7–14, 1998.
209. Smith R, Athanasou NA, Vipond SE. Fibrodysplasia (myositis) ossificans progressiva: Clinicopathological features and natural history. *Oxf J Med* 89:445–456, 1996.
210. Soriano-Guillen L, Coste J, Ecosse E, et al. Adult height and pubertal growth in Turner syndrome after treatment with recombinant growth hormone. *J Clin Endoc Metab* 90:5197–5204, 2005.
211. Sparkes RS, Graham CB. Camurati-Engelmann disease. Genetics and clinical manifestations with a review of the literature. *J Med Genet* 9:73–85, 1972.
212. Spranger M, Schapera J. Anomalous inheritance in a kindred with split hand, split foot malformation. *Eur J Pediatr* 147: 202–205, 1988.
213. Stanley D, Seymour N. The Larsen syndrome occurring in four generations of one family. *Int Orthop* 8:267–272, 1985.
214. Stephan MJ, Hall BD, Smith DW, et al. Macrocephaly in association with unusual cutaneous angiomatosis. *Pediatrics* 87:353–359, 1975.
215. Stern HJ, Graham JM, Lachman RS, et al. Atelosteogenesis type III: A distinct skeletal dysplasia with features overlapping atelosteogenesis and oto-palato-digital syndrome type II. *Am J Med Genet* 36:183–195, 1990.
216. Stevenson DA, Carey JC, Palumbos J, et al. Clinical characteristics and natural history of Freeman-Sheldon syndrome. *Pediatr* 117:754–762, 2006.
217. Stevenson RE, Jones KL, Phelan MC, et al. Vascular steal: The pathogenetic mechanism producing sirenomelia and associated defects of the viscera and soft tissues. *Pediatrics* 78:451–457, 1986.
218. Stone JA, Castillo M (Letter) MR in a patient with Zellweger syndrome presenting without cortical or myelination abnormalities. *AJNR* 19:1378–1379, 1998.
219. Stroustrup Smith A, Grable I, Levine D. Case 66: Caudal regression syndrome in the fetus of a diabetic mother. *Radiol* 230:229–233, 2004.
220. Surana RB, Fraga JR, Sinkford SM. The cerebro-oculo-facioskeletal syndrome. *Clin Genet* 13:486–488, 1978.
221. Sweeney E, Fryer A, Mountford R, et al. Nail patella syndrome: A review of the phenotype aided by developmental biology. *J Med Genet* 40:153–162, 2003.
222. Sybert VP. Adult height in Turner syndrome with and without androgen therapy. *J Pediatr* 104:365–369, 1984.
223. Takebayashi T, Yamashita T, Yokogushi K, et al. Scoliosis in Proteus syndrome. *Spine* 26:e395–e398, 2001.
224. Temtamy SA, Aglan MS, Nemat A, et al. Expanding the phenotypic spectrum of the Baller-Gerold syndrome. *Genet Counsel* 14:299–312, 2003.
225. Thanemozhi G, Santhiya ST, Chandra N, et al. Trisomy 4p and partial monosomy 18q due to paternal translocation t (4; 18) (p11; q21.3). *Ind J Pediatr* 67 B:601–604, 2000.
226. Thorey F, Jäger M, Seller K, et al. How to prevent small stature in Rett syndrome-associated collapsing spine syndrome. *J Child Neurol* 22:443–446, 2007.
227. Tissières P, Didier D, Dahoun S, et al. Turner syndrome with complex mosaic monosomy and structural aorta anomalies. J Pediatr 142:341, 2003.
228. Tosi LL. Osteogenesis imperfecta. *Curr Opin in Pediatr* 9:94–99, 1997.
229. Trevatham E, Moser HW. Diagnostic criteria for Rett syndrome. *Ann Neurol* 23:425–428, 1988.
230. Trusen A, Beissert M, Collmann H, et al. The pattern of skeletal anomalies in the cervical spine, hands and feet in patients with Saethre-Chotzen syndrome and Muenke-type mutation. *Pediatr Radiol* 33:168–172, 2003.
231. Tumolo M, Moscatelli A, Silvestri G. Anaesthetic management of a child with fibrodysplasia ossificans progressiva. *Br J Anaesth* 97:701–703, 2006.
232. Turra S, Santini S, Cagnoni G, et al. Gigantism of the foot: Our experience in seven cases. *J Pediatr Orthop* 18:337–345, 1998.
233. Valentine GH, McClelland MA, Sergovich FR. The growth and development of four XYY infants. *Pediatrics* 48:583–594, 1971.
234. Van Keirsbilck J, Cannie M, Robrechts C, et al. First trimester diagnosis of sirenomelia. *Pren Diagn* 26:684–688, 2006.
235. Vismara L, Romei M, Galli M, et al. Clinical implications of gait analysis in the rehabilitation of adult patients with "Prader-Willi" syndrome: A cross-sectional comparative study ("Prader-Willi" syndrome vs matched obese patients and healthy subjects). *J Neuroengineer Rehab* 4: 1–12, 2007.
236. Warkany J, Passarge E, Smith LB. Congenital malformations in autosomal trisomy syndromes. *Am J Dis Child* 112:502–517, 1966.
237. Weisz B, Achiron R, Schindler A, et al. Prenatal sonographic diagnosis of hemivertebra. *J Ultr Med* 23:853–857, 2004.
238. West LA, Ballock RT. High incidence of hip dysplasia but not slipped capital femoral epiphysis in patients with Prader-Willi syndrome. *J Pediatr Orthop* 24:565–567, 2004.
239. Wong HB. Genetic aspects of foot deformities. *J Singapore Paediatr Soc* 29:13–22, 1987.
240. Wong V. The spectrum of arthrogryposis in 33 Chinese children. *Br Dev* 19:187–96, 1997.
241. Wood VE, Rubinstein J. Duplicated longitudinal bracketed epiphysis "kissing delta phalanx" in Rubinstein-Taybi syndrome. *J Pediatr Orth* 19:603–611, 1999.

242. Wynne-Davies R. Genetic and congenital musculoskeletal disorders. *Obstet Gynecol Annu* 6:247–260, 1977.
243. Yakish SD, Fu FH. Long-term follow-up of the treatment of a family with nail-patella syndrome. *J Pediatr Orthop* 3:360–363, 1983.
244. Yamada K, Matsuzawa H, Uchiyama M, et al. Brain developmental abnormalities in Prader-Willi syndrome detected by diffusion tensor imaging. *Pediatr* 118:e442–e448, 2006.
245. Yamada K, Miyamoto K, Hosoe H, et al. Scoliosis associated with Prader-Willi syndrome. *Spine* 7:345–348, 2007.
246. Yamamoto T, Kurosawa K, Masuno M, et al. Congenital anomaly of cervical vertebrae is a major complication of Rubinstein-Taybi syndrome. *Am J Med Gene. Part A* 135:130–133, 2005.
247. Yatziv S, Erickson RP, Epstein CJ. Mild and severe Hunter syndrome (MPS II) within the same sibships. *Clin Genet* 11:319–326, 1977.
248. Yunis JJ, Sanchez O. A new syndrome resulting from partial trisomy for the distal third of the long arm of chromosome 10. *J Pediatr* 84:567–570, 1974.
249. Zampino G, Conti G, Balducci F, et al. Severe form of Freeman-Sheldon syndrome associated with brain anomalies and hearing loss. *Am J Med Genet* 62:293–296, 1996.
250. Zeitlin L, Fassier F, Glorieux FH. Modern approach to children with osteogenesis imperfecta. *J Pediatr Orthop* 10B:77–87, 2003.
251. Zlotogora J, Nubani N. Is there an autosomal recessive form of the split hand and split foot malformation? *J Med Genet* 26:138–140, 1989.

CHAPTER 33

Adult Consequences of Pediatric Foot Disorders

Sig T. Hansen

INTRODUCTION

I am pleased to have been asked to add a postscript to this book, a commentary on the types of problems I have seen in my full-time practice consisting of secondary and tertiary orthopedic care of adult foot and ankle problems. Prior to narrowing my focus exclusively to foot and ankle reconstruction, my practice was split equally between acute Level 1 trauma care and an elective foot practice where I saw both children and adults.

At the start of my career, I did general medicine in the Navy, mostly pediatrics, for three years after completing a rotating internship. Following that, I completed four years of general orthopedic residency training, including one year at the Spokane Shriners Hospital. In 1970, I spent six months at the Sheffield Children's Hospital in Sheffield, England, doing primarily neuromuscular pediatric orthopedic reconstruction but also seeing all the acute pediatric orthopedic trauma occurring in a relatively large portion of the city.

On return to Seattle and the University of Washington Orthopedic faculty, I ran a Congenital Defects Clinic and Foot Clinic at the Seattle Children's Hospital and Medical Center (previously Children's Orthopedic Hospital) and started an adult foot and ankle clinic, which included a podiatrist, at Harborview Medical Center. This was followed by nearly 18 years as the Orthopedist-in-Chief at Harborview, when it was becoming a Level 1 trauma center. Harborview had a very active fire department-based paramedic team and we initiated a program of very early and aggressive operative care of multiply injured patients that included extensive rigid internal fixation of both open and closed fractures, eventually using primarily Arbeitsgomansilaft for Osteosysthoserfergen (AO)/Association for Study of Internal Fracture (ASIF) implants. During this time, I ran a traumatology fellowship that started with one Fellow per year and worked its way up to about five. In about 1990, I reduced my involvement in trauma a bit and increased my foot practice. At the same time, I switched from being the head of the traumatology fellowship to running a foot and ankle fellowship. This program also began with one Fellow per year and has increased to about three one-year Fellows and three faculty members doing primarily foot and ankle surgery.

I mention all of this as a way to explain my admitted biases on a number of care issues. I am unashamedly biased toward surgical treatment. This is perhaps the result of timing, as several important advances in surgical care occurred in the years during my early career. We were emboldened when prophylactic antibiotics became a reality in the early 1970s, anesthesia became progressively safer, and operative technology and implants (at the time particularly from AO-ASIF, now Synthes) were improved. These technologies are much more common today they were 30 years ago.

My approach to the foot, in particular, was considered controversial early on. I was more likely to operate on children's "flatfoot," femoral anteversion, tibial rotational problems (particularly external torsion), and even at first on clubfoot abnormalities, than were my contemporaries. I changed my mind after a few years only about clubfoot, where I backed off to very early (two to four months) posterior release consisting of an open heel cord lengthening and posterior capsulotomy, particularly posterior tib-fib ligament excision. When followed by casting or splinting and further surgery as needed, this produced much better results in my hands.

About 10 years into practice, I became convinced that too much of our standard treatment was based on the presenting symptoms and not enough on the underlying cause of the pathologic presentation. Some time later, I read Morton's 1935 textbook on *The Human Foot* (6) as it fit perfectly with my still undeveloped philosophy from my college course in comparative anatomy. I now absolutely believe that many if not most foot and ankle problems, more so in adults, are caused primarily by atavistic traits, predominantly gastrocnemius equinus and, Morton's favorite, excessive mobility of the first metatarsal at the tarsometatarsal and/or naviculocuneiform joints. He noted this leads to overload of the second or lesser metatarsals and to secondary midfoot and hindfoot disorders. It follows that treatment must include correction of these underlying traits as well as dealing with their sequelae, which are often the presenting problems.

Having confessed my bias, I will discuss my observations about problems commonly seen in a pediatric foot and ankle practice, their treatment, and what happens to these patients after age 16.

THE EXCESSIVELY PRONATED OR "FLATFOOT" DEFORMITY

An area of mutual interest in pediatric orthopedics and adult reconstruction that no doubt includes the greatest number of patients and is a very important problem is "flatfoot." This is not the common simple flatfoot of childhood that firms up with growth and development and becomes perfectly normal. My concern lies with the 2% to 10% of flatfeet that become symptomatic fairly early and/or flatfeet with a tight heel cord and valgus heel. Left untreated into adulthood, so many go on to have significant symptoms and increasing deformity with posterior tibial tendon failure, that this problem in its various forms is the most discussed difficult problem in adult foot and ankle orthopedics.

The deformity is marked by dorsal and lateral subluxation of the calcaneus and navicular under the talus. I coined the term "dorsolateral peritalar subluxation" to differentiate this type of foot from the routine "flatfoot." Computerized axial tomography confirms that there is, indeed, subluxation in the subtalar joint. The problem is associated with posterior tibial tendon failure and the degrees of deformity are categorized into four grades, with grade 4 having the greatest amount of lateralization so that the talus tilts into valgus in the mortise and causes marked arthrosis and symptoms. I do many mid-foot and hindfoot reconstruction procedures as well as ankle replacements and fusions and this late-stage so-called flatfoot, which is actually much more than that, is an enormously challenging situation that when left untreated is extremely disabling to the patient.

Theories of causation and favorite solutions vary, but in my opinion, the primary cause is gastrocnemius equinus. Contributing causes are congenital valgus in the heel, a mobile first ray (or Morton's foot problems), or ligamentous laxity involving the entire medial column. Rarely, injury to the medial ligaments is at fault. All are aggravated by excessive weight and aging of the soft tissues. We were taught in the past that the Achilles tendon is an inverter of the heel, so some surgeons feel it cannot be the cause of a valgus heel and posterior tibial tendon failure. It seems obvious to me that the Achilles tendon can invert the heel but only when the posterior tibial tendon first begins inversion, bringing the heel cord past the midline. The test for posterior tibial tendon function is a single-leg heel rise, and the posterior tibial tendon is declared non-functional when the heel fails to invert. In this case, of course, the Achilles is perfectly normal. Therefore, if the heel is not inverted by the posterior tib or it is in fact in anatomic valgus, tension on the heel cord becomes an eversion force. This type of heel valgus can be a result of a weak or mobile medial column that allows excessive pronation and is the opposite of the plantarflexed first metatarsal which causes heel varus as demonstrated by the Coleman Block Test.

Once breakdown of the medial column begins, the medial plantar ligaments or posterior tibial tendon continue to stretch out the spring ligament, the anterior deltoid ligament, the long and short plantar ligaments, the plantar fascia, etc. With time, weight, and activity the arch collapses and the talar head or navicular virtually makes contact with the ground. Symptoms are always present on the lateral side as well. The sinus tarsi closes down with the foot and heel rotating laterally and posteriorly under the talus until the anterior beak of the calcaneus pushes against the lateral shoulder of the talus. The heel tilts laterally and can become impacted under the lateral malleolus in later stages and, especially in older osteopenic women, a stress fracture of the fibula can develop about four or five centimeters above the distal tip of the fibula.

This progression of problems can be stopped by very simple measures in the earliest phases, e.g., by a gastroc slide or Strayer procedure and possible augmentation of the posterior tibial tendon by the flexor digitorum longus. If there is greater failure in the medial column, particularly at the first tarsometatarsal joint identified by Morton, this joint can be appropriately realigned and fused. Often the break in the medial column is in the naviculocuneiform joint and here, the classic Miller procedure is the treatment of choice but always with a gastroc slide. It is interesting to note that in a classic long-term follow up of the Miller procedure from Melbourne by Menelaus et al., around 2000 (5), the authors did not mention heel cord lengthening in the title or abstract, but in the body of the paper, they noted that 90% of their patients incidentally needed heel cord lengthening. Their overall success rate was 90%. When the heel is in anatomic valgus, a medializing calcaneal osteotomy can also decrease stress on the posterior tibial tendon. In a slightly later phase, this medialization can be very helpful in relieving a damaged and weakened posterior tibial tendon.

Without surgical intervention, the problem progresses and eventually salvage becomes more difficult. In late stages, a difficult triple arthrodesis called a "medial triple" may be required. This procedure does not usually include the calcaneal cuboid joint but only the naviculocuneiform joint, leaving the tilted ankle mortise and arthrosis. If the deltoid ligament is significantly stretched a pantalar arthrodesis may be needed, and if the deltoid is still relatively intact, total ankle arthroplasty may be possible in conjunction with complete realignment of the foot.

These problems are seen so commonly in adults that I would strongly recommend that more gastroc slides with an added Miller or Evans procedure be done in the pediatric age group. Then again, the newly introduced calcaneal z-osteotomy that lengthens and medializes the calcaneus and moves the sustentaculum tali forward to give more support to the talar head may prove to be more effective. The bottom line is that a symptomatic flatfoot that has a tight gastroc and is developing increasing heel valgus and a shortened lateral column must be differentiated from a simple, supple, asymptomatic true pediatric flatfoot and treated accordingly. A gastroc slide can be done through a very short medial incision at the gastrocsoleus junction and the downside of the procedure is virtually negligible. The patient will experience a short period of weakness followed by return of near normal strength within four to six months.

It would be difficult to prove that a gastroc slide is effective and that the condition would not resolve spontaneously when both sides are done in childhood. Interestingly, I had the opportunity to follow two or three patients who for non-medical reasons had only one side lengthened in childhood. Usually, the patient was brought in by a mother who requested that only one side be done at a time and then did not come back for social or situational reasons. Two of these patients showed up at my practice later on as adults and wanted their opposite feet treated. In each case, the foot that had had a gastroc slide was completely normal, while the one that had not had deteriorated to a significantly symptomatic flatfoot.

TALIPES EQUINOVARUS OR CLUBFOOT AND OTHER CAVOVARUS FEET

The problems seen in adults after childhood treatment of clubfoot are much less common than symptomatic arch collapse in adult practice and they are seldom discussed at AOFAS meetings. My experience, however, is consistent with that of others with large foot and ankle reconstruction practices judging from casual conversations and comparisons of cases.

The first consistent finding is that many of the feet treated apparently successfully by aggressive posteromedial releases in childhood went on to serious overcorrection into marked valgus when the patients got heavier in late adolescence or young adulthood. I assume this is the reason for the current return to much less aggressive surgical treatment for clubfoot in children. Frequent findings include absence of a functional posterior tibial tendon, stretching of the anterior deltoid and spring ligament, and possible absence of the long toe flexors. The navicular and/or the first metatarsal often are markedly elevated above the desired alignment with the axis of the talus, apparently due to an unopposed tight or contracted anterior tibial tendon and without the plantar flexing support of the posterior tibial tendon and possibly the plantar ligaments. The only successful treatment seems to require at least a medial triple arthrodesis, often with added lateral transfer and/or lengthening of the anterior tibial tendon.

If the flexor hallucis longus is still intact and the first metatarsal is elevated by a reaction to strong flexion of the first metatarsophalangeal joint, the flexor hallucis longus can be transferred back to the neck or a more proximal shaft of the first metatarsal to pull it down to the ground. It is interesting that this procedure was also described by Lapidus. Careful selection of tendon balancing and necessary fusions can improve things significantly, but if the subtalar joint has to be fused, late changes in the ankle can create the need for total ankle arthroplasty.

The converse situation is a patient treated by strong casting against rigid equinus. This causes enough damage to the talar dome with flattening etc. that again, ankle fusion or replacement will be needed. Rarely, patients are also seen with avascular necrosis from circulatory damage of the talus apparently related to overaggressive release of the subtalar capsules, etc.

My observations after 12–15 years of operating on clubfeet and over 20 years of providing major tertiary care are that both aggressive surgery with complete posteromedial release and pure manipulation and casting leave major long-term residuals that become disabling after 30+/-10 years. In my opinion, the best alternative seems to be the Iowa approach (1) consisting of early heel cord lengthening (or in my hands, an open heel cord lengthening and posterior capsulotomy at two to four months) and then manipulation and splinting until the need for further surgery arises. An alternative approach, which I understand is used in South Africa, is to do early surgery with medial and posteromedial lengthening but lengthening both the anterior and posterior tibial tendons above the ankle so they are not lost. This procedure bears more evaluation.

The next interesting observation in talipes equinovarus and in cavovarus feet seen in Charcot-Marie-Tooth (CMT) disease is the association of external tibial torsion. I am not sure which is the cause and which is the effect, but an association definitely exists. It is frequently noted that during complete straightening of a severely supinated foot, e.g., by a triple arthrodesis for severe cavovarus deformity with marked internal rotation, severe (about 45 degrees) of external tibial torsion occasionally is discovered in late teens and adults. I follow this surgery with an internal rotational osteotomy of the tibia. Moreover, many of my adult patients who are around 50 years of age or so have severe midfoot and hindfoot arthrosis with a tendency toward varus and lateral ankle instability. The primary cause appears to be external tibial torsion. It seems that external tibial torsion can cause or aggravate cavovarus but also that cavovarus may cause or aggravate external tibial torsion. It appears that the powerful posterior tibial tendon causes inversion and/or internal rotation in a foot with a weak or absent peroneus brevis. The often powerful peroneus longus seen in CMT not only does not help but apparently aggravates the problem by plantar flexing the first metatarsal and causing a forefoot-driven hindfoot varus.

We see entirely too many patients in young adulthood with progressively worsening cavovarus feet that were treated nonoperatively with various braces. In keeping with my aforementioned bias, it makes no sense to me to not treat a patient with marked muscle imbalance that causes increasing deformity that will absolutely and predictably becomes fixed. The type of muscle balancing needed here is easy to accomplish and generally is quite successful when done before the deformity becomes more rigid and fixed in the bone and ligaments. Strong deforming forces which can be reduced include: the posterior tibial tendon working against a weakened peroneus brevis, a long peroneal tendon working against a weakened or absent anterior tibial tendon, or the gastrocsoleus working against a weakened anterior tibial muscle.

Releasing the overly powerful deforming muscles always produces a favorable result. Only the attempt to transfer them in order to make them work as a constructive force is less predictable, as the muscles are often out of phase. The thing that seems to deter some surgeons is the prospect of transferring muscles out of phase, as if this were not at all possible. In actual practice, however, it frequently works relatively well. The fact is, muscles can adjust to this more frequently than not. For example, removing the posterior tibial tendon and putting it through the interosseous membrane and attaching it not to the dorsum of the foot, which makes it too tight, but to the extensor digitorum communis above the ankle and then tenodesing the long toe extensors in the midfoot almost always results in an active working dorsiflexor. The extensor digitorum longus can be attached by tenodesis into the midfoot at about the second or third cuneiform. It is not necessary to try to bring the tendon down to the midfoot bones, where it will be so tight it sometimes pulls out or does not allow any plantar flexion. Posterior tibial tendon function is easily replaced by transecting the flexor digitorum longus at the Master Knot area and placing it into the stump of the posterior tibial tendon, where the distal centimeter or two can be left intact if one is not trying to run the posterior tibial tendon all the way to the bone when transferring it anteriorly (2).

The strongly deforming peroneus longus can be used very simply to replace the always weak or absent peroneus brevis by simply transecting it under the base of the fifth metatarsal, removing some paratenon, and suturing it into the distal peroneus brevis through a stab wound. If the extensor hallucis longus is causing a cock-up deformity in the great toe and also plantar flexion of the first metatarsal, it can be attached by tenodesis to the distal first metatarsal in a manner similar to the Jones procedure. Clearly, if the plantar fascia is tight a proximal partial plantar fasciectomy can be done and, if necessary, a gastroc slide. These procedures can be easily done together, have a minimal downside, and allow early full weight bearing.

With the aid of a neutral positioning night splint (clamshell splint, not a posterior splint with straps) the foot may remain un-deformed for a long time, if not indefinitely. If weakness causes instability, appropriate fusions, including a triple arthrodesis, can be done. In my experience, this is more often necessary in female patients who have more generalized weakness than men, while men have more rigid cavovarus deformity, seemingly from the overpowering force of the long peroneals.

The essential point is, I see no reason to delay this surgery in late childhood because delay will only cause increased deformity and difficulty for the patient that will require later treatment.

ADOLESCENT BUNION OR HALLUX VALGUS

As in most adults, "bunion" or "bunionectomy" is a totally inappropriate term in adolescents. The medial deformity of a so-called "bunion" is from hallux valgus angulation and not from osteophytes or a growth on the bone. No "ectomy" should be done: no medial exostectomy or any form of adult bunionectomy is indicated here in my opinion. Distal or even proximal osteotomies, Akin osteotomies, and adductor releases or transfers are all non-anatomic procedures and do not address the true problem.

In adolescents, one must determine the etiology of the problem. Generally, it cannot be chalked up to high-heeled shoes, which these patients usually have not been wearing. In my opinion, high heels have nothing to do with this deformity, even in adults. As I noted, I am a believer in Morton's philosophy about foot deformity and certainly this applies to virtually all adolescent "bunions." He theorized that the primary cause of "bunions" is excessive mobility at the first tarsometatarsal and/or intercuneiform joints and that this is an atavistic trait. He did not mention it specifically, but I think it also may occur with gastrocnemius equinus, the other major atavistic trait that affects the foot.

Lapidus published his paper recommending stabilization of the hypermobile first metatarsal in 1934 (4), one year before the publication of Morton's book. Both worked in Manhattan but at different institutions. Unfortunately, he was ahead of his time and catgut fixation was not adequate for him to carry out his operation accurately enough to validate his operation, and it fell out of favor. After some abject failures treating adolescent bunions with the standard technics early in my career in the 1960s, I adopted the Lapidus technic but integrated my internal fixation skills from traumatology and got markedly better results. We published our early results in adolescents in a Hospital for Joint Diseases Bulletin which was a tribute to Lapidus in about 1987 (3). I now have over 35 years' experience with this operation and I consider it a forefoot reconstruction, not a bunionectomy. We continue to have good long-term results.

The reason that I mention this here is that my primary forefoot reconstruction practice is over 75% revisions of previously failed "bunionectomies." Whether done during adolescence or a bit later, this distal osteotomy unfortunately included excessive medial head removal and often an adductor release. Fortunately, fibular sesamoidectomy is rare today. In that the primary problem was at the unstable first tarsometatarsal joint, all this surgery was rarely successful over the long term. Revisions with a Lapidus procedure are quite successful when the original surgery did not remove so much normal medial head that there is no place to retrack the medial sesamoid and when the adductor and medial capsular release was not so excessive that we risk hallux varus by properly realigning the first metatarsal. Obviously, my advice to pediatric orthopedists who choose to do a forefoot reconstruction is to consider waiting until the epiphysis is closed and then perform a Lapidus procedure.

ACCESSORY NAVICULAR WITH PRONATION

We still see a number of patients who have had the accessory navicular removed with nothing else being done. This usually results in a painful, excessively pronated foot. Kidner FC, The One Hallux and its relation to Flatfoot, JBJS II, 831–37, 1929, original paper indicated that the attachment of the posterior tibial tendon was normally quite extensive beyond the navicular. We know from general anatomic studies that it attaches to the first cuneiform and the bases of the middle metatarsals. For this reason, he recommended advancing and firmly reattaching the posterior tibial tendon after removing the prominent accessory navicular rather than just removing the bump.

Early in my adult practice, I saw several patients with significant early failure after both simple excision and the classic Kidner procedure with at least an attempt to reattach the posterior tibial tendon. Invariably the patients had gastrocnemius equinus and major sag at the naviculocuneiform joint or evidence of inadequate distal attachment of the posterior tibial tendon. In that I already had a tendency to relate flatfoot and gastrocnemius equinus, I treated these patients with augmentation of the posterior tibial tendon with the flexor digitorum longus. I advanced both to attach to the first cuneiform by lifting up tendon and periosteum on the underside of the cuneiform and drilling holes for sutures from this area with some grooving of the bone and suturing the tendon minus some paratenon to the underside of both bones. The gastrocnemius was always lengthened. Occasionally, I even lengthened the Achilles if Silfverskiöld's test indicated that more than the gastroc was tight. This virtually always salvaged the situation.

Consequently, I designed what has become a very successful protocol for patients with accessory navicular: to remove the accessory as well as any other projecting bone on the medial side of the navicular and extend the denuded area under the medial side of the first cuneiform. A secondary 2.0-cm drill is used to make four to six drill holes from this denuded plantar medial bone out the dorsal surface of the bone and both the detached posterior tibial tendon and the transected flexor digitorum longus are advanced and sutured here. The gastroc is routinely released and the patient treated for six weeks in a neutral cast followed by gentle inversion strengthening until return to activity. This procedure provides excellent results in resections of accessory navicular in terms of both removing the prominence and relieving the excessive pronation.

We must never assume that the problem is simply an extra bump of bone that should be removed but look the whole problem and determine what underlying causes need to be treated. If basic foot reconstruction principles are always followed, long-term results are much more likely to be gratifying to both patient and surgeon. The goals are proper alignment, including rotational alignment, and muscle balancing, including relieving gastroc equinus. Rigid internal fixation is used with compression screws and plates as appropriate for fusions and osteotomies.

A difficult problem in evaluating pediatric orthopedic foot and ankle care is that the results of treatment may not become apparent for many years after the treatment has been carried out. This is the reason, I assume, why I was asked to shed a little light on what we see later on in just a few of the more common problems.

REFERENCES

1. Jacon Tech for Club Foot LAAVG Sd Pousole Ignasio *JBJS* 62: pp23–31, 1980.
2. Sigvard T, Hansen P. Functional Reconstruction of the Foot and Ankle, Lippincott Williams & Wilkins 2000.
3. Clark Herbert R, Robert G, Venti Sigvard T, Hansen MD. Adolesecnt Bunions Treated by the Modified Lapidus procedure. *Bulletin of the Hospital for Joint Decisoion Orthopedic Institution.* 47, 2: 109–122, 1987.
4. Lapidus Paul W. MD, FRCS. Operation Correction of the Metathasthius Varus in Hallux Valgus. *SG & O* LXIII: 183–191, 1934.
5. Fraser RK, Menelans MA, Celestians RF, Cole WG. The Miller Procedure for Mobile Flat Foot. *JBJS.* 778: pp 2396–399, May 1995.
6. The Herman Foot, Dudley & Morton, Columbia University Press, 1935.

INDEX

Note: Page numbers referencing figures are followed by an "f". Page numbers referencing tables are followed by a "t".

B

D

H

I